# Women's Health During the Childbearing Years

## A Community-Based Approach

# Women's Health During the Childbearing Years

## A Community-Based Approach

**Peggy Sherblom Matteson, RNC,PhD**

Associate Professor,
Northeastern University,
Bouvé College of Health Sciences,
School of Nursing,
Boston, Massachusetts

*With 430 Illustrations*

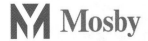

A Harcourt Health Sciences Company

St. Louis  London  Philadelphia  Sydney  Toronto

*Vice-President and Publishing Director, Nursing:* Sally Schrefer
*Senior Editor:* Michael S. Ledbetter
*Developmental Editor:* Lisa P. Newton
*Project Manager:* Catherine Jackson
*Production Editor:* Jodi Everding
*Designer:* Amy Buxton

**NOTICE**
Pharmacology is an ever-changing field. Standard safety precautions must be followed, but as new research and clinical experience broaden our knowledge, changes in treatment and drug therapy may become necessary or appropriate. Readers are advised to check the most current product information provided by the manufacturer of each drug to be administered to verify the recommended dose, the method and duration of administration, and contraindications. It is the responsibility of the treating physician, relying on experience and knowledge of the patient, to determine dosages and the best treatment for each individual patient. Neither the publisher nor the editor assumes any liability for any injury and/or damage to persons or property arising from this publication.

Mosby, Inc.
*A Harcourt Health Sciences Company*
11830 Westline Industrial Drive
St. Louis, Missouri 63146

Printed in the United States of America.

International Standard Book Number 0-323-00915-8

01 02 03 04 05  GW/KPT  9 8 7 6 5 4 3 2 1

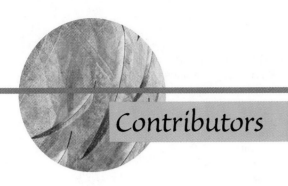

# Contributors

**Anne-Marie Armstrong, MSNc**
South Shore Women's Health PLC,
Scituate, Massachusetts

**Caroline E. Brown, RNC, DEd, WHNP, CCES, IBCLC**
Post-Doctoral Fellow,
The International Center of Research for Women, Children
and Families,
University of Pennsylvania,
School of Nursing,
Philadelphia, Pennsylvania

**Lizabeth (Libby) L. Carlson, ADN, BSN, MSN**
Delta State University,
Coordinator Maternity Nursing,
Assistant Professor,
School of Nursing,
Cleveland, Ohio

**Kathryn V. Deitch, PhD, RNC**
California State University, Long Beach,
Associate Professor,
Department of Nursing,
Long Beach, California

**Carol J. Green, RN, MN, PhD**
Professor of Nursing,
Johnson County Community College,
Overland Park, Kansas

**Jeanne-Marie E. Havener, MS, C-FNP, IBCLC**
Hartwick College,
Assistant Professor of Nursing,
Department of Nursing,
Oyuron Hill,
Onconta, New York

**Janice Hitchcock, RN, MSN, DNSc**
Professor Emeritus,
Sonoma State University,
Rohnert Park, California

**Lori Hoffman, RN, PhD**
Allentown College,
Center Valley, Pennsylvania

**Susan A. Johnson, BSN, MA, PhD**
Assistant Professor,
College of Mount St. Joseph,
Cincinnati, Ohio

**Susan Kendig, RNC, MSN, WHCNP**
Coordinator, Women's Health Nurse Practitioner Program,
Barnes College of Nursing,
University of Missouri—St. Louis,
St. Louis, Missouri

**Ermalynn M. Kiehl, RN, BSN, MSN, PhD, ARNP**
Assistant Professor,
School of Nursing,
University of Central Florida,
Orlando, Florida

**Patricia A. Kiladis, MS, RN,**
Clinical Nurse Specialist,
School of Nursing,
Northeastern University,
Boston, Massachusetts

**Jeanette H. Koshar RN, NP, PhD**
Associate Professor,
Department of Nursing,
Sonoma State University,
Rohnert Park, California

**Jeanne M. Leffers, RN, PhD**
Assistant Professor,
University of Massachusetts—Dartmouth,
College of Nursing,
North Dartmouth, Massachusetts;

**Evelyn Lengetti, RN, MSN**
Clinical Nurse Specialist, Neonatology,
The Children's Hospital of Philadelphia,
Philadelphia, Pennsylvania

**Linda Adams Leslie, RN, CS, MS, FNP**
Clinical Assistant Professor,
MGH Institute of Health Professions,
Boston, Massachusetts

**Judith A. Lewis, BS, MS, PhD**
Associate Professor,
Maternal Child Nursing Department,
School of Nursing,
Virginia Commonwealth University,
Richmond, Virginia

**Catherine O'Connor, RN, CNM**
Certified Nurse Midwife,
South Shore Women's Health,
South Weymouth, Massachusetts

**Jeanne P. Westcott, BS, MA, MS, PhD**
Certified Nurse Midwife,
Bassett Healthcare,
Cooperstown, New York

**Judith M. Wilkinson, RN, PhD**
Nursing Educator and Consultant,
Shawnee, Kansas

**Delaine Williamson, MS, MPH, RD**
Associate Professor,
School of Nursing,
Northeastern University,
Boston, Massachusetts

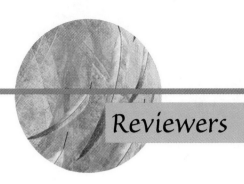

# Reviewers

**Louise Aurilio, RNC, MSN, CNA**
Instructor,
Department of Nursing,
Youngstown State University,
Youngstown, Ohio

**Janet C. Brookman, DSN, MSN, BSN**
Clinical Associate Professor,
College of Nursing,
University of Alabama in Huntsville,
Huntsville, Alabama

**Kathy Brown, RN, BSN, MS, WHCNP, LCCE**
Assistant Professor,
RN to BSN Advisor,
Department of Nursing,
University of Southern Colorado,
Pueblo, Colorado

**Penny DeRaps, PhD, FNPc**
Adult Nurse Practitioner,
President of Maine Nurse Practitioner Association,
University of Southern Maine—Graduate Program;
Pittsfield Health Care Center;
Pittsfield, Maine

**Mary Louise Drake, RN, SCM, DPH, MA, BA, BScN, EdD**
Associate Professor,
School of Nursing,
University of Windsor,
Windsor, Ontario, Canada

**Shari Gould, ADN**
RN-Education Coodinator,
Gonzales Healthcare Systems;
Memorial Hospital,
Gonzales, Texas

**Deborah Greener, RNC, CNM, PhD**
Associate Professor and Assistant Chairperson,
Department of Nursing,
Towson University,
Towson, Maryland

**Louise K. Martell, RN, PhD**
Associate Professor of Family and Child Nursing,
School of Nursing,
University of Washington,
Seattle, Washington

**Barbara S. Migliore, BSN**
Professor of Nursing,
Pierce College,
Woodland Hills, California;
Los Angeles Community College District,
Los Angeles, California

**Susan K. Myers, BSN, RN**
Department of Nursing,
Yakima Valley Community College,
Yakima, Washington

**Stephanie Oetting, MSN, RN**
Director, BSN Program,
Associate Professor,
University of St. Francis,
Fort Wayne, Indiana

**Nicole Robert, RN, MSN**
Instructor,
College of Nursing,
McNeese State University,
Lake Charles, Louisiana

**Ruby Salewski, BSN**
Assistant Professor,
College of Health Sciences,
School of Nursing,
University of Texas at El Paso,
El Paso, Texas

**Patricia Sullivan, BSN, MS, RN**
Instructor,
Midland College,
Midland, Texas

This book is dedicated to the women who allow us into their lives
and trust us to collaborate with them for the benefit of their
health and well-being. Each one has a story to tell and
much to teach if we will only listen.

This book is also dedicated to the students of nursing practice.
You are the hope for the future. We encourage and empower you to
practice with your heads and your hearts, providing the type of care
women deserve and desire—no matter what the location.

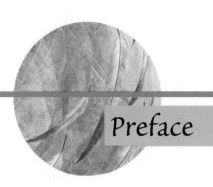

# Preface

*Women's Health During the Childbearing Years: A Community-Based Approach* developed out of the need to have a textbook that presented the information necessary to provide holistic women's health in partnership with women from diverse populations, across all environments. The community-based approach to nursing education provides an expanded and effective model to prepare students to support women's desire for health and well-being, whether encountered in community sites, outpatient facilities, inpatient facilities, or at home (Matteson, 1995, 2000). As an active participant in the development of a community-based educational program and the teacher of undergraduate nursing students in the area of women's health during the childbearing years, I became aware that a new textbook was required to adequately support the students' expanded learning experiences.

*Women's Health During the Childbearing Years* presents a holistic view of maternity and women's health care that moves beyond the biomedical approach to include the concepts of totality, centrality, and diversity. Based on the concept of totality, women are viewed as inextricably connected with their families and communities—not separate from their multiple roles as mothers, sisters, wives, workers, and caretakers. Developing a successful intervention with a woman becomes dependent upon considering not only her individual efforts but also her family and community.

The focus of centrality implies care that is woman-centered, with the woman supported as the active decision maker in her own health care. The woman is viewed and valued as the expert in her self-care. Assessment is based on what is normal for women and, when the information is available, what is normal for women of a certain age and ethnic group. Interventions include screening, diagnosis, and management of conditions that are unique to women, more common in women, or more serious in women.

Diversity entails meeting the needs of all women. It requires recognizing not only women's different social roles but also their different histories, ages, races, economic conditions, sexual orientations, and cultures and how these relate to their health. We can assist women in finding and using their own power to create a life that is physically, mentally, emotionally, and spiritually healthy and fulfilling. We can encourage women to reclaim their own authority about their bodies.

*Women's Health During the Childbearing Years* supports the actualization of empowerment for students, faculty, and clients. It strives for the emergence of consciousness and critical intervention based on the revealed reality of all participants. Integrating both the cognitive and experiential aspects of learning, this text exposes students to values and beliefs that include egalitarianism, cooperation, valuing of personal experiences, balancing personal responsibilities, and mutual empowerment (Freire, 1986). With community-based clinical education, participants may learn to deal critically and creatively with reality and discover how to participate in the transformation of their world.

## Features

*Women's Health During the Childbearing Years* has a full-color, contemporary design throughout to enhance overall visual appeal and provide a logical and consistent presentation of material. There are four units organized to present chapters in a rational way to heighten understanding and learning. Each chapter begins with opening questions and vignettes designed to stimulate critical thought. Every chapter includes key terms alerting students to important vocabulary; these terms are boldfaced and defined within the glossary. More specific features are presented throughout the text and are summarized as follows:

- A *community-based approach* focuses on providing a woman with nursing care through the childbearing years. This emphasizes providing nursing care for the woman within her family and her community in a partnership framework that is community-based and community-responsive, because most of the care takes place in the community.
- A *holistic/humanistic approach* specifically places the focus on the care for the woman as a partner in her own health care. This allows students to expand their knowledge base to provide a humanistic, holistic approach to care.
- *Care of the adolescent and older woman* is integrated throughout the text. This content provides important

age-related considerations within each corresponding content area because age-based considerations occur on a continuum.

- *Complementary therapies* are current, integrated wherever appropriate, and indicated in the margin by this logo. They stress the importance of understanding culturally based and therapeutic care alternatives to allopathic interventions.
- *Nursing care plans* use NANDA nursing diagnoses and NIC priority interventions and include NOC suggested outcomes. These plans guide students in selecting the nursing activities and NIC priority interventions for specific conditions.
- *Nutritional* considerations are integrated throughout to provide important information on how to assess, intervene, and evaluate the woman's nutritional needs across the continuum of care.
- *Abuse, ethical, and legal issues* are included where appropriate within the text. These issues alert students to important information to be aware of and guide them in effective questioning techniques when assessing the care needs of the woman.

- *Client/family teaching* considerations are integrated throughout the text and indicated by this logo. These considerations provide the student with the necessary tools to effectively teach the woman and her family about self-care.
- *Cultural considerations* integrate cultural sensitivity and assessment content. This will ensure that the student understands and is aware of the complete image of a woman's life in order to provide effective, holistic care.
- *Case Studies* and *Scenarios* are included at the end of every chapter. Each is designed to promote critical thinking while testing knowledge of the material just completed.

An *Interactive CD-ROM* is included with the text. This CD includes critical thinking case studies and care plan exercises, review study questions in NCLEX format, a vocabulary review with sound pronunciations, and examples of forms for charting care. The focus is placed on testing the students' knowledge of the content and their critical thinking skills.

A *MERLIN Website,* designed to enhance both teaching and learning, is also provided. MERLIN—Mosby's Electronic Resource Links and Information Network—is a valuable website that provides additional up-to-date tools and resources to expand content knowledge. This website contains web links for each chapter, author information, key features, content updates, links to lecture outlines, and links to community-based resources. In addition, the website contains links or references to the following resources:

NANDA—Approved Nursing Diagnoses
NIC—Nursing Interventions Classifications
NOC—Nursing Outcomes Classifications
Medications and Drugs Commonly Used During Pregnancy
Immunizations During Pregnancy
Relationship of Drugs to Breast Milk and Effect on Infant
Summary of the Hazards of Infant Formula

You will find the passcode to enter this valuable website, http://www.harcourthealth.com/MERLIN/Matteson, inside the front cover of your book.

## References:

Freire P: *Pedagogy of the oppressed*, New York, 1986, Continuum.

Matteson P: *Teaching nursing in the neighborhoods*, New York, 1995, Springer.

Matteson P: *Community-based nursing education*, New York, 2000, Springer.

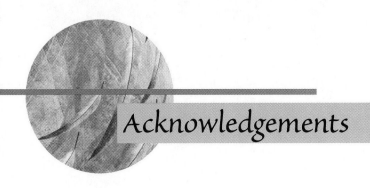

# Acknowledgements

Creating a book is a journey into the unknown. On some days, remarkably smooth progress is made across seemingly wide-open vistas, while on other days, you can't see far enough ahead to put one foot in front of the other. On this journey, I have been guided, encouraged, and assisted by two very talented and dedicated people: Michael Ledbetter, Senior Editor, Nursing Division and Lisa Newton, Developmental Editor, Nursing Division. The synergy that developed between us created not only this book but also special friendships for which I will always be grateful.

Thank you also to the rest of the members of the Harcourt team, especially Jodi Everding, Production Editor, and Catherine Jackson, Project Manager, who guided the manuscript through the production process; and Amy Buxton, who guided the design for the book. A special thanks to John Denk of Graphic World Illustration Services and the other artists who created the illustrations for the book. The process of developing a new book was complicated, but the outcome was worth it. Thank you all.

Starting with a belief in an idea, the journey toward a book was nourished by the materials provided by the contributors. These knowledgeable and dependable professionals—Ann Marie Armstrong, Caroline Brown, Kathy Deitch, Jeanne-Marie Havener, Janice Hitchcock, Lori Hoffman, Sue Johnson, Sue Kendig, Ermalynn Kiehl, Trish Kiladis, Jeanette Koshar, Jeanne Leffers, Linda Leslie, Judith Lewis, Evie Lengetti, Kay O'Connor, Jeanne Westcott, and Delaine Williamson—provided some of the basics needed to start the journey. In addition, Caroline Brown also used her expertise to capture the humanness of our clients' experiences on film. Thanks, also, to Carol Green and Judith Wilkinson for developing the nursing care plans and the case studies and review questions for the interactive CD-ROM. The reviewers provided insight on how the information was perceived and the direction of the next steps of the journey, which was very appreciated.

Ongoing encouragement throughout the journey came from a variety of people, including family members Bill, Jenny, Jeff, Cole, Eric, Elizabeth, and Ryan; and friends Val and Carl Benker, Sue Burr, Ellen Christian, and Cynthia Johnson-Smith.

A variety of experiences and encounters prepared me to make this particular journey. I will be forever grateful to my mentors: Joellen Hawkins, who introduced me to both the joys of women's health and writing; Maureen Hull, who first brought me into the community; and Eileen Zungolo, who provided me with the challenge and support to develop my piece within a community-based educational program. Equally important have been my colleagues in the Center for Community Health, Education, Research and Service and the people of Codman Square.

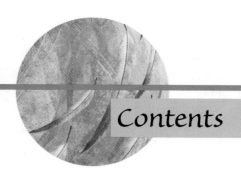

# Contents

# Women's Lives

*"A sphere is not made up of one, but of an infinite number of circles; women have diverse gifts and to say that a women's sphere is the family circle is a mathematical absurdity."*

— MARIA MITCHELL

*Who defines the concept of health for a woman?*

*What are the gender differences between the health of women and men?*

*What determines the health of women?*

*What are the differences in the health across ethnic/racial groups?*

*How does the history of the women's health movement affect health care today?*

*How can nurses influence women's health?*

Women's lives are about more than having babies! The lives of women are diverse—filled with experiences influenced by cultural beliefs and societal expectations, as well as political, economic, and environmental factors. To provide nursing care that is responsive to women's diverse needs, we must understand how women develop both their personal expectations and perspective on health.

People operate as physical, psychologic, and social entities and are constantly influenced by their constitutional makeup, physical and social environments, past experiences, present perceptions and reactions, and even future aspirations. This configuration is brought to every life situation encountered (Perlman, 1957 as cited in Whittaker and Federico, 1997).

What is a healthy person? Health is defined by people throughout their everyday lives and is measured within the totality of their experiences and the context of their personal expectations. **Holistic health** exists when the mind, body, thoughts, and feelings of a person are connected.

**Women's health care** is more than a euphemism for maternal-child health care. "Caring calls for a philosophy of moral commitment toward protecting human dignity and preserving humanity" (Watson, 1988). Nurses working with women support each one on her unique journey to attain, maintain, or regain an optimal sense of well-being throughout life. With discovery and sharing of knowledge and skills, nurses help women to influence their own health destinies.

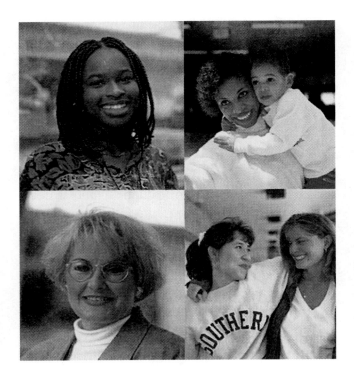

Health care encounters can be effectively positive when they support self-determination and individual power and control and are conducive to holistic healing and nurturing of positive self-images for both clients and practitioners (Heide, 1985; Oakley, 1993). Appropriate and supportive care can occur when providers understand the historical, cultural, ethnic, social, economic, and political factors that influence not only women's health but also their health care.

 **CONSIDERING DIVERSE PERSPECTIVES**

The United States is home to the most diverse, multicultural society in the world, and this diversity is increasing. A **culture** is the set of beliefs and life practices that a group of individuals follow and pass down from generation to generation. Cultural beliefs may evolve over time in response to the needs of the group.

Individuals differ not only in culturally based health beliefs and practices, class, race, and/or ethnicity but also in their responses to biologic factors. The following cultural phenomena vary among cultural groups: (1) expected response to health-related experiences; (2) biologic variations—both physical and genetic; (3) variations in social organization, (4) communication differences including language differences, verbal and nonverbal behaviors, and silence; (5) personal space and attitude toward space around them; and (6) time

orientation (e.g., oriented in the present, past, or future) (Table 1-1) (Giger and Davidhizar, 1995).

## Communication Differences

To learn a woman's beliefs and practices, we must communicate with her. **Communication** between people of the same culture—or even the same family—often presents difficulties. It can be even more difficult for a nurse and client to communicate when they are from different cultures and may be most articulate and comfortable speaking in the language of their own culture.

People from different cultural backgrounds learn to communicate in specific ways. Communication occurs primarily through body language and paralinguistic cues (e.g., how the voice is used), with the use of actual words having the least effect. How body language is interpreted varies from culture to culture. For Anglo-Americans, eye contact is expected when speaking with someone. "Asian, Native American, Indochinese, Arab, and Appalachian clients may consider direct eye contact impolite or aggressive, and they may avert their own eyes when talking with a nurse" (Andrews and Boyle, 1995).

## Physical Differences

People from different cultures have different "body builds and structure, skin color, enzymatic and genetic variations, susceptibility to disease, and nutritional variations" (Spector, 1996). More specifically, there are **biocultural** variations in people's bodies. For example, the number of vertebrae varies from 23 to 25 based on racial and sex differences; 11% of black females have 23 vertebrae, and 12% of Eskimo and Native American males have 25 vertebrae. The presence or absence of muscles also varies. For example, the peroneus tertius muscle in the foot is absent in as many as 10% of Asians, Native Americans, and whites and 15% of blacks. Genetic traits and disorders also vary by population or ethnic group. Blacks have a higher frequency of sickle cell disease and lactase deficiency. People of Anglican descent have a higher rate of cystic fibrosis. Irish persons have phenylketonuria and neural tube defects more often. Japanese have a higher frequency of cleft lip and/or palate. Mediterranean persons (i.e., Italians and Greeks) have more ß-thalassemia and familial Mediterranean fever. Navaho Indians have more ear abnormalities, and Eskimos have a higher frequency of congenital adrenal hyperplasia (Schrefer, 1995).

## Responding to Health Concerns

Each woman comes from a family, a community, and a culture that has taught her how to respond to health

## TABLE 1-1    Variations among Selected Cultural Groups

| Concept | African Americans | Asians | Hispanics | American Indians |
|---|---|---|---|---|
| **Verbal Communication** | Asking personal questions of someone that you have met for the first time is seen as improper and intrusive | High respect for others, especially those in positions of authority | Expression of negative feelings is considered impolite | Speaks in a low tone of voice and expects the listener to be attentive |
| **Non-Verbal Communication** | Direct eye contact in conversation is often considered rude | Direct eye contact with superiors may be considered disrespectful | Avoidance of eye contact is usually a sign of attentiveness and respect | Direct eye contact is often considered disrespectful |
| **Touch** | Touching another person's hair is often considered offensive | It is not customary to shake hands with persons of the opposite sex | Touching is often observed between two persons in conversation | A light touch of the hand instead of a firm handshake is often used when greeting a person |
| **Family Organization** | Usually have close, extended family networks. Women play key roles in health care decisions | Usually have close, extended family ties. Emphasis may be on family needs rather than individual needs | Usually have close, extended family ties. All members of the family may be involved in health care | Usually have close, extended family ties. Emphasis tends to be on family rather than individual needs |
| **Time** | Often oriented in the present | Often oriented in the present | Often oriented in the present | Often oriented in the present |
| **Perception of Health** | Harmony of mind and spirit with nature | When there is a balance between the "yin" and "yang" energy forces | Balance and harmony among mind, body, spirit, and nature | Harmony of mind, body, spirit, and emotions with nature |
| **Alternative Healers** | "Granny," "root doctor," voodoo priest, spiritualist | Acupuncturist, acupressurist, herbalist | Curandero, espiritualista, yerbero | Medicine man, shaman |
| **Self-Care Practices** | Poultices, herbs, oils, roots | Hot and cold foods, herbs, teas, soups, cupping, burning, rubbing, pinching | Hot and cold foods, herbs | Herbs, corn meal, medicine bundles |
| **Biologic Variations** | Sickle cell anemia, mongolian spots, keloid formation, inverted T waves, lactose intolerance | Thalassemia, drug interactions, mongolian spots, lactose intolerance | Mongolian spots, lactose intolerance | Cleft uvula, lactose intolerance |

Compiled from Giger JN and Davidhizar RE: *Transcultural nursing,* ed 2, St Louis, 1995, Mosby.

concerns and follow practices for health and healing. Examples of implied or explicit **cultural teachings** are as follows: men never complain about pain, women should receive care from female providers, culturally specific remedies (i.e., chicken soup, garlic, herbs, coining) are to be tried first, and a doctor/clinic/hospital should be sought only as a last resort.

The traditional and contemporary ways of healing do not have to be in conflict with each other but can be complementary and work together toward healing the sick and maintaining the health of the well (Perrone, Stockel, and Krueger, 1990). When we strive for synergy between the two perspectives, our clients benefit. They cannot only reap the benefits of both types of care but

**TABLE 1-2**  *Guide to Cultural Assessment*

| Component | What to Assess |
|---|---|
| **Background** | Primary language, religion, cultural identification |
| **Health beliefs** | Definition of wellness and illness |
| | Attitudes about conventional medicine |
| | Attitudes about mental illness, pain, birth defects, disability, chronic disease, death, dying |
| | Relationship between illness and religion (e.g., illness is punishment or sickness is spiritual disharmony) |
| **Health practices** | Identification of family, religious, or cultural remedies for cure of illness (e.g., eating garlic for a cold or applying heat to cure an ear infection) |
| | Identification of rituals to ward off sickness (e.g., wearing amulets or religious medals, praying or performing dances) |
| | Use of alternative health care providers (e.g., medicine person, herbalist, folk healer, or witch) |
| **Dietary practices** | Preparation rituals |
| | Forbidden foods |
| | Food taboos (e.g., mixing certain foods) |
| | Foods for cure of illness |

also will be more apt to tell contemporary providers about simultaneously using traditional methods. The possibility of negative and sometimes harmful interactions between different but simultaneous therapeutic interventions can then be reduced.

Traditional methods of healing are based on centuries of care giving and are the original methods of healing. These traditions use a variety of ways to help the human body maintain homeostasis. The basis of care is the premise of a partnership between the healer and the person seeking assistance. The pair agrees on a purpose, and then works together to achieve it. Other members of the family and community may also be involved in the process.

We provide care to a heterogeneous group of persons with different cultural perspectives, religious beliefs, social and behavioral expectations, economic resources, and personal goals. Health and healing occur when we listen to and learn about our clients' experiences, expectations, and needs and work in collaboration with them. A cultural assessment is vital to this process (Table 1-2).

## SEXUAL DIFFERENCES

Women and men are biologically similar but also very different. Sex-based biology is the field of scientific inquiry that examines the biologic and physiologic differences between men and women. Findings about sexual differences are changing the way scientists conduct research and health professionals care for patients.

**Gender** is the masculine or feminine category to which an individual is assigned by self or others based on sex. Persons assume a pattern of behavior based on a gender role, defining masculine or feminine in terms accepted by their culture. In some cultures, gender roles are distinctly defined with no overlap, but in other cultures there is a great deal of overlap between the roles men and women may or are expected to assume (Spalding, 1998).

### Differences in Perspective

Researchers have spent years studying human behavior. Most of the subjects studied by Freud, Erikson, Piaget, Kohlberg, and others, however, have been middle class males. The findings therefore give preference to the development of the male as the norm or standard applied to both men and women. With this expectation, women often appear to be abnormal or inadequate—not the equal but different people that they are.

"Research focused on understanding the nature of the female world—its structure, its culture, its functioning—can counteract the tendency to see the female component in societies as somehow deficient, deviant versions of the male world" (Bernard, 1981). Female researchers have determined the life experiences and viewpoints of women may be very different from those of men. Women grow up with a female perspective as their personalities develop (Horney, 1967) and can find forms of strength based on their own life experiences (Miller, 1976); formulate their own definitions of self, view of relationships, and determination of morality (Gilligan, 1982); and cultivate and value ways of knowing that develop the power of their minds (Belenky, 1986). A shortcoming of this research is that it has generally been limited to white, middle class

## TABLE 1-3  Leading Causes of Death (1995)

| Rank | All Persons | Males | Females |
|------|-------------|-------|---------|
| 1 | Diseases of the heart | Diseases of the heart | Diseases of the heart |
| 2 | Malignant neoplasms | Malignant neoplasms | Malignant neoplasms |
| 3 | Cerebrovascular diseases | Cerebrovascular diseases | Cerebrovascular diseases |
| 4 | Chronic obstructive pulmonary diseases | Unintentional injuries | Chronic obstructive pulmonary diseases |
| 5 | Unintentional injuries | Chronic obstructive pulmonary diseases | Pneumonia and influenza |
| 6 | Pneumonia and influenza | Pneumonia and influenza | Diabetes mellitus |
| 7 | Diabetes mellitus | Human immunodeficiency virus infection | Unintentional injuries |
| 8 | Human immunodeficiency virus infection | Diabetes mellitus | Alzheimer's disease |
| 9 | Suicide | Suicide | Nephritis, nephrotic syndrome, and nephrosis |
| 10 | Chronic liver disease and cirrhosis | Homicide and legal intervention | Septicemia |

USHHS: *Health, United States, 1998,* Washington, D.C., 1998, U.S. Government.

women, although the findings do broaden our perspectives and reinforce the need to continue to explore and develop information about women's lives.

## Differences in Health and Illness

Men and women have different **patterns** of health, illness, and death. The extent to which these differences may be attributed to sex or the role of the assigned gender are just starting to be studied.

Women appear to be more endowed with genes that contribute to their durability. Around the world, more females survive from the time of conception through old age. Men have a higher mortality rate for every year of life with more frequent deaths from almost all causes at all ages. As a result, women have a longer life expectancy at birth than males (Montagu, 1992; Moss, 1996).

### Life Expectancy Rates

In the United States, the **life expectancy** for all women is 76.5 years. A difference in life expectancy remains, however, between whites and blacks and males and females. White females have the highest life expectancy at birth (79.9 years), followed by black females (74.7 years), white males (74.3 years), and black males (67.2 years). Both white and black men have been gaining in life expectancy, narrowing the gap between men and women to 5.8 years (National Center for Health Statistics, 1999).

### Physical Differences

As a group, the **physical differences** of women enable them to endure starvation, exposure, fatigue, shock, illness, and other devitalizing conditions better than males. The overall subcutaneous fatty layer in women's bodies renders them better insulated against the cold and provides extra reserves for energy when necessary. Women's body temperatures can rise 2° or 3° above men's before they begin to sweat, but because women have more sweat glands that are distributed more uniformly over their bodies, they perspire more evenly (Montagu, 1992).

Women's bodies also deal better with microorganisms and illness than men's. Women possess an immunologic system that provides greater immunity against infection and a faster recovery rate. Statistics from the public health services of various countries, including the United States, show that after the age of 15 the illness rate is higher among females; however, more recover (Montagu, 1992). Although they have fewer episodes of sickness, men experience more fatal conditions. A combination of genetic, hormonal, neuroendocrine, and immunologic function probably creates the differences in mortality. Ongoing research will determine how much of the difference is related to biology and how much is related to environmental influences (Table 1-3).

Conditions such as high blood pressure, heart disease, and many types of cancers affect women and men in equal numbers but have been studied almost exclusively in males. Other diseases such as lupus, rheumatoid arthritis, and scleroderma primarily affect women. Women's gender-specific organs also provide the possibility of a variety of reproductive disorders, infections, or cancers that cause disability and death.

Until recently, research on medical conditions and therapeutic interventions has been focused on men. The manifestation and course of diseases and infections in

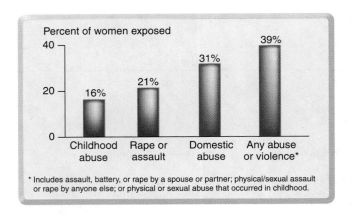

Percent of women exposed

* Includes assault, battery, or rape by a spouse or partner; physical/sexual assault or rape by anyone else; or physical or sexual abuse that occurred in childhood.

FIGURE 1-1 • Women's lifetime experience with violence and abuse, 1998. *(The Commonwealth Fund 1998 Survey of Women's Health.)*

women and the type and dose of therapeutic medications required by women are just starting to be explored (Hubbard, 1995). Men and women may have dramatically different reactions to medications, but very few drugs have been studied to determine the proper dose and safety warnings according to sex. New research is uncovering startling—even life-threatening—differences. It is now apparent that risk factors, indicators of disease, and therapies used to treat conditions or infections may be different for women and men.

## Differences in the Lived Experiences

Women are more likely then men to participate in **self-care** and self-protective practices. Many daily health factors, however, depend upon personal safety and money, so in our society, some people can take better care of themselves than others. Men move though our society with less risk for physical harm and more financial security than women. When a woman manifests a lack of health, she does not necessarily lack interest in being healthy.

### Personal Safety

Violence, as well as fears and threats of violence, are significant health problems that affect women of all social groups, ages, and races (i.e., including rural and urban women, heterosexuals, lesbians, bisexuals, rich and poor women, able and disabled women). Violence is the second leading cause of injury to women of all ages and the leading cause of injury to women between the ages of 15 and 54 (Schnitzer and Runyan, 1995). Thirty-nine percent of women report violence or abuse in their lifetime (Figure 1-1) (Collins and others, 1999).

Women are safer on the streets than in their own homes because of **domestic violence.** Ninety-five percent

of domestic assaults are experienced by women. Estimates indicate that each year in the United States, 1 million women are assaulted by a family member, with a woman being battered every 15 seconds. "Assaults by husbands, ex-husbands, and lovers cause more injuries to women than motor vehicle accidents, rape and muggings combined" (Rodriguez-Trias, 1992). Twenty-two to thirty-five percent of women seen in emergency rooms are there for injuries inflicted by a partner.

Nationwide, the risk of being murdered by a family member is four times greater than being murdered by a stranger (Campbell, Harris, and Lee, 1995). Male intimates kill 30% of the female homicide victims—a rate that has held steady over the last 30 years.

Violence or threats of violence create serious health problems that result in increased visits to health care providers, physical and emotional trauma, and use of alcohol and drugs that can further disrupt the physical and psychologic health of women.

Domestic violence often leads to unemployment because abusers interfere with or sabotage women's work lives or employers fail to grant sufficient time off to attend civil or criminal legal proceedings or are unwilling to deal with the outcomes of violence, dismissing women once they learn about an abusive relationship. Other times, a woman must leave a job to enter a shelter or otherwise hide from the abuser.

A woman can get caught up in a cycle of violence against her by her partner (Figure 1-2). Abusers have periods of time when they are loving and caring, showering the woman with attention and gifts. The tension gradually builds, however, and is then released with a verbal or physical attack. Even though abused by her partner, the woman remembers the feelings of attachment she developed before the abuse started. She wants to believe that each violent incident is the last so that they can return to the loving relationship.

### Poverty

In 1996, women made 75 cents for every dollar men made. This disparity leads to a greater risk of **poverty** for women.

There are great variations in the wage gap in different occupations. The gap between male workers and female workers is the widest in medicine and sales and the lowest in professional nursing and clerical work. Education increases the earning potential for both women and men, but in general, higher education adds less to a woman's earnings than to men's (Bureau of the Census, 1996). With retirement, the average annual Social Security income received by men and women differs, with men receiving $14,134 and women receiving $13,219. This disparity is due to women's lower salaries and years of employment lost for child rearing and taking care of elder parents (Estes and Close, 1994). Social security, pension plans, and health insurance are all based

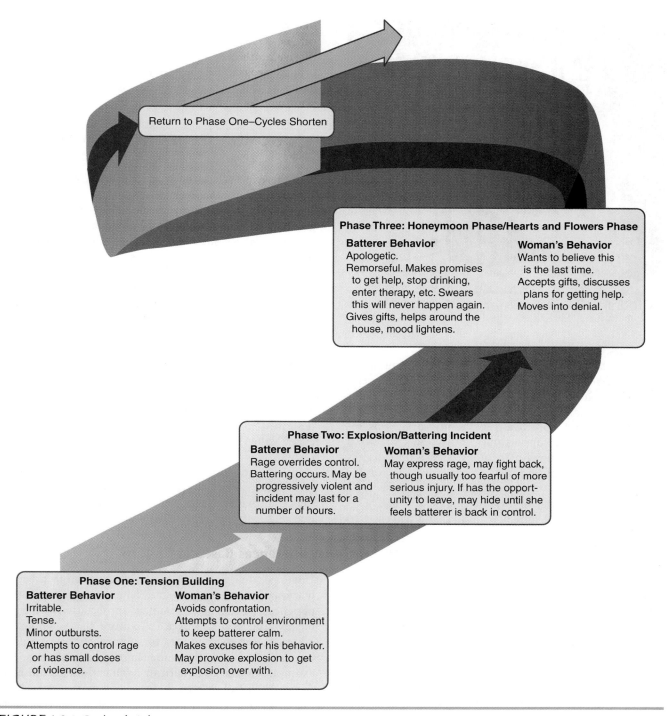

Return to Phase One–Cycles Shorten

**Phase Three: Honeymoon Phase/Hearts and Flowers Phase**

**Batterer Behavior**
Apologetic.
Remorseful. Makes promises
 to get help, stop drinking,
 enter therapy, etc. Swears
 this will never happen again.
Gives gifts, helps around the
 house, mood lightens.

**Woman's Behavior**
Wants to believe this
 is the last time.
Accepts gifts, discusses
 plans for getting help.
Moves into denial.

**Phase Two: Explosion/Battering Incident**

**Batterer Behavior**
Rage overrides control.
Battering occurs. May be
 progressively violent and
 incident may last for a
 number of hours.

**Woman's Behavior**
May express rage, may fight back,
 though usually too fearful of more
 serious injury. If has the opportunity to leave, may hide until she
 feels batterer is back in control.

**Phase One: Tension Building**

**Batterer Behavior**
Irritable.
Tense.
Minor outbursts.
Attempts to control rage
 or has small doses
 of violence.

**Woman's Behavior**
Avoids confrontation.
Attempts to control environment
 to keep batterer calm.
Makes excuses for his behavior.
May provoke explosion to get
 explosion over with.

FIGURE 1-2 • Cycle of violence.

on the concept that a family has a male wage earner and a spouse at home.

More women than men live in poverty, and women remain poor for longer periods of time. Reasons for poverty include: loss of a job and/or career due to relocation of the family, chronic illness, job-related injuries, less access to regular full-time work with prospects for seniority and benefits, divorce, less access to high paying professions, functioning as single heads of households, retirement with minimal benefits, and loss of income or retirement benefits after the death of a spouse (Figure 1-3).

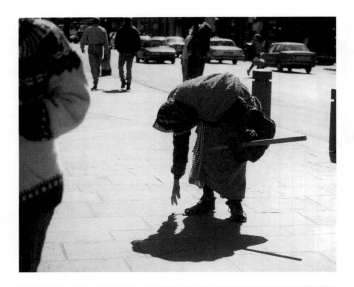

FIGURE 1-3 • Homeless woman.

### Relationship between Poverty and Health

There is a tie between overall health and economic security. Good health and access to health care often depend on having a good job, but keeping a job depends on not only the woman staying healthy but also the people within the family. Poor health or family care-giving responsibilities reduce opportunities to work. Half of all nonworking women with incomes of $16,000 or less have a disability limiting their capacity to work or are caring for a sick or disabled child, spouse, parent, or other family member (Collins and others, 1999).

Poor women have difficulty finding and traveling to health services and then paying for care. They habitually live with illness and pain, for which women of the middle class suffering the same ailments receive care (Figure 1-4).

In addition, women are often left with the responsibility of caring for children without the same access to health benefits or financial resources as the other parent. Nine percent—more than 9 million women—are currently caring for a sick or disabled family member, often spending at least 20 hours per week at this task. Time burdens and lack of paid help have a heavy effect on women with below-average family incomes (Collins and others, 1999).

Although most uninsured women are working or married to a full-time worker, they do not have health insurance. In 1998, the proportion of working women without insurance increased. Of women who earned less than $16,000 per year, 35% were uninsured in 1998 compared with 29% in 1993. During that same 5-year period, the uninsured rate among women earning between $16,001 and $35,000 rose from 15% to 21%. Twenty-six percent of women ages 18 to 64 were either uninsured or had spent some time in the past year without insurance. Lack of insurance greatly increases the likelihood of not being able to attain care (Collins and others, 1999). Many poor women and children cannot receive heath care if it is not provided by a government-funded program. Policymakers have failed to develop and advocate policies that address the diverse needs of poor women.

##  WOMEN OF THE UNITED STATES

The life expectancy for women in the United States is shorter than in 18 other countries. In addition to this poor status, the health of women in America varies a great deal among groups and individuals (Table 1-4).

There is no such thing as a "typical" American woman, but there are similarities in the health needs and concerns of all women. Each woman's experience varies by regional heritage and national origin, rural or urban lifestyle, occupation, and sexual partner preference, as well as how her ancestors were treated within the history of the country (Bair and Cayleff, 1993).

### Psychologic Strength

The healthy functioning of a woman is often based on an inner strength, a **psychologic strength.** Women have described this as the ability to simultaneously experience "vulnerability with safety, tenacity with flexibility, resolution with ambiguity, movement with stillness, and emotion with logic" (Rose, 1990). Balancing between these interrelated behaviors, attitudes, beliefs, and experiences provides their inner strength and helps them attain and maintain a healthier state.

### Differences Based in Culture

Understanding cultural differences can lead to the affirmation of the multiplicity and richness of our distinct experiences, as well as bring a new appreciation and a better awareness of American culture as a whole. In addition, an exploration of cultural beliefs held by women often finds that they share common views. For example, Mexican-American women and Southeast-Asian-American women share the common view of striving for balance in order to achieve health. Native American women and African-American women share a historic perspective as healers and midwives and the spiritual sense brought to lay medical practice (Bair and Cayleff, 1993). Affirming cultural variations encourages the sharing of knowledge and positive health practices within and across cultural groups.

### Differences in Sexual Preference

In addition to diverse racial and ethnic groups, women also have different experiences and health needs based on their sexual preference. **Lesbians** are women whose

| TABLE 1-4 | Life Expectancy of Women at Birth and 65 Years of Age in Selected Countries | |
|---|---|---|
| **Country** | **At birth** | **At 65 years** |
| Japan | 83.1 | 21.3 |
| France | 82.3 | 21.1 |
| Switzerland | 81.7 | 20.4 |
| Canada | 81.4 | 19.5 |
| Sweden | 80.8 | 19.6 |
| Australia | 80.8 | 19.3 |
| Spain | 80.7 | 19.2 |
| Norway | 80.5 | 19.2 |
| Netherlands | 80.5 | 19.4 |
| Italy | 80.5 | 19.2 |
| Greece | 80.4 | 18.7 |
| Finland | 79.6 | 18.0 |
| England and Wales | 79.5 | 18.5 |
| Austria | 79.5 | 18.5 |
| Germany | 79.3 | 19.3 |
| New Zealand | 79.2 | 18.8 |
| Puerto Rico | 78.9 | 19.4 |
| Singapore | 78.9 | 18.5 |
| **United States** | **78.8** | **18.9** |
| Northern Ireland | 78.7 | 17.7 |
| Israel | 78.5 | 17.6 |
| Ireland | 78.2 | 17.3 |
| Portugal | 77.9 | 17.3 |
| Denmark | 77.9 | 17.6 |
| Costa Rica | 77.8 | 17.6 |

Data are based on reporting by countries for 1992 or the most recent year available. Rankings are from highest to lowest life expectancy based on the latest available data for countries or geographic areas with a population of at least 1 million.

USHHS: *Health, United States, 1998,* Washington, D.C., 1998, U.S. Government.

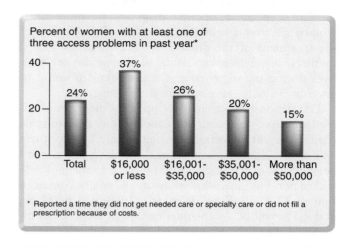

FIGURE 1-4 • Health care access problems by income, 1998. *(The Commonwealth Fund 1998 Survey of Women's Health.)*

are members of multiple and diverse groups that differ by age, race, ethnic origin, social class, sexual preference, and so forth.

Women of color include Native American, Hispanic, black, and Asian women. For this group, definitions of "health" or "illness" are often inextricably tied to their family history, their status within a dominant society that only affords them a secondary role, and their place within their own communities. Communities of color, which are sometimes matriarchal, can provide women a source of strength on which to lean, as well as a history of activities that promote self-empowerment and a tradition of community caring (Bair and Cayleff, 1993). Each of these resources may have a positive effect on a woman's health and sense of well-being.

### Census Data

Within the United States, census data is collected every 10 years. On census forms, people are expected to identify themselves as members of one of eight racial/ethnic groups with Hispanic and non-Hispanic categories provided for each of the following four races: white; black; American Indian, Eskimo, and Aleut; and Asian and Pacific Islander. Persons of Hispanic origin may be of any race and may also identify themselves as "other." When a person identifies him- or herself as being of one race/ethnic group, it does not mean that he or she does not have ancestors from other groups. Keep in mind that going back five generations gives a person 32 ancestors. The **ethnicity** or race of some of these ancestors may be known; that of others may not be known.

Data provide quantitative measures about groups and can give us statistics such as how many women have been treated for a certain disease or how long

emotional, social, and sexual relationships are primarily with other women. Lesbians include the following: women who identify themselves as homosexual or bisexual; women who are sexually attracted to women; and women who have had sex with other women. Lesbians face greater barriers to health care than heterosexual women, often finding that providers are prejudiced against them or unaware of their needs.

### White Women and Minority Women

A host of factors (e.g., class, ethnic and/or racial identification, sexual preference, age, and geographic location) shapes women's lives (Ware, 1980). Statistics are often given to differentiate between the experiences of white and **minority** women or white and black women, but these simplified designations don't start to account for the variances in women's lived experiences. Women

women in a certain group live. Data cannot, however, tell us things such as how many women did not receive the care necessary to obtain a diagnosis; how individual women felt about being ill; the effect of the disease or the treatment of the disease on their roles as sisters, mothers, wives, workers, etc.; or the quality of their lives during the experience. Census data are useful to develop estimates about future developments.

**Population projections** developed by the Census Bureau are based on assumptions about future demographic trends. Current projections are that by July 1, 2005, there will be 146,196,000 women in the United States, composing 51% of the population. Of these women, 69.6% will be non-Hispanic white women, 1% will be American Indian, 12.3% will be Hispanic, 12.8% will be black, and 4.5% will be Asian-American. (U.S. Dept. of Commerce, 1998). These projections are useful in planning for the future health care of women (Table 1-5).

## Differences between Women

Each ethnic group of women, including Euro-Americans, shares some health issues that differentiate it from other ethnic groups. Differences in the cause of death, as well as the occurrence of certain diseases, occur across race and ethnic groups. New understandings about past disparities in care, however, have led to recent federal initiatives that are attempting to eliminate racial and ethnic disparities not only in health risks but also in the approach to health care for women.

Many minority women are chronically put in positions that endanger their health and offer improper recourse for their illnesses (e.g., scrubbing floors, walking long distances between buses, performing repetitive tasks on assembly lines, using emergency rooms as clinics, and/or speaking with practitioners who do not know their language or grasp the full meaning of their concerns). These women are less likely to have access to elective procedures, fertility services, and other forms of

high technology or to receive intensive care treatment when ill. They are also less likely to have a personal provider or quality health insurance coverage, or be treated with respect and understanding when dealing with healthcare facilities (Bair and Cayleff, 1993).

Socioeconomic status has a direct influence on insurance coverage and access to care for both preventive services and regular visits. As a group, women of color are disproportionately represented among the total U.S. population of people without health insurance (National Women's Health Information Center, 1999).

### Non-Hispanic White Women

Non-Hispanic white women are generally of European descent; some are recent immigrants and others are descendents of women who arrived as early as 1620. As the major colonizers of what became the United States and the establishers of the current government, this group is currently predominant, and its traditions dominate most areas of our lives (Benitez, 1998).

Most resource information about women's lives is recorded in two categories: white female and other. Researchers of women's issues have tended to focus on the white female as the major concern, considering them the standard by which "normal" is determined.

Only since 1993 have researchers been required to include females and minorities in their studies. Therefore when most of the published information refers to women as a group, it generally represents the experience of non-Hispanic white women. What we know in general about "women" refers to this group.

### African-American Women

"African American is a term that represents a people who are a spectrum of colors and experiences; therefore, there can be no presumption of uniformity" (Taylor, 1998). American women of African descent come from a variety of cultures that are different in terms of language, beliefs, values, and learned behaviors. They have

**TABLE 1-5** *Resident Population of the United States: Middle Series Projections, 2001-2005\**

|  | July 2001 | July 2002 | July 2003 | July 2004 | July 2005 |
|---|---|---|---|---|---|
| **Both Sexes** | 276,918 | 279,189 | 281,452 | 283,713 | 285,981 |
| Median age | 35.9 | 36.1 | 36.3 | 36.5 | 36.6 |
| Mean age | 36.6 | 36.7 | 36.9 | 37.0 | 37.2 |
| **Females** | 141,606 | 142,754 | 143,899 | 145,045 | 146,196 |
| Median age | 37.1 | 37.4 | 37.6 | 37.8 | 37.9 |
| Mean age | 37.9 | 38.0 | 38.1 | 38.2 | 38.4 |
| **Males** | 135,312 | 136,436 | 137,553 | 138,668 | 139,785 |
| Median age | 34.7 | 34.8 | 35.0 | 35.2 | 35.3 |
| Mean age | 35.3 | 35.4 | 35.6 | 35.8 | 35.9 |

\*Numbers in thousands.
USHHS: *Health, United States, 1998,* Washington, D.C., 1998, U.S. Government.

not only descended from the African continent but also from the English-, French-, Dutch-, Portuguese-, and Spanish-speaking nations of the Caribbean (McBarnette, 1996). The leading causes of death in this census group of women are heart disease and cancer, followed by cerebrovascular disease, diabetes mellitus, unintentional injuries, pneumonia, influenza, human immunodeficiency virus infection, chronic obstructive pulmonary disease, kidney disease, and conditions related to pregnancy and childbearing (Table 1-6).

In general, blacks have more undetected diseases, higher disease and illness rates, more chronic conditions, and a shorter life expectancy than whites. Morbidity and mortality rates for blacks for many conditions exceed those for whites even though black women report fewer health-risk behaviors, such as smoking cigarettes, consuming alcohol, or using other substances.

Across all ethnic groups, working class and poor women are at greater risk for hypertension than affluent women. When comparisons are made for ethnic groups within each income level, black women are more likely to be hypertensive than white women (Moss, 1996).

Fifty percent of African-American women are considered obese by white, American standards. Obesity (i.e., 20% over desirable body weight) is associated with increased risk for diabetes, hypertension, cardiovascular disease, respiratory disorders, arthritis, and some cancers.

Diabetes, a major contributor to the death and disability of American women of African descent, is 60% more common in this population than white women. Diabetes increases the risk of kidney disease, heart disease, and eye and foot problems. The death rate from diabetes for African-American women is two and a half times that of American women of European descent.

The incidence of cervical cancer, although dropping in both white and black women, remains twice as high in African-American women. Black women are less likely to survive than white women diagnosed at the same stage. Although more white women develop breast cancer than black women, more black women die from it. Although not life-threatening, uterine fibroids—resulting in pain, excess bleeding, and pregnancy problems—are

## TABLE 1-6  Leading Causes of Death for Women (1995)

| Rank | White | Black | American Indian or Alaskan Native | Asian or Pacific Islander | Hispanic |
|---|---|---|---|---|---|
| 1 | Diseases of the heart | Diseases of the heart | Diseases of the heart | Malignant neoplasms | Diseases of the heart |
| 2 | Malignant neoplasms | Malignant neoplasms | Malignant neoplasms | Diseases of the heart | Malignant neoplasms |
| 3 | Cerebrovascular diseases | Cerebrovascular diseases | Unintentional injuries | Cerebrovascular diseases | Cerebrovascular diseases |
| 4 | Chronic obstructive pulmonary diseases | Diabetes mellitus | Diabetes mellitus | Unintentional injuries | Diabetes mellitus |
| 5 | Pneumonia and influenza | Human immuno-deficiency virus infection | Cerebrovascular diseases | Pneumonia and influenza | Unintentional injuries |
| 6 | Unintentional injuries | Unintentional injuries | Chronic liver disease and cirrhosis | Diabetes mellitus | Pneumonia and influenza |
| 7 | Diabetes mellitus | Pneumonia and influenza | Pneumonia and influenza | Chronic obstructive pulmonary diseases | Human immuno-deficiency virus |
| 8 | Alzheimer's disease | Chronic obstructive pulmonary diseases | Chronic obstructive pulmonary diseases | Suicide | Chronic obstructive pulmonary diseases |
| 9 | Nephritis, nephrotic syndrome, and nephrosis | Nephritis, nephrotic syndrome, and nephrosis | Septicemia | Nephritis, nephrotic syndrome, and nephrosis | Certain conditions originating in the perinatal period |
| 10 | Septicemia | Certain conditions originating in the perinatal period | Homicide and legal intervention | Congenital abnormalities | Congenital abnormalities |

Data are based on the National Vital Statistics System—Causes of death.
USHHS: *Health, United States, 1998,* Washington, D.C., 1998, U.S. Government.

more common in African-American women (National Women's Health Information Center, 1999).

Lupus is an **autoimmune disease** in which the body attacks its own healthy tissues and organs. It is over twice as common in African-American women than in white women.

### Asian and Pacific Islander Women

Asian and Pacific Islander Americans compose one of the most diverse populations in the United States. Up to 48 separate Asian and Pacific Islander ethnic populations have been counted as residents. The major Asian groups are Chinese, Filipino, Japanese, Asian-Indian, Korean, Vietnamese, Laotian, Cambodian, Thai, and Hmong. The major Pacific Islanders are Hawaiian, Samoan, Chamorro (Guamanian), Tongan, and Melanesian. Speaking a vast array of languages, some are fourth and fifth generation Asian-Americans, although 75% are recent immigrants and refugees (True and Guillermo, 1996). Cultural and language differences, as well as cost, are their major barriers to receiving health care.

Asian beliefs place the responsibility for health and illness within the individual, yet Asian-Americans have culturally distinct patterns of illness interpretation such as are found between women of Chinese, Japanese, and Filipino origin. Chinese-Americans have been found to view health skeptically and as problematic. Maintaining good physical health focuses on food choices and cooking styles, while remaining concerned about the development of the unexpected. Japanese-Americans may see health as a matter of will; that is, if you think about getting sick, you will. Illness prevention occurs by ignoring the symptoms of illness while continuing to perform daily responsibilities. Filipino-Americans consider health to be a moral statement that is created by fulfilling social responsibilities. Health occurs when there is a strong relationship between body and soul rather than body and mind (Ito, Chung, and Kagawa-Ainger, 1997).

Even though the focus is on individual responsibility, Japanese women are held responsible for both the health of everyone living in their household and the occurrence of most illnesses within the family. They are expected to nurture other family members, even at the expense of their own health. They are also expected to be stoic about any suffering they experience so as not to disrupt the household (Lock, 1998).

Asian-American women have the highest life expectancy (85.8 years) of any ethnic or racial group in the United States, but there are wide disparities between the women in this group. Note the following life expectancies of Asian-American women: Samoan (74.9 years), native Hawaiian (77.2 years), Filipino (81.5 years), Japanese (84.5 years), and Chinese (86.1 years). In addition, Asian-American women have the highest suicide rates among women ages 15 to 24 and those over age 65.

Heart disease and cancer are the leading causes of death among Asian-American women. Other common health problems are tuberculosis, hepatitis B, and cervical cancer. The rate of tuberculosis is 13 times more common in Asian-American women—especially among immigrants from China, Korea, India, Vietnam, Laos, Cambodia, and the Philippines. Hepatitis B is 25 to 75 times more common than the U.S. average among Samoans and immigrants from Cambodia, Laos, Vietnam, and China, which is a significant concern for Asian-American women because it may be transferred from mother to child during birth. Although the overall cancer rates are lower among Asian-American women, incidence rates of cervical cancer among Vietnamese women are nearly five times those of white women. In regard to breast cancer, native Hawaiians have the highest mortality rate for any racial/ethnic group in the United States—37.2 per 100,000. Chinese- and Japanese-American women have higher occurrence rates of breast cancer than their ancestors in China and Japan (National Women's Health Information Center, 1999).

Osteoporosis, a preventable condition, is a particular risk for this group of women because of their relatively lower bone mass and density, smaller frames, and lower intake of calcium compared with other population groups (National Women's Health Information Center, 1999).

### Native American Women

In traditional American-Indian cultures, the women were valued biologically for being mothers and raising healthy families. Spiritually, they were considered extensions of the Spirit Mother and keys to the continuation of their people. Socially, they served as transmitters of cultural knowledge and caretakers of their children and relatives (Figure 1-5). The process of forced acculturation to the "white man's ways" decreased the status, power, and role flexibility enjoyed by women in many tribes (LaFromboise, Heyle, and Ozer, 1990).

The surviving Native American women come from more than 550 tribes, ranging in size from 20 to 250,000 people. Descending from early inhabitants of this land, American Indians and native Alaskans face health risks created by cultural dislocation and the tremendous loss of the knowledge and skills that sustained Indian societies for thousands of years. Over half of the total population no longer resides on reservations, with many living in urban settings. Health care services are provided by the Indian Health Service (IHS) based on annual appropriations from Congress. The per capita expenditure for this population is less than the per capita health expenditure for other U.S. citizens, forcing care to be rationed. In addition, the distribution of services is inequitable, with some tribes receiving full-service care and others obtaining very little.

Native American cultures believe that health is the balance or beauty of all things physical, spiritual, emotional, and social. Sickness occurs when there is an absence of harmony or balance. Within American-Indian societies, women were historically considered to be the center of the extended family system, providing an integral force for balance and harmony. With the experience of cultural dislocation, women have faced a loss of the traditional role within their native society and support systems.

The health status of Indian women is affected by the fact that rates of poverty and unemployment are higher among American Indians than other U.S. ethnic populations, with 27% living in poverty. The major health concern among American-Indian women is heart disease. As a group, they are at higher risk than all other U.S. women are due to their rates of obesity, diabetes, and cigarette and alcohol use. Native American women have some of the highest smoking rates in the country (44%) compared with white (29%), African-American (23%), Hispanic (16%), and Asian women (6%)(National Women's Health Information Center, 1999).

For American-Indian women, the rate of death due to alcoholism is 10 times that of U.S. women of other ethnicities. Services for alcohol-related problems are one of the unmet health care needs of American-Indian women. The traditional medical model for prevention and treatment of alcoholism has had little effect. Strategies that work to regain "balance" may provide the key (Kauffman and Joseph-Fox, 1996).

Other causes of death among American-Indian women are cervical cancer, tuberculosis, accidents, and suicide. Survival rates from cervical cancer are the lowest of all the ethnic groups. Native American women die from tuberculosis at five times the national rate. Their rate of accidental deaths is nearly three times the national average. The suicide death rates for young Native American women are nearly twice the national average but are lower than average in older women (National Women's Health Information Center, 1999).

Within the Native American population, there are also differences in disease rates. Native Americans have the highest prevalence of gallstones in the United States. Among the Pima Indians of Arizona, 70% of the women have gallstones by age 30. Diabetes rates range from 5% to as high as 50% in different tribes (National Women's Health Information Center, 1999).

### Hispanic Women

"Hispanic" is the designation most commonly used in government documents, and "Latino" and "Latina" are the self-identifying terms of choice among some Hispanics born in the United States. In this book, *Hispanic* refers to all persons of Hispanic origin who live in the United States, regardless of where they were born; the

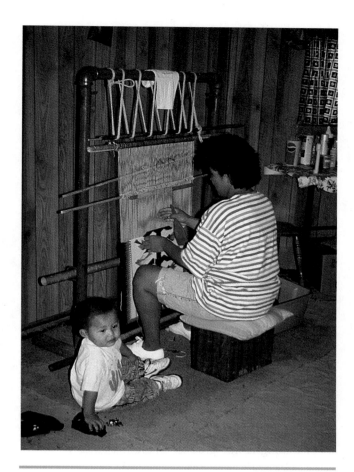

**FIGURE 1-5** • Woman at work. *(From Potter P and Perry A: Basic nursing, ed 3, St Louis, 1995, Mosby.)*

terms *Latino* and *Latina* refer specifically to those born in the United States.

The Hispanic culture has a holistic view of health and illness in which good health means that a person is behaving in accordance with his or her conscience. There is no separation between the psychologic and physical well-being of an individual. Illness is the result of psychologic states and environmental or natural causes and supernatural causes.

There are nearly 14 million Hispanic women in the United States. They are a diverse group, defined by the U.S. Census Bureau as persons who consider themselves to be Mexicans, Mexican-Americans, Puerto Ricans, or Cubans or persons who are born or descended from those born in Central or South America, Spain, or selected locations in the Caribbean. By this definition, the category *Hispanic* encompasses a diverse group of people who may come from more than 20 countries (Giachello, 1996).

Like other women, heart disease and cancer are the leading causes of death among Hispanics. Within other disease categories, lung, cervical, colorectal, and breast cancer are the types of cancer most frequently reported. Although the incidence of breast cancer is lower when compared with white, non-Hispanic women, Hispanics are more likely to die of breast cancer than white women are because it is usually detected in a more advanced stage.

Deaths from diabetes are twice the rate for non-Hispanic whites. Demonstrating the range of difference in manifestation of disease within this group, Cuban-Americans develop diabetes at half the rate of whites, and Mexican-Americans and Puerto Ricans experience up to 112% higher rate compared with whites. Many of the cases of diabetes in the Hispanic population are undiagnosed.

Health care access is difficult for Hispanic women. There is a higher percentage of uninsured Hispanic women (33%) than in any other race/ethnic group, even though many Hispanic women are employed or live with someone who is employed (National Women's Health Information Center, 1999). Difficulties with language, transportation, child care, immigration status, and cultural beliefs are further barriers to care.

### Differing Risks and Rates within and between Groups

The patterns of risks for and rates of a condition may differ among ethnic groups. There may also be differences within ethnic groups of women. The risks for hypertension of Hispanic women vary by national origin, with Mexican women having the lowest risk, Central American women at higher risk, and Puerto Rican and Cuban women at the highest risk. Mexican-American women have a higher risk for hypertension than white women, despite actually experiencing hypertension at lower rates. The rate of hypertension in Asian and Pacific Island women also varies. The few studies of Japanese and Chinese women in the United States show them to have low rates of hypertension. Filipino women coming from the same area have high rates, almost equal to those of African-Americans. Within groups of Native American women, rates also vary. Those who live in the northern plains have higher rates of hypertension than those in the southwest (Moss, 1996). We can conclude that there is considerable variation in the risk for developing hypertension and the rate at which it occurs within and between groups of women.

### Assisting Individual Women with Their Health

Even with the recent increase in information about women's health in general and the diverse health issues of specific groups, getting information that is relevant to individual women is an ongoing challenge. Not all information or recommendations are based on the needs or experiences of specific ethnic groups, not to mention

variations within the groups. Providers and clients must be vigilant in determining if there has been sufficient research within specific ethnic groups to support specific recommendations for health education, screening, diagnosis, and treatment of a particular condition. The most individually specific source of information available to determine a woman's health risks is the woman herself.

 **WHAT IS HEALTH?**

Conceptualizations of health are dynamic, changing across both history and cultures. The literature contains numerous definitions developed by sociologists, physicians, policymakers, and other professionals. In addition, individuals have their personal definitions of health. Therefore the definition of health varies among individuals, cultures, and governments.

### Definitions of Health

Health is not an absolute condition but a comparative term. We feel healthier at one time or another, or we say that someone is healthier than someone else.

What a person learns to recognize as illness or disease is what has been labeled as such by their society. Every society delineates what is normal and therefore healthy, yet what is normal is not universal. For example, "Women who are obese may be seen as 'strong' and 'healthy' in one culture and as 'weak' and 'unhealthy' in another" (Andrews, 1995).

#### Personal Definition

In order to help persons to attain health, as they define it, we must learn and understand their personal definition and goals. In addition, we must identify the factors that are helping or impeding their achievement of these goals. What type of assistance do they think we in health care can provide?

The categories of health and illness describe a continuum of experiences. The way we feel often fluctuates from one moment to the next depending on what else is attracting our attention. At what point on the continuum we decide that we are ill, at what point we decide to seek advice from someone else, and whom we turn to depends on our personal beliefs about health, our cultural practices, our finances, and the resources available to us (Hubbard, 1995). Understanding what makes persons decide that they are ill or that someone they care for is ill, and when, where, and from whom they seek care is important information for health care providers.

#### Models of Health in the Literature

The following distinctive models or contexts are used to describe health in the literature, each considering it on a health-illness continuum: "(1) clinical model, (2) role

## BOX 1-1 *The Health-Illness Continuum*

|  | **HEALTH** | **ILLNESS** |
|---|---|---|
| Clinical Model | Absence of signs or symptoms | Conspicuous presence of signs or symptoms |
| Role-Performance Model | Maximum expected performance | Total failure in performance |
| Adaptive Model | Flexible adaptation to environment | Total failure in self-corrective response |
| Eudaimonistic Model | Exuberant well-being | Enervation, languishing debility |

From Smith J: *The idea of health: "The health-illness continuum,"* New York, 1983, Teachers College, Columbia University Press.

performance model, (3) adaptive model, and (4) eudaimonistic model. Each of these models can be defined by the way the extremes of the health-illness continuum are characterized" (Smith, 1983) (Box 1-1).

Within the context of the clinical model, persons are considered to have health when they do not have disease. This is the model most often used in the field of medicine as a cure is sought to eradicate disease (Smith, 1983). As a result of following the clinical model, Western-trained professionals have been taught to recognize disease. What is not taught is the ability to recognize the more important, culturally conditioned concepts of illness and wellness and how to treat each.

A concept more often used by lay people to explain if they are healthy is the role performance model. Health is defined by the ability to fulfill one's central roles, which are usually those associated with family responsibilities and income production. When persons cannot do what they expect to do, they consider themselves to be toward the illness end of the continuum (Smith, 1983).

In the adaptive model, there are two types of adaptation to consider: biologic, which involves coping with environmental change, and social, which leads to successful interpersonal relationships. Adaptation is an active response when persons modify or change their environment to better meet their needs. "The achievement of a stable condition of optimum health is viewed as impossible. What can be achieved is the development of adaptive responses in order to meet the continuous threats to health" (Smith, 1983).

The eudaimonistic model provides the broadest focus on the physical, social, aesthetic, and moral conditions of a person. "Health is the condition of complete development of the individual's potential. Illness is the condition that interrupts or obstructs this development" (Smith, 1983). Health within the context of the three

previously described models can be viewed as the building blocks towards the eudaimonistic model of health (Smith, 1983).

### World Health Organization

The attempt to provide a global definition of health has been undertaken by a number of groups. Most prominently, the World Health Organization (WHO) has endeavored to create a universal definition that governments could use to determine if their people are healthy. In 1947, WHO defined health as "a state of complete physical, mental, and social well-being not merely the absence of disease and infirmity." This definition presented the idea that health is more than the absence of disease. Individuals were to be considered in a holistic manner that included their biologic functions and mental functioning, as well as their social interactions.

In the summer of 1978, the definition was altered and expanded to include individuals' ability to participate in their community. Health was defined as "a state of enough physical, mental and social well-being to enable people to work productively and participate actively in the social and economic life of the community on which they live" (WHO, 1978).

In 1986, WHO again altered the definition of health to position it as a resource from which people may participate in life. Thus health was defined as "the extent to which an individual or group is able, on the one hand to realize aspirations and satisfy needs; and, on the other hand, to change or cope with the environment. Health is therefore, seen as a resource for everyday life, not the objective for living; it is a positive concept emphasizing social and personal resources, as well as physical capacities" (WHO, 1986). Persons or groups within a community are considered healthy when able to satisfy their aspirations and effectively deal with their environment.

## Measuring Health

Even as the definition evolves, health still remains a difficult concept to measure directly. As a result, studies are designed to quantify its opposite: disease, disability, and death. The data is derived from official documents or population surveys. Conclusions about the health status or health situation of a group—rather than individuals—are then made. Whether there is a direct connection between declines in ill heath, disease, disability and death, however, and an increase in health is debatable.

## The Lived Experience of Health

The definitions of health developed by WHO, although meaningful to governments and the development of their programs, are not based on people's lived experiences and vary in emphasis from definitions provided by individuals. In a study conducted in France to distinguish between the health conceptions of lay persons compared with those of persons in the medical profession, 11,000 men and women identified the factors they saw as creating health. The items picked by more than 80% of the people were cleanliness, safe living and working conditions, and feeling well in a psychosocial sense. About 20% believed that their health—or its absence—was a matter of luck. This belief was most common among the socially disadvantaged (Oakley, 1993).

In a recent survey in the United States that asked individuals to define their health, most individuals related it to their ability to perform desired functions (Edelman and Mandle, 1998). Expanding the idea of health beyond the physical state, individuals include a positive mental state and the abilities to think, feel, be spiritual, and foster self-esteem. In addition, individuals included the ability to perform life roles, adapt successfully to the surrounding environment, and carry out activities of daily living.

## Health in the United States

Vast inequities in the experience of health exist around the world. Within the United States, people of all ages and every race and ethnic group have better health today than a decade ago, yet considerable disparities remain (Satcher, 1999). Not all Americans have the same access to knowledge, resources, or services that support a healthy life experience. Good health is the product of many different kinds of investments that include housing, education, exercise, proper diet, self-esteem, healthy lifestyles, social supports, and acceptable health care services (Bayne-Smith, 1996).

There are a number of measures used to judge the health of the residents of the United States. Epidemiologists determine the status of groups based on vital statistics—data obtained from official registrations such as death certificates and birth certificates—and the health statistics—data listing incidences of accidents, disease, and other occurrences that affect people's health.

Recent findings have led to the conclusion that our nation's health is improving, but with socioeconomic disparities. A strong relationship has been documented between socioeconomic status and health in the United States for every race and ethnic group studied. Americans with low incomes or less education are not as likely to benefit as those who are more educated or economically advantaged. For almost all health indicators considered, an increase in education or income heightened the likelihood of being in good health. Adults with less education tend to die at younger ages than those who are more educated. Across all races and ethnic groups, less educated adults have higher death rates from all major causes of death, including chronic diseases, communicable diseases, and injuries.

A person's socioeconomic status has a direct influence on insurance coverage and access to care—for both preventive services and regular visits. In 1998, the National Center for Health statistics reported that almost 200,000 of the people who died in 1993 needed but had not received health care. The primary reasons were problems in paying bills or finding or getting treatment. Low income adults are seven to eight times as likely to be uninsured as their high-income counterparts, with fewer poor women insured than men (USHHS, 1998).

 **WOMEN'S HEALTH**

Women live in households, neighborhoods, and communities and in times, places, and circumstances that support their health or disease, life or death. The health of women is deeply implanted in their status and roles. Complex societal factors are the basic determinants of women's health.

Women cannot separate their own health care from their roles as workers, caretakers, mothers, sisters, partners, family stabilizers, and heads of households. Each day, women are forced to make choices about others' needs that affect their own health. Wives and daughters are often expected to care not only for children but also care for the sick or disabled within the family.

Although medical care sometimes helps women when they are sick, it does not keep them healthy. The factors that make women healthy or unhealthy are as follows: how they are able to live their daily lives; what they eat; how they exercise; how much rest they get; how much stress they live with; how often they use alcohol, cigarettes, or drugs; how safe or hazardous their workplaces are; and whether they experience the threat or reality of sexual violence. Some of these things are under a woman's control, but many are not and can only be changed by collaborating with others. Nurses have the opportunity to play a large role in assisting women with factors under their individual control, as well as working with groups to bring changes (Sanford, 1992).

## The Health of an Individual Woman

The actual state of an individual woman's health is tied to the culture in which she lives and her position and responsibilities within it, as well as in the way she views herself and lives her life as an individual (Northup, 1995). For a woman, the concept of being healthy is bound with her experiences in everyday life and can be best understood through the lived experiences of the woman herself. Sociologist Jocelyn Cornwell has asked working-class people about their perceptions of health, and—surprisingly—the women repeatedly describe themselves as healthy even though they are experiencing chronic or acute medical conditions. As the women talk about their lives, the concept of coping is embedded in their personal accounts. Whatever their state of health or illness, the women find themselves obliged to carry on and care for their families (Oakley, 1993). If the woman is able to perform the functions required of her, she considers herself to be in a state of health.

## Improving a Woman's Health

Obtaining a general education improves a woman's health. Research findings suggest that what is important for a woman's health is not health-specific education but literacy and access to education in a more general sense. Instead of being told what to do, women benefit more when their education supports the process of self-determination, coping, and the dimensions of power and control. These are far more crucial to women's health than learning to do what the health authorities say (Oakley, 1993).

### Role of a Support System
Families, friends, and community provide the environment in which a woman functions. Families enhance or compromise a woman's health through a delicate balance of supporting her and demanding services from her. Social groups provide support for health practices or sources of health-endangering behavior. Even the neighborhood or community, as it promotes or restricts women's opportunities, influences a woman's health potential (Woods, 1985). When working with a woman, we must listen to her individualized experiences. Over time, she will explain her health needs, as well as the roles and responsibilities she is balancing.

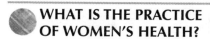

## WHAT IS THE PRACTICE OF WOMEN'S HEALTH?

The practice of women's health is devoted to the preservation of wellness, prevention of illness, and restoration of the whole person through women-centered practice. Women's health includes education for self-care, screening, and diagnosis and management of conditions that are unique to women; more common in women; more serious in women; and have manifestations, risk factors, or interventions that are different for women (Ruzek, Clarke, and Olsen, 1997).

An emphasis on preservation of wellness implies that women have a state of wellness to preserve, but what is not considered is from where that state of health comes or what is to be done if women do not have health. Poverty, the single most important factor affecting health and well-being, continues to affect a growing percentage of the population. As a woman's income rises, so does her receipt of screening for breast and cervical cancer.

Violence also persists as a major cause of disability and death among women (Moss, 1996). Women can only improve their health and obtain a level of wellness if they have the resources available to them within a supportive and safe environment.

Historically, women have been valued for their capacity to bear children. When the medical specialty of obstetric and gynecologic care developed, it focused on women's reproductive capacities and how to facilitate, diminish, or repair those capacities. These specialists supported the patriarchal and erroneous notion that all women's problems stem from the reproductive processes of her body (Webster and Lipetz, 1986). Even now when a woman has a health concern, her reproductive anatomy and physiology are still often the first area explored. The philosophy of women's health in practice provides a broader focus than a woman's reproductive capacities. Women are considered in a holistic manner, with consideration given to the interaction of their minds, bodies, thoughts, and feelings.

## ADVOCATING FOR WOMEN'S HEALTH CARE

Women have always provided care and healing within their families and neighborhood, and this continues today. Women have particular characteristics—that are not necessarily unique to women—that have led to them assuming the healing role. When culturally appropriate, touching, hugging, talking, and paying attention to another person and verbal and nonverbal communication skills support the process of caring. Women bring empathy and attention and a sense of connectedness, caring, and community (Perrone, Stockel, and Krueger, 1990). Historically barred from

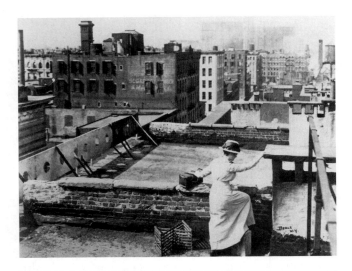

FIGURE 1-6 • Nurse walking across the rooftops to reach her next patient. *(From Mosby:* Nursing reflections, *St Louis, 2000, Mosby. Courtesy Instructive Visiting Nurse Association of Richmond, Richmond, VA.)*

books and formal education, women have learned from each other and passed that knowledge along to others across generations. When medical doctors assumed the role of experts in women's health, many of the normal biologic process of women's bodies (e.g., menarche, menstruation, pregnancy, birth, and menopause) became medicalized conditions to be "fixed" (Ehrenreich and English, 1973). Desiring knowledge and participation in their own care, the self-care women's health care movement grew and changed health care.

American women became health care reformers. Projecting the standpoint of women with authority of their own knowledge and voice, they have worked to change both their health status and the services offered to them (Smith, 1987). The movements have occurred in waves with periods of high levels of pressure for change, followed by times of acceptance. Women have formed self-help groups and educational programs, changed social policy, and created new forms of health care services for women and their families.

Nurses, seeing the need for a holistic approach, have responded with new models of care (Figures 1-6 and 1-7). It is important for today's nurses to understand how the providers and consumers of care have arrived at this period in our history. Many of the practices and health care interactions of individual women are still influenced by the prior experiences of other women.

The success of the women's health movement has changed the scope and type of care offered to women today. Challenges remain, however, with barriers to appropriate health promotion services and appropriate illness care still existing.

## 1830s and 1840s— The Popular Health Movement

During the 1830s, an assault on medical elitism and an affirmation of traditional medicine occurred. The popular health movement was not just an attempt to get more or better health care, but an effort to get a different kind of health care—preventive care and gentle treatments. Viewed as the caretakers of their families, women were the strength and the focus of the popular health movement. "'Ladies Physiological Societies,' the equivalent of our know-your-body courses, sprang up everywhere, bringing rapt audiences simple instruction in anatomy and personal hygiene" (Ehrenreich and English, 1973). The emphasis was on preventative care so health reformers, often overlapping with activists in other movements, advocated self-help in such forms as frequent bathing, loose fitting clothing, whole grain cereals, vegetarianism, temperance, exercise, and a number of other issues important to women. They sharply criticized the exclusively male medical profession, which frequently inflicted damage with cures such as bleeding, leeching, and amputation.

The peak of the popular health movement coincided with the beginnings of an organized feminist movement that sought equality for women. In the 1800s, a woman's legal status was largely defined by her marital status. Women were subject to physical and economic domination by their husbands with little recourse in the courts. Unmarried women with or without children often faced social ostracism and were in legal limbo. Women were unable to sue or be sued, own property, or pursue a career of choice. Women could neither vote nor hold political office, and it was not until the 1960s they were able to serve on juries. Poor and minority women suffered even more deprivations (Jarvis, 1998).

On July 19 and 20, 1848, in Seneca Falls, New York, a women's rights convention was organized to promote women's desire for equality under the law. Attended by more than 200 women and about 40 men, they took issue with a woman's loss of all financial or personal independence upon marriage, their lack of voting rights, and the inability of a woman to legally refuse her husband access to her body. (The phrase "voluntary motherhood" would later be used.) The resulting *Women's Rights Declaration* claimed women's rights as full citizens.

This beginning crusade for women's rights proposed that to address both the cause and effect of poor health in women, the status of women's lives had to be taken into account. The struggle for women's rights and many of the early women's health issues continued until the 1970s.

## Post-Civil War Era

After the Civil War, more women started to change the way they lived their lives. Looking and acting more self-reliant and dressing with more freedom, women increasingly participated in education, athletics, reform, and the job market. By the late nineteenth and early twentieth centuries, a slightly higher proportion of girls than boys were attending school. Against the advice of physicians, some even went on to college. Medical experts warned that the strain of a college education would make a woman an invalid and that diverting blood to the brain for the purpose of study could leave young female graduates incapable of performing their normal reproductive functioning. These experts were proved wrong. As one woman recounts, "Now that we have tried it (college), and tried it for more than a generation, we know that college women are not only not invalids, but that they are better physically than other women in their own class of life" (Thomas, 1908).

After successfully completing college, the growth in professional careers provided avenues for gainful employment and a viable alternative to marriage. When women who wanted to become physicians were blocked from training and working in hospitals, some founded their own for the educational benefit of both physicians and nurses. These were the first institutions created by women to provide women's health care.

In many ways, the late nineteenth century was a golden age for single women. "Approximately ten percent of the cohort of women born between 1860 and 1880 remained single—one of the highest rates recorded. Choosing not to marry did not mean, however, giving up a fulfilling emotional life, for many of these new professional women chose to share their lives with other women in lifelong relationships" (Ware, 1989).

Married women—especially urban, white, middle class homemakers—also experienced important changes in their lives. Central heating, electricity, indoor plumbing, and kitchen appliances decreased their work efforts and improved their living conditions. Store-bought goods and commercially prepared foods (e.g., bread and milk) lessened the time required for housekeeping and provided free time for participating in the activism of the women's associations increasingly prevalent in the next era.

## 1890 to 1920—The Progressive Era

Historians usually refer to the period between 1890 and 1920 as the progressive era. This became a time of reform and activism, confronting the problems raised by recent industrialization, massive immigration, and the increasing concentration of the population in the cities. Humanitarians and social reformers raised the issues of

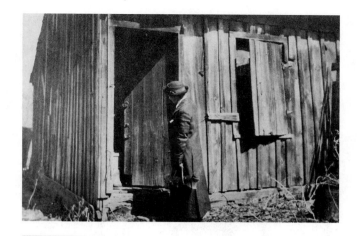

FIGURE 1-7 • The visiting nurse would provide care wherever needed. *(From Mosby:* Nursing reflections, *St Louis, 2000, Mosby.)*

child labor; unhealthy conditions in city apartments; and long hours, low pay, and unsafe conditions in factories or sweatshops. Settlement houses and women's reform associations consolidated the collective power of female voluntarism in efforts to offer help. They brought middle class women together, furnishing a base of expertise from which to shape public policy and address the health needs of all women.

### Settlement Houses

The plight of urban, white, lower class women was made public through the development of settlement houses. In Chicago, Jane Addams and Ellen Gates Starr opened Hull House in 1889. Understanding that improving health is based on improving individual people's quality of life, these college graduates lived and worked among immigrant settlers, sweatshop workers, unwed mothers, the hungry, the aged, the injured, and the sick. They decreased the health risks for individuals by rescuing girls from the streets, provided safe places for children to play after work, and taught reading and writing. They simultaneously worked in the political arena to change labor laws and slum-clearance policies and protect the rights of the poor (Addams, 1910).

In New York in 1893, Lillian Wald and Mary Brewster founded the Henry Street Settlement House and the Visiting Nurse Service of New York. The nurses "provided professional care in the home at low or no cost to countless patients who otherwise would have been completely neglected. They also offered each family they visited information on health, education, sanitation, and disease prevention" (Coss, 1989). The concept of settlement houses eventually spread to most major cities. Living in the poorest sections, the city-educated, middle-class women provided assistance to residents and pushed social and civic reform (Figure 1-8).

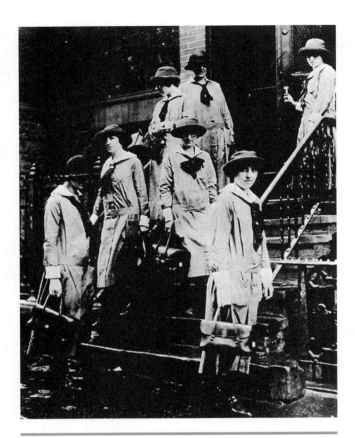

**FIGURE 1-8** • Nurses leave the Henry Street Settlement House founded by Lillian Wald and Mary Brewster to help the poor and needy. *(From Donahue P: Nursing: the finest art, St Louis, 1996, Mosby.)*

### Women's Associations

"Women are vital to the creative cultural process of social change" (Gilkes, 1994). During this time, more than a thousand women's clubs were formed by middle class women with newfound leisure time. Organized around a variety of issues, most clubs focused on issues affecting women and children, such as child labor laws and women's pensions. There was no solidarity, however, among the reformers. These groups of white women, although interested in providing assistance, were deeply imbued with class bias. They focused on helping the poor survive rather than helping them change their status.

Minority women approached this reform work with a different philosophy. In the black community, professional women and middle-class housewives formed their own clubs with a different focus. The motto of the National Association of Colored Women was "Lifting as we climb." Viewing it as a component of their family role, minority women as a whole worked to assist their community in addition to their work in the household and the labor force (Gilkes, 1994).

Emphasizing self-help and community responsibility, the club movement provided classes, recreation, welfare institutions, kindergartens, orphanages, homes for the elderly and working girls, and public health campaigns. Settlement houses were created within black communities to provide a full range of services (Evans, 1989) (Figure 1-9).

### Changes within the National Government

Many practitioners and healers at the time—including **allopathic** medical physicians, **homeopaths, osteopaths,** naturalists, and midwives—used and sold a whole spectrum of nostrums, tonics, and patent medicines. Many were targeted at women, especially for problems "peculiar to her sex." In 1906, the national Food and Drug Act took a first step at protecting the health of women by prohibiting false and misleading statements on medicine labels. This act, however, failed to require safety testing and regulate drug advertising (Johnson and Fee, 1997).

Between 1900 and 1930, approximately 60 white women and more than 100 black women died for every 10,000 live births. In 1912, in response to pressure from settlement house leader Lillian Wald, the Department of Labor created the Children's Bureau. Directed to help children, it developed a number of activities including the creation of two widely read pamphlets, "Infant Care" (1913) and "Prenatal Care" (1914). These brochures offered mothers scientific information, as well as common sense advice, on how to keep themselves and their children healthy (Ware, 1989).

## 1920 to 1960—A Period of Calm but Not Dormancy

With the onset of World War I in 1917 to 1918 and the Great Depression that followed, this cycle of reform wound down. On August 20, 1920, women won the right to vote and became a legitimate voice in the politics of health. Women attained new roles, greater opportunities for employment and education, and a better understanding of self-care—and they took advantage of these gains. The young women of the 1920s turned their backs on the political activities of their mothers and grandmothers. Instead, they wanted to have fun, emphasizing pleasure, consumption, sexuality, and individualism.

Activities with the potential to affect women's health grew in response to the changing beliefs about women's roles and rights. During this time, the Comstock Law prevented the dissemination of obscenity by mail or in person. Contraceptive information and devices were considered obscene, so sharing the information was illegal. Margaret Sanger recalls, "Early in the year 1912 I came to a sudden realization that my work as a nurse and my activities in social service were entirely palliative

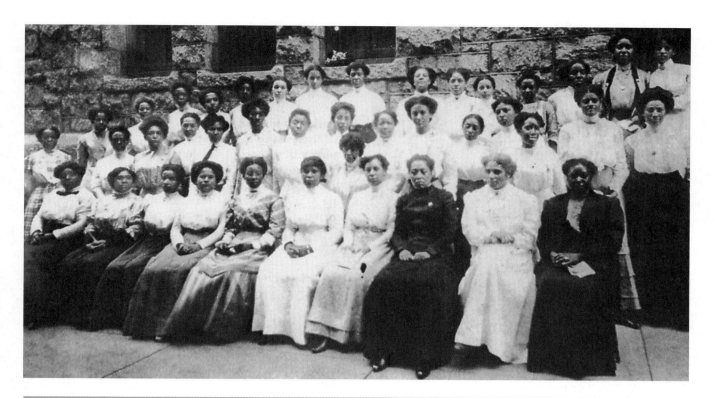

FIGURE 1-9 • First convention of the national association of colored graduate nurses. *(From Donahue P:* Nursing: the finest art, *St Louis, 1996, Mosby. Courtesy Schomburg Center for Research in Black Culture, The New York Public Library, New York.)*

and consequently futile and useless to relieve the misery I saw all about me. . . . Many of the women had consulted midwives, social workers and doctors at the dispensary and asked a way to limit their families, but they were denied this help, sometimes indignantly or gruffly, sometimes jokingly; but always knowledge was denied them. Life for them had but one choice: either to abandon themselves to incessant childbearing, or to [risk death] and terminate their pregnancies through abortions" (Sanger, 1931) (Figure 1-10).

Proclaiming that women have a right to voluntary motherhood without sacrificing their sexuality, Sanger initiated the fight to legalize the sharing of knowledge and use of methods of contraception. Attracting growing support for the individual freedom of women, in 1921 Sanger founded the American Birth Control League (ABCL). Momentum grew, and in 1938 a federal court decision made it possible for physicians to import, mail, and prescribe birth control devices. Sanger opened a chain of over 300 birth control clinics (Borysenko, 1998). In 1942 the ABCL, changing the focus to family planning, became The Planned Parenthood Federation of America, emphasizing family stability rather than individual freedom.

Parallel to the birth control movement were the maternal and child health efforts led by public health professionals, women from the settlement houses, and a number of women's associations. Rather than try to prevent pregnancies, this group was trying to promote healthy motherhood by improving and expanding pregnancy and child-health services. In 1921, Congress passed the Sheppard-Tower bill for maternal and infant health education. This bill was intended to lower high infant death rates by educating mothers in prenatal and early childhood nutrition, sanitation, and child care practices. Careful to avoid encroaching on the growing professional power of physicians, the bill had public health nurses, under the supervision of the Children's Bureau, provide education but no direct medical services. The program met sustained opposition from two sides: (1) those philosophically against government-supported health and welfare programs, and (2) physicians who did not want nurses to practice autonomously or government programs that might compete with their practices. By the 1930s, the funds had been entirely eliminated (Evans, 1989).

## 1960 to 1970—The Women's Health Movement

The next major wave of activity occurred in the 1960s and 1970s as political reorganization occurred on the national level and the grassroots activity of women's health groups increased. Women shared their collective

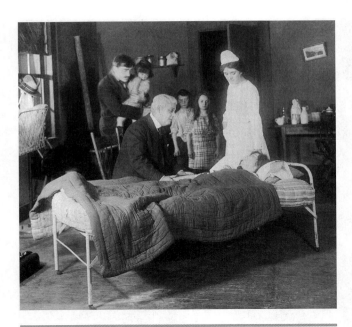

**FIGURE 1-10** • Margaret Sanger, nurse and founder of the American birth control movement. *(From Sophia Smith collection, Smith College, North Hampton, MA.)*

knowledge and challenged the assumed medical authority. With initial activity around women's reproductive rights of fertility control and access to abortion, the movement expanded to include women's health issues over a lifetime. Some of the key contributions of this movement included women's health advocacy, women-centered health services, and the sharing of information that was written by women for women. This revival of national interest in women's issues and health was brought about by several events.

### On the National Level

On December 14, 1961, President John F. Kennedy established the Presidential Commission on the Status of Women as a compromise move with those in support of and those against women's rights. Support for the Equal Rights Amendment (ERA), which was first proposed by the National Women's Party (NWP) in 1923, had grown during the 1950s. With the National Consumers League, the American Civil Liberties Union (ACLU), and other powerful unions and groups against the ERA, the newly elected Kennedy was seeking an alternative way to cope with the pressure.

The final report of the Commission titled, *American Women,* was released on October 11, 1963. Although the final recommendations were limited, the creation of the Commission caused many women to begin to think about their status. The commission's final report confirmed their suspicions that U.S. women were discriminated against both overtly and subtly (Ware, 1989; Linden-Ward and Green, 1993).

An Equal Pay Act, first proposed in 1945, finally passed in 1963. For the first time, a federal law addressed sex discrimination, requiring that women doing the same work as men be paid the same wages. This eventually led to the court decision that nurses aides (women) and orderlies (men) doing essentially the same work should be paid the same wage. Certain areas, such as domestic and agricultural work, and executive, administrative, and professional workers, were excluded from protection. Unprotected women trying to support a family on their own had to endure the stress of working more hours to earn the same amount of money as men in the same field.

In 1964 the Civil Rights Act (Title VII) was passed, outlawing discrimination on the basis of race, color, religion, national origin, or sex. The word *sex* was included at the last minute in an effort to kill the bill. This amendment was greeted with laughter on the floor of the House, yet the bill passed due to crucial behind-the-scenes work. Sections of this act prohibited discrimination in public accommodations, federally funded programs, employment, and other areas. Women now had expanded access to a variety of programs and an important tool to challenge discrimination. The law now stated that employers could not discriminate in hiring, firing, compensation, benefits, privileges, and conditions of employment (Linden-Ward and Green, 1993).

A five-member Equal Employment Opportunities Commission (EEOC) was formed to enforce the provisions of the Civil Rights Act, but it was lax in addressing sex-discrimination issues. Dissatisfied with the work of the EEOC, the National Organization for Women (NOW) was founded in 1966 to push for the civil rights of women. NOW's statement of purpose asks that women be fully included into the mainstream of American society. Rather than be antagonistic toward men, NOW desired that women be included in a truly equal partnership. A *Bill of Rights for Women* was developed, supporting change that would affect the health and well-being of women of all ages.

From 1970 to 1974, Wilma Scott Heide served as president of NOW, as the organization grew to over 40 thousand members. As a nurse, Heide recognized that "personal and social factors represent 90% of health indices that determine the underlying health status of people: housing, nutrition, fair employment opportunities, humane interrelationships, a single standard of mental health for both sexes, realization of social and economic justice" (Heide, 1985). Women's health is not possible without women's rights.

The activities of the 1960s and 1970s brought changes in both the legal and societal constraints on women's health and well-being. Women's health advocates began to address a variety of issues such as abortion rights, childbirth reform, product safety, self-help, lesbian health needs, and the high numbers of women undergoing hysterectomies and oophorectomies, mastectomies, and cesarean sections. The National Women's Health Network, established in 1976, monitored and influenced national health policy, while serving as a clearinghouse and resource for information. In 1977 a bimonthly academic journal, *Women and Health,* was initiated by the network to publish the growing body of new research available to both women and the media.

## Obstetrics and Gynecology

Women's groups, health and medical providers, and other activists came together in the late 1960s to organize a nationwide effort to legalize abortion. Although Margaret Sanger originally presented birth control as a woman's right, she had changed the legalistic strategy after 1915, downplaying the demand for women's autonomy. Instead, she gained the support of the conservative male medical community by making the ability to prevent pregnancy a medical issue. Sanger stated that women's lives could be saved if access to reproductive medical services was legalized. This politically astute move not only contributed to the process of pregnancy control becoming accessible in some states but also set the stage for the successful reasoning later employed to legalize abortion. In using this strategy, however, control of the process of reproduction was given to the medical establishment (Ware, 1989). The American Medical Association labeled women's health care as the care of the uterus and a woman's reproductive potential. Eighty-six percent of the women who sought healthcare during this era, for both general and female-specific concerns, now entered the system of services via their reproductive organs (Heide, 1985).

## Gaining Reproductive Choice

The sexual pleasure of heterosexually active women has long been influenced by the risk of pregnancy. Three major court cases, *Griswold v. Connecticut* (1965), *Eisenstadt v. Baird* (1972), and *Roe v. Wade* (1973), gave women the ability to control their fertility and the outcome of pregnancy. No health care actions have given women as much control of their lives as the legalization of reproductive choice (Matteson, 1995).

In 1961, the head of the Planned Parenthood League in Connecticut and a physician at New Haven's public clinic were arrested as "accessories" for giving information about contraception to married persons. For sharing this information, they faced 60 days to a year in jail or a $50 fine. Connecticut law made it a crime not only "to aid, abet, or advise someone" in the process of preventing pregnancy but also for individuals to use "any drug . . . or instrument for the purpose of preventing conception. In 1965, the Supreme Court decision in *Griswold v. Connecticut* broke new legal ground and removed legal restrictions in all states on birth control for married couples. Using the "right to privacy" in the Bill of Rights as the basis for decisions on marital intimacy, the Supreme Court struck down prohibitions on distribution and use of contraception (Linden-Ward and Green, 1993).

Unmarried women did not obtain the legal right to prevent pregnancy until 1972 with the *Einsenstadt v. Baird* decision. Bill Baird, a birth control activist, gave a package of spermicidal foam to an unmarried female Boston University student. Under Massachusetts law, this was a felony, so he was arrested and prosecuted. The resulting Supreme Court decision provided unmarried women with the same rights to privacy and contraception as married women (Linden-Ward and Green, 1993).

Fifty percent of all pregnancies are unplanned. The third Supreme Court decision, *Roe v. Wade* (1973) provided both married and unmarried women with a safe option when an unplanned pregnancy occurs. With the legalization of abortion on demand, women no longer had to risk the prospect of injury and death with "back alley" abortions. Trained providers could now make services available in sanitary conditions.

## On the Grassroots Level

During the 1960s, it was incredibly hard for a woman to access medical information unless she was a doctor—and most doctors were men. A patronizing attitude prevailed: women need not worry themselves about anything. The doctor told them what they needed to know and made the decisions about their care. If there were situations to be discussed, the conversation about the course of treatment and what the woman should be told about her situation would often occur between the doctor and the woman's husband or father.

At the grassroots level, women began to meet and share their growing knowledge. Some participants were health professionals, but most were not. As they collected information, they took a more critical stance towards the provision of health care and acted to create change. This collective rise of a feminist consciousness demystified important knowledge and allowed for a rejection of condescending attitudes toward women, as well as toward the poor and ethnic and social minorities (Heide, 1985).

Women began to rebel against the male-generated model of health care with its lack of holism and concern about preventive care. They started to believe in the value of their own experiences and tell the truth about their lives. Increasingly influenced by this broader feminist consciousness, nurses began to reject the handmaiden role that had developed over the past 40 years and began asserting themselves as the best guides to preventive practices.

No longer willing to be defined as "normal" or mentally healthy only when they married and had children, women changed the definitions for themselves. They assisted women providers in starting therapy clinics that supported the broader view of women's roles.

Dissatisfied with the lack of clear information about sexuality, menstruation, pregnancy, childbirth, and menopause, women set up self-help educational programs. In community-based educational programs, with "assertive nurturance," women taught each other how to perform breast and cervical self-examinations, shared self-help treatments, established advocacy groups to pressure institutions and providers to be responsive to their needs, joined local health-planning boards, and worked to change medical education (Boston Women's Health Book Collective, 1973).

They developed women-controlled health centers with the collaborative support of the Federation of Feminist Women's Health Centers. Contrary to most health care facilities, most of these health centers were organized in a non-hierarchical fashion. If doctors were hired to provide care, they were given little or no role in setting policy because that responsibility remained with the women clients (Heide, 1985).

### Changes in Childbirth Care

During the first half of the twentieth century, the process of childbirth had moved from the home and the care of midwives to the hospitals and the care of doctors. "In that transfer the woman giving birth became isolated from the support and proximity of other women who traditionally attended the birthing mother at home. Although the experienced midwives, particularly those who trained in Europe, had far lower maternal and infant mortality than most physicians could report, the hospital birth became the socially acceptable form" (Evans, 1989).

Some women felt depersonalized or ignored during hospital-based childbirth and developed alternative services that provided home births. When doctors pressured states to pass laws preventing nurse-midwives from conducting home births, women found lay midwives to help them. For women who still desired a hospital-birth experience, community-based childbirth preparation and self-advocacy classes developed so women could negotiate their birth experiences. When a provider or hospital was unable or unwilling to meet a woman's expectation for care, she often exercised her prerogative to change providers or facilities.

Physicians and hospitals, concerned about the potential loss in revenues, responded to the competition and offered some of the options their consumers desired. Hospital-based childbirth classes, family members at births, and birthing rooms were offered as hospitals competed for patients.

### Resource Development

One of the major goals of the women's health movement was to make information about women's bodies and health accessible to all women in demedicalized, clear language. In 1969, 12 white, middle-class, lay women—the Boston Women's Health Book Collective—met to discuss health issues and their experiences with the system. What emerged from this process was the book *Our Bodies, Ourselves.* The New England Free Press published the first edition—a 112-page, newsprint book—in late 1970. This "underground" publication sold over 250,000 copies as women spread the information about the existence of the book by word of mouth. Commercial publication began in 1973, and after numerous updates and translation into seven other languages, more than 3 million copies have been sold worldwide. The Boston Women's Health Book Collective remains a non-profit organization devoted to education about women and health. Their projects and services now include a Women's Health Information Center, distribution of free materials to women and organizations in the United States and abroad, several midwifery and reproductive health projects, and a speaker's bureau.

### Results of This Era

The activities of these 40 years had a profound and lasting effect on women and their expectations. They found that they were able to learn equally from professional sources—textbooks, medical journals, doctors, and nurses—and from their own experiences. They also assumed a capacity to evaluate the institutions designed to meet their health care needs. From their collective knowledge grew a sense of individual and collective power that women could create change. This learning provided a basis for growth in other areas of their lives. Finally, body education became core education. Women's bodies are the vehicles that move them out into the world. Learning to understand, accept, and be responsible for their physical selves allows women to be more self-confident and autonomous, stronger, and more whole (Ware, 1989).

Women reclaimed the right to actively participate in decisions affecting their health and the quality of their lives. A holistic, phenomenologic approach to care, with women perceived as clients to be served instead of passive patients, gained popularity. Women shopped for providers who would listen to their concerns and take their needs seriously, and then collaborate with them in decisions affecting their health and the quality of their lives.

This shopping around for providers began as individual women seeking to gain control over their health care coalesced into a movement that helped to bring about changes in the way women viewed themselves, as well as what they expected from health care (Boston Women's Health Book Collective, 1973; Heide, 1985). Some of the more tangible innovations that occurred during this period were package inserts explaining the risks and benefits of contraceptives, the creation of the National Women's Health Network, and the development of information services provided by women's advocacy organizations.

In addition to addressing particular health issues (e.g., contraception, abortion, cancer, gynecologic problems, childbearing, and menopause), the Women's Health Movement (WHM) recognized that other policy factors are central to the overall health and well-being of women. The WHM agenda broadened to include the following: safer, cleaner, and less stressful living and work environments; adequate food and housing for all; reduced violence against women, recognizing that such violence substantially contributes to women's health and medical problems; and a national health program that would guarantee universal access to care (Norsigian, 1996).

## The 1980s and 1990s

The grassroots energy of the WHM dropped off in the 1980s, but efforts continued in certain areas. In 1981, health activist Byllye Avery founded the National Black Women's Health Project, which established local chapters with more than 150 self-help groups for African-American women. In 1994, *Body and Soul,* the first book specifically written to address black women's health concerns, was published. The National Latina Women's Health Organization, the Native American Women's Health Education and Resource Center, and the National Asian Women's Health Organization were also organized during this time.

Women of color health organizations developed agendas that not only included reproductive rights but also continued to push to increase access to medical care for low-income women. They sought ways to pay for abortions no longer covered by Medicaid and focus on diseases and conditions that disproportionately affect women of color (e.g., lupus, fetal alcohol syndrome, hypertension, obesity, drug addiction, and stress). These organizations focused on conditions related to racism and poverty—areas that are not always understood or seen as priorities by the largely white and middle-class movement groups (Ruzek, Olsen, Clarke, 1997).

Identifying additional health needs, other groups added to the health agenda. Lesbians, rural women, working women, and women with disabilities made their health concerns evident. Demonstrating a sense of collaboration, both individually and collectively, women continued to press for issues important not only to their own groups but also for women as a whole.

The concerns of the women during the popular health movement of the 1830s and 1840s arose again during this time. The medical profession came under fire for suggesting to women that their risk for cancer could be reduced by performing prophylactic mastectomies and hysterectomies. Activists pointed out that no prophylactic testectomies were being offered to men at risk for testicular cancer.

## Commercialization of Women's Health Care

In the health care marketplace, executives of traditional health care programs started to adopt the language of the WHM in order to gain female clients, although most programs remained focused on institutional objectives, not the desires of women. Today, "women's health care" does not necessarily mean that women have developed the program or that the program is responsive to the needs articulated by women. It is increasingly difficult to perceive whether a particular women's health center or service is truly women-centered or just marketed as such (Worcester and Whatley, 1988).

A national trade association, originally formed as The National Association of Professionals in Women's Health, changed its name in 1999 to The National Association for Women's Health. As a trade association, it brings together the stakeholder groups that have the most to gain or lose financially in the field of women's health to influence the business environment and marketplace. The consumer's voice (i.e., women's voices) is easily lost as the business of women's health grows, affecting government policy and health care payment policies.

## The Effect of Federal Policies on Women's Health Care

Historically, women have generally been excluded from health research. In addition, the specific health problems of women have been given less serious attention in the areas of research and treatment than the problems of men. The result is a serious deficit in knowledge about the health problems women experience. This lack of information has diminished the competency of health providers to identify health problems and impairs their ability to deliver effective care to all women.

## Implications of Male-Centered Research

Heart disease kills more women than any other condition, but women were excluded from two large, randomized clinical trials on the subject. The findings that taking an aspirin every other day and lowering cholesterol levels reduce the risk of heart disease are based on research with men and are only known to apply to men. Women are also underrepresented in cardiovascular drug trials, even though there is a known gender difference in drug response.

Another example of following the male model in research became apparent with the AIDS crises. Until recently, AIDS, as defined by Centers for Disease Control and Prevention (CDC), did not include gynecologic symptoms. As a result, women—who often first manifest the virus infection in gynecologic symptoms—were not being identified and receiving treatment early in the course of the infection. Because insurance reimbursement was tied to the male-based definition, women who were HIV-positive but lacked male symptoms were denied access to services. Being excluded from consideration led to delayed treatment—and hastened death—for women with AIDS. The definition of AIDS symptoms was not changed until January of 1993 (Johnson and Fee, 1997).

### Changing Research Policy

The process of policy change was instigated by a series of public disclosures. In 1989, the General Accounting Office reported that the NIH had failed to implement its 1986 policy of including women as subjects in clinical research. Under intense pressure, the NIH placed renewed emphasis on its policy to require the inclusion of women and minorities in studies. The NIH also created a new office—the Office for Research on Women's Health—to coordinate activities and ensure that women's health research concerns would be adequately addressed in the future.

In 1993, the FDA reversed its policy excluding women of childbearing age from research trials (Johnson and Fee, 1997). In 1994, the FDA's Office of Women's Health was established to ensure that women are appropriately represented in clinical trials, as well as to seek to correct gender disparities in drug-, device-, and biologic-testing policies (Merkatz and Summers, 1997). The Public Health Service (PHS) agencies also expanded their Offices of Women's Health, and the Department of Defense allocated research funds for women's health programs.

Women began to achieve prominent leadership roles in health administration at the national level. Having two female surgeon generals and the first female director of the NIH helped to solidify the idea that women's health concerns must be considered.

##  LOOKING TO THE FUTURE

Women's health research is now clearly established within the biomedical research model. With this commitment, new biomedical treatments for breast cancer, autoimmune diseases, depression, and other diseases that disproportionately affect women may be found. The socioeconomic and cultural aspects of women's health and healing continue to need analysis along with the needs of millions of underserved women.

Women's health services must be responsive to the actual needs of women—not just the requirements of the business arena. Many of the factors that determine a woman's health (e.g., domestic violence, poverty, maintaining multiple roles, pregnancy and childbearing, experiencing female-specific health risks and conditions) do not lend themselves to quantitative data collection and analysis. We must hear women's voices in order to learn of their individual lived experiences and how to appropriately respond to their health care needs.

### Minority Groups

By the year 2030, women identified as being from a minority ethnic group/race will increase in proportion from one in four to two in five American women and differences across ethnic groups will become a more prominent issue. One in five American women will be of Hispanic heritage, one in eleven will be Asian, and one in four will be African-American. By the year 2050, women of color will represent at least half of the adult female population in America.

As a broad spectrum of people live together in the United States, there will be more generations of people with more than one ethnic/racial heritage. Health-promotion activities and assessment of health risks will have to become broader in scope.

### Longevity of Women

As a group, women live longer than men do but not necessarily live better. Women now live 30 years longer on average than they did in 1900. By 2030, one in four women will be over the age of 65. As women live longer, they face more chronic diseases and conditions that accompany old age.

The aging population will come from an ever-increasing variety of cultural and economic backgrounds. The quality of the life that they will live in 2050 will in large part be determined by the risk factors they can reduce in their lives now. Health promotion and disease prevention are vital parts of preparing for the future. Nursing research is essential to determine how to meet the needs of this diverse population

### Models for Women's Health Care

Health care for women must incorporate the social—not just biologic—dimensions of health and illness. In addition, the psychologic and spiritual dimensions of health and healing must be considered because they have particular significance to women. If we visualize women's health as *embedded in communities*, not just in women's individual bodies, we can start to imagine models of care that are very different from those that now predominate. Attention to the broader base of what actually *produces health*—as contrasted with managing disease—stimulates social investments in a variety of areas necessary to promote the health of women. When we look closely at the variations in women's health statuses and lived experiences, the need for attending to the broader base of health promotion becomes clear (Ruzek, Clarke, and Olsen, 1997).

Health maintenance and access to sensitive and appropriate supportive health care remain an illusive quest as many American women experience economic, social, and cultural barriers to adequate health care. When women do get to care services, providers may not speak their language, understand or value the traditional methods of healing, or know how to integrate treatment options into the woman's life. The unique barriers that women face when seeking health services must continue to be explored and integrated into health care practices. Integrating this knowledge as it develops into our practice creates the possibility of improving women's lives.

## THE NURSE'S ROLE IN WOMEN'S HEALTH

Women's lives are diverse. "Human care can begin when the nurse enters into the life space or phenomenal field of another person, is able to detect the other person's condition of being (spirit, soul), feels this condition . . . , and responds to the condition . . ." (Watson, 1988). Professional caring allows us to learn what matters to a woman and also reveals what they experience as stressful and what options are available for coping. Caring for someone creates possibilities (Benner, 1989) for improved health and well-being.

There are seven subconcepts of professional nurse care, as follow: being there, support, empathy, communication, helping, time, and reciprocity. The process of *being there* for a woman provides her with comfort and security. It can be expressed both verbally and nonverbally but depends upon a demonstrated, predictable, and nonjudgemental presence toward the woman. In this way, you transmit *support* by providing nurturance, advocacy, and access to health information. Such involvement requires that you have *empathy* for the woman. Empathy enables you to understand and accept the woman and enter into her reality without attempting to influence or change her.

Your caring is transmitted to others through interpersonal *communication*—verbal or nonverbal. Touching can be a powerful way to communicate caring. By being there for a woman and using the empathetic self to communicate support, you can effectively *help* her attain health or therapeutic care goals. Develop your practice in a way that caring remains within your interactions. Reducing nursing practice to just the delivery of technical tasks without connecting with the woman negates the holistic practice of nursing. To maintain or recharge our caring capacity, *reciprocity* of caring with our clients and colleagues is fundamental (Green-Hernandez, 1991).

Health for women is a holistic state in which their minds, bodies, thoughts, and feelings are connected. In women's health care, we support each woman on her unique journey to attain, maintain, or regain an optimal sense of well-being throughout her life. Health care encounters support self-determination and individual power and control. They are conducive to holistic healing. A holistic assessment evaluates the woman's total state of being.

### Nursing Process

The **nursing process** is a way of gathering information from a woman by observing her signs, symptoms, and subtle cues; synthesizing and analyzing the data; drawing conclusions and developing nursing diagnoses; validating these conclusions and diagnoses with the woman; collaborating in the development of a plan of care; implementing the plan; and then evaluating how the plan worked with the women. The process is circular and ongoing until the health care relationship is terminated (Box 1-2).

#### Human-Response Patterns

The current taxonomy, or classification schema, of nursing diagnoses is based on the nine **human-response patterns.** Health, a pattern of energy exchange that enhances a person's integrity to move toward life's potential, is manifested by the nine human-response patterns that are interrelated and reflective of the whole person. By collecting data in terms of the nine human-response patterns, we can be thorough in our assessments (Dossey and others, 1988).

Changes that occur in one response pattern always influence change in other dimensions. For example, if a woman develops the diagnosis "Latex allergy response" in the "Exchanging" pattern, it has implications for her health in "Pattern 5: Choosing," because she now has to cope with how that affects her life—and possibly her work choices; in "Pattern 7: Perceiving," because it affects how she views herself; and in "Pattern 9: Feeling," because of how she feels about this in her life (Box 1-3).

#### Nursing Diagnosis

A **nursing diagnosis,** as defined by the North American Nursing Diagnosis Association (NANDA), is "a clinical judgement about individual, family, or community responses to actual or potential health problems/life processes. A nursing diagnosis provides the basis for selection of nursing interventions to achieve outcomes for which the nurse is accountable" (1999). The nursing diagnosis may describe a human response to a level of wellness that has the potential for being improved, or a risk to a client's health condition and/or life processes, or an actual unhealthy condition and/or life process that needs nursing intervention (NANDA, 1999) (Box 1-4).

#### Levels of Prevention

This process of providing nursing care to women is covered in detail in the rest of the book. When we hear a woman's voice through the assessment process and

---

**BOX 1-2** *Using the Nursing Process to Develop a Plan of Care*

### DEVELOPING THE DATA BASE
**COLLECT THE DATA.**
* Develop a rapport (or relationship) with the woman so that she will feel comfortable.

* Interviewing is the primary way to collect subjective information.

* Observation is the primary way to collect objective data.

**Validation of assessment data**
* Review your findings with the woman as you go to be sure that you are hearing the data correctly.

**ORGANIZE THE DATA.**
* Categorize the data into subjective and objective information.
    Subjective—"I can't use my tools."
    Objective—Right arm is in a full cast.

* Cluster the data to identify gaps in information or areas that need clarification.

### NURSING DIAGNOSIS
**Choose appropriate nursing diagnoses.**
Write nursing diagnoses in problem/etiology/signs and symptoms format.

*Problem:* Altered role performance

*Etiology:* related to broken arm

*Signs and symptoms:* interfering with finger manipulation

**Validate the diagnoses with the woman. If she doesn't agree with them, the plan will not make sense to her.**

### PLAN INTERVENTIONS WITH YOUR CLIENT
**SET PRIORITIES.**
* What problems must be taken care of immediately?

* What problems may be easily taken care of now?

* Is there a problem that needs to be resolved before any others?

**COMPOSE GOAL STATEMENTS WITH THE WOMAN, DEVELOPING BOTH SHORT- AND LONG-TERM GOALS.**
Each goal statement must have the following five components:

* Subject: Who is to achieve this?

* Verb: What actions must be performed?

* Condition: Under what circumstance?

* Criteria: To what degree?

* Specific time: By when?

### INTERVENTION
**PUT THE PLAN INTO ACTION.**

### EVALUATION
**BOTH YOU AND THE WOMAN MUST DETERMINE IF THE GOALS HAVE BEEN MET.**

**MODIFY THE PLAN OF CARE AND SET NEW GOALS BASED ON THIS EVALUATION.**

**IF ALL GOALS WERE MET, TERMINATE CARE.**

---

develop nursing diagnoses and **interventions** in an inclusive manner, we can provide supports for her primary, secondary, and tertiary health needs across the life span.

*Primary Prevention.* A nursing intervention that focuses on preventing a problem or illness before it occurs is at the **primary level of prevention.** "It takes in health promotion, illness prevention, and health protection activities such as regular exercise, a balanced diet, good hygiene, rest and relaxation, adequate shelter, meaningful employment, immunization, smoking cessation, family planning and the use of seat belts" (Ayers, Bruno, and Langford, 1999). Unfortunately, there is little funding available to specifically pay for these types of nursing interventions so they must be incorporated into other nurse-client encounters. As nurses develop programs of research that demonstrate the cost effectiveness of disease prevention, more funding will become available.

*Secondary Prevention.* Activities that provide early detection of health problems and interventions to treat the disease or injury to promote recovery and prevent complications are at the **secondary level of prevention.** Examples of this level of prevention are as follows: hearing and vision examinations; pregnancy testing; breast examinations and mammography screening to detect breast cancer; and Papanicolaou (Pap) smears to detect abnormalities in the cervix or sexually transmitted infections. Such interventions do not prevent the start of the health problem but are intended to detect it so that intervention or treatment may be started. This illness care consumes the greatest amount of time and money in the current health care system.

*Tertiary Prevention.* When an activity is designed to reduce or limit the progression of a disease or the disability after an injury, it is considered a **tertiary level of prevention.** "Rehabilitation is used to enhance remaining

---

**BOX 1-3   Human Response Patterns**

1. *Exchanging*—mutual giving and receiving
2. *Communicating*—sending messages
3. *Relating*—establishing bonds
4. *Valuing*—the assigning of relative worth
5. *Choosing*—the selection of alternatives
6. *Moving*—activity
7. *Perceiving*—the reception of information
8. *Knowing*—the meaning associated with information
9. *Feeling*—subjective awareness of information

North American Nursing Diagnosis Association: *NANDA nursing diagnoses: definitions and classification, 1999-2000,* Philadelphia, 1999, The Association.

---

**BOX 1-4   Examples of Nursing Diagnoses**

The following are examples of accepted wellness, risk, and actual nursing diagnoses in the Pattern 4: Valuing.

**Wellness nursing diagnosis:** A level of wellness that has the potential to be improved.
• Potential for Enhanced Spiritual Well-Being

**Risk nursing diagnosis:** A human response that describes a risk to the client's health condition/life processes.
• Risk for Spiritual Distress

**Actual nursing diagnosis:** An actual unhealthy condition/life processes.
• Spiritual Distress (Distress of the Human Spirit)

From NANDA, 1999.

---

capacities, improve abilities to carry out daily routines, and provide alternatives to cope with functional losses" (Ayers, Bruno, and Langford, 1999). Examples of the tertiary level of prevention are as follows: teaching a woman with diabetes how to correctly administer her insulin and change her patterns of diet and exercise or helping a woman recently confined to a wheel chair to increase her ability to care for herself with exercises to strengthen her arms and physical changes to her living space. Even though interventions in this area can prevent the incidence and expense of further treatments for disease and disability, these types of activities are currently underfunded within our system of care.

### Evaluation

The value of our nursing interventions is evaluated from the perspective of both the needs and desires of the woman and our professional standards. The **evaluation** is measured based on the goals statements on which the interventions were developed. Is the client able to do what the goal stated? Has the goal been completely met? Has the goal been partially met? Has the goal been met at all? When discussing the goals with the client, encourage expression of thoughts and feelings about the achievement. If the goal was easily met, were the expectations of the goals too easy? If the goals were only partially met or not met at all, determine what factors contributed to success and what factors impeded progress. Evaluation is an ongoing process that cycles back with further assessment, possible new nursing diagnoses, and reestablishment of goals.

### Improving Women's Lives

With our expertise in health promotion and disease prevention, we have the opportunity to have the greatest effect on helping women to improve the quality of their lives. Working simultaneously with individual women, women's groups, and neighborhoods, we can reduce the social and economic barriers to access, collaborate in the development of services, and respond in new ways that meet their actual needs. By acknowledging and responding to their diverse perspectives, we can begin to reduce the racial and ethnic gaps in health care for women. We can collaborate to develop culturally sensitive educational and communication initiatives that help women take steps to create their own health and wellness. We can also work with the community to address the family and community risk factors that have a negative impact on women's lives.

Community-based models of care offer a holistic, collaborative process that values self-care and wellness. Whether old or young, rich or poor, partnered or single, women must be cared for within the patterns of their connectedness. They will only be able to move toward the positive end of the health continuum to the degree that their family moves with them.

---

## CASE STUDY

Jennifer Hernandez has come to the Women's Health Center for her annual examination. She is a petite, 29-year-old financial analyst for an investment firm. Her husband Carlos has accompanied her. He tells you that he came because he is concerned because Jennifer has not been herself lately. He says, "Her moods keep changing. She will yell at me 1 minute, then cry the next. Other times, she is quiet and won't talk to anyone at all. She doesn't let me touch her. It has been weeks since we have been intimate. But even though she is detached

*continued*

## CASE STUDY

from me, she is also afraid to leave the house without me." Jennifer sits there as he talks and does not say anything. No other problems are revealed as you complete the intake history with this couple.

Jennifer then follows you in silence to the examination room. She sits on the table and gazes at the floor, appearing reluctant to make eye contact. When you ask her what she is feeling, she says that she does not know; she is confused. "I can't understand what is going on with me. I keep trying to get on with my life, but I just can't seem to do it. I can't even sleep without nightmares." She then bursts into tears.

You reach out and hold her hand as she cries, and place a box of tissues next to her. She eventually begins to speak and explains that 2 months ago she was attacked in the parking garage as she left work and was raped in her car. "No matter how many times I bathe, I can't stop feeling dirty. I can't tell the police because I can't stand to have my husband know. The thought of ever having sex again makes me want to vomit."

Working with women from a holistic perspective, the nursing process provides a framework through which problem identification and mutual problem solving may occur. We are able to empower women and facilitate their responses to health and illness and their relationships with others. You will empower Jennifer through your interpersonal relationship to develop interventions that enable her to improve her health and well-being.

Use the nursing process to work with Jennifer:

- What subjective data do you have?
- What objective data do you have?
- What nursing diagnoses might apply to Jennifer's health care needs? How would you validate these?
- Do you need more information? If yes, why? How will you obtain it?
- How will you prioritize the nursing diagnoses?
- Develop a plan of care, listing the interventions and client-centered goals.
- How will you evaluate if your nursing care has made a difference in Jennifer's health status?

# Scenarios

1. Your grandmother, proud of her country says, "People in the United States have access to the best health care in the world. If anyone needs health care they can get the care they need."

- What information do you have about this issue? What information do you need?
- How will you respond?
- What will you say about the factors that enhance women's access to heath care?
- What will you say about the factors that restrict women's access to health care?
- How will you respond so that your grandmother may relate to this issue?

---

2. Your aunt says, "I'm glad that I live in the United States because with our health and safety programs, immunization clinics, and good nutrition we must live longer than anybody else."

- What information do you have about this issue? What information do you need?
- How does our life expectancy compare with that of women living in other countries?
- Why factors do you think may affect our longevity?
- How will you respond so that your aunt may relate to this issue?

---

3. You and your roommate, an engineering major, are discussing the events of your day. You mention that you discussed domestic violence in your nursing class. Your roommate says, "Domestic violence doesn't happen that often. I don't understand why you would spend a whole class on it. Besides, what does that have to do with a woman's health?"

- What information do you have about this issue? What information do you need?

- What potential repercussions do you have to be sensitive to?
- What will you say to your roommate?
- What facts will you give to support your view?

---

4. Keisha has come to you at the college health service looking for information. She has just learned that her aunt—her mother's sister—has been diagnosed with breast cancer. Keisha wants to know what her risk is of getting breast cancer.

- What nursing diagnosis could apply?
- What subjective data would you need to know about Keisha to start to formulate an answer to her question?
- Will her ethnicity influence her relative risk of developing the disease?
- Will her ethnicity influence her relative risk of dying from the disease?
- What will you tell Keisha?
- How will you evaluate if your intervention is successful?

---

5. Annie, a married woman of Japanese descent, has come to the Women's Center for her annual physical examination. You notice that her appointment has been rescheduled seven times. In talking with Annie, you learn that she had to reschedule her appointment four times because each time someone else in her family needed her to do something for them.

- What else do you need to learn from Annie?
- What nursing diagnoses might apply to Annie?
- What interventions can you develop with Annie that may meet her cultural expectations, as well as our expectations for meeting her health care needs?
- How will you plan to evaluate if the interventions work?

---

6. Juanita is a deeply religious woman who has come from Puerto Rico. She has been seeing a *santero*, a folk healer, about her stomachaches. She has now come to the clinic for additional assistance.

- How would you describe her ethnicity?
- How would you respond to her use of a *santero*?
- What data do you need to collect from Juanita?

- What are possible diagnoses?
- What goals and interventions might you develop with Juanita?
- How will you plan to evaluate their success?

---

7. Karin complained to you a month ago of extreme stress in her life. She is the major caretaker of her children, who are ages 2, 4, 6, and 8, as well as her husband and her in-laws, who live next door. She says that she has no time for herself but is anxious that she is not doing enough. She has headaches and is tired all the time. You suggest that she reprioritize her life, assert herself and make her husband help, and start using time-management skills to be more efficient.

She has returned to you today to say that she is no better. If anything, she feels worse.

- What assessment data do you have?
- What else do you need to know?
- Why do you think the interventions you gave her last month might not have worked?
- What will you do differently this time?
- What are possible diagnoses?
- What goals and interventions might you develop with Karin?
- How will you evaluate their success?

---

8. You are assigned the task of designing a program of nursing care at a new women's health clinic in a multicultural community predominated by Hispanics and Asians. The services must reflect the cultural beliefs and needs of the women you will serve.

- What assessments do you need to do?
- What objective data do you have about the health needs of these groups?
- What subjective data do you need to gather? How will you do this?
- What nursing diagnoses may be based on the data?
- What process will you use to develop a program of interventions? Why?
- What will you do to move these theoretic plans into a realistic plan of care that will help the women in the community?
- How will you evaluate whether the plan of care is working?

# REFERENCES

Addams J: *Twenty years at Hull House,* New York, 1910, Macmillan.

Andrews MM, Boyle JS: *Transcultural concepts in nursing care,* ed 2, Philadelphia, 1995, Lippincott.

Ayers M, Bruno AA, and Langford RW: *Community-based nursing care,* St Louis, 1999, Mosby.

Bair B, Cayleff SE: *Wings of gauze,* Detroit, 1993, Wayne State University Press.

Bayne-Smith M (ed): *Race, gender, and health,* Mill Valley, CA, 1996, Sage.

Belenky MF and others: *Women's ways of knowing,* New York, 1986, Basic Books.

Benitez M: Hispanic women in the United States. In Costello CB, Miles SE, Stone AJ, editors: *The American woman 1999-2000,* New York, 1998, Norton.

Benner PE: *The primacy of caring,* Menlo Park, CA, 1989, Addison-Wesley.

Bernard J: *The female world,* New York, 1981, Free Press.

Borysenko J: *A woman's book of life: the biology, psychology, and spirituality of the feminine life cycle,* New York, 1998, Riverhead.

Boston Women's Health Book Collective: *Our bodies, ourselves,* New York, 1973, Simon and Schuster.

Campbell J, Harris M, Lee R: Violence research: an overview, *Scholarly Inquiry for Nursing Practice: An International Journal* 9(2):105, 1995.

Collins KS and others: *Health concerns across a woman's lifespan: the commonwealth fund 1998 survey of women's health,* New York, 1999, Commonwealth Fund.

Cornwell J: *Hard-earned lives,* London, 1984, Travistock.

Coss C, editor: *Lillian D. Wald: progressive activist,* New York, 1989, The Feminist Press.

Dossey BM and others: *Holistic nursing,* Rockville, MD, 1988, Aspen.

Edelman CL, Mandle CL: *Health promotion throughout the lifespan,* ed 4, St Louis, 1998, Mosby.

Ehrenreich B, English D: *Witches, midwives, and nurses: a history of woman healer,* New York, 1973, Feminist Press.

Estes C, Close L: Public policy and long-term care. In Abeles R, Gift H, Ory M, editors: *Aging and quality of lfe,* New York, 1994, Springer.

Evans SM: *Born for liberty: a history of women in America,* New York, 1989, Free Press.

Giachello AL: Latino women. In Bayne-Smith M, editor: *Race, gender, and health,* Thousand Oaks, CA, 1996, Sage.

Giger JN, Davidhizar RE: *Transcultural nursing assessment and intervention,* ed 2, St. Louis, 1995, Mosby.

Gilkes CT: "If it wasn't for the women . . .": African American women, community work, and social change. In Zinn MB, Dill BT, editors: *Women of color in U. S. society,* Philadelphia, 1994, Temple University Press.

Gilligan C: *In a different voice,* Cambridge, MA, 1982, Harvard Press.

Green-Hernandez C: Professional nurse caring: a conceptual model for nursing. In Neil RM, Watts R, editors: *Caring and nursing,* New York, 1991, NLN.

Heide WS: *Feminism for the health of it,* Buffalo, NY, 1985, Margaretdaughters.

Horney K: *Feminine psychology,* New York, 1967, Norton.

Hubbard R: *Profitable promises,* Munroe, ME, 1995, Courage Press.

Ito KL, Chung, RC, Kagawa-Ainger M: Asian/Pacific American women and cultural diversity. In Ruzek S, Olesen V, Clarke A, editors: *Women's health: complexities and differences,* Columbus, OH, 1997, Ohio State University.

Jarvis SJ: Women and the law: learning from the past to protect the future. In Costello CB, Miles SE, Stone AJ, editors: *The American woman 1999-2000,* New York, 1998, Norton.

Johnson TL, Fee E: Women's health research: a historical perspective. In Haseltine FP, Jacobson BG, editors: *Women's health research,* Washington DC, 1997, Health Press.

Kauffman JA, Joseph-Fox YK: American Indian and Alaska Native women. In Bayne-Smith M, editor: *Race, gender, and health,* Thousand Oaks, CA, 1996, Sage.

LaFromboise TD, Heyle AM, Ozer EJ: Changing and diverse roles of women in American Indian cultures, *Sex Roles* 22 (7/8):455, 1990.

Linden-Ward B, Green CH: *American women in the 1960s changing the future,* New York, 1993, Twayne Pub.

Lock M: Situating women in the politics of health. In Sherwin S, editor: *The politics of women's health,* Philadelphia, 1998, Temple University.

Matteson P: *Advocating for self—women's decisions concerning contraception,* New York, 1995, Harrington Park Press.

McBarnette LS: African American women. In Bayne-Smith M, editor: *Race, gender, and health,* Thousand Oaks, CA, 1996, Sage.

Merkatz RB, Summers EI: Including women in clinical trials: policy changes at the Food and Drug Administration. In Haseltine FP, Jacobson BG, editors: *Women's health research* Washington DC, 1997, Health Press.

Miller JB: *Toward a new psychology of women,* Boston, 1976, Beacon.

Montagu A: *The natural superiority of women,* New York, 1992, Macmillian.

Moss KL, editor: *Man-made medicine: women's health, public policy, and reform,* Durham, NC, 1996, Duke University.

National Center for Health Statistics: *Deaths: Final Data for 1997,* 19:99-120, 1999.

National Center for Health Statistics: *New Study of Patterns of Death in the United States,* 1998, http://www.cdc.gov/nchswww/releases/98facts/98sheets.

National Women's Health Information Center: 1999, http://www.4women.org/faq. The U.S. Public Health Service's Office on Women. Department of Health and Human Services.

Norsigian J: The Women's Health Movement in the United States. In Moss KL, editor: *Man-made medicine,* Durham, NC, 1996, Duke University Press.

North American Nursing Diagnosis Association: *NANDA nursing diagnoses: definitions and classification,* 1999-2000, Philadelphia, PA, 1999, Author.

Northup C: *Women's bodies, women's wisdom,* New York, 1995, Bantam Books.

Oakley A: Women, health, and knowledge: travels through and beyond foreign parts, *Health Care for Women International* 14:327, 1993.

Perrone B, Stockel HH, Krueger V: *Medicine women, curanderas, and women doctors,* Norman, OK, 1990, University of Oklahoma Press.

Rodriguez-Trias H: Women's health, women's lives, women's rights, *American Journal of Public Health* 82:663, 1992.

Rose JF: Psychologic health of women: a phenomenologic study of women's inner strength. *Advances in Nursing Science* 12(2):56, 1990.

Ruzek SB, Clarke AE, Olsen VL: Social, biomedical, and feminist models of women's health. In Ruzek SB, Olsen BL, Clarke AE, editors: *Women's Health: Complexities and Differences.* Columbus, OH, 1997, Ohio State University Press.

Sanford W: Introduction. In The Boston Women's Health Book Collective: *The new our bodies, ourselves,* New York, 1992, Simon and Schuster.

Sanger M: Awakening and revolt. In *My fight for birth control,* New York, 1931, Farrar and Reinhart.

Satcher, D: *New Report Documents Improvements in Americans' Health,* June 10, 1999, http://www.cdc.gov/nchswww/releases/99news.

Schnitzer P, Runyan C: Injuries to women in the United States: An Overview, *Women and Health,* 23 (1):9, 1995.

Schrefer S: *Quick reference to cultural assessment,* St Louis, 1995, Mosby.

Smith DE: *The everyday world as problematic,* Boston, 1987, Northeastern University Press.

Smith JA: *The idea of health,* New York, 1983, Teacher's College.

Spalding AD: *Taking sides: clashing views on controversial issues in gender studies,* Guilford, CT, 1998, Dushkin/McGraw-Hill.

Spector R: *Guide to heritage assessment and health traditions,* Stamford, CT, 1996, Appleton and Lange.

Taylor JY: Womanism: a methodologic framework for African American women, *Advances in Nursing Science* 21(1):53, 1998.

Thomas MC: Present tendencies in women's college and university education, *Educational Review* 30:64, 1908.

True RH, Guillermo T: Asian/Pacific Islander American women. In Bayne-Smith M, editor: *Race, gender, and health,* Thousand Oaks, CA, 1996, Sage.

U.S. Dept. of Commerce, Bureau of the Census: *Statistical abstract of the United States 1998,* Washington DC, 1998, U.S. Government.

USHHS: *Heath, United States, 1998.* Washington DC, 1998, U.S. Government.

Ware S: *Modern American women: a documentary history,* Belmont, CA, 1989, Wadsworth.

Watson J: *Nursing: human science and human care,* New York, 1988, National League for Nursing.

Webster D, Lipetz M: Changing definitions; changing times, *Nursing Clinics of North America* 21(1):87, 1986.

Whitaker W, Federico R: *Social welfare in today's world,* Boston, MA, 1997, McGraw Hill.

Woods NF: New models of women's health care, *Health Care for Women International* 6:193, 1985.

Worcester N, Whatley MH: The response of the Health Care System to the Women's Health Movement: the selling of women's health centers. In Rosser SV, editor: *Feminism within the science and health care professions: overcoming resistance,* New York, 1988, Pergamon.

World Health Organization: Constitution of the world health organization, *Chronicle of the World Health Organization* 1: (1-2): 29-43.

World Health Organization: *Report of the International Conference on Primary Health Care, held in Alma Ata, USSR,* Geneva, Switzerland, 1978, Author.

World Health Organization: A discussion document on the concept and principles of health promotion, *Health Promotion* 1:73, 1986.

# CHAPTER 2

# Women Within Their Families

> "The family unit plays a critical role in our society and in the training of the generation to come."
> — SANDRA DAY O'CONNOR

*What is a family?*

*What is the difference between viewing a woman as a client in the context of the family vs. viewing a woman as part of a family client?*

*What is the possible impact on a woman when a society expects her to be part of a nuclear family?*

*How can a home visit affect a family's health?*

*What potentially useful health information about a woman can be obtained from a genogram and ecomap of her family?*

*What are some examples of primary, secondary, and tertiary prevention activities for families that will benefit the females in the family?*

*How may a woman's health be affected by living in a vulnerable family?*

The family is the oldest human institution. It is socially constructed, not merely a biologic arrangement but a product of specific historic, social, and material conditions. The family is closely connected with other structures and institutions in society and cannot be understood in isolation. The family experience is different for people in different social classes and of different races and sexes (Zinn, 1994).

"The term family comes from the Latin familia, which means 'household.' Originally the term referred to all of the people who shared the same domicile, including successive generations and servants" (Mahowald, 1993).

Although the connotation has changed, the human family is still deeply rooted in a sense of responsibility toward biologically and legally related others who may need our assistance (Whitaker and Federico, 1997).

The term *family* labels a concept created by humans to define boundaries and generally incorporates the description of a relationship in which there is a history of concern and caring and the potential for continued commitment. To collaborate in providing the most effective care for one or more individuals within a family, we must understand the components, values, and beliefs of their family system.

## THE STRUCTURE OF THE FAMILY

The word *family* conjures up different images for different individuals based on our personal experiences. The structure of family units differs based on cultural beliefs and societal expectations, as well as the political, economic, and environmental factors that have an effect.

### The State Defines Marriage

The legal definition of family emphasizes relationships through blood ties, adoption, guardianship, or marriage. The institution of **marriage** was created and is defined by state law in the United States. Only a representative of the state can marry people. Clergy are granted the right to officiate at a religious wedding ceremony by the state in which it is performed. The state decides who can marry, as well as at what age and under what conditions they may marry. The state determines what biologic tests have to be done, if there is a waiting period, and the type of licenses that must be obtained. The state determines the terms of the marriage contract and generally no private agreement between a husband and wife—besides agreements respecting property rights—are legally binding. The married couple are covered by the laws of the state in which they reside. If they move to another state, the contractual terms for marriage may be different and they have to abide by the laws of that state. Only the state may declare a marriage as over (Sapiro, 1999).

### Definitions of the Bureau of Census

The Bureau of the Census has determined that the legal definition of marriage does not adequately categorize the information desired in their survey. The bureau has constructed specific definitions to enhance the value of the data collected through that survey.

- A **household** comprises all persons who occupy a housing unit (i.e., a house, apartment or other group of rooms, or a single room that constitutes separate living quarters). A household includes the related family members and any unrelated persons (e.g., lodgers, foster children, wards, or employees) who share the housing unit. A person living alone or a group of unrelated persons sharing the same housing unit are also counted as a household.
- A **householder** is the first adult household member listed on the questionnaire. The first person listed must be one of those in whose name the household is owned or rented.
- A **family** is a group of two or more persons related by birth, marriage, or adoption and residing together in a household. The householder is included as a family member.
- A **married couple** is a husband and wife living together in the same household, with or without children and other relatives.
- A **subfamily** consists of a married couple and their children, if any, or one parent with one or more never-married children under 18 years of age living in a household, but the adults are not the householder (U.S. Census Bureau, 1998).

### Expanding the Definition

Professional disciplines construct their definitions of family to focus on their aspect of interest. Biologists view a family as members with a common genetic network. Sociologists emphasize the concept of people living together in the same household. Psychologists focus on people with strong emotional ties (Hanson and Boyd, 1996) (Figure 2-1).

Within the discipline of nursing, we have also constructed definitions. For clarity, most textbooks define the concept of family at the beginning of the book. In *Family Health Care Nursing*, "family refers to two or more individuals who depend on one another for emotional, physical, and/or economic support. The members of the family are self-defined" (Hanson and Boyd, 1996).

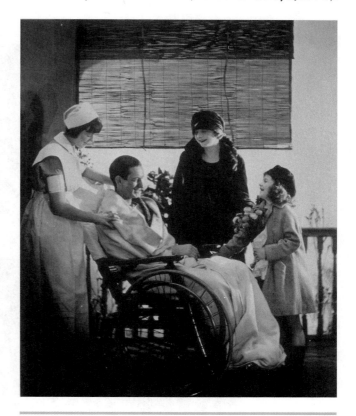

*FIGURE 2-1* • Nurse helping a family. *(From* Nursing reflections: a century of caring, *St Louis, 2000, Mosby.)*

In *Family Nursing,* Friedman (1998) defines a family as "two or more persons who are joined together by bonds of sharing and emotional closeness and who identify themselves as part of a family." In *Community-based Nursing Care,* Ayers (1999) recognizes that "the definition of family is evolving, but is generally viewed as two or more persons in a relationship who are joined by close emotional ties and who identify themselves as a family. These persons have an identifiable structure and defined roles or functions, decision making patterns, and patterns of daily living."

Within each of these definitions, the requirement of having two individuals may be met by an adult and a child or two adults. The relationship may be between heterosexual and homosexual adults. Within lesbian couples, one or both of the adults may choose to experience the relationship of biologic motherhood through pregnancy.

Variations in **family structure** become apparent as soon as we interact with clients and patients (Johnson, 1998). There is no single framework for family that encompasses all cultures, age groups, and time frames. Within the United States, the variety of cultures, religious attitudes, legal expectations, and lifestyles makes it impossible to develop a single definition of family (Table 2-1).

The following two commonalities run through all definitions of *family*: (1) a family does not exist unless there is at least one adult present, and (2) the family is composed of who they say they are (Williams, 1999; Wright and Leahey, 1994). No one type of family is superior to another. Being raised in a two-parent family is not necessarily better than in a one-parent family. Each family unit has strengths and the ability for positive adaptations that will raise its level of health and well-being (Figure 2-2) (Table 2-2).

## Definitions Differ across Cultures

The meaning of family and the household group changes over time and varies with social conditions. "What counts as family, how families operate, and the relative importance of family within larger cultural movements are all under scrutiny" (Bredin, 1998).

Political and economic conditions have created comparable family histories for people of color in the United States, but every group has family arrangements and patterns that are different from those of white Americans. Although each group is distinguishable from each other, black; American Indian, Eskimo, and Aleut; Asian and Pacific Islander; and Hispanic families also share some important commonalties. Such commonalities include an extended **kinship** structure and **informal support networks** that may spread across multiple households (Zinn, 1994).

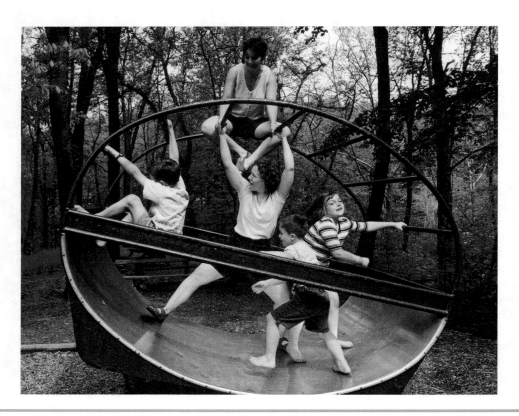

*FIGURE 2-2* • Nuclear family with same sex parents. *(Courtesy of Caroline E. Brown.)*

## Non-Hispanic White Family

The **nuclear family** (i.e., father, mother, and birth children) is thought of as the traditional Western European-American family. In the United States, white women have participated in and received a certain level of protection within the confines of such a patriarchal family. According to state laws, husbands are legally the decision-makers, determining where the family lives, how money is spent, and if the wife should work outside the home. This has created numerous constraints on individual women, but created a family system that was socially valued in the dominant society. The desire to create and maintain a nuclear family has been a vital element in the social order (Zinn, 1994).

---

**TABLE 2-1   *Examples of Family Structures***

| Structure/Form | Composition |
|---|---|
| Nuclear dyad | Two adults (married or unmarried, same or opposite sex). |
| Nuclear family | Two adults (married or unmarried, same or opposite sex) with children (biologic, step, adopted, foster). |
| Single parenting | One adult (separated, divorced, widowed, never married) with children (biologic, step, adopted, foster); adult may have sole or shared custody of children. Children may be members of two households, one of each parent. |
| Extended family | More than two adults with or without children who may or may not be biologically related. |
| Multigenerational | Any combination of adults and children spanning more than two generations. |

---

**TABLE 2-2   *Marital Status of the Population by Sex, Race, and Hispanic Origin, 1990 and 1997****

| MARITAL STATUS, RACE, AND HISPANIC ORIGIN | Total % 1990 | Total % 1997 | Male % 1990 | Male % 1997 | Female % 1990 | Female % 1997 |
|---|---|---|---|---|---|---|
| **TOTAL†** | | | | | | |
| Never married | 22.2 | 23.5 | 25.8 | 27.0 | 18.9 | 20.2 |
| Married | 61.9 | 59.7 | 64.3 | 61.5 | 59.7 | 57.9 |
| Widowed | 7.6 | 7.0 | 2.7 | 2.9 | 12.1 | 10.9 |
| Divorced | 8.3 | 9.9 | 7.2 | 8.7 | 9.3 | 11.0 |
| **WHITE** | | | | | | |
| Never married | 20.3 | 21.0 | 24.1 | 24.7 | 16.9 | 17.5 |
| Married | 64.0 | 62.1 | 66.2 | 63.8 | 61.9 | 60.4 |
| Widowed | 7.5 | 7.1 | 2.6 | 2.8 | 12.2 | 11.2 |
| Divorced | 8.1 | 9.8 | 7.2 | 8.7 | 9.0 | 10.9 |
| **BLACK** | | | | | | |
| Never married | 35.1 | 39.1 | 38.4 | 41.5 | 32.5 | 37.2 |
| Married | 45.8 | 42.4 | 49.2 | 45.3 | 43.0 | 40.0 |
| Widowed | 8.5 | 7.2 | 3.7 | 3.3 | 12.4 | 10.4 |
| Divorced | 10.6 | 11.3 | 8.8 | 9.9 | 12.0 | 12.4 |
| **HISPANIC‡** | | | | | | |
| Never married | 27.2 | 30.6 | 32.1 | 35.7 | 22.5 | 25.3 |
| Married | 61.7 | 58.1 | 60.9 | 56.9 | 62.4 | 59.3 |
| Widowed | 4.0 | 3.8 | 1.5 | 1.5 | 6.5 | 6.1 |
| Divorced | 7.0 | 7.6 | 5.5 | 5.8 | 8.5 | 9.3 |

*In percentages. As of March 1997. Persons 18 years old and over. Excludes members of the armed forces except those living off post or with their families on post. Based on Current Population Survey.

†Includes persons of other races and not of Hispanic origin not shown separately.

‡Hispanic persons may be of any race.

From the U.S. Department of Commerce, Bureau of the Census: *Statistical abstracts of the United States,* 1998, Chart No. 61.

Most of the common assumptions about the mythical family ideal are based on this cultural belief of the white, middle-class, non-Hispanic population. After slavery, whites still expected African-American wives to leave their homes and work for them. If an African-American woman stayed home to take care of her own family, whites considered her lazy. The ideal of the stay-at-home wife was only expected to apply to white middle-class women (Lehrer, 1999).

In 1970, 29% of white mothers were in the paid labor force; and the percentage rose to 49% in 1997 (U.S. Census Bureau, 1998). This current perspective has evolved, and white women are choosing to work outside the home.

Unless otherwise labeled, most past research on families has been with the white, non-Hispanic population. The cultural bias of some studies is apparent when the nuclear family is assumed to be the norm to which families in other cultures are compared.

## African-American Family

Black married women, of both the middle and lower classes, have always worked in proportionately greater numbers than white wives. The figures for 1997 show that 59% of African-American mothers are in the paid labor force (U.S. Census Bureau, 1998). Black women have simultaneously cared for their family at home, as well as for people outside their home (e.g., often others' families). Because of discrimination in the workplace, most jobs open to black women have traditionally been low paying and required long hours away from their families. Unemployment and underemployment are higher for African-American women than for any other group in this country.

One of the strengths of the African-American community has been the existence of informal support networks. Many first generation African slave women, even when married, were forced to raise their children without a lot of male assistance or even presence. This reinforced the cultural emphasis on motherhood that was prevalent in their homeland of Western Africa (White, 1995). Beginning in the slave era, the family obligations of wives and mothers overlapped with a concept of community welfare because they not only nurtured their own families but also others around them.

At the end of slavery, racial discrimination prevented equal access to education, training, jobs, and housing. Black men were now expected to provide adequately for their families but were not allowed access to the education, skills, and opportunities that would enable them to do so. Policies of the government-assistance programs (e.g., Aid to Dependent Children) denied assistance if a father was present in the home. Discouraged, some men in low-paying jobs without health insurance left their families so that their children could receive the govern-

ment benefits and experience a higher standard of living (Franke, 1997).

About 47% of African American families are currently maintained by women (U.S. Census Bureau, 1998). In 1997, 39.7% of African-American women had never been married (U.S. Census Bureau, 1998), partly because the number of marriageable African-American men is declining. For individuals between the ages of 25 and 55, there is a ratio of 86.5 black men to 100 black women. In the same age group, there is a ratio of 100.5 white men to 100 white women (Spalding, 1998).

As heads of households, African-American women have been glorified as strong "black matriarchs." They are not necessarily happy, however, when they find themselves without a partner, thrust into the undesired role of primary provider and protector of their children. Being strong is not easy or even a choice for these woman; they do what is necessary for the survival of their families (Franke, 1997). As one mother explains, "We share similar past experiences of poverty, mental torment and physical abuse, self doubt and confusion. But now we are heading our households and raising our children in well-functioning families" (Omolade, 1986).

## American Indian, Eskimo, and Aleut Families

The survival of American Indian families during 200 years of rule by an external government attests to the resilience of Indian women. Despite continuous role readjustments, value conflicts, and economic pressures, the family has endured. Before contact with Europeans, traditional Indian family life was based on egalitarian systems of reciprocity in which separate, complementary, and equally essential tasks were assigned to each sex. The acculturation to "white man's ways" led to a breakdown of the complementary nature of male-female relations and a general increase in Indian male dominance and control over the family and Indian women (LaFromboise, Heyle, and Ozer, 1990).

American Indian families are generally poor, with the median family income of American Indians less than half that of the nation as a whole. Because less than 1% of American Indian families live in urban areas, many families encounter health problems because of the difficulties of social isolation and access to care.

## Asian and Pacific Islander Families

Asian and Pacific Islander Americans are Chinese, Filipino, Japanese, Asian Indian, Korean, Vietnamese, Laotian, Cambodian, Thai, and Hmong. The major Pacific Islanders are Hawaiian, Samoan, Chamorro (Guamanian), Tongan, and Melanesian. Asians have officially been in the United States for over 140 years, with some Asian families having been residents for more than seven generations. The patterns of immigration and the establishment of families and their expectations—once settled—have differed over time.

Through education and hard work, some immigrant families have become successful. Many poor Asian-American families are uncounted, however, because they are too proud to access public assistance and welfare.

In Asian families, relatives are generally of great importance, and family sharing is a strong obligation. Reciprocity and generosity are highly valued. Respect for family, elders, and those in authority is vital. Respect is demonstrated by seeking and valuing the opinions of family members and maintaining close, **multigenerational** family ties (Andrews, 1995).

In the Japanese family system, the human relationships within a household group are more important than all other human relationships. The wife and daughter-in-law living within the home are more important than blood relatives who have gone to live in another home. Family members care for each other with personal care, financial support, and whatever else is needed (Mizuno, 1999).

For the followers of Confucius, the idea of patriarchy and gender inequity is supported within the home. The Rule of Three Obedience emphasizes women's subordination to men. A woman is instructed to obey her father before marriage, her husband during marriage, and her son(s) after her husband's death. The principle of Distinction between Wife and Husband demands separate living and work spheres and accents the power differential of the genders. Men risk losing face by helping their wives in the home. Some women who immigrated to the United States are challenging male domination in the home and the unequal division of family work (Lim, 1997), but they are facing strong resistance. Because their husbands will not help, Korean women living in the United States work at both unpaid family work and paid work the equivalent hours of 2 months a year more than men. These extra hours of housework are double compared to American women, who work 1 month a year more than American men (Hochschild, 1998).

## Hispanic Families

Hispanic Americans are mistakenly categorized generically and incorrectly as one ethnic or cultural group of Spanish origin or descent, although most Hispanics are aware of the distinct cultural differences within the Hispanic culture. These "subcultural differences are determined by social and economic status, education, country of origin, place of residence, and religious and political affiliation" (Castillo, 1996). In 1997, 37% of Hispanic mothers were working outside the home (U.S. Census Bureau, 1998).

Hispanics originate from more than 20 countries, so there is a great deal of diversity in the family experiences both within and between the people of these countries.

Most Hispanics speak Spanish—although there are regional differences in the Spanish, but some speak Portuguese. Most Hispanic families raise their children in the Roman Catholic Church, although others are members of Protestant or Pentecostal churches.

Because of the large number of Mexicans and Puerto Ricans within the United States, much of the research about Hispanics focuses on people of these cultures. Although these cultures are more easily studied, we cannot assume that what is true in these cultures is equally applicable in other Hispanic cultures.

In Mexican-American families, there is an orientation toward an extended kinship network—which may include godparents (*compadres*) and other nonbiologic kin—and distinctly different roles for men and women. The literature has often stressed the dominant role of men in Mexican and Mexican-American families, but recent studies suggest that the male/female, dominance/submission patterns are much less universal than previously assumed.

In some Mexican-American marriages there is an **egalitarian relationship,** with husbands and wives sharing decisions about where the family lives, how money is spent, and if the wife should work outside the home. Either the dominant male role never existed, or these couples are creating a radical change (Hawkes and Taylor, 1975).

The family is the most important Hispanic institution for Mexican-American migrant farm workers, who form close family bonds and migrate in multigenerational family groups. Within the family group, paid work, cooking, and child care are shared across subfamily groups and generations. Separation from the family group (e.g., with a hospitalization) can be devastating to family members (Hibbeln, 1996).

Puerto Ricans also have a strong family-oriented culture. As with many other Hispanic cultures, a family is not considered a "real family" until after children are born. For Puerto Rican families, a healthy baby—especially a male baby—can be seen as a symbol of the father's virility and the fertility and strength of the mother. When the baby is less than perfect, however, it can threaten the stability of the family, and they will need support. Informal support may be provided by friends and relatives, as well as spiritualists or *curanderos*. This type of cultural support may be more important to the family than the formal support of the community health care services (Crouch-Ruiz, 1996).

## Beyond Specific Cultures

Although it is helpful to understand the beliefs and values of the families, we must also recognize and allow the individual uniqueness of the family to become evident. For example, families from rural areas are different from urban families within the same culture, and

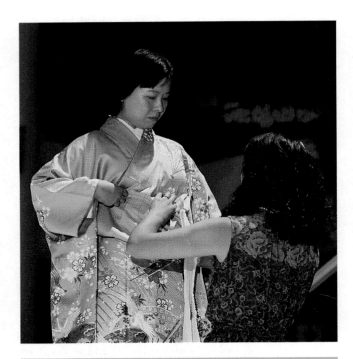

FIGURE 2-3 • Diversity within a culture. *(From Potter P and Perry A:* Basic nursing: a critical thinking approach, *ed 3, St Louis, 1995, Mosby.)*

| Race and Origin of Spouses | Total (in thousands) |
|---|---|
| Married couples, total | 54,666 |
| **RACE** | |
| Same race couples | 51,489 |
|   White/white | 47,791 |
|   Black/black | 3,698 |
| Interracial couples | 1,264 |
|   Black/white | 311 |
|   White/other race (excluding white and black) | 896 |
|   Black/other race (excluding white and black) | 57 |
| All other couples (excluding white and black) | 1,912 |

**TABLE 2-3    *Married Couple of Same or Mixed Race and Origins, 1997****

*In Thousands. As of March 1997. Persons 15 years old and over. Persons of Hispanic origin may be of any race. Except as noted, based on Current Population Survey.

Source: U.S. Department of Commerce, Bureau of the Census: *Statistical abstracts of the United States*, 1998, Chart No. 67.

some families may have more in common with each other across cultural lines than they have with families of their own culture. In addition, the adults in a family may come from different cultures. A growing number of marriages are between couples of different races and cultures. The cultural milieu resulting within the family will develop out of the blending of the beliefs and patterns of the families of origin (Table 2-3) (Figure 2-3).

## Cultural Health Practices

The ways in which health is maintained or restored varies from culture to culture. In families where different cultures are represented, there may be many variations of health beliefs and practices. Spector (1996) notes that "ethnic beliefs and practices related to health and illness of the family are more in tune with the mother's family than with the father's" because the nurturer of the family tends to be the mother.

Knowledge of factors such as family health, socioeconomic status, political and historic aspects, and migration patterns can help us to balance the general understanding of the family culture with the unique patterns and experiences of the actual human network. Be wary of believing you have expertise simply because you have a cognitive understanding of a particular culture's traditional value. This can be especially tempting if the family is from an ethnic and/or socioeconomic

background that is similar to yours. Some knowledge can be helpful, but without the openness to learn about the uniqueness of a particular family from the family itself, the cognitive knowledge can become a barrier and deterrent (Figure 2-4).

Families are not immune to the development of their own stereotyping of the expected beliefs and behaviors of the health care provider. They may enter the relationship with many preconceived ideas based on their own or others' past experiences with people of a certain culture, socioeconomic background, education, or profession.

## Effect of Immigration

A large share of the nation's population growth is due to immigration. The largest 10-year wave in U.S. history occurred during the 1980s, with the arrival of almost 9 million people. By 2020, immigrants will have more influence on U.S. population growth than the reproduction of residents within the country. These patterns of immigration will continue to produce an emerging array of family groups in need of care (Zinn, 1994).

A family's migration experience is an important dimension to consider. For some, the move is the result of a lengthy planning process, but for others it is a rapid uprooting necessitated by turmoil and crisis in their native land. These and other factors affect the process and problems a family experiences in their new environment.

"Immigrants are constantly attempting to balance the values of their cultural heritage with those of the new host society" (Meleis, 1991). Opinions on the place of the new host society's beliefs in their family life may differ across generations. Children and grandchildren of immigrants tend to adopt many of the values and attitudes of the dominant culture, which can be in conflict with the cultural beliefs of the parents. For example, the decision of a child to marry an individual from another cultural or ethnic background can create a great deal of conflict and concern for the future of the family and potential children.

 ## THE FUNCTION OF FAMILIES

Families exist as the basic unit of society and function as the first social structure of which the child is a member. The family is the place in which humans are nurtured, develop a sense of significance and meaningfulness, and learn how to function in ways acceptable to society (Kolander, Ballard, and Chandler, 1999). Each family member—both children and adults—has one or more roles within the family that define the obligations, rights, and behaviors expected of him or her. Role fulfillment within families prepares us for interactions within society as a whole.

### Family Prepares Individuals for Society

In many instances, it is our family that meets our needs for warmth, food, and shelter, as well as for love, acceptance, companionship, and comfort. We learn how to socialize both within our family and with others as a family. Our first encounter with limit setting and understanding what is right and wrong usually develops within the family. Our sense of responsibility for others often comes from our family experience. Families also serve as our first—and often most significant—health teachers.

**Family functions** are connected with roles and refer to "how families go about meeting the needs of individuals and meeting the purposes of the broader society" (Hanson and Boyd, 1996). Friedman (1998) has identified five major functions for families, which are as follows: (1) affective (i.e., affirmation, support, and respect for each other), (2) socialization (i.e., shared cultural and moral values), (3) reproductive (i.e., choosing to procreate or not), (4) economic (i.e., the financial resources available to the family either by family wage-earners or community and governmental resources), and (5) health care (i.e., the provision of physical necessities).

The specifics taught to children within a family vary from culture to culture. Just like language, however,

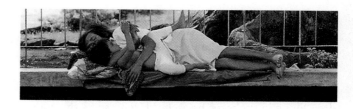

FIGURE 2-4 • Homeless family. *(Courtesy of Caroline E. Brown.)*

lessons learned before the age of 5 become an integral part of a person's thoughts and behavior. A child may learn to eat with a fork, knife, and spoon; or with chopsticks; or with the right hand. They learn the rules of when and how to speak to an adult and when—if ever—to make eye contact (Andrews, 1995).

### Society Affects Family Functioning

Culture affects family functioning in a variety of ways, including the selection of mates, marriage forms, postmarital residence, role expectations, family kinship systems, rules governing inheritance, household and family structure, family obligations, family-community dynamics, and the development of alternative family formations (Andrews, 1995). Every family works both implicitly and explicitly to pass cultural beliefs and practices from one generation to the next. Within each family unit, however, the members modify the culture in ways that are uniquely their own. Some beliefs, practices, and customs are maintained, whereas others are altered or abandoned.

 ## HISTORICAL CHANGES IN THE FAMILY

Historically, the family has often been thought of as patriarchal, consisting of a male head-of-household, his wives or wives and concubines, all of their children and unmarried daughters, and servants with their children. It has also been patrilineal, which means that offspring are genetically related to the patriarch, and the family surname is that of the father.

Although the patriarchal aspects of family have declined in much of modern society, laws and customs sometimes take for granted that husbands and fathers are heads of households. Prior to 1980, the U.S. census assumed that the husband was always the head of the household in married-couple households. This assumption was problematic for couples who believed that marriage should be an equal partnership. Currently, however, if a home or apartment is owned or rented jointly by a married couple, either the wife or the husband may be listed first on the census questionnaire and considered as the head of the household (U.S. Census Bureau, 1998).

## Research on the History of Families

The lack of consensus about what a family is has led to research on the history of families. As a result, two common myths have been revealed. The first untruth is that the nuclear family, composed of the parents and the children living in the same household, represents the majority of families. This is not true today because only 34% of American households are married couples with their children and resources, which indicates that nuclear families may never have been the majority (Johnson, 1998; Lehrer, 1999).

The second myth is that before the industrial revolution, families lived in large extended groups with each member laboring to support the larger unit. In reality, the small family units predate by many years the industrial revolution of the 1900s in many cultures (Cowan, 1976). In 1997, the groups living together remained small, with the average size of a household at 2.64 people and the average size of a family 3.19 members (U.S. Census Bureau, 1998).

## Changes Continue for Families

Most women, both single and with a partner, now work both outside and within the home. In families with two adults with careers, many women still expect to do a "second shift" of housework after a day of work outside the home. Men share housework equally with their wives in only 20% of dual-career families. These extra hours of work create chronic exhaustion, low sex drive, and more frequent illnesses in the women. This work also puts a strain on the relationship and threatens the intactness of the family (Hochschild, 1989). The trend appears to be changing as more males are participating in the maintenance of the home and care of the children.

For the first time in history, a mother knows that all of her children are likely to live to maturity. "Before the nineteenth century, only about three of every 10 newborn infants lived beyond the age of 25. Of the seven who died, two or three never reached their first birthday, and five or six died before they were 6. Today, in developed counties fewer than one in 20 children die before they reach adulthood" (National Center for Health Statistics, 1998).

Infant deaths still occur in American families even though the overall infant mortality rate continues to decline and is now at 7.2 infants per 1,000 births. In general, 1997 mortality rates are lowest for infants born to Asian and Pacific Islander mothers (i.e., 5 per 1000 live births), followed by white (i.e., 6 per 1000 live births), American Indian (i.e., 8.7 per 1000 live births), and African-American mothers (i.e., 13.7 per 100 live births). Among Hispanic mothers, infant mortality rates are higher for Puerto Rican infants (i.e., 7.9 per 1000) than for Mexican (5.8 per 1000), Cuban (5.5 per 1000), and Central and South American infants (5.5 per 1000) (www.cdc.gov/nchswww/releases/99facts).

The average family will have about two children per couple, although racial and ethnic differences are evident. On average in the United States, Hispanic women have the highest number of children (i.e., 3.0 per woman), followed by black women (i.e., 2.2), white women (i.e., 2.0), and Asian women (i.e., 1.9) (Costello, 1998).

Technologic advances to assist in reproduction have created cultural changes in the roles assigned to women and the definition of who is part of the family. Services available to those with health insurance coverage or disposable income (e.g., artificial insemination, surrogate motherhood, in vitro fertilization, and the freezing of human eggs and embryos) have rearranged the boundaries of motherhood (Bredin, 1998). With an increasing ease with which to control fertility, a greater assurance that children will survive, and the continued migration from living in rural to urban areas, the structure and function of families will continue to evolve.

## SOCIAL POLICY ISSUES AND THE FAMILY

In 1994, the gap between the rich and the poor was the widest since the Census Bureau began keeping track in 1947—and this gap has continued to widen. Proportionately, more children live in poverty in the United States than in any other industrialized nation.

Millions of working Americans are struggling to survive and raise a family while working in low-level service jobs in health care, retail, and telemarketing. Jobs pay less than $7 per hour and usually do not offer health insurance or other benefits. Some employers hire people for only part-time work (i.e., 30 to 34 hours per week) so that they do not qualify for the benefits accompanying full-time status. According to the Bureau of Labor Statistics, 3.2 million people are involuntarily working at part-time jobs. The inequality in income has had a polarizing effect, intensifying racial, ethnic, and class differences (Schorr, 1997) (Table 2-4).

### Family Welfare Support

During the twentieth century, the federal government established numerous public programs to assist the poor. Among the most important to families were Aid to Families of Dependent Children (AFDC), Medicaid (i.e., health-care aid for the poor, begun in 1965), and food stamps.

The term *welfare mother* is often substituted with the term *black welfare mother* in the minds of many people. This underlying racism is present, even though white women compose the largest percentage of welfare recipients (Jensen, 1999).

## Aid to Families of Dependent Children

AFDC began in 1935 as a program to aid impoverished children cared for by one-parent families (e.g., by the mother after the death or disability of the male head of the family). The cultural expectation at the time was that women should stay home with their children. AFDC provided women with the financial assistance they required to stay home with their children and not work or, if employed, not be gone for long hours. It is estimated that about 25% of all American children received AFDC at some time in their lives.

The AFDC program grew until Reagan began cutting it in 1981. By that time, the public had become less sympathetic with the poor and were frustrated with rising taxes. An analysis of the Texas AFDC program determined that the state annually spent $15,000 on a family of four to provide only $3,600 in services that included cash, food stamps, child care, and medical costs. Of this $15,000, 66%—or $11,400—went for the administrative costs of salaries of people who generally were not poor or women.

Poor women were accused of having children in order to obtain or increase their welfare payments, which was an erroneous belief. A study of recipients of AFDC, food stamps, and Medicaid revealed that this charge was baseless. After controlling for factors such as race, education, and age, analysis showed that women on welfare had substantially fewer children than other women, as well as that the longer they remained on welfare, the lower their fertility rate became (Sapiro, 1999).

Many Americans also erroneously believed that past efforts to reduce poverty and provide support to families had created the national deficit. This was not true because AFDC accounted for only about 1% of the federal budget, although Social Security took 22%, defense took 18%, interest on the national debt took 15%, and Medicare took 10% (Schorr, 1997).

In response to public pressure, however, President Clinton signed the Personal Responsibility and Work Opportunity Act in August of 1996. This act cut spending on Food Stamps and Supplemental Security Income (SSI) by 22% over the next 6 years and eliminated the AFDC program. At the time, two thirds of the 13 million people receiving AFDC were children; the average monthly payment was about $414 per family (Jensen, 1999).

## Temporary Assistance for Needy Families (TANF)

The Temporary Assistance for Needy Families (TANF) program was designed to replace AFDC. TANF removes the guarantee that needy families will receive financial assistance, provides incentives for the states to spend less money than they did for AFDC, puts a 60 month lifetime limit for assistance, and requires states to force a substantial percentage of all adult recipients into paid or unpaid jobs.

This action removed a system of support without determining if welfare recipients were employable, there were sufficient jobs available, the work paid a living wage, and child care existed and was affordable. TANF did nothing to strengthen collection of child support from absent fathers.

States have now undertaken the initiative to design programs that move people from welfare to work, but TANF provisions make it more difficult for states to help people climb out of poverty. Job-training programs, when available, only prepare women for minimum-wage jobs that will never allow them to support their families.

There are three main groups of welfare recipients, and each has different needs and abilities. Therefore programs must be developed that provide the appropriate assistance.

**TABLE 2-4** *Persons and Families below Poverty Level According to Selected Characteristics, Race, and Hispanic Origin, 1995**

| All Persons | Percent below Poverty |
|---|---|
| All races | 13.8 |
| White | 11.2 |
| Black | 29.3 |
| Asian or Pacific Islander | 14.6 |
| Hispanic | 30.3 |

| Related children under 18 years of age in family | |
|---|---|
| All races | 20.2 |
| White | 15.5 |
| Black | 41.5 |
| Asian or Pacific Islander | 18.6 |
| Hispanic | 39.3 |

| Families with female householder, no husband present, and children under 18 years of age | |
|---|---|
| All races | 41.5 |
| White | 35.6 |
| Black | 53.2 |
| Hispanic | 57.3 |

(Data not available for Asian or Pacific Islander)

*The race groups, white and black, include persons of both Hispanic and non-Hispanic origin. Conversely, persons of Hispanic origin may be of any race. Poverty status is based on family income and family size using Census Bureau poverty thresholds.

From the U.S. Department of Health and Human Services: *Health, United States 1996-1997.*

*Families in Transition.* This is the largest single category of people receiving assistance. They experience economic difficulties because of losing a job; death, divorce, or abandonment of a wage earner; or the illness of a child (requiring a parent to leave work) or a parent. "Historically, half of all recipients have left AFDC within a year of becoming eligible. Three quarters left within two years. Three quarters of those reentering welfare exited again, fifty percent within twelve months" (Schorr, 1997).

*Families where the Adults Choose Not to Work.* In some families, the adult breadwinners are not motivated or willing to do what is necessary to prepare for, obtain, and keep a job. Taxpayers get the most angry about these people, yet they are a very small percentage of recipients. Most women on welfare with skills to earn a living wage are already working, and the rest generally face health-related obstacles to steady employment. "Single mothers do not turn to welfare because they are pathologically dependent on handouts or unusually reluctant to work. They do so because they can't get jobs that pay better than welfare" (Schorr, 1997) or offer health insurance for their children.

*Families where the Adults Cannot Keep a Job.* Some adult breadwinners lack the skills, support, or capacity to find and keep a job that pays enough to get the family out of poverty. "You can have someone who really wants to work, but if Grandma gets sick, or child care falls through, or you get a flat tire...all those things can throw a person out of a job" (Schorr, 1997). Many long-term welfare recipients lack the education or interpersonal skills needed to hold a job at a decent wage. Low cognitive ability also prevents some from getting and holding a job. It is estimated that up to one quarter of welfare recipients have chronic mental and physical health problems, lack of basic skills, or serious language deficiencies that present insurmountable barriers to employment (Schorr, 1997).

Care of the children when the mother works is an ongoing issue. The high-quality child care that is essential to enable most women to work is not always available or affordable. The hours may not coincide with jobs that are outside the 9 to 5 time slot. If a child is sick, the child care facilities usually do not allow him or her to attend, so the mother must miss work. Texas and California, two states that keep track of the availability of care, have had waiting lists for subsidized day care of 40,000 and 225,000 poor children respectively (Schorr, 1997).

Making poor women work outside the home has always been promoted as this country's solution to poverty. This strategy does not work well because the lack of education and support (i.e., proper clothes, dependable transportation, and availability of child care) restricts these women to low-paying positions. Minimum wage pay scales are too low to support a family alone.

The TANF legislation will reduce the number of families on welfare, but unless new initiatives or federal laws are put into place, poverty will increase.

## Family Leave Policies

Another major area of legislation that affects families is job protection when a person has to leave their job for a period of time due to a family issue. Until 1993, the United States had no national family leave policy. States or individual companies developed their own policies, if any. "While all the Fortune 100 companies had maternity leave, most of these companies gave leave only to women during the time they were physically disabled by childbirth rather than offer both men and women time to care for a newborn. Only 28 percent gave disability or parenting leave to mothers; 22 percent to fathers; and 23 percent to adoptive parents. And these large companies, employing only 5 percent of the nation's workers, were providing the most generous benefits. Small and middle-sized businesses tended to offer even less family leave" (Bravo, 1999).

The Family and Medical Leave Act (FMLA) is a federal law that went into effect in August 1993. It guarantees workers "a twelve-week unpaid leave—with no risk to their job—to take care of a newborn or newly adopted child or a sick family member or to deal with personal illness" (Bravo, 1999). The law provides some comfort to working families because they cannot lose their job when leaving for these types of family events, although it has some serious shortcomings.

The law only applies to companies with 50 or more employees and employees that work at least 25 hours a week and have been at their job for at least a year. With these limits in place, more than 95% of all businesses and more than half of all workers are not covered by the protection of this law. Even some employers who are mandated to provide the leave violate the law and fire the women instead. Employees may not know their rights or lack funds to sue the company. There is little monitoring to ensure compliance (Bravo, 1999).

Even when allowed to take the 12 weeks off, many women cannot afford to lose their pay. In 1993, approximately 25% of American families lived on $20,000 or less. Working women contribute one third to one half of the total income in a dual-earner household. They are the sole income providers in single-parent families and in some families with two adults (Bravo, 1999).

Poor women often do not even take the medically advised minimum of 6 weeks time off after a child is born. About 77% of women work in lower-paying, nonprofessional jobs. Less than 40% of working women have sufficient savings to go 6 weeks without pay. The leave is taken at a time when expenses are increasing for the family either because of a new child or illness (Bravo, 1999).

Women who can afford to leave often find themselves reluctant to do so. They most often work in corporate positions and are considered less serious about their careers when they let issues of children and family interfere with their jobs. The persistent corporate expectation that a job should have a higher priority than parenting has also minimized the number of men taking parental leave (Bravo, 1999). As a result of these issues, FMLA has had a limited practical effect.

 **A HEALTHY FAMILY**

Individual differences, changing norms over time, degree of acculturation, the length of time a family has lived in this country, and other factors make it necessary to view each family on an individual basis. In addition, the individual family members experience the same family very differently. If we stereotype a family, we assign a relatively fixed and stable view of attributes and behaviors to them, which leads to overgeneralization and misinformation. Such stereotyping misrepresents the realities of a family's life (Friedman, 1997).

Most families experience a variety of physical and psychosocial health problems. It is important to place families in the context of a continuum of healthy and unhealthy families. Pratt's (1976) classic work identified the following six characteristics of healthy families: (1) members facilitate an interactive process; (2) members enhance individual development: (3) role relationships are structured effectively; (4) members actively attempt to cope with problems; (5) members promote healthy lifestyles, including the home environment; and (6) members establish regular links with the broader community. A healthy family is not devoid of problems, but there is a structure within the family to cope with problems as they arise while also supporting continued family development.

Although it is important to understand these healthy characteristics, it is equally important to remember that each family is unique and addresses these components in its own way. We must not be quick to assume dys-function in a family because their interactions seem different from our own family. On the other hand, we should not normalize behavior because it seems familiar or represents what we believe to be "good" behavior. For example, an interpretation of conflict avoidance as family harmony prevents us from exploring a family's concerns about conflict.

## Women in the Family

The role of the woman within a family varies from one family to the next and from one time period to another. A woman is essential to the production of offspring for a family, but beyond that she may occupy any number of roles (Bredin, 1998). Women decide whether they will marry or cohabitate with a partner based on their individual and family expectations. Many women never marry, and those who do tend to have only one husband or cohabiting partner (Table 2-5).

The range of life choices that are easily available to women are generally those endorsed by the society within which she lives, but other options—both chosen and imposed—also affect a woman's life. How a woman responds to these factors can determine her level of self-esteem, self-confidence, and feelings of pleasure.

## Mastery and Pleasure

The results of the Lifeprints Study were first published in the early 1980s. Among other things, it reported which roles led the women in the study to have the greatest sense of "mastery" and "pleasure." The six groups of women compared in the sample were as follows: (1) never married and employed; (2) married without children and employed; (3) married with children and employed; (4) divorced with children and employed; (5) married with children, at home; and (6) married without children, at home.

Mastery, the measure of self-esteem and confidence, was highest among the groups of working women, who scored much higher on average than the homemakers. The women who scored the lowest on the mastery scale

| TABLE 2-5 *Women 15 to 44 Years of Age by Number of Husbands or Cohabitating Partners\** | | | | | |
|---|---|---|---|---|---|
| Race | Never married and never cohabited | Number of Husbands or Cohabitating Partners | | | |
| | | One | Two | Three | Four or more |
| White (non-Hispanic) | 24.7 | 50.9 | 16.7 | 5.4 | 2.2 |
| Black (non-Hispanic) | 39.7 | 42.3 | 13.1 | 3.6 | 1.3 |
| Other (non-Hispanic) | 33.2 | 51.7 | 12.1 | 2.3 | 0.7 |
| Hispanic | 28.2 | 51.8 | 16.0 | 3.1 | 0.9 |

\*In percentage. Based on the National Survey of Family Growth, a sample survey of women 15 to 44 years of age in the civilian, noninstitutionalized population.
Source: U.S. Department of Commerce, Bureau of the Census: *Statistical abstracts of the United States,* 1998.

were the married women without children who stayed home. The divorced women who had children and were employed, having coped with a difficult situation, scored the highest on the mastery scale.

The married women with children, whether they worked or not, scored highest on the pleasure scale. The women who scored the lowest on the pleasure scale were married women without children who stayed home, unmarried women who worked, and divorced mothers who worked. When the authors looked at the group of women who scored the highest on both mastery and pleasure, they were the employed, married women with children (Borysenko, 1998).

## Health Care Consumer

Women make three fourths of the health care decisions for their families, spend approximately two thirds of the health care dollars, make about 80% of the of the visits to health care providers (HCP), and purchase 60% of the medication in the United States (Smith Barney Research, 1998). Women serve as the "gatekeepers" when their families are interfacing with the health care system (Jacobs Institute of Women's Health, 1997). As women participate in the workforce more equally economically and in policy-setting, their role in making health care purchasing decisions for themselves and their families will become more influential (Phillips, Himwich, and Fitzgerald, 1999).

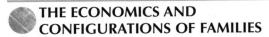 ## THE ECONOMICS AND CONFIGURATIONS OF FAMILIES

Family configurations and economics for women continue to change over time. More women over the age of 30 are starting families but are unmarried (Allen and Phillips, 1997). This change may be due in part to the recording of marital status. In some states, if the mother and father do not have the same last name, this is considered an "out of wedlock" birth, when they may actually be married and have elected to maintain their family names (Sapiro, 1999) (Table 2-6).

The Bureau of Labor Statistics estimates that, overall, women make 75 cents for every dollar men make when all jobs are compared. Additionally, when divorce or separation occurs, the income of women and their children drops 23%, which is one of the reasons that women and their children constitute the fastest growing percentage of homeless people (Youngkin and Davis, 1998).

Social security, pension plans, and health insurance are all based on the concept that a family has a male wage earner and a spouse at home. Women provide most of the paid and unpaid family care for their own young children, as well as for their aging parents. The term, the "sandwich generation," is used to describe the position many women find themselves in when they simultaneously have to provide care to both younger and older family members. More than 70% of the caregivers of the

---

**TABLE 2-6** *Female Family Householders with No Spouse Present, 1997\**

| Characteristic | White | Black | Hispanic |
| --- | --- | --- | --- |
| Female family householder | 8,339,000 | 3,947,000 | 1,617,000 |
| **MARITAL STATUS** | | | |
| Never married | 20% | 46% | 39% |
| Married, spouse absent | 16% | 19% | 23% |
| Widowed | 20% | 13% | 11% |
| Divorced | 44% | 22% | 27% |
| **PRESENCE OF CHILDREN UNDER AGE 18** | | | |
| No own children | 40% | 34% | 30% |
| With own children | 60% | 66% | 70% |
| One child | 30% | 30% | 31% |
| Two children | 21% | 21% | 24% |
| Three children | 7% | 10% | 10% |
| Four or more | 2% | 6% | 5% |
| Average number of children per family | 1.01 | 1.22 | 1.40 |

\*As of March 1997. Covers persons 15 years old and over. Based on Current Population Survey.
From the U.S. Department of Commerce, Bureau of the Census: *Statistical abstracts of the United States*, 1998, Chart No. 82.

elderly are wives and adult daughters, although sisters and daughters-in-law are also enlisted (Olesen, 1997).

 **THEORETIC FRAMEWORKS FOR WORK WITH FAMILIES**

Theories provide the basis for our nursing practice. As you gain experience working with families, theoretic perspectives will allow you to build a sound foundation of knowledge and increase your effectiveness when working with families. Many theories address how to assess and then develop a plan of care based on the strengths and weaknesses of the family unit. Relevant theories address the transitions families experience and the role changes clients will undergo as families enlarge or contract and move thorough a continuum of physical, social, and/or psychologic illness and wellness.

The following three theories are most commonly used: developmental, systems, and role theory. Although they provide a useful framework for nursing care, they are not fundamentally inclusive of all cultures, so cultural and ethnic differences must also be given equal consideration.

## Developmental Theory

Developmental Theory, which is also known as the life cycle approach, describes how families evolve through typical developmental stages similar to how individuals experience growth and development (i.e., each stage is characterized by specific issues and tasks). How the tasks at each stage are resolved helps determine a family's capability for handling the challenges that may present themselves in the next stage. The two developmental models most commonly used were developed by Duvall (1977) and Carter and McGoldrick (1989). Table 2-7 provides a comparison of these models.

Many of the concepts and theories used to understand changes in family structure and function were developed based on the concept of a two-parent nuclear family model and may have limited applicability to single-parent families, blended families, women choosing to remain childless, or families headed by homosexuals. More recent models are used to examine family change over time, designed to examine relationships among family members, and do not cover non-family aspects of individual development (Friedman, 1998).

### Duval's Developmental Model

Duval's eight-stage nuclear family cycle model is one of the more commonly used family developmental models to "measure" family development of a "normal" family. This model begins with the marriage of a couple and ends with retirement for the couple. Although the model appears linear, it develops full circle, starting and ending with the adult dyad.

Duvall's family stages are based on the changes that occur as a family progresses from a two-person married

**TABLE 2-7** *Comparison of Duvall and Miller and Carter and McGoldrick Family Life Cycle Stages and Tasks*

| STAGES | | TASKS |
|---|---|---|
| **Duvall and Miller (1985)** | **Carter and McGoldrick (1989)** | |
| No stage identified although Duvall considers this the time of "being launched" | 1. The unattached young adult | Successful separation of parent and young adult from one another |
| 1. The beginning family or the stage of marriage | 2. The newly married couple | Committing to a new family system |
| 2. Childbearing families | 3. Families with young children | Accepting new members into the system |
| 3. Families with preschool children | | |
| 4. Families with school-aged children | | |
| 5. Families with teenagers | 4. Families with adolescents | Allowing the children independence through boundary modification |
| 6. Families launching young adults | 5. Launching children | Accepting many exits or entrances into the family |
| 7. Middle-aged parents (empty nest up to retirement) | | |
| 8. Retirement to death of both spouses | 6. Families in later life | Accepting shifting generational roles and death |

Adapted from Friedman MM: *Family nursing: theory and practice*, ed 4, Englewood Cliffs, NJ, 1998, Appleton & Lange; Danielson CB, Hamel-Bissell B, and Winstead-Fry P: *Families in health and illness: perspectives on coping and intervention*, St Louis, 1993, Mosby; Duvall EM and Miller BC: *Marriage and family development*, New York, 1985, Harper & Rowe; Carter B and McGoldrick M: The *changing family life cycle*, Needam Heights, MA, 1989, Allyn & Bacon.

couple to the addition of children, and then to the "launching" of these children into their own families, and finally to old age with the return to just the original couple. The family's stage is determined by the age of the oldest child.

Duval designed this model with the understanding that there did not need to be a rigid pattern to the stages (Duval, 1977). For example, married children may be living with their parents for economic reasons or childbearing may be occurring later when couples choose to launch their careers first.

### Carter and McGoldrick's Developmental Model

Carter and McGoldrick's six stages of development begin with an unattached adult and proceed through marriage, the addition and raising of children, and then the launching of the children with the parents then adjusting to new roles (Vaughn-Cole and others, 1998).

These theories of development provide a perspective of continuity with a logical flow through the stages. "However, there has been little validation of any cluster of family characteristics by family stage" (Vaughn-Cole and others, 1998). In addition families, other than nuclear families, may not follow the pattern of these developmental models.

Individuals may belong to different family structures throughout their lifetimes. A person may be born into a nuclear family, be a part of a single parent family upon the divorce of his or her parents, and then be a part of a family as an unmarried parent. Individuals bring their beliefs about family and health to each new family configuration (McCarthy and Mandle, 1998) (Table 2-8).

### Developmental Tasks in the Marriage Relationship

Wallerstein (1995, 1996) and Wallerstein and Blakeslee (1995), from their research designed to "illuminate the interior domains of happy marriages," suggest seven psychologic tasks that couples must address early in their marriage and again during the developmental milestones of their life together. These tasks are as follows:

1. Separate psychologically from their families of origin and begin to create a new and different kind of connectedness that will maintain the generational ties;
2. Build a marital identity with a sense of we-ness;
3. Establish a sexual life as a couple;
4. Create a marriage that is a zone of safety and nurturance;

---

**TABLE 2-8**   *Stages of Family Development and Examples of the Nurse's Role in Anticipatory Guidance*

| Stage | Anticipatory Guidance |
|---|---|
| Couple | Facilitator in interpersonal relationships (e.g., with in-laws), role adjustment, managing finances |
| | Counselor about childbearing (e.g., preconception care, remaining childless, adoption) |
| | Counselor on sexual adjustment, contraception |
| Child | Counselor on prenatal care and antepartum, intrapartum bearing, and postpartum options |
| | Referrer to community resources, social services |
| | Facilitator in adjustment to parenting roles |
| Family with preschool and school-age children | Coordinator of health care services for all family members |
| | Provider of information on developmental stages and enriching environment |
| | Teacher of home safety |
| | Counselor on balancing parents' multiple roles |
| Family with adolescents | Facilitator of interpersonal communication skills |
| | Teacher of problem-solving techniques |
| | Assessor of risk behaviors |
| | Referrer for STD and/or contraception care |
| Family with young/middle-age adults | Screener for accessing health screening |
| | Facilitator in linking families with service agencies |
| | Counselor on role adjustment, death of parents, retirement |
| Family with older adults | Counselor on role adjustment, interpersonal relationships |
| | Referrer to community-assisted living programs |
| | Monitor of changing health needs, medications |
| | Counselor on bereavement and advanced directives |

Adapted from Mccarthy and Mandle: Health promotion in the family. In Edelman C and Mandle C, editors: *Health promotion throughout the lifespan*, ed 4, St Louis, 1998, Mosby.

5. Expand to psychologically accommodate children while safeguarding their own private sphere;
6. Build a relationship that is fun and interesting;
7. Confront and master life crises and maintain the strength of the marital bond during adversity;
8. Provide nurturing and comfort to each other; and
9. Maintain a vision of the other that combines early idealizations with a firm grasp of the present reality (Wallerstein, 1995).

## Systems Theories

Two theories, General Systems Theory and the family as an ecosystem, are both useful when working with families. Systems theories view the family as nesting within larger systems that actively influence the family and are influenced by the family.

### General Systems Theory

General Systems Theory, which is also called cybernetics, was introduced in 1950 by Ludwig vonBertalanffy to describe how units interact with larger and smaller units. The theory is used to explain how a family interacts with its individual members and with the larger group, society.

This theory is useful in family assessment because it emphasizes the interdependence of the family's parts and asserts that the whole of the family is greater than the sum of these parts, as well as that whatever affects the family as a whole, affects each of its parts. Therefore one cannot understand the family by simply knowing each of the members. The interrelationship of the members of the family with each other and with the larger society must also be considered.

As originally conceived, systems theory is mechanistic in that it suggests that an individual can observe the system in interaction from outside the system. More recently, the theory has been expanded to emphasize that the nurse and family are themselves a system. There is a mutual connectedness between them as each takes on the role of observer and the observed. The system becomes the "interaction of the two systems as they both exist within a larger context" (Becvar and Becvar, 1996).

This concept is important because it highlights the notion that we cannot work with the family system (or any other system) without being influenced by the system and also influencing the system. It is a delusion to think that when interacting with a family you are not being affected by the family either positively or negatively (i.e., that you are "seeing" the family objectively).

### Ecosystem

Bronfenbrenner (1977) has developed a view of the family as an ecosystem that is composed of four systems. The microsystem is the immediate setting in which a person fulfills his or her roles (e.g., family, school, business, etc.). The mesosystem is the system of interrelationship. The exosystem is composed of the larger community (i.e., mass media, all levels of government) in which the families live even though they may not have direct contact with those community entities. The final system is the macrosystem, which encompasses the general cultural, social, legal, political, economic, and cultural values. Together these four systems create the ecosystem that encompasses the family. This approach provides an explanation of the extremely complex nature of the relationship between a family and its community (Figure 2-5).

## Role Theory

Every person holds a position within a social system, whether small like a family or large like a community. "For each position a number of roles exist, each of which is composed of a more or less related homogeneous set of behaviors culturally defined as expected of those in that position or status" (Friedman, 1998).

### Women within the Family

Much of the research on women's roles within a family has focused on the effect that employment has on family and the potential allocation or reallocation of roles. Family roles can be described as the "repetitive patterns of behavior by which family members fulfill family

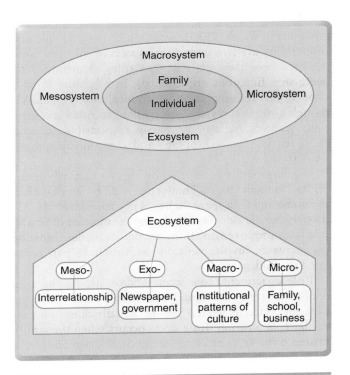

FIGURE 2-5 • Ecosystem. *(From Muuss R: Theories of adolescence, ed 5, New York, 1988, McGraw-Hill.)*

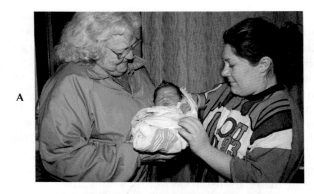

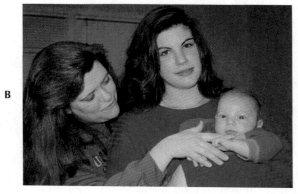

FIGURE 2-6 • Multigenerational family with three generations—grandmother, mother, and newborn.

functions" (Walsh, 1993). Role allocation and role accountability are two important aspects of role functioning (i.e., how the family assigns roles to members to make sure functions are fulfilled). In a healthy family, allocation is reasonable and accountability is clear. Although a move toward more egalitarian roles is occurring, women are still primarily responsible for the child rearing, housekeeping, and community obligations (Friedman, 1998).

In a large study conducted by Hakins and colleagues (1995), women spent 37 hours per week on work within the home and men spent 20 hours in such endeavors. Although there is a disparity between the number of hours, this is an improvement from previous decades. Most of the increased involvement on the husband's part is related to childcare.

Role enactment, role stress and/or strain, and role conflict are terms commonly used in role theory. Role enactment concerns what a person actually does in a particular role position. Role stress occurs when the family creates difficult, conflicting, or impossible demands for a family member. Role strain is generated from the stress and is reflected in feelings of frustration and tension. Role conflict occurs when one is confronted with incompatible expectations (Friedman, 1992). An example of

these concepts is as follows. Julie works full-time, has a 4-year-old child, and is taking classes to become a teacher (role enactment—mother/student). Her husband, Jim, is a fireman who works for several days at a time. When Jim is away, Julie has difficulty taking her daughter to preschool and getting to work on time (role stress). Because she is sometimes late to work, Julie is unable to leave to get to class (role conflict). She is feeling discouraged about passing her course (role strain).

### Role Fulfillment in a Healthy Family

In a healthy family, there must be mutual agreement about a role or modification of a role (role complementarity). The family must be open to shifts in role behavior to keep the family equilibrium (role flexibility). If one member of the family is ill or away, other members must be willing to carry out the functions usually performed by that member. For example, when the mother is ill, the father or a friend will take the children to school and the older children will be enlisted to do some of the household chores usually carried out by mother.

Role expectations can be quite different, depending on the family's culture. Garbarino (1993) notes the wide variability of the role of fatherhood in different cultures. Some cultures encourage interaction and bind fathers to children, and others hardly acknowledge the philosophy of fathers being involved in child care because that role is left to the mother.

All family members, but especially the primary caretaker, should be assessed for role stress, role strain, and role conflict. Learn how roles are allocated. Who does the work when the one to whom it is assigned cannot fulfill the role? Do family members reciprocate in filling in for each other? How could others be empowered to share in the responsibilities? Are family members able to come to an agreement that there are individual differences in how a task may be performed?

Some women are willing to maintain their current roles (i.e., packing her husband's lunch at 4:30 AM before he leaves for work and then returning to bed until 6 AM when she gets the rest of the family up to start their days), even though they may seem unmanageable. Clarification of the congruence between their beliefs about roles and the actual enactment of the role is an important step in the process of evaluating the health status of women and their families (Friedman, 1998).

### Parenting by Other Family Members

It is important to learn about the roles family members outside the home may have in the family's functioning. For example, grandparents may be involved with the family in a variety of ways (Friedman, 1998). They may be considered detached (e.g., see grandchildren once a month or less and have little influence on how they are raised), passive (e.g., see grandchildren at least once a month, but have little influence on how they are raised), or active (e.g., see grandchildren frequently and are actively involved in child rearing) (Figure 2-6).

By choice or by necessity, some grandparents—and even great-grandparents—may be either partially or totally responsible for raising the grandchildren. This occurs when the parents are unable to do so or are deceased. "In 1970, only 3% of children lived with their grandparents. By 1993, this figure rose to 5% of all children (3.4 million)" (Swanson and Nies, 1997) (Table 2-9).

 ## COMMUNICATION WITHIN THE FAMILY

One of the most important tasks of human beings is learning how to communicate with each other. This communication starts within the family group. Language, one form of communication, provides the basis for our existence as social beings, able to act and interact with other people, who are independent and autonomous (Sapiro, 1999).

Language and communication encompass many kinds of nonverbal behavior (e.g., facial grimaces and "body language"), as well as acts of writing and speaking. Language analysis is complicated by the fact that there are many variations within any given natural language (e.g., English, French, or Hindi). Most people are familiar with the concept of regional dialects and language variations resulting from cultural factors (e.g., ethnicity, race, and religion), but language also varies by age, class, occupation, and gender. Situation and context also affect the use of language. People communicate differently when speaking with a friend and a stranger, a parent and a child, a boss and an employee, and a man and a woman (Sapiro, 1999).

Research on the gender differences in communication focuses not only on the gender content of words but also on how men and women speak to each other and interact. Men and women's communication patterns are different, and the way they communicate depends on the sex and status of their audience. Research has shown that in mixed-sex discussions, not only do men talk more and take stronger leads in discussion, but they also employ techniques—often unconsciously—that silence women and diminish their ability to influence the group (Sapiro, 1999). Higher status people talk and interrupt more than lower status people (Sapiro, 1999). There are exceptions and variations, however, to the expected language patterns of race, class, and gender. White males and black females have been shown to be more likely to hold their ground during verbal challenges (Sapiro, 1999).

Internal and external family communication is structured by status relationships. "Although women are central to communication within the family (particularly in the absence of the husband/father) and between the family and outsiders, many of the most important

| TABLE 2-9 | Grandchildren Living in the Home of Their Grandparents, 1997* |
|---|---|
| Total children under 18 years of age | 70,983,000 |
| Children living in the home of grandparents | 3,894,000 |
| With parent(s) present | 2,585,000 |
| Both parents present | 556,000 |
| Mother only present | 1,785,000 |
| Father only present | 247,000 |
| Without parent(s) present | 1,309,000 |

*Based on Current Population Survey.
From the U.S. Department of Commerce, Bureau of the Census: *Statistical abstracts of the United States,* 1998, Chart No. 86.

communications between the family and other institutions are expected to be carried our by either the husband or under his supervision" (Sapiro, 1999).

By understanding patterns of communication, we can better understand the delicate balance between the individual and the family and community (Sapiro, 1999). We can anticipate possible communication problems created by the differences between the health care provider and the family and the individuals within that family.

## NURSE-FAMILY RELATIONSHIPS

### Considering the Family

When we approach the care of people within families we do so with one of two foci of attention. One is the family-as-context, and the other is the family-as-client (Gilliss, 1993). When families are considered as the context or environment within which the individual client or patient functions, the emphasis of assessment and intervention is primarily on that individual. The family is of secondary concern. For example, Nancy, a 33-year-old professional who is married and mother of four young children, has been experiencing a chronic headache for 18 months. Various medical therapies have not relieved the pain. The assessment of Nancy's situation, with the family-as-context, would focus first on Nancy's symptoms, and then on the exploration of any possible connections between her family interactions and her headaches.

In contrast, with the family-as-client focus, the emphasis of assessment and intervention is on the family unit. The primary focus of the assessment is on the whole family, with the family in the foreground, and individual members considered as context. This assessment would focus on the current functioning of the family while Nancy is incapacitated by the headaches. What family needs are not being met? Who is caring for the children? What is the financial and psychologic effect on the family?

## The Therapeutic Relationship

If an effective health care intervention is to take place, you must have a positive interactive relationship with the family. The concepts of caring, family partnerships, cultural considerations, and mutually agreed upon goals are basic to the development of this foundation.

### Providing Care to a Family

Caring indicates connection. When people care about someone or something it is because it matters to them. The worry or threat that they might lose what matters—whether it is their health, a loved one, an object, or something else—causes them stress. Caring creates the possibility of giving and receiving help (Benner and Wrubel, 1989). Caring for a family begins when we enter their "life space" and learn from them (Watson, 1988). We may offer options and support to maintain their health and well-being or, during times of stress, help them develop more effective coping strategies and facilitate the use of appropriate community resources.

Caring must be considered from two different points of view when the focus is the family, as follow: (1) the nurse as caregiver; and (2) the family as caregiver to other family members. Caring encompasses both emotional support and the provision of factual knowledge and skills. Family caregivers need effective support, as well as family behavioral-management skill training to become actively involved in the management of cognitively impaired family members.

Family care giving usually involves a primary caregiver, often a woman, who oversees and organizes responses on a regular basis. In addition, women are generally expected to take on the care of a chronically ill spouse, child, or parent. Care may be intermittent (e.g., shopping or financial management) or include in-home assistance that requires a regular or even full-time commitment. The more time-consuming the care, the less likely that the affective aspects of daily living will be addressed (Pepin, 1992).

In care-giving situations, all family patterns and routines are disrupted—not just those of the caregiver and the person receiving care. You must develop an informed understanding of the family situation and what it means to all the members of the family. In addition, try to evaluate the situation's effect on family dynamics.

### Considering Cultural Variations

The cultural milieu of a family develops from the blending of family beliefs and their place in the context of the larger society. As someone learning to understand the family, you should allow the individual uniqueness of the family to become evident. For example, families from rural areas are different from urban families within the same culture, and some families may have more in common with each other across cultural lines than they have with families in their own cultures.

### Developing a Contract

Clients, whether individuals or families, are responsible for their own lives and capable of making their own decisions. We develop a partnership with the family in which both parties have rights and responsibilities. Creating a contract of partnership makes clear the expectations that each party has of the other, what their mutual goals are, how they will achieve these goals, and when these goals will be achieved. The relationship between the partners—caregiver and recipient—is a complementary one, rather than a supervisor/subordinate one (Hoff, 1989).

A critical component of family care, the family contract, promotes self-care and facilitates a family focus on health needs. This type of contract is not legally binding, but there is an implicit pledge of trust and commitment. A well-developed contract provides a distinct direction for nursing intervention and provides standards for evaluation because it clearly delineates the expected outcomes (Balzer-Riley, 1996).

The most important component to contracting is the concept of partnership (i.e., the shared participation and agreement between client and nurse about the mutual identification of needs and resources, the development of a plan, the decisions regarding the division of responsibilities, the setting of time limits, evaluation, and renegotiation) (Sloan and Schommer, 1991).

Development of the trust that will lead to a fruitful contract begins with the first interaction with the family. In essence, the first contract is, "I will be at your house at 9:30 tomorrow morning to check your blood pressure." When you make an appointment to meet with a family and provide certain services, arrive on time at the agreed upon place and bring the supplies to do what you have said you will. If you do not fulfill such seemingly little agreements, you will never gain the trust of the family.

## THE HOME VISIT

Providing care for clients in the home setting is germane to the concept of the healing art of nurses. A home visit is a purposeful interaction in a home (or any residence) to promote and maintain the health of individuals and the family (or significant others) or to support a family during a member's death (Klass, 1996; Smith and Maurer, 2000). "Home" may be a house, apartment, trailer, shelter for homeless or abused families, or under a bridge.

Almost any nursing service can be accomplished on a home visit (Smith and Maurer, 2000). Home visits are done by health care providers working with visiting nurse associations, hospices, public health departments, home health agencies, school districts, and parish nursing programs. Many hospitals also have discharge programs that employ nurses to provide follow-up care to patients once they leave the hospital.

With a home visit, we enter the domain of the client and her family. We are a guest within their environment and must be respectful of that fact. "The social graces for the community and culture of the family must be considered so that the family is at ease and is not offended" (Smith and Maurer, 2000). Carefully consider things such as when and where you sit and how you will respond if refreshments are offered. You must balance their desire to be courteous and hospitable with your own preferences. We enter the home with permission from the family and may be asked to leave at any time.

There are three phases to the home visit. After the initial contact, you enter the home to become reacquainted and reassess the situation, provide the family with the opportunity to share information with you, review the reason for your visit, and give the family an opportunity to renegotiate what is to be done during this time. In the second phase, you focus on the implementation of the nursing care, as well as on the ongoing data collection and development of your relationship with the family. In the third phase, you bring closure to the visit by summarizing what has been done today, reviewing your expectations and those of the family before the next visit, and setting the appointment for the next visit (Box 2-1).

If you think about the social visits you make with friends, this professional visit follows much the same pattern: (1) "Hi! How are you doing? What's new?" (2) "I came over to . . ." (watch the game, borrow a CD,

---

### BOX 2-1   *Nursing Activities during Three Phases of a Home Visit*

**INITIATION PHASE OF HOME VISIT**

1. Knock on door and stand where you can be observed if peephole or window exists.

2. Identify self as ___(name)___, the nurse from _(name of agency)_.

3. Ask for the person to whom you were referred or the person with whom the appointment was made.

4. Observe environment with regard to your own safety.

5. Introduce yourself to those present and acknowledge them.

6. Sit where directed by the family.

7. Discuss purpose of visit. On initial visits, discuss services to be provided by agency.

8. Have permission forms signed to initiate services. This may be done later in the home visit if more explanation of services is needed for the family to understand what is being offered.

**IMPLEMENTATION PHASE OF HOME VISIT**

9. Complete health assessment database for the individual client.

10. On return visits, assess for changes since the last encounter. Explore degree that family was able to follow-up on plans from previous visit. Explore barriers if follow-up did not occur.

11. Wash hands before and after conducting any physical assessment and direct physical care.

12. Conduct physical assessment as appropriate, and perform direct physical care.

13. Identify household members and their health needs, use of community resources, and environmental hazards.

14. Explore values, preferences, and clients' perceptions of needs and concerns.

15. Conduct health teaching as appropriate, and provide written instructions. Include any safety recommendations.

16. Discuss any referral, collaboration, or consultation that you recommend.

17. Provide comfort and counseling as needed.

**TERMINATION PHASE OF HOME VISIT**

18. Summarize accomplishments of visit.

19. Clarify family's plan of care related to potential health emergency appropriate to health problems.

20. Discuss plan for next home visit and activities to be accomplished in the interim by the community health nurse, individual client, and family members.

21. Leave written identification of yourself and agency, with telephone numbers.

Adapted from Stanhope M and Lancaster J: *Community health nursing: process and practice for promoting health,* St Louis, 1996, Mosby; Smith C and Maurer F: *Community health nursing: theory and practice,* ed 2, Philadelphia, 2000, W.B. Saunders.

---

## BOX 2-2    *Safety and Home Visiting*

1. If possible, obtain the family's permission to work with them by telephone prior to visiting the home. Ask for directions to their road, driveway, building, or apartment.

2. Always leave an itinerary with the agency for each clinical day that includes the name of the family to be visited, their address and telephone number, and the license tag number and make of the automobile you are driving.

3. Do not carry purses or wear jewelry other than engagement or wedding rings. Do not wear rings with large gems.

4. Wear the appropriate dress (e.g., uniform or street clothes) determined by the agency.

5. Carry coins for telephone calls and a small amount of money for emergencies.

6. Carry an identification badge and wear a name pin.

7. Avoid secluded areas (e.g., stairwells, alleys, basements, and empty buildings) or obtain an escort.

8. Avoid areas where persons are loitering or obtain an escort.

9. Use discretion about visiting a family. If you feel unsafe—**do not visit.**

10. If approached on the street by someone requesting a home visit, refer them to the office of the public health or home health agency.

11. Consider whether an escort is needed to avoid visiting a lone male if you are female or visiting a lone female if you are male.

12. Request a nurse partner or escort to a home visit if needed.

13. Avoid entering a home in which fights, drug use, or drug sales are in progress.

14. Always report back to the agency in person or by telephone at the end of the clinical day.

15. Visit only during your scheduled work hours. If you must make an exception to this, permission from your supervisor must be obtained.

Adapted from Stanhope M and Lancaster J: *Community health nursing: process and practice for promoting health,* St Louis, 1996, Mosby; Smith C and Maurer F: *Community health nursing: theory and practice,* ed 2, Philadelphia, 2000, W.B. Saunders.

---

hang out for awhile, or talk); then do what you have said you want to do. (3) "Well I've got to be going. Let's do this again..." Although your professional home visits should reflect a professional demeanor and vocabulary; keep in mind that you have had lots of practice with similar visits.

While in the home, the nursing process is used systematically to ensure that potentially important information is not missed. An assessment incorporating both subjective and objective information is done, nursing diagnoses are made, and a plan is developed. To provide holistic care, we must also consider both the needs of the individual and the needs of the family but focus the care on either the family-as-context for an individual or family-as-client. If the focus is on the family-as-context, we will provide physical and emotional care to the entire family to ensure that the process of recovery continues for an individual client (Boos, 1996).

Assessment and care include individual family member's needs, family subsystems, and the family within the community. Although focusing on multiple individuals (i.e., the family) simultaneously in a setting (i.e., the home) may seem chaotic and overwhelming, using critical thinking skills and the systematic approach of the nursing process allows you to develop your knowledge base and develop mutually agreeable goals with the family. "When the visit ends, it is the family who takes responsibility for their own health, albeit with varying degrees of interest, commitment, knowledge, and skill" (Smith and Maurer, 2000).

### Advantages and Limitations of a Home Visit

The home visit offers many advantages to the partnership of the provider and client. Sitting with the family, you can observe their strengths and the interplay of factors that influence the client's health status. There is more chance of interaction with the various members of the family, as well as with pets, roommates, neighbors, and friends. The family's social environment and family rituals can also be observed (Wright and Leahey, 1994). During these interactions, you can provide immediate reinforcement for positive behaviors, prevent risk factors from developing, understand the client's potential and actual health problems, and intervene before the problems escalate into serious health concerns (Deal, 1993). Environmental resources and hazards that may have a negative effect on the client's health may also be identified and dealt with appropriately. There is an opportunity to assess the client in activities of daily living, provide encouragement, and note health changes.

Families tend to be more comfortable and therefore less anxious in the home environment, so they are more receptive to teaching and able to immediately apply the information. Their motivation to learn new skills is enhanced because they can try them for the first time, with your assistance, in the environment where they will perform the skills. Available family members are drawn into conversations and activities and may become active participants in meeting the health care needs of other family members.

Although home visits provide valuable insights into families, there are also challenges and limitations to be considered. Visiting a client at home generally takes more time than an appointment in the hospital or clinic setting. Home visits prevent group work with clients with similar concerns. Things such as children needing attention or a neighbor's visit are more likely to interrupt the interview. There is no immediate access to emergency equipment or face-to-face consultation with colleagues. Clients may be uneasy about a professional seeing their home setting. Whatever the location of the visit, safety can be an issue (Smith and Maurer, 2000) (Box 2-2).

## Visiting a Home

### Preparing for the Home Visit

Prepare for the visit by reviewing any available records on the family, speaking with other health care professionals involved in the care, obtaining potentially necessary supplies and teaching aids, and arranging the visit with the family. Call the primary client or an adult family member so that a mutually convenient time for the visit can be arranged. On the initial call, introduce yourself, identify the purpose of the visit and the agency you are representing, determine an acceptable time, confirm the address, and request directions both to the building as well as within or around the building (e.g., "Where is the entrance to your building located?") (Box 2-3).

At the first visit, an outline of the approximate plan of visits should be discussed and the next visit should be planned. If the family has a phone, each follow-up visit should be preceded by a phone call to ensure that it is still convenient for the family. Give the family the approximate time of your arrival so they can watch for you. If the family does not have a phone, other arrangements may have to be made. Once having met with the family, a neighbor who can take calls for future contacts may be identified. If the family has the number of your agency, they will be able to contact you if they cannot be home for the planned appointment.

In addition to a nurse, the family may have a social worker, rehabilitation therapist (e.g., physical or speech therapist), and/or a home health nurse or aide who has responsibilities for the same or different members of the family. To prevent confusion or distractions for the client(s), the visits of different providers should be synchronized so that they may overlap but not conflict. Each provider will develop his or her own "piece of the picture" of the family. Working as a provider team can enhance care of the family and its members.

If the family is not home when you arrive, leave a card that provides your name, telephone number, and

---

### BOX 2-3   Planning Before a Home Visit

1. Have name, address, and telephone number of family with directions and a map.

2. Have telephone number of agency where supervisor or faculty can be reached.

3. Have emergency telephone numbers for police, fire, and rescue personnel.

4. Clarify who has referred family to you and why.

5. Consider what is usually expected of a nurse in working with a family who has been referred for these health concerns (e.g., postpartum visit) and clarify the purposes of this home visit.

6. Consider whether any special safety precautions are required.

7. Have a plan of activities for the home visit time.

8. Have the equipment needed for handwashing, physical assessment, and direct care interventions, or verify that the client has the equipment in the home.

9. Take any data assessment or permission forms that are needed.

10. Have the appropriate information and teaching aids for health teaching.

11. Have information about community resources as appropriate.

12. Have gas in your automobile or money for public transportation.

13. Leave an itinerary with the agency personnel or faculty.

14. Approach the visit with self-confidence and caring.

Adapted from Stanhope M and Lancaster J: *Community health nursing: process and practice for promoting health,* St Louis, 1996, Mosby; Smith C and Maurer F: *Community health nursing: theory and practice,* ed 2, Philadelphia, 2000, W.B. Saunders.

---

agency, and write a note asking the client to call to schedule an appointment or indicating a time when you will return. Keep in mind that this will only work if the family can read the information on the card and access a phone. If they have to use a pay phone, there are more barriers to their compliance.

There will be times when the family is consistently unavailable or has moved. Zerwekh (1997) found that knowing how to locate disappearing families is a skill that is foundational to all other work with families in the home. "Effective locating requires community networking, persistence, an extensive map collection, the courage to knock on many doors, and the wisdom to 'sniff out violence' and back away as needed from a threatening household or neighborhood." A reasonable effort should be made to find the family because it may not have been the primary client's idea to move. Also, family stress—not a desire to avoid a visit—may have caused the family to become "lost."

### Beginning the Assessment

As you arrive in the neighborhood, assess the environment for health conditions, including safety. If you think that making a home visit at that time—for any reason—would jeopardize your health and safety, then leave and reschedule the appointment for a different time of day or when someone else can accompany you. Although most home visits do not present a safety risk, some do. Pay particular attention to areas where there is no one on the street or the home is in an isolated area or gang or drug activity may be prevalent. Keep in mind that visiting nurses "are generally known in communities and acknowledged as having skills and relationships

that contribute to the residents' wellbeing" (Smith and Maurer, 2000). This positive view provides a general degree of community protection.

 ## FAMILY ASSESSMENT

A family assessment determines who lives in the family; their relationships, cultural origins, religious preferences, and health practices; the role of each member (i.e., education, occupation); communication patterns among members; material management (i.e., of home, money); goals of the family; relaxation and recreational family activities; and strengths, weaknesses, conflicts, problems, and past patterns and methods of resolution (Youngkin and Davis, 1998) (Table 2-10).

Assessment involves not only the strengths and needs of the referred client's but also those of the family. Begin to establish a rapport and start to gather data. Over time, trust will develop between you and the family. The social skills of being honest, prompt, and quietly confident are important when working with families and will form the basis for the development of the relationship.

### TABLE 2-10    *Guide to Family Assessment*

| Family Component | What to Assess |
| --- | --- |
| Family structure | List of all members of immediate family (names, ages, gender, occupation, school grade, relationships) |
| Family environment | Housing (type, size, room use, utilities) |
| | Transportation (type, availability, reliability) |
| | Available resources (material, financial) |
| | Safety hazards |
| | Community resources (availability, access, use) |
| Daily routines | Eating (number of meals, favorite foods, times eaten, who is present at meals, typical foods) |
| | Sleeping (hours of sleep, times of sleep, sleeping arrangements) |
| | Work/leisure activities (work and school schedules, formal and informal recreation events, frequency of recreation) |
| | Effect of illness of family members on routines |
| | Identification of caregiver(s) in family |
| Family dynamics | Family values and norms (culture, religion, church attendance, family traditions, importance of health) |
| | Positions, roles and functions of each member (roles complementary, flexible, easily traded) |
| | Change in these roles and functions since illness of family member |
| Evidence of role confusion, conflict, overload | Communication patterns among family members |
| | Decision-making patterns |
| Family needs | Identification of family needs, goals |
| | Perception of the current situation |
| | Capacity for self-care |
| | Support available versus support needed |
| | Ways that family is coping with illness of family member |

Adapted from Stanhope M and Lancaster J: *Community health nursing: process and practice for promoting health,* St Louis, 1996, Mosby; Smith C and Maurer F: *Community health nursing: theory and practice,* ed 2, Philadelphia, 2000, W.B. Saunders.

A systematic assessment of the family is important because missing data may impair the client's recovery and place additional strain on the family. Agencies typically have data collection and analysis forms in place to facilitate this process. These forms may or may not be based on a nursing model but are designed to record data and are not necessarily interview tools. Use your professional knowledge and interviewing expertise to gain the necessary information and explore areas that may be necessary but not required on the agency forms.

In addition to assessing the family and the individuals within it, examine the subsystems within the family, which may include two or more family members (e.g., a parent-child or spouse subsystem) (Friedman, 1998). An example of a subsystem with a healthy purpose is a strong mother-infant attachment.

Family assessment includes assessment not only of the internal family functioning but also of the family's relationship to community resources and activities (Reutter, 1991). Family assessment also includes assessment of the effect of the community on the family and the family on the community.

Many assessment models and tools have been developed. Becoming aware of the variety of approaches to data collection enables you to choose an interview approach based on the situation of your clients, the type of practice you are engaged in, and your philosophy of care.

## Gordon's Functional Health Patterns Assessment

A pattern is something that recurs over time. Identifying an individual's, family's, or community's sequences of behavior rather than identifying isolated events helps establish a clearer assessment of activities. The assessment guidelines for families described by Gordon (1995) are a useful tool to determining family functioning. Using the 11 categories as a framework is a comprehensive and useful approach for collecting data. As information is obtained, various patterns begin to emerge. Patterns that may indicate a dysfunctional process are then explored further to identify possible causes. Nursing diagnoses can be formulated, and care planning begun with the family members. Positive reinforcement can be provided for patterns that support healthy behavior (Box 2-4).

## The Family Systems Stressor-Strength Inventory

The family assessment and intervention model is concerned with the family as a system. It is the basis for the family systems stressor-strength inventory, which takes a microscopic look at the family and measures specific family dimensions. For data collection, this survey is given to family members to complete before the interview with the health care provider. Multiple family members should complete the form either separately or together because each of them has a different perspective on the family.

The survey is divided into the following three sections: (1) Family system stressors: general; (2) Family stressors: specific; and (3) Family system strengths. It helps to identify stressful situations occurring in families and the strengths used to maintain the family despite the problems. The interview with the health care provider clarifies the stressors and strengths as identified by the family members. The data is then used to create the family care plan.

## Friedman Family Assessment Model

The Friedman family assessment model uses a structural-functional framework, as well as developmental and systems theory. Viewing families as subsystems of the wider society, the interview form based on this model takes a macroscopic approach to glean more general information. The family is considered an open social system, and the focus is on the family's internal structure and function, as well as on external relationships with other social systems within the context of their community.

Friedman developed the form to provide guidelines for nurses interviewing families so that they might gain an overall view of what is going on in the family. There are six broad categories of interview questions, as follow: (1) identifying data, (2) developmental stage and history of the family, (3) environmental data, (4) family structure, (5) family functions, and (6) family coping. Each of these categories has several subcategories. The interview guide exists in both the short form (see pages 74 and 75) and the long form, which comprises 12 pages (Friedman, 1997). Because the long form is so extensive, not all of the information is gained in the first visit. It may not be important or pertinent to gain information from every category for every family. Professional discretion should be used so that the family does not feel that you are asking for information about them that will serve no purpose.

## Calgary Family Assessment Model

Wright and Leahey (1994) have developed a family assessment model that "blends nursing and family therapy concepts and is grounded in systems theory, cybernetics, communication theory, and change theory" (Hanson and Boyd, 1996). As illustrated in Figure 2-7, the assessment questions are organized into the following three major categories: structural, developmental, and functional. Each category is made up of several dimensions (e.g., external, internal, etc.), each of which has subcategories. The assessment is less specific than the prior two methods, but it focuses on internal relations within the family rather than the interface between the family and the community (Hanson and Boyd, 1996). The model may be used to assess all three areas for a macroassessment of the family, or any part of the model may be selected for a microassessment.

## BOX 2-4    11 Functional Health Pattern Assessment Guidelines for Families

**FAMILY ASSESSMENT**

The 11 functional health-pattern areas are applicable to the assessment of families. Families are the primary client in community health nursing. In some cases, a family assessment may be indicated (1) in the care of an infant or child whose development is influenced by family health patterns, or (2) when an adult has certain health problems that can be influenced by family patterns. The following guidelines provide information on family functioning:

1. Health perception—health-management pattern
   *History:*
   a. How has family's general health been (in last few years)?
   b. Colds in past year? Absence from work/school?
   c. Most important things you do to keep healthy? Think these make a difference to health? (Include family folk remedies, if appropriate.)
   d. Members' use of cigarettes, alcohol, drugs?
   e. Immunizations? Health care provider? Frequency of checkups? Accidents (home, work, school, driving)? (If appropriate: Storage of drugs, cleaning products, scatter rugs, etc.)
   f. In past, has it been easy to find ways to follow suggestions of doctors, nurses, social workers (if appropriate)?
   g. Things important to family's health that I could help with?
   *Examination:*
   a. General appearance of family members and home.
   b. If appropriate: Storage of medicines, cribs, playpens, stove, scatter rugs, hazards, etc.

2. Nutritional—metabolic pattern
   *History:*
   a. Typical family meal pattern/food intake? (Describe.) Supplements (vitamins, types of snacks, etc.)?
   b. Typical family fluid intake? (Describe.) Supplements: type available (fruit juices, soft drinks, coffee, etc.)?
   c. Appetites?
   d. Dental problems? Dental care (frequency)?
   e. Skin problems? Healing problems?
   *Examination:*
   If opportunity available: Refrigerator contents, meal preparation, contents of meal, etc.

3. Elimination pattern
   *History:*
   a. Family use of laxatives, other aids?
   b. Problems in waste/garbage disposal?
   c. Pet animals' waste disposal (indoor/outdoor)?
   d. If indicated: Problems with flies, roaches, rodents?
   *Examination:*
   If opportunity available: Examine toilet facilities, garbage disposal, pet waste disposal; indicators of risk for flies, roaches, rodents.

4. Activity—exercise pattern
   *History:*
   a. In general, does family get a lot of/little exercise? Type? Regularity?
   b. Family leisure activities? Active/passive?
   c. Problems in shopping (transportation), cooking, keeping up the house, budgeting for food, clothes, housekeeping, house costs?
   *Examination:*
   Pattern of general home maintenance, personal maintenance.

5. Sleep—rest pattern
   *History:*
   a. Generally, family members seem to be well rested and ready for school/work?
   b. Sufficient sleeping space and quiet?
   c. Family finds time to relax?
   *Examination:*
   If opportunity available: Observe sleeping space and arrangements.

6. Cognitive—perceptual pattern
   *History:*
   a. Visual or hearing problems? How managed?
   b. Any big decisions family has had to make? How made?
   *Examination:*
   a. If indicated: Language spoken at home.
   b. Grasp of ideas and questions (abstract/concrete).
   c. Vocabulatory level.

7. Self-perception—self-concept pattern
   *History:*
   a. Most of time family feels good (not so good) about themselves as a family?
   b. General mood of family? Happy? Anxious? Depressed? What helps family mood?
   *Examination:*
   a. General mood state: nervous (5) or relaxed (1); rate from 1 to 5.
   b. Members generally assertive (5) or passive (1); rate from 1 to 5.

8. Roles—relationship pattern
   *History:*
   a. Family (or household) members? Member age and family structure (diagram).
   b. Any family problems that are difficult to handle (nuclear/extended)? Child rearing? If appropriate: Spouse/parents (should be included if children are interviewed) ever get rough with you? The children?
   *Family Assessment:*
   a. Relationships good (not so good) among family members? Siblings? Support each other?
   b. If appropriate: Income sufficient for needs?
   c. Feel part of (or isolated from) community? Neighbors?
   *Examination:*
   a. Interaction among family members (if present).
   b. Observed family leadership roles.

9. Sexuality—reproductive pattern
   *History:*
   a. If appropriate (sexual partner within household or situation): Sexual relations satisfying? Changes? Problems?
   b. Use of family planning? Contraceptives? Problems?

**BOX 2-4   *11 Functional Health Pattern Assessment Guidelines for Families—cont'd***

c. If appropriate (to age of children): Feel comfortable in explaining/discussing sexual subjects?
*Examination:* None

10. Coping—stress-tolerance pattern
*History:*
a. Any big changes within family in last few years?
b. Family tense or relaxed most of time? When tense what helps? Use of medicines, drugs, alcohol to decrease tension?
c. When (if) family problems, how handled?
d. Most of the time is this way(s) successful?

*Examination:* None

11. Values—beliefs pattern
*History:*
a. Generally, family gets what it wants out of life?
b. Important goals for the future?
c. Any "rules" in the family that everyone believes are important?
d. Religion important in family? Does this help when difficulties arise?
*Examination:* None

From Gordon M: *Manual of nursing diagnoses,* St Louis, 1995, Mosby.

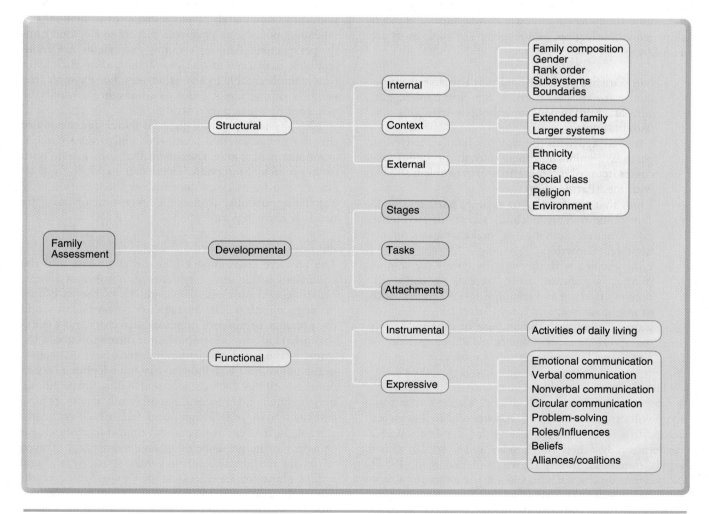

**FIGURE 2-7 •** Calgary family assessment. *(From Wright LM and Leahy M:* Nurses and families: a guide to family assessment and intervention, *ed 3, Philadelphia, 2000, F.A. Davis.)*

### The McMaster Family Assessment Device (FAD)

This tool is a 60-item questionnaire that gathers data on six areas of family functioning. Problem solving, communication, roles, affective responsiveness, affective involvement, and behavior control are measured. Each family member is asked to complete the tool, which takes about 20 minutes. The overall measure of the family's functioning is determined on the general functioning scale. In addition, family members' scores can be compared. Interventions are based on the identification of healthy and unhealthy functional areas (Sawin and Harrigan, 1995).

### Family Apgar

Sometimes you will want to start the assessment process with a quick screening tool. The Family Apgar, which focuses on satisfaction, is one of the quickest ways to screen for family difficulty. The tool uses five statements to explore the following five areas: adaptation, partnership, growth, affection, and resolve. The statements are as follows:

- I am satisfied with the help that I receive from my family (or spouse, partner, significant other, parent, or child) when something is troubling me. (Adaptation)
- I am satisfied with the way my family (or spouse, partner, significant other, parent, or child) discusses items of interest and shares problem solving with me. (Partnership)
- I find that my family (or spouse, partner, significant other, parent, or child) accepts my wishes to take on new activities or make changes in my lifestyle. (Growth)
- I am satisfied with the way my family (or spouse, partner, significant other, parent, or child) expresses affection and responds to my feelings, such as anger, sorrow, and love. (Affection)
- I am satisfied with the amount of time my family (or spouse, partner, significant other, parent, or child) and I spend together. (Resolve)

The client scores each category with a 0 (hardly ever), 1 (some of the time), or 2 (almost always). The total score will range from 0 to 10. A score of 0 to 3 is associated with a severely dysfunctional family; 4 to 6 with a moderately dysfunctional family; and 7 to 10 with a highly functional family (Sawin and Harrigan, 1995). Notice that total satisfaction is not necessary for a family to be considered highly functional.

Each of these instruments for data collection has a different focus and creates a different database and may be used alone or in combination. The key is to ob-

tain the data that is necessary to develop an accurate picture of the family and determine their strengths and limitations.

### The Data-Collection Process

Data collection involves making observations, as well as asking questions. Answers and observations naturally lead to other questions. Validate that the information you are collecting is factual because, taken out of context, many thoughts and actions present a distorted picture.

#### Interviewing

The interview occurs with individuals, families or segments of families—most commonly—committed partners or a parent and child. When individuals in families are interviewed, it is important to remember that each one only represents one point of view. In the process of data collection and validation, make an effort to meet with all family members—as a group or individually—whenever possible to develop a picture of the total family perspective. Although family interviews are more complex than one-on-one interaction, they elicit data that is unobtainable in any other way. For example, the reaction of one family member to another can only be observed in a group interaction.

The physical, psychologic, and social dimensions of the environment within which the family lives are major components of family assessment that incorporate both observation and interview. The degree to which these elements can be assessed depends on whether the nurse has the opportunity to make a home visit or must depend on client report.

#### Physical Environment

The physical environment includes the house and the conditions inside and outside. Size, number of rooms, orderliness, cleanliness, the condition of the yard, furnishings, plumbing, heat, health and safety hazards, and the presence or absence of smoke detectors and fire extinguishers all provide important information about the status of the family. Some families may have a spacious home but cannot buy food or pay for telephone service or basic utilities such as heat and lights. Other homes may be small and crowded, but all family members have sufficient food and clothing and feel secure and comfortable in that environment. An important component to assess is the presence of safety hazards (e.g., frayed wires, no refrigeration, an unvented space heater) and family plans for emergencies such as a fire or earthquake. Box 2-5 provides suggestions on possible hazardous situations. Some hazards are created because of what is present; others are created because of what is absent.

## Social Environment

Significant aspects of the psychologic environment include developmental stages and family dynamics and emotional strengths, as well as communication patterns, including verbal and non-verbal communication both within and outside the family. Family roles and coping strategies also provide important clues to the family's health.

The social environment includes the effect religion, race and culture, social class and economic status, and external resources (e.g., school, church, and health resources) have on the family. Gaining information about these areas helps to clarify the context of the family and provide information about family strengths and resources, as well as deficits.

## Family Strengths

The health provider, as well as the family itself, often tends to look only at the problems and conflicts within a family. In order to know the full extent of how a family functions, however, family strengths must also be assessed. Many years ago, Otto (1963) identified the following family strengths:

1. The ability to provide for the physical, emotional, and spiritual needs of a family.
2. The ability to be sensitive to the needs of the family members.
3. The ability to communicate effectively.
4. The ability to provide support, security, and encouragement.
5. The ability to initiate and maintain growth-producing relationships and experiences within and without the family.
6. The capacity to maintain and create constructive and responsible community relationships in the neighborhood, school, town, and local and state governments.
7. The ability to grow with and through children.
8. The ability for self-help, and the ability to accept help when appropriate.
9. The ability to perform family roles flexibly.
10. Mutual respect for the individuality of a family member.
11. The ability to use a crisis or seemingly injurious experience as a means of growth.
12. A concern for family unity, loyalty, and interfamily cooperation.

These strengths continue to be important to healthy family functioning, but it is unlikely that any given family will have all these characteristics. Encouraging family connectedness—especially during developmental and situational transitions—is important.

---

### BOX 2-5   *Potential Physical Hazards in the Environment*

This is not an all-inclusive list but is provided to start your thought process when assessing safety issues within an environment.

**Presence of:**
- a swimming pool without child-proof barriers to prevent children and animals from falling in
- lead based paint
- a space heater that is not properly vented
- loose throw rugs
- exposed lamp cords crossing a pathway
- broken furniture, stairs, railings, or floorboards
- hazardous materials (e.g., cleaning materials) and medications stored in areas that a child can access
- toys in walkway
- numerous house pets
- exhaust fumes from automobile traffic

**Absence of:**
- working plumbing system
- refrigeration of food
- clean air supply
- smoke and carbon monoxide alarms
- emergency exits and a plan for use that family members know
- lack of poison control phone number and supplies
- barriers to upper story windows, porches, and stairs
- fenced play area for small children
- safety plugs in exposed electrical outlets

## Healthy Relationships

Recent work provides some insight to characteristics of healthy relationships. The Family Formation Project has studied relationships and found that there are subtle patterns of behavior that compromise the quality of relationships. Gottman and associates have determined the following effective indicators of the potential longevity of relationships:

- Healthy relationships are based on kindness. Positive interactions outnumber negative ones at a critical ratio of five to one (i.e., those headed for divorce have more nasty than nice moments).
- Husbands who do housework are happier and healthier, have better sex lives, and are much more likely to stay married.
- Women who are married to belittling, contemptuous men are much more likely to fall ill than those with supportive spouses.

- Disrespectful wives also ruin a marriage. When a wife's face shows disgust four or more times within a 15-minute conversation, it is a silent sign that the couple is likely to separate within 4 years (Borysenko, 1998). Each of these indicators are not causal factors but do provide indicators for possible use in assessment.

## Analyzing Family Data

Work with the family to analyze the data to determine the family health status. It is important to analyze the family structure, function, and process because these dimensions determine the types of decisions made by women and their families. Many families will need to make some crucial decisions related to a member's—or the family's—physical, social, and/or emotional health, so they need to participate in validating the data and nursing diagnoses and developing a plan of care. While doing an analysis of the family, you will also be relating the findings to developmental systems and role theory to guide your understanding of the family's strengths and weaknesses.

Two of the most useful family assessment tools for not only recording data but also teaching the family are the genogram and the ecomap. These tools provide a pictorial representation of complex family patterns and community relationships, allowing both the nurse and family to see the intricacy of the family's relationships within and outside the family (McGoldrick, Gerson, and Shellenberger, 1999).

### Genograms

The genogram provides a graphic picture of an outline of the family's history over a period of time, usually three

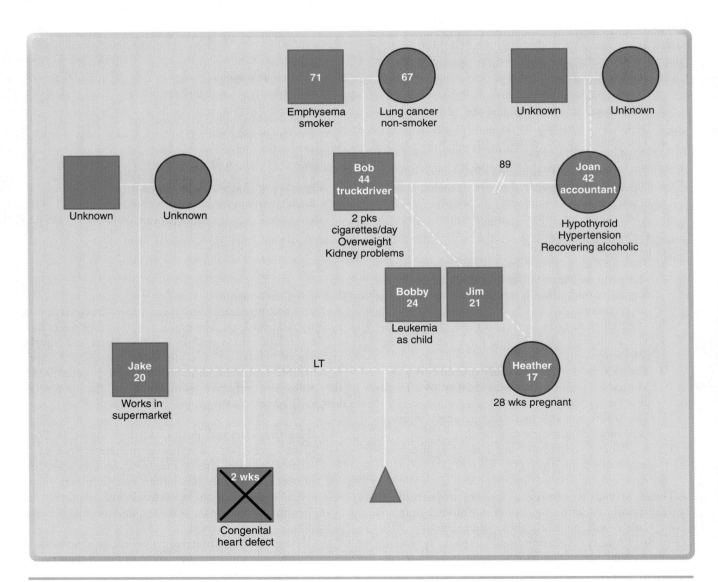

*FIGURE 2-8* • Genogram.

generations (McGoldrick, Gerson, and Shellenberger, 1999). This provides valuable information as the family history unfolds and is a way to map the structure of the family, record family information (e.g., significant life events, cultural and religious identification, occupations, place of residence), and delineate relationships. By adding major dimensions of the family's health history, the genogram becomes a family health tree from which knowledge about genetic and familial diseases can be gained.

Environmental and occupational diseases, psychosocial problems (e.g., obesity, anorexia nervosa, mental illness), and infectious diseases also can be noted. Family risk factors and strengths can be added to the genogram by evaluating how the family manages stress and leisure and how often they have physical exams, pap smears, and exercise. This information can help identify areas of risk and ability, enhance the family's awareness of the situation, and facilitate work with the family in planning appropriate interventions (Friedman, 1992; McGoldrick and others, 1999). Figure 2-8 provides an example of a genogram/family health tree based on the case study described at the end of this chapter. Figure 2-9 identifies the common genogram symbols.

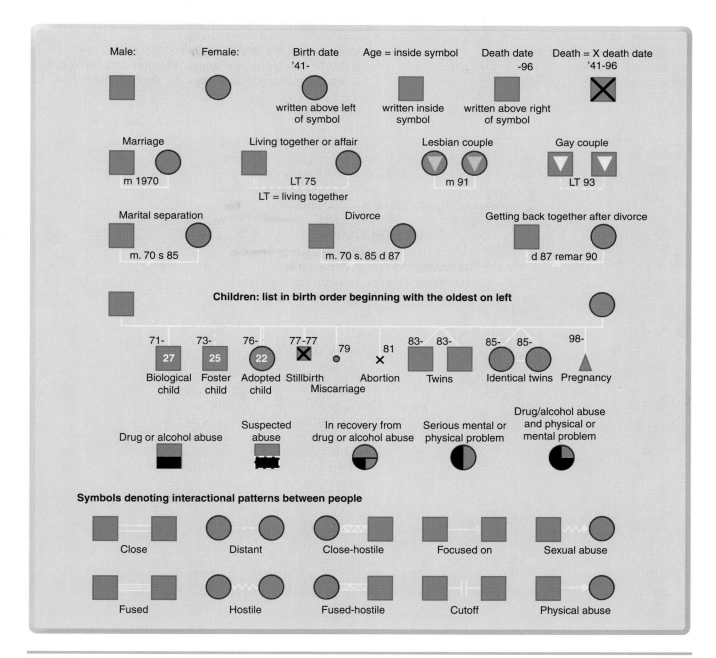

**FIGURE 2-9** • Standard symbols of genograms. *(From McGoldrick M, Gerson R, and Shellenberger S:* Genograms: assessment and intervention, *ed 2, New York, 1999, W.W. Norton.)*

### Ecomap

An equally convenient way of analyzing a family's interactions within the community is through the use of an ecomap. The development of an ecomap with the family facilitates an understanding of the social support and resources identified by the family. An example of an ecomap can be found in Figure 2-5. The ecomap provides a visual depiction of the organizational patterns and relationships of the complex family system in which the balance between the demands and resources of the system can be identified (Clemen-Stone, McGuire, and Eigsti, 1998). Once an ecomap is developed with the family, the information can be used to identify interactive family strengths, conflicts in need of mediation, connections to be made, and resources to be sought and mobilized. Figure 2-10 provides an example of a family's ecomap based on the case study at the end of the chapter.

Both the genogram and ecomap are useful tools during an early interview with a family. The whole family can become engaged in completing each tool so that family involvement in their own health care is facilitated from the beginning of the relationship. Wright and Leahey (1994) note that the visual gestalt conveyed through the use of these tools provides information more simply and usefully than words.

These tools are not static because family functions and relationships change, members roles are altered, and the family structure shifts as members join and leave, are born, or die. Both tools should be updated periodically so that they remain current and useful.

### Family Process

As part of the family analysis, it is also important to describe the family processes. Hanson and Boyd (1996) describe family process as "the ongoing interaction be-

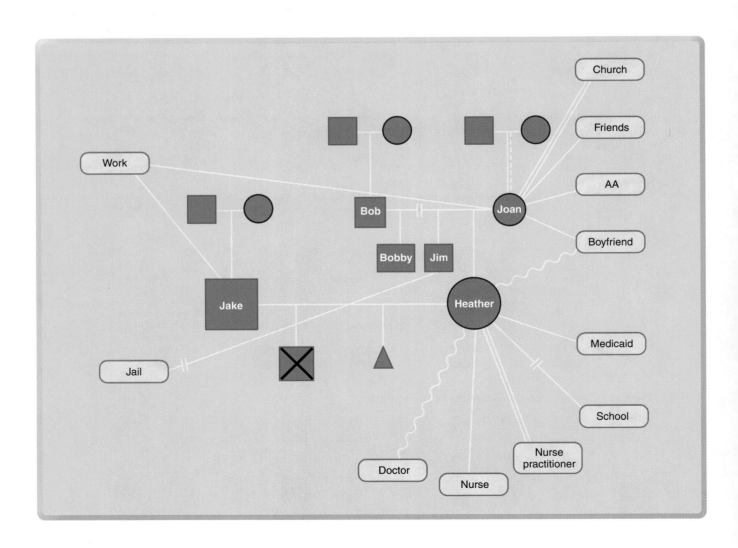

FIGURE 2-10 • Ecogram.

tween family members through which they accomplish their instrumental and expressive tasks." They point out that although families may have similar structure and function in similar ways, they may interact very differently in terms of roles, communication, power, decision making, marital satisfaction, and coping strategies.

***Roles and Communication.*** Negotiation of family roles requires effective and ongoing communication. "Healthy communication is characterized by clear but flexible rules, clarity in the vebalization of thoughts and feelings, and receptivity to and acknowledgement of the other person's communication. The psychological defense mechanisms of projection, denial, blaming and scapegoating are infrequent" (Hanson and Boyd, 1996).

***Power.*** Power within a family is a dynamic and multidimensional process. Men often assume marital power because of the following: (1) the socialization process; (2) the legal marriage contract, which favors men in many states; and (3) economic resources because men are generally better paid. There are variations based on racial differences and where the family lives because the more isolated the woman is from family and friends, the more power the male may assume.

***Decision Making.*** Communication and power are basic to decision making. Family decision making is most successful for the group when it is not always an individual, but a joint effort. Sometimes a collaborative effort develops where "members of the family may have their own spheres of decision making. The father may choose the car, the mother the house, the child the toy. Or the allocation of power may vary from situation to situation" (Hanson and Boyd, 1996). Joint participation in decision making, with the power residing with the parents, is more likely to be satisfactory.

***Marital Satisfaction.*** Satisfaction in the family relationship, especially between the parenting dyad, varies over time. Satisfaction is relatively high among new couples and older couples, with a decrease often occurring during the years of active parenting. The quality of the marital interaction is related to the spouse's involvement and responsibilities both within and outside the household. When the wife's occupational attainment is higher than the husband's, the satisfaction level of the couple generally decreases. Throughout the life cycle, marital interaction promotes marital happiness and marital happiness promotes marital interaction.

***Coping Strategies.*** Each family has its own collection of coping strategies, which may be "classified into three broad categories: (1) responses that change the stressful event, (2) responses that control the meaning of the stressful event, and (3) responses that control the stress itself" (Pearlin and Schooler, 1982). When a stressful event occurs, the family responds based on past experiences and current strengths. Individual family members may also respond differently to an event because of the difference in its meaning to them. Meaningful evalua-

tion of coping strategies is difficult unless they are reviewed long-term.

By understanding the structure, function, and various processes of the family, we can develop a plan of care with them that addresses their unique needs. Cultural and familial variation is to be expected, so the best teachers are the family members themselves. The plan of care must promote the heath of the family by also addressing the health of individual family members because the interactions between the individual and the family group are reciprocal.

## Collaboration in the Development of a Plan

Work together with the family to establish priorities. This process is based on equality, self-value, and empowerment (Youngkin and Davis, 1998). The emphasis of family nursing is on the needs of the family rather than any individual within the family. It is not enough to identify the family member who plays a central role, but the interactions among the members in relation to one another must also be identified.

To provide effective and acceptable care, work in partnership with the family in mutual respect and cooperation. Recognize the "family's rights and responsibilities and their central role in guiding the person's selection and use of health care services" (Boos, 1996). When working on a plan, considerations such as the following must be addressed by the nurse: (1) the immediate health care needs and wishes of the family; (2) constraints caused by time; (3) the availability of community resources available to the family; and (4) constraints caused by money (e.g., insurance coverage) (Boos, 1996).

## Nursing Diagnoses and Planning Care

Based on the assessment and analysis of data, establish the nursing diagnosis. These diagnoses may be for the entire family or individuals within the family. Long- and short-term goals are then established in conjunction with the family. Together, expected outcomes (i.e., including measurable results within a specific timeframe) are set up.

### NANDA Nursing Diagnoses

The North American Nursing Diagnosis Association (NANDA) has developed the most frequently used system of nursing diagnosis. Since the 1970s, nursing diagnostic labels and defining characteristics have been developed and tested on an ongoing basis. Every 2 years, new diagnoses are included and some of the existing diagnoses are revised. The changes reflect the diversity of nursing across populations and settings. In the most recent listing, there are additional diagnoses that address not only the health of individuals but also family system and subsystem health problems. See Box 2-6 for a list of some NANDA nursing diagnoses related to the family.

**Pattern 1: Exchanging**
Altered nutrition: More than body requirements
Altered nutrition: Less than body requirements
Altered nutrition: Risk for more than body requirements

**Pattern 3: Relating**
Impaired social interaction
Social isolation
Altered role performance
Altered parenting
Risk for altered parenting
Risk for altered parent/infant/child attachment
Altered family process
Altered family processes: alcoholism
Parent role conflict
Altered sexuality patterns

**Pattern 4: Choosing**
Ineffective family coping: Disabling
Ineffective family coping: Compromised
Family coping: Potential for growth
Ineffective management of therapeutic regimen: Families
Decisional conflict (specify)
Health seeking behaviors (specify)

**Pattern 6: Moving**
Impaired home maintenance management
Altered health maintenance

**Pattern 8: Knowing**
Knowledge deficit (specify)

**Pattern 9: Feeling**
Dysfunctional grieving
Anticipatory grieving
Post-trauma syndrome
Risk for post-trauma syndrome

This is not an all-inclusive list of diagnoses appropriate for family care. In addition, there are many nursing diagnoses labeling an individual's health problem that affects the well-being of the family.

From NANDA: *Nursing diagnoses: definitions and classification 1999-2000,* Philadelphia, 1999, The Association.

### The Omaha System

The Visiting Nurses Association of Omaha has developed a classification system of client problems that is often used. The problem classification scheme consists of 40 problems that fall into one of the following four domains: environmental, psychosocial, physiologic, and health-related behaviors. For each problem, there may be actual or potential impairments or opportunities for health promotion (Martin and Scheet, 1992).

### Implementing a Plan

Implementing the plan of care with the family is based on the information gathered in the family assessment, data analysis, and plan development. If family members will be providing direct care, assess their skill level and comfort in providing that care. Based on the caregiver's abilities and the needs of the family member(s), assess if it is safe for both the client and the family caregiver for the client to remain in the home (Boos, 1996). Teach new skills, provide periodic supervision, and evaluate the skills performed while providing the family with continued access to resources, materials, and supplies. Throughout the process, assess for additional needs on the individual or family level.

Interventions will incorporate teaching about various health considerations, helping families deal with the stress created by health problems, and making referrals for community services. Interventions are planned, taking into account the family priorities and addressing primary, secondary, or tertiary levels of prevention.

#### Primary Prevention

Primary prevention encompasses health promotion and disease prevention. It identifies actions taken to prevent the occurrence of health problems in families. One of the major nursing activities in this realm is that of anticipatory guidance. Activities might include providing information about normal changes to be expected in a child's growth so that parents are prepared for the changes and are ready to deal with them when they occur. Healthy People 2010 (U.S. Department of Health and Human Services, Public Health Service, 2000) addresses primary prevention for families in most of its objectives. Although the emphasis of the plan is more on individuals, the effect on families is great. For example, the implementation of programs to reduce teenage and unintended pregnancies has important implications on family life and women's health.

#### Secondary Prevention

Secondary prevention has to do with the early recognition and treatment of existing health problems. A family perspective looks at the interactive problems that suggest family dysfunction, as well as the concerns of individuals within the family. Healthy People 2010 (U.S. Department of Health and Human Services, Public Health Service, 2000) emphasizes the use of screening exams (e.g., mammography, pap smears, and fecal occult blood testing) to detect problems early and the avoidance of long-term and costly care that saps families' resources.

#### Tertiary Prevention

Tertiary prevention has to do with the rehabilitative level of health care. In families, the focus is on preventing the problem from returning or ensuring that the family remains intact. An example of tertiary care is helping a homeless mother and child by facilitating their connection to appropriate community services so that they can find permanent housing and employment, allowing them to maintain their home.

In conjunction with the client, nursing intervention begins on the first visit as decisions are made in the planning process about what health needs should be addressed first and what the responsibilities are for both the nurse and client. The time of the next appointment is based on the needs of the client and is mutually agreed on. A visit should be planned to last ½ to 1 hour because the family can only absorb a finite amount of information before they are overloaded and unable to take in more.

Similarly, you are collecting a great deal of information through observation and interview and can easily become overloaded. It is better to arrange a second visit to continue assessment, review what has been taught, and evaluate progress toward goals rather than try to accomplish too much in one visit. Incorporating the family members in the care of the client allows many opportunities for teaching and further assessment of family concerns and needs.

As time passes and the caring relationship between the family and the nurse develops, you will become aware of developing social, emotional, financial and physical problems (Boos, 1996). It is also important to evaluate the strengths that the family members are developing and acknowledge their accomplishments. In addition to the care you are providing, it is equally important to be aware of other resources available within the community. Families may be receiving simultaneous services from a number of volunteer or church-based programs (e.g., Friendly Visitors or a parish nurse). If the family is not receiving other services, you may make the contacts so that the family can take advantage of extended services.

### Evaluation of a Plan

Systematic evaluation of clients is imperative during home visitation. Evaluation of care is done on two levels. The first is the effectiveness of the current interventions, and the second is the nurse's self-evaluation (Boos, 1996). Evaluation is performed for both the individuals and the family as a whole. For example, assessing the skill level progression of primary givers, as well as the well-being of the entire family needs repeated evaluation. Agencies have specific, individual evaluation methods, and nurses should provide input on the usefulness of current tools and suggest ways to improve the quality of evaluation while striving to decrease the amount of paperwork generated. Care paths used in the hospital are being implemented in some home care institutions and will be useful as an interdisciplinary method of evaluation of care (Lowry and others, 1998).

Also, evaluate your ability to help the family implement interventions that are consistent with their wishes and needs (Boos, 1996). Self-evaluation allows you to critique your own work while striving to improve the level of care provided to women and their families.

Documenting each visit is both legally and logically required of nurses. Because of the independent nature of home visits, complete and accurate documentation of the care provided is essential. Third party payers and agencies that are also working with the family may require additional documentation. Charting should include the following: (1) all interventions and services provided and their effects; (2) objective assessments made; (3) progress noted; (4) changes made in the plan of care; (5) teaching provided; and (6) future plans, including revisions (Clark and Hahn, 1996).

 ## CARE OF FAMILIES WITH MULTIPLE PROBLEMS

Vulnerable families are those whose physical and/or mental health, environmental, economic, and emotional resources are insufficient, threatening critical tasks and family functions. Words used to describe these families reflect the labeler's view when describing the quality of family function, which is not necessarily the view held by the family members. Terms often used are marginal, disorganized, and dysfunctional.

All families lose their equilibrium from time to time, often due to illness or disability. The occurrence of a serious illness does not just affect the patient, but the entire family. We must consider how an illness in a specific family member creates family problems (Jassak and Knafl, 1990). The crisis can sometimes be overwhelming for even the healthiest family. Healthy families can take the appropriate actions to return to equilibrium. For example, a healthy family who has a child diagnosed with leukemia would be more apt to reach out to community resources and friends and be assertive in seeking out needed support. Vulnerable families, however, have few resources to help them maintain balance when faced with a crisis. Attempts to offset their difficulties when they have few reserves or resources makes it harder for them to return to a state of equilibrium (Janosik, 1994).

A family might be described as marginally stable if a crisis would consume all of their family resources. Family members might assume the care needed by another member and do a good job, but they may hesitate to use community resources or, in many cases, be unaware of what is available to them and tend to burn out before they try other things.

## Dysfunctional Family

Disorganized or dysfunctional families occur in all levels of society. Members are unable to maintain a healthy environment for themselves. In these families, addiction, low stress tolerance, and impulsiveness may strain the family unit (Janosik, 1994). As a result, they live from crisis to crisis, never able to grow beyond their experiences. These families only use community services when their crises reach such magnitude that they must seek outside help or public knowledge of the condition of the family forces them to participate in care.

Friedman (1998) has delineated four dysfunctional family adaptive strategies, noting that these families do the following: (1) deny problems and exploit one or more family members in nonphysical ways (e.g., using scapegoating or threats); (2) deny family problems and use adaptive mechanisms (e.g., family myths, threat, emotional distance, triangling, and pseudomutuality) that impair the family's ability to meet their adaptive function; (3) separate or lose family members (i.e., through abandonment, institutionalization, divorce, physical absence of family members) and exhibit submission to marked domination; and (4) use physical violence. Heiney (1993) has outlined characteristics that are useful for assessing vulnerable families about their functional and dysfunctional dimensions (Table 2-11).

## Interventions

Interventions directed toward reducing family stress require some specific considerations. Because parents are usually the ones who determine how families will cope, it is important to address their anxiety. Although your tendency may be to directly protect vulnerable family members (e.g., children or the elderly), it is important to support and educate the family caregivers so that they can provide appropriate care to the child or other vulnerable persons.

Another intervention is to promote family strengths, allowing the family to respond to their growth-producing dynamics rather than focusing only on the problems. Zerwekh (1997) identifies this approach, emphasizing positives, as one of the dimensions of expert connecting. Although this intervention is important for all families, it is especially important for vulnerable families. You can also reframe negatives to highlight a positive aspect of generally negative behavior so alternatives that can facilitate the positive behavior can be considered. For example, if a client does not stick to the expected schedule for taking medications, the deviation can be depicted as an attempt to maintain autonomy rather than the client's attempt to be "non-compliant" and disregard the help. Emphasizing a positive characteristic supports the client's self-esteem and encourages her to reconsider the medication regime and respond in a way that is in her best interest.

## Referrals

When making referrals, the important issues to be considered are the five As, as follow: appropriateness to the condition, affordability, availability, acceptability, and accessibility. Perhaps the most important consideration is the acceptability of the service. If the client is not willing to use the resource, the other As do not matter. Similarly, no matter how acceptable the service may be to the client, to be useful, it must be accessible—in terms of affordability, available transportation, and client eligibility. In some settings, particularly some rural areas, a service is simply not available, no matter how acceptable it may be to the client or how eligible the client may be for the service.

## Safety as a Health Circumstance for Women and Families

Family violence is one of the most serious manifestations of family dysfunction. Family violence may be the largest hidden health problem for women and is a major contributor to homelessness for women and children. Domestic violence includes physical, emotional, sexual, and economic abuse. Although 95% of the incidences of domestic violence are men abusing women, the reverse can also be true, so both men and women should be screened for domestic violence during a home visit.

Comply with the reporting laws of the state, which generally focus on the safety of the children and the elderly. Support the woman who, for reasons you may not understand, desires to remain in her relationship or returns to the relationship after leaving. She is the only one who can gauge whether she is more at risk in staying or leaving. Be aware of resources for battered women available in the community.

## TERMINATING THE NURSE-FAMILY RELATIONSHIPS

Depending on your role and the needs of the family, you may make several home visits or provide care for an extended period of time. Preparing the family for the last home visit should begin at the initial visit.

At all visits, help the family to find their own strengths and encourage them to learn to be self-sufficient. Termination will occur when the family's outcomes are met or the duration of care has exceeded the monetary reimbursement allowances. Sometimes, the goals are not completely met because you must terminate service before the client is ready. For example, you may have to reallocate time to families who are at higher risk or take another job. In any situation, be sure that the family's transition to another provider is smooth or that an appropriate referral is provided or suggested, when possible.

---

**TABLE 2-11   *Assessment Summary for Functional vs. Dysfunctional Family Characteristics***

| Functional | Dysfunctional |
|---|---|
| **Emotional System** | **Emotional System** |
| Independence is encouraged. | Dependence is encouraged. |
| Positive self-esteem prompted. | One person is "identified" as problem. |
| Positive conflict resolution. | Negative conflict resolution. |
| Adapts to change. | Repetitive, rigid use of ineffective coping. |
| **Differentiation** | **Lack of Differentiation** |
| Relationships foster emotional maturity. | Emotional immaturity encouraged. |
| Thoughts separated from feelings. | Thoughts and feelings are enmeshed. |
| Sense of separateness among family members. | Sense of fusion. |
| Differences of opinion are allowed and encouraged. | Differences of opinion are unacceptable. |
| Problem-solving to generate solutions to concerns occurs. | Family members do not think through alternatives to problems. |
| **Absence of Triangling** | **Triangling** |
| Patterns of interaction among family members are flexible and adaptive to the situation. | Patterns of interaction among family members are fixed and rigid. |

From Heiney SP: Assessing and intervening with dysfunctional families. In Wegner GD and Alexander RJ, editors: *Readings in family nursing,* Philadelphia, 1993, J. B. Lippincott.

---

It is important to review with the family what has been accomplished and reinforce and support their progress. By the end of the relationship, they will have come to value your input and need reassurance that they can make decisions that will positively affect their health care. The focus on partnership emphasizes that perspective and provides the family with the strength to make independent decisions.

Periodically remind the family members of the anticipated date of termination of services (Boos, 1996). Review client progress and discuss any remaining issues to avoid leaving unfinished business. Express and discuss your own feelings about ending the relationship, and allow the clients to express their feelings. In the process, you may learn of concerns not revealed before this time that may necessitate another referral.

Disconnecting the relationship takes time and effort and should not be dealt with hastily. If you and the family both reside in the same community or family members have contact with you in nonprofessional activities, it is sometimes more difficult to bring the therapeutic relationship to a close while maintaining the other relationship. All parties in the partnership must be clear about their roles after termination because there is no longer a provider-receiver health care process or responsibility in place. A successful termination is one in which *both* client and nurse feel satisfied that goals have been met or appropriate referrals made.

## CASE STUDY*

Heather is a 17-year-old woman who is 28 weeks pregnant with her second child. She has been referred to your Visiting Nurses Agency for home visitation, and you have been assigned her care. Even though she has been a client of the agency in the past, you were not her care provider.

During her first pregnancy, Heather attended high school at a special program for pregnant and parenting teens. With this pregnancy, she has been receiving prenatal care from the same nurse practitioner who previously provided her care. You speak with the nurse practitioner, and she believes that they have a fairly good relationship.

Heather has dropped out of school, is not working, and is living with her boyfriend, Jake, the father of both children. He is a 20-year-old high school graduate who is presently working at a local supermarket and does not want her attending school. Heather and Jake do not have a telephone, so she is not easy to contact. Heather uses the bus for transportation.

Heather's first child, Peter, died of a congenital heart defect at 2 weeks of age, which was when your agency had its first contact with Heather.

The events leading up to the death of Peter were as follows. Heather had taken him to the pediatrician's office for a 3-day-old well child check. The physician noticed a slight murmur, but in every other way, the baby was perfectly normal. He had regained his birth weight. The doctor asked Heather to bring Peter back in 3 days for another visit and discussed symptoms of circulatory

*continued*

## CASE STUDY*

problems with Heather. Heather and Peter did not come to that appointment.

A nurse did a home visit, but Heather was not home. No contact was made with Heather for the next week. Shortly before Peter was 2 weeks old, the nurse made a home visit and Heather was there with the baby. Upon an immediate assessment of Peter, the nurse knew he was in cardiac failure. He had generalized cyanosis, his heartbeat was 160, and he was lethargic. Heather said that he had not been interested in eating for a couple of days. The nurse called the pediatrician and then 911 on her cell phone. Peter died in the ambulance on the way to the hospital.

Heather is very pleased that she is pregnant again and hopes this baby is also a boy. She does not know why she didn't start prenatal care earlier in the pregnancy. You think, however, that she is manifesting signs of depression. Because she is not attending school, she is not eligible for public assistance, but she does have Medicaid for health insurance.

Heather's family history includes the following: Joan, her mother, is 42 years old, has mild hypertension, and is hypothyroid. She is proud to be a recovering alcoholic for 5 years and attends AA regularly. She has belonged to a Protestant church for 4 years and enjoys church services and some social contacts. She takes pride in her job and has a few friends. She is also dating a man named Ted, whom Heather does not like very well.

Her father, Bob, who is 44 years old, and her mother have been divorced for 12 years. Her father lives 150 miles away and rarely sees Heather. He is a truck driver, smokes 2 packs of cigarettes a day, is overweight, and has had some kidney problems.

Heather has two older brothers. Jim is 21 and was recently released from jail for his second DUI. He has no known health problems. Her oldest brother, Bobby, is 24 and lives 10 miles away. He is working and attending school part time. He had leukemia as a child but has had no problems since.

Heather's mother was adopted, and her grandparents know nothing about her mother's biologic parents. Heather is close with these grandparents. Her father's parents are alive. Her paternal grandfather is 71 and has emphysema. He is also a smoker. Her paternal grandmother is 67 and has lung cancer now. She was not a smoker.

- What will you do to begin to develop your professional relationship with Heather?
- How will you organize the information about the family using an genogram and ecomap?
- What strengths are presented in this case?
- What concerns do you have about this case?
- What are possible nursing diagnoses?
- What interventions can you offer Heather during this visit?

Prepare for your next visit to Heather:

- What further information do you need to obtain? How will you do that?
- How will you validate your assumptions and nursing diagnoses?

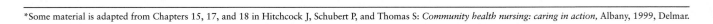

*Some material is adapted from Chapters 15, 17, and 18 in Hitchcock J, Schubert P, and Thomas S: *Community health nursing: caring in action,* Albany, 1999, Delmar.

# Scenarios

**1.** You are scheduled for a home visit with Davida on a referral from child protective services. She has had to leave her 11-year-old son and 6-year-old daughter home alone while she works nights at a local restaurant. This situation was discovered when she brought her daughter into the emergency department for stitches on her hand because of an accident involving a broken drinking glass.

- What additional information would you obtain from other health care providers before making an appointment with Davida and her family?
- Using role theory, what kind of role strain might Davida be experiencing?
- What type of information might be helpful to Davida?

- What family nursing diagnoses might apply?
- What interventions would you consider offering to Davida?

---

2. In your community, there is a large apartment complex that is mainly inhabited by legal immigrants from Russia. When doing a home visit to a client in the building, she tells you that many of these residents will not seek prenatal care even though they have Medicaid. Instead they either have a Russian immigrant with midwifery experience deliver their children at home or go to the emergency department of the hospital in active labor. Their rationale for not receiving care is that they have heard that if an immigrant uses too many medical services, when that person applies for citizenship, he or she will be denied for this reason.

Your client is concerned about her cousin, Galena, who is pregnant and lives next door. She asks what you might do to help Galena.

- What is the first thing you would do?
- What family nursing diagnoses might apply?
- What goals would be appropriate?
- What factors will help to develop a successful plan of intervention?
- What factors will inhibit the success?
- What will you do that will increase the chance of success?

---

3. A family has been referred to your care because their 3-week-old newborn is being released from the hospital where she was treated for pneumonia. The infant was born preterm (i.e., 34 weeks). You are asked to see the family to determine if the home environment seems adequate for this infant. There are 13 family members living in the 3-bedroom apartment.

- What observations would you make related to the physical environment?
- What aspects of the psychosocial environment will you assess?
- What other factors will you want to assess?
- What family nursing diagnoses might apply?
- What interventions will you develop with the family?
- What strengths within this situation might help to make interventions work?

---

4. Jackie has been in a battered women's shelter for 2 weeks. She was able to leave her home with $734, some clothes for herself and her two children, their social security cards, and her driver's license. For the family's safety, she has enrolled her kids in a different elementary school and has taken a new job in the back room of an auto parts store. She is trying to find a place to live with relatives out of town. She is eager to accept any help available to her.

- What strengths does this family appear to have?
- What family nursing diagnoses might apply?
- When meeting this family for the first time, what would you do to establish a therapeutic relationship with this family?
- What problems do you anticipate that Jackie might want to discuss?
- What might you do to help?

---

5. You are doing a home visit with Rachel and Anna, a lesbian couple. Two weeks ago, Rachel gave birth to a girl, whom she named Ruth. Ruth was conceived through artificial insemination of sperm from a male friend, Jim. Jim plans to be part of the family, although Rachel will be the primary parent. You are there doing a well-baby postpartum home visit. The baby is healthy and gaining weight. Anna tells you that Jim wants to take Ruth with him for the weekend. Although Rachel is willing, Anna wonders if it is too soon for Ruth to leave her mother.

- What further assessment information do you need?
- What strengths does this family appear to have?
- What family nursing diagnoses apply?
- What might be the goals of this family?
- What interventions are possible at this time?

---

6. You are working at a clinic at a homeless shelter as a case manager. One of your clients is a 36-year-old woman, Dorian, who has been staying at the shelter for several days with her 10-year-old son, Jess. Dorian has been having severe abdominal pain and needs to be hospitalized for tests. She has no money or health insurance. Her ex-husband is an alcoholic, and she does not know where he is. She has no other family to whom she can turn. She has no idea about how to care for Jess if she goes to the hospital.

- What are the issues in this situation?
- What family nursing diagnoses might apply?
- What type of interventions can you offer that might help Dorian and Jess?
- How would you manage this situation?

---

7. Joan has three children. Her husband, Barry, is the CEO of a large company. He works long hours, but when he comes home, he expects his dinner to be ready and the children to be in bed. He is quick-tempered and has yelled at and hit Joan several times for not getting dinner ready quickly enough or other infractions of his "house rules." Over the years, Joan has dropped most of her friends because Barry does not like them and want them in his home. She only goes out with Barry to business social functions, because he demands that she go with him.

Their life is a cycle of his being angry and abusive to her then being very apologetic and bringing her flowers and candy, so their life is calm and good for a while. One night Barry loses his temper with the 3-year-old and picks her up by her arm, dislocating it. While the child is being seen in the emergency room, Joan starts to cry and tells you that she can't take it any more. She doesn't know what to do because she has no money of her own and has never held a job outside the home.

- What is your initial response?
- What would be your first responsibility?
- What other assessment data do you need?

- What family nursing diagnoses might apply?
- What interventions can you offer Joan?

---

8. Margo and Frank are married and in their mid-40s. They have two children, Jon and Barbara, who are 16 and 14 respectively. Frank's 70-year-old frail mother, Amy, who is a widow, has recently moved in with them so Margo can care for her. You are making a home visit for the Senior Center.

Amy is unhappy with the move and complains about how Margo runs the house. She also criticizes the fact that Jon has been staying out late and is belligerent when his parents express their concern.

Because Frank is at work all day and is tired when he gets home, Margo is the one who has to deal with most of the family issues. When Amy leaves the room to get some papers, you have a chance to speak with Margo. She tells you about the situation of Amy moving in and says she has not been sleeping well and is losing her temper much more than usual. She's not sure why she's having these problems.

- What developmental stage is this family in, and what is one of their tasks?
- What is the term used to describe an adult like Margo who is caring for both younger and older family members?
- What other information do you need to obtain?
- What family nursing diagnoses might apply?
- What interventions might be helpful?

## REFERENCES

Allen K and Phillips J: *Women's health across the lifespan,* New York, 1997, Lippincott.

Andrews MM: Transcultural perspectives in the nursing care of children and adolescents. In Andrews MM and Boyle JS, editors: *Transcultural concepts in nursing care,* ed 2, Philadelphia, 1995, Lippincott.

Ayers M, Bruno AA, and Langford RW: *Community-based nursing care,* St Louis, 1999, Mosby.

Balzer-Riley JW: *Communications in nursing,* ed 3, St Louis, 1996, Mosby.

Becvar DS and Becvar RJ: *Family therapy: a systematic integration,* ed 3, Needham Heights, MA, 1996, Allyn & Bacon.

Benner P and Wrubel J: *The primacy of caring,* Menlo Park, CA, 1989, Addison-Wesley.

Boos S: Home visits 101: a simple framework for practice, *Kansas Nurse* 71(7):3, 1996.

Borysenko J: *A woman's book of life: the biology, psychology, and spirituality of the feminine life cycle,* New York: 1998, Riverhead.

Bravo E: The job/family challenge today. In Kesselman A, McNair LD, and Schniedewind N, editors: *Women—images and realities,* ed 2, Mountain View, CA, 1999, Mayfield.

Bredin RM: Togetherness: family and community. In *Perspectives: women studies,* Boulder, CO, 1998, Coursewise.

Bronfenbrenner U: Toward an experimental ecology of human development, *Am Psychol* 7:513, 1977.

Carter B and McGoldrick M: Overview: the changing family life cycle: a framework for family therapy. In Carter B and McGoldrick M, editors: *The changing family life cycle,* Boston, 1989, Allyn & Bacon.

Castillo HM: Cultural diversity: implications for nursing. In Torres S, editor: *Hispanic voices,* New York, 1996, NLN.

Clark M and Hahn P: *Nursing in the community,* ed 2, Stamford, CT, 1996, Appleton and Lange.

Clemen-Stone S, McGuire SL, and Eigsti DG: *Comprehensive community health nursing,* ed 5, St Louis, 1998, Mosby.

Costello CB: Introduction. In *The American woman 1999-2000,* New York, 1998, Norton.

Cowan RS: The "industrial revolution" in the home: household technology and social change in the twentieth century, *Technology and Culture* 17:1-23, 1976.

Crouch-Ruiz E: The birth of a premature infant in a Puerto Rican family. In Torres S, editor: *Hispanic voices,* New York, 1996, NLN.

Deal LW: The effectiveness of community health nursing interventions: a literature review, *Pub Health Nurs* 5:315, 1993.

Duvall EM: *Marriage and family development,* Philadelphia, 1977, J.B. Lippincott.

Franke NV: African American women's health: the effects of disease and chronic life stressors. In Ruzek SB, Olesen VL, and Clarke AE, editors: *Women's health complexities and differences,* Columbus, OH, 1997, Ohio State.

Friedman M: Teaching about and for family diversity on nursing, *J Fam Nurs* 3(3):280, 1997.

Friedman MM: *Family nursing: research theory and practice*, ed 4, Stamford, CT, 1998, Appleton & Lange.

Garbarino J: Reinventing fatherhood: families in society, *J Contemp Human Serv* 74:51, 1993.

Gilliss CL: Family nursing research, theory and practice. In Wegner GD and Alexander RJ, editors: *Readings in family nursing*, Philadelphia, 1993, J.B. Lippincott.

Gordon M: *Manual of nursing diagnosis*, St Louis, 1995, Mosby.

Hakins A, Marshall, and Meiners K: Exploring wives' sense of fairness about family work, *J Fam Issues* 16(6):693, 1995.

Hanson SMH and Boyd ST: *Family health care nursing: theory, practice, and research*, Philadelphia, 1996, F.A. Davis.

Hawkes G and Taylor M: Power structure in Mexican and Mexican American farm labor families, *J Marriage Family* 37(4):807, 1975.

Heiney SP: Assessing and intervening in dysfunctional families. In Wagner GD and Alexander RJ, editors: *Readings in family nursing*, Philadelphia, 1993, J.P. Lippincott.

Hibbeln JA: Special populations: Hispanic migrant workers. In Torres S, editor: *Hispanic voices*, New York, 1996, NLN.

Hochschild A: *The second shift*, New York, 1998, Avon.

Hoff LA: *People in crisis: understanding and helping*, ed 3, Menlo Park, CA, 1989, Addison-Wesley.

Jacobs Institute of Women's health: Women's health and managed care in California, www.jiwh.org, 1997.

Janosik EH: *Crisis counseling: a contemporary approach*, ed 2, Boston, 1994, Jones and Bartlett.

Jassak PF and Knafl KA: Quality of life: exploration of a concept, *Sem Oncol Nurs* 6(4):298, 1990.

Jensen RH: Exploding the stereotypes: welfare. In Kesselman A, McNair LD, and Schniedewind N, editors: *Women—Images and Realities*, ed 2, Mountain View, CA, 1999, Mayfield.

Johnson MA: Who is the Family? In Vaughn-Cole B and others, editors: *Family nursing practice*, Philadelphia, 1998, Saunders.

Klass CS: *Home visiting: promoting healthy parent and child development*, Baltimore, 1996, Paul H. Brookes.

Kolander CA, Ballard DJ, and Chandler CK: *Contemporary women's health*, Boston, 1999, McGraw-Hill.

LaFromboise TD, Heyle AM, and Ozer EJ: Changing and diverse roles of women in American Indian cultures, *Sex Roles* 22(7/8):455, 1990.

Lehrer S: Family and women's lives. In Kesselman A, McNair LD, and Schniedewind N, editors: *Women—images and realities*, ed 2, Mountain View, CA, 1999, Mayfield.

Lim I: Korean immigrant women's challenge to gender inequality at home, *Gender and Society* 11:31, 1997.

Lowry L and others: Care paths: a new approach to high-risk maternal-child home visitation, *JOGNN* 23(6): 322, 1998.

Mahowald MB: *Women and children in health care*, New York, 1993, Oxford University Press.

Martin K and Scheet N: *The Omaha system: applications for community health nursing*, Philadelphia, 1992, Saunders.

Mccarthy N and Mandle C: Health promotion in the family. In Edelman C and Mandle C, editors: *Health promotion throughout the lifespan*, ed 4, St Louis, 1998, Mosby.

McGoldrick M, Gerson R, and Shellenberger S: *Genograms: assessment and intervention*, ed 2, New York, 1999, W.W. Norton.

Meleis AI: Between two cultures: identity, roles and health, *Health Care for Women International*, 12:365, 1991.

Mizuno M: The changes and strategies adopted by the Public Health Services and medical society in Japan. In Zhan L, editor: *Asian voices*, Sudbury, MA, 1999, Jones & Bartlett.

National Center for Health Statistics: *National Vital Statistics Report* Vol 27(9):51, Hyattsville, MD., 1998, The Center.

Olesen VL: Who cares? women as informal and formal caregivers. In Ruzek SB, Olesen VL, and Clarke AE, editors: *Women's health: complexities and differences*, Columbus, 1997, Ohio State University Press.

Omolade B: *It's a family affair: the real lives of single black mothers*, Latham, NY, 1986, Kitchen Table.

Otto HA: Criteria for assessing family strength, *Family Process* 2:329, 1963.

Pearlin LI and Schooler C: The structure of coping. In McCubbin HI, Cauble AE, and Patterson JM, editors: *Family stress, coping, and social support*, Springfield, IL, 1982, Thomas.

Pepin JI: Family caring and caring in nursing, *Image* 24:127, 1992.

Phillips C, Himwich D, and Fitzgerald C: The business of women's health, *AWHONN Lifelines* 3(2):23, 1999.

Pratt L: *Family structure and effective health behavior: the energized family*, Boston, 1976, Houghton-Mifflin.

Sapiro V: *Women in American society*, Mountain View, CA, 1999, Mayfield.

Sawin K and Harigan M: *Measures of family functioning for research and practice*, New York, 1995, Springer.

Schorr L: *Common purpose: strengthening families and neighborhoods to rebuild America*, New York, 1997, Doubleday.

Sloan MR and Schommer BT: The process of contracting in community health nursing. In Spradley BW, editor: *Readings in community health nursing*, ed 4, Philadelphia, 1991, J.B. Lippincott.

Smith Barney Research: The New Women's Movement: women's health care: 1998, www.smithbarney.com/index.html.

Smith C and Maurer F: *Community health nursing: theory and practice*, ed 2, Philadelphia, 2000, Saunders.

Spalding AD: Is finding a husband a major concern for African American women? In *Taking sides: clashing views on controversial issues in gender studies*, Guilford, CT, 1998, Dushkin/McGraw-Hill.

Spector RE: *Cultural diversity in health and illness*, ed 4, Stamford, CT, 1996, Appleton & Lange.

Stanhope M and Lancaster J: Community health nursing: process and practice for promoting health, St Louis, 1996, Mosby.

Swanson JM and Nies MA: *Community health nursing: promoting the health of aggregates*, ed 2, Philadelphia, 1997, Saunders.

U.S. Department of Commerce, Bureau of the Census: *Statistical abstract of the United States 1998*, Washington, D.C., 1998, U.S. Government Printing Office.

U.S. Department of Health and Human Services, Public Health Service: *Healthy people 2010: summary report*, Pittsburgh, 2000, U.S. Government Printing Office.

Vaughan-Cole B and others: *Family nursing practice*, Philadelphia, 1998, Saunders.

VonBertalanffy L: The theory of open systems in physics and biology, *Science* 111:25, 1950.

Wallerstein JS: The early psychological tasks of marriage: part 1, *Am J Orthopsychiatry* 65:640, 1995.

Wallerstein JS: The psychological tasks of marriage: part 2, *Am J Orthopsychiatry* 66:217, 1996.

Wallerstein JS and Blakeslee S: *The good marriage: how and why love lasts*, New York, 1995, Houghton-Mifflin.

Walsh F: Conceptualization of normal family processes. In Walsh F, editor: *Normal family processes*, ed 2, New York, 1993, Guilford.

Watson J: *Nursing: human science and human care*, New York, 1988, National League for Nursing.

Whitaker W and Federico R: *Social welfare in today's world*, ed 2, Boston, 1997, McGraw-Hill.

White DG: The nature of female slavery. In Kerber LK and DeHart JS, editors: *Women's America—refocusing on the past*, ed 4, New York, 1995, Oxford University Press.

Williams R: The family and culture. In Lowdermilk DL, Perry SE, and Bobak IM, editors: *Maternity nursing*, ed 5, St Louis, 1999, Mosby.

Wright LM and Leahey M: *Nurses and families: a guide to family assessment and intervention*, ed 2, Philadelphia, 1994, F.A. Davis.

Youngkin E and Davis M: *Women's health: a primary care clinical guide*, Stamford, CT, 1998, Appleton & Lange.

Zerwekh JV: Making the connection during home visits: narratives of expert nurses, *Int J Human Caring* 1(1):25, 1997.

Zinn MB: Feminist rethinking from racial-ethnic families. In Zinn MB and Dill BT, editors: *Women of color in U.S. society*, Philadelphia, 1994, Temple University Press.

# The Friedman Family Assessment Model (Short Form)*

The following form is shortened for ease in assessing families.

Before using the following guidelines in completing family assessments, two words of caution are noted: First, not all areas included here will be germane for each of the families visited. The guidelines are comprehensive and allow depth when probing is necessary. Every subarea does not need to be covered when the broad area of inquiry poses no problems to the family or concern to the health worker. Second, by virtue of the interdependence of the family system, redundancy is unavoidable. For the sake of efficiency, the assessor should try not to repeat data, but to refer the reader back to sections where this information has already been described.

 **IDENTIFYING DATA**

1. Family Name
2. Address and Phone
3. Family Composition (Table A-1)
4. Type of Family Form
5. Cultural (Ethnic) Background
6. Religious Identification
7. Social Class Status
8. Family's Recreational or Leisure-time Activities

 **DEVELOPMENTAL STAGE AND HISTORY OF FAMILY**

9. Family's Present Developmental Stage
10. Extent of Family Developmental Tasks Fulfillment
11. Nuclear Family History
12. History of Family of Origin of Both Parents

*From Friedman M: *Family nursing,* ed 4, Stamford, Conn., 1998, Appleton & Lange.

 **ENVIRONMENTAL DATA**

13. Characteristics of Home
14. Characteristics of Neighborhood and Larger Community
15. Family's Geographical Mobility
16. Family's Associations and Transactions With Community
17. Family's Social Support System or Network
    Ecomap is helpful here. Family Genogram is also useful here.

 **FAMILY STRUCTURE**

18. Communication Patterns
    *Extent of Functional and Dysfunctional Communication (types of recurring patterns)*
    *Extent of Emotional (Affective) Messages and How Expressed*
    *Characteristics of Communication Within Family Subsystems*
    *Extent of Congruent and Incongruent Messages*
    *Types of Dysfunctional Communication Processes Seen in Family*
    *Areas of Open and Closed Communication*
    *Familial and Contextual Variables Affecting Communication*
19. Power Structure
    *Power Outcomes*
    *Decision-making Process*
    *Power Bases*
    *Variables Affecting Family Power*
    *Overall Family System and Subsystem Power (Family Power Continuum Placement)*
20. Role Structure
    *Formal Role Structure*
    *Informal Role Structure*
    *Analysis of Role Models (optional)*
    *Variables Affecting Role Structure*

## TABLE A-1  Family Composition Form

| Name (Last, First) | Gender | Relationship | Date/Place Of Birth | Occupation | Education |
|---|---|---|---|---|---|
| 1. (Father) | | | | | |
| 2. (Mother) | | | | | |
| 3. (Oldest child) | | | | | |
| 4. | | | | | |
| 5. | | | | | |
| 6. | | | | | |
| 7. | | | | | |
| 8. | | | | | |

21. **Family Values**
    Compare the family to American or family's reference group values and/or identify important family values and their importance (priority) in family.
    *Congruence Between the Family's Values and the Family's Reference Group or Wider Community*
    *Congruence Between the Family's Values and Family Member's Values*
    *Variables Influencing Family Values*
    *Values Consciously or Unconsciously Held*
    *Presence of Value Conflicts in Family*
    *Effect of the Above Values and Value Conflicts on Health Status of Family*

 **FAMILY FUNCTIONS**

22. **Affective Function**
    *Family's Need-Response Patterns*
    *Mutual Nurturance, Closeness, and Identification*
    Family attachment diagram is helpful here.
    *Separateness and Connectedness*
23. **Socialization Function**
    *Family Child-rearing Practices*
    *Adaptability of Child-rearing Practices for Family Form and Family's Situation*
    *Who Is (Are) Socializing Agent(s) for Child(ren)?*
    *Value of Children in Family*
    *Cultural Beliefs That Influence Family's Child-rearing Patterns*
    *Social Class Influence on Child-Rearing Patterns*
    *Estimation About Whether Family Is at Risk for Child-rearing Problems and If So, Indication of High Risk Factors*
    *Adequacy of Home Environment for Children's Needs to Play*
24. **Health Care Function**
    *Family's Health Beliefs, Values, and Behavior*
    *Family's Definitions of Health—Illness and Their Level of Knowledge*
    *Family's Perceived Health Status and Illness*

*Susceptibility*
*Family's Dietary Practices*
Adequacy of family diet (recommended 3-day food history record).
Function of mealtimes and attitudes toward food and mealtimes.
Shopping (and its planning) practices.
Person(s) responsible for planning, shopping, and preparation of meals.
*Sleep and Rest Habits*
*Physical Activity and Recreation Practices* (not covered earlier)
*Family's Drug Habits*
*Family's Role in Self-care Practices*
*Medically based Preventive Measures* (physicals, eye and hearing tests, and immunizations)
*Dental Health Practices*
*Family Health History* (both general and specific diseases—environmentally and genetically related)
*Health Care Services Received*
*Feelings and Perceptions Regarding Health Services*
*Emergency Health Services*
*Source of Payments for Health and Other Services*
*Logistics of Receiving Care*

 **FAMILY STRESS AND COPING**

25. **Short- and Long-term Familial Stressors and Strengths**
26. **Extent of Family's Ability to Respond, Based on Objective Appraisal of Stress-producing Situations**
27. **Coping Strategies Used** (present/past)
    Differences in family members' ways of coping
    Family's inner coping strategies
    Family's external coping strategies
28. **Dysfunctional Adaptive Strategies Used** (present/past; extent of usage)

# CHAPTER 3

# Women Within Their Communities

*In the search for solutions, we should not overlook the fact that women everywhere are actively involved in working against social, cultural, racial, economic, and political discrimination. It seems therefore just as important to ask the question of "how do women stay healthy in difficult circumstances" and "how can we strengthen those processes" as to ask the question "what makes them sick?"*

— RICHTERS, 1992

*What is a community?*

*Why is it important to consider the role of community in women's health?*

*What role do social factors play in the health of women?*

*Why use frameworks to assess a community?*

*How can nurses develop partnerships in the community?*

*What strategies can the nurse employ to develop effective interventions with women in communities?*

Women are relational and interconnected to others. As noted in the previous chapter, women's lives are both influenced by and strongly influence families. Historically, however, women have had profound interrelationships within their community. "Women everywhere are actively involved in working against social, cultural, racial, economic and political discrimination. It seems . . . as important to ask the question of 'how do women stay healthy in difficult circumstances' and 'how can we strengthen those processes' as to ask the question 'what makes them sick?'" (Richters, 1992).

As noted in Chapter 1, women collaborated to establish and build the women's health movement over the last 100 years in order to increase self-care and control of their health experiences. Relationships and collaboration are central to women's lives and are often linked to the caretaking of others and, for some, to the biologic role of motherhood and nurturing. Within their families, women are most often expected to be the caregivers of not only children but also parents, spouses, and partners (Muller, 1990; Glazer, 1993; McGuire and Freund, 1995). This expectation places them in a position of advocating for the health of others as they become aware of the needs of those they are caring for within their families, homes, or communities.

Feminists explain that women's affiliation strengths can become sources of empowerment (Miller, 1976; Gilligan, 1982; Belenky and others, 1986). Relationships between women provide the means for them to look beyond themselves and address issues that affect not only them and their families but also their communities. "A large part of public problem solving is done by people active in their own communities, where issues about education, land use, and the availability of other services are most focused" (Sapiro, 1998).

 WOMEN AS COMMUNITY ACTIVISTS

Women's social roles are vital to their interconnectedness with others. Women engage in community action directly (e.g., politics as elected officials, lobbyists, and voters), as well as indirectly (e.g., through churches, clubs, and other organizations). Women constitute the majority of people performing volunteer work (U.S. Census Bureau, 1992). They are aware that their lives are influenced by their roles in the labor force, their families, and the community—and they respond.

### Women's Roles Within the Community

Chinn and Wheeler (1991) identify feminine approaches to group and community work (e.g., sharing, holism, collectivity, and diversity) as sources of power and peace for women. Women's organizational efforts and grass-roots political activities have activated more than white middle-class women; women of different classes and ethnic and racial groups have organized for community action and problem solving. "Part of the historical and current importance of women's community participation is that it is so embedded in the large variety of circumstances of women's individual lives and their communities. Although levels and types of participation may differ, there are issues and organizations in which all types of women have participated from the different communities of the United States" (Sapiro, 1998).

Women have worked to change the work environment for themselves outside the home by forming or joining unions in support of clerical workers, textile workers, farm workers, and workers in other areas of employment. "The words of Maria Varela, a Chicana woman from the Southwest, suggest the common struggle that unites people of color and women's role in it, 'When your race is fighting for survival—to eat, to be clothed, to be housed, to be left in peace—as a woman, you know who you are. You are a principle of life, of survival and endurance. . . .'"(Ware, 1989).

There are many instances of women organizing boycotts and other consumer-related political actions in U.S. history. In fact, there have been few major social movements in American history in which women were not the leaders or involved in large numbers (e.g., the temperance, health care reform, world peace, civil rights, and welfare rights movements (Figure 3-1).

Because of their desire to have relationships with others, women are more likely than men to establish support networks. Examples are Candy Lightner's Mothers Against Drunk Driving (MADD) and the many disease- and condition-related support groups (e.g., Reach for

Recovery for women after a mastectomy and the March of Dimes for raising money to fund research on infant disease and death).

Lois Gibbs of Love Canal, NY and Anne Anderson of Woburn, MA are examples of women initiating local community action for health concerns they have identified. Love Canal was a housing development in upstate New York that had been built on a toxic waste dump. When higher than expected rates of miscarriages and birth defects occurred, Lois Gibbs became concerned, spoke with other women, pressured for the initiation of investigations, and applied political pressure. The homes in the most dangerous sections were eventually bought by the government and destroyed, and the families relocated. More recently, Anne Anderson's concerns in Woburn, MA involved the occurrence of cancer in her young son, as well as in others in her neighborhood. Convinced that the waste products she observed in the nearby river had something to do with it, Anderson sought information and raised the awareness of her community. The story of the events in this community are chronicled in the book, *A Civil Action* (Harr, 1996), which was made into a movie of the same name.

Commonly cited reasons for women's ability to initiate such actions are their community-based **social networks** that sustain the necessary communication, their ability to identify their neighborhood health problems, their role as the primary caretaker for their children's health, and their disagreement with many businesses and corporations that disease is a necessary risk of economic growth (Brown and Mikkelson 1990).

Rusek, Olesen, and Clarke (1997) contend that women's health is embedded in communities, requiring us to examine social factors in any conceptualization of more "inclusive models of health that can mobilize social forces

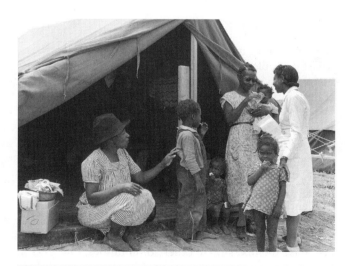

FIGURE 3-1 • Nurse helping in a community setting. *(From Mosby: Nursing reflections: a century of caring, St Louis, 2000, Mosby.)*

for caring, curing, and concern." Activities such as Take Back the Night walks enable women to increase public awareness of the legitimate concern for their safety when venturing out alone at night, whether in their neighborhood, in a parking lot of a store, or on a college campus. Such activities have led to the creation of escort services and better lighting in public places. The importance of relationships to women provides the impetus for women's health care providers to go beyond the biomedical model and consider the environment where women live.

### Women's Use of Community Resources

Much research attention has been paid to the relationship of social support and the role, extent, and quality of social relationships that affect human health (House, Landis, and Umberson, 1994). Women are often thought to have stronger **affiliation** capacities based on their family connections and friendship networks. Research indicates that women are more likely than men to use senior centers and meal sites and, when disabled, use more supportive services (e.g., community and home health services).

Women are most often caregivers to children, parents, and spouses (Muller, 1990; McQuire and Freund, 1995) and provide important social support in such roles. Also, as creators and participants in many support groups, women counsel and mentor other women. Health care providers often ask women who are breast cancer survivors to contact newly diagnosed women for support and guidance. In such activities, women's community roles—both as providers and receivers of community support—are extended and strengthened.

 **UNDERSTANDING COMMUNITY**

### Defining a Community

A **community** can be defined as a social group characterized by people within a certain geographic place and/or having common goals and interests. The members of a community know and interact with one another.

Definitions vary across disciplines and texts, although most definitions include the following key components: a collection of people, common characteristics or interests, and social interaction between members. The common features of a community may be common rights and privileges as members of a city or common ties of identity, values, norms, shared communication, or social support. Most definitions indicate that communities may overlap and members of a given community may also have membership in other communities. One person may be part of many communities in the course of daily life (Figure 3-2).

In this example, Anne Green works at the Visiting Nurses' Association, which is a collection of people who

have the common characteristic of all working within the same organization and being in communication with each other. She lives in Anderson Way Apartments, which is also a collection of people who share the common characteristic of living in the same complex and interacting with each other to some degree as they move about their buildings or come and go. Anne is a graduate student at the University of Massachusetts, which places her in a community of people working on furthering their education. She attends Smith Mills Church, which is another collection of people who share the characteristic of participating in church programs together. Her social communities are created by her participation in the Parent-Teacher Association at her children's elementary school and participation in the programs at the YWCA.

### Types of Communities

There are two broad types of communities: geopolitical and relational. **Geopolitical** communities are those with geographic boundaries (e.g., a town or city) but can also be legal demarcations (e.g., particular locations that have governing bodies to confer rights upon and protect the members). Geopolitical communities include communal living arrangements, such as apartment complexes, condominiums, and public housing units. Examples of Anne's geopolitical communities are the town where she lives, the fire district that covers her part of the town, and the apartment complex where she resides.

**Relational** communities are those that are developed with common goals or interests as the focus. These include social units that develop for social action or problem solving (e.g., of environmental concerns, safety hazards, and improved access to health care). Examples of

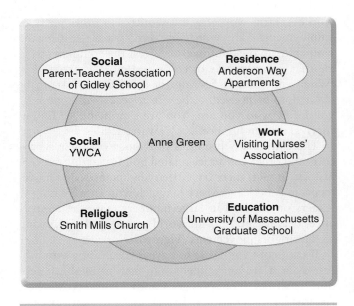

*FIGURE 3-2* • Membership in multiple communities.

Anne's relational communities are her work, school, church, the YWCA, and the Parent-Teacher group at her children's school (Table 3-1).

## Defining a Neighborhood

A **neighborhood** is a specific type of community. In current American culture, this term might seem to be an anachronism because many people claim to not know the people who live next door to them or anyone in their neighborhood. The geographic proximity, however, closely links those who live together in neighborhoods. The term itself means "near dweller."

In many areas, particularly urban locations, a neighborhood may take on significance for those who live there, linking them in communal ways that distinguish them from other neighborhoods in the city. With the urbanization and industrialization of the past 100 years, neighborhoods have often come to define themselves ethnically, as well as socially. Other neighborhoods are created because of natural divisions (e.g., rivers, mountains) that keep people from living near each other or easily communicating or other physical barriers (e.g., major highways) that divide residential areas. Whether the neighborhood is created by natural or man-made divisions, many people identify themselves in relationship to their own neighborhood. When asked where they are from, most people often state the name given to the neighborhood instead of the name of their city or town.

The difference between whether an area is described as a community or a neighborhood is often based upon the history of an area and who is doing the defining. Outsiders, rather than those who dwell there, often apply the label of "community" to an area. The title of "neighborhood" reflects the perspective of the members, indicating factors of acquaintance if not companionship. For example, although an individual may not know a neighbor by name, there is often a familiarity as they greet one another en route to work or in the local market. Also, a neighborhood's history often explains relationships and issues of importance to consider. What caused the neighborhood to form and grow there?

Were all the homes built at the same time? Is there a social or business center that links the members? Do residents move to this neighborhood for ethnic or religious connections? When we work in community settings, the important fact to remember is that the members of a community—whether it is a neighborhood or other type of community—are best able to articulate the nature and boundaries of the community.

 ## COMMUNITY AS CLIENT

Individuals who have one or more common characteristics reside within each community. These individuals are referred to as an **aggregate**. The aggregate may share the same relative age (e.g., elementary school children or the elderly) or have the same economic status, cultural background, gender, area of residence, or medical condition (Figure 3-3). Each individual in a community is a member of numerous aggregates. This term *aggregate* is one we will use in our work to label the part of the community with which we are concerned at the time. That is, it is not generally a term that our clients will use when referring to themselves.

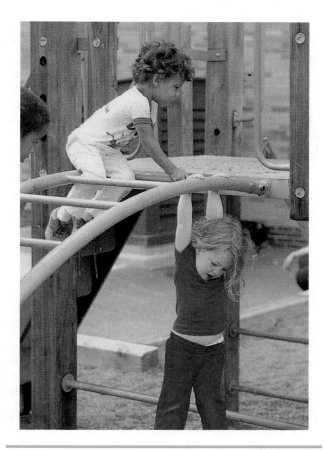

FIGURE 3-3 • Children at a playground. *(From Potter P and Perry A: Basic nursing, ed 3, St Louis, 1995, Mosby.)*

| TABLE 3-1 *Types of Communities* | |
| --- | --- |
| **Geopolitical** | **Relational** |
| Territorial | May cross territorial boundaries |
| Political | Ideologic |
| Geographic boundaries | Shared concerns and interests |
| Legal jurisdictions (e.g., town, neighborhood) | Common goals (e.g., Mothers Against Drunk Driving [MADD]) |

*Group* is a term our clients are more apt to use. When two or more interacting individuals within a community come together around a common purpose or activity, they are labeled a **group.** To fulfill the purpose of the group, the size should be small enough to allow for direct communication between members. Key components of the definition are their shared purpose or goal and the interaction between members. Groups can be formal, informal, or established, as well as learning groups, support groups, socialization groups, psychotherapy groups, or task-oriented groups (Spradley and Allender, 1996; Stanhope and Lancaster, 1996).

A **population** is all of the individuals occupying a geographic area or composing a whole. Populations can have common personal or environmental characteristics. They are more loosely connected than groups and often have no well-defined goals or interests in common. For example, a population could comprise all the residents in a town or all of the children in the public school system (Table 3-2).

Whether providing care at the individual or family level, the **domain** within the community must be considered. Individuals have an effect on the neighborhood and groups in which they interact, while the community simultaneously provides the environment within which these individuals strive to live.

The ability to determine the needs of a community is vested in learning from the community. Health care providers function as **consultants** working in partnership with community residents and other providers within the community. As **partners,** we join with and learn from the people of the community, with each person actively participating and bringing their own expertise to develop a mutual learning experience (Matteson, 1995). This process strives for the emergence of consciousness and critical intervention based on an understanding of the reality of the concerns of all of the participants (Friere, 1989). Through a partnership model, the actual—not the assumed—needs of the residents become the focus of care.

A **partnership** is "the negotiated sharing of power between health professionals and individuals, family, and/or community partners" (Courtney and others, 1996). Our role within a community may be at least one of the following: advocate, caregiver, care manager, case finder, counselor, educator, epidemiologist, group leader, health planner, and/or manager.

Participating in a proactive change process while building on community strengths facilitates community **empowerment,** which encourages people and organizations to use their skills and resources collectively to improve the quality of life within the community (Israel and others, 1994). To ensure that our help is useful and will be sustained after we leave, we should always combine empowerment with the care.

## Collaborating with Different Cultures

Cultural considerations are as important when working with a community as in planning care for individual women. The United States continues to become more diversified as thousands of immigrants come to this country each year. Health care providers often lack sufficient knowledge of the cultural beliefs and health care practices of people from diverse populations with whom they work. Differences in role, status, communication, and dietary patterns among immigrant groups profoundly affect their interaction with providers and subsequent acceptance of health care recommendations. Women become particularly vulnerable as they bear and raise children, maintain their households, and provide resources for themselves and their families. Many have no health insurance, limited access to health care, and distrust or fear of the American health care system. When these women do overcome their reluctance and seek medical assistance, they are often misunderstood because of language and cultural differences and become more reluctant to repeat the experience. Immigrant women often relied upon local healers and herbal medicines in their home countries, so they seek care

**TABLE 3-2** *System Levels*

| Client/Partner | Characteristics | Example |
|---|---|---|
| Individual | Individual person | Juanita Perez |
| Family | Family system with individual members | Juanita's family |
| Group | Two or more people with common interests, problems, or goals; communicate with each other, are interconnected | Breast cancer support group |
| Aggregate | Individuals in a community who have one or more common characteristics | Women with asthma |
| Organization | Organized group with structure and governance | Women's Health Center |
| Community | Aggregate of people with common goals, interests, or geography | Fishing village |
| Population group | Total individuals who share one or more characteristics in common; not interconnected | Residents of a town |

from similar healers in this country. For refugees, the adjustments to living in this country are particularly difficult. These women often suffer profound grief at the many losses they have endured, feel isolated in their new culture, and struggle economically for the survival of their families (Fox, Cowell, and Johnson, 1995). When working with multicultural populations in this country, we must gain the trust of community women before attempting to plan any health interventions.

The following example demonstrates how we must do things the women are comfortable with, gradually develop their interest in the health care topic to be presented, and then proceed in a manner and at a pace that are comfortable to them. Sokhary is a nurse working with a community program for Southeast Asian women. The community organizers have requested that she present an educational program about common cancers in women and the medical services available. Since Sokhary is a Cambodian woman, she is culturally competent in her knowledge of factors related to Southeast Asian culture. She plans her presentation keeping in mind the fact that most Asian women are very private about their bodies and less likely to seek preventive health services in the United States because of their mistrust of health services and the focus on acute care. Therefore Sokhary plans activities that are common to the women in attendance before showing films or demonstrating breast self-examination on a breast model. She facilitates a discussion of health risks that encourages the women to develop an interest in health screenings before discussing the importance of these activities. Using culturally appropriate dress, language, touch, and strategies, Sokhary is able to engage the women in the educational program. Because of the respect she has demonstrated for them, they request that she return to present another health program.

## USE OF THE NURSING PROCESS IN THE COMMUNITY

The use of the nursing process to plan client care within a community involves the same steps as for the individual and the family, but the focus is broader. We assess the community with our partners to learn its strengths, as well as actual and potential health problems, and then develop primary, secondary, and tertiary prevention interventions (Box 3-1).

To be both comprehensive and inclusive and allow the broadest picture possible, an organizing framework must guide our data collection. The data gathered from a community perspective will be broad enough to include all aspects of the community, yet manageable enough to provide an organizing framework for synthesis and analysis. Depending on the purpose of our assessment, we may choose to use one or a combination of the community health frameworks that follow. The

assessment tools can be used to gather data for both a neighborhood and a wider community.

## Community Frameworks

The community is an organism studied by professionals from many disciplines. As a result, a variety of perspectives and organizing frameworks have been developed. When we collaborate with the residents and other professionals interested in the same geographic areas, an interdisciplinary focus for assessment is required. Educators and practitioners often develop community assessment tools that reflect a combination of these frameworks. An awareness of other perspectives and assessment tools, in addition to ones developed in nursing, will facilitate our work.

### A Developmental Framework

The developmental perspective of community assessment examines the history of a community to understand its important influences over time. Changes such as development of rural land into housing and industry, urban decline or gentrification, and demographic change by age and ethnicity greatly affect the present community. Trends such as governmental neglect or attention to an area, funding of community programs and community participation over time are central to community assessment and analysis. For example, "Southside" is an area of a larger city to which history is important to its current status. Originally settled as pasture land in the 17th century, the population expanded to more than 100,000 residents during the industrial revolution. The area was first built as housing for the Irish immigrants who came to work in the factories of the growing city. Workers could travel to other areas by foot, horse, car line, and then trolley line. The growth of industry led to ongoing residential development. As each wave of immigrants came through, the ethnic diversity changed. From the 1940s to 1970s, the neighborhood saw the migration of a large number of African-Americans from the southern

---

**BOX 3-1** *Levels of Prevention*

**PRIMARY LEVEL**
*Example:* Health-education program for women focusing on healthy lifestyles, exercise, nutrition, and relaxation

**SECONDARY LEVEL**
*Example:* Mobile van brought to neighborhood for mammography screening for breast cancer

**TERTIARY LEVEL**
*Example:* Implementation of home-safety strategies for physically disabled women

states. By the 1970s, both Southeast Asian refugees and island migrants from Puerto Rico and the Dominican Republic arrived in larger numbers. Today, almost 20% of the neighborhood residents are foreign-born. Depending on whom we consult, the answer to "Whose neighborhood is it?" might vary. Some churches serve only a particular ethnic group within the larger city, while others have older Irish men and women worshiping with immigrants newly arrived from Southeast Asia and the Caribbean. Now the neighborhood is developing pride in its diversity, with more than 20 countries of origin represented.

Without considering the history of this neighborhood, we might have an inadequate understanding of its ethnic ties, how some groups of teen activity and gangs have emerged there, or where public services have been built. Such focus upon change over time and the life history of the community, however, is only one part of the analysis.

### An Epidemiologic Framework

**Epidemiology,** which is derived from the Greek word epidemic, is the discipline that studies the relationship of various factors that affect health as well as determines the frequency and distribution of diseases in the human community. Epidemiologists use research to try to identify the patterns and frequency of health and illness in a population. With a systematic investigation, they can sometimes identify the factors creating or contributing to the development of the situation. The study and control of infectious diseases (e.g., polio, smallpox, scarlet fever, autoimmune disease syndrome [AIDS], and Ebola-Marburg) have occurred because of epidemiologic studies.

The epidemiologic approach to community assessment integrates the principles of epidemiology with the collection of data, the analysis of that data, and the diagnosis for the community. A model developed by Finnegan and Ervin (1989) gives the definition of community as "people and the relationships that emerge among them as they develop and use in common some agencies and institutions and a physical environment" (Moe, 1977). Epidemiology focuses on the determinants of disease in human populations to identify peoples' risk factors for that disease. In the epidemiologic framework for community health assessment, the epidemiologic triangle of host, agent, and disease is adapted to include the following considerations: who, what, where, when, how, and why (Figure 3-4).

This model identifies *people factors*, such as age, sex, race or ethnicity, income, occupation, education, and health status, as the host. *Place and time factors*, such as environment, resources and services, and temporal relationships, compose the environment. The *agent factors* ask why and how and can be examined as the interplay of forces such as power, authority, and commu-

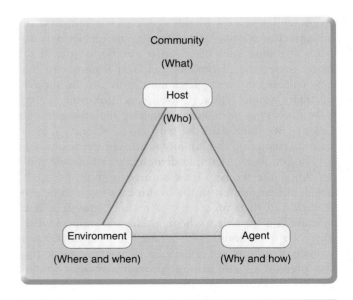

FIGURE 3-4 • Epidemiologic triangle.

nication (Finnegan and Ervin, 1989). Together, the data collected and analyzed within this model will lead to a community diagnosis identifying specific risks for the community being studied.

A limitation of this model is that the focus upon the risk for disease emphasizes the deficits rather than the strengths of the community, thus reducing the significance of many social factors. For example, statistics for low-income families (e.g., high teen pregnancy rates) may oversimplify the dynamics of communication, networks, and social support, as well as social structural concerns (e.g., inadequate access to care and racism). The epidemiologic triangle often oversimplifies complex causative factors by its focus upon the specific determinants.

### Web of Causality

The links and complex interrelationship of many factors are more accurately depicted using a model called the web of causality. Heart disease is a major killer in the United States. Figure 3-5 displays the links of relevant biologic, environmental, and social factors that increase the risk for cardiovascular disease. Interventions that effectively disrupt causal pathways decrease a person's risk for cardiac disease (Stanhope and Lancaster, 1992).

### Asset Mapping

Communities are composed of people and have problems just like people. Every community has needs and deficits that ought to be corrected. When we do a community assessment, we too often focus on the needs and deficits and forget to learn and consider the role of the assets. The assets and strengths are what can be used to meet community needs and improve life in the community. When we start looking closely at health or

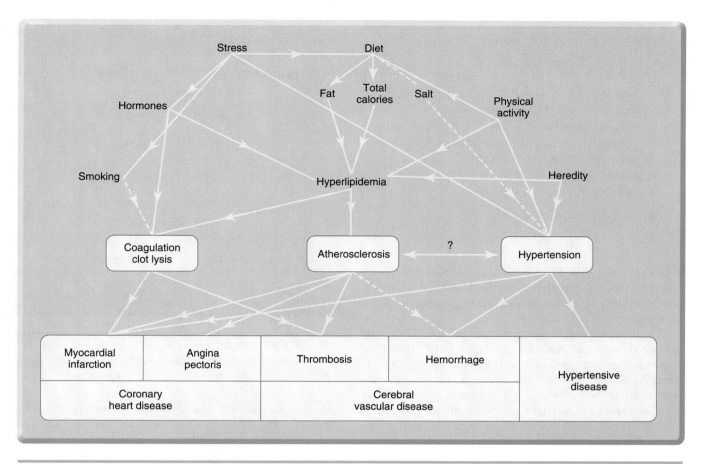

FIGURE 3-5 • An example of a web causality for cardiovascular disease. *(From Stallones RA. In* Cerebrovascular disease epidemiology: a workshop, *Public Health Monograph No 76, 1966, US Public Health Service, Pub No 1441.)*

community-development issues, we must know the needs of the individuals and the organizations that serve them, as well as the available resources.

A **need or problem** is a gap between what a situation is and what it should be. It can be as basic as the need for clean water or as abstract as developing a sense of a cohesive neighborhood. Examining needs helps us to discover what is lacking and sets the direction for future improvement. A community may have several needs or problems such as arson, child abuse, corruption, crime, domestic violence, elder care, emergency services, graffiti, health, housing, noise, racism, rats, safety, schools, stress, and trash collection. Each community has its own unique list based on the criteria of frequency, duration, scope or range, severity, legality, and perception of the problem (www.ctb.lsi.ukans.edu.ctb, 1999) (Box 3-2).

Of all of the criteria, the last one—perception—is perhaps the most important. If people perceive that there is a problem, whether it exists or not, it becomes a factor for the community (www.ctb.lsi.ukans.edu.ctb, 1999) (Figure 3-6).

A community **asset or resource** is anything that can be used to improve the quality of community life. It can be a person (e.g., the master mechanic down the street who can fix any car or the stay-at-home mom or dad who organizes the playgroup), a physical structure or place (e.g., a school, church, library, social club, town landmark, or park), or a business that provides jobs so that people in the community can earn an income (www.ctb.lsi.ukans.edu.ctb, 1999).

**Asset mapping,** based on the work of Kretzmann and McKnight (1993), is the process of locating and making inventories of the **gifts and capacities** of individuals, of citizens' associations, and of local institutions. Surveys are used to collect the information from individual residents and people within organizations. "Every single person has capacities, abilities, and gifts. Living a good life depends on whether those capacities can be used, abilities expressed, and gifts given. If they are, the person will be valued, feel powerful and well connected to the people around them. And the community around the person will be more powerful because of the contribution the person is making" (www.tcfn.org, 1999).

The capacities that an individual offers may have been gained through experience in the home or at work, through work in the church or other groups, or in the community.

The interactions between the people—whether they belong to the same extended family, work together, play softball together, are active in the historical society, attend Alcoholics Anonymous meetings, or serve on the school council—provide a web of human connectedness that increases the strength of the community. Gatherings are considered citizens' associations and may range from three neighbors meeting over coffee to plan a community event to a full-fledged community meeting. The residents can best identify these groups within the neighborhood (Figures 3-7 and 3-8).

Other assets may be located within the community but are essentially controlled by others outside the community. These assets may be businesses, schools, parks, and public services (e.g., police and fire departments, hospitals, and social service agencies).

There are also potential building blocks that originate outside the neighborhood, such as initiatives developed by government programs or foundations to help in a variety of areas to neighborhoods seeking change. If a case can be made for funding to address a specific program, a grant of money can be made to start the program.

Through assessment, the capacity inventory of community assets and needs is developed, which is the first step to creating community ownership and mobilizing community residents for change. Solutions may be derived more quickly and with more pride when community problems are identified and addressed with the skills, experience, resources, and organizations already present.

### Structural Functional Perspective

This approach is often used to assess families (Wright and Leahy, 1994) but can also be applied to communities. Originally described in sociology (Parsons, 1951),

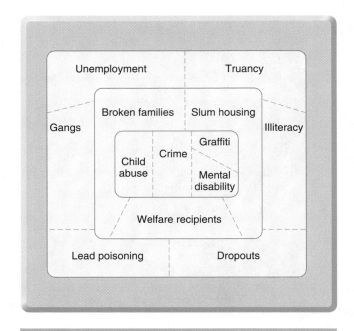

FIGURE 3-6 • Neighborhood needs map. *(From Kretzmann J and McKnight J: Building communities from the inside out, Evanston, IL, 1993, Institute for Policy Research.)*

the assessment is based upon the following two components: the structure or parts of the system and function (i.e., what the family does). **Structure** is the organization of parts within the whole. **Functions** are those activities that a group, organization, or community use to achieve goals. Structural elements (e.g., composition, ethnicity, social class, environment, and religion) and functional elements (e.g., socialization, communication, roles, problem solving, alliances and coalitions, and influences) are components of this perspective. A critique of this framework is that when used alone it limits the ability to reveal the complexities that politics and many other broader agendas place upon the structures being examined.

### Systems Theory Perspective

The **systems theory perspective** is the perspective most commonly used by community health nurses. Based upon general systems theory by von Bertalanffy (1973) in biology as a way to examine organisms, this perspective focuses upon community interaction and organization. It is a hierarchical model, moving from simple units to larger units of relationships. For example, a community can be identified as a system with inputs, outputs, feedback, and boundaries. A **subsystem** is smaller elements of the system (e.g., the family unit). A **suprasytem** is the larger unit or context of the system. When using the community as a system, the county, a statewide organization, or national association can be viewed as the suprasytem. **Inputs** are information, environmental influences, or diseases that affect the community. **Outputs**

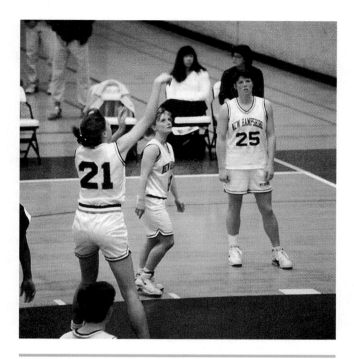

FIGURE 3-7 • Group of women playing basketball.

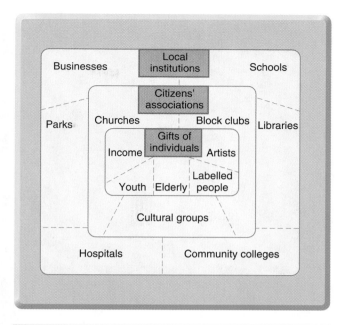

FIGURE 3-8 • Community assets map. *(From Kretzmann J and McKnight J: Building communities from the inside out, Evanston, IL, 1993, Institute for Policy Research.)*

are the effects of any community influences upon the other units. **Boundaries** are the borders of the system that serve to separate the community and the environment, while maintaining autonomy of the community. **Feedback** refers to the mechanisms where the system gains information that aids in establishing equilibrium within the system.

In community health, the community is considered a social system composed of interdependent subsystems (e.g., economics, education, religion, health, social services, politics, recreational and legal agendas, and safety programs). It is important to remember that this perspective considers the system to be more than the sum of its parts because the dynamics of the relationships create the system as much as the components do.

Nursing theories have primarily been developed with a focus on the care of individuals. Theories that are based in part on general systems theory are those by King (1971), Johnson (1980), Neuman (1982), and Roy (1984) and may be used when the community is viewed as an environmental system that influences individuals and families (Smith and Maurer, 2000).

Anderson, McFarlane, and Helton (1986) expanded on Neuman's system model to create a community-as-client model for practice. In this model, the community has eight major subsystems, as follow: recreation, safety and transportation, communication, education, health and social services, economics, politics and government, and the physical environment. The core of the commu-

nity is its people and their values, beliefs, culture, religion, laws, and mores. Stressors in the community produce stimuli that may cause disequalibrium. The degree of reaction is how much disequalibrium or disruption occurs. The primary, secondary, and tertiary prevention interventions have been developed to prevent actual or potential disruption of equalibrium. The evaluation process leads us to further assessment (Figure 3-9).

## Theoretic Perspectives

In order to understand the concepts of collaborative nursing care, a participatory approach to community health, empowerment, and a philosophy of "upstream" thinking, several theoretic perspectives are explained here. These conceptual approaches are used throughout the rest of this chapter.

### Community Nursing Care

Programs are more likely to succeed and be sustained over time when they are developed with full participation of community members. This does not mean that every individual in the community must play a role in the development of programs but that health professionals must embrace community members as equal and full partners in all phases of the program. This is based on a process of collaboration where the community members provide the expertise about the community and its internal factors and health professionals provide

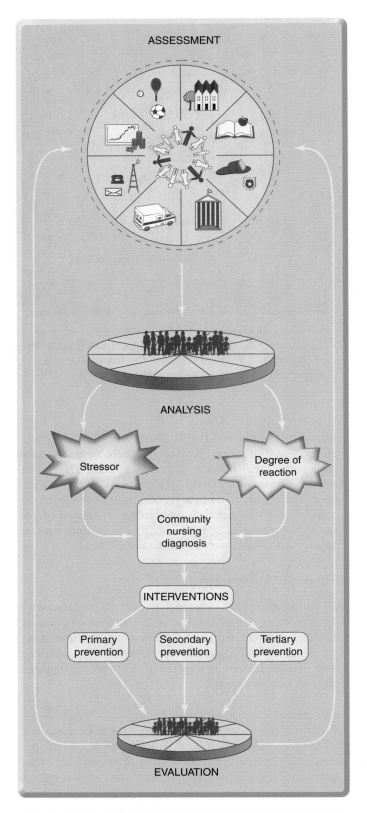

FIGURE 3-9 • The community-as-client model. *(From Anderson E and McFarlane J: Community as partner: theory and practice in nursing, ed 2, Philadelphia, 1996, Lippincott.)*

expertise on the epidemiology of health issues, community health planning, and external resources.

**Partnership** is the "informed, flexible, and negotiated distribution (and redistribution) of power among all participants in the processes of change for improved community health" (Shuster and Goeppinger, 1996). This requires the active participation of community members to identify the needs and resources of their communities. Potential partners are individuals and citizen associations located in churches, neighborhood centers, and among parents seeking improvements for their families. Although they may not have the specific knowledge and expertise that health professionals bring, partners know their own circumstances and what their needs are. By working as partners, they are more likely to implement effective strategies because they know the history of what has worked in the community before and the current priorities of the community. For health care providers who are not used to sharing their professional power with clients, the partnership model may be difficult in the beginning. Participants in successful partnerships must maintain a flow of information, monitor their progress, be inclusive of the perspective of all members, and maintain flexibility (U.S. Department of Health and Human Services, 1998).

Health professionals must also serve as advocates for the residents of the community. **Advocacy** is pleading another's cause or speaking on behalf of someone to help them achieve what they desire. Advocacy enhances the autonomy of the community by helping community members make their own voices heard in health care arenas. Health professionals can also serve as advocates for clients by making the health care system more responsive to their needs, as well as use their expertise to bring attention to inadequacies in the care of clients (e.g., inaccessibility, unacceptability, and expense of health services). To accomplish this, health professionals must be committed, assertive, aware of resources, risk-takers, and good communicators (Spradley and Allender, 1996).

A natural progression from partnership and advocacy is **empowerment** for the community members. Empowerment is a socialization process that promotes the participation of people, organizations, and communities in gaining control over their lives in their community and larger society. Empowerment is not characterized as the power to dominate others, but rather the power to act with others to effect change (Wallerstein and Bernstein, 1988). This term is grounded in the social justice approach of Paulo Freire (1989), in which change must be not only at the individual level but also at the social structural level. To accomplish this, Freire employs a participatory model of education. First, conscientization takes place when oppressed people become aware or conscious of the power imbalances that create domination. Participants become empowered by their own efforts to gain knowledge rather than continuing their passive roles. Community members are supported in posing their own questions and determining solutions to their problems through information, communication, and health education. Community members are considered the best resources for community change (Freire, 1989).

Nursing care of population aggregates in the community is preventive in nature in efforts to promote health and prevent disease. Recent health policy concerns about cost-containment are driving health care professionals to implement programs that increase health and reduce the sequelae of disease and disabling conditions. Public health measures aimed at smoking cessation, safe automobile use, and immunizations affect population health. Based upon the analogy of rescuing drowning victims from a river, McKinley (1981) suggests that looking **"upstream"** to where the victims are falling into the river and figuring how to prevent that from happening is ultimately more effective than constantly rescuing individuals.

Rather than plan interventions at the individual, family, or social network level, McKinley recommends that the manufacturers of illness (i.e., the large corporate profit-making institutions that pollute the environment and market unhealthy foods and tobacco products, thereby contributing to the ill health of many people) must bear responsibility for its effect. The term *upstream* is used to promote a political-economic approach to changing social structural conditions affecting the health of women in the community, not simply prevention strategies aimed at changing behavior or treating illness in individuals.

 ## USING NURSING PROCESS IN THE NEIGHBORHOOD OR COMMUNITY

The steps of the nursing process can be adapted for use in working with community aggregates. We enter community settings, follow the steps of the community nursing process, and care with and for residents in community. Assessment of a community is vital before selecting sites and developing programs of care. City or town governments often have some documentation describing the historic background of their neighborhoods. Viewing the public buildings, centers, and signs for programs also often indicates important services for a community. Churches, educational resources for adults, and community centers often serve as hubs of community life and places to interact with residents. The use of assessment tools such as participant observation, interviews with key informants, and communication sources (e.g., the newspaper and local television), as well as formal data available in documents, is essential. For example, we might read in the local newspaper about an upcoming community event, then attend the event as a participant observer, noting the leadership in the community, the availability of a neighborhood newsletter, and some issues that residents express as concerns. We then have some informal conversations with area residents and determine that community members perceive a need for better access to health care information and services.

## Assessing a Community/Neighborhood

In order to understand the health needs of a community, use a systematic approach to assessing the community. Not unlike other assessments (e.g., physical assessments of clients and family assessments), the community assessment provides the necessary **primary sources**—the people themselves—from which to collect data to identify both needs and strengths within the community.

### Community Assessment Tool

The **community assessment tool** (Box 3-3) provides an organizing framework for collecting data. Various strategies may be used to identify important data. By using a variety of techniques, the data should be more accurate and complete. Potential problems identified by one source should be verified through discussion with another source. The best way to begin an assessment is to use "self" as the observer.

### Windshield/Walk Assessment

A common tool is called a **"windshield survey"** (Box 3-4) because we can identify many important characteristics of a community by being a careful observer when driving through a geographic area. This approach is useful if the community is large geographically or comparisons with nearby communities are to be made. The best way to make oneself an observer is to walk about the community and interact with the members.

### Participant Observation

The "self" may also be used as an assessment tool by **participant observation** in key settings. For example, we may attend a community meeting or neighborhood event. This may be an annual summer street fair. During our visit, we can identify the interests, concerns, and activities of community members. Key leaders and communication patterns may be noted, which is often a way to identify community strengths and cohesiveness.

### Other Possible Strategies

A **survey** is a useful strategy to collect data if the residents choose to participate and see it as something that will benefit them. This data, if reliable and valid, can supplement the official data available through governmental sources. Survey questions might address demographic characteristics, health service use, perceived health needs, health-related behaviors, or health knowledge. In order

*(Text continued on p. 90.)*

## BOX 3-3  *Community Assessment Tool**

The following guidelines will help you assess the community you are working with this semester. With your clinical instructor, determine how you are to summarize and analyze your findings. Supplement your observations from the windshield survey with data collected from resources described at the end of this assessment. You may wish to cooperate with others in your clinical group to gather the necessary data.

Is the community a city, town, neighborhood, island, or special community (e.g., the university community or a fishing community)?

### LOCATION
- Is the area urban or rural?
- *Boundaries*—What are the boundaries? Are they physically determined (e.g., by waterways, highways, railways)?
- *Geography*—What is the size in square miles?
- What are the climate and average temperature? How do these affect health?
- What emergencies result from weather patterns?
- What types of flora and fauna are present? Do these affect health in any way?
- *Locale*—What types of industry or businesses are there (i.e., urban or rural community)?
- *Housing*—What types are available? What is their condition? What percent are owned? What percent are rented? What is the quality or the housing (e.g., presence of lead or other safety hazards)?
- How is water supplied? What type of sewage system is in place? How are waste and water disposed?
- *Environmental hazards*—Are toxic waste and/or pollution a problem? How are air and water quality?
- *Transportation*—Is public transportation available? What is the condition of roads?
- *Location of services*—Where are police, fire, health, and social services located? Where are the nearest grocery store, pharmacy, bank, and laundromat?

### POPULATION
- *Demographics*—What is the size, density, and composition (e.g., age gender, race, ethnicity, religion, SES, educational attainment, income distribution) of the community?
- *Trends/change*—Has there been a growth or decline in population parameters (i.e., implications for health planning)?
- *Mortality*—What is the crude death rate, infant mortality rate, maternal mortality rate, and the leading causes of death?
- *Morbidity*—What is the incidence and prevalence of reportable diseases and other conditions?
- What is the birth rate?
- What is the rate of immunization?

- What is the unemployment rate?
- What are crime rates and rates of other social problems (e.g., school dropout rate)?
- What are the patterns of mobility and migration?

### DYNAMICS
- How stable is the community?
- How do various population groups in the community interact? Is there unity or disunity among community members?
- Are community action programs in place?
- How does the community celebrate (e.g., festivals, parades)?
- What are the strengths of the community?
- What are the concerns of community members?
- What activities are available for residents? Are illegal activities taking place?
- How is communication within the community?
- Who are the community's key informants? Are there community representatives?
- What is the history of the community? How was it developed? Has it declined? Has the population changed?

### SOCIAL SYSTEM
Determine the functions of each system listed here, as well as how these functions are implemented in the community. Identify specific subsystems and organizations of the community.

*Health*
- Public and private
- Services available
- Location and access

*Family*
- Predominant family forms
- Unrelated family members

*Economic*
- Major industry and business
- Banks and other resources

*Education*
- Public and private schools
- Postgraduate programs
- Libraries

*Transportation*
- Public sources
- Private sources

*Legal*
- Crime rate
- Location of legal facilities

*Public Services*
- Types
- Location

*This tool is used at the University of Rhode Island College of Nursing.

## BOX 3-3   Community Assessment Tool—cont'd

**Religious**
- Specific denominations
- Resources

**Welfare**
- Official agencies
- Voluntary agencies
- Services for particular populations

**Political and Governmental**
- Community resources
- Accessibility to constituents
- Representation

**Recreation**
- Location and types
- Common recreational activities

**Communication**
- Resources
- Formal and informal

For each of the above systems, determine what the functions are and how they are implemented in your community. Identify specific subsystems and organizations of the community.

## BOX 3-4   Windshield or Walking Community Assessment*

The following may be used as a guide for a quick and general assessment of the community from your tour on foot and by automobile. Use all of your senses when conducting this assessment.

### LOCATION
- *Boundaries*—What are the boundaries of the community? Are they clearly defined? Are they physical (e.g., waterways, train rails, highways), political (e.g., designation as a city or town), economic, or cultural (e.g., ethnic enclaves)?
- Does the community have an identity?
- *Common areas*—Are there places where people congregate? Are these "commons" or park areas, stores, restaurants, bars?
- *Housing and zoning*—What is the layout of the community housing? What is the density of the housing? Is the housing in good repair? Are the homes rental or privately owned? Can you determine the age of the homes? Is commercial property mixed with residential property?
- *Open space*—Are there park areas? Are there vacant lots? Do you see many trees or much greenery? Who uses the open space, and for what?
- *Environmental hazards*—Do you see animals around? Are there any activities that could harm the environment of this community? How are air and water quality? Do you see peeling paint in housing? What about toxic waste?

### SERVICES
- *Service centers*—What services are available?
- Are there social agencies (e.g., police, fire department, health clinics, hospitals, private doctors, dentists, lawyers, banks, recreation)?

- *Educational*—Do you see schools? How well are they maintained?
- Are there institutions of higher learning? Libraries?
- *Stores and merchants*—Are there grocery stores nearby? What special types of foods are offered?
- What types of restaurants are there? Is there any area to park?
- What about pharmacies and laundromats?
- *Churches*—Where are the churches or other places of worship located?
- What do they tell you about the population?
- *Transportation*—What types are available? What is their frequency? What is the condition of the roads?

### PEOPLE
- *Demographics*—Who do you see on the street? What can you tell about their age, ethnicity, and race? What are they doing? Can you identify what type of work they do?
- *Health*—Can you determine factors about their health? (Consider factors such as climate, environmental hazards, safety, and evidence of chronic diseases.)
- *Politics*—Do you see any signs of political activity?
- *Communication*—What newspapers and magazines do you see? What language are they written in?
- Do you hear radios? What types of stations?
- What informal means of communication do you see (e.g., posters, flyers)?

*This tool is used at the University of Rhode Island College of Nursing.

to be effective, the survey must be congruent with the population's literacy, culture, age, gender, and interest levels.

Personal **interviews** with key informants are often most helpful and time-efficient. In a partnership model, we recognize the knowledge base of the community members as a valid source of data about community needs. This method should not be used alone, however, until the community has come to trust us. Initially informants may be careful about disclosing private information to a stranger; until we have developed a partnership in the community, use key informants.

We often participate in **community forums** as invited guests. Such forums can serve as important sources of data to identify leadership, group dynamics, and important community concerns. We might then elect to invite a focus group of community members to discuss health concerns, which can also be an effective assessment strategy.

**Secondary sources** of information (i.e., obtained not from people but from existing data sources) can be very important sources of information. For example, women may be very concerned about the rates of asthma among the community members. Epidemiologic studies and health department records can provide the necessary verification and documentation for substantiating their concerns. Such supporting documentation is usually necessary as evidence of community needs or problems for funding sources. Our ability to access official documents is an important way we can share expertise with community partners. Once the assessment data is collected, the partners develop goals and plan interventions.

## Planning for Community Change

### Health-Planning Models

Health planning is a crucial component of community health programs. Without partnering with the community and adequate planning, interventions are unlikely to be successful. Rothman (1972) describes three models for organizing community health that illustrate the various roles that community health providers can take. The three approaches are social planning, social action, and locality development.

In the **social planning** approach, model change is based upon the role of "expert" planners who are generally members of health departments, organizations, or nursing groups. The emphasis is upon rational decision making based upon factual documentation of needs. The social planning approach is used when the goal is fast, direct action for a problem, and the health care providers take on the role of program implementers (e.g., immunization campaign during an outbreak of meningitis).

The **social action** approach relies upon the polarization of community members around an issue or issues.

This locates the center of power within the community members as they develop support for their own viewpoint. In this model, the role of the health professional is often as social activist or negotiator. Policy decisions and the development of programs often result from such visible debates.

The **locality development** approach is also called community development. This model emphasizes the self-direction of community members as they determine their own needs and solutions to problems. Strong community involvement relies upon problem-solving skills and cooperative strategies. Initiatives of locality development are referred to as "grass roots" organizing. In this model, health professionals serve as facilitators and strive to empower the community members in this project.

Health planning may not be limited to one of these models, but they are useful for understanding how program development may be structured with regard to the roles of both community members and health care providers. The best planning most often involves some of each model. The community's ownership, with health care professionals sharing their expertise to facilitate goal attainment, is particularly important.

### Women in the Community

When we work with women in a community, it is very important to recognize that many aggregates of women (e.g., those in prison, the homeless, victims of domestic violence, lesbians, women in war zones and refugees, and migrants) are particularly vulnerable to health problems because of their social problems or lack of visibility in the broader community. In some instances, specialized assessment tools have been developed to collect data more appropriately.

Women in prison may only receive secondary prevention for acute and chronic health problems and lack the information and resources for health promotion and maintenance not only while they are imprisoned but also when they return to the community. Homeless women are at higher risk for disease and are often without the resources to access care for their problems. They face increased risks for alcohol and substance abuse, psychiatric disorders, sexually transmitted infections, cystitis and otitis media, as well as chronic health problems (e.g., hypertension and diabetes). Homeless women tend to be socially isolated with fewer support networks (Hatton, 1997).

We may have a positive effect not only by providing care for clients but also by advocating and developing social and political changes to improve health care for all women. Many women are the victims of neglect and violence—both in their homes, as well as in other settings. They may suffer a similar lack of resources as women who are in prison or homeless, but they hide in their communities due to fear of the abuser or shame that they may be to blame for their abuse. Working in the community, we must be vigilant in assessment so as to not overlook the special needs of these women. Raising the topic of violence serves not only to allow the victim the opportunity to identify herself but also to educate her about available help (Dickson and Tutty, 1996).

Lesbians as aggregates have been victimized in society, as well as in the health care system. Many describe hostile and humiliating health encounters, isolation and lack of support during times of illness, exclusion of their partners from their care, lack of health insurance and access, and inadequate health assessment due to the practitioner's assumption of heterosexuality (Haas, 1994). Our attention to vulnerable and frequently overlooked aggregates of women can enable them to improve their health status and quality of life. We must use our community health skills to work with population groups and share our skills with the underserved not only to improve care at the individual level but also to change policy and improve their lives.

Worldwide, women are at risk because their social status magnifies their vulnerability to disease, diminished allocation of resources, and violence. Conditions that particularly affect women are female infanticide, malnutrition and anemia, genital mutilation (Morris, 1996), early marriage and childbearing, high fertility patterns, maternal mortality, sexually transmitted disease, violence, incest, and rape. In war zones, women are frequently victims of rape and violence. For many women, their movement from a war zone into a refugee resettlement fails to improve their health or support services. Because they are not part of a system of providers, many refugees have no access to health services in their resettled homes (Kramer, 1999).

Professionals with cultural expertise have led the development of specific tools for assessment, screening, or analysis. For example, Urrutia-Rojas and Aday (1991) developed a framework for community assessment for use in a Hispanic and refugee community. In addition, cultural and language adaptations were made to a well-established framework developed by Aday and Anderson (1981) to identify problems in heath care access for the Hispanic and refugee community. Another example is the assessment of the HIV prevention needs of Asian and Pacific Islander women developed by Jemmott, Maula, and Bush (1999). In an effort to identify culturally specific assessment and intervention strategies, adaptations were made to the health belief model (Becker, 1974) for use with this population. A final example is Baldwin's model (1996) to assess the participation of low-income African-American women in breast and cervical cancer early detection and screening. Focus groups and interviews were used to test the use of culturally relevant content on breast and cervical

health teaching on the importance of these screenings. The identification of African-American women's decision-making practices can guide interventions with this population.

Places of employment are often not environments that are conducive to health. More often than men, women are employed in factory assembly lines, as migrant farm workers and clerical help, and in nursing. Hazards such as chemical pollutants used in manufacturing processing, radiation therapy in health care, and pesticides used in farming affect women in their places of work. Injuries and accidents often occur in manufacturing and hospitals, as well as with farming equipment. Ergonomic factors for women in assembly lines—bending, lifting, and sitting at video display terminals—create work-related health problems. Stress-related factors, both in the workplace and at home, further reduce women's health (Chavkin, 1984). Women also take on the disproportionate burden and risk of the "second shift" at home by providing household care and handling the many solvents and cleaning materials used (Hochschild, 1989).

## Steps for Program Planning

Before beginning any intervention plan, a thorough assessment using community-assessment tools must be completed. Part of this assessment is the careful synthesis and analysis of data by the partners.

*Step 1: Synthesize.* During this step, information is combined into charts, figures, and tables to allow for comprehensive examination. This might involve the categorization of the data into topics such as demographic, geographic, socioeconomic, and health resources and services or other categories, depending on the focus of analysis. For example, if we hope to understand issues related to adolescent health in a local high school, we might elect to categorize the information in the following ways:

1. Demographic components of the population (e.g., gender, race/ethnicity, and socioeconomic status);
2. Community resources available to adolescents;
3. Economic factors (e.g., employment opportunities and salaries);
4. Educational opportunities (e.g., post-secondary resources available to students); and
5. Health status indicators.

*Step 2: Analyze.* This step can also be considered the final phase of assessment in which we examine the synthesized data collected from the community health assessment, compare the findings with information gathered from the literature, and review this to establish deviations from norms and focus upon potential areas for intervention. We must be careful to select accurate data that include diverse populations in the analysis. Differences in ethnicity and socioeconomic status are as important to examine as commonalities among groups (Rusek, Olesen, and Clarke, 1997).

Sources such as health information, statistics, and other research reports identify national and statewide trends for comparison. For example, the data collected in a neighborhood in a moderate-sized city may indicate that rates of asthma, lead poisoning, and malnutrition in children are high; that many women have been treated for breast cancer; and that a high rate of teenage pregnancy exists. By comparing these rates with the city and state averages, we can confirm that the rates in the target neighborhood are indeed higher than the city or state rates. In fact, we may find that the rate of lead poisoning is among the highest noted in the country. Such statistical comparisons often lead to grant funding of programs to address the health problem.

The assessment should suggest not only potential problems, however, but also highlight the strengths of the community (e.g., how the members deal with difficulties, who the leaders are, and where potential sources of help are available). Identification of community strengths facilitates planning because any program's success is built upon the participation of community members.

*Step 3: Develop Community Diagnoses.* We use nursing diagnosis to identify both problems and health issues in the community. The naming process is important for identifying a focus for intervention because the label describes a situation and may imply a cause. A nursing diagnosis in community health nursing may be problem-oriented or have a wellness emphasis.

Because an "upstream" and prevention focus rests upon building on strengths, a diagnosis at the community level often identifies a wellness response—not simply a deficit focus. The diagnosis should have a three-part focus: population, aggregate, or group involved; healthful, actual, or potentially unhealthful response; and related factors. For example, the diagnosis may address the following: (1) The target population of women in a particular neighborhood (2) who are at risk for developing respiratory diseases (3) due to the poor air quality of the neighborhood, the high rates of tobacco smoke (both from personal smoking and second-hand smoke), and amount of crowded, poorly heated, and insulated housing units. Common diagnoses for community health include mortality and morbidity concerns, inaccessible and unavailable services, environmental hazards, and populations at risk.

North American Nursing Diagnosis Association (NANDA) diagnoses have applications to the community as a whole, as well as to determining women's inclusion within an aggregate. For example, the diagnosis of stress incontinence places a woman within the aggregate of other women with the same diagnosis. Interventions could be developed to assist all the women in the

community with the same diagnosis. Examples of diagnoses applicable to the community as a whole are as follow: Potential for Enhanced Community Coping, which provides a positive focus, and Ineffective Management of Therapeutic Regimen: Community, which has a problem-oriented focus (NANDA, 1999).

The **Omaha Classification System** was developed by the Visiting Nurses Association of Omaha, Nebraska to provide a framework for the client problems they diagnose in their work with family and communities. There are three major components in the system, as follow: a Problem Classification Scheme, an Intervention Scheme, and a Problem Rating Scale. In the problem classification scheme, the 40 client problems are grouped into the following four domains: environmental, psychologic, physiologic, and health-related behaviors. Problems may relate to health promotion, or a potential or actual impairment. The problem rating scale helps us to evaluate client outcomes on a Likert type of scale. The intervention scheme consists of nursing activities to address the identified problems. The four categories of intervention are as follow: health teaching, guidance and counseling, treatments and procedures, case management, and surveillance (Clemon-Stone, McGuire, and Eigsti, 1998).

Outcome and Assessment Information Set for Home Care (OASIS) is a data set that include the following categories: demographics and client history, living arrangements, supportive assistance, body systems, activities of daily living and/or independent activities of daily living, medications, equipment management, and emergent care. The data are assessed at the following three points: upon admission, at some time during care, and on discharge to measure outcomes between two or more points (Clemon-Stone, McGuire, and Eigsti, 1998).

*Step 4: Validate with the Community.* At this point, confer again with the community partners to validate the identified diagnosis and determine if we have missed anything of importance to the community. This may be done by using a questionnaire, thorough personal interviews, or by consultation with the planning groups. Once the analysis determines that the nursing diagnoses are relevant and appropriate to the community, planning continues. The next step involves prioritizing the nursing diagnoses and developing appropriate goals and interventions.

*Step 5: Prioritize.* Collaborate with the community members to prioritize needs and problems. Interventions seldom succeed when they are supported solely by the health professional, rather than emerging from the felt need of the community itself. Various frameworks may be used to assist in prioritizing. Leavell and Clark's (1958) levels of prevention encourage health promotion and prevention by addressing primary prevention strategies that help people avoid becoming sick (i.e., falling into the stream). Health-education programs are an example of primary prevention. The nature of the identified problem, however, may also require secondary or tertiary approaches (i.e., pulling people from the stream and providing care for them). Common interventions at this level are health screenings at the secondary level and exercise programs for cardiac rehabilitation at the tertiary level. Cardiac disease is the most common killer of women.

An important factor for prioritizing is the potential for change in the target population. There are many theoretic perspectives for changing human behavior, but the most commonly used model in community health is Lewin's (1947) change theory. Change refers to a planned or unplanned alteration in an individual, group, or organization. In systems theory, this means that change disturbs the equilibrium of the system and must be reestablished or recreated. Change can occur when a disaster such as a tornado hits an area or can be an innovation such as a smoke-free policy in a place of employment. For us, however, change most often relates to the desired outcome of changing behavior, health policies, or social structure.

Lewin (1947) describes three stages of change: unfreezing, changing, and refreezing. During the unfreezing phase, the need for change causes the disequilibrium in the system, which is necessary for people to become motivated to make the necessary change. During the changing phase, people actually try the innovation and decide what they think about it. The innovation may be new behavior, policy, or structure. In the refreezing phase, the system returns to equilibrium, and it is hoped that the innovation has been accepted and will become part of the system. This involves the integration of the change into the system so that it is maintained once the people who have empowered the change have left. Any planned change should consider the importance of readiness for change. If any change is to occur, the target population must recognize the need for change and participate in the disequilibrium of the unfreezing phase.

The following criteria provide a guide for prioritizing. For each identified problem, the criteria are ranked in order of importance (e.g., on a scale of 1 to 5 stars) and then both importance and likelihood of success are ranked in order to prioritize (Table 3-3).

## Goals and Objectives

Goals and objectives are developed collaboratively with the community partners to ensure appropriateness and acceptability. Using a systems framework, goals can be developed for each level of system intervention (i.e, individual, families, aggregates, or community). **Goals** are general statements of intent and purpose that should help focus the planning project toward long-range outcomes.

### TABLE 3-3   *A Tool for Prioritization*

| Criteria | Rating |
|---|---|
| Degree of community concern and awareness | |
| Community motivation for change | |
| Aggregate preferences | |
| Degree to which it threatens the population | |
| Severity of the problem or consequences | |
| Practical considerations: | |
|    Cost | |
|    Skills or expertise required | |
|    Time involved | |
|    Available resources (e.g., supplies, facilities, equipment) | |
| Ease of solution | |
| Availability of alternative potential solutions | |

**Objectives**, however, are more specific and should be measurable and criterion-referenced. The objectives can be short or long-term, and often both are stated. Objectives may focus only on the outcome of the interventions, or may focus on the process of reaching the objectives. **Outcome objectives** direct the program toward changes in health status or behaviors. **Process objectives** focus upon implementation activities and necessary strategies of health care delivery. **Management or structure objectives** define the structures needed to carry out process objectives such as funding, personnel, or program support. Objectives should be measurable, stating what portion of the population is expected to achieve the outcome, the timing of that achievement, and the actual outcome measure to be used to determine that the outcome has been achieved.

## Develop Interventions

Intervention is the action phase of the process where the community partnership puts the community health plan into action. The goals and objectives lead to the strategies to be followed. The appropriate means—especially in terms of cost and benefits—to achieve the goals should be set. Criteria must be established for goal attainment. During this phase, the collaboration maintained throughout the partnership leads to ownership of the program by the community members. Full participation in the planning phase is essential for the community members to truly feel a sense of ownership. This requires us to work *with* instead of *doing for* the clients involved (Box 3-5).

In order to proceed effectively with an intervention plan, the community partnership should ask the following questions: What needs to be done? How can it be accomplished? What resources are needed to carry it out? When will it occur? How much time will it take? Where should it occur? Who is responsible for what

---

**BOX 3-5** *Common Types of Interventions*

Health-education programs
Screening programs
Establishment of health services
Policy development and implementation
Collaborations in the development of community health
  coalitions
Support of community empowerment

---

activities, materials, and tasks? After collaboratively answering these questions, the plan can be put into process. Be careful to retain the role as facilitator and advocate and not to take charge of the intervention (Anderson and McFarlane, 1996).

Scheduling is important in order to maximize participation in any program. Validate practicality issues and consider barriers to successful implementation. The community partners will be extremely helpful in identifying barriers (i.e., women do not come out in the evening, or there is no public transportation to the site), as well as planning interventions that are culturally acceptable. In many cultures, health-promotion projects are more readily accepted when incorporated into another community celebration or festival. Our community partners will help us learn how to do this.

### Implement Interventions

Assisting as a facilitator within the community by collaborating and coordinating the components of the plan can be stressful. Remember that the change process is stressful for all involved.

Health care implementations in communities often involve health education. Because education is a primary prevention strategy, we often begin with education in order to prevent disease and problems from occurring. Freire's empowerment model of education is very effective. In this model, the community members take ownership of their future. Knowledge is power, and for many women in the community, knowledge is the first step to independence.

***Peer Health-Educator Project.*** A peer health-educator project is an example of the empowerment process. Various women (and an occasional man) elect to become health educators for peers within their community. These persons are all students at the Genesis Center, a center for immigrants and refugees in Providence, Rhode Island, where they learn English and job-training skills. This program, which is funded by the state health department, brings participants from countries such as Cambodia, Laos, Liberia, Haiti, Cape Verde, Guatemala, and the Dominican Republic together to learn about various health conditions and prevention strategies. The classes are student-centered, with each student develop-

ing teaching presentations to share with the group and with other students before taking them to churches, community centers, and their homes to educate peers. This training has led some students to become skilled enough to obtain jobs as community health workers. Such empowerment education can transform lives.

The focus "upstream" on prevention and risk reduction may begin with attempts to change behavior to more healthy lifestyles and participation in early screenings but may extend beyond that effort to more structural changes. One of the women in the peer health-education group focused her interest on diabetes in the Hispanic community. Once she became involved in promoting healthy dietary and exercise lifestyle issues, she recognized that the neighborhood's lack of safe walking areas prevented her neighbors from getting needed exercise. Now she is eager to lobby for a cleanup of a nearby park and more lighting so that residents can feel safe walking at night. Such structural, "upstream" change may have the greatest positive health effect upon her neighbors.

***De Madres a Madres.*** An example of a collaborative intervention is the "*de Madres a Madres*: A Partnership for Health" program developed in 1989 in Houston. The name of the program translates to "from mothers to mothers." The program is a collaborative effort by local residents, businesses, and volunteers to identify Hispanic women at risk for not starting early prenatal care. Responding to a Texas health plan priority that low-income women receive prenatal and maternity care, the local March of Dimes chapter sponsored a community health nurse to initiate the program. This nurse completed a community health assessment of a poverty stricken, socially isolated residential neighborhood in Houston that included the identification of 31 key community leaders, many of whom were Hispanic. Individual meetings with these leaders, formal presentations, and her assimilation into community activities helped the nurse to establish trust in the community. The nurse and the community women formed a partnership to improve the health status of women and children in the community. Most of the 13,000 residents identified themselves as Hispanic but came from various cultures from Central America. Therefore the nurse recruited volunteers from the various groups to serve as volunteer outreach mothers. These volunteers completed an 8-hour training session that included topics such as their advocate role, community resources, communication and support techniques, aspects of quality prenatal care, health resources, causes of low birth weight in infants, family dynamics, interpersonal relationships and social support, and issues of pregnancy. As the community volunteers increased their role and visibility in the program, they established camaraderie and a growing enthusiasm for their work. Community awareness led to community ownership. This strengthened the reception of the program and its success in meeting the goals.

After several years, the volunteers had provided visits to hundreds of high-risk women, referred eligible women to sources of health care funding, and provided outreach to thousands of residents. Since its inception, no low–birth-weight infant has been born to a mother followed by a *de Madres a Madres* volunteer and the infant mortality rate for the neighborhood has dropped.

Other indicators of the success of the *de Madres a Madres* program relate to the women's growth and development in community work. Their increased sense of empowerment has led them to lobby successfully for policy changes in health care eligibility for women and programs to further their own education, as well as attain growing entrepreneurship in small business ventures. The program has become a model for similar community partnerships for health throughout the country (Mahon, McFarlane, and Golden 1991; Anderson and McFarlane, 1996).

Most certainly, the key to the success of programs such as *de Madres a Madres* is the collaboration between health professionals and community members. The formation of such community coalitions can achieve improved health outcomes and stability by community ownership, and can enhance the growth and development of community members.

Once we, along with the community partners, have established the interventions, we must develop several strategies to ensure that the most effective and efficient intervention is selected. Using the systems perspective, consider possible interventions at system, subsystem, and suprasystem levels. In the *de Madres a Madres* example, if the neighborhood is defined as the system, the original plan targeted subsystem strategies by personal interventions with community women. Several suprasystem initiatives began, however, when the volunteer mothers began to lobby for health policy changes.

## Evaluation

Throughout the planning of the program strategies, maintain careful consideration of how evaluation will be done. Factors such as the adequacy, efficiency, effectiveness, outcome attainment, appropriateness, cost-effectiveness, relevancy, and impact of the program must be considered. Possible outcome measures are as follows: knowledge, behaviors, skills, attitudes, emotional well-being, health status, the presence of health care system services, satisfaction, the presence of policy, and an altered relationship with physical environment

The evaluation phase can be divided into the following broad areas: (1) process and (2) product, or outcome. In the **process** evaluation, issues such as how the planning and interventions occurred, how effective the communication between parties was, and how timely and efficient each step was are examined. The appropriateness of the intervention and a careful cost-benefit analysis are of particular concern. Include time and resources as costs. Identify the strengths and weaknesses of

each stage of the nursing process (e.g., in the planning stage, evaluate how well the goals fit the assessed needs).

To evaluate the product or outcome evaluation of the program, ask what measurable change occurred (e.g., knowledge or skills gained, behavior change, or the development of new services) and the effect of the program upon morbidity or reduction in symptoms. Another outcome measure is participant satisfaction, which can be accomplished through formal satisfaction surveys or an informal feedback session with participants and key community planners. The product evaluation should also identify unintended consequences of the intervention, which may be both positive and negative in nature. The current focus on outcomes for funding and health care financing drives the inclusion of evaluation measures that focus upon outcomes. The evaluation should highlight the role of nursing care in the program, as well. We often neglect to take credit for our important role as a partner to and advocate for vulnerable and underserved groups.

***Building in Evaluation.*** The following is an example of the development of a program without careful consideration of evaluation. Undergraduate students in a community health clinical practicum responded to an invitation to work in establishing a wellness center in a high rise apartment building for older adults in an urban area. The students were eager to plan and carry out what they perceived as important activities for the residents. They established a consultation clinic for blood pressure and glucometer follow-up, for teaching and referrals, and resource information. They planned and implemented several relevant educational sessions. They collected large amounts of educational materials, advertised, and decorated the facility. By their enthusiasm and caring, they developed active participation in the project. However, they neglected to give careful enough attention to two phases of the nursing process, assessment and evaluation. Their nursing assessment of the apartment community failed to identify several important client factors and scheduling issues that affected attendance at the educational and wellness center sessions. More importantly, as the enthusiasm for the project has grown, important outcome measures as well as client satisfaction data is necessary in order to apply for external funding to continue and expand the project. If outcome measures were built in to the initial intake information gathered from clients, and if client satisfaction data had been formally collected, then there would be more comprehensive measures of success to include in funding applications.

Finally, at the completion of a program or project, a final report documents the intervention for future reference and provides a resource for other planning endeavors. The development and implementation of a community health program—whether successful or not—becomes part of the history of the community. Residents will remember it when the next person comes along and respond accordingly.

Another example demonstrates how the measurement of outcomes can be built in from the start. Community women are most active in advocating for their children. In a neighborhood where drug dealers were targeting adolescents, the mothers became concerned about the safety of their children and sought interventions that led to a successful partnership. They approached a nurse at the neighborhood health clinic for assistance in this initiative. Together, they established goals for safety on the streets, having regular police patrols, better lighting, and safer recreational facilities. They approached the police department and requested assistance, and their initial goals were met. As the women worked together, their program goals expanded. A partnership with the housing authority led to a well-supervised after school program in the community, educational activities for adolescents and children, and a greater sense of community connectedness. Measurable outcomes were as follows: the neighborhood became safer, the teen pregnancy rate declined, the high school retention rate increased, and the use of drugs by neighborhood youth declined. By measuring these outcomes, the residents ensure that the funding for these programs will continue.

 **CONCLUSIONS**

Community nursing intervention for women's health must seek models of care that are collaborative, holistic, and relevant to women's lives. Stein (1997) proposes a utopian model of women's health in the community. This model includes the social and environmental resources necessary to promote wellness for all women (Figure 3-10).

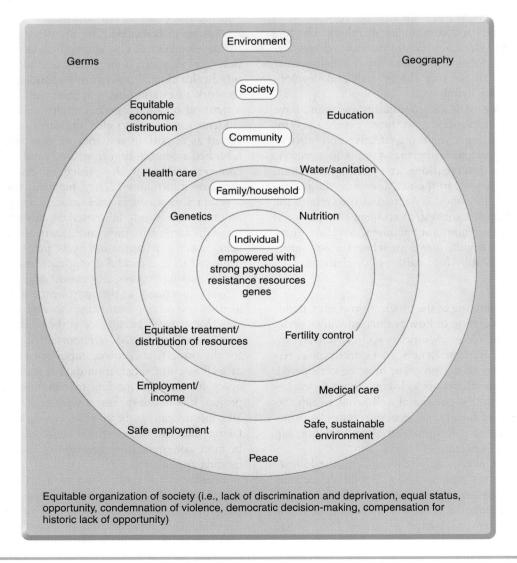

**FIGURE 3-10 •** Utopian model of women's health. *(From Stein J:* Empowerment and women's health: theory, methods and practice, *ed 2, London, 1997, Zen Books.)*

New models of care shift the focus of care to client needs, recognize that the context of environment is very important to women, and consider emotional well-being and prevention (Harrison, 1993). Future health care policy must not only build upon the strengths of women as architects of community health change but also protect them from becoming overburdened with caretaking demands in an age of cost containment.

## CASE STUDY

The Glendale Neighborhood Association is an independent community organization comprising white, African-American, and Jamaican families. Although of diverse racial and economic background, the community shares a common interest—care of the children. After an association meeting to discuss the summer recreation programs for the children, some women began to talk about their friends who had recently been diagnosed with breast cancer. As they compared notes, the number of women with breast cancer seemed alarmingly high. The women decide to find out more about the problem. Two of the women are nurses, and three know home care nurses assigned to their neighborhood.

Tamika Johnson, a community health nurse working at a nearby health center, hears about the women's concerns. She talks with the health center staff to determine what measures they can take to address the problem. The staff suggests that Tamika schedule a breast cancer awareness program to encourage the women to seek early screening exams.

Tamika schedules a class on breast cancer awareness for Tuesday at 4 PM at the health center and puts a notice in the newspaper. Three women come to the program. Tamika provides them with the information and answers their questions. Disappointed with the low turnout, Tamika decides to collaborate with the women of the community and other providers.

The women of the community and the providers meet and develop a joint strategy, dividing the work. Because the nurses' expertise involves working with agencies, they gather information from the health department and other secondary sources. One of the nurses helps the women construct a questionnaire to bring door to door throughout the neighborhood. While all the data collection is occurring, two more women are diagnosed with breast cancer. Several women wanted to quit the assessment process and "just do something" before they heard of another woman who was ill. After all, they said, "How much assessment is necessary?"

Several other women, however, voted to continue the assessment. After 2 months and many hours of work, the women identified several important findings. The rate for breast cancer was indeed five times the state rate and seven times higher than the national rate. A large number of other types of cancer also exceeded the local and national rates. The group also identified other concerns such as neighborhood safety, teenage substance use, and asthma among their children. The nurses helped to develop community-nursing diagnoses for each problem identified.

- Why are nursing diagnoses for the community important?
- How should community nursing diagnoses be prioritized?
- What would the group have to do to take an "upstream" approach?
- Why is it important to identify outcomes during the planning phase?
- Why should the objectives be measurable?
- What primary prevention efforts might occur?
- What secondary prevention efforts might occur?
- What tertiary prevention efforts might occur?

# Scenarios

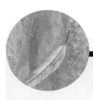

1. A state survey of public schools indicates increasing rates of alcohol and tobacco use among middle school students. The leaders of the parents' group and the school administrators say that the state report does not accurately reflect the behavior of the students at Lakeside Middle School. You are the school nurse for the community of students that attend this school.

- How will you determine if students are using tobacco and alcohol?
- How will you do this without angering the community or school leaders and endangering your job?
- What community diagnoses might apply? Why?
- How will you validate the diagnoses?
- How will you then proceed?

---

2. You are of Irish-American descent and grew up in a large city. You are making a well-child visit to a family of Haitian descent to assess the growth and development of a 6-week-old infant. The family lives in a section of the community that has a high number of Haitian families. This is the first client you have had from this ethnic background.

The grandmother, the matriarch of the family, has raised 14 children. She is now the primary caretaker and health care decision maker for the infant because the mother works. While talking with the grandmother, you observe her chewing ground beef and sharing the beef juice mouth-to-mouth with the infant. This is a practice with which you are unfamiliar.

- What information would you obtain?
- How you would phrase the questions so that they will not be threatening or insulting?
- Give an example of how the conversation might go.
- What if your findings reveal that prechewing meat and giving the juice to an infant by mouth are seen as vital to the growth of a strong infant? How would you respond or not respond? How would you intervene or not intervene?
- If you are not sure what to do, where might you seek information?

---

3. You are a nurse of African-American descent. When making a follow-up well-child visit to a 5-year-old in a Hispanic family, the mother asks you to look at her toddler. The mother says that the child has been lethargic. You touch the toddler's forehead, and it feels hot. The mother agrees with your request to take a rectal temperature. While examining the child, you notice several round, quarter-size marks that look like second degree burns.

- What information would you obtain?
- Describe how you would phrase the questions so that they will not be threatening or insulting.
- Give an example of how the conversation might go.

You learn from the mother that when the child first became ill she called her neighbor who is a curandero or healer. The curandero recommended the traditional remedy, burning lemon slices and applying them while still hot to the child's abdomen. This practice is expected to "draw out" the fever.

- How would you respond or not respond?
- How would you intervene or not intervene?
- If you are not sure what to do, where might you seek information?

---

4. Jane and her partner, Susan, have lived together for 6 years in a diverse neighborhood of professionals, laborers, families, and single people near a large university in the Midwest.

Their neighbors are generally accepting of their lesbian relationship, but Jane and Susan find that they derive their social support by meeting with a group of lesbian friends. Susan has experienced discrimination and insulting phone messages at her place of work. Her stress level has led her to experience stress-related health problems, such as hypertension and headaches. Susan has come to the health center seeking care for these problems.

- What additional information would you obtain during your intake interview?
- What nursing diagnoses might apply to Susan?
- What nursing diagnoses might apply to her community?
- How would you validate these diagnoses?
- How might you intervene?

---

5. Each morning on your way to work at a community health center, you see a woman and her three children come out of an alley between two warehouses and walk down the street. They are each carrying a backpack, and the woman also carries a large canvas bag. Today, a few hours after arriving at work, you notice them sitting in the waiting room, their bags surrounding them. You do the intake interview and learn that the woman has come because her 4-year-old daughter, Rose, has experienced vomiting and diarrhea for the last 3 days and is not interested in eating.

- What additional information would you try to obtain during your intake interview?
- What nursing diagnoses might apply?

- How would you validate these diagnoses?
- What interventions might be necessary for primary, secondary, and tertiary prevention?
- How would you develop or find the resources to provide this care?

---

6. Alice, a nursing student, volunteers for 10 hours a week at a shelter for women who have been victims of domestic violence. This transitional housing site shelters 18 women and their children in a homelike atmosphere in a residential neighborhood. During the day, most women go to work or attend classes. A fully staffed day care center is available on site to care for all the children while their mothers are gone. The women share the responsibility of shopping for food and cooking the meals. You are a community health nurse assigned to visit the shelter for 1 hour a week.

- How would you start collecting data to determine the needs of the families living in the shelter?
- To whom would you talk? What questions would you ask?
- What observations would you make at the facility?
- What nursing diagnoses might apply?
- How would you validate these diagnoses?
- What interventions might provide appropriate measures of primary, secondary, and tertiary prevention?
- How would you develop or find the resources to provide this care?

---

7. Florence and many of her friends are of British descent and have lived in this community for their whole lives. Florence, who is 78 years old, has been an active participant in the weekly activities of the community senior center for the last 23 years. Among other things, the senior center provides a hot lunch program; flu immunization clinic; and periodic health screenings for vision, hearing, and skin conditions.

A number of Hispanic families, originally from Santo Domingo, have recently moved into the community. There are generally three generations of a family living together, grandparent(s), parents, and children. The elderly members of these families have started to attend the senior center, especially on days when health screening programs are offered. You are the nurse sent by the Department of Health to do the health screenings. During today's visit, you notice that not all the participants in the hot lunch program eat their food.

- How would you determine why this is occurring? To whom would you talk?
- What questions would you ask?
- What other observations do you think you will be able to make?
- What nursing diagnoses might apply?
- How would you validate these diagnoses?
- What interventions might provide appropriate measures for primary, secondary, and tertiary prevention?
- How would you develop or find the resources to respond to this need?

---

8. You are the nurse in a prenatal clinic in an inner city neighborhood. There are a number of women in the area, both married and single, who do not come in for prenatal care on a regular basis. You find this frustrating because you think that the clinic offers excellent programs. You ask some of the women who you do see why the other mothers are not coming. They each share their thoughts but because they are coming they cannot really be sure why the rest are not.

- How could you learn more about why women are not coming? Outline the strategy you would use. Why do you think that strategy would be successful?
- How would you validate the information you receive?
- What other resources might you need?
- What would you do with the information and resources?

## REFERENCES

Aday L and Andersen R: Equity of access to medical care: a conceptual and empirical view, *Medical Care* 19(12), 1981.

Anderson E and McFarlane J: *Community as partner: theory and practice in nursing*, ed 2, Philadelphia, 1996, Lippincott.

Anderson E, McFarlane J, and Helton A: Community-as-client: a model for practice, *Nursing Outlook* 34(5):220-224, 1986.

Baldwin D: A model for describing low-income African American women's participation in breast and cervical cancer early detection and screening, *Adv Nurs Sci* 19(2):27, 1996.

Becker MH: The health belief model and personal health behaviors, *Health Education Monographs* 2:324, 1974.

Belenky M and others: *Women's ways of knowing: the development of self, voice, and mind*, New York, 1986, Basic Books.

Brown P and Mikkelsen E: *No safe place: toxic waste, leukemia and community action*, Berkeley, CA, 1990, UCLA-Berkeley Press.

Chavkin W: *Double exposure: women's health hazards on the job and at home*, New York, 1984, Monthly Review Press.

Chinn P and Wheeler C: *Peace and power: a handbook of feminist process*, New York, 1991, NLN Press.

Clemon-Stone S, McGuire SL, and Eigsti DG: *Comprehensive community health nursing*, ed 5, St Louis, 1998, Mosby.

Courtney R and others: The partnership model: working with individuals, families, and communities toward a new vision of health, *Pub Health Nurs* 13:177, 1996.

Dickson F and Tutty L: The role of public health nurses in responding to abused women, *Pub Health Nurs* 13(4):263, 1996.

Finnegan L and Ervin N: An epidemiological approach to community assessment, *Pub Health Nurs* 6(3):147, 1989.

Freire P: *Pedagogy of the oppressed*, New York, 1989, Continuum.

Gilligan C: *In a different voice: psychological theory and women's development*, Cambridge, MA, 1982, Harvard University Press.

Glazer N: *Women's paid and unpaid labor: the work transfer in health care and retailing*, Philadelphia, 1993, Temple University Press.

Haas A: Lesbian health issues: an overview. In Dan A, editor: *Reframing women's health*, Thousand Oaks, CA, 1994, Sage.

Harr J: *A civil action*, New York, 1996, Random House.

Hatton D: Managing health problems among homeless women with children in transitional shelter, *Image* 29(1):33, 1997.

Hochschild A: *The second shift: working parents and the revolution at home*, New York, 1989, Viking.

House J, Landis K, and Umberson D: Social relationships and health. In Conrad P and Kern R, editors: *The sociology of health and illness: critical perspectives*, ed 4, New York, 1994, St. Martin's Press.

Israel BA and others: Health education and community empowerment: conceptualizing and measuring perceptions of individual, organizational and community control, *Health Educ Q* 21(2):149, 1994.

Jemmott L, Maula E, and Bush E: Hearing our voices: assessing HIV prevention needs among Asian and Pacific Islander women, *J Transcult Nurs* 10(2):102, 1999.

Johnson D: The behavioral system model for nursing. In Riehl J and Roy C, editors: *Conceptual models for nursing practice*, ed 2, New York, 1980, Appleton-Century-Crofts.

King I: *Toward a theory for nursing: general concepts of human behavior*, New York, 1971, John Wiley & Sons.

Kramer E, Ivey S, and Ying Y: *Immigrant women's health: problems and solutions*, San Francisco, 1999, Jossey-Bass.

Kretzmann J and McKnight J: *Building communities from the inside out: a path toward finding and mobilizing a community's assets*, Evanston, IL, 1993, Institute for Policy Research.

Leavell HR and Clark EG: *Preventive medicine for the doctor and his community*, New York, 1958, McGraw-Hill.

Lewin K: Frontiers in group dynamics: concept, method, and reality in social science; social equilibria and change, *Human Relations* 1(5):4-41, 1947.

Mahon J, McFarlane J, and Golden K: *De madres a madres*: a community partnership for health, *Pub Health Nurs* 8(1):15, 1991.

Matteson P, editor: *Teaching nursing in the neighborhoods*, New York, 1995, Springer.

McGuire M and Freund P: *Health, illness and the social body: a critical sociology*, Englewood Cliffs, NJ, 1995, Prentice Hall.

McKinley J: A case for refocusing upstream: the political economy of illness. In Conrad P and Kern R: *The sociology of health and illness: critical perspectives*, New York, 1981, St. Martin's Press.

Miller J: *Toward a new psychology of women*, Boston, 1976, Beacon Press.

Moe EO: Nature of today's community. In Reinhart AM and Quinn ML, editors: *Current practice in family-centered community nursing* 1:117, St Louis, 1977, Mosby.

Morris R: The culture of female circumcision, *Adv Nurs Sci* 19(2):43, 1996.

Muller C: *Health care and gender*, New York, 1990, Russell Sage.

Neuman B: *The Neuman systems model: application to nursing education and practice*, Norwalk, CT, 1982, Appleton-Century-Crofts.

North American Nursing Diagnosis Association: *Nursing diagnoses: definitions and classifications 1999-2000*, Philadelphia, 1999, The Association.

Parsons T: *The social system*, New York, 1951, Free Press.

Richters A: Introduction, *Soc Sci Med* 35(6):747, 1992.

Rothman J: Three models of community organization practice. In Zaltman G, Kotler P, and Kaufman I, editors: *Creating social change*, New York, 1972, Holt, Rinehart, and Winston.

Roy C: *Introduction to nursing: an adaptation model*, ed 2, Englewood Cliffs, NJ, 1984, Prentice-Hall.

Rusek S, Olsen V, and Clarke A (eds): *Women's health—complexities and differences*, Columbus, OH, 1997, Ohio State University Press.

Sapiro V: *Women in American society*. Mountain View, CA, 1998, Mayfield.

Shuster G and Goeppinger J: Community as client: using the nursing process to promote health. In Stanhope M and Lancaster J: *Community health nursing: promoting health of aggregates, families, and individuals*, ed 4, St Louis, 1996, Mosby.

Smith C and Maurer F: *Community health nursing: theory and practice*, ed 2, Philadelphia, 2000, Saunders.

Spradley B and Allender J: *Community health nursing: concepts and practice*, ed 4, Philadelphia, 1996, Lippincott.

Stanhope M and Lancaster J: *Community health nursing: promoting health of aggregates, families, and individuals*, St Louis, 1996, Mosby.

Stein J: *Empowerment and women's health: theory, methods and practice*, ed 2, London, 1997, Zen Books.

USDHHS: *Healthy people in healthy communities: a guide for community leaders*, Washington, DC, 1998, The Department.

U.S. Department of Commerce, Bureau of the Census: Statistical abstracts of the United States, Washington, DC, 1992, U.S. Government.

Urrutia-Rojas X and Aday L: A framework for community assessment: designing and conducting a survey in a Hispanic immigrant refugee community, *Publ Health Nurs* 8(1):20, 1991.

von Bertalanffy L: *General systems theory*, New York, 1973, George Braziller.

Wallerstein N and Bernstein E: Empowerment education: Freire's ideas adapted to health education, *Health Educ Q* 15(4):379, 1988.

Ware S: *Modern American women—a documentary history*, Belmont, CA, 1989, Wadsworth.

Wright LM and Leahy M: *Nurses and families: a guide to family assessment and intervention*, Philadelphia, 1994, F.A. Davis.

# CHAPTER 4

# Assessment of a Woman's Health

*"Doing to" involves hands.*
*"Doing for" involves intellect or head.*
*Neither is minimized; both are essential.*
— BREWER, MOLBO, AND GERBIE, 1966

*What might a woman expect from a health encounter with you?*

*How would you encourage a woman to tell you about her life and health?*

*How might a woman's physical health affect her daily life?*

*How might a woman express her psychologic or emotional concerns to you?*

*What emotions might a woman feel prior to her health examination?*

*What ongoing support services might a healthy woman need or want?*

*How do you want a woman to feel after an encounter with you?*

Well-woman care consists of screening programs and health examinations designed to provide anticipatory guidance and early identification of threats to women's health. We may provide well-woman services at community health fairs or screening programs, through periodic programs in churches or other gathering places, or through programs of ongoing care in homes, community health centers, clinics, or private offices.

As health care providers, we are responsible for setting the relational tone that fosters a positive, effective, empowering health partnership (Yoder-Wise, 1999). Nurses who have positive attitudes about others and are aware that a collaborative relationship with clients is a privilege are better able to develop partnerships that significantly influence care (Carlson-Catalano, 1994).

This chapter focuses on the role of the nurse in an assessment of a woman's health. Many of the health education opportunities that may occur in the process are identified. Educational information that may be offered is covered in detail in Chapter 5.

 **DEVELOPING A SUPPORTIVE PARTNERSHIP PROCESS**

### The Role of the Nurse

We strive to connect with women to help them attain, maintain, or regain their health. Our professional practice skills of presence and therapeutic listening enable us to connect with clients and develop the necessary client-centered practice. These communication

**101**

skills are potentially powerful tools through which women can learn to promote their own health, cope with illness, or adjust to loss, to reach levels of maximum well-being.

### Presence

**"Presence** is a process of being available with the whole of oneself and open to the experience of another through a reciprocal interpersonal encounter" (Moch and Schaefer, 1998). By "being there" and "being with" we are available to develop a personal relationship with a client (Gardner, 1992). This type of relationship can reduce barriers and allow us to experience each woman's uniqueness and, in turn, allow the women to experience our uniqueness (Carson, 1989) (Box 4-1).

 Being fully present with another person is basic to providing holistic, humanistic, collaborative care and requires authenticity, honesty, self-disclosure, and vulnerability.

*Authenticity.* To be **authentic** is to be genuine, true to oneself and one's word, not pretending to be someone or something different. Being trustworthy, showing respect, and appropriately sharing information are actions through which authenticity is displayed. To establish authenticity with a client, we must be fully present in body, mind, and spirit. Smiling warmly, listening attentively, and conveying confidence in oneself and the woman seeking care are nonverbal behaviors that promote authenticity.

*Honesty.* Honesty is required when we are unfamiliar with a finding or procedure. We acknowledge uncertainty by saying, "That's an excellent question. I don't know the answer, but I will find out." By admitting in this way that we do not know, we maintain our accountability and demonstrate confidence in our abilities and respect for a woman's right to know.

*Self-disclosure.* More than simply "being yourself" with a client, self-disclosure involves respectful and sincere communication with another person, in a manner that is therapeutic or helpful (Slunt, 1994). Self-disclosure occurs when we acknowledge non-obvious personal experiences, attitudes, and emotions. For example, you might say, "As a woman, I have also experienced . . . ," or "As a parent, I have also lost sleep over. . . ." The therapeutic effects of provider-initiated self-disclosure may increase your ability to be understood, enhance the level of trust, decrease the client's sense of loneliness, and reduce a perception of role distance (VanServellen, 1997).

*Vulnerability.* Being able to accept vulnerability as an aspect of being human means we accept that both we and our clients are **vulnerable,** capable of being physically, psychologically, and spiritually harmed. Our clients may feel powerlessness in the midst of illness, suffering, and loss. Simultaneously we may feel incapable and have to confront our own tension, self-doubt, and spiritual distress as we care for them.

Before initiating a client contact, we must first take a "period of quiet attention to self before a planned encounter; for example, simply taking a deep breath and closing one's eyes in order to center self and detach from other distractions. The centering process promotes openness and readiness for caring" (Moch and Schaefer, 1998) and only requires a few seconds. After centering ourselves, we are ready to focus on the client

---

#### BOX 4-1  Experience of "Presence"

Because of the reciprocal nature of presence, how much presence comes through affects both the woman and the provider.

The woman could be asked to answer "yes" or "no" to statements such as the following:
- I felt understood.
- I decided what to talk about at least once during this encounter.
- I felt cared about.
- At least one member of the health care team took time for me and my real needs.

We can evaluate the interaction by asking ourselves to answer "yes" or "no" to the following:
- Did I learn what was important to the woman?
- Do I have awe and respect for her?
- Do I feel connected to her?
- What did I learn about myself from this encounter?

Adapted from Moch and Schaefer, 1998

---

#### BOX 4-2  Examples of Active Listening

**WOMAN**
"I live alone and don't eat right, and now I haven't had my period for 2 months."
**[What she is saying.]**

*Nurse*
"You haven't had a menstrual period for 2 months, and you think it might be because of your diet?"
**[Paraphrase the message heard.]**

*Woman*
"That's right."
**[Validation of accuracy.]**

*Nurse*
"What concerns you about not having a menstrual period?"
**[Asking about what she is feeling.]**

*Woman*
"I don't know; it just worries me."
**[Statement of feeling.]**

*Nurse*
"What is it about not having a menstrual period that worries you?"
**[Asking for clarification.]**

with our professional skills of listening, observation, and feeling.

### Listening

Listening, which is both an art and a learned skill, is a method of obtaining information and meaning. We quiet our own thoughts and responses and attend to the woman with open ears, eyes, and mind. "**Active listening** is the skill of understanding what another is saying and feeling" (Ryden, 1998). After the client speaks, an active listener paraphrases the message heard back to the speaker to clarify that it was heard and understood accurately (Box 4-2).

Observation reveals the client's nonverbal messages. Facial expressions communicate additional information beyond the verbal messages. Six of the basic human emotions—happiness, sadness, anger, fear, surprise, and disgust—are expressed with a limited number of facial muscle movements. These facial expressions are generally interpreted as having the same meaning across different cultures (Ryden, 1998). When the verbal and nonverbal messages that we receive from a client are contradictory, we rely on facial expression and tone of voice for additional information (Mehrabian, 1971). By being present and using the skills of active listening, our therapeutic relationship with clients is improved and our collaboration towards health and wholeness is more effective.

### Empowerment

A person is **empowered** when he or she believes that he or she has the authority or power to control what happens to himself or herself (Robertson, 1997). Empowered nurses have a vision of collaboration with

clients and accept responsibility for realization of that vision, viewing themselves as primary facilitators for a woman's connection to the health care system (Carlson-Catalano, 1994).

Our collaborative relationships with women are intended to empower each of them to make choices about their health and determine the extent of the role they wish to play in their health care. Some women may want health care providers to assume full responsibility for all decision making. Others may want to make the decisions themselves concerning their care. Most women develop some degree of collaborative arrangement for anticipatory guidance and care with the health care providers whom they select.

Women who come to think of themselves as empowered develop the physical, psychologic, and social strengths that enable them to more fully participate within their family, support networks, and community (Figure 4-1). Even though we may collaborate with a woman on her health issues, the time we spend with her and our sphere of influence are small. Where the woman lives and who she interacts with on a daily basis have much more influence on her health and well-being. The woman's family and community form her "life partnerships," which are relationships that both promote and detract from health.

### The Effect of the Health Care Setting

The setting in which we encounter the woman plays a role in the process of "inviting, establishing, and maintaining" the connection with the woman. A health care environment may be conducive to collaboration and the

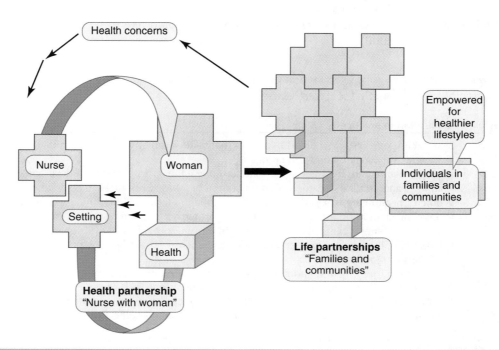

*FIGURE 4-1* • Collaborating with women: health and life connections.

development of connections, or it may be structured around the needs of providers, with rules, routines, and regimens that leave woman feeling objectified, tense, misunderstood, and powerless. Clinical environments are most effective when the environment is nurturing, power is shared, mutual decision-making is encouraged, and collaborative care actually occurs (Hultgren, 1994). Review the principles for woman-centered care in Table 4-1. By evaluating the clinical reality for women in the places where we provide care, the constructive or constraining elements within the setting can be identified and, if necessary, addressed (Phillips, Himwich, and Fitzgerald, 1999).

### Inviting Connection

A variety of factors will either invite or discourage a woman's participation in her health care. For example: Is the location accessible? Is the neighborhood known to be safe? Are the hours convenient? Does the facility have a reputation of being welcoming to all women? If a woman does not speak or understand English, are there translation services to ensure that she will be understood? Box 4-3 provides examples of considerations that invite connection.

### Establish Connection

The physical environment and routines may or may not embrace and empower those who enter the setting (Kerfoot and Neuman, 1992). Are the entrances to the facility clearly identified so clients can easily find their way into the facility without feeling rushed or stressed? Is it easily wheelchair accessible? Are the waiting rooms and examination areas safe, warm, clean, and comfortable? How does the facility smell? Through the diffusion of essential oils into the air, unpleasant odors can be kept to a minimum (Fontaine, 2000).

Is the process of client care efficient? Is privacy maintained during the interview and in the examination area? Are teaching materials adequate and convenient? If a woman does not read English, is the written information available in her language? If a woman cannot read, is the information provided through pictures or a pictogram format?

Are the examining rooms comfortable? Are they warm enough for a woman who has to take off her clothes? When a woman has to remove some or all of her clothing for the examination, does she have culturally appropriate options available as to what to wear? All women appreciate soft, concealing gowns or two-piece examination outfits in attractive prints and/or colors—whether in cloth or paper.

Is the equipment sufficient and well-maintained? If a woman has limited mobility or a disability, does the table adjust to a lower level to accommodate transfer from a wheelchair or stretcher (Sulpizi, 1996)?

Are personnel competent and committed? What other resources are available to meet the needs of women? Can various needs be met within the facility so that a woman does not have to visit multiple sites? Box 4-4 provides examples of considerations that establish connection.

### Maintain Connection

After a woman's health visit is finished, does a nurse, nurse practitioner, nurse-midwife, or physician verify her understanding of the findings with her before she leaves? If follow-up care has been suggested, does someone review the rationale with her and help her make arrangements? Is the woman told how long it will take to get the lab results? Is the woman asked how she would like to be contacted about the results? Will the nurse, nurse practitioner, nurse-midwife, or

---

### TABLE 4-1  *Principles for Woman-Centered Care*

| Underlying principle | Application to practice |
|---|---|
| Mission | Health care practices are guided by beliefs that value women's special and multidimensional biologic, psychosocial, and spiritual needs. |
| Continuum of care | Women require care throughout a continuum of wellness (or illness) with developmental, economic, and cultural considerations for community-based resources. |
| Practices | Women's health care is based on competent, collaborative, multidisciplinary providers. |
| Decision-making | Women have an important role in the health partnership and are respected for their decision-making abilities—even when differing from those of providers. |
| Access | Health care programs are convenient and comprehensive, based on the preferences and recommendations of those served. |
| Education | Programs offer information and guidance that are based on research or evidence, culturally appropriate, and allow women to make independent decisions with confidence. |
| Evaluation | The organization values qualitative results of care, including women's satisfaction, regard of the program, and clinical considerations, in addition to economic outcomes. |

Adapted from Phillips and Fenwick: The business of women's health: building a successful women's practice, In Phillips CR, Himwich DB, and Fitzgerald C: *Lifelines* 3(3):32-36, 1999.

physician share the results of diagnostic tests with her within 24 to 48 hours of their completion?

Does a woman have the opportunity to share her view of the facility and the experience? Collecting the woman's view of the interaction through evaluation is one way that she may feel empowered and valued as a partner in the health care process. Such collection also provides valuable information on how the facility and services are perceived. Box 4-5 provides a sample of an evaluation tool that may be used at the close of a health visit to give each woman the opportunity to evaluate the services of the facility from her perspective.

Box 4-6 describes some nursing practices that are designed to maintain or restore a woman's connections within the collaborative health partnership.

After learning from women what they expect and desire in a health care setting, we may work to establish a clinical reality that supports women-centered care. Factors to pay attention to initially are communication of a warm welcome, provision of clarifying information, respect of individuality, and concern about client satisfaction. Examples of such supportive clinical realities are given in Table 4-2.

---

### BOX 4-3 Considerations that Invite Connection

To invite a connection with the woman the staff should do the following:

- Learn from the woman what would make her comfortable during this health visit.
- Determine the type and gender of health care provider she wishes to see.
- Document whether a non-English interpreter or written information will be needed.
- Ascertain if there is an impairment of speech or hearing.
- Learn if children or others will accompany the woman for support.
- Offer advice on how to access the health setting, especially if woman has mobility needs.
- Learn her full name and how she likes to be addressed.
- Clarify her address and other contact information essential to the health care follow-up.
- Encourage her to call in advance of her visit with any questions.
- Ask her to bring information on all teas, tonics, or medications she currently takes.
- If she has health records or laboratory or other diagnostic test results, ask her to bring them.
- Just before the appointment, contact her with a reminder notice or telephone call.
- Provide individualized information on transportation or parking if necessary.

---

### BOX 4-4 Considerations that Establish Connection

To establish a connection with the woman the staff should do the following:

- Provide an attractive and welcoming exterior with well-marked parking and entrances.
- Ensure that the woman's needs for safety and security are met.
- Be hospitable, greeting the woman and her companions warmly and personally.
- Offer information about the status of her appointment.
- Create a pleasant interior that is warm, clean, and comfortable.
- Have clear guidelines on how to access interpreting and/or translating services.
- Provide bilingual resources as appropriate.
- Recognize that medical concepts and terms may be unfamiliar to all women.
- Accommodate the interests of the woman and her significant others.
- Provide adequate space for the woman to maneuver, particularly when special equipment is needed.

---

### BOX 4-5 An Evaluation Tool

We were pleased to have served you at  (the facility) . It is extremely important to us that you were satisfied, and we welcome any constructive comments you have. On the form below, please circle the "Faces" that best reflect how you feel about the visit.

1. I received enough information before the visit. ☺ ☺ ☹
2. The staff made sure I understood what I needed to learn. ☺ ☺ ☹
3. My waiting time was enjoyable. ☺ ☺ ☹
4. I felt safe and secure. ☺ ☺ ☹
5. The areas were clean and attractive to me. ☺ ☺ ☹
6. It was not hard to find where I needed to be. ☺ ☺ ☹
7. My needs were given special attention. ☺ ☺ ☹
8. The results of my exam were reviewed with me. ☺ ☺ ☹
9. Follow-up health care resources were explained. ☺ ☺ ☹
10. I'll come back here for care again. ☺ ☺ ☹

There is something else that I have to say:

_____

_____

Note: "Faces" scale adapted from Rafferty EA: *Choices program: curriculum evaluation tool* [unpublished], Bethlehem, PA, 1999, Abstinence Council of the Lehigh Valley Coalition to Prevent Teen Pregnancy.

## The Woman Seeking Care

There may be a variety of factors that require a woman to have a health visit for screening or a full examination. Therefore it is important for us to individualize our interactions and ensure that each woman's contact is a positive experience. When we know the thoughts or concerns that have caused a woman to require care, our professional energies can be better focused on related key elements in the health assessment.

In practice, well women have been generally encouraged to seek out annual examinations that focus on the care of their reproductive organs. Women's rates of cardiac disease, respiratory disease, diabetes, mental health, and acute and chronic illnesses, however, indicate that they need to seek care with health care providers who provide attention to all dimensions of their health.

---

### BOX 4-6   Considerations that Maintain Connection

To maintain a connection with the woman the staff should do the following:

- Explain her health assessment findings in relation to health status and health promotion.
- Validate any of her concerns about her health status and follow-up.
- Provide as much information as possible on diagnostic results (whether or not complete) within 24 to 48 hours.
- If possible, give results immediately to women with high levels of concern for them (e.g., results of mammograms before leaving the facility).
- Verify that support is available to a woman when results are negative or difficult.
- Contact the woman after the visit with health resources, support, and encouragement.
- Offer the woman an opportunity to evaluate her experiences at the setting.

---

### Why Women Do Not Seek Health Care

There are many reasons why women do not seek the assistance of a provider within our health care system. A woman's views about her health and the health care system; beliefs about whom to see for assistance with health problems; and lack of insurance or money, transportation, or someone to care for her children may discourage a timely entry into the health care system. In order for health promotion or early disease detection activities to be truly effective, early and ongoing access to health care is critical and we must find ways to engage the woman in the process (Box 4-7).

##  WELL-WOMAN ASSESSMENT

The women who meet with us for care are multidimensional human beings, each dealing with more than just a physical self. Their health statuses depend upon how they think about themselves, what they do, and where they live. The health assessment encourages the discovery of the significant elements of a woman's self and allows insight into her concerns, her work, and her world. Health-related needs are mutually determined. Findings may require direct care, screening, health education, social support, and/or referral services. Effective use of the nursing process can lead to the development of an effective provider-consumer health care partnership.

Our goal of care is to meet with women in their homes and neighborhood facilities to mutually develop a plan to respond to actual or potential health problems that are identified by either the woman or ourselves. No matter where the encounter occurs, at the beginning of the health care visit we must use the skills of both presence and active listening to initiate a partnership (Lashley and others, 1994; VanServellen, 1996). These techniques will promote the exchange of vital information with women. It is important for a client to share her story during the health history and physical examination.

Verbal communication with a mutually understood language facilitates development of the health partnership. Even when the woman speaks English, it is some-

---

### TABLE 4-2   A Supportive Clinical Reality

| Supportive Factor | Example of a Supportive Statement |
| --- | --- |
| Welcome communication | "Hello. It's nice to see you." (Smile) <br> "I know this is your first time at this center. Did you have any problems getting here?" |
| Clarifying information | "This is not easy to understand. I'd be happy to answer any questions or go over it again." <br> "I gave you a lot of information. This pamphlet goes over the key points." |
| Individualization | "Will you need an appointment while your daughters are in school?" <br> "There is a support group at the church near your apartment." |
| Client satisfaction | "If there is anything you think we need to do to make your visit easier, just let us know." <br> "Are you satisfied with how you were treated here?" <br> "Is there anything else I can do for you?" |

times difficult for her to understand the meaning of the terms we use. Examples of some words that are unfamiliar are cervix, vulva, endometrium, perineum, or follicle. We can clarify concepts and teach by using pictures and models as we talk.

When we do not speak the patient's language, we must find someone to translate for her. Appropriate written information should also be available. Bilingual health resources are increasingly available online. For example, "Ask NOAH" (New York's Online Access to Health) is a website that provides up-to-date and comprehensive health information in both English and Spanish (NOAH, 1999).

As a basis for ongoing care, the well woman's health assessment includes the health history, as well as appropriate screening measures and the physical examination. In order to be thorough, the assessment must be organized with adequate time allotted. Sometimes a full assessment for a new client will entail two visits in order to be complete. After the initial visit(s), the woman's chart is updated at each subsequent visit. The importance of an unhurried approach and individualized attention during an assessment process is that it leaves the woman feeling that her needs have been addressed.

There are five desired outcomes of the well woman's health assessment. Through the process we interact with the woman to (1) learn her health concerns or health problems; (2) provide screening for actual or potential threats to her health; and (3) provide the appropriate health education and resources. After identifying areas where a woman could use information, we also (4) provide the appropriate information, enabling her to accomplish better health problem-solving. Through interactive communication, we (5) provide a woman with reinforcement for positive behaviors for better health (Box 4-8).

## Enabling the Woman to Tell Her Story

The first part of a formal health assessment involves having the woman tell her story. This story includes what it was that made her come for the visit, prior health events in her life and the lives of family members, and her hopes for what she might gain from this encounter. Our communication techniques will enable her to fully share her relevant life experiences. If the woman feels safe, she may also voice her more private concerns.

The health interview is a complex, sensitive process of not only asking questions but also encouraging the woman to ask some difficult questions of herself at the same time. Although the primary goal of the health history is to obtain information that allows us to collaborate with the woman, there are other interpersonal benefits from taking a thorough, sensitive health history. "The health history is a conversation with a purpose" (Bickley, 1999). The conversational aspects involved in taking the health history facilitate the therapeutic relationship with the hope that mutual trust and rapport develop. With good history taking, information that is personal and precious is gathered. When used effectively, this information fosters individualized care based on the actual context of a woman's life (Box 4-9).

### Prepare for the Interview

The most important skill required in taking the health history is being able to communicate well during the interview. Be well-acquainted with the instrument used to collect historic data. Forms for history taking can

---

### BOX 4-7   *Reasons Women May Not Seek Health Care*

Some of the reasons that a woman may not enter the health care system are as follows:
- Satisfied with self-care.
- Satisfied with cultural healers.
- Uncomfortable with sharing private information.
- Difficulty accessing health care (e.g., timing, transportation, money).
- Concerns about being understood (e.g., non-English speaking, cultural differences).
- Embarrassment about conditions (e.g., weight, disability).
- Dissatisfaction with health care providers.
- History of bad experience with the health care system.
- Fear of having to leave family and/or community for care.
- Disavowal of health concerns.
- Fear of cancer.
- Fear of being pregnant.
- Belief that nothing can be done.

---

### BOX 4-8   *Positive Outcomes of a Well Woman's Health Assessment*

- Connection between the woman and the health care system
- Location of a safe haven where personal expressions and concerns can be heard
- Identification of areas of personal health concern
- Screening procedures completed
- Receipt of appropriate health education and related resources
- Collaboration and mutual problem-solving for her health
- Recommendations for management of actual or potential health problems
- Social supports that complement her immediate social context

be found in health assessment manuals, and several commercial assessment forms are also available. A setting may also create a specialized form that raises questions and addresses issues that are important for collaboratively working with the women it serves.

Prepare for the health interview by reviewing any available documentation about the woman's prior health, medical and surgical experiences, family circumstances, and psychosocial situation.

From the time we call the woman's name and she stands and walks toward us, she is providing information about her physical well-being. The ease with which she stands and walks, the way she interacts with the environment and the people around her, and the manner in which she responds to us provide preliminary information that helps us determine how to relate to her. This preliminary assessment also influences how we will structure the interview and the areas of concern we will include in the interview.

During the history taking, a woman who is fully dressed will relax and talk more freely. The environment for taking the health history should be quiet and private, free from distractions and intrusions. We convey a sense of equality and mutual goal setting by conducting the interview with the woman comfortably seated at eye level. When the woman is speaking, we must focus on her, listen attentively, and use appropriate eye contact and display body language that indicates our interest and concern. Do not write or read as she speaks. The woman will provide the information we request if she feels that we are interested, she can trust us, and she can see a direct relationship between the information she gives and the care she thinks she needs (Figure 4-2).

Trust is conveyed by the way we introduce ourselves and explain our role, as well as where and how we conduct the interview. Many women will not provide accurate information or in-depth answers unless they understand the purpose of a line of questions. The woman may think that it is none of our business how often she has intercourse, what type of protection she uses against sexually transmitted infection, and/or if she is satisfied with her sex life. She may also feel it is not relevant to tell us about the illnesses of her friends or family members.

We increase trust when we provide the woman an explanation before asking a question (e.g., "Immunizations provide you with protection against some diseases. So that we know what diseases you are protected against, could you tell me what immunizations you have received and when?"). The information we gather through the data-collection phase of the nursing

---

**BOX 4-9** *Purposes of the Health History*

- To obtain information that is unique and special about the person
- To develop mutual trust and rapport between the woman and nurse
- To provide necessary health interventions and information
- To offer counseling and support

---

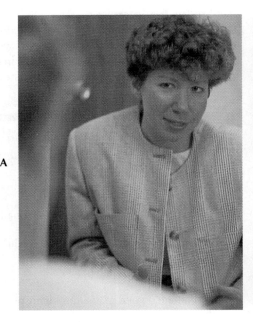
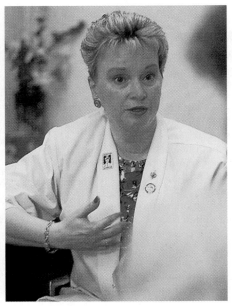

FIGURE 4-2 ● **A,** In a positive relationship, the client can communicate freely with the nurse. **B,** Nurse uses therapeutic communication skills to attend to the client's expressed needs. *(From Potter P and Perry A: Basic nursing, ed 3, St Louis, 1995, Mosby.)*

process is used to guide the diagnoses, interventions, and evaluation activities for the woman.

### The Use of the Self-Administered History Form

Some facilities have clients complete a self-administered history form while they are waiting to be seen, which can be useful to start the woman thinking about the factors associated with her health. The written history form is not used to the exclusion of the person-to-person history but may provide the basis for further assessment questions. The interview portion of the health history is still conducted systematically for verifying and further clarifying the information reported on the written form. Figure 4-3 provides an example of a self-administered history form.

### Health History Interview

Whether the woman is accessing the system for a wellness check-up or because of a specific health problem, a comprehensive health history interview is generally done the first time she enters a health-care setting. Taking a comprehensive health history is extremely im-

---

**Women's Clinic**

I.D. #: _____
NAME: _____
PHONE: _____
DATE: _____

**Confidential:** to be completed by patient

Reason for visit _____

First day of last menstrual period _____ | Drug allergies _____ | Present medications _____

**REPRODUCTIVE HISTORY:** Age at 1st period _____ Date of Last Pap _____

Number of: Live births _____ Pregnancies _____ Abortions _____ Miscarriages _____

Have you ever had: Breast abnormality _____ Uterus/tube infection _____ Sexually transmitted disease _____ Abnormal Pap _____

Other OB/Gyn problems: _____

Did your mother take DES (a hormone) while pregnant with you? ❏ Yes ❏ No ❏ Unsure

Do you have: Flow: ❏ excessively heavy ❏ missed periods
❏ painful periods ❏ excessively light
❏ spotting between periods
❏ unusual discharge/infection
❏ sexual concerns

Are you sexually active? ❏ Yes ❏ No
Current contraception? (Specify) _____ Are you in need of contraception? ❏ Yes ❏ No
List any problems you are experiencing: _____

**FAMILY HISTORY:**

Have any members of your immediate family (i.e., grandparent[s], parent[s], sibling[s]) ever had:

❏ high blood pressure ❏ heart attack or stroke ❏ anemia ❏ depression
❏ diabetes ❏ cancer, type _____ ❏ inherited disorder, type _____

**MEDICAL HISTORY: (Please check any that apply to you)**

❏ heart disease ❏ anemia ❏ gallbladder disease ❏ kidney or bladder infections
❏ high blood pressure ❏ asthma ❏ cancer ❏ thyroid disease
❏ migraine headaches ❏ epilepsy ❏ high cholesterol ❏ liver disease/jaundice
❏ blood clots (leg or lungs) ❏ diabetes ❏ sickle cell disease ❏ surgery, type _____
❏ eating disorders ❏ depression ❏ other _____

**HEALTH BEHAVIORS:**

Do you: (please check all that apply)
❏ smoke ❏ eat a well-balanced diet
❏ have a weight problem ❏ exercise regularly
❏ have a history of alcohol or other drug use ❏ perform monthly self-breast examinations
❏ have more than 2 sexual partners in the past 6 months ❏ have Rubella immunization

*FIGURE 4-3* • Self-administered history form.

portant, not only for the initial visit but also as a basis for future health visits. At subsequent visits, it may only be necessary to update personal facts and to conduct a focused review of systems.

Skill in taking a health history involves more than just asking questions and recording the answers. It is the ability to discover meaning in a woman's verbal and nonverbal messages and requires a critical analysis of the woman's story while she tells it. Any situation in which we are taking a health history also becomes an opportunity for a supportive and therapeutic communication.

At subsequent health visits, it is essential to review the woman's previous health histories and ask about her current status. This allows us to then focus the interview with a clearer understanding of who the woman is. Validate all conclusions about her status with the woman. Statements such as, "Do you still live at . . ." provide not only the chance to update contact information but also for her to offer information about changes in her living accommodations. We should also ask the woman about her health in reference to her last visit. For example, "You were here 3 months ago with ear pain and were given medication for it. How did it work? Is it still a problem?" Tying this visit to her previous encounter will demonstrate a continuity of care and may strengthen the health partnership. It will also provide an indication of her evaluation of prior interventions.

### Adjustments due to Children

No matter how busy a setting is, find a way to create a good situation for conversation. For example, if a woman has to bring her children with her, arrange for them to be cared for away from her for 5 minutes. When present, they will distract her and possibly prohibit her from revealing certain things. If removal is not an option, engage them in quiet play.

### Adjustments due to Age

Age is a factor to consider before initiating the interview. Taking a thorough history from an adolescent is not an easy task. The girl may not know the answers to many of the questions asked and may not have been accompanied by an adult who could provide this information. Conversely, an adult may accompany her and wish to be included in the entire health assessment. In this case, the adolescent and the adult must be diplomatically separated so that the girl can speak for herself about her life situation, feelings, and concerns.

### Adjustments due to Individual Needs

Some women are accompanied to the visit because of their high anxiety, language difficulties, developmental levels, physical disabilities, or abusive relationships. It is essential that the woman herself participate as much as possible and is the focus of our care (Coulehan and Block, 1997). For example, if the woman needs a trans-

lator, speak directly to the woman and then watch her face as the translator relays your words. Then listen carefully as the woman replies, watching her facial expressions and body language to reveal additional data. Sometimes a woman may not feel comfortable speaking English but will understand enough to determine if the translator is being accurate. Her face and body language will reflect the accuracy.

### Responding to Revealed Behaviors

If the woman reveals behaviors such as those in Table 4-3, consider how these may affect her health. Follow-up questions should be used to investigate the possible problem areas such behaviors often reflect or create.

## Screening for Potential or Actual Heath Issues and Problems

During the health assessment interview, you will learn about the woman and recognize the significant age-appropriate screening procedures that may be beneficial to her. These procedures may be primary, secondary, or tertiary prevention measures. **Primary prevention** involves activities directed toward decreasing the probability of becoming ill. **Secondary prevention** focuses on screening for disease so that early treatment may be given. **Tertiary prevention** interventions minimize a disability that the woman has already encountered. We provide the information about the potential benefits and possible harm of screening procedures, explain what is known and not known about the sensitivity and specificity of the screening tests, and explain the possible consequences of choosing whether or not to participate. Each woman reaches her own decision about the best course for her to follow.

The **sensitivity** of a screening test is defined as the proportion of persons with a condition that will be correctly identified as having it when screened. If a test has poor sensitivity, a proportion of the people tested will be told that they do not have the condition when they actually do have it (i.e., **false negative** results).

**Specificity** is the proportion of people without the condition who correctly test negative when screened. If a test has poor specificity, some people are identified as having the condition when they actually do not (i.e., **false positive** results). Because a positive test result often leads to further tests and procedures, a person with a false positive is unnecessarily put through the expense, psychologic stress, and risks of further testing. Client preferences are important in all clinical decisions. This becomes even more apparent in screening because the issues of test accuracy and an individual's relative risk for the condition being screened for are evaluated by the provider and client.

Offering clinical preventative services is an important part of what is done during a well-woman or annual ex-

TABLE 4-3  *Women's Behaviors and Health Problems: Reflected or Created*

| Behavior | Possible problem area reflected | Possible problem area created |
|---|---|---|
| Cigarette smoking | Stress | Pregnancy complications |
| | Depression | Respiratory illness (self and others) |
| | | Oral and respiratory tract cancer |
| | | Lung cancer |
| Substance use or abuse | Stress | Pregnancy complications |
| | Depression | Fetal alcohol effects/syndrome |
| | Low self-esteem | Legal stressors |
| | |    Underage drinking |
| | |    Driving under the influence |
| | | Alcoholism |
| | | Loss of self |
| | | Loss of control over life events |
| | | Financial distress |
| Eating disorders | | |
|   Overeating | Low self-esteem | Obesity |
| | Social isolation | Illnesses (e.g., cardiac disease, osteoarthritis, diabetes, cancer) |
|   Anorexia/bulimia | Low self-esteem | Cardiac arrhythmia |
| | Social isolation | Poor oral/dental health |
| Avoidance of exercise | Powerlessness | Obesity |
| | Hopelessness | Musculoskeletal problems |
| | Anxiety/stress | Cardiovascular disease |
| | Depression | Diabetes |
| | | Osteoporosis |
| | | Cancer |
| Violent actions | Victimization (i.e., of women, children) | Family crises |
| | Powerlessness | Spiritual distress |
| | Hopelessness | Rape |
| | Anxiety/stress | Physical injury |
| | Depression | Legal stress |
| | | Homicide |
| | | Suicide |
| Poor sleep habits | Anxiety | Chronic fatigue |
| | Stress | Frequent illness |
| | Depression | Abuse of medications |
| | Obesity/sleep apnea | Inadequate role performance |
| Unsafe sexual activities | Substance use (e.g., caffeine, nicotine) | Sexually transmitted disease |
| | Poor self-concept | Pelvic inflammatory disease |
| | Powerlessness | Infertility |
| | Hopelessness | Abortion |
| | Anxiety/stress | Pregnancy complications |
| | Depression | Rape |
| | | Victimization |
| | | Abortion |
| | | Unplanned/neglected children |

amination. Specific responses and interventions are provided in Chapter 5. In the United States, the Department of Health and Human Services, through the Office of Disease Prevention and Health Promotion, has initiated a program titled "Put Prevention Into Practice." The intent of the program is to provide guidance to clinicians so that they will incorporate early detection of disease, immunizations, prophylaxis to prevent disease, and counseling to modify health risks into all health care visits. The *Clinician's Handbook* provides the standards for preventive care for the general population based on the recommendations of major authorities (U.S. Department of Health and Human Services, 1998). The primary and secondary clinical preventive services target asymptomatic persons based on their individual risk profiles. Because of the specialty nature of tertiary prevention interventions, pre- and perinatal care, and preventive care for certain high-risk groups, these areas are not included in the screening program (Figure 4-4).

All adults are considered to be at risk for obesity, hypertension, coronary artery disease, elevated cholesterol, diabetes mellitus, malnutrition, dental disease, alcohol-related problems; injuries—either intentional, unintentional, or related to the use of drugs and alcohol; and measles and mumps if born after 1956 and should be screened in these areas whenever possible. Appropriate primary and secondary preventative services and referrals can then take place to improve the health and quality of the individual's life. Before they become pregnant, women of childbearing age may take the preventative steps of reducing the occurrence of neural tube defects and congenital rubella syndrome in future infants. The precautions of having a sufficient level of folate in their diet and being immunized against rubella are two simple steps, based on primary prevention services.

## Learning Her Story: The Health History

Common components of a comprehensive health history are described in the following paragraphs. We progress from general, noninvasive questions about a woman to the more personal or private issues that she may not be comfortable discussing until she feels comfortable and understands the need for us to know. Some questions are asked more than once in different sections. This is purposeful in order to offer the woman several occasions to remember or choose to share what is often difficult or painful to report. Descriptions of the structural elements of a health history, as well as key considerations in the process of data collections, follow for each part (Box 4-10).

Before we start to ask the woman questions, we tell her our name and specific role in her health care. She has the right to know who is asking her questions and what our role is within the health facility. As our questions touch on more personal topics, the woman may

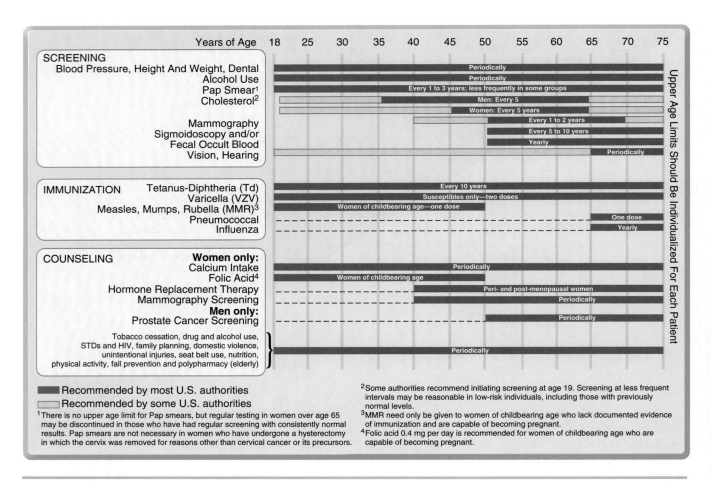

FIGURE 4-4 • Clinical preventative services for normal risk adults. *(From USDHS, Public Health Service, Office of Public Health and Science, Office of Disease Prevention and Promotion: Clinician's handbook of preventative services, ed 2, Washington, D.C., 1998, US Government Printing Office.)*

need reassurance about what happens with the information she provides us.

If we take her history and an advanced practice nurse or physician then performs the extensive physical examination, the woman needs to know who the additional people are that she will be interacting with and how the information will be shared between providers.

We should also outline the time frame for the interview and physical exam, indicating the steps that will be followed, and ask the woman if she has time constraints (i.e., has to get back to work or to her children) or can stay for the anticipated time period. If the appointment times are running late or the visit will take longer than the woman expected, we must reconfigure the appointment or arrange for her to leave after a portion and return at a later date. Unless we address her time constraints, the woman may answer questions in a way that is only intended to make the visit move more rapidly.

### Identifying Data

The hardest part of an interview is getting started. A question like, "I would like to start by asking you some general questions about yourself; could you please give me the correct spelling of your full name?" (Barkauskas and others, 1998) may break the ice.

The **introductory section** of a health history includes the date and time for the health visit and identifies who conducted the interview. Information that identifies the woman, including her legal name, the name she prefers to be called, her age and date of birth, as well as her complete address and the community where she resides, is used for both identification purposes and a beginning assessment of her life events. The information about supportive persons and dependents and where and when the woman works (if she works outside the home) helps us to understand the woman within the context of her life and also alerts us to some of the possible issues that she confronts daily.

The source of this information (i.e., if it comes from the woman or from another source) must be documented because, if the woman is unable or unwilling to speak for herself, the validity and reliability of the data from another source must be evaluated. The information may have come from a partner, a family member, an interpreter, or another provider's notes (Box 4-11).

### Reason for Seeking Care

The reason that the woman came in today—not yesterday and did not wait until tomorrow—is sometimes identified as her **chief complaint.** Opening questions might be as follows, "What is it we can help you with today?," "Do you have any symptoms that are troubling you that I can help you with?," or "Can I help you with anything in particular today?" Such questions encourage her to share her concerns so that collaboration can begin.

We record the reason for her visit in her own terms (e.g., "I am really worried about this lump I found in my breast yesterday," "I am just so tired all of the time since my baby was born," or "I hadn't had a Pap smear in 5 years and I figured I was due") (Box 4-12). With this information, we can focus the interview on the chief complaint that appears to be of primary importance to her. Because these are her stated reasons for initiating the health partnership, they are then clarified, validated, and addressed.

Be aware that sometimes what is identified as the "chief complaint" by the woman when making the

---

**BOX 4-10**   *Components of a Woman's Health History*

1. Data identification
2. Reason for visit or chief complaint
3. Current health status or illness
4. Past medical history
5. Personal health information
6. Family health history
7. Psychosocial history
8. Review of systems
9. Developmental assessment
10. Family assessment
11. Stress/risk assessment
12. Occupational assessment
13. Nutritional assessment

---

**BOX 4-11**   *Identifying Data*

**IDENTIFYING DATA**

**Setting Information**
Interviewer
Date/time

**Biographic Information**
Woman's full name (nickname or personalizing name)
Supportive others
Dependents
Birth date
Social security number
Current address
Permanent address
Telephone numbers (e.g., home, work, other contacts)

**Source of Information**
Client
Parents
Interpreter
Others (e.g., family, friends)

appointment or while starting the interview may become less important as the interview progresses. As the woman becomes more comfortable, she may reveal that something else is bothering her. She may have felt too embarrassed to tell the unknown stranger on the phone or was not sure how we would respond if she mentioned it in the beginning. As the interview continues, a chief complaint of a sore throat—which is socially acceptable—can become secondary to a request for a pregnancy test. Understanding such changes in focus and supporting the woman as she reveals additional concerns show her that we value her concerns and that she can trust us.

### Current Health Status or Illness

During this part of the health history, the woman is asked to give details about what she is experiencing. Describing her **current health status,** or **present concern,** allows the woman to express in her own words any alterations in health or symptoms of illness that she is experiencing.

We should listen carefully to her story of the symptoms she is experiencing, because they may provide a focus to the physical examination and its findings. Encourage her to describe the symptoms that are troubling her and provide information about their onset and characteristics.

Ask what she has done to treat the condition or feel more comfortable. Most people respond to a pain or discomfort by changing their level of activity or "taking something for it." The woman may take aspirin for a headache or sit down and put her feet up because her ankles are swollen. Another type of self-care measure might be a traditional remedy, herbal medication, over-the-counter drug, prescription left from a prior episode that was similar, or a drug that worked for a friend.

Alternative and complementary therapies can be loosely defined as those alternative health practices that are not readily used or prescribed in conventional Western medicine. At least one third of the population in the United States currently uses alternative or complementary therapies, and that number is rising (Tiedje, 1998). As providers, we need to be concerned because 70% of those incorporating alternative practices into their health care do not consider discussing their alternative treatments with us—their traditional Western medical care providers (National Women's Health Resource Center, 1998). We must ask directly about the use of herbs in teas, tinctures, or capsules and other culturally based interventions—but not to criticize the woman for using them. They can be a viable part of a self-care plan. The information about use is important to reduce the risk for

---

**BOX 4-12** *Reason for Visit (or Chief Complaint)*

**REASON FOR VISIT**
Use her exact words.
When does it affect her?
Why did she come for care today?

---

**BOX 4-13** *Current Health Status or Present Illness*

**CURRENT HEALTH STATUS OR PRESENT ILLNESS**

***Symptom Analysis***
*Onset of symptoms (i.e., date, gradual or sudden, duration)*
*Causes, precipitating factors, or factors associated with symptom*
Factors that improve symptom
Factors that worsen symptom
*Description of symptoms*
Location
Quality
Quantity
Effect on life roles (e.g., family, home, work, play)

***Gynecologic History****
Menstrual characteristics
*Onset of menarche*
*Last menstrual period (menses)*

*Menstrual experience (i.e., frequency, duration, amount of bleeding)*
*Occurrence of midcycle bleeding*
Menopause
  Date of last menses
  Desire for hormone supplementation therapy (i.e., hormone replacement therapy [HRT])
Sexual concerns
Sexual preference
Partner information
Desire for contraception

***Obstetric Information***
*Gravida (times pregnant)*
*Para (e.g., full-term, pre-term, spontaneous or induced abortions)*
*Childbirth experience (e.g., vaginal, cesarean, complications)*

*Unless the woman brings up the topic, some or all of the following questions may be delayed until later in the interview when she is more comfortable with the interviewer and surroundings.

potential harm from a drug interaction with medication the woman might be given as a result of this visit.

We must also determine how the symptoms the woman is experiencing have affected her ability to cope with the daily events in her life. A reported change in her activities of daily living is an important finding of her assessment.

Part of a woman's health history also includes her gynecologic history, which includes at what age her menses started (menarche), the date of her last menstrual period (LMP), and if she has stopped ovulating and menstruating (menopause) or has concerns about the expression of her sexuality. These areas may be explored now if that is the focus of the woman's chief complaint or delayed until later in the interview when she may be more comfortable with us and the interview process (Box 4-13).

## Past Medical History

Prior experiences with **health problems** and crisis events influence a woman's current health state. Ask the woman about other health conditions that are ongoing (e.g., asthma, diabetes, hypertension) or health problems that she has been treated for in the past. Most facilities have a form listing the conditions most commonly occurring in people living in the community that we can show or read to the woman. If the woman is receiving treatment for other problems at the time of the interview, the question "Are you currently taking any kind of medication?" may help her remember to identify other health-related problems.

We should also ask about both childhood and adult events of injury or trauma. If the woman has mental health concerns—either from the past or that are ongoing—she may share it at this time. Recognizing that violence can be associated with injuries, hospitalizations, and disruptions in mental health for the woman, we might also ask about the presence of violence in her life if she gives an indication of this type of problem. Otherwise, questions about violence will be asked later when the woman is more comfortable (Box 4-14).

Based on the answers the woman provides to some of the questions in this category, we may identify that she is at risk for certain conditions. Share recommended primary prevention interventions and secondary prevention screening initiatives with her. By integrating teaching into the taking of the health history, we make the process more interactive, offering information to the woman as we recognize a need for it. Sometimes only preliminary information can be given during the interview, but further discussion and/or written materials should be shared with the woman before she leaves (Table 4-4).

Due to their age, activities, and developmental status, adolescent females are at risk and require screening for certain conditions. More accurate answers may be given if the adolescent understands what will and will not be shared with adults in her family. For an adolescent who is participating in sexual activity, the questions asked of adult women must also be included. Depending on the status of the adolescent, prevention services and/or referrals for care often depend on the action of an adult in her life. For example, few adolescents can access dental care (Table 4-5).

## Family History

This section focuses primarily on the woman's **family history of medical diseases** and allows her to consider her risk for certain kinds of health problems. We should also use this part of the interview to interpret how the woman views her current health situation with relation to her family's overall health experience. The presence of significant illnesses in her family could affect both her emotional and physical health as she copes with her own anxiety, as well as with her family members' needs for care. In

---

**BOX 4-14** *Past Medical History*

**PAST MEDICAL HISTORY**

**Other Health Problems**
Chronic illnesses
Current medications

**Allergies**

**Childhood Diseases and Immunizations**

**Previous Illnesses and Surgeries**
Dates
Treatments
Outcomes

**Previous Hospitalizations**
Dates
Reasons

**Accidents or Injuries**
Precipitating event
Any resultant disability
Outcomes (i.e., counseling, treatment)

**Risk Behaviors**
Sedentary lifestyle
Caffeine use
Cigarette smoking
Alcohol
Drugs (i.e., over-the-counter or prescription)
Unsafe sexual practices

**History of Violence/Abuse**
Assault injuries
Rape experience
Outcomes (i.e., infection, pregnancy, counseling, treatment)

## TABLE 4-4    Examples of Risk Factor Categories Identified with Medical History

| Risk Factor | Prevention Target Condition | Prevention Service and/or Referral |
|---|---|---|
| Obesity | Coronary heart disease | Obesity screening |
| | Hypertension | Blood pressure screening |
| | | Cholesterol screening |
| | | Nutritional screening |
| | | Exercise counseling |
| | Diabetes | Fasting glucose |
| Radiation exposure to head and neck during infancy or childhood | Thyroid cancer | Palpation of thyroid |
| | Hypothyroidism | Thyroid function tests |
| Down syndrome | | |
| History of dysplastic congenital nevi | Skin cancer | Avoidance of sun exposure between 10:00 AM and 3:00 PM |
| History of immunosuppression | | |
| History of severe sunburn in childhood | | Protective clothing, sunscreen |
| Poor tanning ability (i.e., light skin, hair, or eyes; freckles) | | Consider dermatology referral for those at high risk |
| Depression | Suicidal ideation | Question regarding preparatory actions |
| | | Mental health counseling referral |
| Diabetes mellitus | Influenza | Influenza vaccine |
| | Pneumococcal disease | Pneumococcal vaccine |
| | Early retinopathy and glaucoma | Referral for screening |
| | Early nephropathy | Urine screening for microalbuminuria |
| | Coronary heart disease | Obesity screening |
| | | Blood pressure screening |
| | | Cholesterol screening |
| | | Nutrition counseling |
| | | Exercise counseling |
| | | Smoking cessation counseling |
| Ulcerative colitis, duration >10 years | Colorectal cancer | Referral for colonoscopy |

Adopted from Table A.7 Risk Factor Category: Personal Medical History—All Ages. U.S. Department of Health and Human Services, Public Health Service, Office of Public Health and Science, Office of Disease Prevention and Promotion: *Clinician's handbook of preventative services,* ed 2, Washington, D.C., 1998, U.S. Government Printing Office.

## TABLE 4-5    Examples of Risk Factor Categories for Adolescents

| Risk Factor | Prevention Target Condition | Prevention Service and/or Referral |
|---|---|---|
| Adolescence | Dental hygiene | Counseling regarding daily care |
| | | Counseling regarding regular dental examinations |
| | Hypertension | Blood pressure screening |
| | | Exercise counseling |
| | | Nutritional counseling |
| | Obesity, malnutrition | Obesity screening |
| | | Exercise counseling |
| | | Nutritional counseling |
| | Scoliosis | Visual inspection following state guidelines |
| | Tobacco-related complications | Counseling regarding tobacco use (e.g., cigarettes, cigars, and chew) |
| | Unintentional injury | Counseling regarding use of seat belts; use of appropriate safety equipment when participating in activities |
| | Intentional injuries | Counseling regarding protection of self from injury from others either inside or outside the family |

taking the family history, it is useful for both the woman and the interviewer to construct a personalized genogram. (See Chapter 2 for details on constructing a genogram.)

Do not be surprised if the woman says, "No, no, no . . ." as you ask about each condition, then later says, "Oh yeah, my grandmother had diabetes." Illnesses and conditions within the family are often such common knowledge they are easily forgotten until each family member is thought of individually. We should also be aware that a negative response does not mean that a condition is nonexistent. A woman may not be aware of the health conditions of some family members—either because they were never diagnosed or the family member never shared the information (Box 4-15).

We should consider not only the woman's risk for hereditary diseases but also that for any potential or actual offspring. In families that experience inherited disease, it can create a high level of anxiety among family members who worry about having the same problem (e.g., a young woman with breast pain thinks about her mother's death from breast cancer, or a woman with numbness in her fingers thinks about her sister who has multiple sclerosis). If the disorder does not have a familial tendency, you can reassure the woman that she is at no greater risk than anyone else. If the condition is something with a familial tendency, then it is relevant to share recommended primary prevention interventions and secondary prevention screening initiatives with her (Table 4-6).

---

## BOX 4-15  Family History

### FAMILY HISTORY

**Hereditary Diseases**
Anemias (e.g., thalassemia, sickle cell)
Genetic disorders (e.g., Down syndrome, Huntington's chorea)

**Acute and Chronic Familial Illnesses**
Cardiac disease
Cancer (e.g., breast, colon)
Diabetes

**Mental Illnesses**
Types of health problems (e.g., mood disorders, alcoholism)
Effect on family functioning

**Current Illnesses in Family**
Communicable diseases (e.g., HIV, tuberculosis)
Other health problems (e.g., cancer, cardiac problems)
Caregiver stress

**Family Genogram**
Family tree over 3 generations
Living and deceased family members
Types of health problems

---

## TABLE 4-6  Risk Factor Categories Identified with Family History

| Risk Factor | Prevention Target Condition | Preventive Service and/or Referral |
|---|---|---|
| Diabetes mellitus | Diabetes mellitus and subsequent complications | Fasting glucose<br>Obesity screening<br>Nutritional counseling<br>Exercise counseling |
| Glaucoma | Glaucoma | Referral for screening |
| Hereditary childhood sensorineural hearing loss | Hearing impairment | Refer for auditory brainstem response or otoacoustic emission testing |
| Breast cancer | Breast cancer | Clinical breast examination<br>Mammography |
| Hereditary polyposis or hereditary non-polyposis colorectal cancer | Colorectal cancer | Referral for colonoscopy |
| Colorectal cancer prior to age 50 | Colorectal cancer (patients aged 40 to 60 years) | Fecal occult blood testing<br>Sigmoidoscopy |
| Ovarian cancer, especially ovarian cancer syndrome (HCS) | Ovarian cancer | Ultrasound<br>Pelvic exam<br>CA-125 measurement |
| Skin cancer (e.g., familial atypical moles, melanoma) | Skin cancer | Consider dermatology referral for those at highest risk |

Adopted from Table A.8 Risk Factor Category: Family Medical History—All Ages. U.S. Department of Health and Human Services, Public Health Service, Office of Public Health and Science, Office of Disease Prevention and Promotion: *Clinician's handbook of preventative services*, ed 2, Washington, D.C., 1998, U.S. Government Printing Office.

## Psychosocial History

Although it is not necessarily easy to construct, the **psychosocial history** is important as it includes many facets of a woman's family role, work, education, recreation, and cultural interests. This part of the health history can be very interesting as you encourage the woman to share the colorful and unique story of herself in her world. She is invited to describe her family of origin, as well as her current network of family and friends. One valuable approach is to request that the woman describe a "typical day" or relate meaningful events in her life over recent days and weeks. Another approach is to ask her what she had to do to arrange to make it to the scheduled appointment.

This area in the health assessment usually reveals the essential personal and social facets of a woman's life that affect her well-being. With this information, we can examine with the woman the mechanisms of social support and daily coping that may be supportive to her.

The woman may also share her spiritual base and participation in organized religion. When asking about these areas, we should be sure to differentiate between spirituality and religion because they are not necessarily synonymous. **Spirituality** is "the core of one's being; a sense of personhood; what one is and what one is becoming. [It is] concerned with bringing meaning and purpose to one's existence; what or who one ought to live for" (Carson, 1989). Every person—whether religious, atheist, or humanist—has a dimension of spirituality. This sense of inner being is the basis of many of a woman's decisions. A **religious framework** is a system of belief, worship, or conduct that may be followed to help satisfy a person's spiritual needs. A woman may identify that she follows the practices of a specific religious denomination, which is important to know because some religions place restrictions on their members (e.g., the Roman Catholic Church does not support the use of contraception).

It is difficult to gather extensive psychosocial data about a woman's world, considering staffing and time constraints within current health care settings. The sensitive nature of some of the information also requires that a relationship be developed before the information is shared by the woman, if ever. Especially if she is visiting a new provider or the interviewer is a novice, the woman may not be ready to discuss some personal issues of her life (e.g., mental illness or domestic violence). Interviewers often find that crucial subjective findings are unveiled with the physical exam or at the end of a session, once rapport and trust are better established (Box 4-16 and Table 4-7).

## Sexual History

Questions about her reproductive and sexual history may occur whenever the woman raises a question in this area or as the final part of the review of systems. Because these are very direct questions about such personal topics, both the woman and the interviewer may be uncomfortable. The comfort level of the woman will increase in proportion to the comfort level of the interviewer.

State the purpose of asking questions about her sexual history and activities; for example: "I have asked you a number of questions about your lifestyle in order to identify areas in which you would like me to provide assistance. Your sexual activity is part of your lifestyle. How satisfied are you with your sexual activity? What

---

### BOX 4-16 *Psychosocial History*

**PSYCHOSOCIAL HISTORY**

***Culture/Ethnicity***
Birthplace
Race
Culture or ethnicity

***Relationships/Friendships***
Living arrangements
Support persons

***Education***
Last grade completed
Continuing education

***Occupation***
Current employment arrangements
Job security/economic aspects
Job satisfaction
Effects on health

***Risk for Domestic Violence***
Ask the woman directly:
- Do you feel safe in your home?
- Has anyone threatened to physically harm you?
- Has anyone hurt you?
- Have you been forced to have sex against your will?
- How can we help you be safe?

***Individual Coping***
Self-awareness and self-esteem
Stress management
Substance use (e.g., alcohol, smoking, drugs)

***Health Maintenance***
Use of traditional or complementary health strategies
Use of health care system

***Health Patterns***
Nutrition
Sleep hygiene
Activity and exercise
Recreation

***Spiritual Strengths***
Religion
Spiritual care practices

## TABLE 4-7    Examples of Risk Factors Identified with Psychosocial History

| Risk Factor | Prevention Target Condition | Prevention Service and/or Referral |
|---|---|---|
| **CULTURE/ETHNICITY** | | |
| African-American, Hispanic, Pacific Islander | Tuberculosis | PPD |
| Native American, Hispanic, African-American | Diabetes mellitus | Fasting glucose |
| | | Obesity screening |
| | | Nutritional counseling |
| | | Exercise counseling |
| Immigrants from areas with a high prevalence of tuberculosis, hepatitis B, or HIV (i.e., most countries in Africa, Asia, or Latin America) | Tuberculosis | PPD |
| | Hepatitis B | Hepatitis B vaccine |
| | STI/HIV | STI/HIV counseling |
| | | STI/HIV screening |
| African-American | Glaucoma (≥40 years of age) | Ophthalmology referral |
| Asian Indians who use chewing tobacco or betel nut | Oral cancer | Oral exam |
| | | Cessation counseling |
| | | Regular dental examinations |
| **OCCUPATIONAL AND RECREATIONAL** | | |
| Health care workers | Tuberculosis | PPD |
| | Hepatitis B | Hepatitis B vaccine |
| | Influenza | Influenza vaccine |
| Multiple sex partners; commercial sex workers; illicit drug use | Hepatitis B | Hepatitis B vaccine |
| | Hepatitis C | Hepatitis C vaccine |
| | STI/HIV | Gonorrhea and chlamydia screening |
| | Pelvic inflammatory disease | RPR for syphilis |
| | Chronic pelvic pain | HIV serology |
| | Unintended pregnancy | STI/HIV counseling |
| | Ectopic pregnancy | Unintended pregnancy counseling |
| | Infertility | |
| Employed in dye, leather, tire, or rubber industry | Bladder cancer | Smoking cessation counseling |
| Exposure to dusts and fumes related to work in welding, construction, shipyards, or foundry | Respiratory problems | Smoking cessation counseling |
| | | Counseling on use of personal protective equipment |
| Lead exposure related to work or hobby (e.g., radiator repair, metal worker, construction, bridge painting, shooting gallery) | Lead poisoning | Blood lead level |
| | | Occupational/residential lead hazard control |
| Exposure to excessive noise related to work or hobby (e.g., construction, maintenance, manufacturing, aerospace, musicians) | Hearing impairment | Refer to work site program for audiogram |
| | | Counsel on use of personal protective equipment |
| **SOCIAL CIRCUMSTANCES AND LIVING CONDITIONS** | | |
| Low-income household or community | Tuberculosis | PPD |
| Institutionalized persons (e.g., persons living in correctional facilities or chronic care facilities) | Tuberculosis | PPD |
| | Hepatitis B | Hepatitis B vaccine |
| | Influenza | Influenza vaccine |
| | Pneumococcal disease | Pneumococcal vaccine |
| Homeless | Tuberculosis | PPD |
| | Hepatitis B | Hepatitis B vaccine |
| | Influenza | Influenza vaccine |
| | Pneumococcal disease | Pneumococcal vaccine |
| Resident of American Indian reservation or Native Alaskan community | Tuberculosis | PPD |
| | Hepatitis B | Hepatitis B vaccine |
| | Hepatitis A | Hepatitis A vaccine |
| | Influenza | Influenza vaccine |
| | Pneumococcal disease | Pneumococcal vaccine |

*Continued*

**TABLE 4-7**   *Examples of Risk Factors Identified with Psychosocial History—cont'd*

| Risk Factor | Prevention Target Condition | Prevention Service and/or Referral |
|---|---|---|
| **SOCIAL CIRCUMSTANCES AND LIVING CONDITIONS—cont'd** | | |
| Settings where large numbers of young adults congregate (e.g., colleges, military bases, health care settings) | Rubella | Rubella vaccine |
| Recent divorce or separation; unemployment; bereavement | Depression | Referral for mental health counseling |
| **SUBSTANCE ABUSE** | | |
| Use of tobacco products | Lung cancer | Smoking cessation counseling |
|  | Oral cancer | |
|  | Chronic obstructive pulmonary disease | |
|  | Asthma | |
|  | Coronary heart disease | Obesity screening |
|  | Stroke | Blood pressure screening |
| Excessive alcohol use | | Cholesterol screening |
|  | | Nutritional counseling |
|  | | Exercise counseling |
|  | | Alcohol counseling and referrals |
|  | Injuries and violence | Injury and violence counseling |
|  | STI/HIV | STI/HIV counseling |
|  | | STI/HIV screening |
|  | Tuberculosis | PPD |
| Illicit drug use, especially intravenous | Liver disease | Hepatitis B vaccine |
|  | Cardiomyopathy | |
|  | Malnutrition | Nutrition counseling |
|  | | Consider also influenza vaccine and pneumococcal vaccine |
|  | | Drug counseling and referrals |
|  | Tuberculosis | PPD |
|  | STI/HIV | STI/HIV counseling |
|  | | STI/HIV screening |
|  | Hepatitis B | Hepatitis B vaccine |
|  | Hepatitis C | |
|  | Malnutrition | Nutrition counseling |
|  | Depression | Assess for depression |
|  | Suicide | Question regarding preparatory actions |
|  | | Mental health counseling referral |

Adopted from Tables A.3 Risk Factor Category: Social Circumstances and Living Conditions—All Ages; A.4 Risk Factor Category: Geographic and Ethnic Background—All Ages; A.5 Risk Factor Category: Occupational, Recreational, Residential and Environmental Exposure—All Ages; and A.6 Risk Factor Category: Substance Abuse. U.S. Department of Health and Human Services, Public Health Service, Office of Public Health and Science, Office of Disease Prevention and Promotion: *Clinician's handbook of preventative services*, ed 2, Washington, D.C., 1998, U.S. Government Printing Office.

concerns or questions do you have about sex? How many different sexual partners have you had? Do you have sex with men, women, or both? Do you or one of your partners use intravenous drugs? Does your partner have other partners?"

If the woman is experiencing difficulties, you might ask, "Has your pleasure from sex changed? Why do you think this is? How would you or your partner like it to be different? How have you tried to change the situation? Have you participated in any sexual activity that makes you uncomfortable?" (Table 4-8).

### Review of Systems

During the **review of systems,** we ask about problems a woman may have experienced in each of the main body systems. This line of questioning provides a way to direct a woman's thoughts to each segment of her bodily functions. Such a subjective review of systems may be asked as part of the health history or included while the examiner conducts the objective physical examination (Box 4-17).

The review of systems begins with a general overview and then proceeds with questions about past and present problems that may have occurred in each body system.

TABLE 4-8  *Risk Based on Sexual History—Adolescent and Adult Females*

| Risk Factor | Prevention Target Condition | Prevention Service and/or Referral |
| --- | --- | --- |
| Multiple sex partners<br>Prior STI | Hepatitis B<br>STI/HIV<br>Pelvic inflammatory disease<br>Chronic pelvic pain<br>Ectopic pregnancy<br>Infertility<br>Unintended pregnancy | Hepatitis B vaccine<br>STI/HIV prevention and screening<br><br><br><br><br>Unintended pregnancy counseling<br>Substance abuse counseling |
| Ever sexually active | Cervical cancer | Papanicolaou smear |

Adopted from Table A.2 Risk Factor Category: Age and Gender Profile and Table A.10 Risk Factor Category: Sexual History—Adolescent and Adult Females. U.S. Department of Health and Human Services, Public Health Service, Office of Public Health and Science, Office of Disease Prevention and Promotion: *Clinician's handbook of preventative services*, ed 2, Washington, D.C., 1998, U.S. Government Printing Office.

We generally want to learn about the woman's general health, fatigue, exercise tolerance, episodes of unusual weight loss or gain, interest in life, and ability to fulfill her activities of daily living. Can she do everything she expects of herself? Can she fulfill the roles she has taken on with regard to the care of others? Is this because too much is expected of her or because she is unhealthy?

Her psychologic status may range from anxious or irritable to the more lethal problems of suicidal or homicidal thoughts. Based on your observations and the woman's comments, we review her psychologic status with her. "It seems like you are depressed. How does it feel to you?"

Fatigue may be brought on by illness or lack of sleep from a variety of causes. Explore with the woman if she is having difficulty sleeping. Identify if she has experienced a change in medications, alcohol, substance abuse; the onset of an illness; or a lifestyle change before the onset of the difficulties? Determine with her if a change in the time, place, or position of her sleep is possible or would be helpful. Work with the woman to do some preliminary problem solving. Determine if there are times during the day when she may take short rests or have some conscious relaxation or a nap. If her fatigue persists with an unknown cause, a sleep study assessment may provide a better understanding of her actual stages of sleep (Sims and others, 1995).

After the general review is complete, we then ask specific questions about each system. It is customary to move from the top to the bottom of the body, while simultaneously considering the woman's broad concerns and specific complaints. The systems to consider are as follows: integumentary, musculoskeletal, head and neck, eyes, ears, endocrine, neurologic, cardiovascular, pulmonary, gastrointestinal, genitourinary, and reproductive. See Box 4-17 for a review of systems for a guide on how to start to investigate each system with the woman.

Begin with a general question associated with the body system and then seek details about signs or symptoms mentioned with more direct, focused questions. A

client may remember significant factors while answering these questions.

Anticipate that some questions may illicit more emotionally laden responses than others. A woman's skin, hair, and nails are major components of how she presents herself to others and in some cultures determine her value as a woman, so she may be very sensitive to what she perceives as deficits. We must be sensitive in how we ask the questions and our verbal and nonverbal responses. What might seem insignificant to us may be of great significance to the woman.

A woman's daily activities and expectations of her own physical performance determine how she evaluates her musculoskeletal system. Any recent changes in her level of activity should be investigated for a possible cause of pain.

The region of the head and neck requires a major portion of the time allotted for this part of the history. Ask about the head (skull) and the neck that supports and moves it. Ask if the woman experiences headaches. Have her describe the affected areas, the factors she experiences before the onset of a headache, how long a headache lasts, and how she treats it. Then ask about each of the prominent features located in the head: the eyes, nose, mouth, and ears.

Changes that may occur in the endocrine system are less obvious. With questioning, the woman may reveal signs and symptoms that indicate that the endocrine system is not functioning correctly. Her report of a change in shoe size or in her skin or hair texture can be helpful in this assessment.

Our assessment of her neurologic system started when the woman first responded to her name, stood, and walked toward us. The questions in this part of the general survey focus on limitations that the woman may have noticed about herself or that others have pointed out to her. If she reports a loss of memory (e.g., "I keep losing my keys," or "I can't remember anything anymore"), learn more details. How often? In what circumstances? Is she overwhelmed with other concerns?

## BOX 4-17 *Review of Systems*

When performing a review of systems, ask the woman about each of the following areas, obtaining both a past and current history of each system. Explore each positive response in more detail (e.g., date of occurrence, treatment, outcome, and any other relevant data). Remember that this line of questioning is used to stimulate the woman's memory, so provide enough time for her to think and answer.

### A. GENERAL

Perception of health, level of fatigue, exercise tolerance, and unusual weight gain or loss; despair or depression

Ability to carry out activities of daily living, fulfill expected roles

Sense of anxiety or irritability, apathy, mood swings, depression, sleep disturbances, appetite disturbances, suicidal or homicidal thoughts

### B. INTEGUMENTARY SYSTEM

Skin lesions or discolorations; easy bruising; itching or flaking; changes in skin texture, moisture, color, or temperature

Hair breakage or loss; rapid color change

Nail breakage or discoloration

### C. MUSCULOSKELETAL SYSTEM

Movement limitations, range of motion, ease of walking

Tendon, ligament, or muscle strain or pain

Muscle weakness or strength, muscle cramping

Joint stiffness, swelling, or pain

Backaches or pains

Experience with fractures or other injuries

### D. HEAD AND NECK

Head injuries and treatment; headaches (description of occurrence)

Neck stiffness or pain, loss of range of motion, enlarged nodes

Ability to smell; breathing difficulties and treatments; nosebleeds; nasal congestion, discharge, and infections

Mouth lesions, condition of teeth (any loose or missing) and date of last examination, ability to perform routine care, bleeding gums

Sore throat or hoarseness, change in voice; problems with chewing, swallowing, or taste

Date of last vision exam, change in vision, use of corrective lenses, redness of eyes, discharge

Date of last hearing exam, change in hearing, loss of hearing, ringing, vertigo, infection, discharge

### E. ENDOCRINE SYSTEM

Changes in height, weight, glove, or shoe size

Excessive thirst, hunger, or urination; intolerance of heat or cold; weakness or fatigue; excessive sweating

Changes in skin or hair (e.g., loss, excessive growth, change in texture)

### F. NEUROLOGIC SYSTEM

Loss of coordination; weakness; numbness; tremors; paralysis

Cognitive changes with loss of memory

Fainting spells, blackouts, or seizures

Loss of judgement; mood swings or hallucinations

### G. CARDIOVASCULAR SYSTEM

Chest pain or palpitations; "blue" lips or fingers; swollen or tingly fingers; shortness of breath when lying flat; excessive urination at night; varicose veins; limb pain when exercising

Diagnosed with high blood pressure (hypertension), heart murmur, bruits, irregular heartbeat, or rheumatic fever

Blood type and Rh factor; prior diagnosis of anemia; bleeding tendencies; transfusions

Date and results of last cholesterol and lipid screening

### H. PULMONARY SYSTEM

History of tobacco use

Date of last chest radiograph and results; date of last tuberculosis (TB) test and results

Difficulty breathing; wheezing, shortness of breath, or pain when breathing; amount of sputum, bloody sputum

Diagnosed with asthma (type), bronchitis, pneumonia, TB, emphysema

### I. GASTROINTESTINAL SYSTEM

Heartburn, food intolerances, loss of appetite, pain when swallowing, belching, indigestion, nausea, vomiting, reflux, use of antacids

Abdominal pain; distention; changes in stool color, consistency, or frequency; fecal incontinence; hemorrhoids; use of laxatives

### J. GENITOURINARY SYSTEM

Changes in urine or urination; sensation of urgency; incontinence any time or when coughing or sneezing; frequent need to urinate, urge to urinate, disturbing sleep

Pain upon urination; pain in flank, blood in urine

Prior diagnosis of cystitis or pyelonephritis

From Mosby: *Expert 10-minute physical examinations,* St Louis, 1997, Mosby; Youngkin and Davis: *Women's health: a primary care clinical guide,* Stamford, CT, 1998, Appleton and Lange).

---

**BOX 4-17**   *Review of Systems—cont'd*

---

**K. FEMALE REPRODUCTIVE SYSTEM**

Breast self-exam; changes in breasts during menstrual cycle; date of last clinical breast exam and findings

Date of last mammogram (if age appropriate)

Pain or discharge

Date of last menstrual period and frequency, duration, and amount of flow; age menses started, experience in week before monthly menses; tampon or pad use, and number used per day; medications for pain; treatment used if pain during menses

Date of last pelvic exam and Pap smear, results and follow-up; vaginal discomfort or discharge; protection from sexually transmitted infections; method of contraception used in past; current need for contraception; sexual satisfaction (this may be an especially difficult area for a woman to discuss)

---

Women often believe that cardiac problems happen only to men. Remind her that cardiac disease is the top killer of women. Help her evaluate her cardiac risk and learn how to prevent cardiac disease. This is an area of ongoing research especially with regard to the signs of a heart attack and the role of cholesterol and lipids in a woman.

With the increase of adult-onset asthma and lung cancer in women, the pulmonary system review is also vital. Tuberculosis is also on the rise within both developed and undeveloped countries. Questions about shortness of breath, breathing difficulties, and sputum are necessary.

Gastrointestinal problems are difficult to evaluate. Questioning during the general survey will start to reveal if the woman is having any difficulties. Generally forms do not ask specifically if the woman is experiencing anorexia or bulimia, so be alert and ask about these.

The review of the genitourinary system is relatively simple but not without challenge. A woman may be very conscious of how often she has the urge to urinate but not report it because she thinks it is normal. She may say, "But I've had three kids so that is to be expected." Teach her that this is not necessarily the case. An infection in her genitourinary system can cause pain in one of several different sites. Pain with urination may be more familiar to the woman, and she may report it more quickly than pain in her flank. Further assessment may reveal a cause for the pain that can be treated.

Changes in comfort with sexual stimulation and activity, as well as discomfort, discharge, or pain, may also be revealed at this time.

## Special Assessments

### Developmental Assessment

**Growth and development** do not just occur in children but continue throughout our lives. The process is both universal, in that everyone goes through it, and unique, in that every individual progresses differently. All aspects of our growth and development are interrelated because the physical, mental, social, emotional, sexual, moral, and spiritual components come together to create the whole individual.

Because of the complexity of development we cannot learn everything about a client's developmental accomplishment during one interview. A complete assessment is accomplished over time as the woman gradually reveals more about herself.

Help a woman understand her own development by first having her review her past and then compare it with the present. Then explore her expectations and plans for the future. Ask about her thoughts and feelings about her family, work, and other activities. Record the assessment data the woman has reported to you in a brief, descriptive paragraph.

If a more focused or in-depth assessment is necessary, there are specific tools developed to assess the client's perception of various aspects of adult change. The recent life changes questionnaire and the life experiences survey are two commonly used tools. Both are used to try to determine the recent experiences in a client's life and her or his view of these events (Sarason and others, 1978) (Box 4-18 and Table 4-9). After a woman has completed these tools, review the findings with her.

### Family Assessment

A woman may live alone or with one or more people. Who a woman lives with, her relationship with the household members, the ethnicity and religious preference of the household members, the role each family member fulfills, the goals of the family, and the health practices followed are important to learn. Each family will have strengths and weaknesses and a pattern of conflict development and resolution. The Family APGAR is a quick screening tool that may identify areas where the woman is not satisfied with her interactions with family members and indicate possible family difficulties. This tool looks at the areas of **A**daptation, **P**artnership, **G**rowth, **A**ffection, and **R**esolve within the family and the members' perceptions of satisfaction (Barkauskas and others, 1998) (Box 4-19, page 129).

For a more in-depth assessment, the McMaster Family Assessment Device (FAD) may be used. This device investigates the six family functioning areas of problem solving, communication, roles, affective

## BOX 4-18 *Recent Life Changes Questionnaire*

We all experience life changes events. These changes may be in five major categories: health, work, home and family, personal-social, and financial events. Read the list of life changes below and place a check (✓) next to those that you have experienced during the past year.

| LIFE CHANGES | ✔ | (1–100) | LIFE CHANGES (cont.) | ✔ | (1–100) |
|---|---|---|---|---|---|
| **A. HEALTH**—Within the past year have you experienced: | | | 19. The death of a: | | |
| 1. An illness or injury that: | | |    (a) Child? | | |
|    (a) Kept you in bed a week or more, or took you to the hospital? | | |    (b) Brother or sister? | | |
|    (b) Was less serious than described above? | | |    (c) Parent? | | |
| 2. A major change in eating habits? | | |    (d) Other close family member? | | |
| 3. A major change in sleeping habits? | | | 20. The death of a close friend? | | |
| 4. A major change in your usual type or amount of recreation? | | | 21. A change in marital/relationship status of your parents: | | |
| 5. Major dental work? | | |    (a) Divorce? | | |
| | | |    (b) Remarriage? | | |
| **B. WORK**—Within the past year have you: | | | 22. Marriage? | | |
| 6. Changed to a new type of work? | | | (Note: Questions 23 to 33 concern marriage or committed relationships. If this does not apply to you, go to item 34.) | | |
| 7. Changed your work hours or conditions? | | | 23. A change in arguments with your partner? | | |
| 8. Had a change in your responsibilities at work: | | | 24. In-law problems? | | |
|    (a) More responsibilities? | | | 25. A separation from partner: | | |
|    (b) Less responsibilities? | | |    (a) Due to work? | | |
|    (c) Promotion? | | |    (b) Due to relationship problems? | | |
|    (d) Demotion? | | | 26. A reconciliation with partner? | | |
|    (e) Transfer? | | | 27. A divorce? | | |
| 9. Experienced troubles at work: | | | 28. A gain of a new family member? | | |
|    (a) With your boss? | | |    (a) Birth of a child? | | |
|    (b) With co-workers? | | |    (b) Adoption of a child? | | |
|    (c) With persons under your supervision? | | |    (c) A relative moving in with you? | | |
|    (d) Other work troubles? | | | 29. Partner beginning or ceasing work outside the home? | | |
| 10. Experienced a major business readjustment? | | | 30. Wife/partner becoming pregnant? | | |
| 11. Retired? | | | 31. A child leaving home: | | |
| 12. Experienced being: | | |    (a) Due to marriage? | | |
|    (a) Fired from work? | | |    (b) To attend college? | | |
|    (b) Laid off from work? | | |    (c) For other reasons? | | |
| 13. Taken courses by mail or studied at home to help you in your work? | | | 32. Wife/partner having a miscarriage or abortion? | | |
| **C. HOME AND FAMILY**—Within the past year, have you experienced: | | | 33. Birth of a grandchild? | | |
| 14. A change in residence: | | | **D. PERSONAL AND SOCIAL**—Within the past year, have you experienced: | | |
|    (a) A move within the same town or city? | | | 34. A major personal achievement? | | |
|    (b) A move to a different town, city, or state? | | | 35. A change in your personal habits (your dress, friends, lifestyle, etc)? | | |
| 15. A change in family "get-togethers"? | | | 36. Sexual difficulties? | | |
| 16. A major change in the health or behavior of a family member (e.g., illness, accidents, drug or disciplinary problems, etc.?) | | | 37. Beginning or ceasing school or college? | | |
| 17. A major change in your living conditions (e.g., home improvements or a decline in your home or neighborhood)? | | | 38. A change in school or college? | | |
| | | | 39. A vacation? | | |
| | | | 40. A change in your religious beliefs? | | |
| 18. The death of a spouse? | | | 41. A change in your school activities (clubs, movies, visiting)? | | |

Adapted from Rahe RH: Epidemiological studies of life changes and illness, *Int J Psychiatr Med* 6(1-2):133-146, 1975

**BOX 4-18    *Recent Life Changes Questionnaire—cont'd***

| LIFE CHANGES (cont.) | ✔ | (1–100) |
|---|---|---|
| 42. A minor violation of the law? | | |
| 43. Legal troubles resulting in your being held in jail? | | |
| 44. A change in your political beliefs? | | |
| 45. A new, close personal relationship? | | |
| 46. An engagement to marry? | | |
| 47. A "falling out" of a close personal relationship? | | |
| 48. Girlfriend or boyfriend problems? | | |
| 49. A loss or damage of personal property? | | |
| 50. An accident? | | |
| 51. A major decision regarding your immediate future? | | |
| **E. FINANCIAL**—Within the past year, have you: | | |
| 52. Taken on a moderate purchase, such as a television, car, freezer, etc.? | | |
| 53. Taken on a major purchase or a mortgage loan, such as a home, business, property, etc.? | | |
| 54. Experienced a foreclosure on a mortgage or loan? | | |
| 55. Experienced a major change in finances: | | |
| (a) Increased income? | | |
| (b) Decreased income? | | |
| (c) Credit rating difficulties? | | |
| TOTAL SLCU Score | | |

**SUBJECTIVE LIFE CHANGE UNITS (SLCU)**

Persons adapt to their recent life changes in different ways. Some people find the adjustment to a residential move, for example, to be enormous, while others find very little life adjustment necessary.

Next to each recent life change that you marked with a ✔, indicate the amount of adjustment you needed to handle the event. Use both your estimate of the intensity of the life change and its duration.

Your scores can range from 1 to 100 "points". For example, if you experienced a recent residential move but felt it required very little life adjustment, you will choose a low number and place it in the column to the right of the check. On the other hand, if you recently changed residence and felt it required a near maximal life adjustment, you will place a high number in the column to the right of the check. For intermediate life adjustments you will choose a number more in the middle between 1 and 100.

Add up the numbers to determine your SLCU score. This provides a rough estimate of your risk of illness during the coming year.

SLCU 130 – at increased risk for minor illness
SLCU 164 and above – at increased risk for major illness

Adapted from Rahe RH: Epidemiological studies of life changes and illness, *Int J Psychiatr Med* 6(1-2):133-146, 1975.

responsiveness, affective involvement, and behavior control (Sawin and Harrigan, 1995).

### Stress and/or Risk Assessment

Everyone experiences **stress.** Being seen for a health assessment can make a woman more anxious. If a woman seems nervous or overly apprehensive, we should help her to relax by using conscious abdominal breathing rather than chest breathing (see Chapter 13 for more details on how to teach and use relaxation breathing). Once learned, the woman can use this relaxation technique to help her relax in a variety of stressful situations, including the dentist's chair, vaginal examination, and labor.

Distress occurs when a woman experiences stress overload. Heavy loads of stress and ineffective coping can lead a woman to experience illnesses such as hyper-

tension, coronary artery disease, headache, back pain, gastrointestinal upset, depression, and decreased immunity. The Social Readjustment Rating Scale was one of the first tools developed to assess the major life events and predict a relationship between a person's level of stress and his or her chance of developing a major physical or psychologic illness (Holmes and Rahe, 1967) (Table 4-10).

### Occupational Assessment

The environment in which a woman spends her time will affect her health. **Working** outside and/or inside the home may expose a woman to a number of environmental factors that may be hazardous. Assess the type of work, the number of hours, the physical labor involved, the rest breaks allowed, the possible environmental hazards, and

## TABLE 4-9 The Life Experiences Survey

Listed below are events that sometimes bring about change in the lives of those who experience them, necessitating social readjustment. *Please check the events that you have experienced in the recent past and indicate the time period during which you experienced each. Be sure that all check marks are directly across from the items they correspond to.*

For each item checked below, *please also indicate the extent to which you viewed the event as having either a positive or negative effect on your life at the time the event occurred. That is, indicate the type and extent of impact that the event had.* A rating of −3 would indicate an extremely negative impact. A rating of 0 suggests no impact either positive or negative. A rating of +3 would indicate an extremely positive impact.

| | 0 to 6 mo | 7 mo to 1 yr | Extremely negative | Moderately negative | Somewhat negative | No impact | Slightly positive | Moderately positive | Extremely positive |
|---|---|---|---|---|---|---|---|---|---|
| 1. Marriage | | | −3 | −2 | −1 | 0 | +1 | +2 | +3 |
| 2. Detention in jail or comparable institution | | | −3 | −2 | −1 | 0 | +1 | +2 | +3 |
| 3. Death of spouse | | | −3 | −2 | −1 | 0 | +1 | +2 | +3 |
| 4. Major change in sleeping habits (much more or much less sleep) | | | −3 | −2 | −1 | 0 | +1 | +2 | +3 |
| 5. Death of close family member: | | | | | | | | | |
| a. Mother | | | −3 | −2 | −1 | 0 | +1 | +2 | +3 |
| b. Father | | | −3 | −2 | −1 | 0 | +1 | +2 | +3 |
| c. Brother | | | −3 | −2 | −1 | 0 | +1 | +2 | +3 |
| d. Sister | | | −3 | −2 | −1 | 0 | +1 | +2 | +3 |
| e. Grandmother | | | −3 | −2 | −1 | 0 | +1 | +2 | +3 |
| f. Grandfather | | | −3 | −2 | −1 | 0 | +1 | +2 | +3 |
| g. Other (specify) | | | −3 | −2 | −1 | 0 | +1 | +2 | +3 |
| 6. Major change in eating habits (much more or much less food intake) | | | −3 | −2 | −1 | 0 | +1 | +2 | +3 |
| 7. Foreclosure on mortgage or loan | | | −3 | −2 | −1 | 0 | +1 | +2 | +3 |
| 8. Death of close friend | | | −3 | −2 | −1 | 0 | +1 | +2 | +3 |
| 9. Outstanding personal achievement | | | −3 | −2 | −1 | 0 | +1 | +2 | +3 |
| 10. Minor law violations (traffic tickets, disturbing the peace, etc.) | | | −3 | −2 | −1 | 0 | +1 | +2 | +3 |
| 11. *Male:* Wife/girlfriend's pregnancy | | | −3 | −2 | −1 | 0 | +1 | +2 | +3 |
| 12. *Female:* Pregnancy | | | −3 | −2 | −1 | 0 | +1 | +2 | +3 |
| 13. Changed work situation (different work responsibility, major change in working conditions, working hours, etc.) | | | −3 | −2 | −1 | 0 | +1 | +2 | +3 |
| 14. New job | | | −3 | −2 | −1 | 0 | +1 | +2 | +3 |
| 15. Serious illness or injury of close family member: | | | | | | | | | |
| a. Father | | | −3 | −2 | −1 | 0 | +1 | +2 | +3 |
| b. Mother | | | −3 | −2 | −1 | 0 | +1 | +2 | +3 |
| c. Sister | | | −3 | −2 | −1 | 0 | +1 | +2 | +3 |
| d. Brother | | | −3 | −2 | −1 | 0 | +1 | +2 | +3 |
| e. Grandmother | | | −3 | −2 | −1 | 0 | +1 | +2 | +3 |
| f. Grandfather | | | −3 | −2 | −1 | 0 | +1 | +2 | +3 |
| g. Spouse | | | −3 | −2 | −1 | 0 | +1 | +2 | +3 |
| h. Other (specify) | | | −3 | −2 | −1 | 0 | +1 | +2 | +3 |

From Sarason IG, Johnson JH, and Siegal JM: Assessing the impact of life changes: development of life experiences survey, *J Consult Clin Psychol* 46(5):932-946, 1978.

TABLE 4-9   *The Life Experiences Survey—cont'd*

| | 0 to 6 mo | 7 mo to 1 yr | Extremely negative | Moderately negative | Somewhat negative | No impact | Slightly positive | Moderately positive | Extremely positive |
|---|---|---|---|---|---|---|---|---|---|
| 16. Sexual difficulties | | | −3 | −2 | −1 | 0 | +1 | +2 | +3 |
| 17. Trouble with employer (in danger of losing job, being suspended, demoted, etc.) | | | −3 | −2 | −1 | 0 | +1 | +2 | +3 |
| 18. Trouble with in-laws | | | −3 | −2 | −1 | 0 | +1 | +2 | +3 |
| 19. Major change in financial status (a lot better off or a lot worse off) | | | −3 | −2 | −1 | 0 | +1 | +2 | +3 |
| 20. Major change in closeness of family members (increased or decreased closeness) | | | −3 | −2 | −1 | 0 | +1 | +2 | +3 |
| 21. Gaining a new family member (through birth, adoption, family member moving in, etc.) | | | −3 | −2 | −1 | 0 | +1 | +2 | +3 |
| 22. Change of residence | | | −3 | −2 | −1 | 0 | +1 | +2 | +3 |
| 23. Marital separation from mate (due to conflict) | | | −3 | −2 | −1 | 0 | +1 | +2 | +3 |
| 24. Major change in church activities (increased or decreased attendance) | | | −3 | −2 | −1 | 0 | +1 | +2 | +3 |
| 25. Marital reconciliation with mate | | | −3 | −2 | −1 | 0 | +1 | +2 | +3 |
| 26. Major change in number of arguments with spouse (a lot more or a lot fewer arguments) | | | −3 | −2 | −1 | 0 | +1 | +2 | +3 |
| 27. *Married male:* Change in wife's work outside the home (beginning work, ceasing work, changing to a new job, etc.) | | | −3 | −2 | −1 | 0 | +1 | +2 | +3 |
| 28. *Married female:* Change in husband's work (loss of job, beginning new job, retirement, etc.) | | | −3 | −2 | −1 | 0 | +1 | +2 | +3 |
| 29. Major change in usual type and/or amount of recreation | | | −3 | −2 | −1 | 0 | +1 | +2 | +3 |
| 30. Borrowing more than $10,000 (buying home, business, etc.) | | | −3 | −2 | −1 | 0 | +1 | +2 | +3 |
| 31. Borrowing less than $10,000 (buying car, TV, getting school loan, etc.) | | | −3 | −2 | −1 | 0 | +1 | +2 | +3 |
| 32. Being fired from job | | | −3 | −2 | −1 | 0 | +1 | +2 | +3 |
| 33. *Male:* Wife/girlfriend having abortion | | | −3 | −2 | −1 | 0 | +1 | +2 | +3 |
| 34. *Female:* Having abortion | | | −3 | −2 | −1 | 0 | +1 | +2 | +3 |
| 35. Major personal illness or injury | | | −3 | −2 | −1 | 0 | +1 | +2 | +3 |

*Continued*

### TABLE 4-9 The Life Experiences Survey — cont'd

| | 0 to 6 mo | 7 mo to 1 yr | Extremely negative | Moderately negative | Somewhat negative | No impact | Slightly positive | Moderately positive | Extremely positive |
|---|---|---|---|---|---|---|---|---|---|
| 36. Major change in social activities, e.g., parties, movies, visiting (increased or decreased participation) | | | −3 | −2 | −1 | 0 | +1 | +2 | +3 |
| 37. Major change in living conditions of family (building new home, remodeling, deterioration of home, neighborhood, etc.) | | | −3 | −2 | −1 | 0 | +1 | +2 | +3 |
| 38. Divorce | | | −3 | −2 | −1 | 0 | +1 | +2 | +3 |
| 39. Serious injury or illness of close friend | | | −3 | −2 | −1 | 0 | +1 | +2 | +3 |
| 40. Retirement from work | | | −3 | −2 | −1 | 0 | +1 | +2 | +3 |
| 41. Son or daughter leaving home (due to marriage, college, etc.) | | | −3 | −2 | −1 | 0 | +1 | +2 | +3 |
| 42. Ending of formal schooling | | | −3 | −2 | −1 | 0 | +1 | +2 | +3 |
| 43. Separation from spouse (due to work, travel, etc.) | | | −3 | −2 | −1 | 0 | +1 | +2 | +3 |
| 44. Engagement | | | −3 | −2 | −1 | 0 | +1 | +2 | +3 |
| 45. Breaking up with boyfriend/girlfriend | | | −3 | −2 | −1 | 0 | +1 | +2 | +3 |
| 46. Leaving home for the first time | | | −3 | −2 | −1 | 0 | +1 | +2 | +3 |
| 47. Reconciliation with boyfriend/girlfriend | | | −3 | −2 | −1 | 0 | +1 | +2 | +3 |
| *Other recent experiences that have had an effect on your life. List and rate.* | | | | | | | | | |
| 48. _____ | | | −3 | −2 | −1 | 0 | +1 | +2 | +3 |
| 49. _____ | | | −3 | −2 | −1 | 0 | +1 | +2 | +3 |
| 50. _____ | | | −3 | −2 | −1 | 0 | +1 | +2 | +3 |

the possibility of stress overload in her roles. Be alert to possible problem areas such as "prolonged standing or sitting, heavy lifting, excessive noise, excessive heat or cold, exposure to toxins, exposure to chemicals or radiation, excessive hours on the job, boredom, low pay, low recognition, and little or no control over work" (Youngkin and Davis, 1998).

### Nutritional Assessment

"Nutrition is a key component in the maintenance of health and in the prevention or treatment of disease" (Barkauskas and others, 1998). Before developing a dietary plan with a client, we must learn information about her circumstances. Some of the necessary data includes information about her family unit, living environment, food storage and preparation facilities, cultural-ethnic food practices, and special dietary practices.

The primary influence on how an individual decides which foods to eat is his or her culture. "In France, corn is considered animal feed not fit for human consumption, whereas in the United States, corn is a popular vegetable. Due to religious beliefs, some Jewish, Muslim, and Seventh Day Adventists clients consider pork inedible, whereas members of many other religions would eat it without hesitation" (Andrews and Boyle, 1995).

Culture also determines meal patterns. In the Anglo-American culture, the pattern of eating is generally breakfast in the morning, lunch between 10:00 AM and 1:00 PM, and the large meal of the day in the early evening. "Among many Native American and Latin American groups, two meals a day are usually eaten. In Spain, four meals a day plus frequent snacks are customary. In some nomadic African tribes, one meal is

## BOX 4-19   *Family APGAR*

**DEFINITION**

*Adaptation* is the use of intrafamilial and extrafamilial resources for problem solving when family equilibrium is stressed during a crisis.

*Partnership* is the sharing of decision making and nurturing responsibilities by family members.

*Growth* is the physical and emotional maturation and self-fulfillment that is achieved by family members through mutual support and guidance.

*Affection* is the caring or loving relationship that exists among family members.

*Resolve* is the commitment to devote time to other members of the family for physical and emotional nurturing. It also usually involves a decision to share wealth and space.

**FUNCTIONS MEASURED BY THE FAMILY APGAR**

How resources are shared, or the degree to which a member is satisfied with the assistance received when family resources are needed.

How decisions are shared, or the member's satisfaction with mutuality in family communication and problem solving.

How nurturing is shared, or the member's satisfaction with the freedom available within the family to change roles and attain physical and emotional growth or maturation.

How emotional experiences are shared, or the member's satisfaction with the intimacy and emotional interaction that exists in the family.

How time (and space and money) is shared, or the member's satisfaction with the time commitment that has been made to the family by its members.

**OPEN-ENDED QUESTIONS TO ASK**

• How have family members aided each other in time of need?

• In what way have family members received help or assistance from friends and community agencies?

• How do family members communicate with each other about such matters as vacations, finances, medical care, large purchases, and personal problems?

• How have family members changed during the past year?

• How has this change been accepted by family members?

• In what ways have family members aided each other in growing or developing independent lifestyles?

• How have family members reacted to your desires for change?

• How have members of your family responded to emotional expressions such as affection, love, sorrow, or anger?

• How do members of your family share time, space, and money?

Modified from Smilkstein G: The Family APGAR: a proposal for a family function test and its use by physicians, *J Fam Pract* 6:1231-1239, 1978.

---

consumed every other day" (Andrews and Boyle, 1995).

What constitutes a meal also differs between cultures. "For example, in India, a meal is only a meal if rice or another traditional grain food (such as flat bread) is served. Although other foods may be eaten in large quantities, they are considered snacks if no rice or bread is consumed" (Andrews and Boyle, 1995).

Culturally related food patterns and food choices should be identified. Methods of cooking and storing food, along with any food taboos within the culture of the family, should be explored. We should determine how strongly the family follows ethnic food practices when making food choices because to some degree this influences where food is purchased and the possible financial effect it may have on the family's resources. Food from some small grocery stores and markets catering to specific ethnic food preferences are more costly than if the food is purchased at a larger supermarket.

The convenient location of such stores, however, may outweigh the disadvantage and expense of traveling to a larger store with lower food prices.

Explore the roles of family members with regard to food. Identify who purchases the food and who prepares the food as these are both critical factors in family nutritional status.

The general socioeconomic status of the household is also helpful information before developing a customized food plan. Does the person and/or family receive food assistance (e.g., food stamps) or need food assistance? What are the food practices of the family and their beliefs about food? What options do they have for cooking food? What options do they have for storing food?

The observance of religious food laws and the required restrictions (e.g., Jewish, Muslim, Catholic) should be determined. Food preferences based on vegetarian diets, weight loss diets, and other special diets developed because of food allergies or gastrointestinal

## TABLE 4-10  *Social Readjustment Rating Scale*

Holmes and Rahe developed this scale to rate the amount of stress caused by many changes in life: major and minor, pleasant and unpleasant. To obtain your score, circle the ones that apply to you and then add up the total. Follow-up studies show that people who accumulate more than 200 points in a year are high risks for physical or psychologic stress-related illnesses.

| Life event | Mean value |
|---|---|
| 1. Death of spouse | 100 |
| 2. Divorce | 73 |
| 3. Marital separation from mate | 65 |
| 4. Detention in jail or other institution | 63 |
| 5. Death of a close family member | 63 |
| 6. Major personal injury or illness | 53 |
| 7. Marriage | 50 |
| 8. Being fired at work | 47 |
| 9. Marital reconciliation with mate | 45 |
| 10. Retirement from work | 45 |
| 11. Major change in the health or behavior of a family member | 44 |
| 12. Pregnancy | 40 |
| 13. Sexual difficulties | 39 |
| 14. Gaining a new family member (e.g., through birth, adoption, oldster moving in) | 39 |
| 15. Major business readjustment (e.g., merger, reorganization, bankruptcy) | 39 |
| 16. Major change in financial state (e.g., a lot worse off or a lot better off than usual) | 38 |
| 17. Death of a close friend | 37 |
| 18. Changing to a different line of work | 36 |
| 19. Major change in the number of arguments with spouse (e.g., either a lot more or a lot less than usual regarding child rearing, personal habits) | 35 |
| 20. Taking out a mortgage or loan for a major purchase (e.g., for a home, business) | 31 |
| 21. Foreclosure on a mortgage or loan | 30 |
| 22. Major change in responsibilities at work (e.g., promotion, demotion, lateral transfer) | 29 |
| 23. Son or daughter leaving home (e.g., marriage, attending college) | 29 |
| 24. Trouble with in-laws | 29 |
| 25. Outstanding personal achievement | 28 |
| 26. Wife beginning or ceasing work outside the home | 26 |
| 27. Beginning or ceasing formal schooling | 26 |
| 28. Major change in living conditions (e.g., building a new home, remodeling, deterioration of home or neighborhood) | 25 |
| 29. Revision of personal habits (dress, manners, associations, etc.) | 24 |
| 30. Trouble with the boss | 23 |
| 31. Major change in working hours or conditions | 20 |
| 32. Change in residence | 20 |
| 33. Changing to a new school | 20 |
| 34. Major change in usual type or amount of recreation | 19 |
| 35. Major change in church activities (e.g, a lot more or a lot less than usual) | 19 |
| 36. Major change in social activities (e.g., clubs, dancing, movies, visiting) | 18 |
| 37. Taking out a mortgage or loan for a lesser purchase (e.g., for a car, TV, freezer) | 17 |
| 38. Major change in sleeping habits (a lot more or a lot less sleep, or a change in part of day when asleep) | 16 |
| 39. Major change in number of family get-togethers (e.g., a lot more or a lot fewer than usual) | 15 |
| 40. Major change in eating habits (a lot more or a lot less food intake, or very different meal hours or surroundings) | 15 |
| 41. Vacation | 13 |
| 42. Christmas | 12 |
| 43. Minor violations of the law (e.g., traffic lights, jaywalking, disturbing the peace) | 11 |
|  | TOTAL |

From Holmes TH, Rahe RH: *J Psychosom Res* 11:213, 1967.

difficulties (i.e., including lactose intolerance) should be explored. Many adults have lactose intolerance; it is especially prevalent among people of African descent.

A woman's individual preferences and choices are also important. Learning her personal eating habits provides a basis for screening her risk for developing chronic heart disease or obesity. Encouraging her to make healthy food choices provides her with an opportunity to reduce her health risks.

*Dietary Assessment.* For a dietary assessment, we must learn a woman's overall nutrient intake, as well as her need for nutrition education and support. Additional information may be gained from biochemical tests, clinical observations, weight history, and anthropometric tests.

Methods for dietary assessment may be used alone or in combination. Some of the most commonly used methods are a 24-hour recall, a food record, or a food frequency questionnaire. With the **24-hour recall,** the woman is asked to recall specific foods—including amounts—eaten over the previous 24-hour period. Methods of food preparation, descriptions of ethnic dishes, and notations of sauces, gravies, and dressings should be included. An advantage of this method is that it is fast and inexpensive and offers a beginning picture of food habits and intake. The disadvantages of this method is that it represents only one point in time and the ability to recall all intake in the previous 24 hours is usually faulty.

Asking a person to do a **food record** for a period of time, generally for 3 or 7 days, is another technique. The woman is instructed to record all foods eaten, as well as estimate the amounts she consumed. We must explain the reasons for the food record in order to expect the woman's full participation. The advantages of this method are that it tends to provide more information than the 24-hour recall. The disadvantage is that the woman may find it tedious and not do a complete record. Sometimes using a combination of 24-hour recall and a 3-day food record such as a Food Diary is suggested (Table 4-11).

The **Food Frequency Questionnaire (FFQ)** helps to identify food intake over a specific period of time (e.g., during a large weight gain or recent illness, such as anemia, coronary heart disease, diabetes mellitus, or hypertension). The FFQ provides a list of foods and a scale for identifying how often each is consumed over a given period of time (e.g., a day, week, or month). The food list may be all-inclusive for an overall food intake picture or may focus only on foods specifically related to the particular chronic illness. For example, if a woman is newly diagnosed with coronary heart disease, the FFQ questionnaire may ask only about foods high in fat and cholesterol. The facility may have a specialized Food Frequency Questionnaire for the medical diagnoses in which food consumption is a factor. Advantages of this questionnaire are that the woman is provided with items to respond to, so it does not totally depend on recall. The disadvantage is that the record may still be incomplete.

*Diet Analysis.* Analysis of a woman's food-intake information may be done one of two ways, depending on time and resources. Some facilities—or women themselves—have a recommended diet analysis software computer program so that they may enter the information and receive a printed analysis. Most often, we provide an overall nutrient check using the food pyramid guide. Analysis by either method provides an excellent basis for beginning diet counseling and nutrition education.

When available, a computer program that performs diet analysis provides a more complete record for the woman. Sources of energy intake and fat energy and comparisons with recommended intakes can be printed out and shared with the woman. Any nutrient intake concerns may be noted and discussed with the woman. Alternate food choices and/or increasing or decreasing intake from the targeted food group(s) may be discussed. Therefore this method offers us excellent follow-up opportunities for additional nutrient intake checks while we are working with the woman to determine alternate food choices within her ethnic and socioeconomic parameters. This method also provides excellent opportunities to educate a woman on the functions of particular nutrients and their roles in making her healthier.

## Transitioning to the Physical Assessment

The health history and the physical examination create a health assessment. The health history provides insight into the woman's perspective about her health. The data obtained with a health history are subjective. For the full picture to emerge, we must combine these data with the objective findings of the general survey and the physical examination. Part or all of the physical assessment may occur, depending on the purpose of the interaction.

The transition from health history to physical examination is smooth if a woman knows at the outset that both an interview and examination are necessary for a comprehensive health assessment. Once the health history has been completed, we must review the preliminary findings and establish the focus for the physical examination. The woman should validate the accuracy of the information and purpose. Encourage the woman to share anything more she wants to mention; she may have one more thing to tell you (e.g., something that she remembered during the interview or that she was hesitant to say earlier).

### Preparing for the Physical Examination

Which health care provider does the physical examination is determined by the site of the care, the purpose of the examination, the abilities of the available providers, and the expectations of the person or insurance company reimbursing the cost of the procedure. Professional nurses, nurse practitioners, nurse-midwives, and

## TABLE 4-11 Food Diary

Name _____ Date _____

| Time | Food type and amount | Where eaten and with whom | Other activity while eating | How you feel before eating (e.g., anxious, bored, tired, angry, depressed) |
|---|---|---|---|---|
| | | | | |

physicians may each provide this service. If you are not performing the remainder of the examination, describe to the woman what will happen next, explaining the purpose of each procedure and answering her questions about what each procedure might feel like.

Be sensitive to a woman's personal comfort level, possible prior history with abuse or assault, or cultural or religious beliefs because any of these may limit who may touch her or be with her for the physical part of the data collection. Learn her preferences before beginning to touch her. Remember that every client has the right to refuse care from a specific provider. Because of a prior experience, some women do not feel comfortable having a particular provider do their examination. This concern must be addressed to the satisfaction of the woman. If a woman is coerced or pressured into an undesired physical assessment, this not only violates her trust but also is considered assault and battery—an illegal offense.

Because being viewed and touched by another person—even a professional nurse or physician—makes women uneasy, provide some relief for her pre-exam anxiety by giving her information and options. For example, describe who will have a role in the examination and what they will be doing. If she wants a friend or family member to be with her, include them. If the woman is to have a pelvic examination, explain the procedure to her, how you will assist her, and how she may watch the examination with a mirror if she wishes. Deep breathing and conscious relaxation techniques can be reviewed with the woman and/or done with her during intrusive acts of the examination.

Explain to the woman what clothing she must remove for the examination and give her the appropriate garments to put on. If she is to put on a shirt or "johnny," explain whether it is to open in the back or front. Some facilities have created user-friendly clothing that maintains the woman's modesty while allowing the examiner access to the parts of the body being examined. Loose fitting and held in place with plastic gathers, the clothing resembles a bolero top and skirt.

Tell the woman to pull the curtain or lock the door while she changes. Give her a way to indicate to you when she is ready. One of the reasons many women feel awkward getting undressed for an examination is that they fear someone will walk in on them before they are covered and ready. Box 4-20 describes some guidelines to use prior to the actual examination.

## Positioning for the Physical Examination

Most women being seen for a physical sit on the examining table for the beginning of the physical examination, making both the anterior and posterior aspects of their upper body available for examination and placing them at an easy height for the examiner. The woman then reclines on the examining table for the clinical breast examination and the abdominal examination. To prepare for the genital-rectal examination, the woman

---

### BOX 4-20   Prephysical Examination Preparation

Encourage the woman to express her concerns or desires about the examination.

Introduce others who will assist with the examination, and obtain her approval.

Obtain assistance for her according to her wishes.

Explain the procedures that will be used (e.g., palpation of the thyroid, auscultation of the chest, palpation of the breasts, percussion of the abdomen).

Use pictures and other audiovisual materials as appropriate.

Determine if she has known allergies to Betadine or latex.

Encourage her to use the bathroom to empty her bladder.

Provide the easy access clothing and a drape for her to wear.

Indicate what clothing and jewelry she may keep on.

Protect her privacy as she changes her clothing.

Leave the room or draw the curtain, according to her wishes.

Return when she is ready.

---

is generally expected to place her heels in the metal stirrups at the foot of the examination table and slide her buttocks to the edge of the table. Having cloth covers (some facilities use "hot mitt" potholders) over the stirrups helps to keep a woman's feet warmer and makes the experience more comfortable for the woman.

### Meeting Special Needs

There are a number of things that may be done to promote a comfortable physical examination for a woman who needs special accommodations. They are based on the needs of the woman and include how we speak to her, adjustments made within the environment, and the expectations of the woman. Decisions such as who helps the woman undress for the exam, should a sign language interpreter stand in the exam room, or how to transfer a woman who uses a wheelchair to the examination table must be made collaboratively. All necessary adjustments should be considered both before and during the physical examination. Keep the following points in mind:

- A woman with mobility impairment (e.g., spinal cord injury, polio, or cerebral palsy) may appreciate being able to bring a urine sample with her rather than having to negotiate the use of a bathroom within the facility.
- Each disability affects each person differently. Our knowledge about a disability and sensitivity to ask only pertinent questions about her disability will increase a woman's comfort and cooperation.

- Speak directly to the client. We sometimes unconsciously address the attendant, interpreter, friend, or family member accompanying the woman, negating her presence.
- Specialized educational materials (e.g., information in Braille or on audiotape) are appreciated by the hearing impaired. Three-dimensional models that can be touched during an explanation help the visually impaired.
- If a special communication system must be used by a hearing- or speech-impaired woman (e.g., a sign language interpreter, word board, or talk box), we must learn about this and accommodate our interactions to the woman's needs. If a translator or interpreter is necessary, he or she must be placed in a position in the room where the woman can give and receive communication.
- Conserve the woman's time and energy by having her remove only the clothing that absolutely must be removed for the examination.
- The examination room must be able to accommodate the wheelchair, and the table should be able to be lowered for an easier transfer. If the table cannot be lowered, other arrangements are necessary.
- The woman is the expert on how best to transfer her from her wheelchair or have her climb onto the table. "Transfers are relatively simple if the woman, assistants, and clinician all understand the method that will best suit the woman's disability, room space, and exam table" (Ferreyra and Hughes, 1984). Most examination tables are covered with paper to facilitate cleaning between patients, but this may need to be removed if it interferes with the process of positioning.
- The foot stirrups may need to be equipped with straps to secure a woman's foot when she cannot control it herself because of her condition.
- Everyone should identify themselves as they enter the examination room. Encourage the woman with a visual impairment to specify the orientation and mobility assistance she desires. Keep her cane or guide dog where she places them (Ferreyra and Hughes, 1984).

## Learning about Her Body: The Physical Examination

A nurse, nurse practitioner, nurse-midwife, or a physician may do the general survey and physical examination in part or whole. If our role is to assist the woman when another provider is doing the physical examination, we must still have an understanding of the examination process. When we have a clear understanding of what and why aspects of the examination are performed, we can anticipate a woman's needs and provide supportive and appropriate information before, during,

and after the examination. For information to provide to a woman in response to an identified risk factor, see Chapter 5.

During the physical examination, we pay special attention to the areas of concern that the woman shared during the health history, especially when there is a strong family tendency or individual risk factors for specific disease processes (e.g., cardiac disease, breast cancer, diabetes). Most of the concerns mentioned by the woman during the history may be explained with objective findings during her physical examination. Other symptoms she described may not be so easily explained. When this is the case, we support her report of symptoms and continue to seek the factor or factors that are causing her concern.

### General Survey

The general survey is a general overview of the woman (Box 4-21). The gathering of physical information requires the use of vision, hearing, smell, and touch. We begin to develop an overall impression, and begin the woman's physical examination when we first observe her (e.g., What is her posture?). This process continues as she looks up when she hears her name (an indication that she can hear), stands (an indication that she has lower body strength), and walks toward us (an indication that she has balance and strength). It continues as we watch her facial expressions (i.e., muscle movements are symmetrical and of appropriate affect) as she talks. "Note the woman's speech, the pace at which she speaks, her ability to answer/speak spontaneously, clearly, logically, and with appropriate inflection" (Youngkin and Davis, 1998). Does talking make it more difficult for her to breathe?

When we are near the woman, we can start to assess the self-care areas of grooming and hygiene. Keep in mind that "different cultures have different customs regarding hygiene. For example, the use of deodorant is unheard of and shaving of a woman's axillary hair is rare in some cultures" (Mosby, 1997). Unusual odors may alert you to possible physical problems such as

---

### BOX 4-21    *General Survey*

**GENERAL OVERVIEW OF THE WOMAN**
Orientation to time, place, and person
Age
Height and weight
Body type
Body positioning
Gait and posture
Overall hygiene
Emotions expressed (e.g., nervousness, sadness)
Vital signs (i.e., temperature, pulse, respirations, blood pressure [both arms, sitting and supine])

tooth decay, infection, incontinence, or a malignancy (Table 4-12).

The woman's height (without shoes) and weight (without shoes and heavy clothing) are necessary baseline data. Noting in the chart the amount of clothing the woman has on when her weight is obtained allows a more accurate comparison to be made when she weighs in the next time.

The ratio between height and weight determines if the woman falls within the appropriate weight parameters for someone of her age, height, and bone structure. The woman's body type and whether she is slender, average, or stocky should be noted in her chart.

When comparing the woman's height and weight with those on standardized charts, keep in mind the variations determined by age and race. Adolescents may not have reached their peak height. "African Americans tend to be heavier and taller than Caucasians; Asians tend to be slighter and shorter than Caucasians" (Youngkin and Davis, 1998).

In some settings, once a baseline height and weight are obtained and the woman is no longer changing in height, she measures and records her own weights on her chart. By including the woman as an active participant in this evaluation, the philosophy of collaboration is encouraged.

As an ongoing measurement, a woman's weight can alert us to possible problems—either physical or psychosocial—that may result in a weight change. Such problems are of special concern when evaluating the weight of a woman who may be experiencing anorexia or bulimia.

### Vital Signs

The woman's vital signs may be taken at the beginning of the interview or delayed until now at the start of the physical examination. There are a variety of ways to take a client's blood pressure, temperature, and pulse. The method selected depends on where and why the woman is being seen. Always recheck abnormal findings.

The woman's temperature may be measured with a standard glass thermometer, a disposable paper thermometer, a battery powered or electronic thermometer, or a tympanic thermometer. The instrument chosen depends on what is available, where the temperature will be taken, and how critical the temperature reading is to the woman's care. Depending on the purpose, the temperature reading may be obtained orally, rectally, or tympanically. Informing a woman of her temperature and explaining the variations in the range of normal body temperatures depending on how and when the temperature is taken during the day helps her with her own future assessments.

There are a number of sites at which the pulse may be counted. The radial pulse is generally the first site selected; additional sites are based on the woman's heath concerns and needs. For the most accurate pulse rate, take it for 1 full minute. This enables you to determine if the pulse is irregular and, if so, what the pattern is. If the woman wishes to learn how to take her own pulse, show her how to take it radially and tell her what the range of normal findings is for her.

Consciously or not, some patients change their breathing when they are aware that we are assessing their patterns of breathing (Mosby, 1997). Assessing the rate, depth, and character of the woman's respirations is best done when she thinks you are still measuring her pulse. Count the respirations for 1 minute and note the regularity of the rhythm and the depth of the breathing.

Taking the woman's blood pressure will provide a preliminary assessment of her cardiac output, circulation, state of hydration, and the elasticity of her arteries. Ask

### TABLE 4-12   *Identifying Unusual Odors*

| Odor | Probable cause |
| --- | --- |
| Fruity breath | • Diabetic ketoacidosis |
| Halitosis | • Lack of access to toothbrush and toothpaste |
| | • Dental decay |
| | • Throat or sinus infection |
| Putrid breath or body odor | • Lack of access to bathing |
| | • Infection (e.g., lung abscess or wound infection) |
| | • Malignancy |
| Fishy vaginal odor | • Menses flow without adequate hygiene |
| | • Vaginitis from douching or use of tampons or other potential irritants |
| | • Vaginal infection |
| Urine or ammonia-like odor | • Dehydration |
| | • Incontinence |
| | • Urinary tract infection |
| Fecal breath or body odor | • Bowel obstruction (with fecal breath) |
| | • Incontinence |

Adapted from Mosby: *Expert 10-minute physical examinations*, St Louis, 1997, Mosby.

the woman what her blood pressure reading is normally. Use an appropriate sized cuff for the woman's arm, and take the measurement on her arm while she is comfortable and relaxed in a sitting position. If her reading is higher than normal for her, repeat it later during the examination, either on the same arm or on the other arm and possibly with her lying down. As the interaction continues, the woman will become more comfortable, and her blood pressure may drop. For some women, the reading will not return to their normal range until the physical examination—especially the vaginal examination—is finished.

Share all findings with the woman and write them down for her. For the woman to be knowledgeable about her own body and for continuity of care, we should inform her of the normal range of her vital signs.

## Continuing the Physical Examination

The clinician that performs the physical examination must have an in-depth knowledge of the normal characteristics of the body systems; skill in inspection, palpation, percussion, and auscultation; and the ability to use appropriate equipment to collect accurate data. A valid assessment depends on differentiating normal physical findings and normal variations from abnormal findings.

As the data collection process continues, we may perform some or all of the components of the assessment or help another provider and then teach or review preventive care measures with the woman as needed.

### Integumentary System

The assessment of the woman's skin, hair, and nails provides general insight into her overall health. The examination of the integumentary system is ongoing as different parts of the woman's body are revealed during the evaluation of other systems.

*Skin.* Observe exposed skin for subtle changes in color, texture, moisture, temperature, vascularity, turgor, and thickness, as well as new or healed bruises. Chart all lesions by type, location, and size.

Ask the woman about the cause of any bruises, how she treated them, and how long they took to heal. Keep in mind that multiple bruises in various stages of healing may be an indication that she is being abused. Think about how she would position her arms or legs to protect herself if someone was trying to hit her. Are the bruises in those areas (e.g., underside of arms, back, or sides of thighs)? To evaluate skin color or bruising in a woman with dark skin, it is best to observe her sclera, conjunctiva, buccal mucosa, tongue, lips, nail beds, palms, and soles.

During adolescence, a woman's skin texture changes. As her sebaceous glands become more active and increase in size, she may develop the inflammatory condition of acne. If so, review with her how to care for her face and present available options to her.

Adult women may be embarrassed by a condition that creates pimples that is not acne. Rosacea is a skin disease that occurs most often in fair-skinned adults, especially females between the ages of 30 and 50. It causes redness and swelling on the face, with the most color across the nose. As the disease progresses, small, solid, red pimples or pustules appear and there may be burning and conjunctivitis. A woman may be concerned or embarrassed that she is developing "acne" as an adult. Reassurance, education about the condition, and referral to a dermatologist may be helpful. The diagnosis may be confirmed, her triggers for flare-ups can be determined, and she can receive medication to control this condition.

Look for body piercing or tattoos on the woman, and determine if she has had any problems with them. If she has open lesions, review how she cares for them. Remind her to check her skin for freckles or moles that may change in shape. Review with her how to examine for changes. If she has tanned or sunburned skin, teach her how to select and apply suntan lotion with an SPF of 15 or above.

*Hair.* Assess both the woman's terminal hair (e.g., on her scalp, eyebrows, axillae, and pubic areas) and her vellous hair (e.g., the short, fine hair on her skin). Note the color, quantity, and distribution of the hair on her scalp. How is her hair cared for? Has she suffered adverse effects from dying her hair or using permanent wave solutions or chemical straighteners? Are the hair shafts fragile and easily broken? Is her hair falling out? Does she have areas on her scalp that are without hair? If so, ask her when she noticed any of these. Inspect her scalp for lesions, scaling, infection, or signs of infestation of head lice. A louse may not be visible, but its nits (eggs) are more easily observed attached to the hair shaft.

Note the distribution, color, and quantity of her vellous hair. It is important to determine if the woman's facial hair has changed in density or coarseness. Ask about her observations of these possible changes.

*Nails.* Disease may also affect the shape, color, consistency, texture, and overall condition of a woman's fingernails or toenails. If she is wearing nail polish, we may ask to remove it from one or more nails on her hands or feet. If she is wearing acrylic nails, we must ask her about the condition of her real nails. Why did she have the acrylics put on? Her dissatisfaction with her nails (e.g., brittle, thin, peeling, cracks, or fissures) may provide us with insight to her health. If the woman is wearing acrylic nails, review with her the signs and symptoms of fungal infection and be sure to evaluate her toenails (Box 4-22).

### Head and Neck

With the examination of the head and neck, we are starting the head-to-toe examination. As we progress, we must pay special attention to areas that are the woman's chief complaint, as well as to areas in which she may be at higher risk for problems because of her personal or family history.

***Head, Scalp, and Face.*** Observe the general size and shape of the woman's head. Have her demonstrate the range of motion of her head. Palpate for lumps, deformities, swelling, or masses. Note any lesions, scaliness, abnormal contours, tenderness, or edema. Determine if her face is symmetrical, and ask her about any swelling or edema that she might have noticed. Watch for any involuntary movements.

***Eyes.*** Ask the woman about her vision. Does she wear contacts or glasses? Does she need them for distance or reading or both? Ask when she had her last vision examination.

Inspect her eyes and eyelids for symmetry and obvious abnormalities. Note if she experiences tenderness as you palpate and if lesions or discharge are present. Are the hairs of her eyebrows and eyelashes present and intact? If they seem sparse, ask if she has the hair of her eyebrows removed. If appropriate, a visual acuity and fundoscopic examination are also done.

***Nose.*** The woman's nose should be symmetrical. Ask about her sense of smell. Use a light and, if necessary, a nasal speculum to inspect the nasal mucosa for inflammation or erythema. If either exists, ask if she has had a "runny nose" and what she thinks is the cause. Ask her what she has done to treat it. If she has a nose stud or ring, ask about the occurrence of infection.

***Mouth and Teeth.*** A woman's lips are a good place to assess her skin color. For accuracy, she may need to remove her lipstick, lip pencil, or lip gloss. The woman's lips should be symmetrical, of uniform color, moist, and free of lesions. If she has a lesion on her lip, ask when she developed it and what she has done to care for it. If the lesion is herpes simplex, provide her with information about medications that may increase her comfort and advise her about how to minimize her risks of passing the virus to another person.

Examine the woman's teeth to determine if they are all present and intact or have visible caries. If she has a mouth odor, we must rule out dental caries. The woman's teeth may be her own, be multiple crowns that are permanent, or be dentures. If she has a partial or full set of dentures, we must ask her to remove them so that we can inspect her gums. The request to remove her teeth may be embarrassing to the woman, so inspect the gums as quickly as possible. Her gums should be smooth and intact and free of bleeding or discoloration. Missing or broken teeth may be a sign of poor nutrition or a lack of dental care as a child or an adult, or may be the result of being punched in the mouth.

The oral mucosa, tongue, palate, uvula, and tonsils should be inspected for color and texture. If the woman smokes tobacco or uses tobacco chew, be especially vigilant in inspecting the buccal tissues for early signs of nicotine damage and cancer. Be sure to inspect and palpate the floor of the mouth and the underside of her

---

---

tongue because these are two areas where oral cancer develops.

***Ears.*** The woman's ears should be symmetrical, of equal size, and at the same level on both sides of her head. Examine places where her ears have been pierced to determine if there is irritation or infection. Ear lobes can become stretched and misshapen due to the wearing of heavy earrings. If one ear appears misshapen or larger than the other, it could be an injury from being punched in the side of the head. Is there erythema or discharge? Can the woman hear a whisper? Is the difficulty more prominent on one side than another? We may need to inspect both the external and internal canals to determine if she has more than a small amount of cerumen (ear wax). In an effort to clean their ears, some women use cotton-topped swabs, which can actually compress the cerumen and block hearing. She may also be unable to hear out of one ear if a diving accident or the force of a blow has ruptured her eardrum. If indicated, use an otoscope to view the internal canals and tympanic membranes.

**Neck.** Have the woman turn her head from side to side, as well as tuck her chin to her chest and then raise it as high as possible. Ask her if she experiences any difficulty or pain while doing this. Observe her neck for distended blood vessels, tenderness, bruising, or wounds. Palpate her thyroid gland, carotid arteries, and lymph nodes (Box 4-23).

### Back and Chest

After assessing her thyroid, which is usually done from behind, it is easy to transition to the woman's back, although either her chest or back may be assessed next.

**Back.** Her skin should be warm, dry, and free of lesions. If moles, acne, or other lesions are found, examine them to determine if they should be of concern. Evaluate the contours, symmetry, and shape of her thorax. The anterior-posterior diameter of her thorax should be less than the transverse diameter by almost half.

Ask the woman to stand, and assess the alignment of her spinal column. Her spinal column should be straight and without obvious deformities. Large breasts may cause a woman to hunch forward. Her shoulders should be of even height. The repeated use of a heavy shoulder bag can cause discomfort or irregularities on her frame.

---

### BOX 4-23 *Assessment of Head and Neck*

**HEAD**
Inspect head for:
Size, shape, symmetry; and scalp for deformities or lesions.
Unusual movements.
Palpate head for:
Tenderness, deformities, lesions of the scalp.
Temporal artery pulses.
Temporomandibular joint.
Lymph nodes.

**FACE**
Inspect face for:
Expression, symmetry of structure and features, skin color, involuntary movements.

**NECK**
Inspect neck for:
Symmetry, mobility, range of motion, distended blood vessels, bruising, wounds, tenderness.
Palpate neck for:
Thyroid (size and shape), carotid artery pulses, lymph nodes (enlargement), muscle strength, cervical vertebrae (formation and tenderness).
Auscultate neck for:
Bruits in the carotid arteries and thyroid gland.

**EYES**
Inspect eyes for:
Symmetry, lesions, discharge, tearing.
Palpate eyes for:
Firmness, mobility, texture, and smoothness of eyelids.
Swelling, tenderness, and discharge from lacrimal glands and sacs.
Test visual acuity, visual fields, pupil response, blink reflex, red reflex.
Do ophthalmic exam.

**SINUSES**
Palpate frontal and maxillary sinuses for tenderness and swelling.
Use transillumination if indicated.

**NOSE**
Inspect nose for symmetry, deformity.
Inspect turbinates and septum for symmetry.
Inspect nasal mucosa for:
Inflammation, erythema, swelling, bleeding, drainage.
Palpate nose for tenderness, lesions.
Test for sense of smell.

**MOUTH AND TEETH**
Inspect:
Lips for color, symmetry, moisture, and lesions.
Teeth for number and condition (if she wears dentures, ask her to remove them to examine gums).
Gums for swelling, bleeding, retraction, or discoloration.
Oral mucosa for color, pigmentation, lesions, or infections.
Tongue for symmetry, position, size, color, and texture.
Floor of mouth and underside of tongue.
Hard palate for color and shape.
Soft palate, uvula, tonsils, and posterior pharynx for symmetry, color, exudate, edema, ulcerations.
Palpate floor of mouth and underside of tongue for lesions or masses.
Stimulate the gag reflex.

**EARS**
Inspect ears for symmetry, position, color, integrity, lesions, discharge (cerumen).
Inspect auricles and external and internal canals.
Palpate ears for tenderness, lesions, masses.
Test auditory acuity with Weber and Rinne tests.

From Expert 10-minute physical examinations, St Louis, 1997, Mosby; Barkauskas VH and others: *Health and physical assessment*, ed 2, St Louis, 1998, Mosby.

Scoliosis, which is a lateral curvature of the spine, occurs more often in female adolescents than in males. It may be present at birth or develop due to illness, weak spinal muscles, habitual bad posture, or unknown causes. By asking the woman to bend over, the straightness of her spine may be more easily assessed. While she is standing, also have her demonstrate her ability to flex, hyperflex, and rotate.

As she breathes, the movements of her thorax should be equal and bilateral. The respirations should come easily without the use of thorax muscles and be even and regular.

Palpate her thorax, noting any bulges or depressions, lesions, tenderness, unusual vibrations on inspiration, or unusual movements. Compare symmetric areas of the lungs for tactile fremitus. Measure respiratory excursion. Evaluate the possibility of a kidney infection by palpating the costovertebral angle on each side (Mosby, 1997) (Box 4-24).

**Chest.** The chest is inspected for color; bruises, wounds, or scars; lesions, nodules, or superficial venous patterns. It may be necessary to lift up the woman's breasts to evaluate her chest tissue. Gently hold them out of the way as you continue the evaluation of her respiratory and cardiac systems.

Evaluate the prominence of the woman's ribs. Determine again the respiratory rate, rhythm, and effort of her breathing. Inspect for color and pulsations. Palpate for thrills, masses, and deformities. Assess the location of her apical impulse. Auscultate for abnormal lung and heart sounds.

### Breasts

A clinical breast examination (CBE) is an assessment of a woman's breasts, axilla, nipples, and lymphatic structures. The breast assessment has different meanings for different women, depending on their age, culture, prior experiences, education, and personal or family history. For a young woman, concerns about the development of her breasts (e.g., their size and lack of symmetry) may be paramount. Another woman may be concerned about her breasts and their role in breast-feeding. A woman with a family history of breast cancer may focus on the threat they pose to her of developing breast cancer. Another woman may value her breasts for their effect on her sexual identity or her partner's sexual response and satisfaction with them.

***Understanding the Breasts.*** The lobes and ductal network, blood vessels, nerves and lymphatic structures, and fatty tissue are all in the breasts. The size and shape

---

## BOX 4-24   Assessment of Back and Chest

**BACK\***
Inspect:
  Skin color, condition, irregularities, lesions.
  Chest shape and dimensions.
  Spine and scapula shape and symmetry.
  Anterior-posterior and lateral dimensions of chest.
  Respiratory effort.
  Range of motion of spinal column.
Palpate:
  Temperature and consistency.
  Lesions, masses, or areas of tenderness.
  Spinal column structure for possible deformities.
  Respiratory excursion.
  Tactile fremitus.
  Tenderness at costovertebral angle.
Percuss:
  Resonance over lung fields.
  Diaphragmatic excursion.
Auscultate:
  Breath sounds.
  Vocal resonance.

**CHEST†**
Inspect:
  Configuration and skin.
  Jugular vein distention.
Palpate:
  Skin temperature, consistency, tenderness, and thoracic configuration.
  Tactile fremitus.
Percuss:
  To assess underlying structures.
Auscultate:
  Breath sounds.
  Vocal resonance.
  Heart sounds, bruits.
  Point of maximal impulse (PMI).

\*Standing behind woman.
†Moving in front of the woman as she is sitting and then lying down.
From Mosby: *Expert 10-minute physical examinations,* St Louis, 1997, Mosby; Barkauskas VH and others: *Health and physical assessment,* ed 2, St Louis, 1998, Mosby.

of a woman's breasts are related to the amount of sub-cutaneous and adipose tissue that she has. Breast size, shape, and even symmetry are not related to the lactation process.

The components of the breasts overlie the woman's rib cage, from her second to seventh ribs and from the sternal edge into her axillary region. Breast tissue extending into axilla is often thicker because it contains more glandular tissue than other areas. Because the upper, outer quadrant of the breast is often the site of malignant growth, palpation of the area called the tail of Spence is important during both clinical- and self-breast examinations (Figure 4-5).

Underlying the breasts are the muscles of the chest wall—the pectoralis major and serratus anterior muscles. When women have large or enlarged breasts, the muscles of their chest walls may be strained. Cooper's ligaments connect the breasts to the chest wall muscles, suspending and supporting the breasts in their position. Distension of breast tissue from edema, milk engorgement, or masses may stretch these ligaments, decreasing their supportive ability. Back pain can result when the lateral and spinal muscles then become involved in supporting the suspension of the breasts (Barkauskas and others, 1998).

 To increase a woman's self-understanding and participation in breast self-examination, we explain the anatomy and physiology of the mammary glands during the examination. Have the woman feel her breasts while we identify their components. Breasts are normally a little "lumpy," which may frighten a woman because she may not know what she is feeling. The comfort that may come from knowing what a normal breast feels like can increase her participation in breast self-examination (BSE).

The color of the nipples and areola may be dark pink or brown, depending primarily on the woman's skin color and age, if she is pregnant, and her lactation history. Erectile tissue in the nipples allows them to become firm if they are cold or stimulated, either physically or emotionally. While you are doing the CBE, the woman's nipples may become erect. Unaware that this is a natural response to cold or touch, the woman may be embarrassed. If she appears upset, explain that the nipple response is normal.

Opening onto the surface of the nipple are milk ducts from the 10 to 15 lactiferous sinuses behind the nipples. Unless the woman is pregnant or lactating, it is unusual for discharge to secrete from these openings. Occasionally, a woman who is not pregnant or lactating can manually express a clear, yellowish secretion from her nipples. This hormonal response to estrogen and progesterone may also occur in women who are taking oral contraceptives or are premenstrual or postpartum.

***Clinical Breast Examination (CBE).*** Examination of the breasts and axilla requires the assessment techniques of inspection and palpation. If lesions or secretions of the breast are present during the CBE, universal precautions are required. Assess a woman's level of sexual maturity,

as well as breast symmetry, uniformity of color, and vascular patterns. Note lesions, rashes, unusual pigmentation, edema, nipple retraction, scaling, and nipple discharge. Palpation may reveal thickening, masses, nodules, or abnormal lymph nodes.

The Tanner development levels provide five stages of breast development in females. Based on the size and shape of the woman's breasts as observed from both the side and the front, we can identify and label her age and stage of sexual maturity. Her physical development should be in the range expected of her chronologic age. If sexual development is earlier than expected (precocious puberty) or breast budding is completely absent at age 13 (delayed puberty), a thorough investigation beginning with complete family and personal medical histories is necessary (Youngkin and Davis, 1998) (Figure 4-6).

*Sitting.* While sitting up with her arms at her side, have the woman drop or raise her clothing to expose both breasts simultaneously. As you inspect and palpate her breasts, she can learn how to do breast self-examination (BSE). Information on teaching BSE is provided in Chapter 5.

During the inspection, have the woman put her arms at her side, then place her hands on her hips and press down so that her chest muscles become tight. She may also raise her arms and place her hands behind her head. Assuming these three positions contracts the chest wall muscles posterior to the breasts and increases the possibility of observing retraction or "dimpling," which may indicate a breast mass or disease process. If the woman has large or pendulous breasts, have her lean forward at the waist so that her breasts fall away from her chest. This is also a way to make underlying abnormalities within the breasts more visible (Figure 4-7).

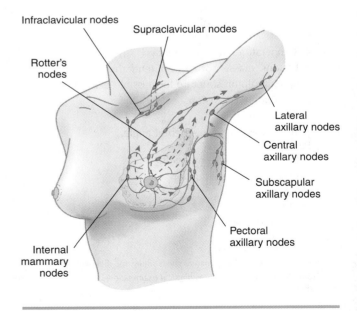

*FIGURE* 4-5 • Areas of breast to palpate.

Palpation of the breasts and axilla is done to determine if there are any areas of thickness or tenderness or lumps in the breasts, axilla, and related lymph nodes. The pads on the index, middle, and ring fingers are used to palpate. The woman's axillary area is initially in-

spected and palpated while she is sitting up. With the woman in a relaxed posture, we support her left arm with our left hand while we palpate the left axillary area. We begin high in the axilla and palpate with small, circular rotations downward and along the axillary line to

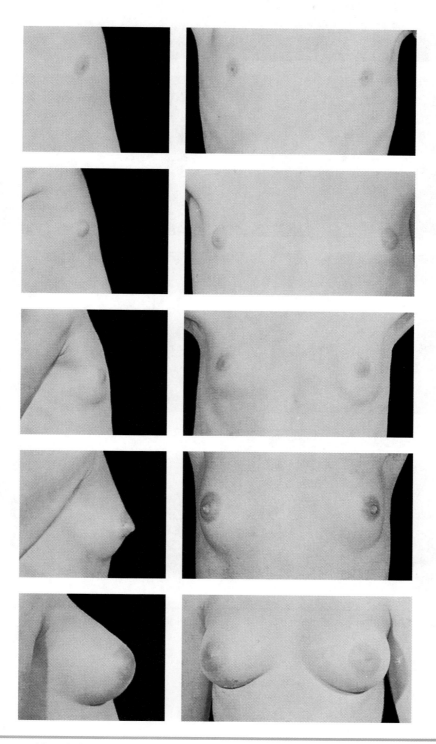

**FIGURE 4-6** • Five stages of female breast development. *(From Barkauskas VH and others:* Health and physical assessment, *ed 2, St Louis, 1998, Mosby.)*

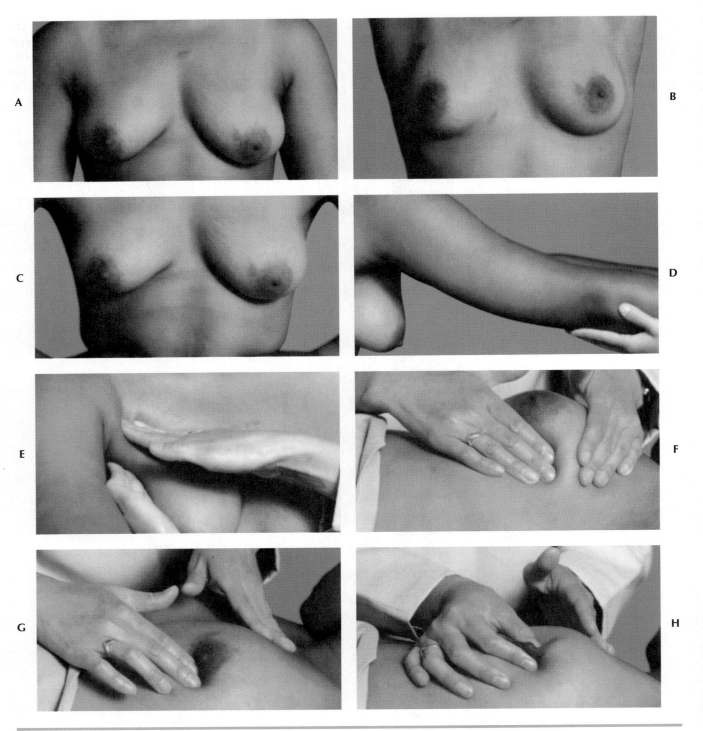

FIGURE 4-7 • Breast examination positions performed by the provider. *(From Barkauskas VH and others:* Health and physical assessment, *ed 2, St Louis, 1998, Mosby.)*

the level of the seventh or eighth rib. The lymph nodes that line the interior aspect of the upper arm are also palpated. After examining her left axilla, the process is repeated on the woman's right side. We support her right arm with our right hand, while thoroughly palpating the axilla with the fingers of our left hand (Box 4-25).

*Arms.* The woman's arms can be examined as a continuation of the exam of the axilla on first one side and then the other. Assess the color, warmth, texture, and edema. Look for bruises, especially on the underside of the lower arm. If there is concern about the woman's circulation, check not only her radial pulse (if not already done), but also her ulnar and brachial pulses, which should be bilaterally equal. Palpate her infraclavicular and epitrochlear nodes. Examine her hands for lesions and check the capillary refill of her nails and her handgrip strength. Evaluate if her body structure, strength, and range of motion are symmetrical (Barkauskas and others, 1998).

*Lying on Her Back.* Palpate the woman's breasts while she is lying down. To examine her left breast and nipple, place a towel under her scapula on the left side to shift the breast structures slightly to the right, making them more accessible. Having the woman lift her left arm and place her left palm beneath her head or neck helps distribute the breast tissue more evenly on that side. Systematically palpate the breast and nipple on that left side. Once the left side is complete, remove the rolled towel, place it under the woman's right side, and repeat the process for the right breast and nipple areas.

There are two systematic approaches to breast palpation that are useful both for us to use and to teach to women for BSE. Both techniques begin in the center of the breast and work outward to cover the entire area of the breast. These techniques are as follows:

1. "The wheel" treats the sections of the breast as if they are spokes on a wheel, beginning with the nipple at the wheel's center. Palpation proceeds outward along each spoke, spinning off into the tail of Spence when palpating that area.
2. "The pinwheel" begins with palpation around the nipple and areola, moving in concentric circles throughout the breast area and up through the tail of Spence.

After using either of these patterns to palpate her breasts, evaluate any discharge from the nipples. Discharge might become apparent when we gently compress behind the nipple with our thumb and forefinger. If discharge is present, determine the color, amount, and odor. Nipple secretions that are blood-tinged or greenish are not normal and require further diagnosis through cytology and culture analyses.

Talk to the woman about the findings while doing the breast examination, as well as when the examination is finished. Discuss relevant physical findings and

guide her hand to feel them. If findings from the breast examination were abnormal, we must be ready to provide guidance and supportive follow-up. When findings are normal, we should review the importance of performing a monthly BSE and have the woman do it with us to evaluate her skill with the technique.

### Abdomen

The woman's knees should be slightly flexed so that her abdominal muscles relax. Sometimes placing a small pillow or rolled up towel under her knees to support them helps her relax (Box 4-26).

Inspect the woman's skin for discoloration, striae (i.e., stretch marks may be caused by more than the stretching of pregnancy), scars, lesions, nodules, or distended veins. Ask about any scars as they may remind the woman about prior problems and surgery. It is always amazing how many times a woman will have

---

**BOX 4-25** *Clinical Breast Examination*

**BREAST**
*When the woman is seated, stand in front of her.*
Inspect:
　Condition of skin.
　Size of breast and areola, symmetry and configuration of the breasts, characteristics of the surface.
　Configuration of nipples, symmetry in position and direction.
　Symmetry of movement of breasts when hands are placed on hips, raised over head, when leaning forward.
　Skin of axilla.
Palpate:
　Axillary nodes and breast; then repeat on other side.

*Have the woman lie on her back and position a small pillow under the shoulder of the side to be examined. With warm hands, do the following.*
Inspect:
　Skin of thorax.
　Surface characteristics of breasts.
Palpate:
　Breasts to determine consistency of tissue and presence of masses.
　Areolar areas for masses.
　Nipples to determine presence of discharge.
Review your findings with the woman.
Have her palpate areas of her breasts and explain what she is feeling.
Review with her how to do breast self-examination.

forgotten a surgical experience and only be reminded when we ask about the scar. Inspect her umbilicus, noting its color, contour, and location. There is some variation in the height of the umbilicus on the abdomen. Inspect the area around the umbilicus for small scars. If a woman has had a laparoscopy, the scar in the umbilicus and a tiny abdominal scar may be the only indications.

Bending down to be level with the surface of her abdomen, inspect the contour, symmetry, and movement. Resuming a standing position, have the woman take a deep breath so that her abdominal muscles tighten. As she holds the breath, look for bulges or masses. After she releases the breath, have her lift her head up slightly and observe her abdomen again for bulges or masses. With the diaphragm of the stethoscope, listen for bowel sounds in all four quadrants. Use the bell of the stethoscope to listen for bruits in the aorta and renal arteries.

Palpating the abdomen for tenderness and masses is the last step. Palpate lightly over all four quadrants, and then repeat the process palpating deeply. If the woman has mentioned that she has been having pain in her abdomen, pay special attention to that region. Check for rebound tenderness.

### Legs

Assessment of the woman's lower extremities started as we watched her walk. Now we assess her legs more closely for color, warmth, texture, edema, and bruising. To evaluate her circulation, we palpate her pulses, which should be bilaterally equal. Note inguinal node enlargement, tenderness or pain, or rigidity.

The woman's muscle development should be uniform and equal. Leg hair should be distributed symmetrically, which may be difficult to evaluate if the woman shaves all or part of her legs. If there is a partial distribution of hair or no leg hair, ask her if she shaves or waxes her leg hair. She can describe what she does and how heavy the distribution of hair appears to her. Examine her feet for lesions, and check the capillary refill of her nails. Her strength and range of motion should be symmetrical and pain-free.

Shoes can cause difficulties for women. In order to be lightweight, many women's shoes do not have a supportive structure built into them. Shoes that are considered stylish often do not conform to the real shape of a woman's foot, which can lead to daily discomfort, as well as the development of calluses and corns. Some women regularly wear shoes with at least 1-inch heels. Over time, their Achilles tendons may shorten, making it uncomfortable for them to stand flat-footed. Wearing shoes that elevate the heel without also providing support can also place women at risk for ankle injuries. Ask the woman about the variety of shoes she wears and if she is experiencing any difficulties with her feet or ankles.

### Preparing for the Pelvic Examination

The pelvic examination requires that the woman empty her urinary bladder and then be positioned on the table so that her perineum and rectum can be seen. A variety of equipment must be close by so that the provider can reach it easily (Figure 4-8).

***Examination Gloves.*** We wear nonsterile exam gloves, unless sterile gloves are required for surgical procedures or wound care. Because an increasing number of women are allergic to latex, ask about this before starting the physical examination. If the woman has a latex allergy, latex-free materials must be obtained. The num-

---

**BOX 4-26** *Assessment of the Abdomen*

**ABDOMEN**

Inspect:

Skin for discoloration, striae, scars, lesions, nodules, or distended veins.

Umbilicus, noting its color, contour, and location.

Contour, symmetry, and movement of abdomen when relaxed and tightened.

Auscultate:

All four quadrants for bowel sounds.

For bruits in the aorta and renal arteries.

Palpate:

For tenderness and masses.

First lightly, then deeply, in all four quadrants.

Check for rebound tenderness.

From Mosby: *Expert 10-minute physical examinations,* St Louis, 1997, Mosby; Barkauskas VH and others: *Health and physical assessment,* ed 2, St Louis, 1998, Mosby.

---

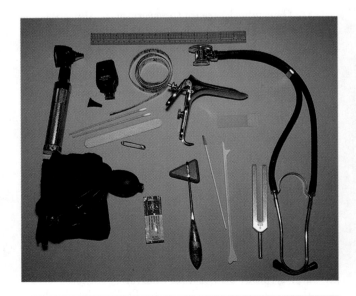

*FIGURE 4-8* • Pelvic examination tools. *(From Potter P and Perry A:* Fundamentals of nursing, *ed 5, St Louis, 2000, Mosby.)*

ber of people with latex allergies is increasing so nonlatex gloves and latex-free equipment must be readily available. Our nails should be trimmed short and we should only wear small, flat rings when doing a pelvic examination so that the gloves are not torn or the woman hurt.

Even when nonsterile gloves are worn, handwashing is of utmost importance before and after the physical examination to prevent spreading infection to the woman or others. Universal precautions require that we wear gloves while examining the urinary, gynecologic, and anorectal areas. Gloves should be changed during the examination when they become contaminated with secretions.

*Speculum.* There are two basic types of specula used to separate the vaginal walls for inspection and to view the cervix. The Pederson has narrow, flat blades that barely curve along the sides, and the Graves has wider, arched blades that curve markedly. To facilitate a woman's comfort, both come in a variety of sizes, including a pediatric size (Klingman, 1999). The Graves specula vary in length from 3.5 to 5 inches and in width from .75 to 1.5 inches. Because of its wider, curved blades, the Graves separates the walls of sexually active and multiparous women. The Pederson is generally more comfortable in women who are young, have not had intercourse, or are postmenopausal (Barkauskas and others, 1998).

The metal specula are reusable, and the plastic specula are disposable. Although both have levers that open the distal and then the proximal ends of the blades and a locking mechanism to keep them open while specimens are obtained, they are somewhat different to use. Examiners tend to favor one type over the other. Some providers are uncomfortable with the locking mechanism of the plastic specula because they sometimes get locked into position and are difficult to release. If a plastic speculum is to be used for a woman's vaginal examination, be aware that the clicking sound of it locking is loud and sharp. The woman may think that the speculum has broken in her, so alert her to the sound before it happens so that she is not frightened. The plastic speculum offers us the advantage of being able to see the vaginal walls through it, providing for a more thorough assessment (Secor, 1999) (Figure 4-9).

Keeping a metal speculum under a warm heating pad and/or running it under warm water to lubricate it before insertion helps to decrease the woman's discomfort. Although they do not feel as cold, plastic

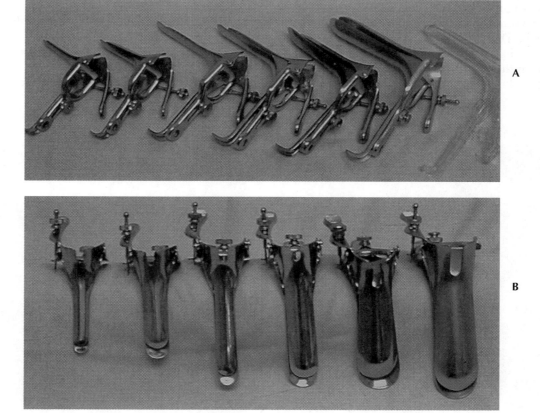

FIGURE 4-9 • Vaginal specula. From left to right: **A,** Short-billed pediatric, pediatric, Small Pederson, Pederson, Small Graves, Large Graves, Plastic Graves. **B,** Short-billed pediatric, pediatric, Small Pederson, Pederson, Small Graves, Large Graves. *(From Seidel HM and others: Mosby's guide to physical examination, ed 3, St Louis, 1998, Mosby.)*

specula are also held under warm water for lubrication before insertion.

In some instances, a gel lubricant may be necessary. Because these lubricants are bacteriostatic and distort cells on a Pap smear, however, their use is generally avoided. Even if a woman has no symptoms indicative of vaginal problems, we will not know if we need to take a specimen until the vaginal walls and cervix are examined, so no lubricant is used.

***Sterile Cotton Swabs.*** Sterile cotton swabs are used to wipe the internal genitalia, removing excess substances. A woman's cervix may normally have mucus on it. Sometimes the cervix is friable (i.e., bleeds easily) when touched by the speculum or there may be a deposit of seminal fluid. Cotton swabs are also used to obtain specimens for gonorrheal culture and chlamydial culture. Sometimes sponge forceps and cotton balls may be used to remove the mucous plug from the os of the cervix before taking a Pap smear.

***Papanicolaou (Pap) Smear Collection.*** The Pap smear is a screening test to detect neoplastic cells in a woman's cervix or vaginal secretions. Depending on the protocol set by the laboratory and the available equipment, the areas from which cell samples are obtained and how the samples are obtained and fixed will vary. Samples are generally obtained from the endocervix, cervix, and vaginal pool. The endocervical specimen is taken from within the cervical os by a small brush or cotton swab. The cervical specimen is obtained from the surface of the cervix and the squamocolumnar junction with the end of a wooden Ayre spatula that is shaped roughly like a thumb and first finger. The

longer projection is inserted into the os and forms the center of the circle as the spatula rotates around the cervix. The sample from the vaginal pool may be collected using the round end of an Ayre spatula to scrape the posterior cervical fornix. Immediately after being obtained and spread on the slide—before the cells are allowed to air dry, they are sprayed with a fixative or immersed in a fixative solution. Each sample must be correctly labeled as to where the cells in the sample were obtained (Figure 4-10).

***Obtaining Other Specimens.*** Sexually transmitted infections (STIs) or vaginitis may require other specimens. Wet mounts are used to obtain vaginal specimens to look for the presence of *Trichomonas vaginalis*, *Candida albicans*, or the "clue cells" of bacterial vaginosis. Normal saline and potassium hydroxide are necessary to prepare a sample of the discharge so that a slide can be examined under the microscope for organisms. To test the pH of the vagina, pH tape is needed.

Samples of fecal material obtained during the recto-vaginal examination are often tested for occult blood. These tests rely on detecting peroxidase as an indication of hemoglobin in the stool specimen. Various reagent substances are used to detect occult blood. The sensitivity of these substances varies according to the following:

1. Orthotoluidine (Hematest, Occultest)—10 times more sensitive than benzidine.
2. Benzidine—10 (or more) times more sensitive than guaiac
3. Guaiac (hemoccult)—the least sensitive reagent

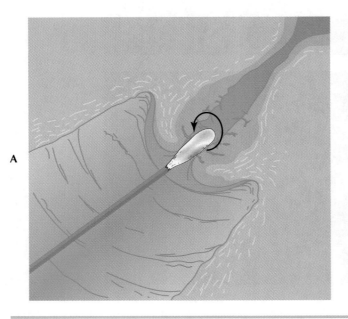
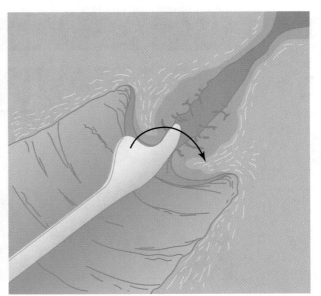

*FIGURE 4-10* • Tools for Pap specimen collection. **A,** Endocervical specimen. **B,** Cervical specimen with Ayre spatula.

If one of these tests is positive, gastrointestinal bleeding is not necessarily present. The test must be repeated at least three times while the woman refrains from eating meat and eats a high residue diet (Barkauskas and others, 1998).

*Seeing the Area.* Adequate lighting is necessary for us to not only see the external tissues but also the vagina and cervix. Some providers prefer a lighted speculum system because it offers a built-in light source and enhanced illumination of the cervix and vagina. During a nonspecific genital examination, the light source is a long-necked floor lamp that may be adjusted to direct light over the shoulder of the provider.

Have a mirror available so that the woman may see her perineum and, when the speculum is in place, her cervix. A woman may express fear about looking at these structures, but encouraging her to view them helps to take the mystery away and enables her to then think realistically of them as part of her body. Knowledge of the anatomy of her female genitalia is fundamental to health promotion and disease prevention, as well as increasing her understanding of how to receive sexual pleasure. Helping a woman find her clitoris is necessary before she can truly understand about clitoral stimulation for pleasure (Box 4-27).

### Initiating the Pelvic Examination

Provide the woman with the opportunity to discuss any of her concerns related to this part of the exam. Normal anxiety about the gynecologic exam may be heightened by prior experiences (e.g., an insensitive examination or a surgical procedure).

Women from 28 of the African nations and the Middle East (e.g., Egypt, Oman, Yemen, and the United Arab Emirates) may have experienced female genital circumcision (i.e., female genital mutilation [FMG]). These women may have had part or all of their external genitalia removed and the tissues brought together so that only a narrow opening remains. If the woman underwent the surgery as an infant, she may not be aware that her body is no longer the normal female anatomy and physiology. See Chapter 7 for more details about this condition and the health problems it creates for the woman. When a woman has experienced any type of surgery to her external genitalia, including a vaginal examination in a well-woman visit is at the least difficult and often inappropriate (Lightfoot-Klein, 1989; Klingman, 1999).

Because of the close proximity of the organs in the pelvis, the woman should be encouraged to empty her urinary bladder before the gynecologic exam. If the woman has a distended bladder, it not only alters physical findings but can make the examination more uncomfortable for her.

If a urine specimen is to be collected as part of the examination, this may be done at this time. Instruct the woman on how to cleanse her perineal area, and then col-

---

### BOX 4-27    *Pelvic Examination*

Verify that there is good lighting and a mirror available.

Set up the necessary supplies for all aspects of the examination (i.e., warmed speculum, nonsterile gloves, supplies for screening [Pap smear, STI tests], vaginal pH paper, wet mount kits, test for fecal occult blood).

Show the equipment, especially the speculum and implements for taking specimens to the woman and explain how they are used.

Determine with the woman what position will be most comfortable for the examination, and help her into that position.

Before proceeding with the examination, ask the woman if she is ready. Let her know that she is in control and may ask at any time for you to stop, especially if she is experiencing pain or severe anxiety.

Be sure that she is told of the procedures as the exam proceeds in a language she can understand (e.g., "I'm going to be touching your thigh and then inserting the speculum. I'm opening the speculum . . .").

Encourage her to express questions, sensations, and concerns as the exam proceeds.

Reassure her as the exam continues.

Help her to stay comfortable and relaxed with deep breathing.

Inspect the external genitalia.

Palpate the external genital area, including the labia and Batholin's and Skene's glands.

Perform the speculum examination to inspect the vagina and cervix.

Obtain necessary laboratory samples.

As the examination moves from the speculum exam, explain the bimanual exam and the rectovaginal examination to the woman.

Inspect the rectal area.

Perform the bimanual vaginal examination, palpating sphincter tone, rectovaginal septum, ligaments, uterus, tubes, ovaries, and cul-de-sac.

Perform bimanual rectovaginal examination, palpating vagina, cervix, uterus, tubes, ovaries, and muscle tone.

Inspect the appearance of fecal matter on the glove.

After the examination is completed, compliment the woman on how well she did.

Provide her with tissues (so that she may wipe the lubricant and secretions from her perineum), and instruct her to get dressed.

After she is dressed, return to discuss the findings of the examination and answer any questions.

Provide her with written materials to take home about the findings, laboratory tests, and/or possible follow-up care.

From Mosby: *Expert 10-minute physical examinations,* St Louis, 1997, Mosby; Barkauskas VH and others: *Health and physical assessment,* ed 2, St Louis, 1998, Mosby.

lect her urine. Also provide her with clear instructions on what to do with the sample after she has voided. It can be embarrassing for her to be left holding a urine specimen cup, without knowing where to put it. The urine dipstick screening test can be done by the woman, or at least in her presence, and the urine analysis is explained to her.

### Positioning for Vaginal Examination

A cooperative approach to the positioning for the pelvic examination allows the woman and the clinician to work together to meet both their needs. Accommodations must be made when a woman is unable to sit up for the physical examination or is uncomfortable or unable to assume the lithotomy (traditional) position with her feet in the foot stirrups. Women with joint stiffness or inflammation; lack of muscle control; paralysis; pain in the hips, knees, or back; muscle weakness or contractions; spasticity; or a lack of balance will have difficulty with the lithotomy position and foot stirrups. A woman who has been sexually assaulted may have a difficult time being put in the same position for a vaginal examination.

***Lithotomy (Traditional) Position with Foot Stirrups.*** The woman lies on her back with her buttocks at the end of the table. Her knees are bent and spread, and her feet are in the foot stirrups (Figure 4-11, *A* and *B*).

***Knee-Chest Position.*** The knee-chest position does not require the use of stirrups to provide comfort and

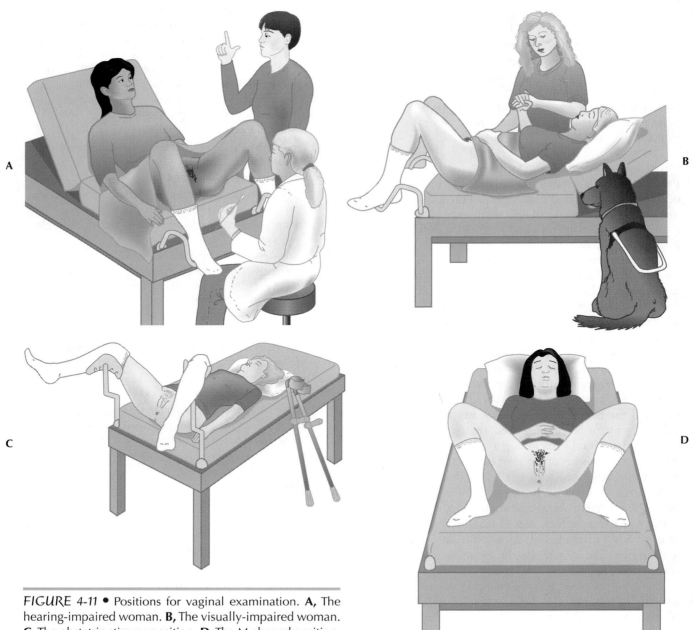

FIGURE 4-11 • Positions for vaginal examination. **A,** The hearing-impaired woman. **B,** The visually-impaired woman. **C,** The obstetric stirrups position. **D,** The M-shaped position.

access for the speculum during the vaginal examination. The speculum is inserted with the handle pointing either in the direction towards the woman's back or abdomen, with the front of the blade angles toward the small of her back. After the speculum examination is completed, the woman must lie on her back for the bimanual examination. Women who feel more balance lying on their sides or who have experienced a frontal approach sexual assault may be more comfortable in this position (Ferreyra and Hughes, 1984) (Figure 4-11, *F*).

***Diamond-Shaped Position.*** The woman lies on her back with her knees bent and her heels together on the table. Depending on her condition, the woman may need help holding her feet together. Pillows may be placed under the woman's thighs to help her support them. The speculum is inserted with the handle up (Ferreyra and Hughes, 1984) (Figure 4-11, *G*).

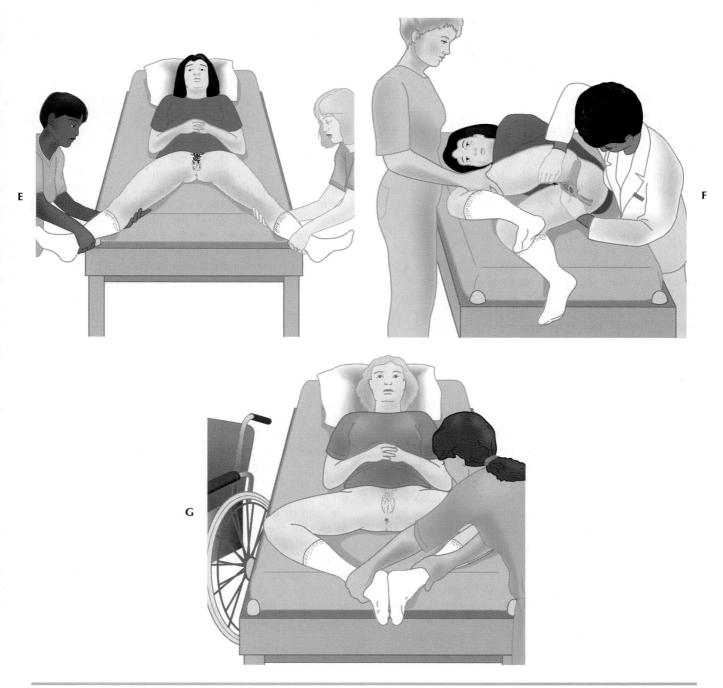

**FIGURE 4-11**, *cont'd* • **E,** The V-shaped position. **F,** The knee-chest position. **G,** The diamond-shaped position. *(Reprinted with permission from Planned Parenthood.)*

*V-Shaped Position.* While she is still lying on her back, the woman's legs are straightened out and spread widely on the table. Her legs must be supported by assistants at both the knee and ankle. The woman may be more comfortable with a small pillow placed under the small of her back and/or coccyx. The speculum must be inserted with the handle up (Ferreyra and Hughes, 1984) (Figure 4-11, *E*).

*M-Shaped Position.* To assume an M-position, the woman lies on her back and places her feet flat on the table with her knees apart. An assistant may be needed to hold the woman's knees and feet so that they feel stable on the table. If the woman has had one or both lower legs amputated, the assistant can hold the woman's leg in the air to stimulate this position. The speculum is inserted with the handle up (Ferreyra and Hughes, 1984) (Figure 4-11, *D*).

*Knee Support Position.* In this position, the woman's buttocks are near the end of the table. Her legs are raised and placed on the obstetrical stirrup supports and then secured in place. This position allows women who have difficulty using the foot stirrups to still achieve the traditional position for a pelvic examination (Ferreyra and Hughes, 1984) (Figure 4-11, *C*).

### Communication Constraints and the Vaginal Examination

*Hearing Impairment.* "A woman with a hearing impairment will most likely want to assume the foot stirrup position. Her head may be elevated so that she can see the clinician and/or interpreter" (Ferreyra and Hughes, 1984). The drape that is used to cover the legs must be lowered so that the woman may see the face of the examiner. Communication may be through lip reading or writing if the woman does not want the interpreter in the room. Because she will not hear what is happening the woman may want to see the examination with a mirror.

*Visual Impairment.* Prior to the examination the woman with a visual impairment may wish to feel the instrument and three-dimensional models so that she understands what is going to happen. During the examination, the woman will probably be able to relax more if constant tactile or verbal contact is made (e.g., a hand on her and/or a continuous description of what the clinician is doing). The woman may feel most secure in a foot-stirrup position (Ferreyra and Hughes, 1984).

### Special Concerns during the Vaginal Examination

Some women with cerebral palsy, spina bifida, spinal cord injury, muscular diseases, multiple sclerosis, polio, or who have had a stroke have other concerns that must also be attended to during a vaginal examination.

*Bowel and Bladder Concerns.* A woman's bladder and bowel routines could affect the pelvic examination. An indwelling catheter—whether urethral or suprapubic—may remain in place because it will not interfere with the exam. The urine, however, is drained into a bag that is strapped to the woman's leg, which should be drained before the examination. If a woman uses an intermittent catheterization system, the tactile stimulation in her pelvic area could cause her to urinate. The pelvic examination should be scheduled around her urinary schedule. If a woman has a bowel movement routine based on physical stimulation, she may experience these same physical sensations during the speculum, bimanual, or rectal examination, causing a bowel movement to occur (Ferreyra and Hughes, 1984).

*Hyperreflexia.* Someone with a spinal cord injury may experience hyperreflexia due to stimulation of the bowel, bladder, or skin below the spinal lesion. Hyperreflexia may also occur as a reaction to a cold, hard exam table or stirrups, insertion and manipulation of the vaginal speculum, swabbing of the cervix for the Pap smear, or pressure during the bimanual or rectal examination. Symptoms of hyperreflexia include high blood pressure, sweating, blotchy skin, nausea, or "goosebumps." Ask the woman if she has had a pelvic examination since the injury, and inquire about her common hyperreflexic symptoms. If a hyperreflexic reaction occurs during the examination, we must immediately reduce her blood pressure and discover the source of the reaction. Sitting the woman up will generally lower her blood pressure. If the symptoms continue, it becomes a medical emergency. If the hyperreflexic reaction ceases, the woman—as expert of her own symptoms and reactions—should be consulted about whether to continue the exam (Ferreyra and Hughes, 1984).

*Hypersensitivity.* Some women experience spasms or pain in response to ordinary touch. To prevent possible discomfort or spasms during the examination, ask the woman about any hypersensitive areas. Once identified, sensitive areas can be avoided or an extra amount of lubricant can be used to decrease friction or pressure (Ferreyra and Hughes, 1984).

*Spasticity.* A woman may experience spasms that range from slight tremors to quick, violent contractions. These spasms may be initiated by movement onto the table or when she is in an uncomfortable or awkward position or her skin is stimulated. The intensity or frequency of the spasm can be reduced when the woman feels physically secure, so someone should always stand next to her and maintain physical contact. If a spasm occurs during the vaginal examination, her body parts should be gently and securely supported so that she is not injured. After the spasm has resolved, the examination may continue (Ferreyra and Hughes, 1984).

### Performing the Pelvic Examination

By explaining the procedures and describing what the woman will experience and how we will assist her during this experience, we may lessen a woman's anxiety. If we ask her how she is feeling while we move through the examination, not only are we able to do a more sensitive and thorough examination but also the woman is recognized as a participant.

It is important to show respectful sensitivity while positioning the woman, inserting a speculum, and performing manual palpation activities. There are many women who are overtly expressive when their genitalia are assessed, especially those who are young or experiencing one of their first exams. There are some women who cry out in pain even during the gentlest of speculum or bimanual exams, and there are others who do not express—either verbally or nonverbally—any pain yet comment later. Because part of our assessment is based on the woman's response to tenderness when we palpate an area, we should encourage a woman to be responsive and describe what she is feeling while we conduct the examination.

The **external genitalia** are collectively termed the vulva or pudendum. We inspect the vulvar area from front to back, looking at hair distribution. Assessment of the female's pubic hair on the mons pubis and labia majora provides a comparative measurement for determining her stage of sexual development (Figure 4-12).

Next observe the color and condition of tissues. Are there rashes; swelling; bruises; lacerations; lesions; parasites; discharge; and scars on the mons pubis, clitoris, and labia majora, or needle marks in the groin? Palpate the groin and vulva for tenderness or masses. Be aware of an unpleasant or "fishy" odor, which may indicate an infection.

To continue the assessment, spread the labia majora to fully visualize the two labia minora, the darker and thinner skin folds that protect the flattened area just beneath them, the vestibule. Continue to assess for abnormalities. Palpate the labia minora for masses or tenderness.

The vestibule has the openings for the woman's urethra and vagina, as well as the openings for the periurethral Skene's glands and the transvaginal Bartholin's glands, which secrete cleansing and lubricating fluids. Look for signs of irritation or infection. Palpate the area for swelling and tenderness. Ask the woman to bear down so that you can assess for the presence of a cystocele, rectocele, or vaginal prolapse.

Some women have a partial covering of connective tissue around the vaginal os called a hymen, but this membrane may also be naturally absent. Having little or

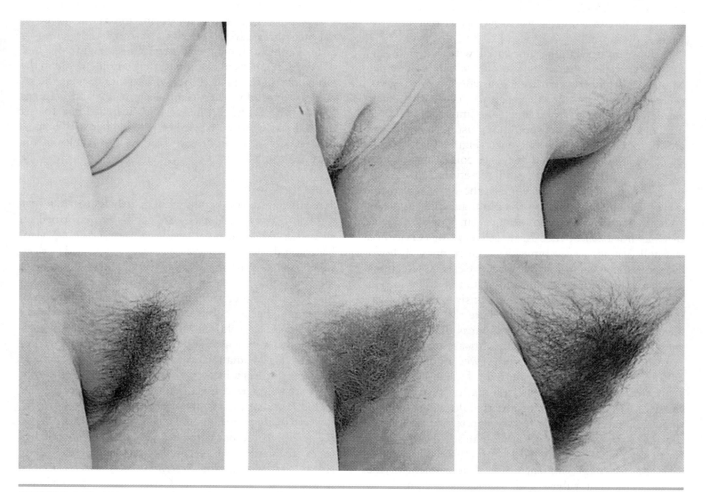

FIGURE 4-12 • Six stages of sexual maturity in females—pubic hair development. *(From Barkauskas VH and others:* Health and physical assessment, *ed 2, St Louis, 1998, Mosby.)*

no hymen can be disturbing to women or their partners who believe that it is an indication of virginity. This myth of a virgin having a hymen has led to the expectation of "blood on the sheets" the first time a woman has intercourse. On rare occasions, a young woman who has not experienced a menses will have a hymen that completely covers the vaginal introitus, thereby blocking the normal monthly flow. She may have been experiencing the hormonal and tissue changes of a menstrual cycle without a monthly bleed.

During this phase of the examination, women can be taught and encouraged to feel comfortable using a mirror to learn how to do a self-examination of the vulva. "The two minutes it takes to provide the woman with a 'tour' of her genital area may save her life. The self-exam should be done monthly" (Youngkin and Davis, 1998), as she looks for changes in her tissues and vaginal discharge.

With a finger inserted into the vagina, assess the vaginal wall. Ask the woman to tighten her vagina around the inserted finger or fingers so that you can evaluate the strength of her pelvic floor muscles. For a quantified assessment, there is a special tool that may be placed in the woman's vagina to measure the pressure with which she tightens those muscles. Next, ask her to bear down so that you can evaluate for a cyctocele, rectocele, or vaginal prolapse.

The warm speculum, lubricated with water, is inserted to reveal the internal genitalia, which include her vagina and the cervix of her uterus. Because the cervix points in different directions during the course of a woman's fertility cycle, it may not immediately come into view. Sometimes the speculum must be inserted several times before the cervix is seen (Figure 14-13).

The cervix is examined for size, color, surface texture, position, appearance, and secretions. In a nonpregnant, premenopausal woman, the diameter of the cervix is 2 to 3 cm, the color is pink, and the surface is smooth. The cervix extends about 2 cm into the vagina. If it has not been opened for a delivery, the cervical os is small, round, and symmetrical. Once opened, however, it assumes a slitlike appearance. Cervical secretions are generally odorless and nonirritating, varying in color from clear to white and in consistency from watery to thick, depending upon where the woman is in her fertility cycle. Any discharge that is discolored, purulent, or has an odor indicates an abnormality and must be investigated further with a wet mount exam or cultures for a sexually transmitted infection (STI). Cervical erosions, cysts, lesions, trauma, or a string from the os (i.e., indicating an intrauterine device) should be noted. Take the specimen for the Pap test as well as indicated cultures based on the woman's history and visual examination (Figure 4-14).

In nonpregnant women, physical assessment of the uterus, fallopian tubes, and ovaries is accomplished with bimanual palpation. The examiner must stand and insert lubricated, gloved index and middle fingers into the vagina. The other hand is placed on the woman's abdomen, above her symphysis pubis. With the external hand on the fundus of the uterus, use the internal fingers to palpate the cervix for consistency, nodules, masses, tenderness, or pain on movement. The texture of the cervix should feel like the tip of a nose. With the uterus gently compressed between the two hands, assess the cervix for position, size, shape, consistency, masses, and tenderness. After this examination of the uterus, the adnexal areas are generally palpated for tenderness or masses. Although this part of the examination is not specific and/or sensitive enough for a screening test, it is still generally included (Frover and Quinn, 1995).

After removing our fingers from her vagina, we change the glove and apply lubricant. We tell the woman that next we are going to inspect the anal area for hemorrhoids and fissures. We then explain that we are putting a finger in her rectum and she may feel a momentary urge to bear down and this is normal. With a finger in the rectum, palpate the sphincter, rectal walls, septum between the rectum and the vagina, posterior surface of the uterus, and the adenexa, looking for tenderness or masses. When we remove our finger from her rectum, the fecal material is tested for blood. If the findings warrant it, additional information about the internal structures can be obtained through ultrasound or radiographic and magnetic imaging (see Figure 4-13).

After the physical examination is completed, help the woman to sit up. Provide her with tissues to wipe the secretions and lubricant from the perineum and help her get off the table, if she desires. Instruct her to get dressed and give her privacy or provide her with help as needed. Once she is dressed, review the results of the examination.

## Laboratory Tests

Screening tests for hemoglobin and hematocrit levels, the Pap test, and urinalysis are generally performed on every woman during a well-woman screening visit. Based on the woman's history and concerns and our observations during the examination, some—or all—of the following may also be included: a gonorrheal culture, chlamydial culture, wet mounts, pH evaluation of the vagina, herpes culture, pregnancy test. If the woman participates in rectal and/or oral intercourse, a gonorrheal culture may also be taken from the rectum and/or throat. If a woman is at least 40 years of age or is younger but has a history of breast cancer in her family, she may be referred for a mammogram.

Explain that the results of her Pap smear will probably not be available for several days or a week. When the results come back, the woman will be informed of them. The nationally accepted reporting system for Pap smears is the Bethesda System, which was developed following a 1988 National Cancer Institute sponsored workshop. This system uses descriptive diagnostic terms rather than class numbers, which were previously used

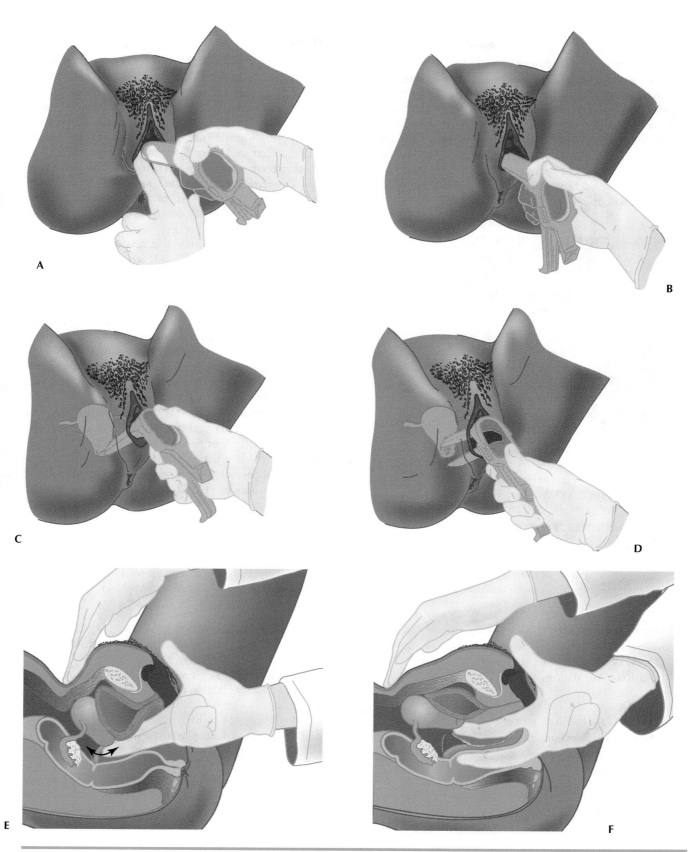

*FIGURE 4-13* • Insertion of speculum. **A,** Opening of the introitus. **B,** Insertion of the speculum. **C,** Positioning of blades. **D,** Opening of blades. **E,** Bimanual palpation. **F,** Rectovaginal palpation.

to report Pap test results. The system of reporting includes an evaluation of specimen adequacy (Box 4-28).

Cells on the surface of the cervix sometimes appear abnormal but are not cancerous. There are several terms, such as **dysplasia,** that may be used to describe abnormal results. Dysplasia is not cancer, although it may develop into a very early stage of cervical cancer. In dysplasia, cervical cells undergo a series of changes in their appearance. The cells look abnormal under the microscope but do not invade nearby healthy tissue. There are three degrees of dysplasia—mild, moderate, or severe, depending on how abnormal the cells appear under the microscope.

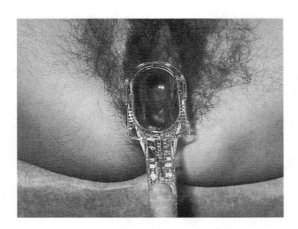

FIGURE 4-14 • Vaginal speculum in place with cervix in full view. *(From Potter P and Perry A:* Fundamentals of nursing, *ed 5, St Louis, 2000, Mosby.)*

The term *squamous intraepithelial lesion (SIL)* is also used to describe abnormal changes in the cells on the surface of the cervix. The word *squamous* describes cells that are thin and flat and lie on the outer surface of the cervix. An intraepithelial lesion means that the abnormal cells are present only in the surface layers of the cells. The SIL changes may be described as being low-grade (i.e., early changes in the size, shape, and number of cells) or high-grade (i.e., a large number of precancerous cells that look very different from normal cells).

Another term sometimes used to describe abnormal cells is *cervical intraepithelial neoplasia (CIN).* *Intraepithelial* refers to the surface layers of the cells. CIN I, CIN II, or CIN III describes how much of the cervix contains abnormal cells.

The term *carcinoma in situ* describes a preinvasive cancer that involves only the surface cells and has not spread to the deeper tissues. **Cervical cancer,** or invasive cervical cancer, occurs when abnormal cells spread deeper into the cervix or to other tissues or organs.

Other results may be termed as **atypical squamous cells of undetermined significance (ASCUS)** or **atypical glandular cells of undetermined significance (AGCUS).** When abnormalities are found in squamous or glandular cells but the changes do not fulfill the criteria for SIL, CIN, or dysplasia, they are labeled atypical.

Human papillomavirus (HPV) are viruses that can cause warts. More than 30 types of HPV may infect the cervix, and about 15 of those are associated with cervical cancer. HPV is a major risk factor for cervical cancer. Nearly all cervical cancers show cellular evidence of HPV. Not all cases of HPV develop into cervical cancer,

---

**BOX 4-28** *The Bethesda System (TBS) for Classifying Pap Smears*

In the past, a number of different classification systems have been used to label the cellular changes seen under the microscope. Because this can be confusing, the Bethesda System was adopted. This system includes an evaluation of specimen adequacy and descriptive diagnoses to tell the provider exactly what the findings are.

**SPECIMEN ADEQUACY**
**Adequate:** Has endocervical cells and either squamous cells or squamous metaplasia
**Unsatisfactory:** Inadequate sample

**FINDINGS**
**Normal:** Class 1—no abnormal cells present
**Inflammatory infection**
**ASCUS:** Atypical squamous cells of undetermined significance
**AGCUS:** Atypical glandular cells of undetermined significance
**Low-grade SIL:** Mild dysplasia; CIN 1; HPV
**High-grade SIL:** Moderate or severe dysplasia; CIN 2 or CIN 3; carcinoma *in situ*
**Cancer**

**UNDERSTANDING ABNORMAL RESULTS**
**Dysplasia:** Abnormal cells; classified as mild, moderate, or severe
**Squamous intraepithelial lesion (SIL):** *Low-grade* (early changes in the size, shape, and number of cells); *high-grade* (a large number of precancerous cells that look different from normal cells)
**Cervical intraepithelial neoplasia (CIN):** *CIN 1, CIN 2,* and *CIN 3* describe how much of the cervix contains abnormal cells
**Carcinoma in situ:** A pre-invasive cancer that only involves the surface cells and has not spread into deeper tissues
**Cervical cancer,** or **invasive cervical cancer:** Occurs when abnormal cells spread deeper into the cervix or to other tissues or organs

but infection with the types of HPV associated with cancer may increase the risk that mild abnormalities will progress to more severe abnormalities or cervical cancer.

Unfortunately, relying solely on manual inspection of the Pap smear slides makes it inevitable that sometimes the results will be false negative or false positive. A false positive result can cause anxiety for a woman and lead to the time and expense of further invasive procedures.

A false negative result occurs when a specimen is identified as normal, but the woman has a lesion. A false negative Pap test may delay the diagnosis and treatment of a precancerous or cancerous condition. One way this has been addressed is through annual screening, because if abnormal cells are missed once, chances are good that they will be detected the next time.

In an effort to reduce the number of false negative readings, the Food and Drug Administration has approved two computerized systems to rescan negative Pap smears for abnormal cells. When an abnormality is detected by the computer, the cells are recorded for a cytologist to reevaluate. These systems will not identify all abnormal cells in every smear but do provide a means of double-checking the negative reading and reducing the risk for false negatives.

If the Pap results show an ambiguous or minor abnormality, the provider may repeat the test to ensure accuracy. If the Pap shows a significant abnormality, a colposcopy may be done to examine the vagina and cervix. A Schiller test (i.e., coating the cervix with an iodine solution so that the healthy cells turn brown and abnormal cells turn white or yellow) can help to determine a more definitive diagnosis. A biopsy of cervical tissue may be obtained for examination by a pathologist to determine the nature and scope of the cellular changes.

### Summarizing the Results

We should review findings and suggested follow-up procedures, share educational materials, and answer all questions. The results of any screening tests that are already determined should be shared with the woman. Explain any follow-up care that may be needed. Help her learn what her insurance will cover and what her possible out-of-pocket expense may be.

If results (e.g., the Pap smear or cultures) take time to come back, the woman should be asked how she would like to be informed of the results. Provide a means for her to have future questions or concerns answered once she leaves the office. The date for a future visit, if appropriate, should be scheduled.

##  SUMMARY

A health assessment is a personally invasive and intensive data-collection session. When a woman is included as a partner in the process, richer data is obtained and the session can be an educational experience for her. Whether through a home visit, a screening program located in the community, or an annual examination in a health facility, the data collected provide the basis for further interactions. Based on the assessment, nursing and medical diagnoses are developed, preliminary goals are established, and the first steps of planning interventions occur. The next three chapters provide the information that is necessary to develop an appropriate plan of care with the woman.

---

## Care Plan · *The Woman Interested in Health Promotion and Illness Prevention*

**NURSING DIAGNOSIS:** **Health-Seeking Behaviors**\* (i.e., screening participation, smoking cessation, weight management, exercise management)

**GOALS/OUTCOMES:** Maintains optimal level of wellness

### NOC Suggested Outcomes
- Adherence Behavior (1600)
- Health Beliefs (1700)
- Health Orientation (1705)
- Health-Promoting Behavior (1602)

### NIC Priority Interventions
- Developmental Enhancement: Adolescent (7052)
- Exercise Promotion (0200)
- Health Education (5510)
- Health Screening (6520)
- Health System Guidance (7400)
- Substance Use Prevention (4500)
- Learning Facilitation (5520)
- Nutrition Management (1100)
- Self-Modification Assistance (4470)
- Smoking Cessation Assistance (4490)
- Weight Management (1260)

\*Note: Wellness nursing diagnoses do not need an etiology.

*Continued*

## Care Plan  ·  The Woman Interested in Health Promotion and Illness Prevention—cont'd

### Nursing Activities & Rationale

- Encourage active participation in screening activities and decisions regarding own health care. *Active participation in health care decisions gives the woman power and authority over her health care.*
- Screen for health problems and teach woman to recognize significant age-appropriate screening procedures (e.g., anemia, hypertension, hyperlipidemia, abnormal sexual maturation or physical growth, body image disturbances, eating disorders). *All women have at least some risk for obesity, hypertension, coronary artery disease, elevated cholesterol, diabetes mellitus, malnutrition, dental disease, and alcohol-related problems. Primary and secondary clinical preventive services target asymptomatic persons based on their individual risk profiles in order to detect and/or prevent disease development.*
- Instruct on rationale and purpose of health screening and self-monitoring. *Knowing the benefits of screening provides motivation to perform.*
- Encourage routine monitoring of blood pressure, weight, percent body fat, cholesterol, blood glucose levels, urinalysis, pap smear, mammography, and vision check as appropriate. *See rationale for screening above.*
- Counsel woman with abnormal findings about treatment alternatives or need for further evaluation. *To encourage early treatment and avoid complications.*
- Provide appropriate immunizations. *Immunizations prevent many viral diseases that can result in serious sequela. For example, women of childbearing age should be immunized against rubella prior to becoming pregnant.*
- Appraise health beliefs and capabilities concerning physical exercise. *To enable the nurse to individualize the plan.*
- Assist with development of an appropriate exercise program to meet needs. *Many clients lack knowledge of how much and what kind of exercise will produce benefits.*
- Inform about different types of health care facilities and types of health care provided by each. *Information is needed for self-care.*
- Inform regarding community resources and contact persons. *Information is needed for self-care and support-seeking.*
- Begin instruction after the woman demonstrates readiness to learn. *Adults learn best when they perceive a need for the information and/or when it has relevance to their situation.*
- Set mutual, realistic goals with the woman. *Active participation promotes adherence to the plan. People are more motivated to achieve goals they perceive as realistic.*
- Tailor content to the woman's cognitive, psychomotor, and/or affective abilities/disabilities. *Individual learning styles and capacities vary; the same approach cannot be used with everyone.*
- Ascertain the woman's food preferences and eating habits. *Adherence to any dietary regimen is enhanced if it includes foods that the client likes and that are readily available. Learning her eating habits provides a basis for screening her risks for developing chronic heart disease or obesity.*
- Assess the woman's nutrient and caloric needs for body type and lifestyle. *To prevent under- or over-nutrition.*
- Encourage the woman to make healthy food choices. *This provides the woman with an opportunity to reduce her health risks.*
- Discuss the relationship between food intake, exercise, weight gain, and weight loss. *Understanding relationships between intake and energy expenditure increases the likelihood of compliance with planned dietary programs.*
- Discuss risk factors associated with being overweight or underweight. *Knowledge increases the woman's power over her own health care and her ability to alter her future in a positive manner.*
- Help the woman identify reasons to quit (or not begin) smoking and barriers to quitting. *Having a valid reason (e.g., increased risk for cardiac or lung disease) may serve as incentive to stop smoking. Once barriers to smoking cessation have been identified, effective strategies for overcoming the barriers can be planned and executed.*
- Help the woman choose the best method for giving up cigarettes when she is ready to quit. *Not all methods are effective for all women. Allowing the woman to identify the method that will best help her to quit smoking will increase the likelihood of adherence to a smoking-cessation program.*
- Help the woman plan specific coping strategies and resolve problems that result from quitting. *If the woman is prepared for problems that may occur and has preplanned strategies for coping with those problems, adherence to a smoking-cessation program is more likely to occur.*

## Care Plan · The Woman Interested in Health Promotion and Illness Prevention—cont'd

- Encourage responsible decision making about lifestyle choices. *This increases the woman's power and control over her future health. Making responsible lifestyle choices will decrease her risk for disease development and increase the probability of remaining healthy.*

**Evaluation Parameters**
- Demonstrates adherence behaviors.
- Reports using strategies to maximize health.
- Performs routine self-screening and self-monitoring.
- Reports using strategies to eliminate unhealthy behaviors

## CASE STUDY*

The Silver Lake Community Church has a health ministry program led by a parish nurse. As part of the services provided to the congregation and community, a health fair is held every year. Community health organizations are invited to set up education and screening booths, and the local hospital sends a mobile mammography unit.

Elizabeth, a 34-year-old mother of two young children and a member of the community has come to the health fair. The expense of health care for the children takes a large chunk of money from the family budget. Elizabeth has been unable to find the time or extra money to have an annual examination herself. She is hoping to learn some things about her own health at the health fair.

When she enters the hall, Elizabeth is given a personal health guide in which she may record and keep findings. At the first booth, Elizabeth learned that her height was 5'6" and her weight was 197 lbs. At a nutrition education table, information about low-fat cooking and samples and recipes were given. At the next booth, she learned that her blood pressure was 149/82, her heart rate was 78 beats per minute, and her respirations were 20 per minute. The booth that provided cholesterol screening was busy when Elizabeth got there, so she skipped that and went on to the next table where there was information about breast self-examination and breast models on which to practice. Elizabeth listened to the description on how to do the examination and tried it on the model. She took the printed instructions to hang in the shower.

You are working at the final station where the results of all the screening tests are reviewed with the woman before leaving.

- What assessment data do you have about Elizabeth?
- What other assessment data do you want to obtain?
- What nursing diagnoses might apply to Elizabeth?
- What goals might you be able to establish with Elizabeth?
- What may hinder the achievement of these goals?
- In anticipation of these difficulties, what problem solving techniques might you be able to offer?
- What interventions can you offer to Elizabeth immediately?
- Based on the information given here, what resources do you know are available to Elizabeth?
- Reputable health-screening programs offer referrals for individuals who have possible health problems. What type of resources and referrals might be available to Elizabeth?
- How will you measure the effectiveness of your nursing care because a health fair does not establish a long-term interaction?

# Scenarios

1. To establish authenticity with a client, we must be fully present in body, mind, and spirit. You work full-time as a staff nurse in a family practice clinic setting and are thinking about going to graduate school. You are not sure how much it will cost or if you will even be accepted. You also don't know how your 15-year-old daughter will react because you will no longer be as available to transport her if you go to school. Today at 4 PM you have an admissions interview at the university, so you are feeling very anxious.

You are thinking about the interview and how complicated your life might become as you pick up the chart and head for the waiting room to call in the next patient. You see from the chart that her name is Theresa, she is 15 years old, and she is concerned that she might be pregnant.

- What is the first thing you will do?
- After you have Theresa settled in a room, how will you proceed?
- What questions will you initially ask her?
- What information might you share?
- What will be the initial focus of the assessment interview?
- What will determine how you proceed with Theresa's health assessment?
- What are two possible focuses?

---

2. Mary is 45 years old and has come to the women's clinic for her annual Pap smear. She is 5'4" tall and weighs 200 pounds. Her blood pressure is 140/90. During the interview, Mary says that she has regular menstrual periods but has not had one for about 6 weeks. She also indicates that she "never got around to going for that mammogram" that the nurse practitioner made the appointment for last year. "I have young children and just couldn't make it. Besides, I'm not sure my insurance will cover it. How often do I really need one anyway?"

- Based on the data provided, what possible nursing diagnoses can you develop concerning Mary's health?
- How will you validate these concerns?

- What primary and secondary screening efforts will you offer during this visit?
- What health-education resources will you make available to Mary?
- What health screening tests would you anticipate being done or ordered by the nurse practitioner? Why?

---

3. Lingyan is a 19-year-old college student who moved to the United States from China with her family when she was 12 years old. She is a sophomore and has come to student health services for the first time. At the start of the interview, she explains that her sorority sisters told her that she needs an annual examination. She says that she has never had one.

- In completing Lingyan's health history, what areas are of special concern? Why?
- What subjective and objective data do you have? What data do you need?
- What tentative nursing diagnoses might apply to Lingyan's situation?
- How will you validate these diagnoses?
- What other information must you obtain before developing goals with Lingyan?
- What are three possible nursing interventions? Why?

---

4. Roberta is a non-English speaking woman who has come to the office because of midcycle bleeding. You are aware from her chart that the results of her Pap smear 4 years ago indicated that she had moderate dysplasia. She has not been seen since. Roberta's cousin, Marie, is acting as interpreter during this visit.

As you update Roberta's health history, you ask her questions that Marie translates for her and then translates the answers back to you. After a few questions, Marie says to you "I need you to explain something to me." You respond, "Sure, what can I help you with?" Marie says, "There are a couple of words I didn't quite understand. First of all, what is this word, 'cervix?'"

- In completing Roberta's health history what areas are of special concern?

- What subjective and objective data do you have? What data do you need?
- What tentative nursing diagnoses might apply?
- How will you validate these diagnoses?
- What other information must you obtain before developing goals with Roberta?
- What are three possible nursing interventions? Why?
- How will you prepare Roberta for the physical examination?

---

5. Tatyana is a 22-year-old blind woman who has become sexually active in the past few months. She and her partner Michael, both in their fourth year of college, have come to student health services.

While giving her health history, Tatyana reveals that she has not previously used any method of contraception. She and her partner now want to choose a reliable method before they have coitus again. She expresses concern about the ease of use and possible side effects of some of the contraceptive methods.

- In completing Tatyana's health history, what areas are of special concern?
- What subjective and objective data do you have? What data do you need?
- What tentative nursing diagnoses might apply?
- How will you validate these diagnoses?
- What other information must you obtain before developing goals with Tatyana?
- What are three possible nursing interventions? Why?
- How will you prepare Tatyana for the physical examination?

---

6. Sara Wolkovich, a 17-year-old high school student, is a below-average student who might best be described as a concrete learner. She has come to the in-school clinic complaining of nausea, vomiting, and fatigue. She states, "For the last few weeks I haven't liked food and when I do eat I throw up. I am falling asleep in my classes."

You ask Sara when her last menstrual period (LMP) was, and she cannot remember but states that "it hasn't been for a while." She tells you that she has been sexually active for about 2 years but has never been pregnant. When you ask her what she uses for

contraception she states, "I leave it up to the guy to stop in time."

- In completing Sara's health history, what areas are of special concern? Why?
- What subjective and objective data do you have? What data do you need?
- What tentative nursing diagnoses might apply to Sara's situation?
- How will you validate these diagnoses?
- What other information must you obtain before developing goals with Sara?
- What are three possible nursing interventions? Why?
- Based on Sara's educational needs, what special interventions might you have to develop?

---

7. Aimee is 32 years old. A new client, she has come to the women's clinic for the first time for an annual examination. She is concerned that she has never had an annual examination that included a Pap smear. You explain to her that an internal examination and Pap smear will be part of today's visit. You ask if she has any other concerns, and she says, "No." In the process of completing her health history, you ask if she is sexually active. She replies, "Yes." When you ask if she is in need of contraception she says, "No."

- What meanings might this response have?
- In completing Aimee's health history, what areas are of special concern? Why?
- What subjective and objective data do you have? What data do you need?
- What tentative nursing diagnoses might apply to Aimee's situation?
- How will you validate these diagnoses?
- What other information must you obtain before developing goals with Aimee?
- What are three possible nursing interventions? Why?

---

8. Genevieve has had an annual examination scheduled for more than 6 months. While skiing 3 weeks ago, she fell and broke her left fibula. Her leg was put in a cast that runs from midthigh to her toes. She is walking with the aid of crutches. Hesitant to postpone her visit and Pap smear because it takes

so long to get an appointment, she has kept her appointment.

- In completing Genevieve's health history what areas are of special concern? Why?
- What subjective and objective data do you have? What data do you need?

- What tentative nursing diagnoses might apply to Genevieve's situation?
- How will you validate these diagnoses?
- What other information must you obtain before developing goals with Genevieve?
- What are three possible nursing interventions? Why?

## REFERENCES

Andrews MM and Boyle JS: *Transcultural Concepts in Nursing*, ed 2, Philadelphia, 1995, Lippincott.

Ask Noah: New York online access to health, 1999, www.noah. cuny.edu.

Barkauskas VH and others: *Health and physical assessment*, ed 2, St Louis, 1998, Mosby.

Bickley LS and Hoekelman RA: *Bates' guide to physical examination and history taking*, ed 7, Philadelphia, 1999, Lippincott.

Carlson-Catalano J: Invest in yourself: cultivating personal power, *Nursing Forum* 29(2):22, 1994.

Carson VB: *Spiritual dimensions of nursing practice*, Philadelphia, 1989, Saunders.

Coulehan JL and Block MR: *The medical interview: mastering skills for clinical practice*, ed 3, Philadelphia: 1997, F.A. Davis.

Ferreyra S and Hughes K: *Table Manners—a guide to pelvic examination for disabled women and health care providers*, San Francisco, 1984, Planned Parenthood-Alameda.

Fontaine KL: *Healing practices*, Upper Saddle River, NJ, 2000, Prentice-Hall.

Frover S and Quinn M: Is there any value in bimanual pelvic examination as screening tests?, *Med J Australia* 162:408, 1995.

Gardner DL: Presence. In Bulechek GM and McCloskey JC, editors: *Nursing interventions: essential nursing treatments*, ed 2, Philadelphia, 1992, Saunders.

Holmes T and Rahe R: The social readjustment rating scale, *J Psychosomatic Res* 11:213, 1967.

Hultgren FH: Being called to care-or-caring being called to be: do we have another question? In Lashley M and others, editors: *Being called to care*, Albany, 1994, State University of New York Press.

Kerfoot K and Neuman T: Creating a healing environment: the nurse manager's challenge, *Nurs Econ* 10(6):423, 1992.

Klingman L: Assessing the female reproductive system, *Am J Nurs* 99(8):37, 1999.

Lashley ME and others: *Being called to care*, Albany, NY, 1994, State University of New York.

Lightfoot-Klein H: *Prisoners of ritual: an odyssey into female genital circumcision in Africa*, Birmingham, NY, 1989, Harworth.

Mehrabian A: *Silent messages*, Belmont, CA, 1971, Wadsworth.

Moch S and Schaefer C: Presence. In Snyder M and Lindquist R, editors: *Complementary/alternative therapies in nursing*, ed 3, New York, 1998, Springer.

Mosby: *Expert 10-minute physical examinations*, St Louis, 1997, Mosby.

National Women's Health Resource Center: Alternative therapies and women's health, *Nat Wom Health Rep* 17(3):1, 1998.

Rahe RH: Epidemiological studies of life changes and illness, *Int J Psychiatr Med* 6(1-2):133, 1975.

Robertson A: *Empowering women—teaching active birth in the '90s*, Camperdown, Australia, 1997, ACE.

Ryden MB: Active listening. In Snyder M and Lindquist R, editors: *Complementary/alternative therapies in nursing*, ed 3, New York, 1998, Springer.

Sawin K and Harrigan M: *Measures of family functioning for research and practice*, New York, 1995, Springer.

Secor MC: The challenging pelvic examination, part I, *Patient care for the nurse practitioner* 36, 37, 40, 43-45, July 1999.

Sims LK and others: *Health assessment in nursing*, Redwood City, CA, 1995, Addison-Wesley.

Slunt ET: Living the call authentically. In Lashley M and others, editors: *Being called to care*, Albany, 1994, State University of New York Press.

Smilkstein G: The family Apgar: a proposal for a family function test and its use by physicians, *J Fam Pract* 6:1231-1239, 1978.

Sulpizi LK: Issues in sexuality and gynecologic care of women with developmental disabilities, *JOGNN* 25(7):609, 1996.

Tiedje LB: Alternative health care: an overview, *J Obstet Gynecol Neonat Nurs* 27(5):557, 1998.

U.S. Department of Health and Human Services, Public Health Service, Office of Public Health and Science, Office of Disease Prevention and Promotion: Clinician's handbook of preventative services, ed 2, Washington, D.C., 1998, U.S. Government Printing Office.

VanServellen G: *Communication skills for the health professional: concepts and techniques*, Gaithersburg, MD, 1996, Aspen.

Yoder-Wise P: *Leading and managing in nursing*, St Louis, 1999, Mosby.

Youngkin EQ and Davis MS: *Women's health: a primary care clinical guide*, Stamford, CT, 1998, Appleton & Lange.

# CHAPTER 5

# Teaching for Self-Care

*"To know how to suggest is the great art
of teaching."*

— HENRI-FRÉDÉRIC AMIEL (1828-1881),
SWISS PHILOSOPHER

*How does a woman develop the capacity for self-care?*

*What information does a woman need to promote her health and prevent disease?*

*What information does a woman need for self-assessment?*

*How does knowledge of the reproductive hormonal events of the life span add to a woman's
ability for self-care?*

*What information does a woman need to decide whether or not to practice contraception?*

*How does a woman use self-assessment to select a contraceptive method?*

American women from all ethnic backgrounds view themselves as active participants in their personal health care but are not always confident that they are making the right choices to take care of themselves (Fishbein and Bash, 1997). "Knowledge deficit related to . . ." is one of the most common nursing diagnoses. The knowledge deficit may be in relation to information about their bodies and how they function, strategies for health promotion and disease prevention, or self-care for diseases that are encountered. A woman's confidence in her abilities to care for herself and her family members increases as she learns self-assessment and self-care activities that are individualized to her personal interests and needs.

 **EXPLORING THE BELIEFS AND PRACTICES
OF SELF-ASSESSMENT AND SELF-CARE**

**Self-assessment,** or self-examination, is a woman's ability to determine and evaluate change in her body. Her breasts, genitalia, skin, hair, and nails are the primary areas she may observe. She may also gauge changes in her patterns of eating and sleeping, her activity level, or her internal responses to things such as foods, medications, or stress.

**Self-care** is how a woman provides for her health promotion needs and responds to the findings of her self-assessment. Each woman takes care of her health needs by herself most of the time. Because we are participants

**161**

in our own experiences, we know what works and what does not work for us. Health care providers can enhance a woman's self-knowledge and support the level of self-care that she chooses and then supply the care that the woman cannot provide for herself (Webster, 1991).

Our success in educating and empowering women to be confident in their self-assessment and self-care largely depends on our ability to communicate effectively. Getting clients to let us know about their wishes and desires and the particulars of their situations requires both knowledge and skill. Once the woman's wishes are known, we can collaborate to develop a specific plan to address those concerns. A safe, private environment must be provided in order to elicit feelings and beliefs from clients, and effective interview techniques are required to encourage self-disclosure. The characteristics of the client's age, cultural background, literacy, emotional state, and readiness for behavior change influence the encounter. Other important considerations of the situation can include the woman's goals, our goals as a provider, and the time available for discussion (Guest, 1998).

## Age-Related Concerns

Mutual empowerment is important in the relationship between an adolescent and her health care provider. By virtue of seeking care, even at the suggestion of someone else, the girl demonstrates a beginning level of trust and confidence that we might be helpful. When we respond by providing personalized care, we validate her right to care (Devine, 1996).

Adolescents may be very indirect in their communication, frustrating us. The initial reason that the girl gives for seeking care may represent only a small portion of her concerns. She may wait until she feels comfortable or

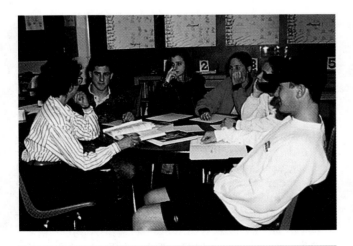

*FIGURE 5-1* • Adolescents sitting around a table with an educator. *(From Dickason EJ:* Maternal-infant nursing care, *ed 3, St Louis, 1998, Mosby. Courtesy Marjorie Pyle, RNC, Lifecircle.)*

is asked directly before sharing her other needs. In response to her vagueness, our communication must be neither patronizing nor condescending. We must use active listening, eye contact, a body language that signals approachability, combined with an appropriate vocabulary that indicates a sincere interest in what she needs or perceives to need (Devine, 1996) (Figure 5-1).

When providing care, the developmental level of the  woman is more important than her chronologic age in determining her educational needs and ability to learn. By virtue of their lived experiences or self-expectations, some adolescents are developmentally older than their years. The developmental age of an individual is one of the first assessments needed.

An adolescent who is 14 or 15 by both chronologic and developmental ages will exhibit certain characteristics. Adolescents in this age group are very involved with their peers and think concretely. They often have idealized and romanticized first love relationships. They are focused on the here and now and cannot foresee consequences to their actions. Experimentation with drugs, sexual activity, and alcohol is common. Interventions to improve self-esteem and healthier self-care must be concrete and focused on immediate gain for the adolescent. Threats to appearance and relationships are more powerful persuaders than the future consequences of actions.

Cognitive development gradually allows the concrete "here and now" thinking to become more abstract. The capacity for abstract thinking typically begins around age 16 years and is accompanied by the ability to think and plan ahead. A person with the ability to do abstract reasoning is capable of higher levels of both self-assessment and self-care. We may relate to a client with abstract reasoning skills as an adult to an adult. But we should not expect that she can implement a plan of care as an adult might be able to because she probably lacks the resources.

## Cultural Considerations

Every society determines for itself what is normal and therefore healthy. The concept of health or what is normal is not universal across race or ethnic groups, nor is the concept of a person's role or responsibility in maintaining his or her health.

### Concept of Health

In a society that believes in the presence of supernatural interventions, people who hear voices of spirits or believe they are controlled by these spirits may not be thought of as ill. A woman who is "thin as a stick" may be seen as emaciated and diseased in one culture, yet held up as a model of health in a culture that values thinness as a sign of beauty. Likewise, a woman who is overweight may be seen as strong and healthy in one culture and weak and unhealthy in another culture (Andrews and Boyle, 1995).

## Personal Responsibility for Health

Cultural beliefs related to who is responsible for health also vary across and within race and ethnic groups. The Asian and Pacific Islander census group includes people of Chinese, Japanese, Vietnamese, and Filipino backgrounds. The Chinese culture presents the belief that a healthy body is a gift from our parents and ancestors and must be cared for by us individually. Illness is caused when the energy forces (yin and yang) get out of balance. The Vietnamese culture also stresses that health comes from remaining in harmony with the universe by pleasing good spirits and avoiding evil ones. The Japanese cultural beliefs rely less on maintaining balance and more on preventing access to outside spirits. Disease is caused by not caring for the body, and illness occurs when outside spirits and polluting agents are allowed to make contact. In sharp contrast to the three other groups, the Filipino culture believes that illness is a punishment from God (Schrefer, 1994).

Similar differences are found across and within the other racial and ethnic groups. As a result of these differences, the mechanisms the people from these cultures use to stay healthy vary in focus and emphasis. In addition, even within a family, there are variations in the beliefs about health and the assumption of responsibility for maintaining health. Although influenced by their culture and their families, individuals come to their own definition of health and determine their own level of responsibility.

## Interaction between Culture and Care

Cultural values influence personal self-assessment and self-care. The values learned during childhood continue to influence every aspect of life. We must assess an individual's personality and beliefs with an understanding of the possible influence of their culture's system of health beliefs.

Culturally competent communication begins with a personal understanding of how we are influenced by our culture and how this differs from the influence of other cultures. Within the Western culture, it is believed that if you want something, you ask for it. For example, if you do not understand directions, you ask about them. People from other cultures often find this behavior unacceptable. They quietly wait to be told what to do or be given the information the "healer" wishes to provide. As providers, if we hold question-asking behavior as the norm and structure our teaching based on the questions asked or offer clarifying explanations only when questioned, we will not be meeting the needs of those who do not ask questions.

## ⬤ EDUCATING FOR SELF-ASSESSMENT AND SELF-CARE

When women come to us for care, part of our nursing role is to provide information that addresses their concerns. We become partners in education, as we collaborate with each woman while addressing her issues of importance. We support the woman's analysis of her experiences and needs and then help her address those needs while building upon her current competencies in self-assessment and self-care.

## Andragogy

Learning theory for adults, "**andragogy,**" differs from the more commonly heard term "**pedagogy,**" which provides more emphasis on the learning of children. Adults seek information and education in a manner and for reasons that are different from children. In presenting information to adults, we must be concerned with the following:

- Changes in self-concept—Adults are generally more self-directed in seeking knowledge.
- Life experiences—Past experiences, both positive and negative, form the basis for new learning.
- Aim of learning—Adults want to learn what is important to them at that particular moment.
- Problem-focused learning—Adults want information and skills that can be applied immediately (Renner, 1994).

## Educational Approaches

A variety of educational approaches are required to meet the individual needs of our clients. However, before we can start to teach, we must understand how people learn.

### Understanding Learning

Learning involves three domains: the cognitive domain, the affective domain, and the psychomotor domain.

***Cognitive Domain.*** Cognition is the process of knowing in the broadest sense and includes memory, recognition, understanding, and application. "The **cognitive domain** deals with the recall or recognition of knowledge and the development of intellectual abilities and skills" (Renner, 1994). With cognitive learning, a woman must first be able to remember something before she can then understand it, apply it, determine its relationship to other information, or judge its value. Each level of cognitive learning builds on the next. To be effective teachers, we must determine the cognitive abilities of the woman with respect to the information we want to provide so that our efforts are directed at the correct level.

***Affective Domain.*** "The **affective domain** describes changes in attitude and values, and the development of appreciations and adequate adjustment" (Renner, 1994). A woman does not simply change behaviors because she is told to do so. For affective learning to occur, a woman must first receive the information, respond to or consider it, value it as useful, make sense of it, organize it within the information she has already learned, and then adopt or take on the behavior. Each level of affective learning builds on the next. It is difficult to adjust or change a woman's values, attitudes, beliefs, and interests. We can only offer the information and then provide support and encouragement.

***Psychomotor Domain.*** Psychomotor skills are the activities we perform based on neuromuscular coordination. "**The psychomotor domain** has to do with the development of manipulative skills, involving tools, machinery, procedures, and techniques" (Renner, 1994). The level of psychomotor learning also progresses from the simple level of reflex movements to the complex level of communicating feelings, needs, and interests to others. Psychomotor learning best occurs when the skills are demonstrated either in person, by video, or through pictures. The learner must have the ability to perform the task, a sensory image of how to carry out the skill (i.e., be able to imagine the process in the mind), and have the opportunity to practice the new skill. Physical or cognitive impairments may prevent a woman from learning a psychomotor skill.

### Basic Sequence of Instruction

In order to teach, a series of events must take place in a prescribed order. Whether teaching one or two persons, a small group, or an auditorium full of people, the sequence remains the same so that the participants will gain as much as possible.

1. Gain the learner's attention.
2. Tell what it is you are teaching.
3. Review prior learning.
4. Present new information.
5. Make new information relevant to the learner.
6. Have the learner repeat or demonstrate new knowledge.
7. Provide encouraging feedback.
8. Evaluate learning.
9. Enhance retention with problem solving (Stanhope and Lancaster, 1996).

## Barriers to Learning

Factors that may influence the capacity to learn and apply information on self-assessment and self-care are literacy and level of emotional distress (Guest, 1998).

### Literacy Level

Handouts, booklets, brochures, instructions, and forms for informed consent must be in the appropriate language and at a reading level compatible with that of the client. Reading materials for clients should generally be at the fifth to seventh grade reading level (Stanhope and Knollmueller, 1997). Tools are available to determine the reading grade level of written materials. Before we hand a woman information that augments what we have already explained, we must be sure that it is in a language she can read and at a literacy level that is comfortable to her. Note that many people cannot read English as well as they can speak it.

Readability formulas are useful in determining the reading level of written information. The SMOG Readability Index is one formula that is often used by educators. It is not specific to literature that provides technical information, as some health care brochures do, but is a way to start determining the readability level of printed materials (Box 5-1).

### Emotional Distress

Before trying to teach a woman, we must determine if she is in a situation where she can learn. Clients experiencing strong emotions—whether anger, euphoria, shock, fear, or disappointment—are not candidates for an educational session. We must address or defuse the emotions before attempting to accomplish anything else. It may be necessary to reschedule a session if a client is too overwhelmed by emotion to learn.

## Facilitating Learning

Individuals learn best and are able to make the most progress "in the absence of threat, when information seems relevant, when teaching takes cultural factors into account, when the learning process is interactive, when having a chance to ask and receive answers to questions, with time to digest, and room for insight" (Guest, 1998).

Presenting information to individuals does not automatically mean that they learn it. Learning occurs because the thought process and resulting activity are reinforced.

- *For a thought process or behavior to continue, it must be rewarded.* If we make eye contact and nod at the woman, smile, or similarly reward her as she shares information about what she has done, we are rewarding her behavior and she is more likely to continue.
- *For behavior to stop, it must be unrewarded.* This is true of both healthy and unhealthy behaviors. If we do not pay attention or minimize the effects of her efforts, she will eventually stop.
- *Incremental steps must be recognized and rewarded.* Whether a woman is trying to increase her level of exercise or decrease the number of cigarettes she smokes, each improvement—no matter how small—must be recognized and rewarded. Just saying, "You are down one cigarette a day; that is great," recognizes and rewards her efforts and encourages her to continue.

BOX 5-1   *The SMOG Readability Formula**

To calculate the SMOG reading grade level, begin with the entire written work that is being assessed and follow these four steps:

1. Count off 10 consecutive sentences near the beginning, in the middle, and near the end of the text.
2. From this sample of 30 sentences, circle all of the words containing three or more syllables (polysyllabic), including repetitions of the same word, and total the number of words circled.
3. Estimate the square root of the total number of polysyllabic words counted (i.e., find the nearest perfect square and take the square root).
4. Finally, add a constant of 3 to the square root. This number gives the SMOG grade, or the reading grade level that a person must have achieved if he or she is to fully understand the text being assessed.

A few additional guidelines will help to clarify these directions:

- A sentence is defined as a string of words punctuated with a period (.), an exclamation point (!), or a question mark (?).
- Hyphenated words are considered to be one word.
- Numbers that are written out should also be considered and, if in numerical form in the text, should be pronounced to determine if they are polysyllabic.
- Proper nouns, if polysyllabic, should also be counted.
- Abbreviations should be read as unabbreviated to determine if they are polysyllabic.

Not all pamphlets, fact sheets, or other printed materials contain 30 sentences. To test a text that has fewer than 30 sentences, do the following:

1. Count all of the polysyllabic words in the text.
2. Count the number of sentences.
3. Find the average number of polysyllabic words per sentence as follows:

$$\text{Average} = \frac{\text{Total \# of polysyllabic words}}{\text{Total \# of sentences}}$$

4. Multiply that average by the number of sentences short of 30.
5. Add that figure to the total number of polysyllabic words.
6. Find the square root of the number you obtained in step 5, and add the constant of 3.

Perhaps the quickest way to administer the SMOG grading test is to use the SMOG conversion table. Simply count the number of polysyllabic words in your chain of 30 sentences and look up the approximate grade level on the following chart.

**SMOG CONVERSION TABLE†**

| Total Polysyllabic Word Counts | Approximate Grade Level (± 1.5) |
| --- | --- |
| 0-2 | 4 |
| 3-6 | 5 |
| 7-12 | 6 |
| 13-20 | 7 |
| 21-30 | 8 |
| 31-42 | 9 |
| 43-56 | 10 |
| 57-72 | 11 |
| 73-90 | 12 |
| 91-110 | 13 |
| 111-132 | 14 |
| 133-156 | 15 |
| 157-182 | 16 |
| 183-210 | 17 |
| 211-240 | 18 |

*Reprinted from Office of Cancer Communications, National Cancer Institute: *Making health communications work,* Rockville, MD, 1989, The Institute.

†SMOG conversion table developed by Harold C. McGraw, Office of Educational Research, Baltimore County Schools, Towson, Maryland. Reprinted from National Clearinghouse for Alcohol and Drug Information: *You can prepare easy-to-read materials,* Technical Assistance Bulletin, Rockville, MD, 1994, The Clearinghouse.

*Continued*

---

**BOX 5-1** *The SMOG Readability Formula—cont'd*

### USING THE SMOG READABILITY FORMULA‡

#### Check Your Weight and Heart Disease I.Q.

The following statements are on a self-assessment test for knowledge of overweight and heart disease.

(1) Being overweight puts you at risk for heart disease. (2) If you are overweight, losing weight helps lower your high blood cholesterol and high blood pressure. (3) Quitting smoking is healthy but commonly leads to excessive weight gain, which increases your risk for heart disease. (4) An overweight person with high blood pressure should pay more attention to a low sodium diet than to weight reduction. (5) A reduced intake of sodium or salt does not always lower high blood pressure to normal. (6) The best way to lose weight is to eat fewer calories and exercise. (7) Skipping meals is a good way to cut down on calories. (8) Foods high in complex carbohydrates (starch and fiber) are good choices when you are trying to lose weight. (9) The single most important change most people can make to lose weight is to avoid sugar. (10) Polyunsaturated fat has the same number of calories as saturated fat. (11) Overweight children are very likely to become overweight adults.

$$\frac{\text{Total \# of polysyllabic words}}{\text{Total \# of sentences}} = \frac{21}{11} = 1.91 \times (30 - 11) = 36.3$$

36 + polysyllabic words (21) = 57

Nearest square root of 57 = 8

8 + constant 3 = 11th grade level

‡From U.S. DHHS: *Check your weight and heart disease I.Q.* Publ. No. 93-3034, Washington, D.C., 1993, U.S. Government Printing Office.

---

- *Provide immediate feedback*. The closer the feedback to the behavior, the more likely the behavior will be affected. Rather than waiting to the end of the visit to provide feedback, do it immediately within the conversation and as often as applicable.
- *To acquire a new behavior, she must participate in the new behavior*. Instead of reading or hearing about a new behavior, a woman must participate in it. For example, have her do a return demonstration of how to do a breast self-examination right after you review it with her (Renner, 1994). This increases the probability she will do it again on her own.

### Expectations for the Learning to Create Change

Self-assessment requires a depth of introspection. Positive self-care often entails changing daily habits to those that foster and promote health. Such introspection and change are difficult and often occur over time. Behavior change is usually incremental, so interventions must be tailored to match the woman's level of comprehension and desire to change (Box 5-2).

For behavior to change, the cognitive domain—with knowledge and awareness—must first be addressed. Change then comes from understanding the consequences of a behavior (i.e., learning in the affective domain). The change must have significance for the woman in order to have a value. Self-efficacy determines the ability to use new knowledge and skills. Women must see themselves as able to have self-control and to change. A woman conducts a cost-benefit analysis when deciding whether to change a behavior. Even a change to a healthier lifestyle (e.g., eating a nutritious diet) has a downside (e.g., giving up sweets or junk food). The benefits of a new behavior must be worth the cost.

Knowledge cannot change behaviors, unless the psychomotor domain becomes involved and new skills are developed. We are in an excellent position to teach new behavior skills. Behavior change takes patience for both the client and us. Such change is likely to occur in fits and starts and requires a series of provisional tries before it occurs with any regularity. To encourage personal change, we must support the positive behaviors while minimizing the backsliding that naturally occurs (Guest, 1998).

### SELF-CARE FOR HEALTH PROMOTION AND DISEASE PREVENTION

In order to provide appropriate information on health promotion and disease prevention to women, we must first understand the major threats to their health. This information enables us to focus our counseling on the most important areas for women in general with selective adaptation to the needs of individual women.

## BOX 5-2    A Model for the Process of Change

Knowledge and awareness
Significance to self
Self-efficacy
Cost-benefit analysis
Capacity building
Provisional tries

From Garrity J and Jones S: *HIV prevention counseling: a training program,* Atlanta, 1993, Centers for Disease Control.

## TABLE 5-1    Leading Causes of Mortality among Women

| Age | Causes |
| --- | --- |
| 15-24 | Accidents |
| | Violence |
| 25-44 | Cancer |
| | Heart disease |
| | Accidents |
| | Violence |
| | Suicide |
| 45-64 | Cancer |
| | Heart disease |
| | Chronic obstructive pulmonary disease |
| | Chronic liver disease and cirrhosis |
| | Diabetes mellitus |
| 65+ | Heart disease |
| | Cancer |
| | Cerebrovascular disease |
| | Pneumonia |
| | Chronic obstructive pulmonary disease |

National Center for Health Statistics: Age-adjusted death rates for selected causes of death, according to sex and race: United States, DHHS Publication No 97-1232, Hyattsville, 1995, The Center.

## Leading Causes of Mortality

Leading causes of mortality among women vary by age. Young women (i.e., those under the age of 25 years) are most likely to die in accidents or by acts of violence. Most of these deaths are from motor vehicle accidents, and alcohol is often a major contributing factor. During the past 20 years, the number of deaths from automobile accidents has decreased, which is probably a result of safer cars—not safer drivers. Violence is the second most common cause of death in young women. Death by homicide, as well as death related to rape, robbery, and assault, has increased. Black women are four times more likely to die by homicide than white women. Suicide is the third leading cause of death among women in this age group, with the largest incidence in the Hispanic community. Deaths from HIV are also rising rapidly.

Women ages 25 to 44 years are most likely to die from cancer (including HIV deaths). Heart disease is the second leading cause of death, with accidents, violence, and suicide also common causes of death in this age group.

Chronic diseases begin to appear as major causes of death in women ages 45 to 64 years. Heart disease, cerebrovascular disease, pulmonary disease, chronic liver disease, and diabetes are the leading causes of death in this age group. Although these diseases manifest during this age span, they start developing earlier in a woman's life. Therefore interventions for disease prevention must be directed at the risk factors of these diseases.

Heart disease is also the leading cause of death in women age 65 years and older, with cancer second. Stroke, pulmonary disease, pneumonia, and diabetes take their toll, and accidents appear again as a major cause of death, primarily as a consequence of falls (Youngkin and Davis, 1998) (Table 5-1).

## Common Risk Factors for All Women

In addition to the major causes of mortality, women are vulnerable to less than optimal health as a consequence of certain common risk factors (Kowal, 1998). These risk factors include use of tobacco and/or alcohol; accidental or violent injuries; sexually transmitted infections; and unintended pregnancy.

### Tobacco Use

Tobacco smoke is associated with lung disease, lung cancer, and heart disease, which are all major causes of death among those aged 45 and older. Women smokers also have a higher risk for osteoporosis, cervical cancer, premature menopause, and impaired fertility. Smoking during pregnancy leads to a higher rate of spontaneous abortion, having a low–birth-weight or stillborn infant, and infant death or disability (Centers for Disease Control and Prevention [CDC], 1989; Stein, 1996). Tobacco use is concentrated among younger women, with one fourth of the women age 18 or older smoking (CDC, 1989). Information to assist young women with the decision not to smoke or to stop smoking is a major factor in self-care for health and prevention of disease.

### Alcohol Use

Use of alcohol is associated with an increased risk for motor vehicle accidents, impaired judgement, increased risk of abuse of other chemicals, liver disease, stroke, hypertension, and osteoporosis (Kowal, 1998). When drugs are used in addition to alcohol, the rates of morbidity and mortality increase. Helping women to limit alcohol and avoid other harmful substances will increase their chances for improved health.

### Injuries

Accidents are a major cause of death among younger and older women. Young women are more vulnerable to motor vehicle accidents associated with alcohol use, and older women are vulnerable to accidental falls that result in disability and death. Younger women can care for themselves by wearing seatbelts, avoiding alcohol when driving, and wearing helmets when riding on bicycles or motorcycles.

Older women can prevent falls by exercising regularly to maintain muscle mass and balance, using ladders and stools appropriately, having regular eye examinations to identify and correct vision problems, removing safety hazards from their homes, and installing safety bars and railings—particularly in the bathroom.

### Sexually Transmitted Infections

Sexually transmitted infections (STIs) are another threat to women's health, resulting in pain, infertility, and even death. Women in the younger age group experience the most sexually transmitted infections, so they are the logical target for an extensive educational plan of self-care. Interventions for self-care should include the choice of abstinence. When sexually active, a woman may reduce her risk for infection by participating in a mutually monogamous relationship in which both partners have had intercourse only with each other or by one partner using a condom (Kowal, 1998).

### Unintended Pregnancy

Unintended pregnancy is a major threat to women's health because nearly half of all the pregnancies in the United States are unintended (Brown and Eisenberg, 1995; Henshaw, 1998). Assisting women with the choice of abstinence or the choice of contraception aids in their ability to take control of their own fertility health. The educational process of helping a woman select contraceptive aids and be successful in preventing pregnancy is covered later in this chapter.

## Guidance in Health-Promotion Activities

An overall sense of well-being and a holistic improvement in a woman's health occurs when she maintains an adequate level of exercise, rest, and sleep.

### Exercise

Regular exercise is an important part of a healthy lifestyle. The benefits of regular exercise go well beyond weight management and include improvement of heart function, improved sleep, changes in body composition (i.e., increased muscle and decreased fat stores), reduced stress, lower blood pressure and blood cholesterol, and improved blood-glucose regulation and psychologic well-being (Cahill, 1995). Exercise improves cardiopulmonary function by increasing the strength of the heart muscle, increasing the diameter of the coronary arteries, lowering blood pressure, lowering resting pulse rates, causing a more healthy lipid profile, and improving the vasculature of the skeletal muscle (Cahill, 1995). Heart disease, a major factor in the death of women as they age, can be prevented or reduced with regular exercise.

Weight-bearing exercise has a significant effect on the development and maintenance of the woman's skeletal system. Women generally have less bone mass than men, so they are more vulnerable to bone loss (osteoporosis). Women who are sedentary are even more vulnerable as they age.

### Strategies for Self-Care

Regular weight-bearing exercise beginning early in life plays a major role in preventing age-related osteoporosis (Birge and Dalsky, 1989). Exercise at any time in life, however, has a positive affect. Along with adequate nutritional intake of calcium and vitamin D, as little as 20 minutes of exercise three times per week has shown positive effects on a woman's health. The 20 minutes of exercise need not be consecutive as long as the activity is performed in short periods that total 20 minutes.

Walking is one of the easiest types of exercising either to begin with or to develop as a lifelong habit. It can be performed by people of all ages and requires only a pair of supportive shoes. Groups of mall walkers have organized in areas with inclement weather or unsafe neighborhoods. Exercise also has a positive effect on psychologic well-being, affecting mood and sleep patterns, increasing circulating endorphins, and improving the quality of sleep.

A woman often states that she has no time to exercise, but we can suggest ways to incorporate exercise during her day. These suggestions may include choosing to take a longer route to get from point A to point B, walking the dog, taking the stairs instead of the elevator or escalator whenever possible, walking during lunch, getting off one stop early when using public transportation, and walking with children.

### Rest and Sleep

Adequate rest and sleep are vital to the promotion of good health. They restore a woman both physically and mentally, helping to ameliorate some of the effects of the stress of daily living. Research has established that the human body requires a minimum number of hours of sleep per day, with adolescents needing a total of 9½ hours and adults needing 8 hours of sleep per day. Consequences of inadequate rest include dozing off while driving, inefficient work patterns, a dysphoric mood (e.g., restlessness or malaise), inadequate coping mechanisms, and a higher chance of risky behavior because of poor judgement.

### Strategies for Self-Assesment

If the woman looks weary or indicates that she is having a problem getting enough rest or sleep, we can help her look at her situation and determine why this is happening and how she might improve her situation. The woman must count the number of sleep periods during the previous 24 hours, as well as the total number of hours of sleep she had—including naps. A sleep diary (i.e., record of when, where, and how long she sleeps) kept by the woman for several weeks provides further information. Perhaps the woman is getting enough hours of sleep but the sleep is not restful. Perhaps the woman is experiencing depression, which is fatiguing her.

### Strategies for Self-Care

Learning how many hours of sleep the human body needs is the woman's first step toward permitting herself to set that many hours aside. Understanding the negative effects of sleep deprivation, both to herself and to those around her, makes it a self-care issue. When she can relate an increase in inefficiency, a sense of restlessness or malaise, an inability to cope adequately, or an increase in risky behavior to a lack of enough sleep, the woman may be able to adjust her own expectations and situation so that she can get more rest. If she has explored her situation and attempted to decrease her level of fatigue herself without success, she needs a more in-depth assessment by a health care provider.

### Nutrition

A woman's culture influences her concepts of healthy eating patterns, and what she eats influences her health, both in the present and in the future. Her food choices, meal patterns, and determination of what constitutes a meal are determined by her culture and family environment, as well as her preferences and choices. We may present her with dietary information, but this will do no good unless she agrees that it is important and she is empowered and supported in her efforts (Table 5-2).

A vegetarian is someone who chooses not to eat animals or animal products. A woman who is a **lacto-ovo vegetarian** (i.e., she eats milk and egg products along with other foods) or a **lacto-vegetarian** (i.e., she eats milk products but not eggs along with other foods) can meet all of her nutritional needs for proteins. If the woman is a vegetarian who also eats fish she is a **pescetarian.** If the woman is a **vegan** (i.e., she eats no food from animal sources), she should consult with a dietician to ensure that her diet has the adequate amount of protein and essential vitamins and minerals.

### Strategies for Self-Assessment

Since 1992, the Food Guide Pyramid has been used to illustrate a research-based food-guidance system developed by the United States Department of Agriculture (USDA) and supported by the Department of Health and Human Services (DHHS) (Figures 5-2 and 5-3). Based on the foods Americans eat, it goes beyond a consideration of the "basic four food groups" to help people make the best food choices (Table 5-2). With suggestions for the number of servings per day, the pyramid helps someone

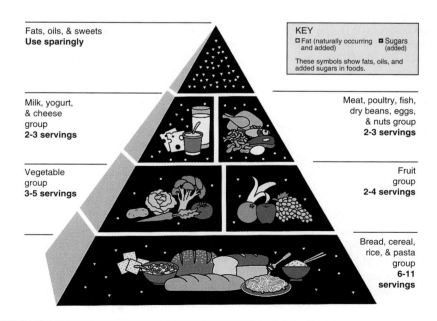

Fats, oils, & sweets
**Use sparingly**

KEY
☐ Fat (naturally occurring and added)   ■ Sugars (added)
These symbols show fats, oils, and added sugars in foods.

Milk, yogurt, & cheese group
**2-3 servings**

Meat, poultry, fish, dry beans, eggs, & nuts group
**2-3 servings**

Vegetable group
**3-5 servings**

Fruit group
**2-4 servings**

Bread, cereal, rice, & pasta group
**6-11 servings**

*FIGURE 5-2* • The food guide pyramid: a guide to daily food choices. *(The Food Guide Pyramid. USDA, Center for Nutrition Policy and Promotion, Home and Garden Bulletin Number 252, 1996, www.nal.usda.gov:8001/py/pmap.htm)*

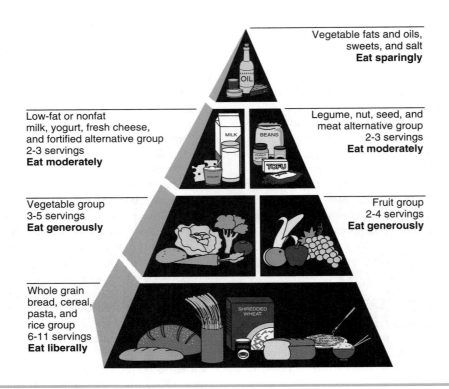

**FIGURE 5-3** • The vegetarian food pyramid: a daily guide to food choices.

**TABLE 5-2** *Ethnic Influences and the Food Pyramid Guide*

| | ETHNIC GROUP | | | |
| FOOD GROUP | Native American | African-American | Hispanic American | Asian-American |
|---|---|---|---|---|
| Breads, cereals, pasta, rice | Corn, many different grains | Biscuits, cornbread, grits | Corn, rice, plantain | Rice, variety of noodles |
| Vegetables | Sweet potatoes, squashes, tomatoes | Dark green, leafy vegetables, okra, sweet potatoes, black-eyed peas | Chili peppers, chayote, cabbage, jicama root | Many different vegetables |
| Fruits | Variety | Variety | Avocado, tropical fruits, plantain | Variety |
| Meats/alternates | Seafood, game meats | Dried peas and beans, pork, chicken (fried meat) | Dried peas and beans | Fish, chicken, pork, beef, soybean products, tofu |
| Dairy | Limited amounts | Limited amounts | Cheese, limited milk | Very little dairy foods |
| Fats/oils | Lard for frying | Lard for frying | Lard for frying | Peanut oil |
| Sweets/desserts | Variety | Pies, cakes | Variety | Variety |

decide not only what foods to choose but also how much to eat from each food group to obtain the necessary nutrients without too many calories, fat, saturated fat, cholesterol, sugar, sodium, or alcohol. A diet low in fat reduces the chances of developing certain diseases and helps a person maintain a healthy weight (The Food Guide Pyramid, 1996).

The pyramid is available in both English and Spanish at www.fns.usda.gov/tn/Resources/sp-middle.html. By following these dietary guidelines, we can enjoy better health and reduce our chances of getting certain diseases. These guidelines provide the best, most current advice from nutrition scientists for self-assessment and self-care (The Food Guide Pyramid, 1996).

There is a suggested number of servings listed for each food group. The number of servings that is right for a woman depends on how many calories she needs, which in turn depends on her age, size, and how active she is. Almost everyone should have the minimum number of servings in each group (Box 5-3).

**Strategies for Self-Care**

Encourage each woman to decide what changes she wants to make and can make for her diet to be healthier. She should start by making small changes (e.g., switching to low-fat salad dressings or adding an extra serving of vegetables). Success will occur if she makes additional changes gradually until healthy eating becomes a habit (Box 5-4).

Women of all ages should be encouraged to drink more milk and less diet soda and consume more dairy products and vegetables that supply calcium. When combined with physical activity, women can enhance their bone structure and be less prone to developing osteoporosis later in life.

## Educating for Self-Care with Common Illnesses

Human beings most frequently experience two types of illnesses—upper respiratory tract infection and gastrointestinal tract infection. These conditions are usually cared for with family or culturally prescribed treatments or rituals. Sometimes the assistance of a traditional or contemporary healing practitioner is sought for recommendations or access to medicinal preparations. These providers may recommend remedies based on the concepts of complementary, alternative, or traditional therapies.

After assistance is provided, a woman must then apply the knowledge and the remedies in a way that has a positive effect on her health. Women are generally expected to be the care providers within their families. They not only are asked what to do but also generally have to provide the remedies and help the person who is sick, deciding when and who they might need to see for further care. When we assist women with self-care, we can affect the health of whole families.

### Respiratory Infections

Infections of the upper respiratory tract are a common cause of mild to moderate illness. The most common episodes are easily managed by self-care, although some require medical attention. Upper respiratory disorders comprise more than half of all acute illnesses, and 20% of these are the common cold. The "common cold" is the household name for acute viral infection of the upper airway. Even though this is considered a minor illness, it occurs at such magnitude that it creates a significant drain on human and financial resources. The common cold is a major cause of medical office visits and a strong contributor to work and school absenteeism. Each year in the United States, 23 million days of work are missed due to colds (Dollemore, 1998). In addition, **over-the-counter (OTC)** products to deal with coughs and colds are a multibillion dollar industry.

---

**BOX 5-3  *What Counts as a Serving?***

**BREAD, CEREAL, RICE, AND PASTA**
- 1 slice of bread
- 1 ounce of ready-to-eat cereal
- $\frac{1}{2}$ cup of cooked cereal, rice, or pasta

**VEGETABLE**
- 1 cup of raw leafy vegetables
- $\frac{1}{2}$ cup of other vegetables, cooked or chopped raw
- $\frac{3}{4}$ cup of vegetable juice

**FRUIT**
- 1 medium apple, banana, orange
- $\frac{1}{2}$ cup of chopped, cooked, or canned fruit
- $\frac{3}{4}$ cup of fruit juice

**MILK, YOGURT, AND CHEESE**
- 1 cup of milk or yogurt
- $1\frac{1}{2}$ ounces of natural cheese
- 2 ounces of process cheese

**MEAT, POULTRY, FISH, DRY BEANS, EGGS, AND NUTS**
- 2-3 ounces of cooked lean meat, poultry, or fish
- $\frac{1}{2}$ cup of cooked dry beans or 1 egg counts as 1 ounce of lean meat
- 2 tablespoons of peanut butter or $\frac{1}{3}$ cup of nuts count as 1 ounce of meat

United States Department of Agriculture, Center for Nutrition Policy and Promotion: *The food guide pyramid,* Home and Garden Bulletin Number 252, 1996, www.nal.usda.gov:8001/py/pmap.htm.

---

### Strategies for Self-Assessment

The common cold is caused by one of 200 different viruses, but the rhinovirus and coronavirus account for half of the cases. Although colds can occur at any time of the year, there is a concentration of illness during the winter months and early spring, when people are crowded together indoors with inadequate ventilation. The average adult has between two and four colds per year. A cold is characterized by rhinorrhea (runny nose), congestion, sneezing, cough, and a sore throat.

### Strategies for Self-Care

Treatment should begin at the first sign of symptoms. Especially with herbal remedies, the earlier response will yield faster results and an earlier recovery. Sleeping at least 12 hours per night and staying well-hydrated are good first steps. Additional home remedies (e.g., hot baths, salt water gargles, and petroleum jelly or other lubricants for noses sore from tissue wiping, and eating chicken soup) have been found to be effective. Comfort will be increased and an earlier recovery may occur with the complementary therapies of aromatherapy (e.g., eu-

---

### BOX 5-4   *How to Rate Your Diet*

You may want to rate your diet for a few days. Follow these four steps.

**STEP 1**
Jot down everything you ate yesterday (meals and snacks).            *Grams of Fat*

_____  _____

(several blank lines for listing foods and grams of fat)

Total ☐

**STEP 2**
Write down the number of grams of fat in each food you list.
- Use the Food Pyramid Guide to get an estimate of the number of grams of fat to count for the foods you ate.
- Ue nutrition labels on the packaged foods you ate to find out the grams of fat they contain per serving.

**STEP 3**
Answer these questions:
- Did you have the number of servings from the five major food groups that are right for you?

| | Circle the Servings Right for You | Servings You Had |
|---|---|---|
| Grain Group Servings | 6 7 8 9 10 11 | ☐ |
| Vegetable Group Servings | 3 4 5 | ☐ |
| Fruit Group Servings | 2 3 4 | ☐ |
| Milk Group Servings | 2 3 | ☐ |
| Meat Group (ounces) | 5 6 7 | ☐ |

How did you do? Not enough? About right?

- Add up your grams of fat listed in Step 2. Did you have more fat than the amount right for you?

| | Grams Right for You | Grams You Had |
|---|---|---|
| Fat | 53 73 93 | ☐ |

How did you do? Too much? About right?

- Do you need to watch the amount of added sugars you eat? Estimate the number of teaspoons of added sugars in your food choices.

| | Teaspoons Right for You | Teaspoons You Had |
|---|---|---|
| Sugars | 6 12 18 | ☐ |

How did you do? Too much? About right?

**STEP 4**
Decide what changes you can make for a healthier diet. Start by making small changes, such as switching to low-fat salad dressings or adding an extra serving of vegetables. Make additional changes gradually until healthy eating becomes a habit.

United States Department of Agriculture, Center for Nutrition Policy and Promotion: *The food guide pyramid,* Home and Garden Bulletin Number 252, 1996, www.nal.usda.gov:8001/py/pmap.htm.

---

calyptus globulus, wintergreen, or peppermint), herbal therapy (e.g., echinacea; goldenseal; ginger; elder, peppermint, licorice, and yarrow tea; garlic), vitamin therapy (e.g., zinc), and homeopathy (Alternative Remedies, 1998; Dollemore, 1998; Nurse's handbook of alternative and complementary therapies, 1999).

Pharmaceutical medications are directed at relieving the most uncomfortable symptoms: rhinorrhea, cough, and congestion, as well as at preventing the development of secondary complications. Nasal sprays with sympathomimetics decrease nasal congestion and rhinorrhea but should be used for a very limited amount of time because excessive use can cause rebound congestion. Antihistamines are of little effect except that they cause drowsiness, which may be desirable when the person has difficulty sleeping. Common over-the-counter antihistamines include diphenhydramine (Benadryl), chlorpheniramine (ChlorTrimeton), and brompheniramine (Bromphen, Dimetane). Analgesics—including acetaminophen, aspirin, or one of the NSAIDs—are useful for fever reduction, as well as reducing symptoms of malaise, muscle ache, and headache. Expectorants are used to increase mucus viscosity, allowing the cough mechanism to move mucus more effectively through the respiratory system. Guaifenesin is the most common expectorant included in combination cold products and cough syrup. Cough syrups act centrally to control the cough reflex at the medullary cough center, or peripherally to anesthetize cough receptors in the respiratory tract. The most common over-the-counter agent used for coughs is dextromethorphan, which is also found in combination cold products and cough syrup.

Teach women to read labels on over-the-counter products for cold symptoms so that they purchase and use products that are intended only for the specific symptoms being experienced, rather than taking ones with chemicals to treat symptoms that they do not have. This is important because the more ingredients a product has, the higher the likelihood of experiencing a drug reaction or interaction. Many of the liquid formulations also include alcohol and sugar, which may not be suitable for people with certain conditions.

Because the common cold and the flu are caused by viruses, antibiotics have no influence on the primary illness (Riggs, 1997). Cold symptoms that last longer than 2 weeks, however, should be evaluated by a health care provider. The development of additional symptoms, such as ear pain (acute viral or bacterial otitis media), sinus pain (sinusitis), or a productive cough with yellow or green sputum (bronchitis), signals the onset of secondary infections and the possible need for an antibiotic.

### Prevention

Cold viruses are spread through the air and through direct contact (hand to mouth) with contaminated surfaces. The incubation period is 72 hours, with the illness lasting 7 to 14 days. The best prevention for the common cold is to avoid crowded places and contact with infected persons. Persons with a cold should cover their mouths when sneezing, and practice good hand-washing techniques. The use of disposable tissues is beneficial.

The number of colds or episodes of flu can be decreased by bolstering natural defenses through the use of herbs, stress reduction, homeopathy, and an annual flu vaccination. Echinacea, garlic, and ginger are three herbs that help boost the immune system. Reducing stress on the body is also helpful because highly stressed people are more likely to catch a cold. Studies show that a simple relaxation technique like slow, deep breathing can help the immune system be more vigilant (Dollemore, 1998). Regular exercise, humidi-

fied air, and avoiding exposure to smoke also help reduce the number of episodes of upper respiratory tract infections.

### Gastrointestinal Infection

The term **gastroenteritis** describes a variety of viral and bacterial infections that affect the stomach, small intestine, colon, and rectum. Most are short in duration, so self-care is appropriate for most of these infections.

### Strategies for Self-Assessment

The most common symptom is diarrhea, but vomiting, muscle pain, fever, dehydration, and abdominal cramping may also occur. Replacement of fluids orally is usually the only treatment necessary. A gastroenteritis may be contagious or noncontagious, caused by bacterial or viral agents. Viral gastroenteritis accounts for 40% of the infectious gastroenteritis seen, and another 40% have no clear cause.

The Norwalk virus causes 40% of the cases of viral outbreaks seen in adolescents and adults in the United States (Moog and Shah, 1997). Transmitted by the oral fecal route, the Norwalk virus causes symptoms within 1 or 2 days of exposure. It presents as a syndrome of acute nausea, vomiting, diarrhea, fever, muscle aches, and headache. Digestion may be affected for up to 2 weeks after infection.

### Strategies for Self-Care

Oral rehydration, using fluids containing water, glucose, and the electrolyte concentration of plasma, is the treatment of choice. Fluids such as Gatorade and other "sports" drinks are ideal, but other clear fluids are equally effective. Diets should also be altered so that fatty, spicy, and high fiber foods, as well as dairy products, caffeinated beverages, and alcohol, are avoided. Juices, noncarbonated drinks, and soft foods are ideal.

Antimotility drugs (e.g., loperamide) may be used to decrease intestinal motility and fluid secretion. Medical care should be sought for explosive, profuse bloody diarrhea; severe abdominal pain; high fever; tenesmus (i.e., ineffectual and painful straining to pass urine or stool); or weight loss (Moog and Shah, 1997).

### Prevention

The basic strategies for prevention are the same as those for upper respiratory infections.

## Educating for Self-Care to Meet Sexual Needs

**Sexuality** is a broad concept that includes sexual orientation, sexual desire, sexual response, view of self, and presentation of self. Sexuality is an expression of the individual's unique personal identity and a component of the human need for closeness and comfort from another person (MacLauren, 1995). Sexual expression includes touching, caressing, looking, teasing, kissing, massaging, licking, sucking, and penetrating. It is not limited by age, attractiveness, sexual orientation, or partner participation (Fogel and Lauver, 1990). Sexuality is a constant of life but is expressed in many different ways throughout the life span.

**Sexual health** is defined by the World Health Organization (WHO) as "the integration of somatic, emotional, intellectual, and social aspects of sexual beings in ways that are positively enriching and that enhance personality, communication, and love" (WHO, 1975). A major component of sexual health is an acceptance of one's self-concept, body image, sexual identity, and sexual orientation (Fogel, 1998). Sexual health is the emotional and physical state of well-being that allows individuals to enjoy and act on sexual feelings (Boston Women's Health Book Collective, 1999). We have a role in promoting sexual health by providing the woman with information about her body and educating her on how she may meet her sexual needs.

### Sexual Equilibrium

Althof and Levine (1993) have described a concept of sexual equilibrium to help in understanding many aspects of sexual life. "**Sexual equilibrium** is the delicate changeable balance of psychological forces between partners and is important because the result of this balance is either sexual comfort or sexual anxiety in each partner" (Althof and Levine, 1993). Sexual equilibrium enhances a person's life, but sexual disequilibrium causes disappointment and diminishing interest in sexual expression. These authors have proposed that there are three aspects of sexual identity and three components of sexual function that contribute to sexual equilibrium.

### Sexual Identity

**Gender identity** is a woman's sense of herself as a female being, which is formed early in childhood and changes throughout life. Examples of factors that can adversely affect a woman's gender identity are illness, disability, unwanted change in employment status, and physical changes brought on by childbirth. Adverse gender identity parallels a negative self-worth and the loss of sexual desire. **Sexual orientation** refers to the choice of sexual partners, which may be totally heterosexual, totally homosexual, totally bisexual, or a sequencing of these choices during a lifetime. When partners have knowledge of and accept the sexual behaviors of the partnership, a state of sexual equilibrium exists. When there is disagreement or lack of knowledge, sexual disequilibrium occurs (Althof and Levine, 1993). The third aspect, **sexual intention,** is how a person chooses to participate in sexual behavior. A woman may choose voluntary celibacy—either all the time or for part of her life, or may provide herself sexual pleasure through

masturbation, or may participate in sexual behaviors with a partner (Kitzinger, 1985). If sexual behavior is used as a manifestation of power over others (i.e., a way to dominate partners) it leads to sexual disequilibrium (Althof and Levine, 1993).

### Sexual Functioning

The three components of sexual functioning are sexual desire or libido, sexual arousal, and orgasm. A person's sexual desire is called his or her **libido.** A woman's libido may be equally aroused all the time or may vary within her monthly cycle. Many women describe feeling peaks of desire immediately before and during menstruation, with a second, less pronounced peak at ovulation. Personal or cultural prohibitions against intercourse during the menstrual flow often prevent women from acting on their desire. Some respond to their sexual desire through masturbation. Others, if they use the diaphragm for fertility control, insert it to act as a barrier to contain the menstrual blood and then remove it after intercourse (Kitzinger, 1983).

A lack of sexual desire or libido may result from a variety of reasons, including confusion over sexual orientation, illness, aspects of the relationship, or disagreements. Women who find sexual intercourse painful, emotionally unfulfilling, or have been assaulted will have their sexual desire affected. For some, the response may last for years following the traumatic event.

Differing **arousal patterns** in a relationship have the potential to contribute to equilibrium or disequilibrium. Partners who have similar and concurrent levels of interest in sexual activity are more likely to experience equilibrium than if they disagree on the timing and frequency of sexual activity. Partners who experience different patterns will have to work harder to maintain a sexual equilibrium (Althof and Levine, 1993).

Different patterns of **orgasmic response** may have the same unsettling effect on a relationship as different arousal patterns. When the activities between partners consistently leave one partner unorgasmic, one or both parties experience frustration and feelings of inadequacy, which may adversely affect their communication patterns in all areas, leading to disequilibrium (Althof and Levine, 1993).

*Sexual Response Cycle.* The **sexual response cycle** is divided into the following two components: (1) the woman's capacity or capability for experiences, and (2) the activity or the current state of experience. Vasocongestion and myotonia (i.e., an increase in muscle tension) are the two basic physiologic responses to sexual stimulation. **Vasocongestion** is part of the process of sexual arousal, occurring as the tissues and blood vessels become engorged. **Myotonia** peaks during orgasm. In a woman, physiologic response to sexual stimuli is not limited to her pelvis but involves her whole body. Changes in cardiovascular and respiratory function occur along with changes in her skin, muscles, breasts, and rectal sphincter.

In *Human Sexual Response*, Masters and Johnson (1966) presented the most widely known approach for identifying the different phases of physiologic change during sexual behavior. This cycle has four stages: excitement, plateau, orgasm, and resolution (Masters and Johnson, 1966).

The **excitement** stage may last from several minutes to several hours and is initially characterized by vaginal lubrication. Lubrication may occur in response to fantasizing, mental imagery, or physical contact and can be prolonged in the continued presence of positive stimuli or interrupted and ended by distracting stimuli. During this process, the uterus moves up in the pelvis and tilts forward, the vagina elongates and opens, the labia minora become larger, and the labia majora separate. In some women, the clitoris becomes erect. Changes also occur in other organs as the nipples harden, the areola become engorged, and breasts increase in size. The woman's heart rate and blood pressure increase, and there is an involuntary tightening of the muscles of the rib cage and abdomen. At first, the skin on her abdomen becomes flushed and mottled and then spreads over her breasts and neck.

The **plateau** phase occurs just before orgasm. The breasts, nipples, and areola continue to enlarge. The sex flush continues to spread up from her abdominal area. Her muscle tone increases, and involuntary shuddering movements may occur. Her heart rate and blood pressure continue to increase, and her breathing gets faster, sometimes becoming irregular and gasping. The uterus becomes fully elevated off the pelvic floor; the cervix rises; the vagina elongates to its fullest; and the tissues of the outer third of the vagina and the labia minora enlarge, creating a response called the **orgasmic platform.** The outer third of the vagina becomes tighter, while the internal two-thirds open up like a balloon. The labia minora become deep purple in color, and a few drops of mucoid fluid are secreted by the Bartholin glands. The hood of the clitoris swells, along with the labia majora, often causing the clitoris to disappear from view.

The third phase is **orgasm** or climax, which is a physiologic and psychologic event. The breasts, nipples, and areola are now firm and large, but the primary response is in the orgasmic platform, where a series of muscle contractions occur in the uterus and the muscles of the pelvic floor. The muscles of the pelvic floor contract against the engorged blood vessels, reducing vasocongestion. "Contractions spread from the circles of muscle which are near the base of the spine and around the rectum, right through to those which form a circle about halfway up around the vagina and deeper inside, in the muscles which are nearer the uterus. These contractions are rhythmic and very fast—each lasts about one eighth of a second" (Kitzinger, 1985). The muscles of the lower abdomen, perineum, and uterus are also involved in the fast rhythmic contractions. The woman's respiratory, blood pressure, and pulse rates peak. This involuntary climax of sexual tension may last only a few seconds, but a woman is capable of multiple climaxes in varying patterns (Kitzinger, 1985).

**Resolution,** the fourth and final stage, involves restoration of organs and tissues to their preexcitement state. The woman's respirations, pulse, and blood pressure slow down within a few minutes. "The lowest part of the uterus, however, the cervix which hangs down in the vagina . . . , remains open for about a half an hour following orgasm. It is not until then that the uterus finally assumes its normal position" (Kitzinger, 1985).

*Sexuality and Life.* A woman's unique experience with sex consists of a whole range of experiences that are not just genital. "Sex involves the whole body and is expressed in different ways at different times in a woman's life, during her ovarian cycle and with the varied and complex biological experiences of pregnancy, childbearing, menopause, and aging" (Kitzinger, 1985).

The focus in adolescence is the development of a sense of sexuality. Dating is an activity that allows adolescents time to try out various expressions by choosing companions, testing ideas about themselves, and eventually experiencing sexual pleasure (Fogel, 1998). Half of all teenagers are sexually active by the time they finish high school. Girls may experience peer pressure to begin sexual activity. However, they may be seeking intimacy rather than the sexual act of intercourse. The earlier sexual intercourse is initiated and the longer a woman participates, the greater the health risks with exposure to sexually transmitted infections and the risk for pregnancy.

During the young adult years, the issues include developing mature and satisfying relationships, completing education, and becoming established in the workforce. Some women choose to find and commit to a life partner. Others choose to maintain a single lifestyle. If a woman chooses to participate in sexual intimacy, she is at risk for a sexually transmitted infection. If she participates in heterosexual intercourse, pregnancy prevention becomes a concern.

During the perimenopausal period, if a woman experiences hot flashes, night sweats, or insomnia, she may become fatigued and experience a loss of libido. If she experiences decreased vaginal lubrication, she may have less desire for intercourse due to dyspareunia (i.e., difficult or painful intercourse). The use of a vaginal lubricant can reduce the effect. After menopause, sexual experiences and activities remain as varied as women themselves. Some women report decreased interest in sexual activity, but others find it more stimulating to be free from the fear of pregnancy.

Patterns of sexuality during the second half of life continue to vary. Fewer persons in the household may mean an increase in sexual expression because there is more privacy. Frequency of intercourse may decline while enjoyment increases (Alexander and LaRosa, 1994). "Masters and Johnson showed in their research that sexual activity does not come to a full stop with increasing age, though the rate of intercourse is often reduced. Seven out of ten couples over age 60 were sexually active" (Kitzinger, 1985). The presence of a partner and the increased chance of chronic illness in one or both partners may make sexual intercourse difficult or impossible.

*Addressing the Barriers.* Myths—Common myths about female sexuality may interfere with women reaching their maximum sexual potential and establishing and maintaining healthy sexual relationships. Many women are not even aware of how such myths have affected their own beliefs and practices. We can help a woman begin to explore her beliefs and separate fact from fiction and personal choice from cultural expectations when taking a sexual history.

Language—Women may not be comfortable talking with us about these sensitive issues. Communication about sex is often hard because they are attempting to convey their nonverbal feelings and activities in words. Clinical or "proper" terms such as vagina, penis, and intercourse may feel formal. Slang words are often avoided because they are degrading towards women, and euphemisms such as "making love" are too vague and open to multiple interpretations (Boston Women's Health Book Collective, 1998).

Role modeling—Basic attitudes are shown by the way we respond to the questions raised during the process of obtaining a sexual history. When and how we respond will show the woman our comfort level with the topic and the value we place on her questions.

PLISSIT counseling model—The **PLISSIT counseling model** can be used to address the sexual needs and concerns of clients and to make appropriate referrals (Annon, 1974). PLISSIT is an acronym for four stages of counseling: permission giving, limited information giving, specific suggestions, and intensive therapy. Even without special training, we should be able to care for clients needing the first two levels of counseling—permission giving and limited information giving. The other two stages—specific suggestions and intensive therapy—require additional training and experience beyond basic nursing skills.

**Permission giving** is different from telling the client what to do. We can give permission for thoughts, feelings, behaviors, and possibly for the woman to do something or not do something. Permission should be given for behaviors that enhance self-esteem—but not at the expense of another person. Permission should not be given for behaviors that may threaten the physical or emotional health of the woman or others. When we give **limited information**, it usually focuses on anatomy and physiology and dispelling common myths.

For example, if a woman asks "How often do most people my age have sex?," we can answer this by giving permission to decide, alone or with a partner, what frequency is appropriate for her relationship. The question "Is it normal to have times when you don't want to have sex?" can be answered with information that assures the woman that sexual desire is variable and affected by other life concerns. "How often is it okay to masturbate?" is another example of a question that can best be answered by giving the woman permission to decide what frequency is appropriate. At other times, women may be seeking assistance with relationship issues that require increased communication skills. A question like, "My partner wants sex more often than I do. What can I do?," can be handled by stressing the variability of individual desires and the importance of communication so that the needs of both partners are met.

### Strategies for Self-Assessment

Many women lack a basic understanding about their anatomy and physiology and the expression of human sexuality. Sharing information and pictures about her genitals and erogenous areas is the first step for self-assessment and self-care. Using a mirror to show her her own body parts helps her to claim them as her own. Other resources can provide information about techniques or positions that are unfamiliar to her.

### Strategies for Self-Care

*Masturbation.* Myths abound that people who masturbate will grow hair on their hands, go blind, or lose their minds. Some religions or cultures have taboos against having sex for pleasure or practicing masturbation.

The woman may need permission to explore what masturbation means for her personally, as well as basic instruction on how to care for herself. **Masturbation** is when a woman is able to give herself sexual pleasure by touching herself or moving her body in a special way. Most women, after they learn how to pleasure themselves, are able to bring themselves to orgasm. An orgasm from masturbation may occur more quickly than from lovemaking with a partner. Some women find it provides an enjoyable physical release.

Some women "only masturbate when other forms of sexual pleasure are missing, a partner is away or if things are going very wrong in a relationship. Others do so at phases of their lives when the sex drive is strong, before there is a regular partner, or when a relationship has split up or a lover has died" (Kitzinger, 1985). Women also choose to masturbate to help with the pain of menstrual cramps, during the last weeks of pregnancy, when they are under stress, to help get to sleep, and just because they like it.

Explain her anatomy and show the woman her genitalia in a diagram or mirror. Answer her questions about her anatomy and the process of masturbating. Have literature and resources available for her.

***Aphrodisiacs.*** Aphrodisiacs are herbs, drugs, or other agents thought to enhance a person's sexual desire or pleasure. Myths and cultural beliefs about the use of such substances are widely shared. Women may have tried some of these substances in an effort to enhance their sexual desire or experience. Caution the woman that there is no research on the efficacy of such agents and that the ingestion of some of them may even be harmful.

## Self-Care for Stress Management

**Stress** occurs when there is an imbalance between the demands of our lives and the resources we have to deal with those demands. It is not the demands themselves, but our reaction to those demands that determines if we feel stressed.

There are many sources of stress for women. Work, family, and personal issues are all potential causes of excessive stress. Many women lead lives that involve multiple roles (i.e., wife, mother, employee) with conflicting demands. Many women not only put in a full shift of 8 hours of work either outside or inside the home but also put in a "second shift" of work in the evening in caring for their families and homes (Hochschild, 1989). Stress management changes the situation so that instead of stress controlling the woman, she takes control of her life.

### Strategies for Self-Assessment

Stress may manifest itself as physical symptoms such as headache, fatigue, insomnia, digestive changes, neck pain, backache, menstrual cycle disturbances, and increased susceptibility to illness. Stress may also be expressed through psychologic symptoms, such as tension or anxiety, anger, reclusiveness, pessimism, cynicism, resentment, guilt, irritability, depression, sleep disturbances, increased tension, and an inability to concentrate.

### Strategies for Self-Care

Stress is how our bodies and minds react to disturbances in our normal balance. On an individual level, the first step to managing stress is to identify the "stressors" that cause stress. The response of choice to the stressors may be either a positive response that helps to manage the stressors or a negative response that increases tension levels. The following basic coping skills deal with stress in a positive way: (1) acceptance of things that are beyond control, (2) attitude adjustment by focusing on the positive side of a situation, and (3) maintaining a perspective that focuses on what is an actual concern, rather than projecting possible concerns.

Beyond that basic, personal response there are many simple, inexpensive treatments to manage stress. A good way to start is to eliminate artificial stress relievers such as alcohol, drugs, and cigarette use and substitute deep breathing, exercise, and walking. Social support is also crucial because relationships with people or pets are key to reducing stress.

A variety of treatment options are widely used, especially activities designed to promote physical and mental relaxation. Aromatherapy (especially essential oil of lavender, Roman chamomile, marjoram, lemon-scented eucalyptus, and lemon balm); aerobic exercise and stretching exercises; herbal therapy (especially teas of chamomile, passionflower, valerian or American ginseng); hydrotherapy; massage; conscious relaxation and meditation; and yoga are most often recommended (Alternative Remedies for Common Ailments, 1998).

Prevention of stress is not possible, but minimizing the level of stress experienced is possible by taking occasional breaks in routine habits, a regular schedule of sleep, unlearning the behaviors of worry and hurry, and facing stressful situations only after taking a deep breath.

## SELF-ASSESSMENT OF A WOMAN'S BODY

### Educating for Self-Assessment of the Breasts

Breast examination plays a critical role in the early detection of breast disease and cancer. There are three types of preliminary breast examinations: breast self-examination, clinical breast examination by a health care provider, and mammography; and all women should have one or more at different times in their lives.

**Breast self-examination** is the regular and systematic assessment of the breast tissue by the woman. It should be done monthly, generally during the week after the menstrual period. When a woman is perimenopausal, menopausal, or pregnant, she should examine her breasts on the first day of the month. During adolescence, women should begin to become familiar with their own breasts, just as they become familiar with other parts of their bodies (Love, 1995). Women who are knowledgeable and comfortable with their own breasts will be more likely to notice a change in a breast that could indicate a significant problem.

Despite recommendations from both the American Cancer Society and the National Cancer Institute that monthly examinations be done, most women report that they do not practice breast self-examination. This is true even with women with a family history of breast cancer (Kash, Holland, and Halper, 1992). Women report that they do not examine their breasts for the following reasons: (1) they do not know how (Dawson and Thompson, 1989); (2) they are fearful of finding a lump; (3) they lack confidence in their ability to perform self-examination correctly; (4) they are uncomfortable touching their breasts; (5) they do not believe they are at risk of breast cancer (i.e., denial); and (6) apathy (Small, 1994).

Despite the lack of general participation in breast self-examination, most breast lumps are still found by the woman herself, usually while showering, or by accident, or by a lover. By then, however, the lumps are usually 2 cm or larger (Love, 1995). In theory, a regular breast self-examination should result in earlier detection of breast cancer, thus giving the woman a greater chance for survival. Although it is not known whether this is true, teaching women to become familiar with their own breasts through breast self-examination is in the best interest of the health of women.

### Breast Conditions

Over her lifetime, a woman can encounter a broad variety of breast conditions, including normal changes that occur during the menstrual cycle, as well as several types of benign lumps. The lobes, lobules, bulbs and ducts of the breasts, as well as the fat tissue and the muscles under the breasts and ribs can sometimes make the breasts feel lumpy, especially in women who are thin or have small breasts. In addition, a woman's breasts generally undergo changes each month until she experiences menopause.

### Types of Benign Breast Changes

Common benign breast changes may be categorized as generalized breast lumpiness, solitary lumps, nipple discharge, and infection and/or inflammation. The menstrual cycle may bring **cyclic breast changes** experienced as swelling, tenderness, and pain before and sometimes during menstrual periods. At the same time, one or more lumps or a feeling of increased lumpiness may develop because of extra fluid collecting in the breast tissue. These lumps normally go away by the end of the menses. **Generalized breast lumpiness,** which is also labeled as **fibrocystic** changes or benign breast disease, may be felt in the area around the nipple and areola and in the upper-outer part of the breast. As a woman approaches middle age, it may become more obvious that the milk-producing glandular tissue of her breasts recedes and soft, fatty tissue increases. Unless a woman takes replacement hormones, this type of lumpiness generally disappears after **menopause.**

Benign breast conditions also include several types of distinct, **solitary lumps,** which can appear at any time and be large or small, soft or rubbery, and fluid-filled or solid (Figure 5-4).

**Cysts** (i.e., fluid-filled sacs) most often occur in women ages 35 to 50 and may enlarge and become tender and painful just before the menstrual period. Some cysts are so small that they cannot be felt, but cysts may also occasionally fill to be several inches across. **Fibroadenomas** are solid, round, benign tumors that are made up of both structural (fibro) and glandular (adenoma) tissues. These lumps are usually painless, rubbery, and can be easily moved around. Fibroadenomas are the most common type of tumors in women in their late teens and early twenties and occur twice as often in African-American women as in other women. **Fat necroses** are painless, round, firm lumps formed by damaged and disintegrating fatty tissues and typically occur in obese women with very large breasts. Fat necrosis often develops in response to a bruise or blow to the breast, even though the woman may not remember the specific injury. Sometimes the skin around the lumps looks red or bruised. **Sclerosing adenosis** is a benign condition involving excessive growth of tissues in the breast's lobules. Sclerosing adenosis often causes breast pain, can produce lumps, and may show up on a mammogram, often as calcifications.

**Nipple discharge** accompanies some benign breast conditions. Because the breast is a gland, secretions from the nipple of a mature woman are not unusual or a sign of disease. Small amounts of discharge commonly occur in women taking birth control pills or certain other medications, including sedatives and tranquilizers. Nipple discharges come in a variety of colors and textures. A milky discharge can be traced to many causes, including thyroid malfunction and oral contraceptives or other drugs. Women with generalized breast lumpiness may have a sticky discharge that is brown or green. Bloody or sticky discharge may be caused by an **intraductal papilloma,** which is a small, wartlike growth that projects into breast ducts near the nipple. Any slight bump or bruise in the area of the nipple can cause the papilloma to bleed. Women nearing menopause may experience a single intraductal papilloma. Multiple intraductal papillomas are more common in younger women. They often occur in both breasts and are more likely to be associated with a lump than with nipple discharge.

Infection and/or inflammation, including mastitis and mammary duct ectasia, are characteristic of some benign breast conditions. **Mastitis** is an infection in the breast. A duct may become blocked, allowing milk to pool, causing inflammation, and setting the stage for infection by bacteria. Mammary duct ectasia occurs in the perimenopausal stage. Ducts beneath the nipple become inflamed and can become clogged. Mammary duct ectasia can become painful and produce a thick and sticky discharge that may be green, milky, serous, serosanguineous, sanguineous, or watery color (Lemcke and others, 1995).

### Strategies for Self-Assessment

Illustrated guides for how to do breast self-examination have been developed and distributed by a variety of organizations and drug companies as a public service. Each guide tends to vary slightly from the others, but they all present the same basic principles. The technique for breast self-examination includes a combination of visual inspection and tactile palpation.

It is important that the entire breast be examined, up into the axilla and under the nipple and areola. The axilla must be palpated for palpable or tender lymph nodes, and the nipple assessed for discharge.

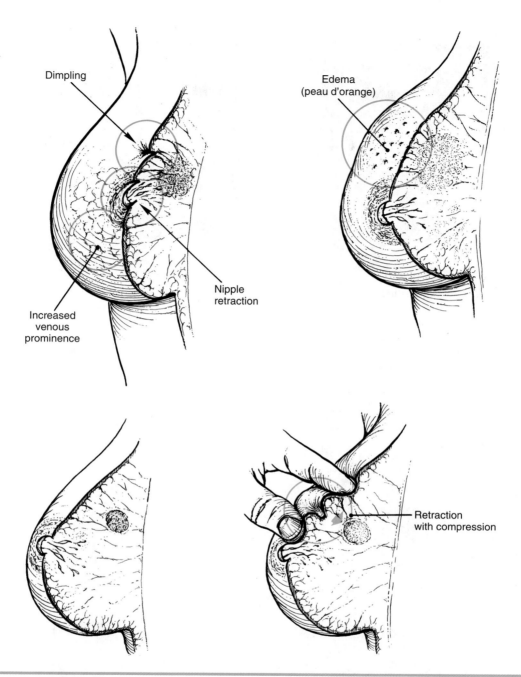

FIGURE 5-4 • Abnormalities of the breast. *(From Barkauskas VH and others:* Health and physical assessment, *ed 2, St Louis, 1998, Mosby.)*

The pads of the fingers—not the fingertips—should be used to do the palpation. The skin should be gently pressed with a firm touch. Some women find it more comfortable to do the palpation in the shower where the water and soap make the skin slippery, making it easier to feel the tissue (Figures 5-5 and 5-6).

 **Strategies for Self-Care**

There is a wide variation of normal in the human breast. Some women normally have smooth breasts,

and others normally have breast tissue that has formed itself in a very clearly lumpy fashion, like a "bumpy cobblestone road" (Love, 1995). Some women have lumpy or nodular breasts only in the upper outer quadrant of the breast while the rest of their breast remains smooth. In other women, one breast may be lumpy, and the other smooth. It is also common for women to have some variation between breasts in size or appearance.

Cyclic changes are also normal in a woman's breast. The hormones estrogen and progesterone secreted by

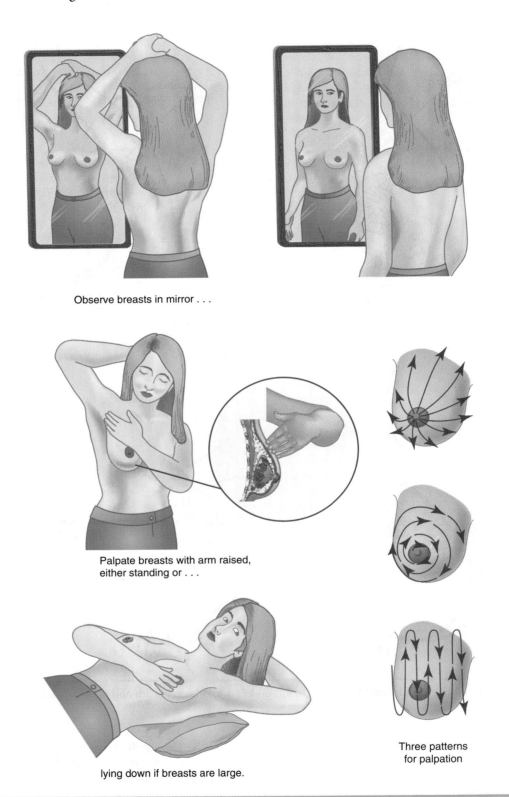

Observe breasts in mirror . . .

Palpate breasts with arm raised,
either standing or . . .

lying down if breasts are large.

Three patterns
for palpation

FIGURE 5-5 • Breast self-examination.

the ovaries cause an increase in ductal and lobular tissue, resulting in the cyclic swelling, pain, and tenderness experienced by women during the 2 weeks before a menstrual period. Because of these common normal variations, it is very important that we teach women how to do breast self-examination using their own breasts as examples. This way, they learn about their own breasts, are able to determine what is normal for them, and are more apt to notice and report change with increased confidence.

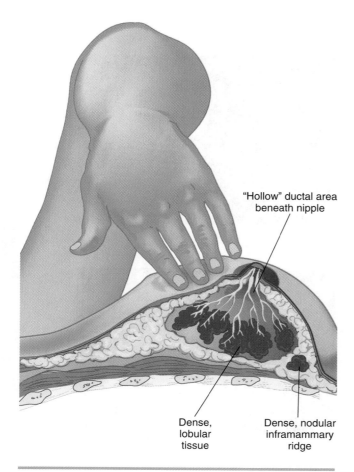

"Hollow" ductal area beneath nipple

Dense, lobular tissue

Dense, nodular inframammary ridge

*FIGURE 5-6* ● Palpation of breasts.

Even though the odds are low, many women fear that any changes in their breasts are indications of breast cancer. When changes in her breasts (e.g., development of a lump or swelling, skin irritation or dimpling, nipple pain or retraction, redness or scaliness of the nipple or breast skin, or a discharge other than breast milk) occur, the woman should see her health care provider as soon as possible for further evaluation. Seeking an explanation and further evaluation will help to keep her anxiety level under control and provide the best chance of successful treatment if it is a serious condition.

Experienced health care professionals can examine the breast and determine whether the changes are probably benign or if they may indicate breast cancer. These professionals will determine when additional tests are appropriate to rule out a cancer and when follow-up exams are the best strategy. If there is any suspicion of cancer, a biopsy will be done.

**Breast augmentation** is an increasingly common surgical procedure that uses silicone sheaths filled with saline to increase the size of a woman's breasts. Incisions are made in the axilla, under the areola, or under the breast. Implants can be placed under the pectoral muscles or under the breast tissue between the breast and the chest muscle (Love, 1995). Breast self-examination

continues to be important for women who have undergone augmentation surgery because they must become familiar with the new feel of their breasts so they can incorporate these changes into their understanding of their own breasts.

## Education for Self-Care of the Skin

Healthy skin does not make many demands for maintenance. All that is required is that it be kept clean, moisturized, and protected from sun and heat. A woman's culture and lifestyle determine the frequency of washing and type of protection that is needed.

### Keeping Skin Clean and Intact

Cleansing the skin removes dirt, sweat, microorganisms, dead skin cells, and body secretions. During winter in cold climates, and during all weather for women with advancing age, bathing should be done less frequently, with soap used only in the axillary and genital areas. Deodorants may be useful in masking the odor of sweat glands, and antiperspirants reduce the amount of sweat produced, but some women are sensitive to the ingredients—especially the fragrances—in these products.

Optimal water content for the first layer of the skin is 10%. In dry weather or in heated rooms, the humidity in the air may not be sufficient to keep the skin hydrated and it may become cracked. Moisturizers are recommended to correct this problem. Moisturizers are emulsions that prevent water loss from the skin and should be applied after drying off from bathing, while the skin is still moist. Products on the market contain water and glycerin, lactic acid, or urea. Products that are more expensive are not necessarily better at maintaining hydration of the skin. Personal preference with regard to the smell, feel, and touch of the skin should be the guide for selection.

### Strategies for Self-Assessment

Self-assessment of the skin surface involves locating and "mapping" moles, freckles, and other benign skin lesions while looking for changes in a wart or mole or the growth of a new lesion. Mirrors should be used for body surfaces not easily seen, and a partner may be helpful in checking the back. Change in an existing lesion or the development of a new lesion warrants further assessment by a health care provider. Individuals over age 50 should have skin examinations as part of the annual examination (Daniel, Dolan, and Wheeland, 1996). If a woman finds a change in any marking on her body, she should have it evaluated by a professional.

The three most common types of skin cancer are **basal cell carcinoma, squamous cell carcinoma,** and **melanoma.** All are the result of acute and chronic exposure to ultraviolet radiation. These cancers from sun

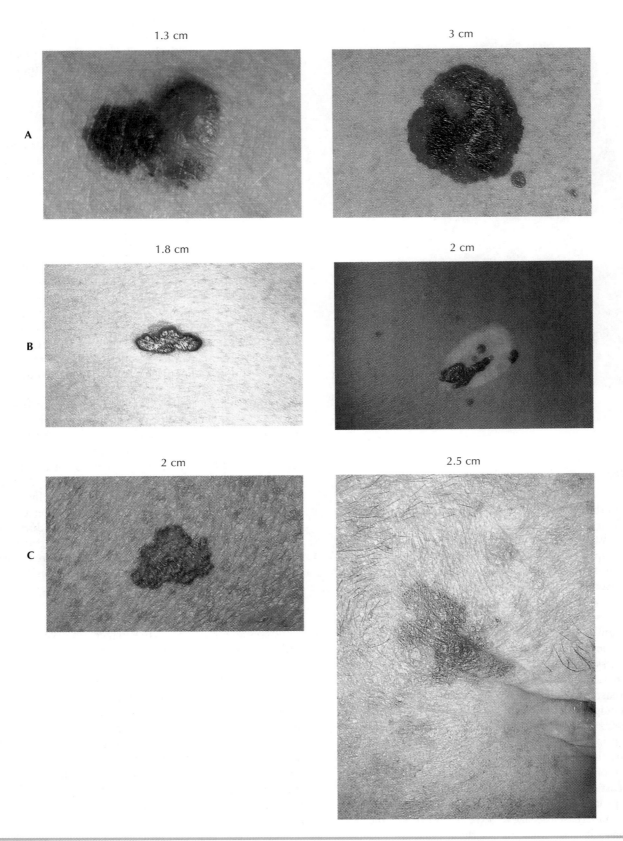

FIGURE 5-7 • Malignant melanomas. Note presence of **ABCD** characteristics (**A**symmetry, irregular **B**order, variation of **C**olor, **D**iameter >6 mm). **A,** Superficial spreading melanomas. **B,** Nodular melanomas. **C,** Lentigo maligna melanomas. *(From Barkauskas VH and others:* Health and physical assessment, *ed 2, St Louis, 1998, Mosby.)*

damage are the most frequent form of cancer in the United States, with an estimated one million new cases diagnosed each year (Brown, 1997).

***Basal Cell Carcinoma.*** **Basal cell carcinoma** is the most common cancer. It is slow-growing, rarely metastasizes, and commonly occurs on surfaces exposed to the sun (e.g., the face, neck, scalp, ears, upper back, and chest). Basal cell carcinoma occurs in fair-skinned people who sunburn easily but is equally frequent among those who work in the sun and live in sunny climates. Basal cell cancer is mainly asymptomatic, but its course is highly unpredictable. A lesion may appear unchanged for many years or may grow rapidly. Symptoms such as enlargement, pain, itching, and change in color warrant prompt investigation.

Basal cell carcinoma usually begins as a small, shiny papule with rolled borders. Over time, it develops temangectiasis and a pearly border and eventually develops a central ulcer that repeatedly bleeds then crusts. Less common basal cell cancers appear as flat plaques or take one of many other forms. The cancer may even appear as a recurrent sty in the eye (Brown, 1997). Basal cell cancers are common in whites and rare in blacks.

***Squamous Cell Carcinoma.*** **Squamous cell carcinoma,** the second most common form of skin cancer, most commonly occurs on the scalp, lower lip, ear, and back of the hand. The lesion usually begins as a reddish papule or plaque with a scaly or crusted surface. The lesion may later appear nodular or warty; then ulceration and invasion of the underlying tissues occurs (Ferrary and Parker-Falzoi, 1998). Squamous cell carcinoma is the most common skin cancer in blacks.

***Malignant Melanoma.*** **Malignant melanoma** is a skin cancer that develops from melanocytes. It may develop anywhere on the body where there is melanin. Malignant melanoma usually begins from an existing pigmented mole. Any change in a mole (i.e., in size, color) should be promptly investigated. Malignant melanoma can be fatal (Figure 5-7).

Malignant melanoma is recognizable in its early stages, so all women should be taught the ABCDs of assessing for melanoma: *A*symmetry of lesion, a *B*order that is irregular, *C*olor that is either blue/black or variegated, and *D*iameter of more than 6 mm (Figure 5-8).

There is a window of opportunity during which the lesion can be excised and survival is more likely, but this window only exists for lesions that are no more than 0.76 mm deep. Melanomas that have grown to more than 4 mm in depth leave the person with a survival rate of only 50% in 5 years (Edwards and others, 1996). Although responsible for only a small percentage of the total number of skin cancers, melanoma causes 75% of the deaths from skin cancer (Daniel, Dolan, and Wheeland, 1996). Suspicious moles are those with variegated color, irregular borders, and where change has occurred (Ferrary and Parker-Falzoi, 1998).

Skin color is the most important risk factor in the development of melanoma, which is rare among blacks. Other risk factors include intermittent, limited but intense sun exposure; fair skin; a tendency to freckle; light hair and eye color; and a history of sunburn, particularly in childhood. A family history of melanoma increases risk, as does the presence of a large number of moles or large congenital moles (Brown, 1997).

### Strategies for Self-Care

Prevention of sun damage is managed by avoiding exposure of skin surfaces to the sun and ultraviolet rays. When this is not practical, the skin can be protected by avoiding exposure between 10 AM and 2 PM and wearing hats, clothing, and sun block products. Tanning booths should be avoided.

Sun block products should be selected to protect the user from both UVA and UVB rays when they cannot be

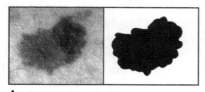

A—Asymmetry of lesion

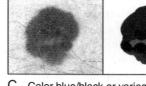

C—Color blue/black or variegated

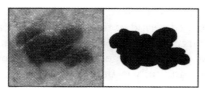

B—Border, irregular

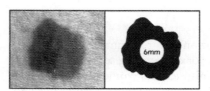

D—Diameter >6 mm

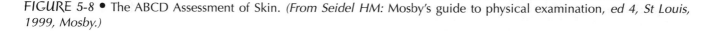

*FIGURE 5-8* • The ABCD Assessment of Skin. *(From Seidel HM:* Mosby's guide to physical examination, *ed 4, St Louis, 1999, Mosby.)*

avoided. The sun protection factor (SPF) is a laboratory-derived figure obtained under strictly defined conditions. "An SPF 2 figure means that 50% of incipient UVB radiation is blocked . . . at SPF 16, 93.75%" (Worobec, 1997) of the radiation is blocked. The degree that these products help to reduce the risk of skin cancer only applies if the woman does not simultaneously increase her length of exposure to the sun. Sunscreen must also be reapplied frequently, especially after swimming or sweating. A sunscreen with an SPF of at least 15 is recommended for everyone. Those with darker skin may use products with an SPF of at least 8 (Ferrary and Parker-Falzoi, 1998).

## Educating for Self-Care of Vaginal Discharge

**Vaginal discharge** is a normal part of a woman's life from a few years before menarche through the postmenopausal period. The characteristics of the discharge vary according to changes in hormone stimulation. A few years before menarche, increasing levels of estrogen cause a thick, viscous, sticky white discharge that stains underwear and is often a source of dismay to the young girl. Around menarche and menopause, when estrogen levels are low, vaginal secretions are minimal. This decrease in mucous discharge also occurs in women who take oral contraceptives. This discharge will not vary from one week to the next. Low estrogen levels lead to thin, inactive mucosa that is more vulnerable to infection.

After menarche when ovulation is well-established, vaginal discharge varies according to the different hormones and their levels throughout the menstrual cycle. Immediately following the menstrual period, hormone levels are low and the vaginal mucosa is thin and inactive, leading to a minimal amount of cervical discharge. At ovulation when estrogen levels are at their highest, vaginal discharge is profuse, stretchy, shiny, and watery. Following ovulation when hormone levels drop again, secretions gradually diminish until just before the next menstrual period.

Women's reactions to discharge vary from lack of interest to extreme concern and anxiety. These reactions vary according to their knowledge and previous experiences together with societal, religious, and cultural beliefs (Fogel, 1998). Women must be helped to understand the normal functioning of their bodies, especially because vaginal discharge is one of the most common complaints of women seeking an office visit.

### Strategies for Self-Assessment

Genital self-examination is recommended for any woman who is at risk for contracting sexually transmitted infections (STI). This includes women who have had more than one sexual partner or whose partner has had other partners. The purpose of genital self-examination is to detect any signs or symptoms (e.g., vaginal discharge) that might indicate the presence of an infection.

Many women who have an STI do not know they have one, and some STIs can remain undetected for years while damaging a woman's health and fertility. Genital self-examination should become a regular part of routine self-care along with breast self-examination.

The benefits and process of genital self-examination  must be explained to a woman and then she must be helped to become comfortable with the process. Instruct her to start by examining her pubic hairs. She may need a mirror so that she can see the entire genital area. The pubic hair should be spread apart so she may look for bumps, sores, or blisters on the skin, which may be red or light-colored, raised or flat, look like pimples, or be a flat, shiny surface. Also instruct the woman to look for warts, which look similar to warts on other parts of her body. Next the woman should spread the vaginal lips and look closely at the hood of the clitoris. Pulling back the hood of the clitoris, she should again look for bumps, blisters, sores, or warts. Both sides of the inner vaginal lips should then also be examined.

Unless a woman is comfortable in using a clear, plastic speculum she will be unable to see the walls of her vagina and cervix. Ask whether she is interested in learning how to do this. Explain that the signs of STIs could also be located in those areas.

If she does not wish to examine herself internally, encourage her to return for an examination whenever she thinks she has been exposed to an STI, even though it is not visible.

The woman should also be aware of other symptoms associated with STIs (i.e., burning or pain on urination, itching or pain on the perineum or in the vagina, pain in the pelvic area, bleeding between menstrual periods, or vaginal discharge). By knowing what her "normal discharge" looks like, she will be better able to determine when she is experiencing an abnormal discharge from an infection. Discharge from an STI may be gray and watery, thick and yellow, green, or white and may have an odor. When the woman experiences one or more of these symptoms, she should seek help with further evaluation from a health care provider (Seidel and others, 1999).

Discharge that does not cause pruritis, odor, or burning is usually physiologic (a normal bodily process). Women are most likely to misinterpret midcycle discharge during the time of ovulation, believing that the obvious changes indicate that they have an infection every month that disappears then recurs.

Women who have been on oral contraceptives for a prolonged period of time and have experienced minimal discharge are often puzzled by the resumption of their physiologic discharge. Such concerns must be taken seriously and fully evaluated.

### Strategies for Self-Care

The normal vagina has a pH of between 3.8 and 4.2. A change in the pH of the vagina and an overgrowth of normally occurring organisms can create an increase in discharge and the possibility of infection.

Women vary in their vulnerability to vaginal infection. Estrogenized vaginal mucosa found during the reproductive years is not as vulnerable to organisms causing infection as mucosa with low levels of estrogen. Women also become increasingly vulnerable to infection if they lack adequate levels of antibodies to the bacteria normally found on the skin surrounding the vagina.

 Women can decrease their risk for infection with good perineal hygiene. Good general hygiene and clean underwear are the first line of defense against infection, along with the appropriate front-to-back wiping technique.

Other simple steps also enhance perineal health and decrease the incidence of vaginal infection. Wearing all-cotton underwear, or at least underwear that has a cotton crotch, increases the natural circulation of air. If pantyhose are to be worn, they should also have a cotton crotch to decrease the amount of moisture retained in that area. Perfumed tampons and/or sanitary napkins should be avoided. Douching is not necessary and may actually result in an increase in discharge, especially when products that contain dye or perfume are used. Women vulnerable to infection may find that using a hair dryer on the low setting to dry the perineum after a shower is helpful. They should avoid perfumed soaps, lotions, perineal sprays, laundry detergent, and fabric softener.

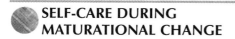

## SELF-CARE DURING MATURATIONAL CHANGE

### Menarche and Menstruation

**Menarche** is defined as the first menstrual period and occurs somewhere between 9.1 and 17.7 years, with a mean age of 12.8 years. Age at menarche has been dropping since the nineteenth century, primarily because of improved nutrition. Sexual maturation occurs earlier in taller and heavier girls (Herman-Giddons and others, 1997). Menarche occurs earlier in girls living in developed nations and later in those living in underdeveloped nations. Age of menarche also varies between ethnic groups. Mexican-Americans develop secondary sex characteristics at an older age (Seidel and others, 1999). One study reported that black girls exhibit an earlier onset of breast and pubic hair development than whites (Herman-Giddons and others, 1997).

The age at which a girl experiences menarche correlates with the age of menarche of her mother and sisters. The timing of menarche is related to the growth of the girl as she must obtain either a critical body mass (i.e., 47.8 kg or 105.16 lbs) or an increase in the percentage of body fat from 16% to 23.5%. The primary factor that allows menarche to occur is the production of estrogen by the ovaries (Woods, 1995).

During the first year of menses, menstrual periods may be very irregular. A regular, predictable pattern does not usually develop until 3 to 4 years after the onset of menstruation. The organs that produce the estrogen and progesterone for a hormonal cycle with ovulation, followed by the menses, require time to mature.

Menarche is one of the physical changes that occurs with puberty. **Puberty** is defined as the period of becoming capable of reproducing and involves maturation of the sexual organs, development of secondary sex characteristics, and menarche. There are several theories describing the trigger for puberty, but none have been substantiated. During early childhood, levels of the hormones GnRH from the hypothalamus and FSH and LH from the pituitary gland are suppressed. With the onset of the process of puberty, the pituitary becomes more sensitive to the influence of GnRH, and the ovaries respond to FSH and LH with the production of estrogen and the development of follicles.

The progression of puberty is predictable, beginning with an increased rate of growth. Breast development (i.e., thelarche) follows the beginning of this growth spurt, with the appearance of breast buds containing a small amount of glandular tissue and an areola. The breasts gradually increase in size as the amount of glandular tissue increases, until the adult contour is reached. The appearance of pubic hair (i.e., adrenarche) occurs after breast budding, with axillary hair occurring about 2 years later. The female growth spurt peaks about 2 years after the development of breast buds. Menarche follows the growth peak in about a year.

### The Female Reproductive Cycle

The **female reproductive cycle (FRC)** is a complex set of events involving the simultaneous occurrence of the ovarian cycle, during which ovulation occurs, and the menstrual cycle, during which menstruation occurs (Figure 5-9). The purpose of the cycle is to achieve pregnancy and if that does not happen, to prepare again. The regularity of a woman's menstrual cycle is influenced by her age, her physical and psychologic health, and factors within her environment.

Menses is the final phase of the menstrual cycle and the end of the female reproductive cycle. Because it is the only external marker of the occurrence of the cycle, however, the first day of the menstrual flow is used to mark the beginning of a new menstrual cycle (the **menstrual phase** comprises days 1 through 5 of the FRC). **Menstruation** is the periodic uterine bleeding that occurs approximately 14 days after ovulation when pregnancy does not occur. This bleeding is composed of blood from the ruptured capillaries, mucin from the glands, and the functional layer of the endometrium that would have supported an implanted ovum if pregnancy

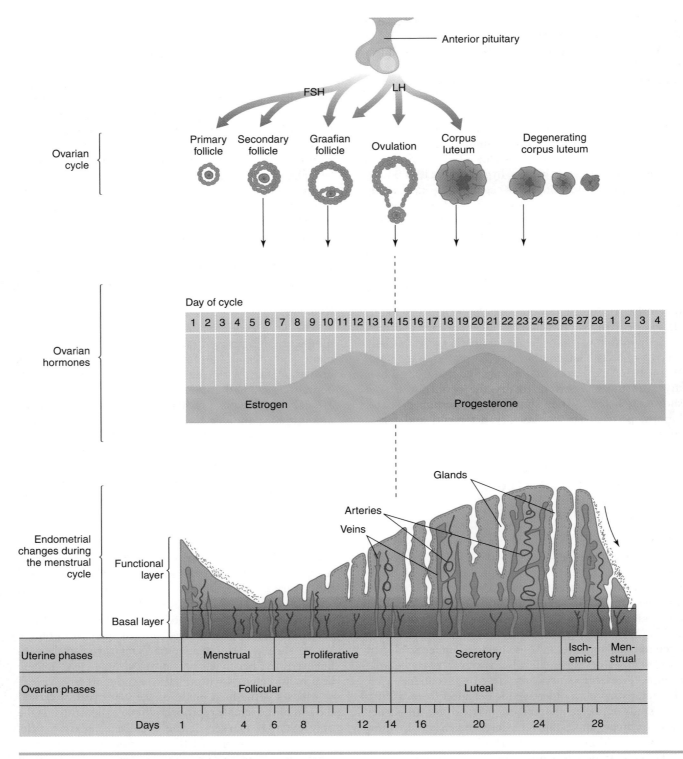

FIGURE 5-9 • Female reproductive cycle. (Adapted from Olds: Maternal newborn nursing care, ed 5, Menlo Park, 1996, Addison Wesley Longman.)

had occurred. During menstruation, estrogen and progesterone levels are low and the cervical mucus is viscous and opaque.

Immediately after the menstrual flow, the woman's body prepares for pregnancy again with the **proliferative phase** (i.e., days 6 to 14). As an ovary begins to form estrogen, the endometrium and myometrium proliferate and thicken. Estrogen levels peak just before ovulation, and the woman's **basal body temperature** drops. On day 14 when ovulation occurs, her basal body temperature increases 0.3° to 0.6° C. Her cervical mucus is clear, thin, and watery and, when stretched between fingers, will demonstrate elasticity (i.e., **spinnbarkheit**). The woman may also experience momentary sharp pains (i.e., **mittelschmerz**) and/or midcycle bleeding.

During the **secretory phase** (i.e., days 15 to 26), estrogen drops sharply and progesterone increases. The uterine endometrium is fully mature, with maximum amounts of blood and glandular tissue providing a luxuriant bed into which a fertilized egg might implant.

If fertilization does not occur, levels of estrogen and progesterone fall, causing the spiral arteries to undergo vasoconstriction. This begins the **ischemic phase** (i.e., days 27 to 28), as the blood supply is cut off and the endometrium becomes necrotic and prepares to slough. The menstrual phase then begins again.

A woman's cycle may be longer or shorter than the FRC just described and still be normal for her. The one constant, whether a woman's FRC is 28 days or 120 days, is that **ovulation takes place 14 days before menstruation.**

## Attitudes about Menstruation

"Cultural, religious, and personal attitudes about menstruation are a part of our menstrual experience and often reflect negative attitudes towards women" (Boston Women's Health Book Collective, 1999). How a woman first learns about menstruation, is prepared for it, or is treated when it occurs will influence her attitude toward it.

In some cultures, women who were menstruating have been considered unclean or in possession of supernatural powers and were therefore limited in their contacts or isolated. Sexual contact during menstruation was, and in many cultures still is, prohibited. Some cultures have menstruating woman go to a central location to be only with other menstruating women, and they are allowed to return to the community after purification rituals once menstruation has ceased (Garrett, 1997). Many women do not consider this a hardship because it gives them relief from the work of the home and provides the company of other women for 5 days.

More common taboos that you may hear in our culture are that a woman should refrain from washing her hair, exercising, showering, and having sexual intercourse during menstruation. It may be expected that a woman keep it a secret when she is menstruating and not refer to the process directly but instead use phrases such as "I have my friend."

In the belief that women are unstable or less capable because of their menstrual cycle, some people deny women certain jobs or treat them as inferior. Both women and men experience mood swings, but for women the mood swings they may experience during the menstrual cycle are predictable, not a sign of instability. Studies have documented that women lose little time from work due to menstrual problems and experience no measurable difference in their thinking capabilities or ability to perform tasks (Boston Women's Health Book Collective, 1999).

## Women's Experiences with Menstruation

Menstruation is a normal, healthy occurrence. Women are different in the way they experience it, and each woman may experience it differently during different times in her life. There are a variety of physical symptoms that may be experienced during different parts of the cycle. We do not know why some women have difficulty and some do not. We also do not know why certain remedies work for some women and others do not.

### Premenstrual Syndrome (PMS)

Some women experience what is termed premenstrual syndrome (PMS), which is a physical condition characterized by a wide range of symptoms that may occur from ovulation to menstruation or at least a period of days before menstruation. These symptoms are resolved with menstruation. "Practically every woman experiences at least one symptom, once in her life. Specific symptoms vary from one woman to another. Although some adolescents suffer from PMS, most women first develop the symptoms during their twenties" (Alternative Remedies for Common Ailments, 1998).

### Strategies for Self-Assessment

The symptoms recur during the same phase of the menstrual cycle each time, usually from 7 to 10 days before menses, and may include any of the following. Breast swelling and tenderness may be caused by increased levels of estrogen. Bloating and fluid retention are common, with the woman gaining as much as 5 pounds. Constipation, followed by diarrhea, may be experienced because of the levels of the hormones progesterone and prostaglandin. Acne, cold sores, and herpes outbreaks may occur. Moodiness, anxiety, depression or irritability; nausea or food cravings; insomnia; drowsiness; or fatigue may also be experienced. The hormone prostaglandin can cause backache and uterine cramping with menses. Use of a premenstrual symptom chart can help a woman track her symptoms (Figure 5-10). Some women are never bothered by these symptoms, and other women find them difficult to manage.

### Strategies for Self-Care

Adequate rest and sleep, stress management, a healthy diet, and regular exercise are useful ways to start providing symptom relief. Remedies may be either hormonal or nutritional, along with lifestyle changes and complementary therapies. Other self-care options in-

**Month**_____

**Severity scale:**
- ☐ = Symptom not present (blank square)
- L = Low severity, not bothersome
- M = Moderately severe, able to cope
- V = Very severe, interferes with activities
- X = Days of menstrual flow

| | 1 | 2 | 3 | 4 | 5 | 6 | 7 | 8 | 9 | 10 | 11 | 12 | 13 | 14 | 15 | 16 | 17 | 18 | 19 | 20 | 21 | 22 | 23 | 24 | 25 | 26 | 27 | 28 | 29 | 30 | 31 |
|---|---|---|---|---|---|---|---|---|---|---|---|---|---|---|---|---|---|---|---|---|---|---|---|---|---|---|---|---|---|---|---|
| Menses | | | | | | | | | | | | | | | | | | | | | | | | | | | | | | | |
| Bloating | | | | | | | | | | | | | | | | | | | | | | | | | | | | | | | |
| Cramps | | | | | | | | | | | | | | | | | | | | | | | | | | | | | | | |
| Acne | | | | | | | | | | | | | | | | | | | | | | | | | | | | | | | |
| Swelling/water retention | | | | | | | | | | | | | | | | | | | | | | | | | | | | | | | |
| Weight gain | | | | | | | | | | | | | | | | | | | | | | | | | | | | | | | |
| Breast tenderness | | | | | | | | | | | | | | | | | | | | | | | | | | | | | | | |
| Joint aches | | | | | | | | | | | | | | | | | | | | | | | | | | | | | | | |
| Headaches | | | | | | | | | | | | | | | | | | | | | | | | | | | | | | | |
| Nausea/vomiting | | | | | | | | | | | | | | | | | | | | | | | | | | | | | | | |
| Loss of appetite | | | | | | | | | | | | | | | | | | | | | | | | | | | | | | | |
| Fatigue | | | | | | | | | | | | | | | | | | | | | | | | | | | | | | | |
| Decreased coordination | | | | | | | | | | | | | | | | | | | | | | | | | | | | | | | |
| Change in urination | | | | | | | | | | | | | | | | | | | | | | | | | | | | | | | |
| Trouble sleeping | | | | | | | | | | | | | | | | | | | | | | | | | | | | | | | |
| Dizziness/faintness | | | | | | | | | | | | | | | | | | | | | | | | | | | | | | | |
| Irritability | | | | | | | | | | | | | | | | | | | | | | | | | | | | | | | |
| Anxiety | | | | | | | | | | | | | | | | | | | | | | | | | | | | | | | |
| Sleeping more | | | | | | | | | | | | | | | | | | | | | | | | | | | | | | | |
| Jittery/restless | | | | | | | | | | | | | | | | | | | | | | | | | | | | | | | |
| Accident prone | | | | | | | | | | | | | | | | | | | | | | | | | | | | | | | |
| Overwhelmed by daily demands | | | | | | | | | | | | | | | | | | | | | | | | | | | | | | | |
| Flare-up of allergies | | | | | | | | | | | | | | | | | | | | | | | | | | | | | | | |
| Depression | | | | | | | | | | | | | | | | | | | | | | | | | | | | | | | |
| Insecurity | | | | | | | | | | | | | | | | | | | | | | | | | | | | | | | |
| Suicidal thoughts | | | | | | | | | | | | | | | | | | | | | | | | | | | | | | | |
| Forgetfulness | | | | | | | | | | | | | | | | | | | | | | | | | | | | | | | |
| Want to stay at home | | | | | | | | | | | | | | | | | | | | | | | | | | | | | | | |
| Impatience | | | | | | | | | | | | | | | | | | | | | | | | | | | | | | | |
| Overtalkative | | | | | | | | | | | | | | | | | | | | | | | | | | | | | | | |
| Decreased self-esteem | | | | | | | | | | | | | | | | | | | | | | | | | | | | | | | |
| Change in interest in sex | | | | | | | | | | | | | | | | | | | | | | | | | | | | | | | |
| Want to be alone | | | | | | | | | | | | | | | | | | | | | | | | | | | | | | | |
| Miss work because of symptoms | | | | | | | | | | | | | | | | | | | | | | | | | | | | | | | |
| Other symptoms not on list: | | | | | | | | | | | | | | | | | | | | | | | | | | | | | | | |
| 1. | | | | | | | | | | | | | | | | | | | | | | | | | | | | | | | |
| 2. | | | | | | | | | | | | | | | | | | | | | | | | | | | | | | | |
| 3. | | | | | | | | | | | | | | | | | | | | | | | | | | | | | | | |
| 4. | | | | | | | | | | | | | | | | | | | | | | | | | | | | | | | |

FIGURE 5-10 • Premenstrual symptom chart.

clude aromatherapy for anxiety, irritability, and breast tenderness; a wide variety of herbal therapies to alleviate many of the symptoms; and mind/body medicine with yoga and meditation. To be successful, it may take trying several different remedies or a combination of remedies.

### Dysmenorrhea

**Dysmenorrhea,** painful menstruation, may occur before or at the onset of the menstrual period. A woman may experience the pain due to either primary or secondary dysmenorrhea. **Primary dysmenorrhea** is caused by a physiologic alteration, the excessive release of prostaglandins. This hormone increases the amplitude and frequency of the uterine contractions, causing severe lower abdominal cramps. The woman may also experience backache, weakness, sweats, gastrointestinal symptoms (e.g., anorexia, nausea, vomiting, and diarrhea) and central nervous system symptoms (e.g., dizziness, syncope, headache, and poor concentration). Primary dysmenorrhea is most common in women in their teens and early twenties. It usually first appears 6 to 12 months after menarche, when the process of ovulation becomes established during the woman's menstrual cycle.

**Secondary dysmenorrhea** is menstrual pain that is typically experienced after age 25 years. The pain is often a dull lower abdominal aching that radiates to the woman's back or thighs. She may also have a feeling of bloating or pelvic fullness. Secondary dysmenorrhea is associated with pelvic disorders such as adenomyosis, endometriosis, pelvic inflammatory disease, endometrial polyps, fibroids, or the use of an intrauterine device (IUD).

### Strategies for Self-Care

Self-care depends on the severity of the problem and on the woman's response to various interventions. Because the uterus is a muscle, relaxation exercises help, as may massage, biofeedback, or acupuncture. Heat, either from a heating pad or a hot bath, reduces cramping by increasing vasodilation and muscle relaxation. Massage of the lower back can reduce pain by relaxing paravertebral muscles and increasing the pelvic blood supply. Yoga and meditation also may be used to decrease menstrual discomfort. Exercise lessens the sensation of pain by stimulating muscles to release endorphins and increasing vasodilation of the uterus.

Dietary changes such as decreasing salt and sugar intake may reduce fluid retention. Natural diuretics (e.g., asparagus, cranberry juice, orange juice, peaches, parsley, or water) may reduce the edema. Some women also find it helpful to change from a high- to a low-fat diet.

The uterine cramping of primary dysmenorrhea may also respond to nonsteroidal antiinflammatory medications (NSAIDs), such as aspirin, fenoprofen, ibuprofen, indomethacin, mofenamic acid, or naproxen sodium, which are available over the counter. For women who need additional assistance, prescription strength medication is sometimes necessary. Oral contraception may be used to artificially regulate a woman's hormones and suppress ovulation when symptoms significantly interfere with normal functioning. Further treatment for secondary dysmenorrhea may require the assistance of a specialist and the removal of the underlying pathologic problem.

### Amenorrhea

**Amenorrhea** is the absence of menses and may be caused by hormonal or physical changes. **Primary amenorrhea** is the term used to describe the absence of menarche and secondary sexual characteristics by age 14 years or the absence of menses by the latest age it usually occurs, age 18. **Secondary amenorrhea** is the cessation of menstruation after at least one menses. The most common causes are pregnancy, menopause, breast feeding, dieting that leads to too little body fat, and use of oral contraceptives.

### Strategies for Self-Assessment

When all of her friends have experienced a menstrual period but a young woman has not, she will probably start to wonder what is wrong with her. She may feel distressed, perhaps thinking she is not a real woman. Her concerns may lead her to seek help from a professional. Although amenorrhea is not a disease, it may indicate a congenital defect, hormonal imbalance, cysts or tumors, an endocrine disorder, or severe stress in her life. She may also be participating in an extreme dieting program or athletic training. Secondary amenorrhea usually leads a heterosexually active woman to seek a pregnancy test as her first level of assessment.

### Strategies for Self-Care

If a woman is experiencing amenorrhea due to dieting, anorexia nervosa, or athletic training, she may not be as concerned about not having a menstrual cycle as she is about meeting her dieting or training goals. When the lack of menses becomes a concern to her or she comes to an understanding that what she is experiencing indicates a possible problem within her body, the woman will seek consultation with a health care provider.

Her anxiety level may be high and her ego may be  fragile, but a sensitive health care provider can conduct a history and physical and pregnancy test to begin to discover the cause. Remember that a woman ovulates before she menstruates, so a teenager who has never had a menstrual period can become pregnant yet exhibit the signs of primary amenorrhea.

## Menopause

**Menopause** is defined by the World Health Organization (WHO) as the cessation of menses for a 12-month period due to changes in estrogen production. The period of time around the menopause (i.e., last menstrual cycle) is labeled the **perimenopausal period,** or the climacteric. The perimenopausal period includes the 2 to 8 years prior to the cessation of menses. The **postmenopausal** period is the time after menopause, including the first 12 months of amenorrhea (WHO, 1981). The perimenopausal period is similar to, but the reverse of, the period of time surrounding menarche and the 6 to 12 months afterward, during which an adolescent's body adjusts to the hormonal changes and moves from an anovulatory cycle (without ovulation) to the establishment of an ovulatory cycle.

Menopause generally occurs around the median age of 51 but may happen at any time between ages 40 and 60 (Boston Women's Health Book Collective, 1999; Speroff, Glass, and Kase, 1994). There is no evidence that the age of menopause has changed over the centuries. Race or parity also do not seem to affect the timing of menopause, but lack of adequate nutrition, smoking, and living at high altitudes may contribute to an earlier menopause. There is also no relationship between the time of onset of menarche and menopause (Achilles and Leppert, 1997).

Menopause results from changes in the functioning of the ovary and a decrease in estrogen levels. The ovaries, adrenal glands, and fatty tissues of the body continue to be sources of small amounts of estrogen for at least 10 years after menstrual periods cease.

 Follicular atresia, the degeneration and resorption of an ovarian follicle before it matures and ruptures, occurs from the age of puberty on. As a woman grows older, follicular atresia becomes a more frequent occurrence, so that after the age of 35 a gradual decline in the production of estrogen by the ovaries begins. As a woman grows older, serum levels of 40 IU/l of estrogen demonstrate that menopause is near (Woods, 1995). In response to the decline in production by the ovaries, the adrenal glands gradually increase production of estrogen by converting a secretion called androstenadione into estrone (i.e., a nonovarian type of estrogen) (Boston Women's Health Book Collective, 1999).

If the woman's lifelong habits of diet and exercise have been poor, the decrease in estrogen may place her at increased risk for osteoporosis and cardiovascular diseases (e.g., artherosclerosis). The decrease in levels of estrogen affects the way the bones absorb calcium and can raise cholesterol levels in the blood.

### Strategies for Self-Assessment

"Although medical and popular literature often discuss numerous menopause 'symptoms,' only three signs can be directly attributed to changes in estrogen production: (1) changes in menstrual cycle, (2) hot flashes and sweats (vasomotor instability), and (3) vaginal changes (decrease of moisture and elasticity in the vagina)" (Boston Women's Health Book Collective, 1999). Some women are bothered greatly by these changes during the perimenopausal period, but other women have few or no signs.

Before the cessation of menses, the characteristics of the menstrual period change. During the perimenopausal period, both short cycles (due to short follicular phases) and long cycles (due to inadequate luteal phases, or anovulation) can occur. As the cycles become more irregular, bleeding may occur at the end of a short follicular phase or after a peak of estradiol in an anovulatory cycle. Menses may be lighter due to less hormonal effect on the endometrium, or may be heavier due to the effect of multiple cycles on the endometrium—causing proliferation, without the secretory effect of progesterone.

Hot flashes and night sweats are caused by vasomotor instability due to a lack of estrogen. Hot flashes begin with a sensation of warmth spreading from the trunk to the face. The skin may redden, and sweating may occur. Flushes typically last several minutes and may occur either rarely or with significant frequency during the day. When hot flashes occur at night, they are followed by night sweats, which can awaken a woman and may interfere with her patterns of sleep, and cause insomnia. Hot flashes and night sweats are temporary and will pass as the body adjusts to less estrogen; however, this may take months.

Vaginal changes also occur in some women at this time. "Thinning of the vaginal walls, loss of elasticity, flattening out of ridges, foreshortening or narrowing of the vagina, and especially dryness or itching (**pruritis**) may make intercourse less comfortable or even painful (**dyspareunia**). These conditions may lead to irritation and increased susceptibility to infection. It is unclear whether these vaginal changes are caused by the decreasing estrogen levels of menopause or simply aging. Some women never have this problem" (Boston Women's Health Book Collective, 1999).

Other changes may also occur during the time of the perimenopausal period. It is difficult to know what is related to hormonal fluctuations and what is related to the events of aging. Some women associate anxiety, depression, increased tension, and short-term memory loss with the perimenopausal period. Urinary problems (e.g., urgency, cystitis, and urethritis) may also occur (Woods, 1995; Achilles and Leppert, 1997; Stewart, 1998).

### Strategies for Self-Care

Before strategies for self-care can begin, an understanding of what a woman generally believes menopause to be and how she thinks it will affect her specifically must be explored. Stereotypical thinking and myths about menopause are pervasive in our society and may cause the woman to have a negative approach to herself and the process. Just like menarche, menopause is an important physical and emotional life transition. With support and information, a woman may be empowered to make the choices that support her and maintain her physical and emotional comfort.

Although many women experience menopausal signs, most are able to handle the changes with nonmedical alternatives. Self-care during the perimenopausal period focuses on general positive lifestyle choices such as adequate rest and sleep, proper nutrition, vitamin supplementation, herbal therapy, stress management, and regular exercise. Many of these interventions will have a positive effect on more than one aspect of the perimenopausal period. When a woman can make these holistic changes, she may experience a variety of benefits.

### Menstrual Changes

 Changes in the menstrual cycle may lead to irregular spacing of periods and a lighter or heavier menstrual flow. Women have found that it is best to be prepared and carry tampons and/or pads with them at all times until they have been a year without a period. The heavy cramping that may occur during some cycles will respond to the interventions suggested for dysmenorrhea. The increased intake of foods containing carotene and some herbal teas may be helpful in reducing heavy menstrual bleeding.

### Hot Flashes and Night Sweats

The discomforts of hot flashes and night sweats are alleviated by using a fan, drinking cold liquids, or applying cold compresses. A variety of herbs and foods containing plant estrogens may help relieve symptoms. Plant estrogens are available in foods such as soybeans, lima beans, sweet potatoes, tofu, and the herb black cohosh.  Herbal combinations such as chaste tree, motherwort, and wild yam, may also reduce the frequency and level of discomfort. A daily intake of 400 to 800 IU of vitamin E will help alleviate the hot flashes and reduce the risk for cardiovascular disease (Alternative Remedies for Common Ailments, 1998). Avoiding personal triggers for flushing (e.g., hot drinks, caffeine, alcohol, and spicy foods) may also decrease the frequency of hot flashes.

### Vaginal Changes

Some women find that interest in sexual activity improves when they no longer need contraception. (Note that a woman is considered at risk for pregnancy until she has had 12 months without a menstrual cycle, so contraception should be used until then.) The decrease of moisture in the vagina can be overcome with saliva, vegetable oil, vaginal lubricants, or estrogen creams. Sexual arousal, masturbation, and intercourse will maintain a comfortable level of lubrication. The muscle tone of the vagina will also be helped by sexual activity, masturbation, and Kegel exercises (i.e., exercises of the pelvic floor).

### Other Self-Care Options

To decrease the risk for osteoporosis, the woman should engage in weight-bearing exercise (e.g., walking) and increase her intake of calcium and magnesium. Premenopausal and perimenopausal women require 1000 to 1200 mg of calcium per day. Postmenopausal women who are not taking hormone replacement therapy need 1500 mg of calcium per day, while women on hormone-replacement therapy require 1200 mg of calcium daily. As much calcium as possible should come from dietary sources, with supplements added as necessary.

To reduce the risk for cardiovascular disease, the woman can follow the same suggestions for all people at risk for cardiac disease. She can exercise, eat a low-fat diet, maintain a healthy body weight, take vitamin E supplements, and get an annual physical that includes a lipid assessment.

Relaxation and stress reduction may be aided with meditation, massage, yoga, and music or herbal therapy. Tension aches and pains may be reduced through chiropractic care or acupuncture. Frequent urination and insomnia may be helped by acupressure, aromatherapy, and herbal therapy.

### Annual Health Examinations

A woman who is no longer menstruating should still be encouraged to seek annual physical examinations. Routine health care for women in the menopausal period should include a complete health assessment, including a pap smear, lipid assessment, colorectal cancer screening (i.e., including stool for occult blood and colonoscopy), a dexa scan for the presence of osteopenia or osteoporosis, mammography, and selective screening for diabetes (Weber, 1997).

### Hormone Therapy

When a woman finds that the symptoms of menopause are interfering with her activities of daily living, she may seek further assistance. Hormone therapy may be useful in restoring a perimenopausal woman's quality of life. Hormone replacement therapy (HRT) may be provided with estrogen, progestin, and/or testosterone administered orally, transdermally, or vaginally. However, HRT is not an option for women with undiagnosed vaginal bleeding, a history of vascular thrombolitic episodes, active thrombophlebitis or thromboembolic disorder, active liver disease, and known or suspected estrogen-dependent carcinomas. Hormone therapy is available, with cautious consideration, to women who are heavy smokers, are obese, or have diabetes; active gallbladder disease; a uterine leiomyomata; peripheral vascular thrombosis or a history of thrombophlebitis, thrombosis, or thromboembolic episodes related to estrogen use; or a family history of breast cancer. The woman and her provider must weigh her risks and benefits of hormone therapy by considering her risks for osteoporosis and heart disease and the presence of indications of benefit to her (Hawkins, Roberto-Nichols, and Stanley-Haney, 2000).

***Therapeutic Regimens.*** There are many estrogen and progesterone products on the market for hormone-replacement therapy. Unless a woman has had a hysterectomy (i.e., removal of the uterus), she will take a combination of progesterone and estrogen. With cyclic therapy the estrogen is taken alone for the first 13 days of the month, and progesterone and estrogen are taken together for the last 12 days. This treatment option will result in monthly withdrawal bleeding in most women. Continuous therapy is provided if the woman no longer wants to experience a monthly "period." Both estrogen and progesterone are taken daily. Side effects may include breast tenderness, bloating, and uterine cramping, but most of these disappear with alterations in therapeutic regimen (Stewart, 1998) (Table 5-3). Estrogen may also be absorbed from a patch. If the woman still has a uterus, oral progestin is taken either continuously or 12 days per month.

The hormone progesterone provides the woman a degree of protection against endometrial cancer. It is also used to manage heavy irregular bleeding. Low-dose birth control pills are particularly effective at relieving

**TABLE 5-3** *Estrogen and Progesterone Therapy, Daily Regimen*

| | |
|---|---|
| Estrogen | 0.625 mg conjugated estrogen or |
| | 1 mg micronized estradiol or |
| | 0.625 mg estrone sulfate |
| Progestin | 2.5 mg medroxyprogesterone acetate or |
| | 0.35 mg norethindrone or |
| | 100 mg micronized progesterone |

From Speroff L and others: *Clinical gynecologic endocrinology and infertility*, ed 5, Baltimore, 1994, Williams & Wilkins.

symptoms of menopause because they provide a substitute for the decline in the body's estrogen production. Birth control pills have the additional benefit of supplying needed contraception because women in the perimenopausal period can still conceive. Combined oral contraceptives can be used safely through menopause in healthy women who do not smoke.

Estrogen decreases the incidence of cardiovascular disease by 56% (Achilles and Leppert, 1997), lowers fibrinogen levels, and decreases lipoproteins. Estrogen prevents bone loss and relieves the symptoms of estrogen deficiency (e.g., hot flashes, sleep disturbances, and urovaginal atrophy). The most clearly documented disadvantage of estrogen therapy is the higher than usual incidence of endometrial cancer, but this consequence can be decreased by adding progesterone to the estrogen taken by postmenopausal women (Speroff, Glass, and Kase, 1994). The understanding of estrogen's relationship to breast cancer is less clear. Multiple studies have been conducted with conflicting results. Major metaanalyses have also shown conflicting results, although several have found a slight increased risk for breast cancer in current estrogen users (Colditz, Egan, and Stampfer, 1993). Women taking estrogen replacement therapy should receive yearly clinical breast exams and mammograms and practice monthly breast self-examinations.

## SELF-CARE IN FERTILITY CONTROL

No single health care development has provided the means to directly alter women's health and lives as momentously as the development of effective methods of contraception. Fertility regulation is a conscious choice with which a sexually active, heterosexual, or bisexual woman can positively affect her physical, educational, economic, and social destiny. When a woman can control her fertility, she has the opportunity to plan her life as she chooses, limiting the size of her family or preventing pregnancy from occurring. The high rate of unintended pregnancies among today's women, however, indicates the complexity of the factors that a woman

must successfully address and the underlying difficulties that may occur (Matteson, 1995).

The primary factor influencing the ability of a woman to consistently use a method of contraception is the ability to integrate the chosen regimen into her life without disrupting her major roles and responsibilities. For a sexually active woman who is at risk for pregnancy, choosing to take action to control her fertility becomes a self-care decision that she must make over and over again. This decision is comprised of five sequential categories that have a degree of overlap and create a circular process of self-assessment and decisions followed by evaluation (Figure 5-11).

The initial stage, **personalizing pregnancy risk**, reflects a self-assessment that the woman is able to become pregnant, and that if she chooses, she has the ability to prevent it. The risk may be made real to her when she has a period that is late or a friend becomes pregnant.

During the second step, **exploring options**, a woman learns about methods of contraception from her partners, friends, sisters, and health care providers. What others say about methods will influence her choices either negatively or positively. The woman will also consider what effect the use of contraception will have on her self-esteem and physical health, as well as on her relationship with her family and current partners. Other factors she will consider are the convenience in obtaining and using the method, the expense and efficacy of the method, safety, and possible cultural or religious constraints. By process of elimination, she will select the method that is least objectionable to her.

The third step, **using an option**, is the next decision. Just because a woman has a method of contraception does not mean that she will feel comfortable when she actually has to use it. The decision to use any self-care method (i.e., excluding an IUD, Norplant, and sterilization) allows the woman to constantly reevaluate her choice and make a change if she does not like it or it is uncomfortable. In general, a fertility control method that requires a woman to take specific actions before intercourse is not as efficient as a method that does not require any specific activities immediately before intercourse.

Once a method is used, the woman enters the fourth step of the cycle, **contending with the ramifications and/or efficacy of use**. Women want to know that a method will actually work for them and prevent an unintended pregnancy. As a woman assesses her protection from a possible pregnancy against the actual way the contraceptive process makes her feel, she decides whether to use it again, decrease the frequency of use, stop use, or reconsider her actual risk for pregnancy and start the decisional cycle all over again (Matteson, 1995).

Controlling one's fertility is a process as individualized as the women themselves, although certain aspects of the self-assessment and self-care process of decision making in fertility regulation are common to many women's experiences. Most women desire to control their fertility and prevent pregnancy for part—if not all—of their fertile years. When attempting to gain this control, they sometimes seek the help of a health care professional. We can be an excellent resource for women to help them learn about the methods available so that they can make an informed choice of a method that is right for them. We can help them obtain the method and learn to use it comfortably so that they may use it consistently. Women often require different methods at different points in their reproductive life span, and we can assist them through these changes (Trussel and Kowal, 1998).

## Assisting in Choice

When a woman consults with you about her contraceptive choice or is investigating changing to a new choice, there are several areas to be explored. If potential problems can be anticipated and resolved before they occur, her chance of success in preventing pregnancy is increased (Box 5-5).

## Expectations of Contraception

Women have questions and concerns about the methods they choose. Three of them are efficacy (i.e., how well it will work), safety (i.e., will it hurt either when I use it or with a future decision to have a child), and cost.

### Efficacy

**Efficacy** is the effectiveness of a given contraceptive method. The use of two methods together, except the male and female condom, greatly enhances the efficacy of contraception. The use of a male condom with most other methods of contraception has become increasingly popular not only for pregnancy prevention but also to reduce the risk for transmission of a sexually transmitted infection.

The most effective methods of contraception are female sterilization, oral contraceptive pills, male condoms, and male sterilization. These methods are also among the most popular methods reported (Abma and others, 1997).

Efficacy is commonly reported in two different categories: the percentage of women experiencing unintended pregnancy in the first year of using the method, and the percentage of women experiencing unintended pregnancy with continued use at 1 year (Table 5-4).

The first year figures are also divided into those women who were typical users of the method, meaning that they occasionally skipped the method, used it incorrectly, or not at all; and the expected effectiveness if the method is used perfectly, meaning that they always used the method and always used it correctly (Trussel and Kowal, 1998).

When helping a woman to determine if a contraceptive will work for her, it is important to remember that contraceptive failure is influenced by many factors

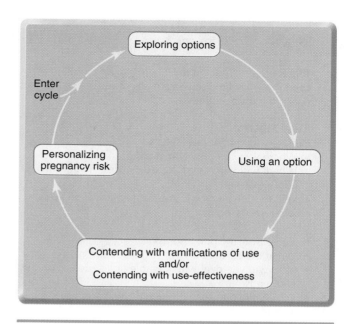

FIGURE 5-11 • Women's process of decisions in fertility regulation. *(From Matteson PS:* Advocating for self: women's decisions concerning contraceptions, *New York, 1995, Haworth Press.)*

(Trussel and Kowal, 1998). Some methods, like sterilization, Norplant, and the IUD, are very effective and are not subject to user error. They do not require the user to do anything to activate or enhance their effectiveness. Therefore pregnancy rates are very low for these methods of contraception. Other methods, such as the pill and Depo-provera injections, are inherently very effective but have a higher rate of user failure. Women can forget to take their pills or fail to return for injections, decreasing the effectiveness of these very effective methods. Periodic abstinence, spermacides, and barrier methods have a lower inherent efficacy than other contraceptive methods and are most vulnerable to sporadic use because they require significant ongoing actions by the user. When explaining the effectiveness of various methods to a woman, the most important point to emphasize is that the correct and consistent use of a method increases its effectiveness.

### Safety

Safety is another factor influencing the choice of contraceptive method. Women want to be safe from harm. Overall, contraception poses much less risk to a woman than if she experienced a pregnancy with related complications. Some methods, however, pose a risk to some users. Myocardial infarction and stroke occur more often in women who use oral contraceptives, especially if they are older than 35 and smoke. Oral contraceptives have protective effects against cancer of the endometrium and ovary, but risk

---

### BOX 5-5 *Assessment Guide to Assist with Choices*

These areas of concern must be explored to enhance success. They may be discussed in any order, but each area of concern must be addressed.

**AVAILABILITY**
Explore with the woman:
- Where will you obtain (method)?
- Where will you store it for easy access and/or for confidentiality?
- Will this location be convenient so it will be available when you need it?

If she is using the pill, also ask:
- When during the day will you take it?
- How will you deal with variable times such as on the weekends?
- What will you use with the pill when you have to take antibiotics?

**COST**
Explore with the woman:
- Do you know how much (method) costs?
- At what point might cost become a problem?
- What other methods do you have available if needed?

**SOCIAL SUPPORT**
Explore with the woman:
- Have any of your family or friends used (method)?
- What did they say about it? Will you tell them you are using it?

- Do your religious beliefs support the use of (method)?
- How does that make you feel?
- How does your partner feel about you using (method)?

**COMFORT LEVEL**
Explore with the woman:
- Do you have any concerns about possible side effects of (method)?
- What effects do you expect?
- How do you think using (method) will affect your sexual pleasure?
- How do you think it will affect your partner's pleasure?
- What will you do if (method) is uncomfortable when you use it?

**LEVEL OF CONVICTION**
Explore with the woman:
- What would happen in your life if you became pregnant?
- What would prompt you to use a back-up system?
- What will it be? Where will you get it?
- Do you anticipate any problems in your starting to use (method)?
- Is there any way that I may help so that it (the process of contraception) is easier for you?

Matteson PS: *Advocating for self: Women's decisions concerning contraception,* New York, 1995, Haworth Press.

---

for cervical cancer is increased in women who use oral contraceptives (Trussel and Kowal, 1998).

Protection of future fertility is also a safety issue for women using contraception. A major cause of infertility is sexually transmitted infections, which are not prevented by hormonal methods, sterilization, or intrauterine devices. Only mechanical methods and chemical barriers reduce the risk of transmission of sexually transmitted infections. Therefore a woman's choice of contraception is influenced by her assessment of risk for sexually transmitted infection. Women who wish to use a highly effective method *and* have protection from sexually transmitted infection will need to use two methods, a hormonal method and a condom, either male or female.

### Cost

Cost is another issue to consider when helping a woman select a method of contraception. Many third party payors do not cover contraception. Private insurers usually pay for sterilization but seldom pay for any other method. Women who receive services in the public sec-

tor are more likely to have contraception methods paid for, but the level of reimbursement for services is low and may limit the number of health care providers who will care for these women.

Of the methods that must be obtained from a health care provider, oral contraceptives cost between $15 and $40 per month while injectable contraception costs $30 per quarter plus the cost of an office visit. Implanted contraceptives and intrauterine devices may cost $400 to $500 dollars for the product and the process of insertion, but can be kept in place for several years without additional cost. When a woman wishes to have such devices removed, the cost is about $100. The diaphragm and the cap have the expense of the device plus the office visit for a fitting, between $50 and $75 and the ongoing expense of spermicidal jelly to use with the device (e.g., about $12 for 10 acts of intercourse).

Of the methods that can be obtained by the woman herself, spermicides and male condoms, the cost is approximately $1.00 each per use. Female condoms are about $3.00 each and can only be used once. The

## TABLE 5-4   *Efficacy of Contraceptive Methods in the First Year of Use*

| Method | % PREGNANT WITHIN THE FIRST YEAR | | % WOMEN CONTINUING METHOD BEYOND 1 YEAR |
| --- | --- | --- | --- |
| | Typical use | Perfect use | |
| Chance | 85 | 85 | |
| Spermicides | 26 | 6 | 40 |
| Periodic abstinence | 25 | 15 | 63 |
| Cap | | | |
|    Nulliparous | 20 | 9 | 56 |
|    Multiparous | 40 | 26 | 42 |
| Diaphragm | 20 | 6 | 56 |
| Withdrawal | 19 | 4 | |
| Condoms | | | |
|    Female | 21 | 5 | 56 |
|    Male | 14 | 3 | 61 |
| Pill | | | |
|    Progestin | | 0.5 | |
|    Combined | | 0.1 | |
| IUD | | | |
|    Progesterone T | 1.0 | 1.5 | 81 |
|    Copper T 380A | 0.8 | 0.6 | 78 |
|    Lng 20 | 0.1 | 0.1 | 81 |
| Depo-Provera | 0.3 | 0.3 | 70 |
| Norplant | 0.05 | 0.05 | 88 |
| Female sterilization | 0.5 | 0.5 | 100 |
| Male sterilization | 0.15 | 0.10 | 100 |

From Hatcher R. and others, editors: *Contraceptive technology*, ed 17, New York, 1998, Ardent Media.

method of periodic abstinence requires the one-time purchase of a basal body temperature thermometer for about $3.00. Withdrawal and the use of no method have no cost (Trussel and others, 1995).

Any discussion of the cost of contraception must be balanced with information about the cost of an unintended pregnancy. An unintended pregnancy is much more expensive than even the most expensive contraceptive methods, ranging from $1680 for care at a publicly funded agency to $5512 for the mother and $3107 for the baby in a managed-care environment (Trussel and others, 1995).

Not to be forgotten in the discussion of cost is the human cost of unintended pregnancy—especially for teens. Each unintended pregnancy creates the possibility that the mother or fetus will experience risks to their health and development during the pregnancy, creating individual and community, human and economic losses.

### Noncontraceptive Benefits

Knowledge of the noncontraceptive benefits of certain methods may help a woman's choice when selecting from several different methods. Fertility-awareness methods provide women with practical knowledge of their own physiology and can later be used to help plan an intended pregnancy. Barrier methods, especially condoms, provide protection from sexually transmitted infections—including HIV. Although more expensive and less readily available, female condoms provide more protection than male condoms. Progestin-releasing intrauterine devices reduce the bleeding and pain of menses (Trussel and Kowal, 1998). Oral contraceptives offer protection from ovarian and endometrial cancer, reduce the occurrence of ovarian and breast cysts, decrease premenstrual symptoms, and reduce the monthly experience of cramping and bleeding. Oral contraceptives are also beneficial in controlling some of the symptoms of the perimenopausal period (Harlap, Kost, and Forrest, 1991).

### Understanding the Choices

The choice of a contraceptive method at any given time in a woman's life is a very personal decision. Many factors, including if she also needs protection from infective diseases, must be considered.

If it is very important to a woman that she not conceive, one of the more effective methods should be selected. On the other hand, if a woman does not mind becoming pregnant but just wishes to delay the process, she can choose one of the less effective methods. Women who are unable or unwilling to touch their own bodies will not be comfortable with barrier methods.

Women whose religious beliefs prohibit the use of artificial means will only be able to consider natural family planning methods. If a woman's partner opposes contraception, methods that cannot be detected should be selected, although these will not protect her from sexually transmitted infections. The most important consideration is that the woman selects a method that makes her comfortable and confident, so that consistent accurate use of the method is most likely to occur.

### Abstinence

The most effective method of contraception and prevention of sexually transmitted infections is **abstinence.** Definitions of abstinence range from no sexual contact at all to complete sexual contact except penile-vaginal intercourse. In order to communicate effectively with clients choosing abstinence, we need to know their individual definition of abstinence. Abstinence may be a difficult method for a partner to accept. When a woman chooses abstinence, we may need to help her develop communication and negotiation skills that will allow her to be successful. Open dialogue between partners before developing the expectation of sexual contact is helpful. Planning in advance what activities are and are not acceptable, then communicating these decisions to a partner helps avoid misunderstanding and the pressure to proceed. Helping women learn to say "no" effectively may be the most important skill to develop. Supporting, encouraging, and respecting a woman's choice of abstinence is part of our role as a health care provider.

### Postcoital Contraception

**Postcoital contraception,** also called emergency contraception or "the morning after pill," is available when unintended, unexpected, or unprotected intercourse has occurred, or the contraceptive method used has failed. It is a phamocologic or mechanical intervention that inhibits fertilization or implantation. The pharmacologic agents are hormones in the form of a high-dose, short-term therapy of estrogen, progesterone, or testosterone. The mechanical agent is an intrauterine device. Postcoital methods should only be used if the woman would terminate the pregnancy if it were to occur because the process is not 100% effective and may leave a developing fetus with abnormalities.

Many women have access to oral contraception and will use emergency contraception as a method of self-care. The process most commonly used is multiple oral contraceptive pills taken within 72 hours of intercourse with a second dose of multiple pills taken again 12 hours later. The number of pills taken depends on the type of oral contraception used (Box 5-6).

This method reduces unintended pregnancy by at least 74% and has no medical contraindications to use (Van Look and Stewart, 1998). Recommend that the woman take the oral contraceptives with an antinausea medication because the ingestion of high doses of hormones may lead to nausea and vomiting. The Yuzpe regimen uses the combination type of oral contraceptive to prevent pregnancy by disrupting or delaying ovulation; if ovulation has already occurred, the oral contraceptives will have no effect on the pregnancy.

Other options for emergency contraception include the progestin-only "mini" pills taken within 48 to 72 hours or the insertion of a copper-releasing intrauterine device up to 5 days after intercourse. The progestin-only pills have the advantage of causing less nausea and vomiting than combined pills, but many pills are required for

---

## BOX 5-6    *Emergency Contraception*

**YUZPE REGIMEN**

Ethinyl estradiol 50 $\mu$g and levonorgestrel 250 $\mu$g pills taken within 72 hours after unprotected intercourse
- First dose as soon as possible
- Second dose *must* be taken 12 hours later

| If you use: | Take: |
|---|---|
| Ovral | 2 white pills + 2 white pills |
| Preven | 2 light blue pills + 2 light blue pills |
| | |
| Levlen | 4 light orange pills + 4 light orange pills |
| Levora | 4 white pills + 4 white pills |
| Lo-Ovral | 4 white pills + 4 white pills |
| Nordette | 4 light orange pills + 4 light orange pills |
| Trilevlen | 4 yellow pills + 4 yellow pills |
| Triphasil | 4 yellow pills + 4 yellow pills |
| | |
| Alesse | 5 pink pills + 5 pink pills |
| Levlite | 5 pink pills + 5 pink pills |

**PLAN B REGIMEN**

Levonorgestrel 0.75 mg taken within 72 hours after unprotected intercourse
- First dose as soon as possible
- Second dose *must* be taken 12 hours later

| If you use: | Take: |
|---|---|
| Ovrette | 20 yellow pills + 20 yellow pills |

This regimen is more effective than Yuzpe regimen and causes fewer side effects.

**COPPER T 380-A**

Insert Copper T 380-A within 5 to 8 days after unprotected intercourse

This is the most effective postcoidal method currently available.

an effective dose. The copper-releasing IUD may have a negative effect on the process of ovulation but is more likely to interfere with the process of implantation. A disadvantage of using the IUD as a method of emergency contraception is the high probability of the woman developing pelvic inflammatory disease if she has been exposed to sexually transmitted infections. For this reason some protocols for IUD use as a postcoidal method require that antibiotics be taken prophylactically (Hawkins, Roberto-Nichols, and Stanley-Haney, 2000).

Sensitivity and compassion are required when dealing with a woman seeking emergency contraception. She may be embarrassed that she did not use contraception; may think she did something wrong that broke the condom or dislodged the diaphragm, cervical cap, or IUD; or may be a victim of rape. Many women will not only be worried about pregnancy but also the possibility of sexually transmitted infections. Emergency contraception alone provides no protection against infection, so women may need additional services (Van Look and Stewart, 1998).

### Strategies for Self-Care

Every woman should be told about the self-care of postcoidal contraception. Because the first dose must be given within 72 hours of intercourse, women do not have a lot of time to find and receive care, which is especially difficult on a weekend. They may use the oral contraception pills of their friends or have a packet on hand for themselves. Women treat themselves as a precaution, but they also should be encouraged to seek care from a provider as soon as possible so that they can receive prophylactic antibiotics if indicated and the necessary follow-up to assist them through this process. If a sexual assault or rape occurred, the woman may want a referral to a rape crisis center or rape counseling. Provide her with information and support and empower her to regain her equilibrium.

## Fertility Awareness Methods

**Fertility awareness methods** are based on the changes that occur naturally in a woman's body and require no medical intervention. "Natural methods of family planning are 75% to 98% effective, depending on the method used and on how well the information about them is learned and followed" (Hawkins, Roberto-Nichols, and Stanley-Haney, 2000). Natural methods use the normally occurring signs and symptoms of ovulation and the entire menstrual cycle to both prevent and achieve pregnancy. The process depends on the woman being able to determine the days that she is fertile and can become pregnant. She ovulates one time in every month so there are only a few days that she may become pregnant. If a couple is using this method to avoid conception, they can either abstain during the most fertile days or use a barrier method at that time.

The three commonly used methods of natural family planning are as follows:

* **Cervical mucus method**—based on detectable changes in the cervical mucus.
* **Basal body temperature method**—based on changes in the temperature of the woman's body at rest, first thing in the morning.
* **Symptothermal method**—based on the cervical mucus, the basal body temperature, and other bodily signs.

Each method requires that the woman understand the changes that occur in her own body in response to shifts in hormone levels. The signs are primarily created by changes in either estrogen or progesterone.

### Cervical Mucus Method

Estrogen, produced in increasing amounts by the developing follicle in the ovary, causes changes in the cervix. After menses when estrogen levels are low, cervical mucus is generally absent. As estrogen levels rise, sticky and thick cervical mucus develops. When estrogen levels peak at midcycle, the mucus becomes copious, clear, slippery, and stretchy (the purpose of this type of mucus is to help transport the sperm through the cervical os and into the uterus). The stretchiness of the mucus is called spinnbarkheit. The degree of wetness and stretchiness increases over several days as the day of ovulation approaches. The last day of clear slippery mucus is the peak day to achieve pregnancy (Hawkins, Roberto-Nichols, and Stanley-Haney, 2000) (Figure 5-12).

After ovulation, the increased levels of progesterone counteract the effect of estrogen on cervical mucus, causing the mucus to "plug" the cervix to prevent further sperm from entering and the cervical os to close. Using assessment of the cervical mucus as the only indicator of fertile days, there is a 20% pregnancy rate for those using abstinence on fertile days (Trussel and Grummer-Strawn, 1990).

### Basal Body Temperature Method

The basal body temperature method requires that the woman take and record her basal body temperature before she gets out of bed each morning when her temperature is the lowest of the day. It is taken with a special thermometer that only records temperature between 96° and 100° F. "As the ova are maturing the temperature is low. At some time shortly before, during, or after the ovum leaves the ovary, the temperature will usually rise about 3/10ths to 1 full degree higher than it has been. This change in temperature tells you that the ovum has left the ovary; that is, ovulation has taken place" (Hawkins, Roberto-Nichols, and Stanley-Haney, 2000). Recording a series of temperatures on the basal body temperature calendar (BBT calendar) helps a woman determine when ovulation occurred (Figure 5-13).

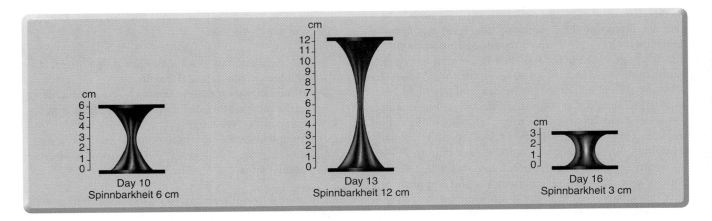

FIGURE 5-12 • Cyclic hormonal changes in the cervical mucus. *(From Garrett C: Anatomy and physiology of the reproductive system. In Lowdermilk D, Perry S, and Bobak I, editors:* Maternity and women's health care, *ed 6, St Louis, 1997, Mosby.)*

FIGURE 5-13 • Basal body temperature record. *(From Hawkins JW, Roberto-Nichols DM, and Stanley-Haney JL:* Protocols for nurse-practitioners in gynecologic settings, *ed 7, New York, 2000, Tiresias Press.)*

If the woman is active before she takes her temperature, becomes ill, has drunk alcoholic beverages, or changes the usual time she takes her temperature, there may be an increase or decrease in temperature unrelated to ovulation.

### Symptothermal Method

The symptothermal method of fertility awareness consists of using the BBT calendar, cervical mucus assessment, and cervical position assessment. Checking the movement and changes that occur in the cervix by palpating it can help a woman differentiate between her fertile and infertile days (Figure 5-14).

Because there is much to learn in order to have natural family-planning methods work effectively, couples should learn together, either alone or in a class, so that they can work together to determine fertile and infertile days. Several rules taught in classes will increase

their success (e.g., the "every other dry day rule," the "rule based on menses," the "peak day rule," and the "thermal shift rule" (Hawkins, Roberto-Nichols, and Stanley-Haney, 2000). Pregnancy rates are 13% to 20% among typical users trying to prevent pregnancy (Jennings, Lamprecht, and Kowal, 1998).

### Additional Advantage

Fertility-awareness methods have the advantage of being acceptable when religion prohibits the use of methods of contraception that prevent fertilization or implantation. These methods are inexpensive and do not require medical intervention. Disadvantages include the fact that these methods offer no protection against sexually transmitted infections, including HIV. They also require a partner who is willing to accept abstinence. Any physical condition that interferes with hormonal function will make these methods more difficult to use. If the woman has recently discontinued a hormonal method of contraception, recently had a child, is currently breastfeeding, has experienced recent menarche or is perimenopausal, the effectiveness of these methods is decreased due to hormonal fluctuations (Jennings, Lamprecht, and Kowal, 1998).

## Barrier Methods

**Barrier methods** of contraception place a physical barrier between the sperm and the ova. In doing so, they also provide a degree of protection against sexually transmitted infection. Barrier methods include male condoms, female condoms, the diaphragm, and the cervical cap.

### Male Condoms

**Male condoms** are an important contraceptive method. They come in various colors, textures (i.e., smooth or

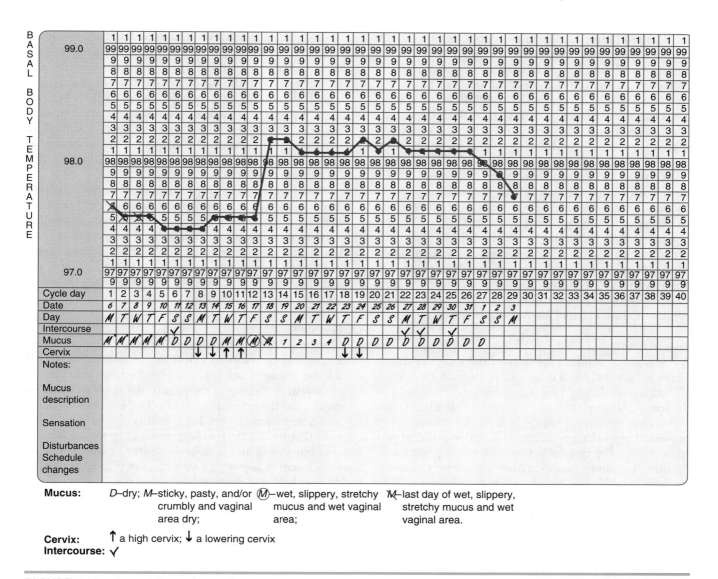

**FIGURE 5-14** • Symptothermal record. *(From Hawkins JW, Roberto-Nichols DM, and Stanley-Haney JL: Protocols for nurse-practitioners in gynecologic settings, ed 7, New York, 2000, Tiresias Press.)*

textured), and prices. They may be plain or lubricated and with or without spermicide. They are relatively effective in preventing pregnancy and protecting against sexually transmitted infections, including HIV. Condoms do not require visits to health care providers because they are readily available without prescription. They are cost-effective and easy-to-use.

Condoms are made from three different materials: latex, natural membrane, and polyurethane. Most condoms used in the United States are made from latex. Latex condoms are effective in preventing pregnancy and sexually transmitted infections. Natural membrane condoms, made from the intestinal caecum of lambs, are not as effective in preventing infection because they contain many small pores that allow viruses and bacteria to pass through the condom. One brand of male condom made

from polyurethane is currently available in the United States, and several others are in development. Polyurethane condoms provide a necessary alternative for couples when one of them has a latex sensitivity or allergy. Polyurethane condoms are thought to be as effective as latex condoms in preventing the spread of sexually transmitted infections (Warner and Hatcher, 1998).

Some condoms are lubricated with a small amount of the spermicide nonoxynol-9. The concentration of spermicide on the condoms is much lower than in vaginal spermicides, making condoms with spermicide no more effective than condoms without spermicide (CDC, 1993). In fact, the spermicide may increase the leakage of allergenic proteins through the latex (Stratton, Hamann, and Beezhold, 1996) causing genital ulceration and irritation in both partners.

"Method failure of the male condom resulting in unintended pregnancy is uncommon, estimated to occur in about 3% of couples using condoms consistently and correctly during the first year of use" (Warner and Hatcher, 1998). Unfortunately, couples do not always use condoms correctly or consistently. With typical use of condoms during the first year, 14% of couples will experience an unintended pregnancy, most often because of a failure to use the condom with every act of intercourse. Other problems with condoms include breakage or slippage during use. Reports of slippage and breakage vary widely from study to study, with reported rates of slippage from 3.4% to 13.1% with acts of vaginal intercourse. Breakage seems to be less likely, occurring in 0% to 6.7% with acts of vaginal intercourse. Because breakage and slippage can occur, it is important that a condom user have multiple condoms available so that a new condom can be used whenever condom failure occurs (Warner and Hatcher, 1998).

### Advantages

Advantages of condom use beyond reducing the chance of pregnancy include a degree of protection from sexually transmitted infections. Condoms are low-cost, easily accessible, portable, have minimal side effects, and allow men to actively participate in the contraceptive process. They offer immediate and visible proof of protection when the ejaculate is held in the reservoir of the condom. Condoms may also help retain an erection and provide benefits for people who do not wish to be touched by genitals or experience postcoital leakage. They may also prevent fertility problems in women associated with their exposure to sperm antibodies (Warner and Hatcher, 1998).

### Disadvantages

Disadvantages of condom use include the need to plan ahead to have it available and then incorporate it into the lovemaking process to place it on the penis. This activity may result in problems with maintaining an erection. Some men and women complain of decreased sensation with condom usage. Men and women may be embarrassed to obtain condoms or suggest their use because of the underlying message of fear of infection. Some men refuse to cooperate with the use of condoms. Latex allergy may be a problem, especially with health care workers. Polyurethane condoms provide a viable alternative (Hawkins, Roberto-Nichols, and Stanley-Haney, 2000).

### Strategies for Self-Care

Education for condom use is vital when condoms are selected as the method of choice. Condoms come in all sizes, and some can stretch enough to fit over a zucchini squash, so there is no truth to a man's comment that "they don't make them big enough for me." We must ensure that a woman understands that the condom is pulled on an erect penis before there is any sexual contact. About an inch of air space is left between the end of the penis and the tip of the condom to contain the ejaculate and prevent breakage. The penis is withdrawn from the woman's vagina before it becomes limp, with the open end held tightly around the penis. A condom may only be used once, so a new condom is required for each act of intercourse (Hawkins, Roberto-Nichols, and Stanley-Haney, 2000).

Consider if it is appropriate to recommend condoms as a method of preventing infection. Stress the personal benefits of condom use, and help the woman explore ways to persuade a reluctant partner. Recommend practicing applying a condom over a penile shaped object (e.g., banana, zucchini, or summer squash) so that she can become skilled in applying the male condom (Warner and Hatcher, 1998).

### Female Condom

Only one brand of **female condom,** the "Reality Vaginal Pouch," is currently available in the United States. It is a loose-fitting sheath made of polyurethane with flexible rings that fit the top of the vagina and form a protective barrier for the external genitalia. This condom is 7.8 cm in diameter and 17 cm long, and is coated with lubricant (Figure 5-15). The polyurethane in the condom is thin but strong and is unlikely to tear or break. The female condom is popular with couples who have used it. Almost half said that they would continue to use it and would recommend it to friends, while only 7% to 8% of those who tried it did not like it (Farr and others, 1994).

The female condom is available over the counter without a prescription. It comes prelubricated, but adding a few more drops of additional lubricant makes the process of insertion easier. It is put in place by pinching the ring at the closed end of the pouch and sliding it up the vagina until it hooks over the cervix. The external ring is adjusted over the labia. The condom may be inserted up to 8 hours before intercourse (Hawkins, Roberto-Nichols, and Stanley-Haney, 2000).

Users have learned that adding 1 to 2 extra drops of lubricant decreases or eliminates a possible squeaking noise and dislocation during intercourse. After intercourse, the woman should remove the condom before standing by squeezing and twisting the outer ring and pulling it out gently (Hawkins, Roberto-Nichols, and Stanley-Haney, 2000). The female and male condoms cannot be used together because they will adhere to each other and possibly tear.

### Advantages

The female condom provides the greatest coverage of a woman's tissues to prevent the transmission of sexually transmitted infections.

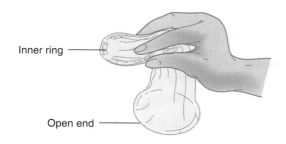

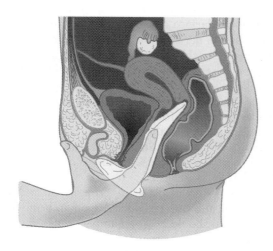

Insertion of the Reality vaginal pouch

FIGURE 5-15 • Female condom. *(Diagrams that show the condom and how it is used may be obtained from the manufacturer: The Female Health Company, 875 North Michigan Ave., Suite 3660, Chicago, IL 60611.)*

### Disdvantages

Some users feel that there is a loss of sensation because the condom does not fit tightly. Some couples have found the occasional "squeaking" noise distracting. Female condoms are more expensive than the male condoms.

### Strategies for Self-Care

In order to use a new product like the female condom, women have to know that it exists, where to get it, and how to use it. Because this product provides a positive alternative for women, we should inform them of its availability and help them be comfortable with its use.

### Diaphragm

**The diaphragm** is another female barrier type of contraception. It is a shallow, round dome of rubber with a semiflexible rim. There are several types of diaphragms made by different manufacturers so one can usually find one that fits well and is comfortable when in place (Figure 5-16).

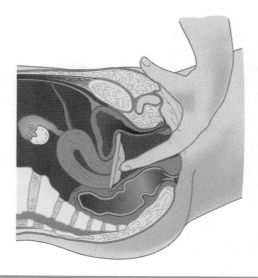

FIGURE 5-16 • A properly placed diaphragm. *(From Foster B: Contraception. In Lowdermilk D, Perry S, and Bobak I, editors: Maternity and women's health care, ed 6, St Louis, 1997, Mosby.)*

The diaphragm is inserted so that one edge of the rim tucks up behind the cervix, the rubber covers the cervix completely, and the other side of the rim rests up behind the pubic bone. "It serves both as a mechanical barrier and a receptacle for the (contraceptive) spermicidal cream or jelly or film which must be used to insure effectiveness" (Hawkins, Roberto-Nichols, and Stanley-Haney, 2000). The spermicide is placed in the dome and around the rim before the diaphragm is inserted. The diaphragm may be inserted up to 4 hours before intercourse but must be left in place for at least 6 hours after intercourse. To slightly extend the time before intercourse or provide protection with multiple acts of intercourse, additional spermicide can be added in the vagina without removing the diaphragm (Hawkins, Roberto-Nichols, and Stanley-Haney, 2000). Wearing the diaphragm for longer than 24 hours is not recommended because of the danger of toxic shock syndrome (TSS).

After removal, diaphragms must be cleaned thoroughly with soapy water and dried before they can be stored. Diaphragms come in several styles and many sizes. The diaphragm is only available with a prescription and must be professionally fitted by a health care provider. Before a woman leaves the office with a diaphragm, she should demonstrate the correct insertion and removal of her diaphragm. The fit should be checked during the woman's annual examination and any time she is having problems using it, as well as when she has gained or lost 10 to 15 pounds (although some experts question the necessity of this), had pelvic surgery, or had her cervix opened with an abortion, miscarriage, or birth (Hawkins, Roberto-Nichols, and Stanley-Haney, 2000).

## Advantages

The advantages of the diaphragm are that it is only used when needed. The diaphragm does not contain ingredients with systemic effects, and the woman is controlling her fertility without having to rely on a partner's cooperation. The diaphragm may be the method of choice for women who are spacing their children or have intercourse infrequently, as well as for older women whose fertility is declining. When used in combination with a male condom, so that there are two barriers, the effectiveness against pregnancy is even greater and the woman gains protection from sexually transmitted infections.

## Disadvantages

The disadvantages are that the woman may feel uncomfortable touching her body in this new way and have difficulty relaxing and performing the correct insertion and/or removal technique. Some women experience an increase in urinary tract infections, which may occur if the diaphragm is in place too long or too often or because of the pressure on the urethra. The incidence of urinary tract infections can be decreased with more frequent urination. If the diaphragm is too large, the woman may experience pelvic discomfort, cramps, and pressure on the bladder or rectum. A woman may experience a local irritation, erythema, or pruritus due to the spermicide nonoxynol-9. Spermicide use may also be associated with the increased rate of urinary tract infections experienced by some diaphragm users (Fihn and others, 1996). If the woman is allergic to the material from which the diaphragm is made, this is not an option for her (Hawkins, Roberto-Nichols, and Stanley-Haney, 2000). Used alone, the diaphragm does not provide protection from sexually transmitted infections.

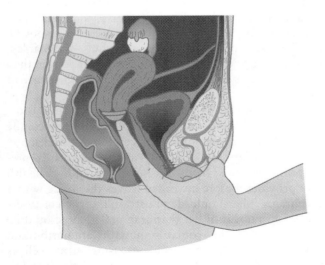

FIGURE 5-17 • A properly placed cervical cap. *(From Foster B: Contraception. In Lowdermilk D, Perry S, and Bobak I, editors:* Maternity and women's health care, *ed 6, St Louis, 1997, Mosby.)*

## Strategies for Self-Care

Many women have used the diaphragm with a great deal of success. If a woman can identify a friend or family member who has been a successful diaphragm user, this will positively affect her adaptation.

## Cervical Cap

The **cervical cap** is a soft rubber thimble with a firm rim. The woman puts spermicide in the cap and then places it snugly over her cervix (Figure 5-17). A groove around the inner circumference of the rim helps create a good seal with the surface of the cervix. Once placed over the cervix, suction develops, helping the cap remain in place and enhancing the barrier against sperm. It generally takes about 3 to 5 minutes for the suction to develop but may take as long as 30 minutes in some women. The cap may be inserted up to 12 hours before intercourse and provides protection for 48 hours. Additional spermicide is not required for further acts of intercourse (Hawkins, Roberto-Nichols, and Stanley-Haney, 2000). The cap should be removed after 48 hours to decrease the possibility of TSS.

The cap is only available by prescription and must be fitted by a health care provider. A woman being fitted for a cervical cap should be given ample time in the office to practice inserting and removing it to increase her confidence in her ability to use this method correctly.

## Advantages

Advantages of the cap are that it does not put pressure on the urethra or bowels, so it is generally more comfortable than a diaphragm and there is less chance of cystitis. This method is also less disruptive of the sexual response because a woman can put it in and then forget about it until the next morning. She does not have to worry about adding additional spermicide, and some partners find it more comfortable than the diaphragm. The cap can also be used to catch menstrual flow when a woman wants to have intercourse during her menses.

## Disadvantages

Disadvantages of using the cap are that it comes in limited sizes and designs, so only 50% to 70% of women who ask for it can be fitted. It is also difficult to fit satisfactorily for women with certain anatomical variations of the cervix or vagina (Hawkins, Roberto-Nichols, and Stanley-Haney, 2000). Although the diaphragm, cap, and condom all provide equal protection in women who have not had children, the cap is less effective in women who have had children. As many as 40% of parous women using the cervical cap experience an unintended pregnancy in the first year of use, compared to 20% of nulliparous women experience pregnancy. A woman may have a reaction to the spermicide or the material from which the cap is made. Some women find that because of the short length of their fingers it is more difficult to insert and remove the cap than the diaphragm. The cap does not provide protection from sexually transmitted infections. The availability of the cap is currently limited by the lack of practitioners trained to fit them.

### Strategies for Self-Care

Many women cannot select caps as an option until more providers learn how to fit them. To improve the ability for women to care for themselves and experience the benefits of using a cap, they must become aware of the method and find providers of this service.

### Barrier Methods of the Future

Several new barrier devices are being developed. One of these is Lea's Shield, which is a device similar to a diaphragm that comes in one size and does not have to be professionally fitted. A silicone cervical cap is also under study, as are polymers that release spermicide, custom fitted caps, and a modified version of a vaginal sponge (Stewart, 1998).

### Strategy for Self-Assessment

TSS is a rare but serious infection associated with the use of the diaphragm or cap (Schwartz and others, 1989). It is caused by toxins released by some strains of *Staphylococcus aureus* and is most often associated with tampon use during menses. Women using barrier methods must be aware of the possibility of developing TSS and the danger signs associated with it. If a woman experiences any of these symptoms while or after using a diaphragm or cap, she should see a health care provider (Box 5-7).

## Vaginal Spermicides

**Vaginal spermicides** are substances used alone or in combination with vaginal barrier methods to prevent sperm from reaching the uterus. The method of insertion, the length of time of effectiveness, and the time required between insertion and intercourse vary with each type of preparation. Spermicides consist of a chemical to kill sperm and a base to hold the chemical. The base may be a cream, gel, foam, film, foaming tablet, or suppository. Products sold in the United States contain the sperm-killing chemical nonoxydol-9, which is a surfactant that destroys the cell membrane. The concentration of nonoxydol-9 within products varies greatly from product to product (Hawkins, Roberto-Nichols, and Stanley-Haney, 2000).

Pregnancy rates from the use of spermicide alone vary widely from 5% to 50% per typical use in the first year (Cates and Raymond, 1998). Spermicides are much more effective when used in combination with a barrier method. Common errors in spermicide use include failure to use the product with every act of intercourse, failure to insert the product in a timely manner, or using too little product to provide adequate protection.

### Advantages

Spermicides are relatively inexpensive, are easily available without prescription, can be used with little advance preparation, and are not associated with the systemic side effects of other methods. Because they come in so many different forms, a woman can generally find one that is comfortable for her to insert. Spermicides offer some protection against sexually transmitted infections, lowering the risk of contracting chlamydia and gonorrhea by 25%, although there is no evidence that nonoxydol-9 has any effect on the transmission of HIV (Cates and Raymond, 1998). The spermicide can act as a lubricant and increase the comfort for a woman when a man uses an unlubricated condom.

### Disadvantages

Spermicide must be inserted minutes before insertion of the penis. Additional amounts of spermicide must be inserted before each act of intercourse. The most common problem with the use of spermicides is local irritation to the vagina, vulva, or penis due to sensitivity or allergy to the chemical component. Women who experience skin irritation can be encouraged to try other forms and brands of spermicide. Jelly may be less irritating but tends to be more viscous than creams or foams. There can be leakage of the spermicide after intercourse, which may be dealt with by wearing a mini-pad (Boston Women's Health Book Collective, 1998).

### Strategies for Self-Care

A woman may easily carry spermicide with her in the form of suppositories or film, allowing her to participate in the process of contraception no matter where she is. When she is in her own home, it is easier to use the preparations that come in larger containers. By carrying a spermicide, a woman will always be able to offer herself some degree of protection, and the level of protection will be improved if her partner also uses a condom.

## Hormonal Methods

**Hormonal methods** of contraception work by altering the hormones within a woman's body. When used

---

**BOX 5-7   *Danger Signals of Toxic Shock Syndrome***

High fever
Rash
Vomiting, diarrhea
Weakness
Dizziness
Fainting

consistently, these methods are among the most reliable forms of pregnancy prevention, with some of the lowest unintended pregnancy rates. Hormonal methods include those combining both estrogen and progesterone (i.e., combined oral contraceptives), as well as those using only progesterone (i.e., progestin-only oral contraceptives, contraceptive implants, injectable contraceptives).

### Combined Oral Contraception Pills

**Combined oral contraceptives,** which are commonly called birth control pills, are considered relatively safe and effective and are among the most studied prescription drugs ever manufactured. Most women can use oral contraceptives for all of their reproductive life, up to menopause; age is no longer a criteria for discontinuing oral contraceptives. In some countries, oral contraceptives are now available over-the-counter without a prescription (Trussel and others, 1993).

Oral contraceptives come in many different formulations. Only two estrogen compounds—ethinyl estradiol and mestranol—are currently used in the oral contraceptives available in the United States. The most frequently prescribed pills contain 35 $\mu$g or less of ethinyl estradiol. Several different progestins are found in oral contraceptives, including norethindrone, norgestrel, norethindrone acetate, and ethyndiol diacetate. The newest progestins in oral contraceptives are desogestrel, norgestimate, and gestodene (not available in the United States). The goal in formulating and prescribing oral contraceptives is to provide the lowest possible hormone dosage that will work for a woman. Sometimes several different formulations must be tried until the right combination is found for an individual.

Oral contraception works primarily through the mechanism of suppressing ovulation by adding estrogen and progesterone to the woman's body. The levels of estrogen and progesterone circulating in the bloodstream mimic pregnancy, so the pituitary gland is not stimulated to produce the hormone that stimulates follicle development, FSH, or the hormone that matures follicular development and fosters ovulation, LH. The lining of the endometrium is also affected, making it incompatible with implantation. Cervical mucus is thickened, and the capacity of sperm to move through the cervix and vagina may be altered (Hatcher and Guillebaud, 1998).

Oral contraceptives are effective when taken exactly as prescribed. In the case of perfect use, the pregnancy rate is only about 1 per 1000 women within the first year of use. Among typical users, or those who occasionally miss pills or take them later than scheduled, approximately 5% will become pregnant during the first year of use (Hatcher and Guillebaud, 1998).

 Women take their first pill on the first day of menstrual bleeding or on the first Sunday after bleeding begins. Back-up contraception is necessary for 7 days with a Sunday start, *except* in those cases when the first day of the pill (Sunday) is also the first day of the menstrual cycle

(Hawkins, Roberto-Nichols, and Stanley-Haney, 2000). Starting the pills on Sunday makes for a pill regimen that is easier to remember and ensures that a woman will probably not have a menses during a weekend.

Pills come in 21-day or 28-day packs. In both cases, hormones are provided for the first 3 weeks (21 days), followed by a week of no hormones so that the woman will have a menstrual bleed. Use of the 21-day packs expects the woman to take a week off from taking pills and then remember to start again with a new package on the correct day. The 28-day packs have a fourth week of inert or nonhormonal pills (e.g., generally sugar pills or iron pills) that are taken on days 22 through 28. This type of packaging helps a woman stay in the habit of taking a pill every day, which may increase her success in maintaining usage.

It is important that the pills be taken at the same time each day. Most women will have fewer problems with nausea if the pill is taken at bedtime. However, this schedule will only work if bedtime is at the same time every night. If pills are missed or delayed for several hours, the circulating level of hormones can drop enough to allow ovulation (and perhaps pregnancy) or the woman may experience **breakthrough bleeding** as the endometrium starts to break down.

Delayed and missed pills occur for a variety of reasons. When a woman starts with oral contraception she needs to know how to respond effectively when this happens. Each time she is seen the protocol should be reviewed with her and she should be given written instructions to help her be successful. This is an important part of her self-care process (Box 5-8).

The physical adjustment time to oral contraceptives is 3 months. During that time, breakthrough bleeding, nausea, and breast tenderness are common. These symptoms generally disappear after three cycles of pills. If the side effects persist beyond this period, the oral contraceptive should be changed to a different formulation that may be more comfortable to the woman.

**Withdrawal bleeding,** the artificial menstrual period while on oral contraceptives, is likely to be short and scanty and may be only a small smudge on a pad or underwear. This counts as a period. Most women are pleased to have lighter and shorter periods, but others are concerned and need to be counseled that this is a normal response to oral contraception.

About 25% to 50% of women discontinue oral contraceptives by the end of the first year, usually due to personal reasons, not medical complications (Hatcher and Guillebaud, 1998). Each woman choosing oral contraceptives should also select a back-up method and feel confident that she can use this method if she discontinues oral contraceptives.

### Self-Assessment

Women who are on oral contraceptives are responsible for performing self-assessment to identify early indications of

---

## BOX 5-8 *When a Pill is Delayed or Missed*

**One pill missed:** Woman should take pill when she remembers, and then take her next pill at the regular time.

**Two missed pills in first 2 weeks:** Woman should take 2 pills at regular time for 2 days, then continue on with her pills on the regular schedule *and use another method of contraception for 7 days.*

**Two or more pills missed in the third week, or 3 or more pills missed any time** (and a woman starts her new package on Sunday): Woman should keep taking a pill each day until Sunday, and then start a new packet on Sunday.

If woman does not start on Sundays, she should throw out that pill packet and start a new packet immediately.

*Either way, she should use another method of contraception until she has taken pills for the first 7 days of the new pill packet.*

Hawkins JW, Roberto-Nichols DM, and Stanley-Haney JL: *Protocols for nurse-practitioners in gynecologic settings,* ed 7, New York, 2000, Tiresias Press.

---

## BOX 5-9 *Early Warning Signs for Pill Users*

**A**  Abdominal pain (severe)

**C**  Chest pain (severe, cough, shortness of breath)

**H**  Headache (severe), dizziness, weakness, numbness—especially if one-sided

**E**  Eye problems (vision loss or blurring), speech problems

**S**  Severe leg pain (calf or thigh)

---

## BOX 5-10 *Conditions Improved with Use of Oral Contraceptives*

- Heavy, painful, or irregular menstrual periods
- Recurrent ovarian cysts
- Premenstrual symptoms
- Family history of ovarian cancer
- Desire for reversible contraception
- Recent delivery (3 weeks) and not breastfeeding
- Endometriosis
- Postabortion contraception
- Acne, hirsutism, or chronic anovulation
- Past experience using oral contraceptives correctly
- Need for emergency contraception

From Hatcher and Guillebaud: The pill: combined oral contraceptives. In Hatcher R and others (eds): *Contraceptive technology,* ed 17, New York, 1998, Ardent Media.

---

 a problem with the added hormones. These women should know how to obtain health care immediately if they experience severe abdominal pain; chest pain; a severe headache; dizziness, weakness, or one-sided numbness; blurred vision or a loss of vision; problems with speech; or a severe pain in the calf or thigh. The acronym ACHES has been developed to help her remember the symptoms that should alert her to seek care (Box 5-9).

### Advantages

In addition to suppressing ovulation, oral contraceptives offer noncontraceptive benefits for women (e.g., improving the common symptoms associated with the menstrual cycle). Women on oral contraceptives have artificially created menstrual cycles that are anovulatory so the menses or bleeding period that a woman experiences is lighter, shorter, and with fewer cramps than women not on oral contraceptives. Because women are not ovulating it eliminates the midcycle pain of ovulation experienced by some women (Hatcher and Guillebaud, 1998). Because the hormonal cycle is altered, the use of combined hormonal therapy may reduce or eliminate premenstrual symptoms such as depression, anxiety, headaches, and fluid retention. The hormones suppress the activity of the endometrium and the ovaries by simulating pregnancy, so they provide protection against the development of diseases such as endometrial cancer, ovarian cancer, benign breast disease, ovarian cysts, and ectopic pregnancy. Because the amount of vaginal bleeding is decreased, women who have a problem with anemia are less likely to experience problems.

The hormones may improve acne, and they have a positive effect on lipids. Sexual enjoyment may improve because the fear of pregnancy is gone (Hatcher and Guillebaud, 1998). Box 5-10 shows conditions that may be improved with the use of oral contraceptives.

### Disadvantages

Oral contraceptives provide no protection against sexually transmitted infections; condom use should be combined with the use of oral contraceptives for women at risk for infection. Pills must be taken daily and at the exact same time every day, so this regimen may not be appropriate for women with widely varying activity or sleep schedules. The expense of oral contraceptives (i.e., $15 to $40 per month) may cause some women to avoid their use.

Nausea, breast tenderness, and unscheduled bleeding are common during the first 3 months of oral contraceptive use. Headaches and depression may begin or worsen for a woman on oral hormones. Her libido may decrease due to falling levels of free testosterone (Hatcher and Guillebaud, 1998). There may also be an increased incidence of chlamydia among oral contraceptive users.

Cardiovascular disease, although rare in healthy women under age 50 who do not smoke, is a serious side effect of oral contraceptives. Women who use oral contraceptives and also have other risk factors are at increased risk for myocardial infarction, stroke, and thrombophlebitis. There is a slightly higher incidence of breast cancer in women who use oral contraceptives, but this risk disappears when a woman has been off of oral contraceptives for 10 years. There is also a slight increase in cervical cancer in oral contraceptive users (Hatcher and Guillebaud, 1998) (Box 5-11).

 There are a number of drugs that can interfere with the effectiveness of the hormones by altering the metabolism of oral contraceptives. Anticonvulsants (e.g., phenobarbitol, Dilantin, and Tegretol) may decrease the effectiveness of the oral contraceptive. If a woman must take these drugs, she may need to be switched to a higher dose pill to increase the effectiveness of the contraception, although this may also increase her experience with side effects (Diamond and others, 1985).

Broad spectrum antibiotics decrease the availability of estrogen in the bloodstream, thus decreasing the effectiveness of the oral contraceptive. Women taking antibiotics should use a back-up method of pregnancy protection during the use of antibiotics and for 2 weeks afterward. We must remind women of this connection each time we see them so that they can protect themselves from pregnancy no matter who gives them a prescription for an antibiotic. Other providers, such as dentists and other specialists, often prescribe antibiotics without asking if the woman is using oral contraceptives.

Oral contraceptives can decrease the clearance of certain drugs (e.g., Benzodiazepines, theophylline, aminophylline, and corticosteroids), increasing the circulating blood levels of these drugs (Hatcher and Guillebaud, 1998). The provider the woman is seeing for the condi-

tions requiring these drugs may need to decrease their dose so that the woman does not experience an overdose. Conversely, faster clearance of common over-the-counter medications (e.g., acetaminophen and aspirin) may mean that the woman has to take higher doses in order to achieve clinical effectiveness (Rizack and Hillman, 1985).

### Progestin Pill

The progestin-only pill, or **"mini pill,"** contains only the hormone progesterone; it does not contain estrogen. Women who cannot use combined pills because of the risk for major side effects may be candidates for the progestin-only pill. Progestin inhibits ovulation, alters the configuration of the endometrium to make it inhospitable to a fertilized egg, and suppresses midcycle peaks of FSH and LH. The mini pill is slightly less effective than the combined pill, with a first year perfect use pregnancy rate of 0.5% (as compared with 0.1% for the combined pills). Pills are taken daily without a week off each month.

### Advantage

Most women taking progestin-only pills have amenorrhea or irregular, light periods. Most of the health benefits of combined pills also apply to the mini pill. Women experience less bleeding, cramping, premenstrual symptoms, and breast tenderness. The progestin-only pill is an appropriate method for breastfeeding women because the progesterone does not alter milk production, and the woman has added protection against pregnancy beyond that provided by lactation (Hatcher, 1998).

A woman may select this pill instead of the combined pill when she is over 35, has certain types of headaches, has controlled hypertension, does not smoke, has varicose veins, chloasma, weight gain, nausea, depression, or persistent acne aggravated by the estrogen in the combination pill (Hawkins, Roberto-Nichols, and Stanley-Haney, 2000).

Contraindications include pregnancy, unexplained vaginal bleeding, breast cancer, or a history of an undiagnosed mass, liver tumors, or thromboembolism (Hawkins, Roberto-Nichols, and Stanley-Haney, 2000).

### Disadvantages

If a woman misses a pill, the risk for pregnancy is much higher than with the combination pills.

### Contraceptive Implants

The **Norplant implant** system consists of six flexible rods made of nonbiodegradable silastic filled with the hormone levonorgestrel, a synthetic progestin. These soft rods are inserted subcutaneously in the inner aspect of the upper arm and provide hormonal contraception for 5 years. The levonorgestrel works by suppressing ovulation, thickening and decreasing cervical mucus, preventing the FSH and LH midcycle peaks, and altering the endometrium so it remains atrophic. Circulating levels of

---

**BOX 5-11   Contraindications to Oral Contraceptives**

- Deep vein thrombosis: pulmonary embolism: or history of stroke, coronary artery or ischemic heart disease, or complicated structural heart disease
- Diabetes with vascular disease of more than 20-year duration
- Breast cancer
- Pregnancy
- Lactation (less than 6 weeks postpartum)
- Liver problems
- Headaches with focal neurologic symptoms
- Major surgery with prolonged immobilization or any surgery of the legs
- Over 35 years of age and smokes more than 20 cigarettes a day
- Hypertension 160/100 or with vascular disease

WHO: *Improving access to quality care in family planning: medical eligibility criteria for contraceptive use,* Geneva, 1996, WHO.

progestin are very low at any one time, and amenorrhea is common. Other women experience irregular and sometimes long periods of vaginal bleeding. Women should be thoroughly counseled about the menstrual changes that may occur before the method is selected.

Over a 5-year period, Norplant is a cost-effective method of birth control, but it has high up-front costs. Norplant requires a minor surgical procedure for both insertion and removal. The set of implants costs $365 to $375, in addition to a surgical insertion fee of $150 to $300. The cost for removal is higher because it takes more time and is more difficult than insertion. In some cases, removal may be very difficult depending on where the implants were placed. Skin irritation or infection may occur at the site. Norplant should not be inserted in women who desire a pregnancy within the next 5 years (Figure 5-18).

### Advantages

First-year perfect use pregnancy rates are 0.05%, making Norplant a highly effective contraceptive. The contraceptive effects of Norplant are readily reversible after removal of the rods. Women are generally satisfied with this method, with 95% of women continuing with the method after 1 year (Sivin and others, 1997). Compliance is a nonissue because the woman has the hormone present at all times.

### Disadvantages

Irregular periods may occur and are the major source of displeasure of Norplant users and the major reason for discontinuing its use. Other disadvantages include lack of protection against sexually transmitted infections, including HIV. Depression, breast tenderness, and headaches may occur. The circulating levonorgestrel is significantly affected by antiseizure medications and the antitubercular rifampin. Women taking these medications should use back-up contraception because Norplant is not effective in the presence of these medications. Finally, ovarian cysts may occur because Norplant is not as effective as combined oral contraceptives in suppressing the production of FSH. These cysts usually resolve without intervention (Hatcher, 1998).

### Injectable Contraception

The synthetic hormone medroxyprogesterone, sold as **Depo-Provera,** is the most commonly used injectable contraceptive. It is given intramuscularly in 150-mg doses every 12 weeks. If the injection was not given during the first 3 days of her menses, the woman must use a back-up method of contraception for 2 weeks after the first injection (Hawkins, Roberto-Nichols, and Stanley-Haney, 2000). Depo is extremely effective, with a perfect use first-year failure rate of 0.3%, in part because the schedule of injection spans a conservative period of time and a degree of protection remains beyond 12 weeks (Mishell, 1996). Depo works by suppressing ovulation and the production of FSH and LH by the pituitary gland. About 50% of

women choose to use it for 1 year (Polaneczky and others, 1996). The cost for 1 year is about $140 in addition to the cost of the woman's annual medical examination.

### Advantages

A woman may control her fertility without the knowledge of her partner. There are no drug interactions with Depo; in fact, this method of contraception actually decreases the number of seizures in women with seizure disorders. Depo may be used by breastfeeding women after lactation is well established. Depo may be used by women who cannot take combined oral contraceptives and older women because of the absence of thrombolitic complications. Women experience decreased blood flow and cramping, as well as decreased anemia, and have a decreased risk for endometrial cancer, ectopic pregnancy, and sickle cell crises (Hatcher, 1998).

### Disadvantages

As with other nonbarrier contraceptive methods, Depo offers no protection against sexually transmitted infections. Menstrual irregularities are common, but amenorrhea is likely to develop after 1 year of using Depo. Some women are disturbed by the weight gain that sometimes accompanies this method. The average weight gain is 5 pounds per year, which some women find unacceptable. Breast tenderness and depression are also factors. When a woman discontinues injections it may take from 6 to 12 months for her fertility to return (Mishell, 1996); so, Depo-Provera is not the contraceptive method of

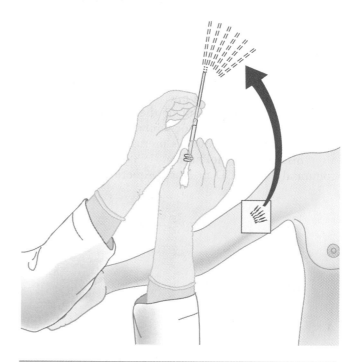

**FIGURE 5-18 ●** Norplant. *(From Foster B: Contraception. In Lowdermilk D, Perry S, and Bobak I, editors:* Maternity and women's health care, *ed 7, St Louis, 2000, Mosby.)*

choice for a woman desiring pregnancy in a few months, or for an older woman whose fertility may already be reduced. In long-term Depo users, decreased bone density (Cundy and others, 1991), as well as decreases in the level of HDL, have occurred (Mishell, 1996). Some women have had allergic reactions to Depo, and others find it inconvenient to return for an office visit every 12 weeks for an injection (Hatcher, 1998).

## Intrauterine Devices

The **intrauterine device (IUD)** is a highly effective method of birth control for some women. There are two IUDs available for use in the United States, with a third pending approval from the FDA. There are additional models available in other countries (Figure 5-19). Pregnancy is prevented through several mechanisms, as follow:

- A local sterile inflammatory response to the foreign body.
- A possible increase in the local production of prostaglandins.
- An alteration in the permeability of the endometrium.
- A decrease in uterine and tubal tonus (Hawkins, Roberto-Nichols, and Stanley-Haney, 2000).

The initial cost of using an IUD is $80 to $200, with insertion costing an additional $70 to $200. The long-term cost of the copper IUD, however, is low. Cost of removal varies.

### Copper T 380

The Copper T 380 (ParaGuard T 380 A®) is manufactured by Ortho Pharmaceuticals. It is made of polyethylene with copper wire wound around the vertical stem of the T and sleeves of copper on each of the two horizontal arms. The bottom of the IUD has a knotted string that is either clear or white. The Copper T 380 may be kept in the woman's uterus for up to 10 years after insertion (GynoPharma, 1988) and is the most commonly used IUD in North America, with 90% of

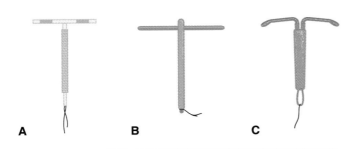

*FIGURE 5-19* • Intrauterine devices. **A,** Copper T 380A. **B,** Progestasert. **C,** Lng. *(From Foster B: Contraception. In Lowdermilk D, Perry S, and Bobak I, editors:* Maternity and women's health care, *ed 7, St Louis, 2000, Mosby.)*

IUD users using the Copper T 380 (Treiman and others, 1995). In the first year of perfect use, the pregnancy rate if 0.6%.

### Progestasert

Manufactured by the Alza Corporation, Progestasert® is made of an ethylene vinyl acetate copolymer with 38 milligrams of progesterone in the vertical stem. It must be replaced each year (Alza Corporation, 1988). This IUD has a blue-black double string that attaches at the base of the T. In the first year of perfect use, the pregnancy rate is 1.5%.

### Lng 20 (Mirena)

The Lng 20 IUD was approved by the FDA on December 6, 2000. It has long been popular in European and Asian countries. This IUD "releases levonorgestrel directly into the uterus at a constant rate of 20 $\mu$g per day for as long as 5 years" (Stewart, 1998). It consists of a polyethylene frame with a cylinder of levonorgestrel mixture around its vertical arm and has a single string. In the first year of perfect use, the pregnancy rate is 0.1%. The Lng 20 is the single most effective reversible contraceptive method available in the world today (Stewart, 1998).

Women who are in mutually monogamous relationships, have had at least one child, and desire an effective method of contraception that is long-acting, may consider this method.

Some women cannot use IUDs because of conditions in their uterus (Box 5-12).

Any woman who has an IUD inserted must understand the early warning signs of a possible problem and  provide self-assessment. If the woman experiences a delayed period, thinks she is pregnant, has abnormal vaginal spotting or bleeding, has pain on intercourse, experiences vaginal discharge, or has signs of a systemic infection (e.g., fever and chills), or there are changes in the string (e.g., it is missing, longer, or shorter), she should be seen. Use the acronym PAINS to help women remember these signs (Box 5-13).

### Advantages

IUDs are advantageous because they do not interfere with lactation. Women who cannot use hormonal methods can use the copper IUD. The progesterone IUD helps reduce menstrual blood flow and dysmenorrhea. The IUD is easy to use, requiring only that the woman check for the presence of a string on a monthly basis to be sure that it is still in place. There are no systemic side effects (Stewart, 1998).

### Disadvantages

The IUD may be spontaneously expelled, and the woman will unknowingly be unprotected from pregnancy. Between 2% and 10% of women expel the IUD within the first year (Stewart, 1998), and this may occur without the woman's awareness.

Women who are with a partner with a sexually transmitted infection are more at risk for contracting the sexually transmitted infection and developing the sequelae of pelvic inflammatory disease (PID) (Caufield, 1998). If pregnancy occurs with an IUD in place, the IUD should be removed immediately as soon as pregnancy is discovered. About 5% of the pregnancies that occur in women with IUDs are ectopic pregnancies, thereby putting the woman at substantial risk and requiring possible surgical intervention. Women using the copper IUD may find that their menstrual flow is heavier and that they have additional cramping when compared with before the IUD was inserted.

## Cultural Response to Changes in Bodily Functions

Each woman holds culturally defined and learned sets of beliefs about her bodily functions. When these functions change, the woman may consciously or unconsciously perceive that the changes indicate that something is abnormal or wrong with her or that she is unhealthy. Many of the hormonal methods and IUDs for fertility control alter the body's usual cycles. As a result, women who use them may become anxious, consider themselves ill, and desire to discontinue the method. They do not know how they will feel until after they have experienced the changes, so education and support are necessary as a woman actually tries to live with the contraceptive process she has chosen.

## Sterilization

Most women ovulate until they are about age 50 or 55. Most people have had their desired number of children before their fertility naturally subsides, leaving a period of years when contraception is necessary. **Female sterilization** is the most popular method of contraception world-wide (Abma and others, 1997). Sterilization is a surgical procedure that alters the pathway of the sperm or the ova.

Female sterilization is the occlusion of the fallopian tubes, which may occur through "excision of a portion of each tube and suturing of the ends; excision of the fimbriated ends; excision of a portion and then the suturing of the proximal end into the muscle of the uterus and the distal end in the broad ligament; banding with silastic bands or clips; ligation of a loop of the tubes with nonabsorbable suture material; occlusion by electrocautery" (Hawkins, Roberto-Nichols, and Stanley-Haney, 2000).

Access to the fallopian tubes may take place at any time through a suprapubic mini-laparotomy. A subumbilical mini-laparotomy may be performed immediately postpartum, or the tubes can be occluded during a cesarean section delivery (Caufield, 1998). Anesthesia is required, and the standard postsurgical complications of infection, hemorrhage, anesthesia complications, and trauma to other organs are a possibility.

Female sterilization is a very effective method of contraception, with a typical first-year pregnancy rate of 0.5%, and a 10-year cumulative pregnancy rate of 0.185% (Peterson and others, 1996). Young women are more likely to become pregnant than older women because they are generally more fertile. Other reasons for detection of a pregnancy following a tubal ligation include a pregnancy already in place at the time of the ligation, a fistula formation or reanastomosis of the tubes, surgical error, or equipment failure (Stewart and Carignan, 1998).

### Advantages

Female sterilization is considered a safe procedure, with a mortality rate that is eight times lower than the mortality rate associated with childbirth. This is an ideal method for women who are sure they do not wish to have future children and still need effective contraception. Advantages include "permanence, high effectiveness, cost-effectiveness, nothing to buy or remember, lack of significant long-term side effects, no need for partner compliance, no need to interrupt lovemaking, and privacy of choice" (Stewart and Carignan, 1998).

### Disadvantages

Because it is considered to be permanent, female sterilization is not recommended for a woman who is unsure

---

**BOX 5-12    *Contraindications to IUD Use***

Active, recent, or recurrent pelvic infection (acute or subacute)
- Postpartum endometritis
- Infection following abortion
- Active sexually transmitted infection

Severely distorted uterine cavity
- Fibroids
- Endometrial polyps
- Cervical stenosis
- Bicornuate uterus
- Small uterus

WHO: *Improving access to quality care in family planning: medical eligibility criteria for contraceptive use,* Geneva, 1996, WHO.

---

**BOX 5-13    *Early warning signs for IUD Users***

| | |
|---|---|
| **P** | Period late, pregnancy, abnormal spotting or bleeding |
| **A** | Abdominal pain, pain with intercourse |
| **I** | Infection exposure, abnormal discharge, any STI |
| **N** | Not feeling well, fever, chills |
| **S** | String missing or shorter or longer |

about her future fertility wishes. It is four times as expensive as male sterilization; is a more complicated procedure that requires anesthesia, an operating room, and a surgeon. Reversibility is rarely effective and is difficult and expensive. If the method fails and the woman becomes pregnant, there is a high probability of ectopic pregnancy (Peterson and others, 1996). There is also no protection from sexually transmitted infections with sterilization.

### Male Sterilization

A woman may decide that she will depend on her partner to undergo sterilization. **Male sterilization** is fourth in popularity following female sterilization, oral contraceptives, and male condoms (Abma and others, 1997). Male sterilization is a simpler procedure than female sterilization and can be performed in an office setting. Local anesthesia is used sometimes with light sedation. Each vas deferens is cut between two ligated sections, thus preventing the sperm from becoming part of the ejaculate.

Male sterilization is easier, safer, less expensive, more effective, and requires less recovery time than female sterilization. The probability of pregnancy in a partner is probably 0.1% in the first year (Stewart and Carignan, 1998).

A so-called "no scalpel" method that reduces the already low complication rate of male sterilization is now in use. The vas is reached through a puncture in the scrotum instead of a surgical incision (AVSC International, 1997). After the sterilization procedure, it generally takes about 20 ejaculations for the vas to be cleared of sperm. Semen analysis is recommended to confirm that the procedure has been effective before the couple may rely on it as contraception. Back-up methods are recommended until the vas has cleared.

### Advantages

Advantages include "permanence, high effectiveness, cost-effectiveness (the most cost-effective of all contraceptive methods), removal of contraceptive burden from the woman, lack of significant long-term side effects, high acceptability, no need to interrupt lovemaking, safety, and quick recovery" (Stewart and Carignan, 1998).

### Disadvantages

Complications such as bleeding and infection can occur. Male sterilization is permanent, although reversal is easier and more successful than reversal of female sterilization. Reversal is a surgical procedure, requiring a surgeon, local anesthesia, and aseptic conditions. Male sterilization is initially expensive, provides protection only for the male, and provides no protection against sexually transmitted infections.

### Possible Long-Term Ramifications

A possibility with both male and female sterilization is regret among those who have undergone the procedure.

Life circumstances change, and decisions that seemed sure and permanent at an earlier age may no longer be desired. Extensive counseling prior to sterilization is essential. Candidates must understand that these methods are permanent because reversals are difficult, expensive major surgeries and offer no guarantee of success. If there are any hesitations, other effective, long-term contraceptive methods (e.g., implants or the IUD) should be offered prior to proceeding with sterilization.

### Informed Consent

As with all contraceptive measures, informed consent is mandatory prior to sterilization. Those using federal or state funds must be at least 21 years old and mentally competent, and must wait 30 days after signing the consent for sterilization (Federal Register, 1978). Components of a consent form should include a description of the procedure to be performed in a language understandable to the client, as well as an explanation of the benefits and risks of surgical procedures. The permanence of the procedure and the fact that the client will no longer be able to have children should be clearly stated. The possibility of future failure must also be stated, because if a woman becomes pregnant after sterilization it is more likely to develop into an ectopic pregnancy and place her life at risk. To ensure that a woman is not being coerced into the surgery by a provider a statement should also be included that says that the woman may decline the sterilization without risking the loss of any financial or medical benefits. In addition, verbal and written preoperative and postoperative instructions should be given and thoroughly reviewed to ensure understanding.

## Future Methods of Fertility Control

Methods of the future include new barrier methods—both mechanical and chemical, new hormonal methods, new IUDs, and a systemic method for men. A one-size-fits-all diaphragm called Lea's Shield is being tested and is intended to be sold over the counter without the need for a prescription or fitting by a health care provider. Femcap is another style of cervical cap that comes in three sizes. A silicone diaphragm is under development and could be easier to insert and remove than currently available diaphragms. Research is ongoing to develop a spermicide that would be less irritating to the mucosa of the cervix and the vagina. Vaginal rings or a single rod to be inserted under the skin, both providing progesterone, are also being developed. New injectables will contain both estrogen and progesterone, a combination that should eliminate the menstrual bleeding disturbances associated with Depo-Provera. A frameless IUD that would eliminate uterine cramping is being tested. Male methods under study include injections that produce oligospermia (Gabelnick, 1998).

## SUPPORTING SELF-ASSESSMENT AND SELF-CARE

Women's lives are busy and full, but their normal physical changes tend to keep them in touch with their bodies and the activities within them. We encourage women to take control of their lives by collaborating with them when sharing information and encouraging them to be experts on what is normal for each of them. Through self-assessment and self-care processes, we enable them to have healthier experiences and more empowered lives.

---

## Care Plan · *The Couple Desiring Self-Care in Fertility Control*

NURSING DIAGNOSIS **Health Seeking Behaviors** related to perceived need for pregnancy prevention

GOALS/OUTCOMES   Will agree on a method of contraception that suits their present and future family goals and is congruent with their lifestyle and sociocultural beliefs; will remain free of sexually transmitted diseases

**NOC Suggested Outcomes**
- Health Seeking Behavior (contraception) (1603)
- Knowledge: Health Resources (1806)

**NIC Priority Interventions**
- Family Integrity Promotion (7100)
- Family Integrity Promotion: Childbearing Family (7104)
- Family Planning: Contraception (6784)
- Fertility Preservation (7160)
- Health Education (5510)
- Self-Modification Assistance (4470)
- Teaching Safe Sex (5622)

**Nursing Activities and Rationale**
- Establish a trusting relationship with woman and partner. *Clients must trust the nurse in order to share personal information and feelings.*
- Facilitate open communications between woman and partner (when client has a partner). *The ability to discuss and agree on contraception methods will increase the likelihood of compliance and strengthen partner bonds.*
- Discuss effects of various contraceptive methods on future fertility. *Women wishing to become pregnant in the future must select contraceptive methods that will not compromise their fertility. Tubal ligations cannot always be reversed, and intrauterine devices increase the risk for pelvic inflammatory disease.*
- Teach prevention of sexually transmitted diseases. *Sexually transmitted diseases can adversely affect a woman's ability to conceive in the future. Condoms are the only effective method for preventing STDs.*
- Inform woman about occupational and environmental hazards to fertility (e.g., radiation, chemicals, stress, infections). *Knowledge of these hazards will help the woman preserve her future fertility.*

**Evaluation Parameters**
- Openly discuss the need for contraception and family planning.
- Identify types of contraceptive methods that meet their specific needs.
- Identify contraceptive methods that preserve future fertility.
- Discuss the need for and methods of avoiding sexually transmitted diseases.
- Discuss the need to avoid occupational and environmental hazards to fertility.

NURSING DIAGNOSIS   **Risk for unintended pregnancy** related to inadequate knowledge or lack of experience with use of contraceptives

GOALS/OUTCOMES   Unintended pregnancy will not occur

**NOC Suggested Outcomes**
- Adherence Behavior (1600)
- Knowledge: Sexual Functioning (1815)
- Knowledge: Contraception Prevention (1821)
- Knowledge: Health Resources (1806)
- Knowledge: Medications (1808)

**NIC Priority Interventions**
- Family Planning: Contraception (6784)
- Self-Modification Assistance (4470)

*Continued*

## Care Plan · The Couple Desiring Self-Care in Fertility Control—cont'd

### Nursing Activities and Rationale

- Determine the need for family planning. *Planning allows the client to control her fertility, limit the size of her family, or prevent pregnancy from occurring. Interventions are effective when the woman has an actual or perceived need for family planning.*
- Assist the woman in identifying a specific goal for change in behavior (compliance with chosen contraceptive method). *Adherence to any contraception method is based on many factors, including the woman's sociocultural beliefs, background and experiences, and ability to obtain or afford the treatment. Identification of goals will foster the needed changes in behavior.*
- Explain the female reproductive cycle to the woman as needed. *Understanding how the reproductive cycle functions will help the woman understand the basis for contraception and facilitate adherence.*
- Explain the reasons for most unplanned pregnancies. *There are multiple reasons why women experience unplanned pregnancy (e.g., lack of knowledge regarding contraception, methods to prevent conception or community resources, inability to integrate chosen birth control method into lifestyle). The woman must understand how to prevent unplanned pregnancy in order to do so.*
- Explain the advantages and disadvantages of various contraceptive methods. *By comparing the various types of contraceptive methods, the woman will be able to make an informed decision about the type of contraception that will be most effective for her particular set of circumstances, wants, and needs.*
- Determine the ability and motivation of the woman and her partner to correctly and regularly use contraception. *Selecting a suitable method increases the likelihood of adherence. Just because a woman selects a method of birth control does not mean that she can appropriately use it, is comfortable using it, or can afford to use it. In general, a method that requires the woman to take specific actions before intercourse is not as effective as a method that does not.*
- Refer the woman to community resources for family planning services as needed. *Many communities have resources available for teaching, physical examination, and provision of birth control medications or devices. Availability of adequate resources helps the woman to obtain and maintain contraceptive behaviors.*

### Evaluation Parameters

- Verbalizes the need for establishing family-planning goals
- Lists advantages and disadvantages of various contraceptive methods
- Identifies local community resources for family planning and contraception
- Uses and reports satisfaction with chosen contraceptive

## CASE STUDY*

Letitia Russo is a 24-year old woman of African-American descent who seeks regular health care. She has three children, ages 2, 4, and 6. Her husband works in construction, which is seasonal work. Unable to find affordable day care and pay for health insurance, Letitia has had to quit her job and the family relies on public assistance for part of their income and the health insurance for the children.

Letitia has two main concerns today: she doesn't want to have any more children, and she wonders why she again has a vaginal discharge. She believes she is in a monogamous relationship. Her family history is positive for diabetes and hypertension, and she had an aunt who died of breast cancer. She has never had any serious illnesses, has never been hospitalized except for the birth of her children, and her last medical care was 6 months ago when she presented with a white discharge that was diagnosed as "yeast." She was treated, and the condition resolved. She is 5'2" tall and weighs 146 lbs. Her blood pressure is 100/70, and her pulse is

## CASE STUDY*

**76.** Her last menstrual period (LMP) was 5 weeks ago; she does not currently use contraception.

- What assessment data do you have about Letitia?
- What other assessment data do you need to obtain?
- What nursing diagnoses might apply to Letitia?
- What health goals might you establish with Letitia?
- What interventions does Letitia need today?

- How will you prepare her for the interventions?
- What factors may limit the interventions Letitia will be able to receive today?
- How will the interventions be prioritized?
- How will you measure the effectiveness of your nursing care?

# Scenarios

**1.** Maria Gonzales, age 16, comes to the high school clinic to find out if she is pregnant. Her pregnancy test is negative, and she is very relieved. She tells you that she has been avoiding having sexual intercourse during the days around her period so she does not get pregnant.

- What nursing diagnoses could apply?
- What subjective and objective data must you know to develop health care goals with Maria?
- What might those goals be?
- What interventions will you provide?
- How will you evaluate the success of those interventions?

**2.** Panagiota, age 18, has come to the Family Health Center with a complaint of continuous "vaginal infections" that occur every month and then go away. She has been evaluated for infection in the past, and no organisms have been found.

- What nursing diagnoses could apply?
- What subjective and objective data must you know to develop health care goals with Panagiota?
- What might those goals be?
- What interventions will you provide?
- How will you evaluate the success of those interventions?

**3.** Haley, age 28, has been seen at the walk-in clinic with complaints of low-grade fever, nasal congestion, and nonproductive cough. She has received a medical diagnosis of having the common cold. She has requested antibiotics for her infection because she doesn't want this to spread to her three young children, but the physician will not give her a prescription because she has a virus and not a bacterial infection. Just before she leaves, she tells you that she's going to take the pills she has left from the last time she was sick.

- How will you handle this?
- What nursing diagnoses could apply?
- What subjective and objective data must you know to develop health care goals with Haley?
- What might those goals be?
- What interventions will you provide?
- How will you evaluate the success of those interventions?

**4.** Yelena, age 20, has come to employee health services seeking care for diarrhea and vomiting that started yesterday. It has been determined that she has simple gastroenteritis.

- What nursing diagnoses could apply?
- What subjective and objective data must you know to develop health care goals with Yelena?

- What might those goals be?
- What self-care measures can Yelena use to treat her symptoms?
- How will you evaluate the success of those interventions?

---

5. Lydia Morales, age 47, has come to the women's clinic requesting medication for anxiety. She says that she feels "uneasy" and her husband has encouraged her to get help. She also reports hot flashes, night sweats, insomnia, mood swings, and depression. Based on her age and her history, you tell her that she is probably entering the perimenopausal period.

- What nursing diagnoses could apply?
- What subjective and objective data must you know to develop health care goals with Lydia?
- What might those goals be?
- What interventions might you offer?
- What self-care measures can Lydia use to treat her symptoms?
- What other treatment options are available to her?
- How will you evaluate the success of your interventions?

---

6. While showering yesterday Crystal, age 45, felt a lump in her right breast and has come to her primary care provider's office for further evaluation. She has never had a mammogram.

- What nursing diagnoses could apply?
- What subjective and objective data must you know to develop health care goals with Crystal?
- What might those goals be?
- What interventions might you offer?
- What techniques will be used to evaluate her breast lump?
- How will you evaluate the success of your interventions?

---

7. Claudia, age 15, has come to see you in the school nurse's office for counseling about sexual activity. She reports that she has a boyfriend who is pressuring her to have sexual intercourse, but she does not think that she is ready for such a big step in their relationship. She wants to know what she should do.

- What nursing diagnoses could apply?
- What subjective and objective data must you know to develop health care goals with Claudia?
- What might those goals be?
- What interventions might you offer?
- How will you evaluate the success of your interventions?

---

8. Marian, age 57, has come to the women's clinic for her annual examination. Her menstrual periods stopped 2 years ago, and her "power surges" (hot flashes) and other symptoms are becoming less intense. Her mammogram is normal. She is thin, weighing 104 pounds, and short, standing at 5'2". Her mother developed osteoporosis and fractured a hip at age 65. She has a sister and a father who developed coronary artery disease before they were 50. There is no breast cancer in her family history. After watching a television show about women and aging, Mary wonders if she should go on hormone augmentation therapy (hormone replacement therapy).

- What nursing diagnoses could apply?
- What subjective and objective data must you know to develop health care goals with Marian?
- What might those goals be?
- What interventions might you offer?
- What will you tell her about the advantages and disadvantages of these hormones?
- How will you evaluate the success of your interventions?

---

## REFERENCES

Abma J and others: Fertility, family planning and women's health: new data from the 1995 national survey of family growth, *Vit Health Stat* 23:19, 1997.

Achilles C and Leppert P: The menopausal woman. In Leppert P and Howard F, editors: *Primary care for women*, Philadelphia, 1997, Lippincott.

Alexander L and LaRosa J: *New dimensions in women's health*, Boston, 1994, Jones and Bartlett.

*Alternative remedies for common ailments*, Alexandria, VA, 1998, Time-Life Books.

Althof S and Levine S: Clinical approach to the sexuality of patients with spinal cord injury, *Urol Clin North Am* 20:527, 1993.

Alza Corporation: *Progestasert intrauterine progesterone contraceptive system*, Product information, 1988.

Andrews MM and Boyle JS: *Transcultural concepts in nursing care,* Philadelphia, 1995, Lippincott.

Annon J: The behavioral treatment of sexual problems, vol 1: *Brief therapy,* Honolulu, 1974, Mercantile Printing.

AVSC International: *No-scalpel vasectomy: an illustrated guide for surgeons,* ed 2, New York, 1997, AVSC International.

Birge S and Dalsky G: The role of exercise in preventing osteoporosis, *Pub Health Rep* 104(suppl):54-58, 1989.

Boston Women's Health Book Collective: *The new our bodies ourselves,* New York, 1998, Simon & Schuster.

Brown M: Skin cancer. In Leppert P and Howard F, editors: *Primary care for women,* Philadelphia, 1997, Lippincott.

Brown S and Eisenberg L, editors: *The best intentions: unintended pregnancy and the well-being of children and families,* Washington, D.C., 1995, National Academy Press.

Cahill C: Exercise. In Fogel C and Woods N, editors: *Women's health care: a comprehensive handbook,* Thousand Oaks, CA, 1995, Sage.

Cates W and Raymond E: Vaginal spermicides. In Hatcher R and others, editors: *Contraceptive technology,* ed 17, New York, 1998, Ardent Media.

Caufield K: Controlling fertility. In Youngkin E and Davis M, editors: *Women's health: a primary care clinical guide,* ed 2, Stamford, 1998, Appleton-Lange.

Centers for Disease Control and Prevention: Update: barrier protection against HIV infection and other sexually transmitted diseases, *MMWR* 42:589-591, 597, 1993.

Centers for Disease Control and Prevention: *Reducing the health consequences of smoking: 25 years of progress—a report of the surgeon general,* Atlanta, 1989, U.S. Department of Health and Human Services.

Colditz G, Egan K, and Stampfer M: Hormone replacement therapy and risk of breast cancer: results from epidemiologic studies, *J Obstet Gynecol* 168:1473-1480, 1993.

Cundy T and others: Bone density in women receiving depo medroxyprogesterone acetate for contraception, *Brit Med J* 303(6793):13-16, 1991.

Daniel C, Dolan N, and Wheeland R: Don't overlook skin surveillance, *Patient care,* 30(11):90-107, 1996.

Dawson D and Thompson G: Breast cancer risk factors and screening, United States 1987, *Vital and Health Statistics,* (Series 10. No. 172. DHHS Publication No. PSH 90-1500), Washington, D.C., 1989, Government Printing Office.

Devine KS: Communication, counseling, and compliance issues. In *Current practice issues in adolescent gynecology,* Fair Lawn, N.J., 1996, MPE Communications.

Diamond M and others: Interaction of anticonvulsants and oral contraceptives in epileptic adolescents, *Contraception* 31(6):623-632, 1985.

Dollemore D: *Natural healing remedies,* Emmaus, PA, 1998, Rodale Press.

Edwards L and others: Melanoma: a strategy for detection and treatment, *Patient care* (30)11:126-153, 1996.

Farr G and others: Contraceptive efficacy and acceptability of the female condom, *Am J Pub Health* 84:1960-1964, 1994.

Ferrary E and Parker-Falzoi J: Common medical problems: cardiovascular through hematological disorders. In Youngkin E and Davis M, editors: *Women's health care: a primary care clinical guide,* Stamford, 1998, Appleton-Lange.

Fihn S and others: Association between use of spermicide-coated condoms and *Escherichia coli* urinary tract infection in young women, *Am J Epidemiol* 144:512-520, 1996.

Fishbein EG and Bash DM: American women and self-care: choices and changes, *J Perinat Educat* 6(3):19-25, 1997.

Fogel C: Women and sexuality. In Youngkin E and Davis M, editors: *Women's health care: a primary care clinical guide,* Stamford, 1998, Appleton-Lange.

Fogel C and Lauver D: *Sexual health promotion,* Philadelphia, 1990, Saunders.

Gabelnick H. (1998). Future methods. In Hatcher R and others, editors: *Contraceptive technology,* ed 17, New York, 1998, Ardent Media.

Garrett C: Anatomy and physiology of the reproductive system. In Lowdermilk D, Perry S, and Bobak I, editors: *Maternity and women's health care,* ed 6, St Louis, 1997, Mosby.

Guest F: Education and counseling. In Hatcher R and others, editors: *Contraceptive technology,* ed 17, New York, 1998, Ardent Media.

Gynopharma: *Paraguard Cu T 380 prescribing information,* 1988, Gynopharma.

Harlap S, Kost K, and Forrest J: *Preventing pregnancy, protecting health: a new look at birth control choices in the United States,* New York, 1991, The Alan Guttmacher Institute.

Hatcher R: Depo-provera, norplant, and progestin-only pills (minipills). In Hatcher R and others, editors: *Contraceptive technology,* ed 17, New York, 1998, Ardent Media.

Hatcher R and Guillebaud J: The Pill: combined oral contraceptives. In Hatcher R and others, editors: *Contraceptive technology,* ed 17, New York, 1998, Ardent Media.

Hawkins JW, Roberto-Nichols DM, and Stanley-Haney JL: *Protocols for nurse-practitioners in gynecologic settings,* ed 7, New York, 2000, Tiresias Press.

Henshaw S: Unintended pregnancy in the United States, *Family Planning Perspectives* 30:24-29, 46, 1998.

Herman-Giddons ME and others: Secondary sexual characteristics and menses in young girls seen in office practice: a study from the pediatric research in office setting network, *Pediatrics* 99:505, 1997.

Hochschild A: *The second shift,* New York, 1989, Avon.

Jennings V, Lamprecht V, and Kowal D: Fertility awareness methods. In Hatcher R and others, editors: *Contraceptive technology,* ed 17, New York, 1998, Ardent Media.

Kash K and others: Psychological distress and surveillance behaviors of women with a family history of breast cancer, *J Nat Cancer Institute* 84:24, 1992.

Kitzinger S: *Woman's experience of sex,* New York, 1983, Penguin.

Kowal D: Abstinence and the range of sexual expression. In Hatcher R and others, editors: *Contraceptive technology,* ed 17, New York, 1998, Ardent Media.

Lemcke DP and others: *Primary care of women,* ed 1, Norwalk, CT, 1995, Appleton and Lange.

Love S and Lindsey K: *Dr. Susan Love's breast book,* ed 2, Reading, 1995, Addison-Wesley.

MacLauren A: Comprehensive sexual assessment, *J Nurse Midwifery* 40(2):104-119, 1995.

Masters W and Johnson V: *The human sexual response,* Boston, 1966, Little Brown.

Matteson PS: *Advocating for self: women's decisions concerning contraception,* New York, 1995, Haworth Press.

Mishell D: Pharmacokinetics of depo medroxyprogesterone acetate contraception, *J Reproduct Med* 41(suppl.):381-390, 1996.

Moog M and Shah A: Gastroenteritis and diarrheal diseases. In Leppert P and Howard F, editors: *Primary care for women,* Philadelphia, 1997, Lippincott.

National Center for Health Statistics: *Age-adjusted death rates for selected causes of death, according to sex and race: United States,* DHHS Publication No. 97-1232, Hyattsville, 1995, The Center.

*Nurse's handbook of alternative and complementary therapies,* Springhouse, PA, 1999, Springhouse.

Peterson H and others: The risk of pregnancy after tubal sterilization: findings from the U.S. collaborative review of sterilization, *Am J Obstet Gynecol* 174:1161-1170, 1996.

Polaneczky M and others: Early experience with the contraceptive use of depo-medroxyprogesterone acetate in an inner-city population, *Family Planning Perspectives,* 29:174-178, 1996.

Renner P: *The art of teaching adults*, Vancouver, 1994, Training Association.

Riggs A: The common cold. In Leppert P and Howard F, editors: *Primary care for women*, Philadelphia, 1997, Lippincott.

Rizack M and Hillman C: *The medical letter of adverse drug interactions*, New Rochell, 1985, The Medical Letter.

Schrefer S: *Quick reference to cultural assessment*, St Louis, 1994, Mosby.

Schwartz B and others: Nonmenstrual toxic shock syndrome associated with barrier contraceptives: report of a case-control study, *Rev Infect Dis* 2:S43-S49, 1989.

Seidel H and others: *Mosby's guide to physical examination*, ed 4, St Louis, 1999, Mosby.

Sivin I and others: Clinical performance of a new two-rod levonorgestrel contraceptive implant: a three-year randomized study with norplant implants as controls, *Contraception* 55:73-80, 1997.

Small E: Psycho-sexual issues, *Obstet Gynecol Clin North Am* 21:771, 1994.

Speroff L, Glass R, and Kase N: *Clinical gynecologic endocrinology and infertility*, ed 5, Baltimore, 1994, Williams and Wilkins.

Stanhope M and Knollmueller RN: *Public and community health nurse's consultant*, St Louis, 1997, Mosby.

Stanhope M and Lancaster J: *Community health nursing*, ed 4, St Louis, 1996, Mosby.

Stein Z: Smoking and reproductive health, *J Amer Med Wom Ass* 51:29-30, 1996.

Stewart F: Menopause. In Hatcher R and others, editors: *Contraceptive technology*, ed 17, New York, 1998, Ardent Media.

Stewart F: Vaginal barriers. In Hatcher R and others, editors: *Contraceptive technology*, ed 17, New York, 1998, Ardent Media.

Stewart G: Intrauterine devices. In Hatcher R and others, editors: *Contraceptive technology*, ed 17, New York, 1998, Ardent Media.

Stewart G and Carignan C: Female and male sterilization. In Hatcher R and others, editors: *Contraceptive technology*, ed 17, New York, 1998, Ardent Media.

Stratton P, Hamann C, and Beezhold D: *Nonoxynol-9 lubricated latex condoms may increase release of natural rubber latex protein* [Abstract Th.C. 433], XI International Conference on AIDS, Vancouver, July 1996.

Treiman K and others: IUDs—an update, *Population Reports*, Series B(6), 1995.

Trussel J and Grummer-Strawn L: Contraceptive failure of the ovulation method of periodic abstinence, *Family Planning Perspectives* 22:65-75, 1990.

Trussel J and Kowal D: The essentials of contraception. In Hatcher R and others, editors: *Contraceptive technology*, ed 17, New York, 1998, Ardent Media.

Trussel J and others: The economic value of contraception: a comparison of 15 methods, *Am J Pub Health* 85:494-503, 1995.

Trussel J and others: Should oral contraceptives be available without a prescription?, *Am J Pub Health* 83:1094-1099, 1993.

United States Department of Agriculture, Center for Nutrition Policy and Promotion: *The food guide pyramid*, Home and Garden Bulletin Number 252:28-29, 1996, www.nal.usda.gov:8001/py/pmap.htm.

Van Look P and Stewart F: Emergency contraception. In Hatcher R and others, editors: *Contraceptive technology*, ed 17, New York, 1998, Ardent Media.

Warner D and Hatcher R: Male condoms. In Hatcher R and others, editors: *Contraceptive technology*, ed 17, New York, 1998, Ardent Media.

Washington A and others: Oral contraceptives, *Chlamydia trachmomatis* infection and pelvic inflammatory disease: a word of caution about protection, *JAMA* 253:2246-2250, 1985.

Weber B: The well woman visit: prevention and screening. In Leppert P and Howard F, editors: *Primary care for women*, Philadelphia, 1997, Lippincott.

Webster D: Mental health: the politics of self-care. In Neil M and Watts R, editors: *Caring and nursing: explorations in feminist perspectives*, New York, 1991, NLN.

Woods N: Women's bodies. In Fogel C and Woods N, editors: *Women's health care: a comprehensive handbook*, Thousand Oaks, CA, 1995, Sage.

World Health Organization: Education and treatment in human sexuality: the training of health professionals, *WHO Technical report series 572*, Geneva, 1975, The Organization.

World Health Organization: *Improving access to quality care in family planning: medical eligibility criteria for contraceptive use*, Geneva, 1996, The Organization.

World Health Organization: Research on the menopause, *WHO Technical Report Series 670*, Geneva, 1981, The Organization.

Worobec S: Everyday skin, hair, and nail care. In Leppert P and Howard F, editors: *Primary care for women*, Philadelphia, 1997, Lippincott.

Youngkin E and Davis M: Assessing women's health. In Youngkin E and Davis M, editors: *Women's health: a primary care clinical guide*, ed 2, Stamford, 1998, Appleton-Lange.

# CHAPTER 6

## Assisting Women with Health Issues

*"I never lose an opportunity of urging a practical beginning, however small, for it is wonderful how often the mustard seed germinates and roots itself."*

— Florence Nightingale 1820-1910

*What environmental and social issues might threaten a woman's health?*

*Why do women need assistance in dealing with these health issues?*

*How can we create a "safe place" for women to discuss these aspects of their lives?*

*What interventions might a woman expect from us?*

*How might we respond to women who are unable to choose behaviors supportive of their health?*

Women's health is influenced by various issues that women must deal with on a day-to-day basis. These issues are related to, but encompass much more than, their physical well-being. To provide a "whole person" approach of supportive health care we must assist the woman with the psychologic, social, emotional, environmental, cultural, spiritual, and lifestyle factors that affect their lives.

Women are the experts regarding their own lives, health needs, and the issues affecting them. Each woman may be coping with multiple health factors in her life, such as mental distress, chemical dependency, depression, domestic violence, homelessness, eating disorders, occupational hazards, and environmental toxins. Unless we assist her with issues such as these, the potential impact of our other health maintenance and disease prevention efforts will be minimized. Because we work where women come together, in homes, schools, churches, neighborhoods, as well as hospitals and health care settings, we are in a unique position to establish the trust necessary to have women reveal the difficult issues that compromise their health. More importantly, we have the expertise in health promotion, risk identification, and referral information necessary to complement the woman's expertise regarding her own life and health needs.

The issues identified in this chapter have a significant impact on women's health. Emotional health issues, chemical dependency, and domestic violence are often challenging to discuss, and even more difficult to assess and address. It is easy to become angry or frustrated when we do not understand or agree with behaviors a client seemingly chooses.

Past experience, personal history, or family history may influence our attitudes and assessments regarding women affected by difficult health and lifestyle issues. It is important to be aware of our personal attitudes and

217

beliefs. The importance of maintaining a nonjudgmental, nonthreatening attitude when conducting an assessment is stressed throughout health care.

Women face multiple stresses, ranging from economic instability to increasing demands on their time from children, aging parents, career, and community responsibilities. The expertise we bring to the nurse-client relationship is essential to understanding the complex issues that affect women's health and complementary to working together toward positive outcomes. Through appropriate assessment, we have the opportunity to open doors to enhanced health and wellness for women.

## EMOTIONAL HEALTH ISSUES AFFECTING WOMEN

Emotional health and mental health care are not the same across ethnic groups. As we in the United States become more attuned to the fact that we live in a diverse culture, new themes supporting diversity in mental health are developing. They are advocacy and empowerment, participatory decision making, and pluralism and multiculturalism. Clients are increasingly being seen within their reference group (the cohort of people around them), and their assessment and care are being matched to their cultural standards (Kavanagh, 1995).

The importance of advocacy and empowerment to help a person maintain his or her cultural values has been demonstrated through observations of Native Americans. "Most Native American populations shared a traditional orientation to being in the present (rather than to doing and to the future, which is more typical of European Americans), to cooperation rather than competition, to giving rather than keeping, and to respect for age rather than youth (Kavanagh, 1995). Silence, a conservative show of interest (i.e., minimizing eye contact), and deference to personal decision making are considered respectful, caring behaviors.

These concepts and conducts are in direct opposition to and have been devalued by mainstream society in the United States, creating the potential for personal confusion among Native Americans. Stress-producing socioeconomic situations (poverty) accompanied by psychologic, cultural, and spiritual stresses have led to perceptions of loss and depression. Those Native Americans who have been the least acculturated to white society and have maintained a strong tribal identity experience fewer mental health illnesses (Kavanagh, 1995).

### Rates of Mental Illness

The American Psychological Association (APA) (1995) estimates that 50% to 70% of primary care visits in the United States have underlying psychologic factors, and 48% of the general population ages 15 to 54 will experience at least one psychologic disorder during their life-

time (Kessler, 1994). Despite the advances in health and social conditions that have lengthened women's lives, women continue to experience excessive stress and mental health problems, many of which are related to alienation, powerlessness, and poverty (Dennerstein, 1995).

"Rates of mental illness and mental diseases do not seem to vary much among groups when social and economic factors are controlled. There is no conclusive evidence that mental illness rates vary with race or other intrinsic human characteristics, although they are clearly associated with low socioeconomic status, low educational level, separation, and loss" (Kavanagh, 1995).

Women are more often diagnosed with major depressive disorders, agoraphobia, and simple phobia, while men are more often diagnosed with antisocial personality and alcohol abuse/dependency (Fogel and Woods, 1995). Because emotional health cannot be separated from physical well-being, it is important for us to understand the nuances of behavioral health problems that may manifest themselves as physical problems. Emotional health screening should be incorporated into every client contact.

### Theories of Risk

Biologic risk factors, self-esteem, victimization, and situational factors within women's lives place their emotional health at a higher risk. Role satisfaction plays an important role in emotional health. Women who are satisfied with the decisions they have been able to make concerning employment, family, and community roles, are less likely to suffer from emotional disorders than their counterparts who are not happy with their life roles. The multiple roles a woman plays can vary in terms of number, type, quality of transition, requirements, overlap of activities, and whether they are freely chosen (McBride, 1989). The lack of choice some women experience in dealing with their lives may combine with other factors to lead to higher rates of depression, dysthymia, seasonal affective disorder (SAD), eating disorders, somatization, panic disorders, anxiety disorders, and suicide attempts (Robins, Locke, and Regier, 1992).

#### Biologic Risk Factors

Genetic factors appear to have a role in risk for mental health disorders. Female relatives of women with anxiety disorders were found to have an increased rate of anxiety disorders (Noyes and others, 1986). Women who have an increased prevalence of depression among first and second degree relatives have a 25% greater risk of developing the disorder themselves. Among twins diagnosed with clinical depression, only 25% of both fraternal twins were affected as opposed to 70% of both identical twins. The biologic relatives of depressed persons were shown to have three times the rate of depression as adopted relatives of depressed persons (Blumenthal, 1994a).

### Self-Esteem

Women with low self-esteem tend to have more emotional health problems than their more self-confident counterparts. Likewise, women with an optimistic life outlook tend to have fewer emotional health problems than women with a more pessimistic view.

### Victimization

A significant number of women have also been victims of physical, sexual, and/or emotional abuse, all of which have been linked to an increased incidence of emotional health problems. A study in England of 286 women with clinical depression found that 64% of the women had been sexually abused before 17 years of age. Posttraumatic stress disorder is more often caused by rape than any other trauma, including combat (Blumenthal, 1994b). Approximately one half of all chronic pain sufferers are female survivors of abuse, with a significant number of women experiencing chronic pelvic pain associated with sexual abuse.

### Situational Factors

Situational factors also influence women's emotional health status. Day-to-day stress of juggling multiple roles, moves, job factors, or displacement resulting in distance from family and lack of social support may have a negative effect on emotional health. The resulting painful separation, loss, bereavement, and uncertainty have made post-trauma syndrome a possible diagnosis for persons of any age and any traumatic background (Kavanagh, 1995).

Poverty has also been linked to an increased risk of depression. This is significant when considering women's health because approximately 75% of the population in the United States at or below the poverty level are women and children. A substantial number of women and children living in poverty experience higher morbidity and mortality rates (Kavanagh, 1995).

Higher rates of depression are associated with problems in areas of family and personal relationships, finances, and living conditions. Marital relations are also a significant factor. In one study, unhappily married women exhibited three times the rate of depression as married men or single women (Blumenthal, 1994a).

## Self-Care by Women

Despite the aforementioned risk factors, women's choices, opportunities, and natural ways of communicating have been shown to be protective against emotional disorders. Women tend to be more likely to express their feelings and seek out friends with whom to discuss their concerns. This allows for processing, and

often diffusion, of the stressful situation. Social supports—friends, colleagues, family members—are an important adjunct to supporting a woman's well-being (Blumenthal, 1994a).

## Common Diagnoses

### Depression

**Depression** is a term applied to mood disorders, including an entire range of illnesses that vary in intensity, duration, and response to psychotherapeutic intervention. Studies suggest that depressive disorders are twice as likely to occur in women as men (Hales, Rakel, and Rothschild, 1994). Generally, this increase in rate of female depressive illness occurs at about 10 to 14 years of age, or coincidentally, with the onset of puberty.

Women demonstrate an increase in vulnerability for depression and other emotional health problems during periods of physical transitions, such as adolescence, pregnancy, postpartum, and the perimenopausal period (Halbreich and Lumley, 1993; Pitula, 1995). How much this is related to situational change or hormonal change is unclear. This increased risk occurs more often among women who have previously experienced emotional health problems or who have other risk factors.

One study suggests that a situational event such as college attendance is a protective factor against depression for women, because no difference in rates of depression was noted between male and female college students. However, women of the same age, but not in college, had higher rates of depression (Blumenthal, 1994a).

*Classification.* The classification of mental health problems includes a range of problems, from the "blues" and adjustment disorders to major clinical depression and bipolar disorders. Symptoms for a diagnosis of major clinical depression, according to the DSM-IV are included in Box 6-1.

*Depressive Symptoms.* We see many women who may be exhibiting depressive symptoms, but do not meet the full diagnostic criteria for a diagnosis of depression. It is important to assess all women and then provide brief interventions and follow-up referrals to help women with the stress or emotional upheaval they are experiencing, and possibly avert a major mood disorder episode. A simple acronym for remembering symptoms of depression is in Box 6-2.

When assessing for signs of depression, remember that physical illnesses, such as hypothyroidism may create similar symptoms. Therefore, it is essential not to assume that "it is all in her head." An integrated assessment must look at both physical and emotional cues.

*Risk for Suicide.* Suicide is a very real possibility for women experiencing severe depression (Hales, Rakel, and Rothschild, 1994). Women tend to attempt suicide more often than men do; however, men's attempts more

---

### BOX 6-1 *Classifying a Major Depressive Episode*

The woman is at risk for experiencing a major depressive episode if (1) at least five of the following symptoms have been present during the same 2-week period and represent a change from previous functioning, and (2) at least one of the symptoms is either depressed mood or loss of interest or pleasure.

**SYMPTOMS**

- Depressed mood most of the day, nearly every day, as indicated by either subjective account or observation by others
- Markedly diminished interest in all, or almost all, activities most of the day, nearly every day
- Significant weight loss or gain when not dieting, or decrease or increase in appetite nearly every day
- Insomnia or hypersomnia nearly every day
- Psychomotor agitation or retardation nearly every day (observed by others)
- Fatigue or loss of energy nearly every day
- Feeling of worthlessness or excessive or inappropriate guilt nearly every day (which may be delusional)
- Diminished ability to think or concentrate, or indecisiveness nearly every day.
- Recurrent thoughts of death (not just fear of dying), recurrent suicidal ideation without a specific plan, or a suicide attempt or a specific plan for committing suicide

**OTHER CRITERIA**

- The symptoms must cause clinically significant distress or impairment in function
- Symptoms are not due to the direct physiologic effects of a substance (e.g., an illegal drug or medication) or a general medical condition (e.g., hypothyroidism)
- Symptoms are not a normal reaction to the death of a loved one (uncomplicated bereavement)

Adapted from the American Psychological Association: *Diagnostic and statistical manual of mental disorders (DSM-IV)*, ed 4, Washington, DC, 1994, Author.

---

### BOX 6-2 *Depressive Symptoms*

**D**—Depressed feeling
**E**— Energy, lack of
**P**— Pleasure, loss of
**R**— Retardation/agitation, motor
**E**— Eating problems
**S**— Sleeping problems
**S**— Suicidal
**E**— Excessive guilt, worthlessness
**D**—Decision-making problems

---

saving help (Pitula, 1995; Schwenk, 1995; Hirschfeld and Russell, 1997). Although it is distressing to have a woman tell you that she has thought of killing herself, that statement alone does not indicate acute suicide risk. Women who have been depressed for a long time may report these feelings, but usually say they would not act on them because of their family, religious beliefs, or the recognition that they are really searching for relief from emotional pain. Because women are often responsible for the care of their children or aging parents, it is also important to assess if their suicide plans include the homicide of persons in their care.

***Assessment Questions.*** Ask the woman specifically if she has ever thought of harming or killing herself and/or someone close. If she answers yes, do not minimize her pain or feelings. Follow up the initial questions with more detailed questions. What kind of plan does she have for suicide? What are the details of the plan? Has she taken steps to execute the plan? Does anyone else know? Has she tried this before?

If you are working with a woman who has a suicide plan and the means to carry it out, she needs a mental health referral immediately. For instance, a woman who admits to having suicidal thoughts and states that she has been saving her mother's sleeping pills and pain pills to use for that occasion and "almost has enough," is at serious, immediate risk and requires immediate attention and possible hospitalization.

Referral to a behavioral health professional is always in order if you are unsure or suspect emotional health problems. Make arrangements with the woman and her provider so that she may be seen immediately by a specialist capable of exploring her feelings and desires in more detail.

### Anxiety

Anxiety is also a significant emotional health problem, experienced by approximately 20% of persons seeking primary care; however, only one fourth receive treat-

---

often result in death. This is because men choose more lethal means, such as guns, to end their lives, whereas women tend to choose pills or asphyxiation as their suicidal method (Petronis and others, 1990).

Often suicidal individuals give cues that indicate they are contemplating suicide. The woman may tell you that she "feels like ending it all;" "life isn't worth living;" her family, friends, children "will be better off without me;" or otherwise verbalize a loss of desire to live. Never ignore a statement regarding suicide.

It is important to develop a series of assessment questions that you feel comfortable with to allow the woman the opportunity to share her feelings and access life-

ment. Most are seen in the general medical setting and are prescribed antianxiety medications. However, non-pharmacologic therapy may be a more effective treatment for lower risk clients.

***Panic Disorder.*** **Panic disorder** is defined as recurrent or unexpected panic attacks consisting of at least one attack followed by 1 month or more of (1) persistent concern about future attacks, (2) worry about the implications and consequences of the attack, or (3) significant behavior change (Diagnostic and Statistical Manual of Mental Disorders [DSM-IV], 1994). Acute anxiety may be evident in the form of panic attacks, during which the woman may experience shortness of breath, chest pain, palpitations, and other frightening physical symptoms. Box 6-3 lists some of the most common recognition cues for anxiety (Valente, 1996).

Assessment for anxiety must also include a thorough physical assessment because many of the symptoms of anxiety are similar to the symptoms of physical illnesses such as thyroid disease and mitral valve prolapse (MVP). A link between thyroid disease and MVP and the expression of panic is being investigated; however, it is unclear if the risk of panic is increased among women as a response to disease symptoms. Because these diseases are more common in women, careful evaluation for the source of a woman's anxiety is essential (Hales, Rakel, and Rothschild, 1994; Weiss, 1994).

***Assessment Questions.*** Ask the woman specifically if she ever feels anxious. Does she ever experience shortness of breath, chest pain, or palpitations when she thinks about doing something or starts to do something? What seems to cause it? How does she handle it?

## Integrated Assessment Strategies

A person's perspectives are shaped by specific values and beliefs rooted in specific cultures, classes, and time periods. Whether or not we understand the practice that a person employs to promote his or her health, people have reason for their behavior. The symptoms of mental illness are dependent on behavioral expression as defined by the society in which the person lives. Assessment of mental illness judges the appropriateness of behaviors within the context of the environment to differentiate what is normal and abnormal. The same phenomena (e.g., visions and dream states, trance states, hallucinations, delusions, belief in spirits, speaking in "tongues," drug or alcohol intoxication, or suicide) may be judged as normal or abnormal, depending on the settings and circumstances within which they occur (Kavanagh, 1995). Diagnosis requires social competence and use of culture-specific criteria.

Mental health and mental illness are more difficult to delineate than physical illness because of the lack of readily observable, discrete, and organic phenomena. An integrated assessment that includes questions about all aspects of health provides us with the most comprehensive picture of a woman's heath status.

---

> ### BOX 6-3  *Symptoms of Anxiety*
>
> Extreme anxiety, apprehension, or worry
> Shortness of breath
> Palpitations, racing, pounding heart
> Shaking, faintness, dizziness
> Tingling or numbness in the hands or feet
> Fear of dying, going crazy, or loss of control
> General restlessness and agitation
> Extreme irritability or impatience
> Phobias that interfere with normal routine
> Recurrent unwanted thoughts or rituals
> Repeated avoidance of particular situations or places
> Fear of being alone

Many standardized behavioral health, self-assessment tools are available for use in various settings. Screening for emotional health problems does not require large amounts of time. It only requires a willingness to ask the right questions and listen to the answers. Two examples are the BATHE protocol (Stuart and Lieberman, 1994) and the Problem Solving Technique (Women's Healthcare Partnership, 1998). Either of these methods may be easily incorporated into the patient interview to provide a guide for further evaluation.

The BATHE protocol is one means of assessment in the primary care setting (Stuart and Lieberman, 1994). It investigates *b*ackground, *a*ffect, *t*rouble, *h*andling, and *e*mpathizing.

***Example of Assessment using the BATHE Protocol.***
**Background:**
  Nurse: "What has been happening in your life since the last time I saw you?"
  Client: "My youngest daughter left for college last fall. She goes to school half way across the country, and I really miss her."
**Affect:**
  Nurse: "How is this affecting you?"
  Client: "I really don't know what to do with myself all day. My husband works all the time. I used to have the cooking and cleaning and laundry to keep me busy and, of course, all of her activities. Now I have nothing to do."
**Trouble:**
  Nurse: "What is it about this situation that troubles you the most?"
  Client: "I feel useless—like I have no purpose in life anymore. I have no one to talk to."
**Handling:**
  Nurse: "How are you handling that?"
  Client: "Not really well. I sleep a lot. Some days I just don't have the energy to get dressed. Sometimes I go to church if my husband is at home to go with me, but that's rare because he travels a lot."

**Empathize:**

Nurse: "That must be very difficult for you."

Client: "Yes it is. I don't know what to do."

As we can see, this method validates the woman's concern, but stops just short of moving into initial problem solving. The following example illustrates how the problem-solving assessment strategy recognizes the problem and also helps the woman begin thinking about possible solutions.

The problem-solving technique recommended by Women's Healthcare Partnership (1998) discourages passivity and helps the client identify useful coping strategies.

***Example of Assessment using the Problem-Solving Technique:***

**Step 1:**

Nurse: "What has been happening in your life since the last time I saw you?"

Client: "My youngest daughter left for college last fall. She goes to school half way across the country, and I really miss her."

**Step 2:**

Nurse: "How are you feeling about this problem?"

Client: ""I really don't know what to do with myself all day. My husband works all the time. I used to have the cooking and cleaning and laundry to keep me busy and, of course, all of her activities. Now I have nothing to do. I feel useless—like I have no purpose in life anymore."

**Step 3:**

Nurse: "What do you want to change about this situation?"

Client: "I would like to find a way to feel useful again, but I really don't know what I would do. We just moved here right before she went to college, so I don't have many friends."

**Step 4:**

Nurse: "What can you do to address this problem?"

Client: "I suppose I could try to find some new friends. I've thought about doing volunteer work, or even going back to school so I can get a job of my own."

**Step 5:**

Nurse: "What can I do to help you?"

Client: "Do you have any recommendations about places that might need a volunteer? I heard something about a new children's program at the library that needed volunteers. I think it might also be helpful for me to talk to someone about how I am feeling." (Box 6-4)

### Brief Intervention Strategies

Most effective behavioral health interventions provide a multifaceted approach. To be helpful, the woman and her health care provider must collaborate and share an understanding about the choice of interventions.

***Education.*** Education is a key component of any intervention. Appropriate guidance helps the woman understand her emotional health concerns, learn coping strategies to minimize or alleviate symptoms, and recognize risk factors that influence the risk of recurrence. It is important that women and their families understand that depression and anxiety disorders are not an indication of personal weakness or flaws, but are medical illnesses, like diabetes or heart disease. As such, recovery is highly likely when suitable interventions are available. There are many effective treatment options, including pharmacologic intervention, psychotherapy, or a combination of both. About 50% of those affected with depression and/or anxiety recover within the first 6 months of treatment. Although the recovery rate is high, recurrence, particularly in stressful situations, is also a reality. Therefore, the woman and her family should learn about the early signs and symptoms of a recurrence and how to access prompt treatment.

***Supportive Care.*** In addition to education, the intervention should also include supportive care. Although physical symptoms may be the direct result of an emotional problem, it is important to address somatic manifestations and to treat underlying medical conditions. Somatic symptoms occur at especially high rates among clients who are Hispanic and Chinese. It would not be unusual to have a client state she is not depressed but report experiencing headaches, backaches, stomach aches, and other physical phenomena prompted by sorrow and suffering.

---

**BOX 6-4** *Comparison of Assessment Questions*

**EXAMPLE OF ASSESSMENT USING THE BATHE PROTOCOL***

Background: "What has been happening in your life since the last time I saw you?"

Affect: "How is this affecting you?"

Trouble: "What is it about this situation that troubles you the most?"

Handling: "How are you handling that?"

Empathize: "That must be very difficult for you."

**THE PROBLEM-SOLVING TECHNIQUE†**

Step 1: "What has been happening in your life since the last time I saw you?"

Step 2: "How are you feeling about this problem?"

Step 3: "What do you want to change about this situation?"

Step 4: "What can you do to address this problem?"

Step 5: "What can I do to help you?"

*From Stuart MR and Lieberman JA: Finding time for counseling in primary care, *Patient Care* 118-131, 1994.

†From Women's Healthcare Partnership: *Depression and anxiety in women: brief assessment and intervention strategies for women's health providers,* Multiple sites.

We can help the woman to understand the intimate mind-body connection and collaborate with her to develop a holistic plan that addresses her condition. Such a plan may include identifying self-care goals, barriers to self-care, and coping strategies. Simple mind-body techniques, such as relaxation, meditation, and visualization are often helpful in reducing physical symptoms.

*Lifestyle Factors.* Lifestyle factors are also an important component of emotional wellness. Women who exercise have been shown to have less depression and more energy than their more sedentary counterparts. This may be due to the natural release of endorphins during exercise. Proper nutrition also supports emotional health. Often, women who are stressed or emotionally distressed undereat or overeat as a means of dealing with their emotional pain. Suggesting that a woman maintain good nutrition, eat at regular intervals, and that she sit down and spend at least 10 minutes with her meal may be a positive step in self-nurturance. Although these are simple interventions, many women find it necessary to have "permission" to begin practicing self-care.

*Complementary Therapy.* Various complementary therapies are used to treat the mental health illnesses of depression and anxiety. Some come from specific cultural traditions, and others are formulations that have been used for years in other countries. Herbs and light therapy lamps are generally available, and the woman may choose to self-treat her symptoms. A specialized therapist must provide other therapies to her.

A common herb in use today is St. John's Wort (British word for herb). St John's Wort has been used since the first century as an antiinflammatory; diuretic; and, most recently, to treat depression and anxiety. It is a monoamine oxidase (MAO) inhibitor with antiviral activity (Nurse's Handbook of Alternative and Complementary Therapies, 1998). "Eighteen double-blind clinical trials in humans indicate that standardized St. John's Wort preparations are safe and effective in the treatment of depression and have far fewer side effects than conventional drugs" (Foster, 1996). St. John's Wort is not recommended for simultaneous use with other antidepressants.

Light therapy may be used to treat seasonal affective disorder (SAD), a condition in which people undergo extreme seasonal differences in mood between the summer and the winter. Light therapy may be used in different ways and may employ different types of light boxes, light visors, and lamps designed to bring extra light to the eyes (Alternative Remedies for Common Ailments, 1998).

Anxiety may be treated with meditation, herbs, therapeutic touch, biofeedback, or transcranial electrostimulation (Nurses Handbook of Alternative and Complementary Therapies, 1998; Snyder and Lindquist, 1998). The woman may learn and use meditation on her own. The herbs she may try are Kava-kava or Valerian. Kava-kava is a preparation from an herb used for symptoms of anxiety, insomnia, and stress. It should not be used to treat depression. Valerian is also a root preparation used to treat menstrual difficulties, anxiety, and insomnia (Foster, 1996). Other treatments sometimes used for anxiety must be sought from a provider trained in the methods of therapeutic touch, biofeedback, or transcranial electrostimulation.

*Pharmacologic Care.* Many pharmacologic interventions are available to address women's emotional health problems. Because women often present in a medical office with vague physical complaints that are difficult to attribute to a specific medical diagnosis, providers respond by offering medication to handle the symptoms. Women are twice as likely as men to be prescribed psychotropic medications. We must provide careful assessment for behavioral health problems and monitor the automatic or exclusive use of medication.

Pharmacologic therapy alone has been shown to be less effective than pharmacotherapy in combination with psychotherapy (Schwenk, 1995).

It is important for us to assess use of over-the-counter (OTC) preparations because they may interact with prescription medications and compromise effectiveness. Also, women who have outdated prescriptions or OTC preparations available may begin taking those when they start to suspect a relapse, rather than report relapse symptoms to their health care provider. Therefore, a frank discussion of therapy options, symptoms of a relapse, and how to handle such a situation is necessary to support wellness.

### Successful Mental Health Referrals

Successful mental health referrals require trust and collaboration between the woman and her health care team. The successful referral process begins with mutual recognition and agreement that an emotional health problem exists. The woman and her health care provider together decide that the problem is serious enough to warrant further explanation. It is important for the woman and her health care provider to begin to try to identify the problem. What are the symptoms? What makes it worse? What makes it better? What coping skills or therapies have worked in the past? When the woman, her significant others, and her health care provider distinguish a problem and agree to seek further care, the referral process can begin (Stuart and Lieberman, 1994).

To make an appropriate behavioral health referral, we need to know what the woman and her family believe will help. In general, mental health providers believe that mental illness occurs because of a relatively impersonal process of natural causation. "In contrast, members of many cultural groups believe that illness is caused by a supernatural being (a deity or god), a nonhuman being (such as an ancestor, a ghost, or an evil spirit), or another human being (a witch or sorcerer). The sick person in such a case is viewed as a victim not responsible for his or her condition or its resolution"

(Kavanagh, 1995). Depending on the perspectives of the woman and her family, different types of referrals may be needed.

We should ask the woman and her family about resources they are aware of and share with them the ones we know of within the community. In addition, women can be given information regarding 24-hour hotlines, emergency services, support groups, and individual counseling services. In making the referral, it is important to provide the woman with basic information, such as the new provider's phone number, the specialty area of the provider, a list of any special information she is to take with her to the appointment, and other pertinent information. A working knowledge of behavioral health services in the community allows us to collaborate with the client in finding the best fit for the woman and her family, in line with her expectations, roles, and responsibilities and within her economic means and in a short time.

***Who Should Be Referred for Emotional Health Problems?*** Women with complex, moderate to severe emotional health problems; those with a diagnosis of major depression or anxiety disorder; or those with a psychiatric emergency, such as suicidal thoughts, should be referred immediately. Sometimes, however, the decision to suggest a referral to behavioral health services may be uncomfortable or confusing. The providers may feel that you are picking up cues that a problem exists, yet the woman seems to be coping well or does not meet all of the DSM-IV criteria. In general, refer any time you feel uncomfortable with the problem. Most importantly, trust your nursing intuition if you have a "gut feeling" that a problem is complicated and should be referred to a specialist (Stuart and Lieberman, 1994).

 **DISORDERED EATING**

Currently in the United States, women tend to want to decrease weight to become more "attractive," whereas men tend to want to increase weight or "bulk up." The desire to change the body through a change in eating habits becomes dangerous when efforts start to have a negative impact on health.

Men are 50% more likely than women to think of themselves as thin and seldom report dieting. Dieting behavior is a major risk factor in the pathogenesis of disordered eating. Both men and women experience disordered eating. **Disordered eating** refers to a spectrum of abnormal eating behaviors, including bingeing; purging; food restriction; prolonged fasting; and unmonitored use of diet pills, laxatives, or diuretics. Disordered eating is more common among women, with a greater prevalence among adolescents and young adults. Prevalence statistics regarding disordered eating are difficult to obtain, largely because of underreporting and missed diagnoses.

Generally, the prevalence of eating disorders among the general population is estimated to be 0.2% to 1.1%, with 90% to 95% of those affected being adolescents. In one study of high school age girls in ninth through twelfth grade, 14% reported inducing vomiting, 21% stated they took diet pills, and 49% reported skipping meals as a means of weight control (Centers for Disease Control and Prevention [CDC], 1991).

## Cultural Values

Culture-bound syndromes develop because of the expectations of that culture. For example, anorexia nervosa occurs only where food is abundant and a thin body is valued (Kavanagh, 1995). Societal attitudes regarding weight and the high value placed on thinness in advertising influence a woman's body image.

The emphasis our society places on external achievement—whatever the cost—breeds individuals who focus on appearance and accomplishment. The effect of this cultural value cannot be discounted because it influences a woman's perception of herself (Robinson, Bacon, and O'Reilly, 1988). Huenemann and others (1966) conducted a study of 900 high school age girls' perceptions of their body image. In this study, the body fat of all participants was measured annually. During the first year, 25% of the participants were overweight based on objective data. However, over 50% described themselves as "fat" and were concerned about weight. At the end of 4 years, the number of overweight participants had remained stable, but the number who perceived they were "fat" had increased.

White and Asian women are more likely to perceive themselves as overweight, and dieting behavior appears to be more common among white women. Among white women, income level appears to be associated with a proportionate reversal of being overweight during the teen years. That is, teens from families with higher income started out heavier but became leaner adults than their counterparts from lower income brackets. White adolescent females also tend to be heavier than their counterparts of African descent, but become leaner as adults (CDC, 1991).

Female athletes appear to have a greater incidence of pathogenic weight control behaviors than the general population. Young women involved in activities that emphasize appearance, such as gymnastics, diving, and ballet, or endurance, such as distance running, swimming, and skiing, tend to be more at risk for disordered eating (Powers, 1996). Additional internal risk factors include a focus on thinness and ideal body weight and type, life stressors without available coping mechanisms, and an abrupt change in body composition. Young women athletes who excel in their sport may experience a change in performance as they go through the normal body changes of puberty. This is a period of potential vulnerability as the young woman attempts to regain her prepubertal body through weight control. External risk factors include a win-at-all-costs mentality among parents or coaches, overly controlling parents and/or coaches, selected training strategies, negative reinforcement related to weight and body changes, social isolation, and a family history of disordered eating or other behavioral health problems.

## Understanding Disordered Eating

### Choices

Eating behaviors, particularly picky eating during childhood, has also been linked to an increased prevalence of eating disorders. Picky eating in early and later childhood often foreshadows extreme symptoms of anorexia nervosa in adolescent women. When extreme pickiness was present in 12- to 20-year-olds, anorectic symptoms increased within 2 years. Problem meals in early childhood, weight loss concerns, and bulimia symptoms were predictive of bulimia nervosa occurring (Marchi and Cohen, 1990).

### Control

Issues of self and control are evident in the manifestation of eating disorders. Women tend to be more vulnerable to disordered eating during life transitions, such as leaving for college or becoming pregnant. These are generally times when women feel the least in control, and what they do or do not put into their mouth may be the only control they feel they have. After the experience of sexual assault, some women develop excessively controlled eating.

### Self-Punishment

Disordered eating may also be a form of self-punishment—a trade-off for something she wanted. An example of this might be the successful young career woman who moves to a large city (immediately out of college), quickly moves up the corporate ladder, and presents with an eating disorder. Her seeming success now is a disappointment to her mother who values a more traditional path of staying close to home and raising a family as a true measure of success. The woman's feelings of unworthiness for her success may have precipitated disordered eating behaviors.

### Disconnection

Some women who experience disordered eating do not seem to live fully in their psyche in the spiritual sense, but rather experience life as drudgery without interest, investment, love, or affection. Behaviors associated with disordered eating are a way to stay connected with life. Food is used to avoid cultivating personal power; exercise is a mode by which to feel alive; and avoidance of eating is a means to push relationships away (Orbach, 1986).

### Body Cleansing

Behaviors associated with disordered eating may also be perceived as a means of cleansing the body of an unwanted experience. Paying attention to purging methods and other behaviors may give important clues to past history. For instance, the woman who uses laxatives as a purging method may actually be trying to cleanse her body of a violent sexual experience or rape (Powers, 1996). Developmental arrest can occur in an adult as a result of trauma, and self-harming behaviors can result from "anger turned inward" or an "inability to mourn."

## Types of Eating Disorders

### Anorexia Nervosa

**Anorexia nervosa** is an eating disorder distinguished by an intense drive for thinness; incessant dieting efforts; and substantial, often dangerous, weight loss. It is characterized by a rejection of maintaining body weight at the level of 85% of recommended weight, an intense fear of gaining weight, undue influence of body shape or weight on self image, and amenorrhea for 3 consecutive months (Figure 6-1).

Anorexia nervosa may manifest as the restricting type or the binge-eating/purging type. With the **restricting subtype**, the woman simply restricts food intake. With the **binge-eating/purging subtype**, the woman may restrict food intake, but she also experiences periods of binge eating followed by purging. Anorexia nervosa has

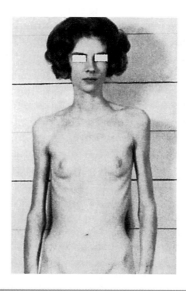

*FIGURE 6-1* • Anorexic woman showing characteristics such as the rib cage. *(From Seidel H and others: Mosby's guide to physical examination, ed 4, St Louis, 1999, Mosby.)*

one of the highest known chronicity and death rates of any psychodynamic disorder (DSM-IV, 1994) (Box 6-5).

Risk factors that may predispose a woman to anorexia nervosa include psychiatric disorders such as obsessive-compulsive disorder (OCD) or schizoid personality traits. Women who have a history of sexual or physical abuse tend to be more at risk, as do women whose families exhibit impaired conflict resolution mechanisms.

Many factors may precipitate the onset of anorexia nervosa or place the woman at a stage of vulnerability. Disruptions in homeostasis, such as a loss in the family or the demands of a new environment resulting from a move, job change, or going off to college, may increase a woman's vulnerability. Likewise, a threat to a woman's self esteem because of job loss, rejection, or relationship problems may be a precipitating event. Some women may respond to the demands of a particular developmental stage, such as adolescence or pregnancy, with increased control issues around food.

Early recognition with appropriate treatment and referral is essential for optimal health outcomes. Physical symptoms may be the most obvious recognition cues. A woman with anorexia may dress in oversized or layered clothing in an attempt to hide her condition or simply to keep warm because her thermoregulatory system may be disrupted by severe loss of body fat. Hands and feet may appear blue as a result of vasoconstriction as the body attempts to conserve heat. The skin may have a yellow tone because of hypercarotenemia caused by the body's diminished capacity to clear carotenoids and decreased tissue storage capacity (Rock and Curran-Celentano, 1996). Hair on her head may be thin because of poor nutrition, and lanugo (fine, downy hair) may appear on the rest of the body. She may report feeling weak or constipated. When eating, she may feel bloated or full early. She may be compulsive about exercise, particularly as it relates to weight loss in comparison to other wellness issues. She may express that she has no friends. This may be a side effect of her efforts to remain thin by distancing herself from food-related activities. On physical examination, she appears emaciated. Assessment may reveal hypotension, bradycardia, evidence of easy bruising, and fractures due to associated osteoporosis (Gidwani and Rome, 1997).

Anorexia affects every body system and may result in several medical conditions. Inadequate iron intake often results in anemia. Renal and cardiovascular problems may occur as a result of electrolyte imbalance. Dental problems may become evident as tooth-building calcium is depleted in the diet. Likewise, osteoporosis may result from the lack of calcium, vitamin D, and other vitamins and minerals necessary for bone regeneration. Recent studies suggest that bone loss resulting from the effect of disordered eating may never be fully recouped (Brooks, Ogden, and Cavalier, 1998).

Women with anorexia may experience alterations in their fertility cycle. As fat stores decrease, estrogen levels and feedback mechanisms are affected, resulting in amenorrhea (Gidwani and Rome, 1997). Ovulation is delayed or ceases, leading to oligomenorrhea (menses occurring at more than 36-day intervals) or amenorrhea (lack of menses) and resultant infertility. In women with severe anorexia, hormonal intervention may be necessary to reinitiate menstrual function (Powers, 1996; Gidwani and Rome, 1997; Mehler, Gray, and Schulte, 1997).

## Bulimia Nervosa

**Bulimia nervosa** is defined as recurrent episodes of binge eating with recurrent inappropriate compensatory behaviors to prevent weight gain and an undue influence of body weight on self-image. It may manifest as a purging or **nonpurging type,** which occurs as binge eating. **The purging type** may take the form of self-induced vomiting and indiscriminate use of laxatives, emetics, and/or diuretics (DSM-IV, 1994) (Box 6-6).

Risk factors that may predispose a woman to bulimia nervosa include obesity during adolescence or previous anorexia nervosa. Women with a history of substance abuse are also at greater risk, as are women with a history of depression. A family history of alcoholism or affective disorder has also been linked to bulimia nervosa. Typically, women who are predisposed to bulimia tend to be high achievers but are passive and nonassertive. Other women may attempt to control their food intake in this way in response to a newly diagnosed illness. Women who are type I diabetics are particularly at risk for this response (Batal and others, 1998).

Often, women who are bulimic do not appear to be underweight. However, other physical symptoms may be evident. She may present with chipped, ragged or discolored teeth, as a result of the stomach acid on tooth enamel during frequent bouts of vomiting. Gingivitis, mouth sores, and parotid gland enlargement may also be present. Calluses may form on the dorsal

---

**BOX 6-5    *Anorexia Nervosa: Diagnostic Criteria***

- Intense fear of gaining weight or becoming fat, even if underweight
- Refusal to maintain body weight at or above minimally normal weight for age and height
- Distorted body image, undue influence of shape or weight on self-evaluation, or denial of seriousness of low body weight
- Amenorrhea for at least three consecutive menstrual cycles in postmenarchal girls and women

Adapted from the American Psychological Association: *Diagnostic and statistical manual of mental disorders (DSM-IV)*, ed 4, Washington, DC, 1994, Author.

surface of the hand, usually at the base of the fingernails (Russell's sign); this is caused by the woman placing her fingers in the throat to induce vomiting. Bloody diarrhea may be present because of gastric irritation from indiscriminate laxative use as a means of purging. Heart burn or chest pain may be related to gastric reflux due to increased gastric acid stimulation. Muscle cramps and weakness may occur because of hypokalemia and electrolyte imbalance. The woman may also experience episodes of fainting, menstrual irregularities, and bruising (Gidwani and Rome, 1997; Batal and others, 1998).

Review of previous medical records usually indicates weight fluctuations. The woman's family or friends may report that she consumes large quantities of food inconsistent with her weight, and/or that she is frequently in the bathroom with the water running immediately after a meal. These are classic cues for actions supporting bulimia. Additionally, family or friends may report large amounts of food or laxatives missing. Money also may be missing, or the woman frequently may have no money. Bingeing is expensive. She may be stealing food and/or money for her binges or spending all of her money on food or medications to aid purging.

The most common medical conditions associated with bulimia tend to be those resulting from fluid and electrolyte imbalance. Metabolic alkalosis, cardiac problems, and sudden death may result from such imbalances. Esophageal rupture is the most significant esophageal complication that can occur. This life-threatening condition results in increased blood loss and requires immediate medical attention. Overuse of laxatives may result in gastrointestinal (GI) problems. Women who use diuretics may experience neuromuscular effects, including weakness (Gidwani and Rome, 1997; Batal and others, 1998).

### Eating Disorders Not Otherwise Specified

Although a woman may present with some of the recognition cues indicative of disordered eating, she may not meet all of the diagnostic criteria for disordered eating. However, it is important to be concerned and provide continued assessment with follow-up care to ensure that her condition improves rather than worsens. This diagnostic category describes disorders of eating that do not meet criteria for a specific eating disorder (Box 6-7).

## Assessment of Disordered Eating

Early detection of disordered eating and risk appropriate interventions can lead to improved health outcomes. If left untreated, all eating disorders can result in serious health problems and death. We must include questions regarding eating patterns in our data gathering, be attentive to warning signs of disordered eating, and aggressively investigate cues that may indicate that the woman has a problem (Box 6-8).

The initial assessment includes general data gathering that may start to provide cues, such as menstrual history, exercise history, 24-hour diet recall, weight history, and body image. The addition of some key

---

### BOX 6-6  Bulimia Nervosa: Diagnostic Criteria

- Recurrent episodes of binge eating in a discrete period of time involving more food than most people would eat
- Sense of a lack of control during eating episodes
- Recurrent inappropriate compensatory behavior to prevent weight gain
- Both binge eating and inappropriate compensatory behaviors occur on average at least twice weekly for 3 months
- Self-evaluation unduly influenced by body shape and weight
- Disturbance does not occur exclusively during episodes of anorexia

Adapted from the American Psychological Association: *Diagnostic and statistical manual of mental disorders (DSM-IV)*, ed 4, Washington, DC, 1994, Author.

---

### BOX 6-7  Eating Disorders Not Otherwise Specified

Diagnostic criteria for females include the following:

- All of the criteria for anorexia are met except that the individual has regular menses
- All of the criteria for anorexia nervosa are met, except that, despite significant weight loss, the individual's weight is still within normal limits
- All of the criteria for bulimia nervosa are met, except that the binge eating and inappropriate compensatory mechanism occur less than twice a week or for a duration of less than 3 months
- The regular use of inappropriate compensatory behavior by an individual of normal weight after eating small amounts of food
- Repeatedly chewing and spitting out (not swallowing) large amounts of food
- Binge eating disorder: recurrent episodes of binge eating without regular use of inappropriate compensatory behaviors of bulimia nervosa

From the American Psychological Association: *Diagnostic and statistical manual of mental disorders (DSM-IV)*, ed 4, Washington, DC, 1994, Author.

---

BOX 6-8 *Warning Signs of Disordered Eating*

- Progressive weight loss to 85% of average weight for height, especially if coupled with persistent concerns of "being fat"
- Enlargement of the salivary glands at the angle of the jaw (parotid glands), resembling mumps
- Deterioration in dental hygiene, especially enamel erosions and caries on upper teeth
- Recurrent complaints of abdominal pain, especially in the area between the navel and breastbone
- Absence of menstrual period for more than 3 months or menstrual periods more than 36 days apart.
- Absence of any sex characteristics by age 14, especially if coupled with failure to gain expected weight associated with growth in height
- Regular use of diuretics, laxatives, or weight loss pills
- Preoccupation with preparing food for family members without eating the prepared foods
- Thinning or loss of scalp hair and increase in downy hair (lanugo) on the rest of the body
- Disappearance of large quantities of food from the house without explanation

From Powers PS: *Initial assessment and early treatment options for anorexia nervosa and bulimia nervosa,* Psychiatr Clin North Am 19(4):639-655, 1996.

---

questions to our intake assessment helps increase our ability to evaluate a woman's risk accurately.

The following key questions introduce topics that may indicate, among other things, disordered eating. The key questions are then followed by examples of more specific probes that may be helpful in gathering additional information and ruling out other causes.

1. Are your menstrual periods regular?
   Have you ever gone for more than 2 months without a period?
   When was your last period?
   Do you take birth control pills or hormones?
2. How much do you exercise in a typical week/day?
   How stressed do you feel if you miss a workout?
3. What did you eat yesterday? or, What do you eat in a typical day?
   Are you satisfied with the way you are eating?
   Is there anything you would like to change about the way you are eating?
   Are there any foods or food groups you refuse to eat?
4. Has there been any change in your weight?
   Are you happy with your current weight?
   If not, what would you like to weigh?
   Are you currently dieting?
   How are you trying to lose weight?

Have/do you ever binge eat? What makes up a binge?
   How much? How often? What ends the binge?
   What do you think makes you start (triggers) a binge?
Have you ever tried to control your weight with vomiting?
   How many times per day?
   Any relation to meals?
   How long has this occurred?
Have you ever tried to control your weight with laxatives, diuretics (water pills), enemas, or diet pills?
   How much? How often? What time frame?
5. Do you have any questions about healthy ways to control weight? (Powers, 1996; Gidwani and Rome, 1997; Kendig and Sanford, 1998)

### Laboratory Assessment

Because disordered eating can affect all body systems and have significant health effects, it is necessary to closely monitor health status. Baseline laboratory data include (1) a CBC and differential to assess for leukopenia and anemias, (2) sedimentation rate to identify occult inflammatory disease, (3) urinalysis to assess for proteinuria and dehydration, and (4) an electrolyte panel. Electrolyte imbalance commonly occurs with disordered eating. The frequency and severity of the electrolyte imbalance depends on multiple factors such as the use of diuretics or laxatives. Because starvation behaviors can affect cardiac function, a baseline electrocardiogram (ECG) is in order, particularly if the woman offers a history of shortness of breath, palpitations, or skipped heart beats.

Additional testing may include (1) thyroid function studies to rule out hyperthyroidism; (2) FSH, LH, serum estradiol, and prolactin levels to monitor hormone status and hypothalamic-pituitary-ovarian axis functioning; (3) prothrombin time (PT) and partial thromboplastin time (PTT) to assess for coagulopathies; and (4) stool for occult blood and stool fat to assess for GI irritation (Gidwani and Rome, 1997; Batal and others, 1998).

## Treatment of Eating Disorders

Disordered eating patterns are psychologically based and once the possibility is identified that a woman is experiencing disordered eating, further evaluation by health care professionals with expertise in the area is necessary. Disordered eating patterns are multifaceted problems requiring a multidisciplinary approach to assessment and treatment. Key team members include the nurse, nurse practitioner, physician, behavioral health specialist, dietitian, patient, family members, and coach if the woman is an athlete (American College of Obstetricians and Gynecologists [ACOG], 1996; Rock and Curran-Celentano, 1996).

Some cases of disordered eating respond well to outpatient treatment and follow-up. Generally, women who have been ill for less than 1 year, who have lost less than 25% of their body weight, do not binge and purge, and have a good relationship with supportive family and friends may obtain treatment on an outpatient basis.

However, more severe cases or cases in which the woman is becoming progressively worse may require hospitalization for a period of time. Women who are at acute medical risk, such as those with cardiovascular or GI complications, require immediate hospitalization. Other indicators that hospitalization is necessary include acute suicide risk and a severe chemical dependency that interferes with maintaining a normal weight, appetite, and eating (Gidwani and Rome, 1997).

The goal of hospitalization is refeeding and weight gain; decreasing morbidity; and, ultimately, improving the woman's quality of life. The American Psychiatric Association (APA) practice guidelines for eating disorders (1993) recommend that the aim of acute care treatment should be to "restore the patient to a healthy weight." However, the shorter hospital stays of today make it difficult to achieve normal weight before discharge. Women who complete inpatient treatment are less likely to relapse compared to women who do not complete the course of treatment (Halmi and Licinio, 1989). Women with anorexia who are still severely underweight when discharged had more severe symptoms and were rehospitalized more frequently (more than 50%) than those who had reached normal weight before discharge (Baran, Weltzin, and Kaye, 1995).

Sometimes it is difficult for families to cope with a diagnosis of disordered eating. They may deny there is a problem or feel that it is only a matter of education, "She only needs to learn what good nutrition is and how to diet safely. Then she will be fine." Others may not understand the severity of the implications of disordered eating and prefer that the primary care provider handle the problem without behavioral health intervention.

We play an important role in providing the information, referrals, and education that may be helpful to families in coming to terms with disordered eating. A nonjudgmental, supportive attitude is essential in working with families. Education must include accurate information regarding health risks and health beliefs surrounding eating patterns. Because many families are familiar with a medical model of primary care, explaining disordered eating in terms of a medical problem is helpful in assisting them to understand. For instance,

> "If Mary had come in complaining of frequent urination, frequent thirst, tremors and dizziness before eating, and had a fasting blood sugar of 225, she would be diagnosed with diabetes. The treatment for that would be a special diet, exercise, and possibly medication. Today, Mary has come in with a large weight loss, a history of eating only animal crackers and water, and vigorously exercising for at least 4 hours daily. She appears very thin, her hair is falling out, and her skin has a yellowish tinge. These are the signs of an eating disorder, which is her diagnosis. The prescribed treatment is a multidisciplinary approach that includes behavioral health intervention, nutrition counseling and follow-up, as well as medical follow-up to monitor her physical health. Just as you and Mary would want to follow all the prescribed treatments necessary to maintain her health if she had diabetes, it is equally important that the prescribed treatment for disordered eating be followed."

Presenting the situation in this manner generally helps a family understand that it is not just that Mary does not want to eat but that she has a medical problem that poses a severe threat to her health. Only multifaceted health care and assistance from her family can help her regain her health and prevent death.

##  UNDERSTANDING ADDICTION

Chemical dependency is an important threat to women's physical and emotional well-being, and it has significant effects on their lives, families, and communities. Women who are chemically dependent encounter multiple, complex health problems, many of which may be attributed to the need to seek drugs (Kendig, 1995). During the years she is fertile, a woman's use of alcohol and other drugs has significant implications for her children. Although the study of teratology and developmental toxicology has been in existence since the early 1900s, it was not until the thalidomide tragedy of the 1960s that the potential harm from medications and other substances crossing the placenta and entering the fetus was fully recognized. Today, we know that the placenta acts not as a barrier, but more as an active transport mechanism, permeable to compounds with a molecular weight of less than 600. Because most medications have a molecular weight of less than 500, approximately 80% of drugs can cross the placenta (Medoff-Cooper and Verklan, 1992).

Addiction is a multifaceted process that is affected by environmental, psychologic, family, and physical factors. Depending on the drug of choice, individuals are affected by two different types of chemical dependency—physiologic addiction and psychologic addiction. **Physiologic addiction** is a result of the body's need for a drug to maintain physical equilibrium. With physiologic addiction, if the drug is not available, the individual will experience physical symptoms, such as tremors, diaphoresis (perspiration), and lacrimation (discharge of tears). Physiologic addiction also includes the phenomenon of tolerance, which is the body's need for increasing amounts of the drug to maintain the same physiologic effects. Drug classifications that result in physiologic addiction include narcotics, opiates, benzodiazepines, and amphetamines.

**Psychologic addiction** is diagnosed when the individual needs the drug to feel normal and to help cope with daily events. A diagnosis of psychologic addiction can be made in the absence of physical symptoms. This type of addiction is most common with cocaine and its derivatives.

## Chemical Dependency

Chemical dependency crosses all racial, ethnic, age, and socioeconomic groups. Approximately 48.6% of women 12 to 35 years of age admit to having used illicit drugs at least once. The incidence of use is relatively similar across ethnic groups, with approximately 35% of white women, 27% of black women, and 24% of Hispanic women surveyed admitting at least one time use (Wetherington and Roman, 1998). Generally, adolescent women tend to use illicit drugs as a result of peer pressure, as a risk-taking behavior, or to deal with emotional pain, whereas elderly women are more likely to self-medicate to help deal with loneliness.

## Gender Differences

There is substantial evidence that women and men use and metabolize the chemicals of abuse differently. Women's physiologic reactions to alcohol, psychosocial factors related to chemical dependency, and socialization regarding alcohol and drug use are unique. Understanding chemical dependency from a woman-focused perspective supports the development of woman-centered prevention, education, and health promotion interventions (Kendig, 1995).

### Alcohol

Physiologically, women metabolize alcohol differently than men do, and these differences make women more susceptible to the effects of alcohol. These physiologic differences in metabolism may explain why women more readily develop cirrhosis and why female alcoholics have significantly higher mortality and morbidity rates than their alcoholic male counterparts (Marshall and others, 1983; Frezza and others, 1990).

***Differences in Metabolism.*** When alcohol enters the stomach, it is oxidized by gastric alcohol dehydrogenase before it enters systemic circulation. Women have less alcohol dehydrogenase than men. Therefore, when a woman drinks, less alcohol is metabolized and more alcohol enters her system. Gastric first-pass metabolism decreases with long-term alcohol use in both men and women, resulting in alcoholic women having virtually no gastric alcohol dehydrogenase. They become unable to digest the alcohol and it enters their system virtually unaltered (Marshall and others, 1983; Frezza and others, 1990).

Women also have less muscle tissue, which contains fluids to dilute the alcohol. Instead, they generally have proportionately more body fat, which retains alcohol. Consequently, women's blood alcohol levels rise faster, and women experience the effects of less amounts of alcohol in a shorter time span than men of the same body weight.

The effect of a woman's normal, daily hormonal fluctuation on the metabolism of alcohol and drugs cannot be discounted. For example, caffeine clearance is slower in the luteal phase of the menstrual cycle, whereas alcohol and salicylate absorption tends to be slower at midcycle (Harris, Benet, and Schwartz, 1995). The use of oral contraceptives may also influence drug and alcohol metabolism.

Conversely, alcohol use affects the metabolism of certain medications. As little as one-half glass of wine has been shown to increase estrogen levels twofold among midlife women on estrogen replacement therapy (Women's Health Advocate Newsletter, 1997).

Elderly women may be more at risk for the effects of alcohol. Decreased body tissue in the elderly results in higher blood alcohol concentrations with alcohol intake. The elderly also experience a slower detoxification time due to a slower metabolism, decreased kidney function, and slower liver function (McMahon, 1993).

***Differences in Health Problems.*** Major alcohol-related health problems occur faster in women, after a shorter history of drinking, and with less alcohol consumption than in their male counterparts. The rate of cirrhosis is higher in women than men, and women who develop liver problems die at a younger age than men (Finkelstein and others, 1990).

Although black women are less likely to drink alcohol than white women are, those who do drink have a higher incidence of cirrhosis than white women do. Native American women have the highest rates of cirrhosis (Finkelstein and others, 1990; National Institute on Alcohol Abuse and Alcoholism [NIAAA], 1990).

***Differences in Treatment.*** Regardless of their socioeconomic status, women tend to have fewer treatment resources available to them than men do. Women are often responsible for their children and their family. The lack of facilities that provide services to women and care for their children is a barrier to treatment for many women. Fear of placing her children in foster care or losing them to "the system" (Department of Social Services), may preclude a woman from seeking chemical dependency treatment. Drug-related behaviors and the tendency to relapse repeatedly may have exhausted her social support network of family and friends, leaving her alone to cope with her addiction.

### Drug Dependency

Chemically dependent women experience more family and relationship problems, and exhibit more codependent behaviors than women who are not chemically dependent. If a woman who is not drinking and drugging is involved with a man who is drinking and drugging, 9 times out of 10 she will stay in the relationship. Conversely, if a man who is not chemically dependent is involved with a woman who is chemically dependent, 9 times out of 10 he will leave the relationship, often leaving her to care for the children as well (Weiner, 1992; Women and Addiction, 1993).

***Differences in Patterns of Use.*** Differences in drinking and drugging patterns may contribute to the difficulty in identifying women who are chemically dependent. Women tend to drink and drug at home, often after the children are in bed. They report "taking the bottle to bed with me and drinking myself to sleep," or "partying after the kids are asleep." Men tend to drink and drug in public, thereby experiencing more barroom fights, driving while intoxicated (DWI) traffic violations, and other behaviors that make their chemical dependency behaviors public knowledge.

Suicide attempts and previous psychiatric histories are more common among women who are chemically dependent (Bigby and Cyr, 1995). Women also tend to have a higher incidence of clinical depression and emotional problems than do men. Factors contributing to a higher incidence of depression, such as low self-esteem, powerlessness, and socioeconomic barriers, may predispose women to substance abuse. Likewise, she may turn to drugs or alcohol to "self medicate" against the effects of depression (Finkelstein, 1990; Weiner, 1992).

***Differences in Assessment.*** Societal attitudes regarding women and chemical dependency may prohibit them from admitting the problem and seeking treatment. Society is reluctant to acknowledge that women, especially mothers, may be chemically dependent. Additionally, society tends to have a stereotypical image of who is using drugs, thereby, labeling a segment of the population, while ignoring the need for assessment and treatment opportunities for all women.

Chasnoff's classic study (1985) of substance-use reporting patterns in Pinellas County, Florida found that while the incidence of positive urine screen for alcohol and illicit drugs among black and white women seeking prenatal care at a public clinic (16%) was statistically similar to those seeking prenatal care in private practices (13%), black women were 9.6 times more likely to be reported for substance abuse than were white women. A study by Moore and others (1989) found that alcoholism was missed by medical staff assessment in up to 93% of patients who had been previously screened positive, with the highest proportion of missed diagnoses among women of higher socioeconomic classes. Buchsbaum and others (1992) found that only 23.7% of female alcoholics were recognized in general medical practice, as compared to 66.7% of men. Societal attitudes, such as "a little drink to calm the nerves or help sleep" may promote the hidden abuse of alcohol or medications by older adults (McMahon, 1993).

## Substances of Abuse

### Licit Drugs

**Licit drugs** are permitted for use by society. They are generally legal to use with some restrictions imposed because of age.

***Tobacco.*** Cigarette smoking is the second leading cause of preventable death in the United States, followed by second-hand smoke exposure as the third leading cause of preventable death (Glantz and Parmley, 1991). Smokers are exposed to 4000-plus chemicals, plus radioactive compounds with each cigarette (Ruppert, 1999). Active and passive exposure to cigarette smoke has been shown to increase liver metabolism of estrogen, thereby decreasing women's estrogen levels, and possibly leading to earlier menopause. Both men and women who smoke have been shown to have an increased risk for cancer of the mouth, esophagus, larynx, bladder, and pancreas; stroke; and lung disease.

Lung cancer is the leading cause of cancer-related deaths among women, since surpassing breast cancer in 1987. This rise in the rate of lung cancer among women was concurrent with the increased prevalence of smoking among women from the 1940s to the early 1960s. Cervical cancer has also been linked to smoking among women, and nicotine has been found in the cervical cells of female smokers on autopsy (Bigby and Cyr, 1995).

Perimenopausal women who smoke are three times more likely to die of coronary artery disease and five times more likely to experience a stroke than women who do not smoke (Rigotti and Polivogianis, 1995). The risk of death from cardiovascular disease, such as stroke, myocardial infarction, or thromboemboli, is increased among women who are over 35 and smoke (ACOG, 1994).

Women who smoke during pregnancy also risk the health of their babies. Helping a woman learn about the risks to a developing fetus may influence her decision to use contraception or decrease her exposure to smoke. Smoking is a major cause of intrauterine growth restriction (IUGR) and is responsible for approximately 30% of all low–birth-weight infants in the developed world. The effects of smoking on infant outcome are so pronounced that in 1985 the CDC labeled fetal tobacco syndrome as a cause of low birth weight. Fetal tobacco syndrome is diagnosed when a term infant with symmetric IUGR is born to a woman who smokes more than five cigarettes per day and no other explanation for the IUGR is evident. Smoking during pregnancy has been linked to an increased risk of maternal hypertension, spontaneous abortion, placenta previa, abruptio placenta, bleeding during pregnancy, and premature rupture of membranes. Fetal and neonatal effects of exposure to maternal smoking include low birth weight and an increased incidence of bronchitis and pneumonia during the first year of life. Sudden infant death syndrome (SIDS) is two to four times more common among infants whose mothers smoke during pregnancy (Rigotti and Polivogianis, 1995; Britton, 1998).

*Alcohol.* Alcohol is the most common substance of abuse in the United States, with an estimated use rate of 8% to 11% among women of childbearing age. Women at risk for alcohol dependence tend to be older; have had children; and are more likely to be single, separated, or divorced (Medoff-Cooper and Verklan, 1992).

Women who are alcoholics have an increased susceptibility to infection, feel unwell more often, and are at greater risk for accidents (O'Neil, 1995). Alcohol consumption has also been linked to cancers of the mouth, esophagus, pharynx, and larynx. Less consistent linkages have been established with liver, breast, and colon cancers (NIAAA, 1990). Recently, the link between alcohol use and increased estrogen levels has received attention as a potential risk factor for breast cancer. Studies have shown that estrogen levels increase twofold when just one-half glass of wine is consumed. Levels rise over 300% with consumption of three glasses of wine (Women's Health Advocate Newsletter, 1997).

Gynecologic health risks associated with alcohol use include amenorrhea, dysmenorrhea, dysfunctional uterine bleeding, significant premenstrual syndrome symptoms, and sexual dysfunction. Studies also suggest a higher prevalence of menstrual dysfunction and accelerated onset of menopause among women who drink heavily. Because repeated, sustained alcohol use interferes with hormonal function, alcohol use may promote the development of osteoporosis. Additionally, alcohol may compound the deleterious effects of other substances. Systolic and diastolic blood pressures of female smokers 49 to 65 years of age become elevated with increased alcohol consumption (1.5 glasses per day) (Bigby and Cyr, 1995).

Helping a woman understand the effects of alcohol on a fetus may influence her to determine how to protect herself from pregnancy or alter her alcohol consumption. The effects of alcohol use during pregnancy are well documented. Fetal alcohol syndrome (FAS) and fetal alcohol effect (FAE) are the leading preventable causes of mental retardation in the United States. FAS is a syndrome consisting of IUGR, organ malformation, cardiac problems, facial malformations, mental retardation, and behavior problems. It occurs in approximately 10% of infants exposed to alcohol. FAE is a condition that has some, but not all of the components of FAS. Maternal alcohol use in pregnancy may also contribute to a low birth weight, neurologic problems, and learning disabilities in the infant.

*OTC Medications.* The woman's report of use of OTC medications provides important clues to her feeling of well-being and addictive behaviors. Frequently misused OTC medications include diet pills, sleeping pills, alcohol-containing preparations such as cough medicine, and antihistamine nasal sprays.

Caffeine, a central nervous system (CNS) stimulant, is found in coffee, tea, soft drinks, and some OTC medications. The cumulative effects of caffeine on women's health are questionable and research continues on this topic (Medoff-Cooper and Verklan, 1992).

*Prescription Medications.* It is estimated that 2 to 4 million women in the United States are addicted to prescription medications. Women, particularly at midlife and older, are at increased risk for addiction to prescription medications. Antidepressants, barbiturates, tranquilizers, and amphetamines are prescribed for women at a rate two to three times more often than for men.

Minor tranquilizers such as Xanax, Librium, and Valium are pharmacologically similar to alcohol. This similarity allows women who are alcohol dependent to "chew" their alcohol in work or social situations, while bingeing on alcohol within the privacy of their home, thus making detection of the problem even more difficult (Finkelstein and others, 1990).

Fatal drug reactions are two times as frequent in women as men and appear to cluster during the fertile years (Blumenthal, 1994b). In the past, many women were given prescription medications during the first trimester of a pregnancy. The Collaborative Perinatal Project Survey of 55,000 women found that 32% were prescribed analgesics, 18% immunizing agents, 16% antimicrobial and antiparasitic agents, and 6% were prescribed sedatives, tranquilizers, and antidepressants during the first trimester of pregnancy (Brill, 1986). With increasing awareness that these drugs may have adverse effects on the developing fetus, the practice has decreased. Now when women are fertile and sexually active, they are advised to avoid taking medications when there might be a possibility that they are pregnant.

Polypharmacy prescriptions (obtaining prescriptions from several pharmacies) can contribute to an overuse of medications or interaction between prescribed medications when a pharmacist is unaware of other medications that the woman may be taking. The elderly are the largest group of consumers of prescription medications, but the prevalence of addiction among this population is unknown. The risk of misuse of medication among the elderly and confusion due to medication interactions can lead to decreased cognitive and motor impairment, resulting in institutionalization (McMahon, 1993).

### Illicit Drugs

**Illicit drugs** are those chemicals that are illegal to obtain or use. Some illicit drugs, such as marijuana, may be legal for research purposes in the United States. Some drugs that are illegal in the United States may be legally used in other countries because the laws vary.

Although both men and women use and abuse illicit drugs, the abuse of drugs by women can create different responses from men and problems that progress differently from men. The effects of these drugs on a pregnancy and fetus are included, so that you will be able to provide a fertile woman engaged in heterosexual intercourse the information relevant to decisions about controlling her fertility.

*Marijuana.* Marijuana (*Cannabis sativa*) is the most commonly used illicit drug in the United States. Recent advances in genetics and growing methods have produced a more potent plant containing stronger substances, particularly of its active ingredient, tetrahydrocannabinol (THC). *Cannabis sativa* is the basis for **marijuana**, which can be smoked in joints or pipes or injected in teas or other foods; **hashish**, which is the dried resin from the flowering and leafy parts of the plant; and **hash oil**, consisting of resins and other juices often spread onto tobacco cigarettes. Depending on the part of the plant used and the way it is prepared, the percentage of THC can vary from 1% in the domestic *sativa* plant to 8% to 14% or more TCH in hashish. The higher the concentration of THC, the greater the risks to the marijuana user (Kolander, Ballard, and Chandler, 1999).

When the smoke is inhaled, the chemicals diffuse into the serum, brain, and throughout the body within 30 minutes and the effects last about an hour. If it is eaten, the effects are usually not felt for 30 to 60 minutes and they last from 3 to 5 hours.

When used for the short term in moderate doses, marijuana produces euphoria and relaxation; however, with the simultaneous altered sense of time, space, and distance, it is unwise to drive or use power tools or devices.

Findings regarding the effect of long-term marijuana use on women's health are inconclusive. However, chronic, long-term use may create several negative consequences on the systems of the body. The effect on the CNS results in reduction of short-term memory, altered judgment, reduced cognitive skills, blurred and impaired vision, altered motor coordination, personality change, and the increased chance of mental illness. Chronic bronchitis, trachea damage, lung damage, pulmonary disease, and lung cancer may develop in the respiratory system because of inhalation. The cardiovascular system may respond to THC intake with increased pulse rate and/or blood pressure, tachycardia, and symptoms of angina. A woman's reproductive system may be altered by disruption of the fertility cycle due to impaired ovulation and menstruation, an increase in levels of testosterone, and possible damage to the female ovum supply (Kolander, Ballard, and Chandler, 1999).

In pregnant women, THC easily crosses the placenta. "Infants born to women who smoke marijuana are likely to weigh less and are shorter in length than infants born to nonsmoking women" (Kolander, Ballard, and Chandler, 1999). In one study, women who used marijuana during pregnancy experienced more prolonged, protracted, or arrested labors than women who did not use marijuana. The marijuana users also had a higher incidence of need for manual removal of the placenta. Marijuana can also be found in the milk of lactating women at concentrations up to eight times higher than maternal serum accumulation (Medoff-Cooper and Verklan, 1992).

*Cocaine.* **Cocaine** is a powder derived from the leaves of a plant, *Erythroxylon coca*. When the effects were first learned it was put into medicines, tonics, and even carbonated drinks. As the developing dependency on this drug became apparent, along with the serious behavioral and health consequences, it was made a controlled substance, with reduced legal availability.

**Crack**, or rock cocaine, is a mixture of cocaine powder and baking soda or ammonia. It is smoked to produce an almost immediate, but brief high (Kolander, Ballard, and Chandler, 1999). The immediate reinforcement results in high addiction potential, compulsive use, and a willingness to do anything to obtain the drug.

Cocaine's ability to decrease a person's natural inhibitions is significantly stronger than that of alcohol, diazepam, and heroin, so its use may release women from inhibitions to engage in sexual activity with multiple partners of both genders, either privately or publicly. A tendency toward high-frequency sex with multiple anonymous partners and the sex-for-drugs phenomenon is more common among women who are addicted to crack (Inciardi, Lockwood, and Pottieger, 1991). This sexual behavior places women at increased risk of sexually transmitted infections (STIs [i.e., sexually transmitted diseases {STDs}]), including human immunodeficiency virus (HIV) infection.

Cocaine may be inhaled, smoked, or injected intravenously. When cocaine is inhaled, it reaches the brain in about 8 seconds, creating a high that lasts for 1 hour. When it is mixed with water and injected intravenously, the woman will experience her high within 30 seconds, and it will last for thirty minutes. If snorted, it takes 3 minutes to reach the brain, and if smoked, it requires 20 minutes. The immediate effects on the body are increases in heart and respiratory rates, blood pressure, and temperature (Kolander, Ballard, and Chandler, 1999).

Physical health risks of cocaine use include hypertension, myocardial infarction, irregular heart rate, stroke, seizures, and intestinal ischemia. Many of the physical problems associated with cocaine use result from its effect on the autonomic nervous system and the resulting vasoconstriction. Fever, respiratory problems, perforated nasal septum, and infections often are related to compromised physical condition. Psychiatric complications and sexual dysfunction are also common (Medoff-Cooper and Verklan, 1992).

Most of the physical and psychologic damage may be reversed when a person stops use. However, permanent withdrawal from use is difficult. Even after the woman is likely to achieve Stage 1 and Stage 2 of withdrawal, the cravings that continue through Stage 3 make it a constant challenge to avoid use (Table 6-1).

| TABLE 6-1 | *Stages of Withdrawal from Cocaine* |
|---|---|
| Stage 1 | (May last several days) |
| | Psychologic depression |
| | Sleeps and eats more than usual |
| | Craves cocaine |
| Stage 2 | (May last several weeks) |
| | Boredom |
| | Anxiety |
| | Lack of motivation |
| | Little pleasure |
| Stage 3 | (May last indefinitely) |
| | Cravings for cocaine when going to places, attending events, or socializing with people associated with former cocaine use. |

From Kolander CA, Ballard DJ, and Chandler CK: *Contemporary women's health—issues for today and the future,* Boston, 1999, McGraw-Hill.

Women should be alerted to the fact that if pregnant, the cocaine will affect her baby within 8 seconds of use. The fetus then experiences the effects of the drug for approximately the same length of time as the mother (Medoff-Cooper and Verklan, 1992). Cocaine's sympathomimetic effects may cause uterine artery spasm during pregnancy and disturb oxygen and nutrient flow to the baby, resulting in preterm delivery and IUGR. Other documented complications of cocaine use during pregnancy include first trimester spontaneous abortion, amnionitis, chorioamnionitis, abruptio placenta, placenta previa, precipitous delivery, and stillbirth.

Fetal and newborn effects of cocaine depend on what stage of fetal development was occurring when the drug was taken, the amount of the drug used, and the substances the drug was "cut" (mixed) with before use. Although there is no clearly defined fetal withdrawal syndrome for cocaine, common clinical signs observed in the cocaine-exposed neonate include irritability, poor feeding, increased heart and respiratory rate, tremulousness, and poor sleep patterns. It is believed that these neurobehavioral patterns are the result of direct CNS insult, rather than cocaine withdrawal.

***Heroin and Opiates.*** **Heroin** is a semisynthetic narcotic produced from chemically changed morphine—a naturally occurring opiate obtained from the opium poppy plant. Heroin was originally marketed as a cough suppressant but was found to be too addictive.

Heroin and opiates are CNS depressants that act on the neurologic centers involved in affective behavior, respiration, and pain perception. The drugs, which are commonly injected, act immediately, resulting in euphoria, a temporary "escape to paradise" within seconds of injection. Just as with other narcotics, it creates a strong physical and psychologic craving for continued use. This may result in other risk-taking behaviors to obtain the drug in increasing amounts as tolerance for smaller amounts develops.

Heroin and opiate use places women at increased risk for poor nutrition, infection, and other health problems. Medical complications associated with heroin and opiate use include infections associated with injectible drug use and shared needles. Intravenous drug users are at greater risk of thrombosis, skin infections, cellulitis, hepatitis, endocarditis, STIs, and HIV.

When drug use is stopped, withdrawal is usually severe and extremely uncomfortable, although not usually life threatening. **Methadone**, a synthetic narcotic developed during World War II as an intended substitute for heroin or morphine, may be taken orally and provides the desired effect for 24 to 36 hours. Methadone clinics have been established to supply the drug to persons addicted to morphine. Although this drug also produces physical and psychologic dependency, as well as tolerance and withdrawal symptoms, the quality and dose of the drug is controlled. With counseling and support, the methadone maintenance programs are intended to reduce the negative physical, social, and legal impact of heroin use while assisting users with rehabilitation of their emotional and professional lives (Kolander, Ballard, and Chandler, 1999).

Because heroin use results in irregular menses, or amenorrhea, a woman who is using may not recognize that she is pregnant. Maternal heroin/opiate use in pregnancy results in fetal/neonatal physiologic addiction. Abrupt withdrawal of the drug may result in fetal death or fetal damage and negative lifelong outcomes. To prevent immediate withdrawal, it is recommended that the woman who is pregnant and addicted to heroin be enrolled in a methadone maintenance program and maintained on the lowest dose of methadone possible to prevent withdrawal and maintain comfort (Hoegerman and Schnoll, 1991).

Heroin and opiate use during pregnancy has been linked to an increased incidence of pregnancy-induced hypertension (PIH), abruptio placentae, preterm labor and delivery, postpartum hemorrhage, and precipitous delivery. Infants exposed to heroin and/or opiates in utero are more at risk for low birth weight, preterm delivery, and lower Apgar scores. These infants also have a tendency toward growth retardation with shorter length and smaller head circumference (Chasnoff, 1985).

Opiates are enzyme inducers that promote the development of surfactant, an enzyme necessary for lung expansion in the newborn. This action results in a decreased incidence of respiratory distress syndrome (RDS) among infants born to women who are heroin or opiate dependent. However, the risk of SIDS among this population is 5 to 10 times greater than that of the general population (Levy and Koren, 1990).

## Assessment Strategies for Alcohol, Tobacco, and Other Drug Use

Prevention of health problems related to the use of alcohol, tobacco, and other drugs begins with the assessment process and identification of use. We must be mindful of the significance of chemical dependency to women and their health, and be willing to look for it and then offer appropriate treatment opportunities.

### Tobacco

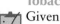

Given the serious effects of smoking on women's health, it is imperative that women seize every opportunity to stop smoking. All health care providers should assess the smoking status of all clients at each health care visit. Strategies for stopping smoking should be discussed with all smokers. The National Cancer Institute (NCI) (1993) has developed a four-step smoking cessation counseling protocol that takes approximately 3 minutes to perform. If the woman is interested in smoking cessation, setting a date to stop smoking and following through is important. We can assist the woman in her efforts to stop smoking through regular contact and support (Table 6-2).

Assisting the woman in developing an individualized plan, which includes identification of goals for number of cigarettes to cut out in a given time frame, time of day each cigarette is to be discontinued, or other explicit goals between visits, may be helpful in supporting cessation efforts (Kendig and Sanford, 1998).

Many local hospitals, health departments, and chapters of the American Lung Association and American Cancer Society offer smoking cessation classes. It is important that we be familiar with community resources (the location, times, contact person, type of program, age of participants, expense, and so on) so that we can make appropriate referrals.

To increase the chance of success, smoking cessation pharmacotherapy is often recommended along with participation in the behavioral smoking cessation programs. However, clients must stop smoking before starting a nicotine replacement regimen. The nicotine may be replaced transdermally with a patch (available OTC and by prescription), with chewing gum (OTC), nasal spray (prescription), inhaler (prescription), or oral tablets (prescription). A woman should be cautioned not to use nicotine replacement products if she has experienced an acute or recent cardiac event, has unstable angina, or serious arrhythmias (Rigotti and Polivogianis, 1995).

### Alcohol and Drug Use

Questions regarding use patterns of both licit and illicit drugs are an essential part of women's general and prenatal health care. Assessing the woman's medical and reproductive health history, psychosocial factors, physical appearance and demeanor, and previous use patterns

| TABLE 6-2 | *Four-Step Protocol for Smoking Cessation* |
|---|---|
| Ask | Routinely ask all patients at every visit whether they smoke and, if so, whether they are interested in quitting. |
| Advise | Send a strong, clear message: "Quitting smoking now is the most important action you can take to live a long and healthy life." |
| Assist | If the client is interested in quitting, set a quit date and provide more information and assistance. If she is not ready to quit, ask what she considers to be the personal benefits and harms of smoking. Discuss short-term benefits and common barriers. |
| Arrange follow-up | This is essential for all clients. |

Adapted from the National Cancer Institute (NCI): *How to help your patients stop smoking (trainer's guide)*, Bethesda, Md, 1993, Author.

may reveal chemical dependency. The CAGE questionnaire is a short assessment tool, without gender bias, that can be administered quickly (Ewing, 1984; O'Neil, 1995). It has been shown to be effective in identifying risk of addiction. The CAGE may be used as a self-assessment tool or added to the routine assessment questions asked during the woman's health visit.

Preceding administration of the CAGE Questionnaire with a statement of invitation, such as "I would like to ask you about your use of alcohol and other drugs," or "May I ask you about your use of alcohol and other drugs?" has been shown to increase the sensitivity of the CAGE Questionnaire to 95% (Steinweg and Worth, 1993) (Box 6-9).

Answering yes to one or more of the questions indicates the need for further evaluation of alcohol and drug use behaviors. Referral for evaluation of alcohol and drug use is indicated by positive answers to two or more of the questions.

***Laboratory Tests.*** Various laboratory tests are also available to assess drug use. Urine testing is the most common. If urine testing is used, it is important to specify which drugs are being tested for and to understand the time frames during which the tests are sensitive. It is also important to take a thorough history to determine if the woman has eaten certain foods such as nuts or seeds, especially poppy seeds, which may confound the test results. It is important to identify legitimate medications the woman may be taking that may show up as positive on the urine test. For instance, Tylenol #3 breaks down into opiate metabolites, which may present as a false-positive for opiates on the urine drug screen.

---

**BOX 6-9** *The CAGE Questionnaire*

The CAGE is a four-item questionnaire designed to assess risk of addictive behaviors.

**C** Have you ever felt that you should CUT DOWN on your drinking/drug use?

**A** Have people ANNOYED you by criticizing your drinking or drug use?

**G** Have you ever felt GUILTY about your drinking/drug use?

**E** Have you ever had a drink or drugs first thing in the morning to steady your nerves or get rid of a hangover? (EYE OPENER)

Ewing JA: *Detecting alcoholism: the CAGE questionnaire*, JAMA 252:1905-1907, 1984.

---

## Woman-Focused Intervention Strategies

Women face unique barriers to obtaining treatment for chemical dependency. Until the late 1980s, most treatment programs were based on a male model of care, and did not address women's need for group support and consensus. Most programs available to women do not address women's additional responsibilities, such as child care, or include counseling for domestic violence and/or sexual abuse, treatment for prescription drug dependence, job training for economic independence, or housing services. Lack of such services, particularly child care, is often cited by women as a barrier to their entering or continuing treatment.

Relatively simple barriers also exist such as program times that are not supportive of the realities of a woman's life. Many outpatient programs require the woman to be present daily from 9:00 AM to 5:00 PM or later. If the woman has school-age children, these requirements may be prohibitive because she will need to be available for her children after school. Because her family may not know of her alcohol or drug use, or it may be the norm in the woman's family and peer group, she often does not have social supports available to help with child care.

It is a misconception that women who are chemically dependent do not care about their children. They care very much and struggle to do what is best for their family. As one woman stated, "I can't go to treatment because I have to be there when my little boy gets off the bus. It isn't safe in our neighborhood, and everyone I know is using (drugs), so I can't trust them not to hurt him. I know I use too, and I may not be much, but I'm the best he's got" (Women and Addiction, 1993).

Important considerations in planning intervention strategies for women include sensitivity to social stigmas and other factors that lead to low self-esteem and feel-ings of guilt related to parenting behaviors. Programs designed to build on women's natural patterns of socialization, women-only groups, female therapists, and contact with women in recovery are most beneficial.

Family therapy is essential in helping the family understand the disease, deal with their feelings, and support recovery. Because the average woman affected by chemical dependency is over 24 years old and has 4 or more children, many women have adolescent or pre-adolescent children who may themselves be at risk for beginning alcohol, tobacco, and other drug use, or early sexual activity. It is important to be attentive to the needs of these children and seek ways to work with the family in providing information and support to avoid high-risk behaviors.

## REALITIES OF VIOLENCE AGAINST WOMEN

Throughout the lifespan, women face the threat of violence. Rape occurs to one in four women, with a peak incidence between ages 18 and 24. Adolescence is a particularly vulnerable time, with teenagers at two times the risk for abuse as children under age 3. It is estimated that 20% of girls are sexually abused, with the peak incidence occurring between ages 8 and 12. Child protective services estimate that 31% of neglect, 42% of child sexual abuse, and 19% of physical abuse cases involve adolescents (Wislows, 1995).

Physical abuse, or battering, is the single most common injury to women, surpassing muggings, rape, and motor vehicle accidents combined, and is the leading cause of violent injury to pregnant women. More than 960,000 incidents of violence against current or former partners are reported annually, and about 95% of the victims are women (Greenfield and others, 1998).

Because acts of violence against women are underreported, it is estimated that over 6 million women are injured annually by their current or former male partner. It is estimated that one fourth of all women in the United States are abused by their partner at some time during their lives (Greenfield and others, 1998). These acts of violence do not occur within any one racial or ethnic group. The three major racial/ethnic groups in this country, Anglo-American, African American, and Hispanic-American, have the same rates of assault from an intimate partner or ex-partner (Campbell and Campbell, 1996).

Although violence is often assumed to occur at the hands of a stranger, the reality is that a woman is more likely to be assaulted by someone close to her—her father, brother, family member, friend, boyfriend, spouse or ex-partner (Crowell and Burgess, 1996). Likewise, the assault is likely to take place in an area where she would typically feel safe, such as her home, school, workplace, or neighborhood. According to the U.S. Department of Justice, three fourths of all incidents of nonlethal violence against women occurs at or near her home (Greenfield and others, 1998).

## Understanding Domestic Violence

Domestic violence is defined as an ongoing debilitating experience of physical, psychologic, and/or sexual abuse in the home, associated with isolation from the outside world and limited personal freedom and access to resources (Flitcraft, 1992). The abusive behaviors are an attempt to gain power and control. They encompass a pattern of intimidating behavior, which may include physical assault; sexual assault; psychologic abuse; emotional abuse with threats against the person, children, or loved ones, and the destruction of personal property; and economic abuse (Flitcraft, 1992) (Box 6-10).

*Physical Abuse.* Battering may include, but is not limited to, hitting, punching, kicking, stomping, shoving, scratching, raping, and any other type of **physical abuse.** A woman is considered battered if she has experienced one episode of abuse at the hands of a partner or ex-partner (Loring and Smith, 1994). Nearly one third of victims of nonlethal violence were victimized at least twice during the previous 6 months (Greenfield and others, 1998). It is important to note that perpetrators of violence against women may be male or female, because lesbians also report battering by their female partners.

Battering is not the only form of abuse inflicted. Emotional and psychologic abuse can also occur, although they are difficult to identify. However, these activities can also be devastating to the victim. Women who have experienced both physical and emotional abuse often report that the psychologic abuse was more distressing than the physical injuries (Loring and Smith, 1994).

*Emotional Abuse.* **Emotional abuse** may include the obvious ridicule, name calling, and verbal harassment or the silent treatment, the manipulations of emotions, repeatedly making and breaking promises, or subverting a partner's relationship with the children. It can also take on more insidious forms, such as restriction of freedom to leave the house, visit friends, or go to church.

*Psychologic Abuse.* Instilling fear, threatening physical harm to self, the children, loved ones, or pets are forms of **psychologic abuse** aimed at controlling the woman's behavior. Violent acts toward pets are often a precursor of escalating violence toward the woman.

*Sexual Abuse.* Sexual abuse, defined as any sexual act by one person on another without that person's consent, is also an important aspect of violence toward women. It may include threats of force or violence, humiliation, or rape. The United States has one of the highest rates of sexual assault in the world, with 25% of women reporting sexual abuse before age 18. The annual incidence of rape is estimated to be 7.1 per

---

### BOX 6-10   *Forms of Domestic Abuse*

**PHYSICAL ABUSE**
- Inflicting or attempting to inflict physical injury and/or illness
- Withholding access to resources necessary to maintain health
- Forcing alcohol or other drug use

**SEXUAL ABUSE**
- Coercing or attempting to coerce any sexual contact without consent
- Attempting to undermine the victim's sexuality

**PSYCHOLOGIC ABUSE**
- Instilling or attempting to instill fear
- Isolating or attempting to isolate victim from friends, family, school, and/or work

**EMOTIONAL ABUSE**
- Undermining or attempting to undermine the victim's sense of self-worth

**ECONOMIC ABUSE**
- Making or attempting to make the victim financially dependent

From Chez N, New York State Office for the Prevention of Domestic Violence: Helping the victim of domestic violence, *Am J Nurs* 94(7); p 37, 1994.

---

1000 adult women. Approximately 13% of women will experience a rape during their lifetime (Crowell and Burgess, 1996). The annual incidence of reported rape in the United States is 80 in 100,000 (Flitcraft, 1992).

Sexual abuse can also include refusal to wear condoms when the woman is concerned about STI transmission or pregnancy. Male partners may fail to inform the woman of HIV infection or other STIs, thus heightening her risk for infection (Flitcraft, 1992).

A *Seventeen* magazine survey of high school age girls found that 83% reported being pinched, touched, or grabbed against their will (Bradway, 1993). This type of sexual harassment and assault accounts for only 16% of sexual assaults that are reported. Sexual abuse is often underreported because of concerns regarding family and friends' reactions to the event, self-blame or feeling that others would blame them, and fear of publicity (National Victim Center, Illinois Coalition Against Sexual Assault, 1992).

Date rape is rarely reported, although it is estimated that one in five women experience sexual assault in a dating situation. The use of the illegal drug Rohypnol (ro-**hip**-nol), also called "Roofies," has increased the reports of date rape. The drug is "colorless and odorless and dissolves quickly in liquid. Within 10 minutes, it can produce a drunklike effect that lasts approximately 8 hours. Effects include loss of inhibition, extreme sleepiness, relaxation, and even amnesia" (Kolander, Ballard, and Chandler, 1999). This drug is being put in women's drinks without their knowing. Once it is ingested, the women are under the influence of the drug and are unable to protect themselves as they are victimized and raped by one or more men.

**Marital rape** is part of the larger picture of domestic violence, occurring as a part of the violence in the relationship. Campbell (1989) found that the majority of women in her study reported that their husbands believed it was their right to have sex whenever, wherever, and however they wanted it, regardless of the woman's wishes or physical condition. Respondents reported forced vaginal and anal intercourse, as well as being kicked, burned or hit during intercourse, having objects inserted into body orifices, or being forced to have sex with animals or while their children watched (Campbell and Alford, 1989). "Wife rape is a significantly negative factor in the lives of clinically depressed and anxious women and is closely tied to a history of child sexual abuse" (Weingourt, 1990).

*Economic Abuse.* Making a woman dependent by maintaining total control over financial resources is **economic abuse**. Examples of this are taking the victim's income or resources, withholding access to money, forbidding access to school or work, harassing her when she is on the job so that her employment is jeopardized, requiring an accounting and justification for all money spent, forcing her to commit welfare fraud, not telling her about family finances, and running up bills that she is responsible for paying.

Currently, no discrete risk factors have been identified as causing battering, although alcohol and substance abuse, low self-esteem, social learning, social stratification, and acculturation have all been explored. Violence against women, like most other issues affecting women's health, crosses all racial, ethnic, and socioeconomic lines.

## Cycle of Violence

The **cycle of violence** continually moves among three stages: the tension building phase, the acute battering episode, and the honeymoon phase (see Figure 6-2). The **tension building phase** describes the time the woman spends anticipating violence. During this phase, conflicts and verbal abuse escalate to the battering episode. An explosion of violence marks **the battering episode**. The **honeymoon period** ensues following the battering phase. During this time, the abuser expresses remorse and promises never to hurt her again. He may shower her with gifts, plan surprises, and be particularly attentive. The batterer's generosity and promises prompt the woman to remain in the relationship, hoping that she can believe his promise that it will never happen again. Unfortunately, the cycle does begin again (Symm-Gruender, 1994). In over 75% of cases, abuse does recur, usually with greater intensity and frequency.

Early in the process, battering may take milder forms, such as hair pulling, pinching, or biting. As the cycle progresses, each episode becomes more violent. Often, the woman can sense the timing of an episode, and arrange for it to occur when the children are away from home or neighbors are not nearby to hear the screams. At other times, she may attempt to avoid the situation by removing herself from the home.

Women who frequently come to the emergency room with vague complaints, bring their children into the emergency room with vague or minor complaints, or present to labor and delivery units with ambiguous complaints, may actually be seeking a safe haven to avoid the violence.

### Abusers

Abusers of women come from all racial, socioeconomic, educational, and professional backgrounds. The abusers tend to be irrationally jealous and patriarchal (Symm-Gruender, 1994). One half of all episodes of violence involve the use of alcohol or other drugs at the time of the act. Abusers and their victims may rationalize the violence because the abuser was "drunk or high" at the time. However, the use of alcohol and drugs does not provoke the attack, instead it lowers inhibitions and allows the person to attack. Often, attacks do not stop even when the perpetrator is sober (McFarlane and Parker, 1994).

### Effect on the Family

Domestic violence affects all family members. Children living in homes where battering occurs are more likely to experience battering or sexual abuse themselves. In 50% of cases where the mother is battered, the same person also injures the children. Even if the child escapes abuse, living in a family in which there is violence between the parents has been linked to increased levels of aggressiveness and antisocial behaviors among the children (Crowell and Burgess, 1996).

Some women think that if they become pregnant their partner will be happy. In fact, abuse during the year before pregnancy was a strong predictor of abuse during pregnancy (McFarlane and others, 1992). In many cases, acts of violence may be initiated or increased during the pregnancy because the woman's changing body does not meet the perpetrator's expectations, or the pregnancy detracts attention from the partner's needs.

### Assessment Strategies

Although abusive relationships and victims of violence share common attributes, the types of relationships and the victims cannot be stereotyped. Women of all educational backgrounds, economic standing, ethnic groups, and relationships report being victimized by abusers who also exhibit diverse backgrounds.

*General Cues.* Women who are victims of battering tend to have chronic illnesses and mental health problems. They may have a history of multiple medical visits for injuries or anxiety symptoms, such as headaches; insomnia; back, chest, or pelvic pain; or choking sensation. In a significant number of pelvic pain cases, the woman will report a history of sexual abuse or relationship problems.

Women who are abused tend to experience a higher incidence of depression and have a higher prevalence of suicide attempts. They may turn to alcohol or other drugs to cope with the abuse. Conversely, women who are chemically dependent tend to experience more violent relationships than women who are not chemically dependent.

Women who are victims of abuse often have low self-esteem and feel powerless to change their situation. Strong feelings of guilt, personal failure, and responsibility for their plight may be overwhelming. As a victim of trauma, the woman who is abused comes to believe that she has no control over the events in her life. Her depression and sense of hopelessness is recognized as a form of post-traumatic stress disorder, similar to that experienced by victims of catastrophe or prolonged captivity (Richards, 1995).

*Screening.* Because every woman is at risk for violence, it is essential that all health care providers assess for domestic violence at each well-woman encounter, at the initial prenatal visit, and at all client contacts when the woman is giving indications or cues of a possible problem. Many health care providers do not screen for domestic violence because of discomfort with the topic, a fear of offending, a sense of powerlessness, a loss of control, and time constraints (Sugg and Inui, 1992). Because we are frequently the first health care providers having contact with a woman, we play a key role in the prevention, detection, and intervention for domestic violence.

All assessments should be done in a private area, away from her partner, children, or friends and family members. This is essential to creating a safe environment that ensures confidentiality and protects her from fear of reprisals or retaliation. Although loved ones may be supportive, they may accidentally let the partner know about the conversation with the health care provider. Children as young as 2 years old may tell the partner what was discussed during the health care visit. When we work in neighborhoods or rural areas we may find this part of the assessment to be especially challenging because of a lack of anonymity. Neighbors are more likely to know one another's daily routines, and often the local authorities may be friends or relatives of the perpetrator, making it difficult for the woman to ob-

tain protection (McFarlane and Parker, 1994). The woman may feel that you know her partner and therefore might not believe that he is a perpetrator. Embarrassment and fear of lack of confidentiality may also be a concern.

Our demeanor and actions can either open the door to help for the woman or establish barriers to disclosing the problem. Because women who are abused often feel powerless, it is important to place her in a position of power as she tells her story. Conducting this interview while the woman is fully clothed and using careful positioning so you are not the dominant person can increase her comfort. For example, in the ambulatory care setting, consider conducting the interview while sitting on a chair opposite the woman, or sitting on the examination stool, looking up at the woman sitting on the examination table. In the hospital setting, sit in a chair next to the woman's bed. Convey concern and believe the woman.

You create a nonthreatening, nonjudgmental atmosphere when you integrate violence assessment questions into all client interviews. Begin this part of the assessment with a general introductory statement such as, "Because abuse and violence are so common in women's lives, I ask all my clients about their safety."

* Do you feel safe in your home? Neighborhood? (Her response may give important clues, not only to domestic violence, but also about the threat of violence from others in the household or her neighborhood.)
* Has anyone you have had a relationship with ever hit, kicked, slapped, or otherwise hurt you? If yes, by whom? How many times?
* Are you currently in a relationship with someone who has hurt you or you are afraid will hurt you?
* Within the last year, has anyone forced you to have sexual activities? If yes, by whom? Number of times?
* Are you afraid of your partner? Are you afraid of anyone else? (McFarlane and others, 1991)

Adjust the questions as necessary to make the woman comfortable. Follow up any cues that indicate she is experiencing a possible problem with questions that help her clarify her situation.

Some health care providers have a woman fill out a self-assessment tool before the interview to be helpful in identifying her risk for domestic violence. It is important to allow her to complete the form privately. While the self-assessment tool may be a convenient method of gathering information in a busy setting, research indicates that it is not as effective as one-on-one questioning by a health care provider. One study found that only 8% of women self-reported abuse on a standardized intake form, as compared to 29% of women who reported abuse when asked the same questions by their health care provider (McFarlane and others, 1991).

In addition to routinely asking questions about violence and/or incorporating a self-assessment tool into practice, it is equally important to be cognizant of cues or signs of domestic violence, and to inquire further if violence is suspected. The following are additional recognition cues that may aid in the identification of domestic violence:

**Injuries** that are recurrent, bruises, scars from blunt trauma, or weapon wounds are typical of physical abuse. Injuries usually begin in proximal, central body areas, such as the chest, breasts, abdomen, pelvic area, and genitalia—areas that could be covered by a bathing suit. The face, head, and neck are also often affected.

In some cases, direct injury may not be apparent, but the woman will exhibit injury sequelae, such as headaches or hearing problems related to head trauma; joint pain; pelvic pain, dyspareunia, or recurrent STIs; recurrent sinus infections or dental problems related to facial trauma; scarring or healed fractures, or other evidence of old injuries.

Injuries consistent with assault that are not adequately explained, such as bruises to the neck, face and upper arms; breast or genital injuries; teeth marks; burns; dental trauma; and clumps of hair missing provide important clues (Figure 6-2).

**Multiple visits for somatic complaints** such as functional GI complaints; chest pain; headache, back, or pelvic pain syndromes; hyperventilation; insomnia; choking sensation; and mood or appetite disorders may be indicative of domestic violence.

**Behavioral health problems** such as depression, anxiety, alcohol or substance abuse; disordered eating; suicidal ideation or suicide attempts may be related to physical abuse.

**Reproductive health concerns,** including unexplained complications of previous pregnancies; recurrent STIs; history of pelvic inflammatory disease; bruising on the pregnant abdomen; frequent missed prenatal care appointments; increase in vague somatic complaints resulting in increased appointments or trips to the emergency room or labor and delivery; and anxiety regarding fetal well-being, could arise from domestic violence–related injuries.

**Situational dynamics,** including the threat of violence, may limit the woman's ability to adhere to health care recommendations and self-care behaviors, thus making her appear irresponsible, unreliable, and ignorant of appropriate health behaviors.

**The behavior of her partner** also can provide clues. Her partner may appear oversolicitous or overprotective, unwilling to leave her side. He may answer questions for her, make her appointments, and otherwise attempt to control contact with the health care provider; he hovers and is conspicuously unwilling to leave her alone with the health care provider. He may also make derogatory remarks about her appearance or behavior (McFarlane and Parker, 1994; Symm-Gruender, 1994; Flitcraft, 1992).

Recognition cues for violence against elderly women may be more difficult to ascertain. Elder abuse or neglect may take the form of physical, sexual, or verbal abuse. Withholding food, care, and other resources, or misuse of the elderly woman's resources or income for personal gain also constitutes abuse. Assessment of the elderly woman for signs of abuse should include: history of the abuse or neglect in the woman's own words, a safety assessment, an emotional and cognitive status assessment, a complete physical examination for evidence of violence, and identification of social or financial abuse (Flitcraft, 1992).

### Interventions

Assessing for abuse carries the responsibility for listening to and following up on a positive response. Disclosure of any type of abuse is both a sign of trust and a cry for help. As health care providers, we serve our clients best not by trying to rescue them, but by appreciating their strengths, being empathetic and supportive, and thereby empowering them. Nonjudgmental listening and psychologic support are the most appropriate interventions when a history of abuse is reported. There is great healing in being able to tell her story. The following three concepts are the most validating to be communicated to the woman at this time:

1. "I believe you."
2. "I am here for you unconditionally."
3. "I am concerned about you." (Personal communication, J. Muerer, Director, The Women's Place, June, 1999).

"Clinical interventions for abused women should be based on four important principles: cultural competence, abuse-stage specificity, childbearing cycle-stage specificity, and empowerment" (Campbell and Campbell, 1996). An attitude of mutual respect and brainstorming together with the woman will help her achieve goals that she must set for herself. She alone can understand and make sense of her situation as it exists and then respond to it. We can offer information, ongoing interest and support, and meet her other health care needs.

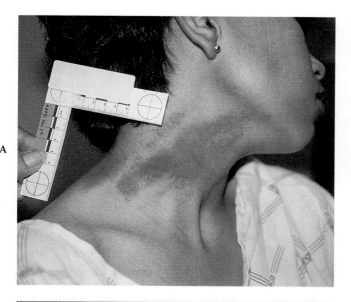

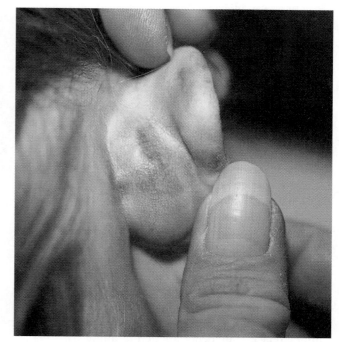

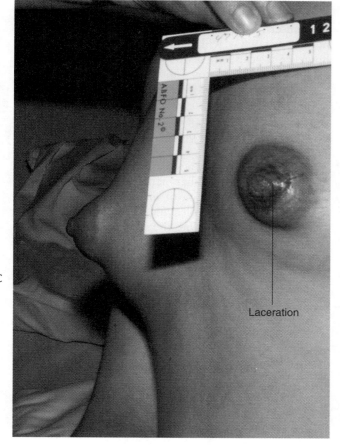

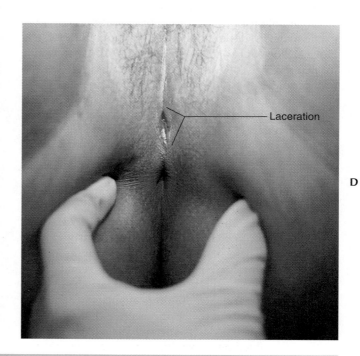

*FIGURE 6-2* • Battered women. **A,** Right neck bruising (ecchymosis); woman was held in a head lock from behind. **B,** Ecchymosis on the posterior aspect of the pinna of the right ear. Ecchymosis is from forceful holding during nonconsensual oral copulation in this white 18-year-old female. **C,** Left nipple and areolar laceration from suction bites in this white 16-year-old. **D,** This white 13-year-old presented with a laceration of the perineum. *(From Girardin B:* Color atlas of sexual abuse, *St Louis, 1998, Mosby.)*

***Treatment of Injuries.*** If the woman has come to us with physical trauma, we must have the injuries evaluated and treated. If other providers are involved in her care, the woman may wish to maintain confidentiality by maintaining a story of walking into a door or slipping and falling down stairs. She must be allowed to do what she feels is necessary to maintain her dignity and safety.

***Documentation.*** If the woman is reporting recent abuse, we must also consider and discuss with her the appropriate collection of evidence to support her case if she decides to report it to the police. Evidence collection may include specimen collection (e.g., pubic hairs and/or semen), physical examination, and photographs of injuries.

If the assessment reveals a positive history of abuse, accurate documentation is essential. Documentation must include details such as frequency and severity of battering; location, extent, and outcome of injuries; with a description of any treatments or interventions. Use direct quotes from the woman in describing the incident, but avoid subjective data that may later be used against the woman, such as "I was so afraid I thought of killing him." Preface statements about the abuse as "(Name) states," and avoid long quotes and descriptions that editorialize or deviate from the problem. Describe any visible injuries, and use a body map (outline of a woman's body) to map where the injuries are.

Obtain photos of the injuries, or document her refusal if the woman declines photos (Braham, Furniss, and Holtz, 1999; McFarlane and Parker, 1994). When asking for permission to obtain photos, it is important to explain to the woman that the photos become part of her confidential patient record and can be released only with her permission. Photos may provide valuable evidence should the woman decide to prosecute now or in the future.

***Safety.*** The primary goals of intervention are to ensure safety and to assist the woman in establishing a feeling of power and control in her life. Her contact with you, a knowledgeable, compassionate health care provider, may be one of the few relationships in which she is validated and respected (Flitcraft, 1992). With mutual regard, you and the client can jointly explore her options. These include remaining in the home and seeking help for herself and her partner; remaining in the home and attempting to avoid situations so as to protect herself and her children against attacks; and leaving her home and the relationship, either temporarily or permanently (McFarlane and Parker, 1994).

Women sometimes have difficulty accepting that this person they have loved and shared their life with may still severely hurt them. Between the acts of abuse the abuser can be very sweet and caring, the person she originally fell in love with. Some women feel pressured to remain with their partner so that the children will not lose a parent, their clothes, toys, home, and friends; financial support; or their health insurance. Others are pressured by the children to "just do better, Mom" or "do what he wants" so they can remain a family. Finding safety by leaving the relationship is a decision only the woman can make. Leaving the relationship is no guarantee that the abuse will stop, and it may actually increase the risk of homicide. One third of female victims of domestic violence were not living with the partner when assaulted (Berrios and Grady, 1991).

Ask her directly about her safety. The current level of abuse may not be life threatening. However, a history of escalating abuse; sexual assault; threats of homicide or suicide; threats or actions against other family members, friends, or pets; gun possession; and the perpetrator's use of drugs or alcohol all place her at increased risk of injury or death (Flitcraft, 1992). A danger assessment tool is useful in helping a woman determine her risk of homicide. The self-assessment tool asks specific questions about the abuser's behavior, how the woman is being treated, if there are weapons (guns or knives) in the home, how the children and pets are being treated, and about the possibility of suicide by either the woman or the abuser (Campbell and Humphreys, 1993). We cannot predict what will happen in each woman's case; however, we can help a woman become aware of an escalating danger and possibility of being killed.

***Escape Plan.*** If the woman plans to return to the situation, it is important to assist her in developing an escape plan. The following key questions will assist in the development of such a plan:

- Can you tell when your partner is nearing a violent episode? What happens during that time? (Early identification of increasing danger can assist the woman in leaving the situation and going to a safe place before the violence occurs.)
- Have you thought about what you will do if he becomes more violent or becomes violent against the children?
- Where does the abuse usually take place? Is there more than one exit?
- If you lock yourself in another room to get away, is there a phone or a window for escape there?
- How will you get away? Where would you go? Is there someone who can help you? (Campbell and Humphreys, 1996)

To reestablish herself away from her abuser she will need copies of documents such as all family social security numbers (his, hers, the children's), birth certificates, pay stubs, bank accounts, insurance policies, marriage license, drivers license, ownership papers of mutual property, and copies of monthly bills. If children are involved she must also have copies of their medical records, birth certificates, school records, and passports or green cards.

Discuss how the woman can hide some money in a safe place to use for immediate expenses if she does decide to leave. If it cannot be hidden in the home, where can she put it so that she has easy access? She will also need to have hidden an extra set of car keys (if she has a car) and house keys, as well as a change of clothing for herself and children.

Having such a safety packet together provides the woman and her children with emergency supplies for the immediate period following escape and a base of information needed to obtain services or to take legal action (Project Safeguard, 1992). One abused woman told of always wearing clothing with pockets and wearing her robe to bed so that she would always have the car key with her in case an immediate escape was necessary.

Because abusers frequently inspect women's personal items and question new information, brochures regarding domestic violence and resources may actually jeopardize the woman's safety. If she feels it is safe to do so, provide her with written information (including phone numbers) for local hot lines and crises intervention services, legal services, shelters, and community resources. Some agencies have very small resource cards that can easily be hidden in the woman's shoe or clothing. Others disguise the information as a friend's phone number, or clinic number. Other sources suggest writing the numbers on a piece of paper that can be rolled and placed in an empty tampon container kept in the woman's purse (McFarlane and Parker, 1994). However, a suspicious abuser may discover the number and call it to find the truth. The woman herself is in the best position to determine how she will remember a phone number and whom she will call for assistance.

### Reporting Abuse

Reporting abuse of nondisabled persons between the ages of 18 and 60 is not mandated in most states. However, at the federal level, health care providers are mandated to report suspected abuse or neglect of persons under 18 years of age; suspected elder abuse, neglect, or exploitation of persons over 60 years of age; and suspected abuse or neglect of any disabled individual. Pregnant adolescents under 18 years old may be considered emancipated minors in some states and are therefore exempt from this law. It is important to understand the mandatory reporting laws regarding abuse in your state and to practice accordingly (Flitcraft, 1992).

Women who are not considered vulnerable because of age or disability have the right to decide what must be done to protect themselves. This option to choose is the opposite of what the abuser has been allowing. Unfamiliar with having choices some women are unsure what to do. Because of the low self-esteem and emotions that are often involved, working with women who are victims of violence can be especially challenging.

Women may be reluctant to report physical, sexual, or emotional abuse because of feelings of embarrassment, guilt, self-blame, or fear of reprisals. It is estimated that a woman who is the victim of domestic violence will return to the abuser seven times before finally leaving the situation. Women who remain in abusive relationships need as much counseling and support as those who choose to leave.

The complexities, emotions, and dangers associated with abusive relationships are difficult to understand. Each woman knows the nuances of her own situation and must be allowed to make decisions in her own time.

## HOMELESSNESS

**Homelessness** is defined as having no permanent residence, which encompasses living on the streets or in a shelter. Women who are "precariously housed" living in poverty, temporarily "doubling up" with friends or family, or living in single room occupancy hotels are also considered homeless. Women and children make up the fastest growing segment of the homeless population in the United States. During the past three decades, the number of women comprising the homeless population has steadily increased from less than 3% before 1970 up to 29% of the current homeless population (Geissler and Braucht, 1999). This is a conservative estimate because individuals who are "precariously housed" are often not identified and counted in studies of the homeless population (Means, 1995).

Homeless women tend to be younger, have fewer legal problems, are more likely to have been previously living with a spouse or children, have higher rates of mental illness, and are more likely to report victimization than homeless men (Geissler and Braucht, 1999). Domestic violence is the most prevalent cause of homelessness for women (Hagen, 1987). While men have criminal records and cite physical illness or injury or job loss as the precipitating cause of their homelessness, women tend to cite family conflict or poverty as their reasons for becoming homeless (Means, 1995).

Homelessness is not synonymous with unemployment or lack of education. Many of the working poor are living at economic margins that force them into homelessness (Mulroy, 1992).

Factors contributing to homelessness are numerous and poorly understood. Prolonged and repeated stressors have been cited as precipitating factors, with homeless individuals reporting up to three times the number of stressful life events during the year preceding initial homelessness than domiciled persons. Profound childhood traumas, such as physical or sexual abuse, foster care placement, and impaired parenting caused by chemical dependency or mental illness, have also been linked to a higher risk of later adult homelessness. Although mental illness is common among the homeless population, not all homeless persons are mentally ill. However, the longer a person is homeless, the higher the risk of developing mental illness.

Women have also been disproportionately affected by events affecting the poor. Societal issues such as high levels of unemployment and lack of affordable housing, coupled with reductions in federal and state day care, housing, and other assistance programs have forced families to pay the majority of their income toward rent, thus making maintaining a household difficult, if not impossible (Bassuk, 1993). Once homeless, women who have their children with them are more likely to be housed earlier than women who do not have children with them.

## Morbidity of the Homeless

Overall, the homeless population has a higher morbidity than the general population. Homeless women have more health problems and less access to care than their counterparts with homes (Geissler and Braucht, 1999). Medical problems in the homeless population include both acute and chronic problems that are both caused and exacerbated by exposure. Gynecologic and reproductive health problems are also more prevalent among this population. Homeless women have an increased rate of sexually transmitted infection, often due to an increased incidence of rape and sexual abuse (Means, 1995). The pregnancy rate among homeless women is twice that of the general population, and they tend to have higher perinatal and infant mortality rates. Inadequate access to prenatal care, malnutrition, and smoking are contributing factors to the poor perinatal outcomes. Chemical dependency, a problem in approximately 30% to 40% of the homeless population, further compromises the health of both the woman and her baby (Hausman and Hammen, 1993). Substance abuse and AIDS occur more frequently among homeless women (Ugarizza and Fallon, 1994).

Chronic illnesses commonly seen in the homeless population include chronic obstructive pulmonary disease, hypertension, congestive heart failure, arthritis, coronary heart disease, liver disease, diabetes, cancer, and seizure disorders (Means, 1995). Offering assistance is a unique challenge for us because the population is transient and health care cannot be a priority when compared with the work of day-to-day survival. Follow-up care with return visits is difficult. Therefore, it is necessary to develop ways for prescribed medical regimens to be incorporated into the client's day-to-day realities. For instance, a diabetic may not have access to refrigeration for insulin, or a safe place to store syringes. Obtaining water to take pills during the day when the shelters are not open may be difficult and results in missed dosages. Access to soap and warm water for cleansing lacerations and abrasions may only be found in a public bathroom.

Other common medical problems include GI problems, urinary tract and other infections, peripheral vascular disease, tuberculosis, skin disorders and infestations, and dental problems. The debilitating effects of situational factors, such as poor nutrition, living in overcrowded conditions or being exposed to the elements, poor hygiene related to inadequate resources, and almost constant walking take a toll on a woman's health in general. Because preventive health care and follow-up are difficult and self-care is next to impossible in the face of more acute day-to-day needs, many homeless women do not seek health care until a situation becomes emergent (Means, 1995; Geissler and Braucht, 1999). Therefore, preventive health care needs, such as Pap smears, should be included in the acute care visit to ensure receipt of these services.

Trauma is the leading cause of emergency room visits by homeless persons. Homeless women suffer from assault, rape, gunshot wounds, fractures, lacerations, burns, and head injuries. Asking a woman how she will care for the wound, who she has to assist her with her care, and where she will go upon discharge may give the first cue of her homelessness (Means, 1995). A plan must then be developed with her that addresses her needs in a way that she feels comfortable. An understanding of and sensitivity to the obstacles presented to the homeless population is necessary to providing the best health outcomes with limited resources.

## Barriers to Care

Homeless women face many barriers to accessing health care. Because they are a transient population, care is accessed at the first available site rather than returning to a prior provider. This creates fragmented care and incomplete medical records. Follow-up is difficult because the woman may not be able to return for visits or have the resources to pay for prescriptions or other recommended regimens. Because homeless persons often are discharged back onto the street, they may require up to 15% to 20% longer hospital stays (Means, 1995).

Sensitivity to the lifestyle of the homeless woman is paramount in providing health care. Think about where she will go to recuperate. Is it a shelter that is open all day so she can rest? Does she have children with her? If so, who will care for them? Is she living in crowded conditions where she may infect others? Can she pay or does she have insurance coverage for a prescription? Is a shower available so she can use Kwell if a lice infestation is diagnosed? If she is living in a shelter, do shelter personnel understand the special needs associated with her condition? Will she be displaced from her current shelter if she fails to appear?

Often, we can intervene to make a difference in the lives of women who are homeless. Because homeless women do not access traditional health care settings, outreach to places where the women live is crucial. Providing services within shelters, soup kitchens, food pantries, and clothing depots can reach the women in need. Many women appreciate the contact, knowledge, and compassion offered by simply talking with them, allowing them to tell their story, and listening to their concerns. Often, we can facilitate referrals to support services, or assist shelter staff to facilitate access to needed services.

 **WORK ENVIRONMENT HAZARDS**

Since the 1950s the number of women in the workplace has steadily increased. Today, women comprise more than 45% of the workforce, and account for approximately one third of occupational injuries and illnesses reported annually (U.S. Department of Labor, Women's Bureau, 1993). In contrast to the 1950s, by 1990 the majority of mothers in the United States worked outside the home. Of those, 75% had children of school age or older and 52% had children less than 2 years old (Atkins, Garbo, and Morse, 1995).

The increasing numbers of women in the workplace has been influenced by economic and relationship issues, as well as social trends. Most working women do so to support themselves or their families. Many are single, divorced, widowed, separated, or have husbands who earn little over minimum wage (Atkins, Garbo, and Morse, 1995). The increased social awareness of women's rights and societal attitudes have changed in favor of full-time careers for women (Roberts, 1995). Despite changing attitudes about being employed, the majority of women continue to work in traditionally female occupations in lower paying jobs than men (Atkins, Garbo, and Morse, 1995; Roberts, 1995). Women tend to be employed in administrative support, health care, education, and service positions. Although more women are entering traditionally male positions, including executive and administrative positions, construction, and skilled labor, they still tend to be the minority.

Although many women work outside the home, they still maintain other roles and responsibilities with primary responsibility for household work and parenting. In addition to work, household, and parenting demands, women may also care for ill, aging, or frail relatives at the end of their workday. King, Oka, and Young (1994) reported negative effects, including increased systolic blood pressures, among older women who worked for pay and also cared for a relative after work.

### Areas of Concern in the Workplace

#### General Health Concerns

Blood-borne pathogens are a special risk to persons involved in jobs that provide direct hands-on care to other individuals, such as health care workers, day care providers, and law enforcement professionals. Service providers, such as laundry and cleaning personnel, housekeepers, and waste disposal workers are also at risk. Because a majority of women are employed in these occupations, this is a significant issue to women's health. Blood-borne pathogens can be transmitted through blood or body fluid exposure via skin punctures and splashes to mucous membranes and nonintact skin. The most concerning infections in this group are hepatitis B, which is transmitted in up to 30% of significant exposures; HIV, which is transmitted in approximately 0.3 significant exposures; and hepatitis C (Atkins, Garbo, and Morse, 1995). Although blood-borne pathogen risks are significant, personnel can take steps to prevent transmission of disease. Universal precautions including use of gloves, face masks, and goggles, as well as appropriate disposal of sharps, can decrease risk. Hepatitis B vaccinations should be available to all at-risk employees. Current legislation in many states requires hepatitis B immunization for children before adolescence because of the risk of sexual transmission. However, many adults have not had access to the immunization outside of the work situation. Boosters should be given to previously immunized persons who have an inadequate antibody response (Atkins, Garbo, and Morse, 1995).

Chemical exposure to dusts, fumes, gases, mists and vapors also poses hazards in the workplace. Dose, concentration, and duration of exposure determine the effects of each substance. Genetic makeup and personal health history may influence the effects of dangerous exposures (Roberts, 1995).

Concerns about video display terminals (VDTs) have surfaced in the past few years, particularly given the increase in use of VDTs in the home and workplace. Evidence regarding physical health problems and adverse pregnancy outcomes due to exposure to electromagnetic radiation is uncertain. However, prolonged use of VDTs has been associated with eyestrain and repetitive motion injuries of the hands and arms. Measures to promote comfort and protect physical health for workers using VDTs for long periods of time include taking hourly rest breaks, access to ergonomically correct chairs, keyboards, and desks, and high contrast screens situated away from sunlight to reduce glare. Exposure to electromagnetic radiation can be decreased by avoiding the sides and backs of terminals and by limiting work to a maximum of 20 hours per week (Atkins, Garbo, and Morse, 1995; Clever, 1999).

Lead is one of the most common chemical exposures for women at work and at home. Exposure can occur in industries, such as battery manufacturing, bridge and steelwork, and automobile repair. More commonly, women are exposed to lead through artistic work or hobbies such as stained glass work, pottery making using lead-based glazes, and home painting or rehabilitation (Clever, 1999). High levels of lead, greater than 25 mg/dL in adults, has been linked to abdominal pain, nervous system dysfunction, joint pain, anemia, and renal problems. Increased spontaneous abortions, preterm labor, fetal death, and damage to the fetal nervous system have been noted with substantially lower parental lead levels (Rempel, 1989).

## Common Illnesses

Contact dermatitis is of particular concern to persons working with chemicals, such as hairdressers, health care workers, and cleaning personnel. The direct effect of irritants such as solvents, detergents, and other irritants or allergens, such as latex and starch powder found in protective gloves, can result in allergic or nonallergic contact dermatitis. Nonallergic contact dermatitis generally presents as a rash that appears within 5 days of exposure. Blistering is more often associated with allergic dermatitis.

Latex allergy has become an increasing problem among health care workers. Symptoms range from contact urticaria to asthma and anaphylaxis. Individuals with symptoms of latex allergies should choose gloves made of vinyl nitrile, polypropelene, or neoprene and avoid other items made of latex such as intravenous tubing (Atkins, Garbo, and Morse, 1995). In their personal life, latex condoms should be avoided. Vinyl condoms are available, although they are more expensive.

As newer buildings are erected for businesses, and many buildings are remodeled for energy efficiency, the risk of "sick building syndrome" has increased. Sick building syndrome presents as irritation of the eyes, nose, and throat; headache; and fatigue, which occurs while working in a particular building (WHO, 1983). An inadequate supply of fresh air; combined with pollutants released from furniture, carpeting, and cleaning materials; cigarette smoking; the entry of outside irritants; and contamination of humidifiers, ductwork, and water-damaged materials with mold and mildew (Atkins, Garbo, and Morse, 1995) combine to make a toxic environment for some people. Those with asthma may become worse when in the building; those without asthma may develop it after being exposed to the environment day after day. Symptoms are usually improved or relieved after being out of the building. Some people may be so seriously affected they must stay out of the building.

## Physical Strains

Low backache is a common source of work disability. Although about 70% of adults experience low back pain at some point, it is more common among persons whose work requires heavy lifting and twisting. Repetitive strain injury (RSI) accounted for a high number of work-related absences by women in 1993. A review of work-related absences showed strains and sprains accounted for 45%, carpal tunnel syndrome for 6%, and tendonitis for 2.1% (Bureau of Labor Statistics, 1995). Carpal tunnel syndrome is characterized by increased pressure in the carpal tunnel of the arm, leading to diminished blood flow and impingement of the median nerve as it passes through the wrist. This syndrome is most common among women whose work requires repetitive flexion and extension of the wrist, particularly if they must use a forceful grip, pinch grip, or vibrating tools (Atkins, Garbo, and Morse, 1995; Clever, 1999). Hobbies, such as macramé, embroidery, and fine needlework can also contribute to carpal tunnel syndrome.

## Work-Related Stressors

Work-related stress can be insidious, producing various physical and psychologic effects. Vague somatic symptoms, such as headaches, GI upset, and chronic pain, and psychologic complaints, such as sleep disturbances, appetite disturbances, and exhaustion, may manifest as a result of stress. It is difficult to separate work-related stress from stress related to other causes. Nevertheless, stress and emotional health issues have a direct effect on the workplace. Mental disorders directly affect the economy through diminished workplace productivity. A recent projection of the economic burden of depressive disorders in the workplace suggests a total cost of $43 million in 1990, with absenteeism alone contributing $12 billion (Conti and Burton, 1994).

## Sexual Harassment

Sexual harassment, any unwanted verbal or physical advances, including sexual comments and suggestions, pressure for sexual favors, career threats, sexual assault and rape, is a concern for women in the workplace. Stress-related psychologic and physical symptoms might result from sexual harassment. Women presenting with symptomatology related to sexual harassment require diagnosis and treatment of physical and emotional problems. An important step in this process is a willingness to listen to the woman and to provide a safe place for her to tell her story. In addition, we can be key in assisting the woman in formulating a plan to address the work situation with the perpetrator, her employer, or the appropriate governmental authorities, and to help her regain a sense of control in her environment. Referral to supportive counseling services may also be helpful for her to regain her sense of self and well-being (Lenhart, 1997).

## Violence in the Workplace

Homicide is the most frequent (41%) cause of women's deaths in the workplace (CDC, 1993). Women are the victims of 56% of nonfatal assaults in the workplace (Toscano and Weber, 1995). Hitting, kicking, and beating are the most common forms of violence endured by women at work, with rape also reported. Women tend to be in lower paying, front-line positions where they are vulnerable to attack because of high visibility, contact with combative clients, and working alone during high-risk hours (Clever, 1999).

### Protecting Reproductive Health

Reproductive health concerns in the workplace affect both men and women. In many families the woman's income and work-related benefits are vital for the support of the family. She may be the head of the household or have a position with higher pay and benefits; therefore, stopping or modifying work may place undue hardship on the family and tremendously increase the woman's stress level. To retain future choices about reproduction, fertility must be protected. A woman is born with all potential ova within her body. Men develop sperm on an ongoing basis. Exposure to toxic agents can affect the nervous system, endocrine function, or sex organs of individuals, resulting in infertility, libido changes, ovulation and menstrual irregularities, and poor pregnancy outcomes (Atkins, Garbo, and Morse, 1995). Several agents in the workplace, such as lead, insecticides, and other chemicals, have been shown to affect spermatogenesis, sexual response, and performance. Likewise, women's reproductive function can also be affected by elements such as lead, mercury, linden, and insecticides (Clever, 1999). Generally, risk is related to the toxicity and dose of the substance.

### Assessing for Occupational Hazards

Although most women do not require a comprehensive occupational health assessment at each visit, simple screening questions can be added to the primary care interview to identify recognition cues warranting further investigation. Atkins, Garbo, and Morse (1995) recommend the WHIP model of assessment. The WHIP consists of the following four questions:

1. What work do you do? (This includes work within the home.)
2. What hazards are you exposed to?
3. What illnesses do you believe you have experienced from these exposures?
4. What protection do you have?

It is important to remember that physical health is not the only aspect of the individual affected by workplace issues. Be sure to also offer opportunity for the woman to discuss any stress or fear of violence she may be experiencing.

Other key elements of the occupational health history include a description of job tasks and current or past use of health and safety practices at work and at home (Hewitt and Tellier, 1996).

In addition to assessment for work-related hazards, it is important for the health care provider to discuss pertinent health issues that may be influenced by work. In the case of suspected toxic exposure, the client may obtain material safety data sheets for review with the provider and otherwise participate in their own care. A discussion of prevention strategies and a reminder to follow work-

place safety guidelines are important parts of client education. Many communities have local teratogen information services that can provide information regarding specific reproductive health risks. We can obtain numbers for local teratogen information services through the local or state health department, or by calling the National Institute for Occupational Safety and Health (NIOSH) information hotline at 1-800-356-4674.

The day-to-day stress of juggling multiple roles, financial concerns, and workplace stressors can combine to overwhelm and emotionally drain women, resulting in increased stress, anxiety, depression, and other behavioral health problems (Clever, 1999).

 ## SUMMARY

Women affected by the health issues discussed in this chapter often feel disenfranchised and disempowered. Working with them around these issues can be challenging because of the multifaceted, interrelated factors that create these challenges to their health. If the negative influences were easy to address the women would have already changed their behaviors themselves. No one enjoys feeling poorly.

Prevention strategies must target facilitating empowered health promotion activities (Kendig, 1995). Basic interactions between ourselves and our clients can foster empowered behaviors. The following steps provide a framework for care that fosters the empowerment process:

1. Discuss personal risk cues.
2. Provide education regarding the physiologic, psychosocial, and relational effects of the at-risk behavior.
3. Express concern for the woman's life situation.
4. Offer referral and assist in reaching needed services (Jessup, 1990).
5. Tell her that she is worth caring about.

Follow the "people first" rule to promote respectful interactions. Remember that the client is a woman first, then a woman who happens to be depressed, chemically dependent, or a victim of domestic violence, rather than a "depressed woman," substance abuser," or "abused woman." This helps place the emphasis of the interaction with the person, rather than the circumstances (Kendig, 1995).

Zerwekh (1992) describes four strategies experienced public health nurses use to foster empowered client behaviors. First, provide the opportunity for small choices to reinforce the belief that the woman does have choices. Second, listen carefully to a woman's story to assist her in determining her needs. Third, discuss realistic possibilities and solutions, and fourth, provide reality-based feedback to promote examination of health-seeking behaviors. This process, which fosters choice among populations who perceive themselves as having little choice or control over their lives, can be applied to nursing care of women in various settings.

Our assistance with risk reduction and health promotion must be based on an understanding of the physical, emotional, socioeconomic, environmental, and spiritual factors unique to women's lives. It is necessary for health care professionals to collaborate with women within an empowerment framework to provide a nurturing, supportive environment that encourages and enables women to gain ownership of their lifestyles and health care decisions.

## Care Plan · The Pregnant Woman Suspected of Being Physically Abused

NURSING DIAGNOSIS  **Risk for Physical Abuse** related to complex etiology*
GOALS/OUTCOMES    Further physical abuse/injury will occur. Woman will leave threatening environment if necessary.

### NOC Suggested Outcomes
- Abuse Protection (2501)
- Family Coping (2600)
- Risk Control (1902)
- Safety Behavior: Personal (2501)

### NIC Priority Interventions
- Abuse Protection Support (6400)
- Abuse Protection Support: Domestic Partner (6403)
- Active Listening (127)
- Anticipatory Guidance (5210)
- Emotional Support (5270)
- Risk Identification (6610)

### Nursing Activities & Rationale
- Establish trusting relationship. *Clients must trust the nurse in order to share personal information and feelings. The nurse's demeanor and actions can open the door or establish barriers to women disclosing information.*
- Provide positive affirmation of worth. *Many women feel that they are at fault and somehow deserve the abuse. Self-esteem is commonly decreased among abused women.*
- Listen attentively when woman begins to talk about own problems. *Disclosure of any type of abuse is both a sign of trust and a cry for help. Assessing for abuse carries the responsibility for listening to and following up on a positive response to questions about abuse.*
- Screen for risk factors (i.e., history of domestic violence, abuse, rejection, excessive criticism). *Because every woman is at risk for violence, nurses must assess for indications of physical, emotional, and sexual abuse.*
- Ask the woman directly about her safety. *It is essential to assess for history of escalating abuse, sexual assaults, threats of homicide, or threats against other family members, pets or friends, gun possession, or use of drugs/alcohol to determine the risk for escalating danger and possibility of being killed.*
- Monitor for signs of physical abuse (e.g., numerous injuries, unexplained bruises, lacerations, welts of the face, mouth, torso) in a private area away from partner. *This provides a safe environment that ensures confidentiality and protects the woman from fear of reprisals or retaliation.*
- With the woman's permission, document evidence of abuse. *It is essential to collect evidence to support the woman's case if she decides to report abuse if it occurs. Evidence includes specimen collections, physical examination findings, and photographs of injuries.*
- Assist with development of an escape plan. *Early identification of increasing danger can assist the woman in leaving the situation and going to a safe place before the violence occurs.*
- Create a "safety packet" in the event escape is required. *Set items such as birth certificates, pay stubs, bank accounts, medical records, money, an extra set of car keys, change of clothing, etc. in an easily accessible location to provide the woman and her children with emergency supplies for the immediate period following escape, as well as with a base of information needed to obtain services or take legal action.*

### Evaluation Parameters
- Acknowledges the threat of physical abuse.
- Relates fears and concerns about possible physical abuse.
- Verbalizes a plan for avoiding abuse.
- Verbalizes a plan for leaving the situation if necessary.
- Identifies safe living environment if abuse occurs or escalates.
- Relates her intent to gather emergency supplies in the event escape is needed.

*The etiology of abuse varies greatly among individuals and is usually complex.

## Care Plan · The Pregnant Woman Suspected of Being Physically Abused—cont'd

**NURSING DIAGNOSIS**   **Risk for Injury: Infant** related to physical abuse
**GOALS/OUTCOMES**   Fetal safety will remain uncompromised.

### NOC Suggested Outcomes
- Fetal Status: Antepartum (0111)

### NIC Priority Interventions
- Risk Identification (6610)
- Surveillance: Safety (6654)

### Nursing Activities & Rationale
- Screen for risk factors. *See rationale preceding nursing diagnosis for screening for risk factors.*
- Prioritize areas for risk reduction. *Prioritizing assists the client with making decisions quickly when the well-being of her fetus is threatened.*
- Teach woman to monitor for alterations in physical status (e.g., change in fetal movement patterns, injuries to abdomen). *She must understand how to monitor for fetal distress in the event that abuse or abdominal injury occur.*
- Assist with development of escape plan. *See rationale for "Risk for Injury: Self."*

### Evaluation Parameters
- Verbalizes the need for protecting fetal safety.
- Monitors fetal movement patterns if abuse occurs.

**NURSING DIAGNOSIS**   **Powerlessness** related to perceived inability to act or to change the situation.
**GOALS/OUTCOMES**   Demonstrates positive control over her situation.

### NOC Suggested Outcomes
- Health Beliefs: Perceived Control
- Health Beliefs: Perceived Resources

### NIC Priority Interventions
- Self-Esteem Enhancement (5400)
- Self-Responsibility Facilitation (4480)

### Nursing Activities & Rationale
- Monitor the woman's statements of self-worth. *Women who refer to themselves in a negative manner or verbalize inability to control the situation are demonstrating their feelings of powerlessness.*
- Encourage the woman to identify own strengths. *Focusing on the areas in which the woman feels in control will increase her sense of power over the current situation.*
- Encourage the woman to accept assistance on others if necessary. *Women need to feel that it is okay to accept help from others in order to protect herself, her children and her fetus.*
- Determine if the woman has adequate knowledge of community resources available to her. *Knowledge of available resources and how to obtain those resources increases the woman's feeling of power and/or control over the situation.*
- Discuss consequences to herself and her fetus of not dealing with her risks and planning escape (escape) if abuse occurs. *Recognition of the possible consequences of abuse (death, loss of fetus) affects the ability of the person to take responsibility for self care and self-protection.*

### Evaluation Parameters
- Verbalizes self-acceptance.
- Verbalizes belief that own decisions/actions control health outcomes.
- Verbalizes perceived support of health care workers/friends/support groups.

## CASE STUDY*

Donna is a 32-year-old woman of Polish descent who has just completed a chemical dependency treatment program. She has been addicted to cocaine and other drugs since her late teens. This is Donna's seventh attempt at recovery. With the successful completion of the program Donna has regained custody of her four children, ages 7, 9, 10, and 13, and they are now living in a women's shelter. The purpose of the program is to

*continued*

## CASE STUDY*

help Donna adjust to regaining her parental role and transition to her own apartment. You are assigned to visit the shelter every week.

Donna likes to "doodle." She shares with you that she had always liked to draw as a child and felt that she was quite good at it. Her family, friends, and teachers were not supportive of her artistic nature, telling her that she would never amount to anything, and it wasn't important. Donna did poorly in school and eventually dropped out. Without an education and a purpose for her life she worked at odd jobs to feed her children and her habit. Each time she has quit drug use in the past, she has been drawn back to drug use by her friends.

- What immediate response will you provide Donna?

- What are her strengths? Where does she face potential problems?

- Because you will be seeing Donna on an ongoing basis for at least 6 weeks, what type of interaction(s) do you want to develop? Why?

- What information do you need from Donna to move forward in support of her?

- What nursing diagnoses could apply? How will you validate these?

- What long-term goals might she have for herself? For her family?

- What short-term goals might the two of you develop for Donna? For her family?

- What interventions may you be able to develop and offer?

- How will these interventions be prioritized?

- How will you evaluate the effectiveness of your interventions?

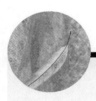

## Scenarios

1. Mary Jo is a 21-year-old woman of African descent who is seeing you for her annual well-woman examination. She has never been pregnant and is taking oral contraceptives. She states that she hasn't had any significant health problems or changes in her personal or family health history since her last visit. Mary Jo currently works at a day care center and is putting herself through college, so "money is tight." She had a boyfriend, but they broke up recently. She is very quiet and controlled during the interview, but does admit to feeling somewhat stressed. She says that she does not feel depressed and is sleeping and eating well. Mary Jo does not make eye contact during the interview process.

However, during the physical examination, Mary Jo appears to become increasingly tense. She keeps her arms folded over her chest, trembles, and then becomes diaphoretic. When questioned further, she begins crying and admits to feeling overwhelmed. She does not want to seek behavioral or mental health care because she does not have insurance and cannot afford to pay for it.

- What will be your first response to Mary Jo?
- What subjective and objective data do you need?

- What nursing diagnoses could apply? How will you validate these?
- What goals might be developed? How will these be prioritized?
- What interventions may you offer?
- How will you evaluate the effectiveness of your interventions?

2. Loretta is a 32-year-old woman of European descent who has had one child. She has come with a chief complaint of pelvic pain for the past 1½ years, ever since the birth of her daughter. She reports that prior providers have told her that nothing is physically wrong, although her pelvic muscles may be a little weakened from childbirth. Each suggested that she do Kegel exercises. You complete Loretta's history, focusing on factors that may be related to this pain. Loretta states that overall her life is pretty hectic. In response to the domestic violence screening questions she states that no one is hurting her. When asked about her sexual activity she says that it is fine.

The nurse practitioner continues the history and does the physical examination. She finds bruises on the back of Loretta's arms. Loretta's pelvic examination is normal. The NP reviewed with Loretta how to do the Kegel exercises and had her tighten her vagina around the NP's inserted finger to assess the strength of the muscles. She has a weak muscle response, so the NP encourages her to continue to do Kegel exercises. The NP tells you of her findings and the interventions she provided. She now wants you to see Loretta before she leaves and to set up future appointments.

- What will be your first response to Loretta?
- What subjective and objective data do you need?
- What nursing diagnoses could apply? How will you validate these?
- What goals might be developed? How will these be prioritized?
- What interventions may you offer?
- How will you evaluate the effectiveness of your interventions?

3. Teri is a 14-year-old Caucasian girl who was brought to the clinic by her mother. Her mother is concerned because Teri is eating very little and is preoccupied with her weight. Teri is dressed in baggy khakis and a sweater with a loose-fitting jacket. During the interview with her mother present, she sits with her shoulders hunched forward, speaks only when spoken to, and does not make eye contact. She lives with her mother, father, older sister, and younger brother. She had a boyfriend, but they broke up about 2 months ago. She states that she is not sexually active. Her 24-hour diet recall, indicates that Teri has been eating about 800 calories per day, or less. Teri says that sometimes she gets sick after she eats and has to vomit. Teri and her mother request nutritional counseling for her "sensitive stomach."

- What will be your first response to Teri?
- What subjective and objective data do you need?
- What nursing diagnoses could apply? How will you validate these?
- What goals might be developed? How will these be prioritized?
- What interventions may you offer?
- How will you evaluate the effectiveness of your interventions?

4. Kelly is a 20-year-old student who lives in university housing. A junior, she has been active in various activities since coming to college 2 years ago. Lately her friends have been concerned because she is going to class less and less. During the past weekend she has not gone to the dining hall to eat. She will not answer the door when someone knocks. Her friends inform the resident hall supervisor who calls student health services. You are sent to the dorm to meet with Kelly and assess her situation. The resident hall supervisor lets you into her room. You find Kelly curled up in blankets on her bed.

- What will be your first action with Kelly?
- What subjective and objective data do you need?
- What nursing diagnoses could apply? How will you validate these?
- What goals might be developed? How will these be prioritized?
- What interventions may you offer?
- How will you evaluate the effectiveness of your interventions?

5. Raeanne has come in for her annual examination and renewal of her prescription for oral contraception. During her health history interview she reports that she is tired all the time, is having problems concentrating, and has frequent mood swings. When you ask if she drinks alcohol, she replies, "just every weekend." Further questioning reveals that her "weekends start on Thursday evenings" and she experiences frequent hangovers. She says that she will probably be leaving school because she has failed her classes as a result of chronic absenteeism.

- What will be your approach with Raeanne?
- What subjective and objective data do you need?
- What nursing diagnoses could apply? How will you validate these?
- What goals might be developed? How will these be prioritized?
- What interventions may you offer?
- How will you evaluate the effectiveness of your interventions?

6. When doing blood pressure screening at the mall you meet Maggy. She is a 27-year-old woman dressed in jeans and a sweatshirt. She is carrying a large shopping bag with her. When you check Maggy's blood pressure you discover that it is 182/89. You

explain what your findings are and the implications for Maggy's health.

You ask her when she had it last checked and she does not remember. You ask who she generally sees for health care and she says she goes to the clinic, but she does not see anyone in particular. She also does not remember when she had her last physical examination.

- What will be your approach with Maggy?
- What subjective and objective data do you need?
- What nursing diagnoses could apply? How will you validate these?
- What goals might be developed? How will these be prioritized?
- What interventions may you offer?
- How will you evaluate the effectiveness of your interventions?

---

7. Ashley works in the office area of an autobody and repair shop. She is seeing you today as part of her annual examination. She mentions that she is having headaches on Monday through Friday at work. She says, "It must be the stress, because they go away on Saturday." You learn that Ashley works at a computer terminal for about 5 hours a day. The rest of her time is taken up by writing up the bills for the day's work with the manager of the body shop, which is right next to her office.

- What will be your first questions for Ashley?
- What subjective and objective data do you need?
- What nursing diagnoses could apply? How will you validate these?
- What goals might be developed? How will these be prioritized?
- What interventions may you offer?
- How will you evaluate the effectiveness of your interventions?

---

8. Amita, a 24-year-old woman, comes to the urgent care facility. She appears anxious and upset. You take her into a private room and ask her how you may help. She tells you, "I've been raped," and starts to cry. You lean towards her in an empathetic manner and wait. She says, "It was probably my fault. My mother told me not to wear this skirt."

- What will be your first response to Amita?
- What subjective and objective data do you need?
- What nursing diagnoses could apply? How will you validate these?
- What goals might be developed? How will these be prioritized?
- What interventions may you offer?
- How will you evaluate the effectiveness of your interventions?

## REFERENCES

*Alternative Remedies for Common Ailments*: Alexandria, VA, 1998, Time-Life Books.

American College of Obstetricians and Gynecologists (ACOG): *Hormonal contraception* (ACOG Technical Bulletin No. 198), Washington, DC, 1994, The College.

American College of Obstetricians and Gynecologists (ACOG): *Nutrition and women* (ACOG Educational Bulletin No. 229), Washington, DC, 1996, The College.

American Psychiatric Association (APA): Practice guideline for eating disorders, *Am J Psychiatr* 150:212-228, 1993.

American Psychological Association (APA): *Practice directorate*, Washington, DC, 1995, APA.

Atkins EH, Garbo MJ, and Morse EP: Occupational and environmental health for women. In Carr PL, Freund KM, and Somani S, editors: *The medical care of women*, Philadelphia, 1995, W.B. Saunders.

Baran SA, Weltzin TE, and Kaye WH: Low discharge weight and outcome in anorexia nervosa, *Am J Psychol* 152:1070-1072, 1995.

Bassuk E: Social and economic hardships of homeless and other poor women, *J Orthopsychiatr*, 63(3):340, 1993.

Batal H and others: Bulimia: a primary care approach, *J Women Health* 7(2):211-220, 1998.

Berrios D and Grady D: Domestic violence risk factors and outcomes, *West J Med* 155:133-135, 1991.

Bigby JA and Cyr MG: Alcohol and drug abuse. In Carlson KJ and Eisenstat SA, editors: *Primary care of women*, St Louis, 1995, Mosby.

Blumenthal S: Women and depression, *J Women Health* 3(6a):467-479, 1994a.

Blumenthal S: Issues in women's mental health, *J Women Health* 3(6a):453-458, 1994b.

Bradway B: *Sexual assault is a hate crime*, Coalition Commentary, Illinois Coalition Against Sexual Assault, Summer 1993.

Braham R, Furniss KK, and Holtz H: *Nursing protocol on domestic violence*, Florham Park, NJ, Jersey Battered Women's Services, Inc, 1999.

Brill JC: Drugs in pregnancy, *Topic Emerg Med* 8:84-88, 1986.

Britton GA: A review of women and tobacco: have we come such a long way?, *JOGNN* 27(3):241-249, 1998.

Brooks ER, Ogden BW, and Cavalier DS: Compromised bone density 11.4 years after diagnosis of anorexia nervosa, *J Women Health* 7(5):567-574, 1998.

Buchsbaum DG and others: Physician detection of drinking problems in patients attending a general medicine practice, *J Gen Int Med* 7:517, 1992.

Bureau of Labor Statistics, U.S. Department of Labor: Profile of women workers: number and percent of nonfatal occupational injuries and illnesses with stays away from work by selected worker and case characteristic, 1993-cont, *The survey of occupational injuries and illnesses*, April 6, 1995.

Campbell J: Women's response to sexual abuse in intimate relationships, *Women Health Care Internat* 10:335-346, 1989.

Campbell J and Alford P: The dark consequences of marital rape, *AJN* 89:946-949, 1989.

Campbell JC and Campbell DW: Cultural competence in the care of abused women, *J Nurse-Midwife* 41(6):457-462, 1996.

Campbell JC and Humphreys J: *Nursing care of survivors of family violence*, St Louis, 1996, Mosby.

Centers for Disease Control and Prevention: Body weight perceptions and selected weight management goals and practices of high school students—United States, *MMWR* 40:741, 747-750, 1991.

Centers for Disease Control and Prevention: Homicide in the workplace, Doc. No. 705003:1-2, Dec 5, 1993.

Chasnoff IJ: Effect of maternal narcotic vs. non narcotic addiction on neonatal neurobehaviour and infant development. In Pinkert TM, editor: *Consequence of maternal drug use*, Washington, DC, 1985, National Institute on Drug Abuse.

Chez N: Helping the victim of domestic violence, *Am J Nurs* 94(7): 33-37, 1994.

Clever LH: Women's work and health. In Wallis LA, editor: *Textbook of women's health*, Philadelphia, 1999, Lippincott-Raven.

Conti DJ and Burton WN: The economic impact of depression in a workplace, *JON*, 36(9):13-18, 1994.

Crowell NA and Burgess AW, editors: *Understanding violence against women*, Washington, DC, 1996, National Academy Press.

Dennerstein L: Mental health work and gender, *Internat J Health Serv* 25(3):503-509, 1995.

*Diagnostic and Statistical Manual of Mental Disorders (DSM-IV)*, ed 4, Washington, DC, 1994, American Psychological Association.

Ewing JA: Detecting alcoholism, *JAMA* 252:1905-1907, 1984.

Finkelstein N and others: *Getting sober, getting well: a treatment guide for caregivers who work with women*, Cambridge, MA, 1990, Women's Alcoholism Program of CASPAR.

Flitcraft AH: *Diagnostic and treatment guidelines on domestic violence*, Chicago, 1992, American Medical Association.

Fogel CI and Woods NF: *Women's health care*, Thousand Oaks, CA, 1995, Sage.

Foster S: *Herbs for your health*, Loveland, CO, 1996, Interweave Press.

Frezza M and others: High blood alcohol levels in women: the role of decreased alcohol dehydrogenase activity and first pass metabolism, *New Engl J Med* 322:95-99, 1990.

Geissler LJ and Braucht N: The health needs of homeless women. In Wallis LA, editor: *Textbook of women's health*, Philadelphia, 1999, Lippincott-Raven.

Gidwani GP and Rome ES: Eating disorders, *Clin Obstet Gynecol* 40(3):601-615, 1997.

Glantz SA and Parmley WW: Passive smoking and heart disease: epidemiology, physiology, and biochemistry, *Circulation* 83:1-12, 1991.

Greenfield LA and others: Violence by intimates: analysis of data on crimes by current or former spouses, boyfriends, and girlfriends, NCJ167237, Washington, DC, 1998, U.S. Department of Justice, Office of Justice Programs.

Hagen JL: Gender and homelessness, *Social Work* 312-316, 1987.

Halbreich U and Lumley LA: The multiple interactional biological processes that might lead to depression and gender differences in its appearance, *J Affect Disord* 29(2-3):159-173, 1993.

Hales RE, Rakel RE, and Rothschild S: Depression: practical tips for detection and treatment, *Patient Care* 60-80, 1994.

Halmi KA and Licinio E: Hospital program for eating disorders. In *CME Syllabus and Scientific Proceedings in Summary from the 142nd Annual Meeting of the American Psychiatric Association*, Washington, DC, 1989, American Psychiatric Association.

Harris RZ, Benet L, and Schwartz JB: Gender effects in pharmacokinetics and pharmacodynamics, *Drugs* 50:222-239, 1995.

Hausman B and Hammen C: Parenting in homeless families: the double crisis, *J Orthopsychiatr* 63(3):358, 1993.

Hewitt JB and Tellier L: A description of an occupational reproductive health nurse consultant practice and women's occupational exposures during pregnancy, *Pub Health Nurs* 13(5):365-373, 1996.

Hirschfeld RM and Russell JM: Assessment and treatment of suicidal patients, *New Engl J Med* 337:910-915, 1997.

Hoegerman G and Schnoll S: Narcotic use in pregnancy, *Clin Perinatol* 18(1):51-73, 1991.

Huenemann RL and others: A longitudinal study of gross body composition and body conformation and their association with food and activity in a teen-age population, *Am J Clin Nutrit* 18:325-338, 1966.

Illinois Coalition Against Sexual Assault: *Ritual sexual abuse*, Coalition Commentary Summer 1992, 12.

Inciardi JA, Lockwood D, and Pottieger, AE: Crack dependent women and sexuality: implications for STD transmission and acquisition, *Addiction & Recovery* 25-28, 1991.

Jessup M: The treatment of perinatal addiction: identification, intervention, and advocacy, *West J Med* 11(4):553-558, 1990.

Kavanagh KH: Transcultural perspectives in mental health. In Andrews MM and Boyle JS, editors: *Transcultural concepts in nursing care*, ed 2, Philadelphia, 1995, Lippincott.

Kendig S: Women at risk for infection: the woman who is chemically dependent, *JOGNN* 24(8):776-781, 1995.

Kendig S and Sanford DG: *Mid-life and menopause: a celebration of women's health*, Washington, DC, 1998, AWHONN.

Kessler RC and others: Lifetime and 12 month prevalence of DSM-III-R psychiatric disorders in the United States, *Arch Gen Psychiatr* 51:8-19, 1994.

King AC, Oka RK, and Young DR: Ambulatory blood pressure and heart rate responses to the stress of work and caregiving in older women, *J Gerontol* 49(6):M239-245, 1994.

Kolander CA, Ballard DJ, and Chandler CK: *Contemporary women's health—issues for today and the future*, Boston, 1999, McGraw-Hill.

Lenhart SA: The psychological consequences of sexual harassment and gender discrimination in the workplace, New York, 1997, Guilford Press.

Levy M and Koren G: Obstetric and neonatal effects of drugs of abuse, *Emerg Med Clin North Am* 8:633-652, 1990.

Loring MT and Smith RW: Health care barriers and interventions for battered women, *Pub Health Rep* 109(3):328-338, 1994.

Marchi M and Cohen P: Early childhood eating behaviors and adolescent eating disorder, *J Am Academy Child Adolesc Psychiatr* 29:112-117, 1990.

Marshall AW and others: Ethanol elimination in males and females: relationship to menstrual cycle and body composition, *Hepatology* 3:701-706, 1983.

McBride AB: Multiple roles and depression, *Health Values* 13(2): 45-49, 1989.

McFarlane J and Parker B: Abuse during pregnancy: a protocol for prevention and intervention. White Plains, NY, 1994, March of Dimes Birth Defects Foundation.

McFarlane J and others: Assessing for abuse: self report versus nurse interview, *Pub Health Nurs* 8:245-250, 1991.

McFarlane J and others: Assessing for abuse during pregnancy: frequency and extent of injuries and entry into prenatal care, *JAMA* 267(23):3176-3178, 1992.

McFarlane J and Parker B: Preventing abuse during pregnancy: an assessment and intervention protocol, *MCN: Am J Matern Child Nurs* 19(6):321-324, 1994.

McMahon AL: Substance abuse among the elderly, *Nurse Practitioner Forum* 4:231-238, 1993.

Means RH: Health care for homeless women. In Carr PL, Freund KM, and Somani S, editors: *The medical care of women*, Philadelphia, 1995, W.B. Saunders.

Medoff-Cooper B and Verklan T: Substance abuse, *NAACOG Clin Iss Perinat Women Health* 3(1):114-128, 1992.

Mehler PR, Gray MC, and Schulte M: Medical complication of anorexia nervosa, *J Women Health* 6(5):533-541, 1997.

Moore RD: Prevalence, detection, and treatment of alcoholism in hospitalized patients, *JAMA* 261:403-408, 1989.

Muerer J: Personal communication, St Louis, June 1999.

Mulroy A: The housing affordability slide in action: how mothers slip into homelessness, *New Engl J Pub Policy* 8(1):203, 1992.

National Cancer Institute (NCI): How to help your patients stop smoking (trainer's guide), Bethesda, MD, 1993, The Institute.

National Institute on Alcohol Abuse and Alcoholism (NIAAA): Alcohol and women, *Alcohol Alert* 10(PH290):1-3, 1990.

Noyes R and others: Relationship between panic disorder and agorophobia: a family study, *Arch Gen Psychiatr* 43:227-233, 1986.

*Nurse's handbook of alternative and complementary therapies,* Springhouse, PA, 1998, Springhouse Corp.

O'Neil C: Identifying alcohol dependence in women, *Advan Nurse Practit* 3(9):43-46, 1995.

Orbach S: *Hunger strike,* New York, 1986, W.W. Norton.

Petronis KR and others: An epidemiologic investigation of potential risk factors for suicide attempts, *Psychiatr Epidemiol* 25:193-199, 1990.

Pitula CR: Recognizing and treating depression in women, *AJN* 16A-16D, 1995.

Powers PS: Initial assessment and early treatment options for anorexia nervosa and bulimia nervosa, *Psychiatr Clin North Am* 19(4):639-655, 1996.

Project Safeguard: *Safety plan: standards for services for battered women and their children,* Denver, 1992, Women and Children's Treatment Committee, Project Safeguard.

Rempel D: The lead-exposed worker, *JAMA* 262(4):532, 1989.

Richards J: Battering/domestic violence. In Star WI, Lommel LL, and Shannon MT, editors: *Women's primary health care: protocols for practice,* Washington, DC, 1995, American Nurses Publishing.

Rigotti NA and Polivogianis L: Smoking cessation. In Carlson KJ and Eisenstat SA, editors: *Primary care of women,* St Louis, 1995, Mosby.

Roberts B: Women in the workplace. In Fogel C and Woods NF, editors: *Women's health care: a comprehensive handbook,* Thousand Oaks, CA, 1995, Sage.

Robins LNG, Locke BZ, and Regier DA: An overview of psychiatric disorders in America. In Robins LN and Regier DA, editors: *Psychiatric disorders in America: the epidemiologic catchment area study,* New York, 1992, Free Press.

Robinson BBE, Bacon JG, and O'Reilly J: Fat phobia: measuring, understanding, and changing anti-fat attitudes, *Int J Eat Disord* 14:467, 1988.

Rock CL and Curran-Celentano J: Nutritional management of eating disorders, *Psychiatr Clin North Am* 19(4):701-713, 1996.

Rost K and others: Measuring the outcomes of care for mental health problems, *Med Care* 30(5):MS266-MS273 (suppl), 1992.

Ruppert RA: The last smoke, *Am J Nurs* 99(11):26-32, 1999.

Schwenk TL: Pairing drug therapy and psychotherapy in primary care, *Consultant* 698-709, 1995.

Snyder M and Lindquist R: *Complementary/alternative therapies in nursing,* ed 3, New York, 1998, Springer.

Steinweg DL and Worth H: Alcoholism: the keys to the CAGE, *Am J Med* 94:520-523, 1993.

Stuart MR and Lieberman JA: Finding time for counseling in primary care, *Patient Care* 118-131, 1994.

Sugg NK and Inui T: Primary care physician's response to domestic violence: opening Pandora's box, *JAMA* 267(23):3157-3160, 1992.

Symm-Gruender NK: Breaking the cycle of domestic violence, *Office Nurse* 10-17, 1994.

Toscano G and Weber W: Violence in the workplace: patterns of fatal workplace assaults differ from those of nonfatal ones, *Compensations and working conditions,* Washington, DC, April 1995, U.S. Department of Labor Bureau of Labor Statistics.

Ugarizza DN and Fallon T: Nurse's attitudes toward homeless women: a barrier to change, *Am J Pub Health* 42(1):26-29, 1994.

USDHHS: Preventing violence against women (fact sheet), Nov 13, 1997, www.waisgate.hhs.gov/cgi-bin/waisgate

U.S. Department of Labor, Women's Bureau: Facts on working women, No. 93-5, Dec 1993.

Valente S: Diagnosis and treatment of panic disorder and generalized anxiety in primary care, *Nurse Practit* 21(8):26-47, 1996.

Weiner S: Perinatal impact of substance abuse. In Raff B and Fiore E, editors: *Nursing issues for the 21st century,* series 3 (module 4), White Plains, NY, 1992, March of Dimes Birth Defects Foundation.

Weingourt R: Wife rape in a sample of psychiatric patients, *Image: J Nurs Scholar* 22(3):144-147, 1990.

Weiss K: Confronting anxiety and depression in primary care, *New J Med* 91(3):157-158, 1994.

Wetherington CL and Roman AB: Drug addiction research and the health of women—executive summary, Rockville, MD, 1998, USDHHS—National Institute on Drug Abuse.

Wislows LS: Child abuse and neglect, *New Engl J Med* 332(21):1425-1431, 1995.

Women and addiction: why/how are they special?, *Addiction treatment forum* 11(1):1,5, 1993.

Women's Health Advocate Newsletter: Alcohol and HRT—drinking boosts estrogen levels: what about breast cancer risk?, *Women's Health Advocate Newsletter* 3(12):1,8, 1997.

Women's Healthcare Partnership: Depression and anxiety in women: brief assessment and intervention strategies for women's health providers, Multiple sites.

World Health Organization (WHO): Indoor air pollutants: exposure and health effects, Copenhagen, 1983, The Organization.

Zerwekh JV: The practice of empowerment and coercion by expert public health nurses, *Image: J Nurs Scholar* 24(2):101-105, 1992.

# CHAPTER 7

# Assisting Women with Health Problems

*"As caregivers, we must know the individuals we are looking after, their strengths and weaknesses. We must also know our own. And we must know how to respond to others' needs."*

— ROSALYNN CARTER

What are the most common health problems that women experience?

What is unique about women's experiences of these conditions?

Over which risks do women have control?

What risks are outside of a woman's control?

What are the major interventions involved?

What diagnostic testing is available to identify these conditions?

What are the primary, secondary, and tertiary areas for intervention?

What major roles do we play when caring for women with these conditions?

Women face common health problems during their reproductive years and beyond. Some illnesses are more likely to appear in women then men. Other problems occur within or as a result of their reproductive organs and capabilities. Women also are more susceptible to some diseases than men, or they respond to them differently than men. Understanding the health problems that women may encounter and the decisions that women face when encountering some of these major health concerns is the focus of this chapter. Our focus of care is to assist the woman in the process of self-care and in her role as possible collaborator in the care others provide to her.

The first part of the chapter provides information on systemic conditions that are generally first suspected through the history taking process and then confirmed by laboratory testing. These are anemia, autoimmune disorders, diabetes, and human immunodeficiency virus (HIV). The remaining health problems are presented in the general order in which a physical examination is performed. The problem may be suspected based on her report of symptoms and then possibly confirmed by physical examination or subsequent laboratory testing. They are conditions of the heart, lungs, breasts, pelvic floor, vagina and vulva, ovaries and uterus, and urinary tract.

**ANEMIA**

Anemia is the most common form of blood disorder, affecting four times as many women as men (Boston Women's Health Book Collective, 1999). The major difference in these numbers comes from higher rates of iron deficiency anemia in menstruating women. In other forms of anemia, men and women are affected in equal numbers.

Anemia should be thought of as the sign of an underlying problem, rather than as a diagnosis (Ferrary and Parker-Falzoi, 1998). Because anemia has many causes, a clinical workup must be done in all cases to determine the precise diagnosis and to ensure an appropriate choice of treatment. Determined by laboratory testing, **anemia** is usually defined as a reduction in hemoglobin concentration, or a reduction in red blood cell (RBC) volume as measured by the hematocrit. **Hemoglobin** is the substance in RBCs that carries oxygen. The **hematocrit** is a ratio measure of the volume of cells versus the volume of plasma in whole blood.

Normal values for these tests depend on age, sex, pregnancy status, and the control values for each laboratory. We must, therefore, research the guidelines used by the laboratories in their settings. In addition, such factors as race, smoking, congestive heart failure, and the altitude of the surrounding geographic area can affect values. The latter is an important factor to keep in mind when assessing immigrant populations.

## Causes of Anemia

Anemia is caused by one of three mechanisms: blood loss, red cell destruction, or decreased red cell production. Laboratory results help determine which mechanism is involved. Once a decreased hemoglobin and/or hematocrit is obtained, supportive tests would minimally include a complete blood count (CBC), which includes the mean corpuscular volume (MCV), mean corpuscular hemoglobin content (MCHC), and mean corpuscular hemoglobin (MCH), and a reticulocyte count. These tests, plus others that might subsequently be ordered, are defined in Box 7-1.

Once the MCV has been obtained, the woman's anemia can be classified as either a microcytic anemia (MCV $<80$ $\mu m^3$), a normocytic anemia (MCV 80 to 100 $\mu m^3$), or a macrocytic anemia (MCV $>100$ $\mu m^3$). Based on this outcome, the possible diagnostic categories for each of these are as follows:

Microcytic anemia: iron deficiency anemia; thalassemias; lead poisoning; anemia of chronic disease
Normocytic anemia: renal disease; bleeding; aplastic anemia; myeloma; hemolysis
Macrocytic anemia: Vitamin $B_{12}$ deficiency; folate deficiency; liver disease; alcoholism; hypothyroidism; drugs

Other tests are then used to refine the diagnostic categories further.

## Iron Deficiency Anemia

The most common cause of anemia in women is iron deficiency anemia (Goroll, May, and Mulley, 1995a), which can be caused by poor nutrition; an increased need for iron; an underlying condition; or by blood loss, often that of menstruation. Iron deficiency anemia is common in infants, children, and pregnant women, and is the most common nutritional deficiency in the world (Ferrary and Parker-Falzoi, 1998). When iron deficiency anemia is found in postmenopausal women, the source is assumed to be blood loss from bleeding in the gastrointestinal (GI) tract, until proven otherwise. Because the human body efficiently recycles and conserves iron (Mitus, 1995), adequate nutritional intake is usually sufficient to replace any iron lost through monthly menstrual losses. The usual loss is about 50 ml of blood;

---

### BOX 7-1 *Laboratory Tests for Anemia*

**MCV (mean corpuscular volume):** a measure of the red blood cell size

**MCHC (mean corpuscular hemoglobin content):** a measure of the concentration of hemoglobin

**MCH (mean corpuscular hemoglobin):** another measure of the concentration of hemoglobin

**RBC (red blood cell) count:** a measure of the number of RBCs

**Reticulocyte (immature RBCs) count:** measure of the reticulocytes

**RDW (red cell distribution width):** a measure of the variation in RBC size

**Peripheral smear or differential (method of staining a sample of blood on a slide):** allows examination of the RBCs for size, shape, color, and variation

**Iron:** a measure of the concentration of iron in the serum

**Ferritin level:** ferritin is a protein that stores iron, and therefore is an indicator of iron stores

**TIBC (total iron-binding capacity):** transferrin is a plasma protein that transports iron; TIBC is a measure of the maximum amount of iron that can be bound to transferrin

From Wilson DD: *Nurses' guide to understanding laboratory and diagnostic tests,* Philadelphia, 1999, Lippincott.

however, women with heavy blood flow can lose up to 5 times this amount (Ferrary and Parker-Falzoi, 1998).

### History

When anemia is gradual in onset, there are usually very few symptoms, and often the problem is found because screening blood tests have been done. However, early symptoms can include fatigue and shortness of breath (SOB) with exertion. Signs and symptoms of more long-standing anemia can include pale mucous membranes, headache, lightheadedness, dizziness, palpitations, poor concentration, pounding in the ears, poor appetite, sore tongue or mouth, nail changes, trouble swallowing, and pica.

History taking should concentrate on assessing for possible sources of blood loss. These include menstrual history, pregnancy history, trauma, blood donations, recent surgeries, rectal or other bleeding, and any family history of anemia. In addition, a nutritional history should be done, as well as an assessment of habits, including smoking, illicit drug use, alcohol use, and exposure to HIV.

### Physical Examination

The physical examination may be completely normal or reveal the following findings:

> General: fatigued, depressed
> Vital signs: tachypnea, tachycardia, and orthostatic BP changes
> Skin: pallor in light-skinned women, grayness in dark-skinned women
> Nails: spooning or ridging of nails
> Mouth: cheilitis, glossitis
> Abdomen: hepatomegaly, splenomegaly
> Nervous system: altered mental status, parethesias
> Rectal: positive guiaic

### Interventions

Treatment of iron deficiency anemia encompasses several interventions. Reassurance that the conditions can be easily treated is important to relate to the client. It will take approximately 6 months for the stores of iron to be replaced, and blood work will be repeated during this interval to ensure that this is happening. Instruct women with this condition to take ferrous sulfate, usually three times a day with orange juice or another source of vitamin C. If she has difficulty with this, other forms of iron that may be more easily absorbed are ferrous gluconate or chelated iron.

In addition, encourage her to increase other sources of iron in her diet: lean meats, leafy dark green vegetables, fortified cereals and bread, blackstrap molasses, fish, egg yolks, raisins, and dried apricots may be suggested. Although these dietary sources will be helpful, without supplementation they are usually insufficient to

correct for the loss of iron stores from heavy menstruation (Ferrari and Parker-Falzoi, 1998).

Iron supplementation can cause side effects, including nausea, constipation, and darkened stools. Starting the dosing slowly and increasing gradually can minimize these side effects. Encouraging women to eat more whole grains, bran, vegetables and fruit, and drinking more water can reduce constipation. Iron can reduce the absorption of vitamin E, and so women should be advised to take these supplements at least 6 hours apart (Boston Women's Health Book Collective, 1999).

In an effort to avoid anemia, or as a "quick fix" when they experience low energy or fatigue, women may begin taking iron supplements on their own. It is important for us to stress to women that they should avoid supplementation, unless diagnostic studies have indicated they require it for their type of anemia. Iron supplementation with some conditions of anemia can cause iron overload, which can be dangerous to the woman's health.

##  AUTOIMMUNE DISORDERS

Several disorders are classified as autoimmune in nature, and another subset of syndromes may be related to disordered immune function. Overwhelmingly, these conditions affect women more than men (Table 7-1).

Researchers hypothesize that the preponderance of women with these conditions is related to an interrelationship between the immune system and the hormones that regulate the female reproductive cycle (Merrill, Dinu, and Lahita, 1996). Exactly how this happens and under what circumstances are not understood; thus, clear etiologies (causes) for these conditions do not exist. This lack of understanding makes it difficult to diagnose these conditions, which often leads to delay, not only in diagnosis, but also in initiating therapy. All are chronic conditions that necessitate lifelong therapy for the woman.

### TABLE 7-1 *Prevalence Rates of Selected Disorders by Sex*

| Disorder | Female:Male |
| --- | --- |
| Scleroderma | 12-15:1 |
| Systemic lupus erythematosus | 3-10:1 |
| Rheumatoid arthritis | 2-3:1 |
| Hyperthyroidism | 3-10:1 |
| Hypothyroidism | 3-10:1 |
| Sjögren's syndrome | 8-9:1 |
| Fibromyalgia | 8-10:1 |
| Chronic fatigue syndrome | female > male (ratio unknown) |

## Types of Diseases and Conditions

The following definitions are provided to help you understand the challenges these disorders present to both the affected women and their health care providers:

**Scleroderma** is a condition that can range from a mild to a systemic disease that can cause death within a few months. It is characterized by degenerative changes and vascular abnormalities of the skin, kidneys, lung, heart, GI system, and musculature and diffuse fibrosis.

**Systemic lupus erythematosis (SLE)** is an autoimmune condition that may cause inflammation in the connective tissue of various systems, especially in the skin, joints, blood, and kidneys. The buildup of immune complexes within these systems is responsible for the inflammation. The course of the disease can be mild to severe.

**Rheumatoid arthritis (RA)** is a systemic, autoimmune disease characterized by symmetric, polyarticular inflammation. The small joints of the wrists and hands are generally involved, but more extensive forms of the condition also exist.

**Hyperthyroidism** refers to a group of diseases all characterized by an overproduction of thyroid hormones. Not all are caused by autoimmune problems; however, the most common form is Graves' disease, which is thought to be autoimmune in nature.

**Hypothyroidism** refers to a group of diseases characterized by an underproduction of thyroid hormones. Again not all are caused by autoimmune problems. The most common hypothyroid condition is Hashimoto's thyroiditis, in which the mechanism is autoimmune, but the original insult to the thyroid has not yet been identified. Viruses, stress, and the process of childbirth have been implicated as causes, among others.

**Sjögren's syndrome (SS)** is an inflammatory disorder characterized by dry mouth (xerostomia) and dry eyes (keratoconjunctivitis sicca). When these are the primary symptoms, the condition is known as **primary SS**; if these symptoms accompany rheumatoid arthritis type of symptoms, then the condition is known as **secondary SS** (Aguirre, 1997).

**Fibromyalgia** is a syndrome of diffuse, chronic musculoskeletal pain with specific trigger points, often accompanied by stiffness, sleep disorders and fatigue. Joints are not usually affected, causing this to be described as a soft tissue rheumatic disease, although no underlying inflammatory component is identifiable. The underlying etiology is entirely unknown.

Unlike fibromyalgia, **chronic fatigue syndrome (CFS)**, has underlying identifiable markers of an activated immune system, thus grouping it with the autoimmune conditions. It is marked by a sudden onset of extreme fatigue that lasts for a minimum of 6 months. Other symptoms that can also accompany CFS, such as myalgias, confusion, mood swings, headaches, and photophobia, make it difficult to diagnose. The cause of the activation of the immune system is unknown, although viral sources are being investigated.

## Differential Diagnosis

The majority of these conditions begin in women during their young adult years. They have courses that are chronic and can cause varying amounts of disability. In almost all of these diseases, one of the major symptoms is fatigue. In addition, each condition can have various symptoms that may help the clinician determine the diagnosis. A good example is Sjögren's syndrome with the unusual and fairly specific symptoms of dry mouth and dry eyes, or RA, which frequently presents with pain and nodularities in the joints of the fingers. For others, the list of presenting symptomatology is so broad and nonspecific that arriving at a specific diagnosis can be a challenge.

## Interventions

### Specific to Condition

Fortunately, for those women diagnosed with thyroid dysfunction, treatment is fairly straightforward. For those with hyperthyroidism, either surgery to remove excess tissue from the gland or chemotherapeutic agents that destroy portions of the thyroid tissues are used so that less of the circulating thyroid hormones are released into the circulation. In the case of hypothyroidism, synthetic forms of the thyroid hormones need to be taken. When circulating levels are within normal ranges, the patient is said to be euthyroid, and in the majority of cases, all symptoms will resolve.

Because the etiologies for the other previously described conditions are unknown, therapy is directed at interference with the inflammatory process. The hallmark for treatment of RA and SLE is the use of various antiinflammatory agents such as nonsteroidal antiinflammatory drugs (NSAIDs), prednisone, or hydroxychloroquine. In the case of Sjögren's syndrome, it is important to replace the lost fluids of the eyes and the mouth through the use of external agents. A number of drug treatment modalities have been found useful in CFS and fibromyalgia, including antidepressants and NSAIDs, among others.

### General Interventions

In all cases, there are a number of important considerations for the health care team providing services to women living with these conditions. The first is to support the woman through the sometimes long diagnostic period that may occur. She may worry that with fatigue as her initial or primary symptom, that health care providers may not believe something serious is wrong with her health.

Once the diagnosis is known, we need to explain the various medications she is to use and their potential side effects. More importantly, we must help the woman through a problem-solving process of identifying ways that she can deal with the fatigue, chronic pain, disruptions in work and family life, and potential disabilities. Women should be encouraged to take advantage of occupational therapy (Schkade and Neville-Smith, 1998) and exercise programs, in particular aquatics (Ferrell, 1997). An openness to complementary forms of health care such as massage therapy, acupuncture, hypnosis, homeopathy, dietary changes, nutritional supplements, and mind-body therapies should also be encouraged because they have been shown to help patients with these conditions (Dalton, 1995; Berman and Swyers, 1997; Chiarmonte, 1997; Margolis, 1997).

Hopefully, as more research is done on these conditions, their etiologic agents will be discovered, and primary prevention techniques will be developed that will reduce the morbidity and mortality associated with them. At the present time, however, our efforts must be concentrated on secondary and tertiary levels of intervention.

 **WOMEN AND HEART DISEASE**

The subject of women and heart disease has received a great deal of attention in the last few years. This well-deserved attention derives in part from two very important facts: (1) heart disease has become and remains the number 1 cause of death for women, and (2) the Society for the Advancement of Women's Health Research (SAWHR) was created in 1990.

Historically, the emphasis in women's health has been on reproductive concerns and maternally related causes of death. Because of risks to the fetus, in the 1970s, the Food and Drug Administration (FDA) forbade any drug testing on pregnant women. To show compliance, researchers excluded women of reproductive age from almost all research trials (Sarto, 1998). Furthermore, the common assumption was that women were not at risk and did not suffer the consequences of heart disease to the extent that men did. As a consequence, not only were they excluded from research studies, but also their symptoms would often go unrecognized, and the treatments offered to men were not as frequently offered to women. Through the leadership of the SAWHR, and the concern for the gravity of the health statistics, there is now an Office of Research on Women's Health at the National Institutes of Health (NIH), and the definition of women's health goes far beyond reproductive concerns. The FDA has now reversed its policy on pregnant women in research trials, and both public and private organizations have increased funding for topics important to women's health (Sarto, 1998). Research on women's health is now getting the attention women so richly deserve, and one of the most impressive areas of research activity is the issue of women and heart disease.

## Risk for Cardiovascular Disease

The statistics are overwhelming. Cardiovascular disease (CVD) kills 500,000 women per year, more women than all those who die from all types of cancer combined. It is estimated that 1 of every 2 women will die from CVD, compared with 1 in 25 for breast cancer (American Heart Association, 1996). CVD is a leading cause of disability in women (Wenger, 1996) and accounts for the largest diagnostic category for the admission of women to hospitals (Howes, 1998). Furthermore, the economic costs of CVD are enormous: between $50 and $100 billion per year in lost wages and health care costs (Haan, 1996).

Risk factors are divided into those over which a woman has no control and those that can be modified. In the first category, factors over which women have no control, are age, race, and family history. There are also lifestyle habits and risk factors that can be modified. The primary prevention interventions of education and counseling concerning physical factors and psychosocial factors can be helpful.

### Unchangeable Risk Factors

*Age.* In the early decades of a woman's life, age is a protective factor, but this dramatically changes at the time of menopause, so that by the age of 65, the rates of CVD for women have caught up with those for men. In general, women have a 10-year lag in the manifestations of CVD as compared with men. The Framingham Heart Study found that the ratio of men to women with CVD was 2.3 to 1 for ages 35 to 64, but then this ratio went down to 1.6 to 1 for those 65 to 94 (Haan, 1996). Because women on average live longer than men do, the actual mortality rates from CVD in those over the age of 85 is twice that of men. Because the population in the United States is aging, these numbers will increase in the years to come.

*Race.* Race is also a risk factor. Although the rates of CVD are the same for white and black men, the prevalence and mortality rates of CVD are greater in black women than they are in white women. Hispanics tend to have lower rates of CVD than the general population, and Native Americans have an increased mortality rate from CVD under the age of 35 (American Heart Association, 1998).

*Family History.* Family history of heart disease has long been known to be a risk factor. The risk is particularly strong if a family member has a history of a significant event, such as a myocardial infarction (MI), at a young age. For male relatives, this is age 55 years, but because of the lag in CVD manifestations in women, this age is 65 years for female relatives (Howes, 1998).

## Modifiable Risk Factors

Although the aforementioned factors cannot be altered, some risk factors can be modified. Health care providers should be aware of all of these risks and provide the primary prevention interventions of education and counseling to those clients who demonstrate the following risk factors: cigarette smoking, lack of physical activity, obesity, estrogen level changes consistent with menopause, elevated cholesterol levels, hypertension, and diabetes. Other researchers include psychosocial factors, such as stress, occupational factors, personality factors, and role changes, while others feel that more research must be done before the actual role of these factors can be determined (Haan, 1996; American Heart Association, 1998).

*Smoking.* Smoking rates are approximately equal in men and women, although if present trends continue, the number of women who smoke will exceed that of men in the not too distant future. This may happen because men are quitting in greater numbers, while women are becoming new smokers in greater numbers (American Heart Association, 1998). Research has shown that the risk of CVD is dose related: the higher the number of cigarettes smoked, the greater the risk of angina, MI, and coronary artery disease (CAD) deaths. Smoking five cigarettes per day increases the risk of CVD twofold (Haan, 1996; Wenger, 1996; Redberg, 1998). Furthermore, cigarette smoking lowers the age of menopause by about 2 years, and lowers the age of first MI in women more so than it does in men (Wenger, 1996). Alternatively, quitting reduces this risk, and within 2 to 3 years, the risk decreases approximately to the level of those who have never smoked (Haan, 1996).

*Hypertension.* Both men and women have an increased risk for CVD when they have hypertension. However, more women over the age of 65 have hypertension than men do (Wenger, 1996). Furthermore, while systolic blood pressure levels in men peak during middle age, women continue to have a rise in systolic blood pressure well into their 80s (Wenger, 1996). Elevated systolic hypertension is associated with an increased risk for stroke, as well as both fatal and nonfatal MI, comparable to the risk from combined systolic/diastolic hypertension. Therefore, systolic levels must be carefully monitored because they are a more important indicator of risk in women (Sharp and Konen, 1997).

Clearly, treatment of hypertension has reduced the incidence of CVD, in particular stroke (Sharp and Konen, 1997). Currently, men and women with hypertension are managed following the same guidelines. However, some conflicting data indicate that women may not benefit as much from this treatment protocol as men do (Howes, 1998; Redberg, 1998). This may be caused by the limited number of women included in clinical trials or may actually reflect variations in benefits depending on physiologic differences, and therefore,

responses to treatment protocols (Redberg, 1998). Ongoing research will be beneficial to women's health care.

*Diabetes.* Diabetes is a very strong risk factor for CVD and is a more important risk factor in women than in men. Furthermore, diabetes eliminates the usual protective effects women enjoy during the childbearing years. Women with diabetes have a threefold to sevenfold increase in risk for CVD, while men with diabetes have a twofold to threefold increase. Fully one half of all those with Type II diabetes will die from CVD (American Heart Association, 1998). Prevention of the onset of Type II diabetes and tight control of the condition are two ways to modify the risk.

*High Cholesterol.* Lipid profiles are known to influence the risk of CVD in both men and women. It is generally accepted that elevated cholesterol levels are an important factor in increased risk for CAD in both; however, this may be more of a risk factor for women before menopause. After menopause, evidence suggests that increased levels of triglycerides and decreased levels of high-density lipoprotein (HDL) cholesterol may have more diagnostic significance for women or may indicate a separate risk profile in addition to that of cholesterol levels (Redberg, 1998). While both men and women who have been diagnosed with CVD benefit from aggressive reduction of elevated lipid levels with medication. The data are less clear concerning the use of these agents for primary prevention of CVD, especially in women who are premenopausal. Treatment, therefore, depends on the total picture of the risk profile for any one individual woman, and the lipid levels she demonstrates.

*Exogenous Hormone Use.* When **oral contraception** (OC) was first introduced, the levels of hormones in the pills were much higher, and an increase in the occurrence of various CVD events, mostly blood clots, stroke, and MI, was noticed in women over 35 taking these pills. It was believed that oral contraceptives (OCs) were to blame. Closer investigation revealed that these events mostly occurred in women who were smokers. Once this factor was controlled for, research studies were able to show that smoking, rather than OC use (Notelovitz and Tonnessen, 1997) increased the risk. Today's OCs have even lower doses of estrogen and use the newer, safer progestogens. Research shows that there is no increased risk of CVD in present or former OC users even those who took the early high-dose forms (Notelovitz and Tonnessen, 1996; Caufield, 1998). It is now common for women to use OC throughout their forties.

However, the risk of both arterial and venous thrombotic events is increased while taking OCs. This risk is dose dependent: the higher the levels of hormones, the higher the risk, with the 20 $\mu$g estrogen pills having a minimal risk profile (Caufield, 1998). As a consequence, a list of health conditions are considered "relative contraindications" for OC use. These include smokers over 35 years of age, diabetic women, obese women, women with dyslipidemia, and women with hypertension. Note that all of these conditions are in and of themselves risk factors for CVD.

The role of **hormone therapy** (HT) in reducing the risk of CVD has taken on enormous importance for women. A variety of studies support the influence of HT on risk reduction, showing decreases in CVD, including decreased risk of MI. Given that a woman's risk for CVD increases dramatically after menopause, use of HT clearly can be of benefit. It is thought that HT works through the favorable effects that the hormones have on lipid profiles and decreases in fibrinogen levels, but there may also be a direct effect on the vasculature of the heart (Redberg, 1998). Even more data will be available once the NIH sponsored Women's Health Initiative studies are completed and analyzed in 2006.

Despite the encouraging results surrounding HT and CVD reduction, there are problems with HT therapy. It is not really known how long women should be on therapy, nor is it clear just how much of a reduction in mortality rates is the direct result of HT. There also is a small increased risk of breast cancer in women who have taken HT, and these small increases, especially for women with a family history of breast cancer, are a cause for concern. In addition, there is also a small increased risk of endometrial cancer, although this risk was reduced when a progestational agent was added to the estrogen component of treatment. The decision to take or not to take HT is an individualized process. All the pros and cons of therapy should be discussed at length and understood clearly before a woman makes a choice. It is hoped that as the data from large research trials become available, this decision will be made easier for women.

## Diagnosis of Cardiovascular Disease

It is becoming clearer that women present differently than men do when they have CVD. Women have more chest pain as the initial sign of CAD than men, and their prognosis associated with this pain is better than it is for men (Sharp and Konen, 1997). Women also present more often with nausea, upper abdominal pain, dyspnea, fatigue, and weakness, and often these symptoms are experienced at rest, rather then during exercise, as is found in men (Judelson, 1997; Redberg, 1998; American Heart Association, 1998). Sharp and Konen (1997) suggest that the differences in presentation of CAD in women may help explain why it goes undetected longer in women than it does in men. Furthermore, women do not do as well after an initial MI—they have higher fatality rates than men do both during hospitalization and during the first year after the MI (Wenger, 1996; American Heart Association, 1998).

Recently, much has been written about the discrepancies in treatment that women receive when they have CVD when compared with men. The first difficulty is

related to the misunderstanding in the community at large about the importance of CVD to women's health. Judelson (1997) sites a Gallup poll done in 1995 that indicated that 80% of the women between 45 and 75 years who were surveyed did not know that heart disease was the number 1 cause of death in women. More astounding yet, 32% of the primary care physicians in the survey also were unaware of this fact. Heart disease is seen as a "man's disease," and therefore may go unrecognized and undertreated in women. In addition, as previously mentioned, women are older when they present, and the symptoms that women exhibit may be different from those of men.

To add to the difficulties, the noninvasive diagnostic tests used to confirm CVD in men may not be as valid in women (Judelson, 1997; Howes, 1998; Redberg, 1998). For example, the exercise electrocardiography (ECG) test varies in its accuracy, depending on a woman's health history and physical status. In the case of thallium stress tests, women's breast tissue may cause artifacts in the results that can be misinterpreted. However, new technologies may improve this picture for both men and women; these include the use of magnetic resonance imaging (MRI) and positron emission tomography (PET) (Redberg, 1998).

There is evidence that women are not referred for invasive diagnostic testing as frequently as men, and because these studies are necessary before surgical interventions such as coronary artery bypass grafting (CABG) can happen, this has tremendous significance for women (Redberg, 1998). Furthermore, women may not do as well as men, even if they have had CABG, or a percutaneous transluminal coronary angioplasty (PTCA). Women die more frequently during these operative procedures, as well as following surgery, and they do not receive as much pain relief from the surgical procedures. Although it is postulated that this is in part due to the smaller vessel size of the coronary arteries of women, it is also believed that women are referred for these types of surgeries when they are sicker, and therefore their level of recovery is compromised (Redberg, 1998).

## Intervention

The major emphasis for health care personnel, therefore, is directed at three areas of intervention with women. The first is primary prevention, as with so many of the health care conditions discussed in this chapter. Women must be encouraged, through a multitude of educational and counseling strategies, to identify and adopt the prevention strategies found in Box 7-2.

The next level is secondary prevention. Both women and health care providers must be aware of the possible presenting signs for CVD in women. Symptoms should not be ignored; CVD should not be seen as "just a man's disease." Women should be referred for evaluation as soon as possible to avoid dangerous sequellae. In addition, diagnostic tests that are most useful in evaluating women must be developed, tested, and made widely available.

Once a woman has a diagnosis of CVD, the various treatment plans should be discussed so she has all options available. Surgical interventions must be done earlier in the disease process, rather than late in the course, when outcomes are less favorable. In addition, women should have access to as many rehabilitation programs as there are for men. These programs must be developed based on the specific needs of women, which are very different from those of men (Conca, 1999).

 ## WOMEN AND DIABETES

In 1996 in the United States, diabetes was the sixth leading cause of death in all women; the fourth leading cause of death in black, Hispanic, and Native American women; and the seventh leading cause of death in white and Asian women (National Center for Health Statistics, 1998). The Pima Indians of Arizona have the highest rates in the world: approximately 50% of the population ages 30 to 64 have Type II diabetes (Edelman and Henry, 1998).

According to the CDC (1999a), in 1998, 15.7 million people were living with diabetes, but only 10.3 million were aware of their diagnosis. Although men and women have equal prevalence rates of about 8.2%, more women than men suffer with the condition: 7.5 million men vs. 8.1 million women. This is because on average, women live longer than men do. Death rates are twice as high in middle-aged people with diabetes than for their counterparts who do not have diabetes (CDC, 1999a).

Not only may diabetes cause premature death, but also it is recognized as being one of the leading causes of disability. Complications include blindness, kidney

failure, vascular problems, heart disease, stroke, neurologic problems, and amputations. The National Institute of Diabetes and Digestive and Kidney Disease (NIDDK, 1999) estimates that diabetes cost $98 billion in 1997—this includes disability payments, time lost from work, premature death, and all of the associated medical costs for diabetic care.

### Understanding Diabetes

Diabetes is a chronic disease in which persistent levels of hyperglycemia are encountered. There are four types of diabetes: (1) **Type I diabetes** is considered an autoimmune disorder in which levels of insulin are very low. In this type, which affects between 5 and 10% of those with diabetes, the immune system attacks the $\beta$-cells (the insulin-producing cells) of the pancreas. Individuals with this form must be given insulin for life. (2) **Type II diabetes** is the most common form of the disease. It usually develops after the age of 40, and most commonly, in those who are obese. In these individuals, the body is still able to produce insulin, but insulin resistance develops, and the insulin cannot be used effectively by cells. Treatment varies from diet and exercise, to oral hypoglycemic agents, to insulin. (3) **Gestational diabetes** develops during pregnancy and is usually resolved after the pregnancy is over. Women who develop gestational diabetes have an increased risk of developing Type II diabetes. (4) **Other forms of diabetes** are those caused by surgery, malnutrition, drugs, genetic syndromes, or other illnesses.

Diabetes requires lifelong monitoring and management. The goal of therapy is to maintain blood sugar levels at normal levels as much as possible. This requires standards of care for the history and physical, as well as counseling and education needs. Specific areas include diet, exercise, choice of medication, blood sugar level monitoring both by the patient and the health care provider, hemoglobin $A_{1c}$ monitoring, and constant evaluation for the potential complications of the disease.

Present research is aimed at determining the most useful blood sugar monitoring schedules and new treatment methods, including painless techniques. Continued development of both oral hypoglycemic and insulin type medications, continued development of both external and surgically implantable devices to deliver insulin, laser techniques to reduce the risk of blindness, and methods of pancreatic transplantation are being explored (NIDDK, 1999). Research is investigating the etiology of type I diabetes, with the hope that in the future vaccines might be available to prevent this form of diabetes (Fantus, Delovitch, and Dupre, 1997; Zechel and Bhagirath, 1998).

### Diabetes in Women

Although there are no differences in the management of diabetes between women and men, and both suffer from the same types of complications, several issues are unique to women. Jaffe and Seely (1995) categorize them as follows: (1) effects on normal female physiology (the menstrual cycle), (2) reproductive concerns, (3) cardiovascular concerns, (4) genitourinary problems, and (5) eating disorders.

## Physiologic Effects

Some women have been shown to have differences in insulin resistance during various phases of her menstrual cycle, with an increase in resistance noted during the luteal phase. Although the cause for this change is unknown, it is postulated that progesterone may have a role to play. Women who have variations in their blood sugar control, regardless of compliance with their management program, should be encouraged to keep records of their blood sugar levels in relationship to their menstrual cycles to determine if this is the cause for the variations. In addition, women with diabetes who are experiencing menopause should be advised that their insulin sensitivity may increase, and therefore they should keep a careful watch on blood sugar levels, which may decrease as a result (Jaffe and Seely, 1995).

Recent research implicates insulin resistance as a factor in polycystic ovarian syndrome (PCOS), with subsequent chronic anovulation and hyperandrogenism (Minchoff and Grandin, 1996). In particular, PCOS is associated with secondary amenorrhea and infertility, among other signs and symptoms. Women with Type II diabetes may be diagnosed with this condition; conversely, women with PCOS should be screened for insulin resistance and counseled concerning ways to prevent the onset of Type II diabetes.

Because of the difficulties in sexuality experienced by men with diabetes, one could postulate that the same sort of problems might be found in women. However, no differences in sexual difficulties have been found between women with and without diabetes (Sawin, 1998).

## Fertility Control

Of special concern is the process of fertility control for women with diabetes. The issue of contraception remains a complex one, especially when considering OC use. Earlier OCs, with the higher levels of hormonal agents, were found to cause varying levels of interference with carbohydrate and lipid metabolism. In recent years, the lower dose forms have been shown to cause little to no interference with carbohydrate metabolism (Jaffe and Seely, 1995; Caufield, 1998). However, women with diabetes who wish to use OC should be counseled to monitor their blood sugar levels more closely, especially when first beginning therapy.

On the other hand, OC use does seem to have an effect on lipids, especially on levels of triglycerides (Johnson, 1995), and therefore these levels should be closely monitored in women with diabetes who choose OC. A choice

other than OC would be indicated for those women with diabetes whose triglyceride levels are elevated. Furthermore, because the risk of cardiac disease is elevated in women with diabetes and OC is known to increase the risk of thromboembolic events, women with diabetes who are older, obese, or who smoke, should not be given OC.

Naturally, there are always exceptions to these recommendations. If the risk for complications from pregnancy is greater for a woman with diabetes than the risk from OC use, and no other method is possible, a woman and her health care provider may make the decision to use OC, as long as the risks are fully understood by both.

Generally, the contraindication profile for Norplant for diabetic women is the same as for OC, since carbohydrate metabolism has been shown to be adversely affected in nondiabetic women who use this method, and progestin levels in OC have been shown to have the greatest effect on carbohydrate metabolism (Caufield, 1998). The same precautions are indicated when considering Depo-Provera (Jaffe and Seely, 1995).

The woman-centered contraceptive method of choice for diabetic women would be barrier methods, such as the female condom, diaphragm, or cervical cap. Intrauterine devices (IUDs) may be used if no risk factors are associated with this method. Tubal ligation may be the indicated choice for those women who have completed childbearing or for those in whom the risks of pregnancy complications are high and unacceptable to the affected woman. For those diabetic women with cooperative partners, male-centered methods may offer the best option of all.

## Cardiovascular Disease

The prevalence of cardiovascular disease (CVD) is higher in women with diabetes as compared with those without diabetes. This risk is estimated to be 3 times higher for women with diabetes for all forms of CVD, and the CVD mortality rate is 4.5 times higher (Jaffe and Seely, 1995). Furthermore, diabetes is a major predictor of mortality after an MI (Ferrary and Parker-Falzoi, 1998). The usual cardioprotective effects that women enjoy in their premenopausal years are severely compromised in women with diabetes (Notelovitz and Tonnessen, 1996). Jaffe and Seely (1995) postulate that the mechanisms involved are those involved with lipid metabolism, hypercoagulability, and hyperinsulinemia, but the exact causes are unknown.

## Genitourinary Problems

Vaginal yeast infections are common in women with diabetes because the organism adheres to the vaginal walls more effectively in the presence of elevated glucose levels. In addition, women with diabetes appear to experience a higher number of urinary tract infections (UTIs).

The precise mechanism is unknown, but glycosuria and neurogenic bladder difficulties have been hypothesized to be involved (Jaffe and Seely, 1995).

### Eating Disorders

Jaffe and Seely (1995) suggest that there may be an increased prevalence of eating disorders in young women with Type I diabetes when compared with their nondiabetic peers. They suggest that women with diabetes may use omission or reduction of their insulin as a special "purge" technique. However, the finding of higher numbers of diabetics with eating disorders may occur because of selection bias—women with diabetes are already highly involved with the health care system and therefore may be identified more readily.

## Interventions

### Early Screening

One important role that we can play is to help identify women with diabetes early in the disease process when there is a greater opportunity to intervene and therefore reduce the risks of serious complications. Two methods help to accomplish this goal: (1) referring women for evaluation who are having the classic signs of diabetes or those who exhibit the known risk profile, and (2) suggesting earlier screening to clients. The guidelines at present suggest screening for Type II diabetes at age 45; however, the CDC Cost-Effectiveness Study Group (1998) provides study data that support screening at age 25. The study shows that this is a cost-effective method, because individuals would be identified on average 6 years earlier. This would save health care dollars; increase life-years; and improve quality of life by decreasing the incidence of end-stage renal disease, blindness, and lower extremity amputation.

### Education for Biophysical Care

Diabetes is a chronic illness that demands a lifelong commitment to a difficult management program to control the biophysiologic aspects of the illness. We can help women be successful in their management of the disease with comprehensive, relevant teaching and individualized support. Since she alone is the person who must deal with it on a moment-by-moment basis, our educational process must meet her needs.

### Psychologic Care

Diabetes poses numerous challenges to women, from body image difficulties to life-threatening illnesses. Not only must we be knowledgeable about the biophysiologic aspects of the illness, but also the enormous psychologic challenges she encounters. Mitchell (1998) suggests that health care professionals must develop a new approach to clients, an approach that emphasizes exploration of the woman's perspective surrounding her quality of life and the decisions that result from an open discussion of this issue. Women must be given nonjudgmental support as they struggle with the restrictions and freedoms involved with coping with this disease.

## WOMEN AND HIV

Until the 1990s, women represented a small proportion of the population with HIV in the United States (Mallory and Fife, 1999). In contrast, according to the World Health Organization (WHO), worldwide women represent 42% of those living with the infection (Burdge and Money, 1996). Of major concern is the fact that in the United States HIV infection is increasing the fastest in women of reproductive age and in children. It is now estimated that around the world, as well as in the United States, the numbers of men and women infected with HIV will soon be equal (Klirsfeld, 1998), and possibly, the numbers of women will surpass those of men (Kazanjian and Eisenstat, 1995). Furthermore, the fastest growing population of patients with newly diagnosed acquired immunodeficiency syndrome (AIDS), the end-stage of HIV infection, is women (Parsey and others, 1996).

Whereas death rates from AIDS in men have been decreasing, the rates in women have been increasing (Mallory and Fife, 1999), and in 1996, HIV/AIDS was the fourth leading cause of death among women ages 25 to 44 in the United States (Centers for Disease Control and Prevention [CDC], 1998a). The CDC estimates that as many as 100,000 women may be infected, yet are undiagnosed, and will not be diagnosed until they show signs of opportunistic infection or deliver an infected newborn (Parsey and others, 1996).

Women of color are disproportionately affected by this epidemic. In 1996, HIV infection was the seventh most frequent cause of death for black women of all ages, and the eighth leading cause of death for Hispanic women of all ages, while it did not appear in the top 10 listing for white women (National Center for Health Statistics, 1998). It was the leading cause of death for black women between the ages of 25 to 44 years (Larkin and others, 1996). Looked at in another way, black women accounted for 68% of HIV infection in women and 56% of AIDS cases between 1981 and 1996, and yet they are only 12% of all women in the population in general. Hispanic women make up 10% of the female population, and yet account for 6% of all cases of HIV and 20% of AIDS cases (NIH, 1998b). Black and Hispanic women together make up just under 25% of the U.S. population of women, yet they make up 76% of the reported AIDS cases reported to date (CDC, 1998a).

Although the focus of this chapter is not to acquaint the reader with the pathophysiology, progression, or management of HIV and AIDS, a brief review provides a valuable baseline to the discussion of why this disease has important ramifications for women and their health.

## Understanding HIV

HIV is a relatively new virus, the effects of which were first individually described in the 1970s and then as a syndrome of symptoms in 1981. The virus itself was identified in 1983. The virus invades and multiplies within T4 lymphocyte cells. It then depletes the number of these cells, reduces the normal functioning of the cells that remain, and interferes with the normal ratio between T4 cells ($CD_4$ helper cells), and T8 cells ($CD_8$ suppressor cells). These changes cause a dramatic decrease in the immune system's capacity to defend against invading organisms, including viruses, bacteria, parasites, and fungi. HIV also invades monocytes and macrophages. As a consequence, a person becomes susceptible to infections from various organisms, and these infections, which cannot be effectively defended against, eventually cause death. At the present time, there is no cure for HIV disease. Treatment programs depend on two major areas of intervention: (1) medications that interfere with the replication of the virus and (2) medications or treatments that help protect against invading organisms. In addition, a great deal of research is being done on vaccines against HIV, including Phase 3 clinical trials. The latest information about these trials worldwide can be found at the United Nations/WHO website.

## Approaches to Disease Management

At present, there are several approaches to dealing with this disease, including (1) prevention, (2) early recognition, (3) continuing development of medications to convert the disease from a life-threatening condition to a chronic illness, and (4) vaccine development. Women are at risk for contracting HIV/AIDS in some ways different from those of men. Also early symptoms present differently in women than in men.

### Primary Prevention

To understand prevention efforts, it is imperative to understand transmission of the HIV virus. It is a sexually transmitted infection, but HIV also may be transmitted through contaminated blood. The known methods of transmission include the following:

1. Contact of infected body fluids with nonintact skin, as in intercourse
2. Transmission from mother to baby during pregnancy and/or childbirth, and possibly through breastfeeding
3. Sharing of injection drug equipment without proper cleansing between uses

4. Infected blood or blood products given intravenously or by organ transplant or injection, including accidental needle sticks suffered by health care personnel

Some of these methods of transmission have been virtually eliminated as risks because of vigilant screening methods. The national blood supply and organ donors are tested, and the system now maintains an impressive safety profile. In addition, regulated artificial insemination programs test donor semen. Also the needle and syringe devices used in health care settings have been improved to reduce or eliminate needle stick injuries.

For women, there are special considerations around transmission, specifically because of their greater risk of infection during heterosexual intercourse and because of the possibility of vertical transmission from mother to fetus or neonate.

***Heterosexual Transmission.*** Heterosexual transmission is the most frequent mode of HIV transmission for women worldwide (Larkin and others, 1996); this is also true of women in the United States (CDC, 1998a). Male-to-female transmission is estimated to be at least two times more common than female-to-male transmission, although other resources have reported even higher numbers (Burdge and Money, 1996). Although the risk depends in part on the viral load of the partner, with higher loads and partners in later stage disease creating a higher risk of transmission, there are also risk factors unique to women. Semen has a higher quantity of lymphocytes to carry the virus than does vaginal fluid (Schaffer, 1998), and occurs in relatively larger volume than vaginal fluids (Larkin and others, 1996). A woman's vagina provides a large mucosal surface susceptible to microscopic abrasions during sexual activity, opening portals for HIV penetration. Furthermore, cervical ectopy, such as that found more frequently in adolescents and those women taking OCs, and cervical friability regardless of the cause increase the ability of the virus to enter her system through breaks in her skin (Larkin and others, 1996; Wang, 1999).

It is therefore imperative for women to protect themselves by using condoms. Condom use has been shown to be a very efficient method for substantially reducing the risk of HIV transmission (Burdge and Money, 1996; Larkin and others, 1996; Johnson, Silberstein-Currier, and Sanchez-Keeland, 1999). However, we must work with women to address the issues that surround condom use. Women do not always have control over the use of condoms. Some men refuse to use them and forbid their female partners to use the female condom. Within married couples, for a woman to say that she wants the man to use a condom implies that she believes he has been unfaithful to her. Some men, either because of individual or cultural beliefs, seek intercourse with women other than their wives. Other men may be actively bisexual and are involved in homosexual relationships. In both instances the nonmonogamous partners may return to their wives carrying the virus.

For some women, role playing the negotiation surrounding condom use may prove helpful; for others, discussions concerning sexuality, control over one's body, and self-esteem enhancement may be more effective. For those women who wish to control their own protection or who cannot rely on a partner to use a condom, the female condom is an option they may be able to negotiate.

When women choose to use OC or other nonbarrier methods of contraception such as Depo-Provera, supportive education must include information about continued condom use for HIV, as well as protection against other sexually transmitted infections (STIs). Unfortunately, diaphragms do not provide protection against HIV transmission. The spermicide nonoxynol-9 has been shown to inactivate the HIV virus in the laboratory; however, it has also been shown to irritate the vaginal mucosa, decreasing the integrity of the skin, which means that it could actually add to the transmissibility of the virus. More research is needed to determine whether women should be encouraged or discouraged from the use of this chemical (Klirsfeld, 1998).

*Intravenous Drug Use.* Intravenous drug use is the second leading cause of transmission of the HIV virus in women. The first step to decreasing these numbers is to convince women not to begin illicit drug use. But for those who do, interventions should emphasize access to appropriate treatment programs so that a woman who wants to stop drug use will have the supports necessary to do so. Those supports include availability of adequate housing, child care, and job training. For those continuing drug use, simple, economically feasible methods to clean syringes should be taught. Some activist groups are attempting to institute changes in local laws so that purchase of syringes without a prescription would be legal; other municipalities have begun free needle exchange programs in which registered intravenous drug users can exchange one used needle/syringe for a new one. Women should also be alerted to the fact that if their male partner is an IV drug user who shares needles, they are at risk for contracting HIV from him.

*Woman-to-Woman Transmission.* Woman-to-woman transmission of the virus has been reported, but is rare. Women who engage in sexual activity with other women should be encouraged to use latex barriers or other products such as dental dams when exposure to potentially infected fluids might occur. They should also avoid shared use of objects during sexual activities; although if they choose to do so, a thorough cleansing before use and between partners is an alternative (Klirsfeld, 1998).

## Secondary Prevention

Secondary prevention techniques emphasize the necessity of early recognition of HIV-positive women. As stated by Parsey and others (1996):

> "The importance of early recognition of HIV and early initiation of treatment cannot be overemphasized. A timely diagnosis of HIV may enable the patient to participate in more AIDS clinical trials and improve her access to medical therapies, such as zidovudine and PCP prophylaxis. Knowledge of HIV infection may decrease the incidence of transmission of the virus to partners and unborn children. Finally, an early diagnosis of HIV allows health care workers to provide social supports for the patient and her family, giving the woman more time for decisions regarding reproduction, child guardianship, and decision-making proxies."

Early identification of HIV-positive women means that we must not overlook the possibility that any woman may be carrying the HIV virus and that the way the disease presents in women is different than in men. Because of the early history of the disease being found primarily in homosexual men, HIV/AIDS may be considered a "men's" disease (Parsey and others, 1996), and women may not be offered testing. Because the fastest growing method of transmission is now heterosexual contact, we must maintain a high index of suspicion, regardless of marital status or socioeconomic class. All women must have thorough sexual histories done, including questions about their number of partners, their beliefs of monogamy from their partners or spouses, and use of condoms.

*Presentation of HIV in Women.* Although, in general, they both suffer from the same opportunistic infections, women with HIV disease present differently when compared with men. The major difference is that in women, gynecologic manifestations may be the first sign and cause significant challenges to the comfort of the woman with the disease. The first signs may include (1) recurrent vulvovaginal candidiasis that may be persistent and difficult to treat; (2) bacterial vaginosis (BV), which also may be recurrent and difficult to treat; (3) recurrent genital herpes simplex infection; (4) human papillomavirus (HPV) infections; (5) aggressive forms of pelvic inflammatory disease (PID); and (6) cervical dysplasia and neoplasia (Larkin and others, 1996).

*Concerns about Pregnancy.* Reproductive concerns become a major consideration for the woman infected with HIV. For women of reproductive age, who are the vast majority, the first decision is whether or not to have a child or more children. Fortunately, in contrast to the early days of the epidemic, research on the treatment of pregnant women has shown that vertical transmission from mother to baby can be greatly reduced with the use of zidovudine, with some studies showing a reduction from 25% down to 8% (Burdge and Money, 1996). It is important for all women to be offered HIV testing, preferably as part of preconceptual planning, but definitely as part of early prenatal care so that if the infection is discovered, drug therapy may be started.

Data suggest that pregnancy does not cause a faster progression of HIV disease for women, nor do there seem to be deleterious effects for the fetus. The exception is in those women with advanced stages of AIDS. In their cases, there are more complications for both mother and infant.

Although transmission may occur prenatally, intrapartally, and during breastfeeding, most cases of transmission are believed to occur during delivery. Although a surgical delivery might seem to be a logical intervention to reduce transmission, no data show that this is an effective option (Burdge and Money, 1996). If a woman has not taken zidovudine during her pregnancy, however, the CDC recommends that she be offered intravenous dosing of this medication during her labor and delivery.

If a woman wishes to delay pregnancy, then she must choose a fertility-control method based not only on her personal preferences, but also on potential medication interactions with drugs she may be taking for HIV treatment, the potential for increased risk for transmission to partners, and the possible side effects of a method. For example, an IUD would not be a recommended choice because of the higher risk of pelvic infections with this method. Oral contraception has a demonstrated decrease in effectiveness when used while also taking protease inhibitors, which are extensively metabolized by the liver (Johnson, Silverstein-Currier, and Sanchez-Keeland, 1999).

Data from the early years of this epidemic showed that women progressed more quickly to end-stage AIDS than men did, and therefore died much more quickly after being diagnosed. It is believed that at that time, women came into care later because their early symptoms were not recognized as being related to HIV infection. In addition, they were less likely to be offered zidovudine and tended to be socioeconomically disadvantaged and in poorer health. As women are identified and treated earlier in the course of their disease, they now seem to follow the same course and progression of the disease as men. In more recent studies, as these and other factors have been controlled, it is now believed that gender does not cause a difference in prognosis.

### Interventions

The face of HIV/AIDS treatment changes from day to day. Although it is not the intention of this section to discuss treatment options, we who care for HIV-infected women must become advocates for them and keep up-to-date with the latest in therapies. Currently, several antiretroviral medications interfere with the capacity of the

virus to replicate. In addition, protocols are available for prophylactic treatment of opportunistic infection.

***Complementary Therapies.*** Women should also be encouraged to research the role of complementary therapies for HIV infection and for dealing with side effects of the treatments. Elion and Cohen (1997) explore the usefulness of nutritional agents, especially in the early stages of the infection, and the role of acupuncture to reduce symptoms such as night sweats, fatigue, and neuropathies; the use of herbal therapies as anti-HIV agents; and the use of massage as a way to calm, energize, and allow patients to tolerate other HIV symptoms.

### Nursing Considerations

We must be aware of the psychosocial sequellae of HIV/AIDS. A diagnosis of HIV puts a woman at a heightened risk for depression and other mental health problems. She may experience grief, fear, or anxiety about the future of her children. Guilt or shame about the source of her infection may make it difficult for her to reveal her diagnosis to family and friends even though she needs a great deal of support. A woman who has attained sobriety, and then is diagnosed with HIV may return to drug use to deal with the psychic pain involved.

Furthermore, she may lose the sense of security she had with her partner because the diagnosis may reveal that her partner has a risk profile she did not know, such as intravenous drug use or having other sex partners. Disturbingly, a woman herself may be at increased risk for violence when she discloses her status to a partner.

Along with the medications that are so vital to her health maintenance, a woman's mental health needs, family dynamics, capacity to work, and social concerns must form an integrated whole to her health care picture. We can help her face the reality of the diagnosis and the treatment options, as well as integrate this into the other aspects of her health care and her life.

##  CONDITIONS OF THE LUNGS

### Asthma

Asthma affects approximately 15 million people in the United States, and the rates are rising (Lammert, 1995). More than 5000 people die each year from asthma, and most of these deaths are preventable (Janson, 1998). There are over 100 million days of restricted activities in both men and women with asthma (Richman, 1997). African-Americans and those who reside in urban areas have higher prevalence rates for the disease. Before the age of 20, more males have the condition; after the age of 20, more females are affected (Lammert, 1995). In addition, women account for almost 75% of the hospitalizations for adults with asthma (Skobeloff and others, 1996).

The exact cause for asthma is unknown. It is known, however, that the condition is a chronic inflammatory disorder of the airways resulting from complicated interactions among inflammatory cells, cell mediators, and normal cells in the airways (Janson, 1998). This inflammation leads to hyperactivity; restrictions in airflow; bronchoconstriction; airway edema; mucous plug formation; and all the symptoms of asthma: coughing, wheezing, dyspnea, chest tightness, and breathlessness.

Multiple triggers or aggravating factors are involved with asthma. Table 7-2 lists only some of these; many others have been implicated. The last factor in Table 7-2, endocrine factors, has particular importance for women. Recent research has supported the role of estrogen in the complex pathogenesis of asthma. Venn and coworkers (1998) suggest that the reversal of prevalence from boys to girls during the adolescent years may be due to the hormonal changes of puberty. Skobeloff and associates (1996) demonstrated a significant relationship between women presenting to the emergency department for asthma exacerbations and the menstrual cycle, with many more women presenting during the perimenstrual portion of the cycle. They postulate that the sustained levels of estradiol found in the earlier portion of the menstrual cycle are somehow protective. The data from Chandler and others (1997) support this preliminary research by demonstrating that administration of estradiol during the premenstrual portion of the cycle to women with asthma improved their pulmonary function test results.

Also of great importance is the recognition of the role of occupational exposure in asthma, either in worsening of symptoms to those who already have the condition or to the development of asthma in those who have never had the problem. Although Table 7-2 lists only a few of the occupational sources according to Chan-Yeung and Malo (1995), over 250 agents have been implicated. These agents may be used by women within their homes or they may be exposed in the workplace outside the home. Considering the large number of women working outside the home, the potential for lost days at work, and lost income, occupational exposure is a factor that must be given high priority.

### Diagnosis

The history and physical examination should focus on description of symptoms, identification of triggers or possible triggers, and a thorough pulmonary and cardiac examination. Diagnostic testing depends on symptoms and the differential diagnoses, but always includes pulmonary function testing. The most common conditions in the differential include tuberculosis, chronic obstructive pulmonary disease (COPD), and lung cancer.

### Interventions

Medical treatment depends on the frequency and severity of symptoms. Nursing interventions focus on assisting the woman in understanding the condition of asthma and problem solving with her about how she will care for herself.

To facilitate understanding of the scope of the disease and the treatment, a step approach to the classification of asthma has been established by the National Heart, Lung, and Blood Institute (1997): Step 1, mild intermittent; Step 2, mild persistent; Step 3, moderate persistent; and Step 4, severe persistent asthma. The mainstays of treatment are inhaled bronchodilators; inhaled corticosteroids or antiinflammatories; anticholinergic agents;

### TABLE 7-2  *Trigger Factors and Aggravating Factors for Asthma*

| | |
|---|---|
| Environmental allergens | Including dust mites, pollens, molds, fungi, cockroaches, animal dander. |
| Environmental irritants | Tobacco smoke and pollution |
| Occupational exposure | Animal sources: dander, shellfish, silkworms |
| | Insects: Moths, mites |
| | Plant sources: wheat, rye, soy, coffee beans, pectin, cotton, psyllium |
| | Wood sources: cedar, oak, mahogany, redwood |
| | Metals: platinum, nickel, cobalt, chromium |
| | Drugs: penicillin, cephalosporins, methyldopa, tetracycline |
| | Chemicals: polyvinyl chloride, urea formaldehyde, freon, latex, glutaraldehyde, dyes, solvents |
| Respiratory infections | Viral infections, bacterial infections |
| Exercise | Jogging, running, lifting and carrying |
| Food additives | Sulfites |
| Environmental changes | Cold air |
| Emotions | Anger, stress, laughter |
| Drugs | Aspirin, $\beta$-blockers, NSAIDs |
| Gastroesophageal reflux | Response to type or amount of food |
| Endocrine factors | Especially lower estrogen levels |

mast cell stabilizers; and the newest treatment group, the leukotriene modifiers. Theophylline, a medication used frequently in the past, is now considered a third- or fourth-line agent. It is a bronchodilator, but has a narrow therapeutic range and a toxic side effect profile, and therefore its usefulness is limited.

*Identification of Condition.* Our role in asthma identification and management is significant. Identification of those women with asthma is the first step to reducing morbidity and mortality. Women may not always seek help when they are having symptoms, may not want to know that they have asthma, or may be unable or unwilling to obtain a health evaluation in a timely way. By the time health care is sought, the symptoms may have subsided, and the diagnosis missed. Any women who mention experiencing symptoms that include chest tightness, shortness of breath (SOB), wheezing, or persistent cough should be encouraged to have a more complete evaluation. Health care providers must have a high index of concern for asthma. According to Janson (1998), underdiagnosis and underrecognition of the severity of asthma on the part of providers are factors in the morbidity and mortality of the disease.

*Triggers.* Once a woman has been diagnosed with asthma, it is important to identify triggers and avoid these as much as possible. Changes in the household and work environments may need to be made. It is also essential to make sure that the client knows the proper use of inhalers and the proper indication for any other medications that have been prescribed. In addition, appropriate therapy choices depend on the use of a personal flow meter. These handheld meters measure the peak expiratory flow rate (PEFR) and are very easy to learn how to use. Normal values depend on sex, weight, height, and age. For women, normal values range from 350 to 500 L/min. We should make sure that patients know how to use this device and that they keep a systematic record or diary of their readings. In this way, use of medications can be based not only on the symptoms that the client is experiencing, but also on her flow meter results.

*Implications of Disease for Women.* Asthma exacerbations can cause enormous disruptions in a woman's life. These disruptions include the inability to perform her usual activities and the time she must spend in health care facilities obtaining assistance. We need to discuss plans ahead of time with our clients, a "what if" approach. The most important point to emphasize is that women should not delay seeking help when their symptoms are worsening—most asthma deaths can be prevented by early intervention, and asthma attacks can be less severe if therapy is started early enough. Plans for child care, communicating with employers and family, and how to get to the nearest health care facility should all be discussed in advance.

*Health Teaching.* The health teaching required when a woman has asthma is time intensive when done in a thorough manner. This requirement adds to the difficulty of a woman managing her condition well. A woman may have the most up-to-date medications, but if she does not know how to use them properly, their effectiveness will be limited. If triggers are not avoided, attacks may be more frequent. Primary care nurse practitioners and physicians may not be able to devote the necessary resources to this education (Gibbons, 1996). As nurses, we have the skills and responsibility to assume this task.

Wieker (1999) encourages that a written treatment plan be developed with the client. This plan is a document that is developed together, outlining the responsibilities of both the client and the nurse. It emphasizes education and understanding about asthma, as well as treatment modalities, and what to do in case of increasing severity of symptoms. It is only with concerted efforts to recognize the condition, assist the woman to self-manage the disease, and promote optimal teaching that asthma will become a more manageable condition.

## Lung Cancer

Although women may be concerned or frightened about the prospect of dying from breast cancer, since 1987 lung cancer has caused greater mortality (Ernster, 1994; Zang and Wynder, 1998). In the majority of cases of lung cancer, cigarette smoking is a factor (Morabia and Wynder, 1991; Harris and others, 1993; Ernster, 1994; Goroll, May, and Mulley, 1995b; Freund and Pastorek, 1996; Dambro, 1998; Feinerman, 1998; Uphold and Graham, 1998c; Zang and Wynder, 1998). Unlike breast cancer, for which little is known about primary preventive strategies, the mortality from lung cancer caused by exposure to cigarette smoke can be greatly reduced if women stop smoking; and in the case of adolescent women, never begin smoking; and avoid passive exposure to smoke by being in rooms or cars with smokers. In addition to lung cancer, smoking has been proven or implicated to be a factor in numerous health problems (Rigotti and Polivogianus, 1995; Dambro, 1998; Feinerman, 1998; Uphold and Graham, 1998c) (Box 7-3).

The longevity of women over men may reflect the very low rates of cigarette smoking in women during the first part of the century. There is concern that as increasing numbers of women began smoking in this century, the incidence of lung cancer rates increased in women. Lung cancer rates in men have leveled off, which is a reflection of the decreased prevalence of smoking. In women, although the rates of smoking have leveled off, the rate of lung cancer continues to rise and may actually surpass those of men, if current trends continue (Travis, Travis, and Devesa, 1995; Zang and Wynder, 1998). These rates reflect an incidence of lung cancer based on earlier use. Current research shows that women may have an increased susceptibility to the carcinogens found in tobacco (Harris and others, 1993; Zang and Wynder, 1998).

---

### BOX 7-3 Health Problems Related to Tobacco Use

Asthma
Chronic obstructive pulmonary disease (COPD)
Coronary artery disease
Stroke
Peripheral vascular disease
Osteoporosis
Earlier menopause
Cervical cancer
Head and neck cancers
Pancreatic cancer
Bladder cancer
Kidney cancer
Stomach cancer
Peptic ulcer disease
Cataracts
Periodontal disease
Bronchitis
Pneumonia
Increased risk of stroke/clots while on oral contraceptives
Premature aging of the skin
Miscarriage
Stillbirth
Neonatal death
Impaired placental function
Premature birth
Fetal growth retardation
Low birth weight
Sudden infant death syndrome

---

### BOX 7-4 Chemicals Associated with the Risk of Lung Cancer

Asbestos
Radon
Chromate
Nickel
Uranium
Halogen ethers
Inorganic arsenic
Radioisotopes

---

Despite the overwhelming evidence that supports smoking as the major risk factor for lung cancer, other risk factors must also be considered. For women, lung cancer without a history of smoking is more common than it is in men (Goroll, May, and Mulley, 1995b). Exposure to second-hand smoke, occupational exposure, and urban pollution appear to be involved, particularly exposure to the agents listed in Box 7-4 (Goroll, May, and Mulley, 1995b; Dambro, 1998).

#### Diagnosis

Unfortunately, chest radiographs and sputum cytology tests are neither sensitive nor specific enough to be used for screening, and often by the time a person with lung cancer is symptomatic, the cancer has become metastatic. The survival rates beyond 5 years for lung cancer are very poor, 10% to 20% at best (Ernster, 1994; Goroll, May, and Mulley, 1995b).

Women may present with symptoms of cough, dyspnea, SOB, chest pain, exercise limitations, hemoptysis, hoarseness, wheezing, weight loss, fatigue, or anemia. In such women, history taking should include a thorough smoking history, occupational history, exposure to second-hand smoke, and any history of living in an urban environment. The physical examination focuses on a complete respiratory system examination, as well as cardiac and skin examination. Preliminary diagnostic studies include a chest radiograph, CBC, ECG, purified protein derivative (PPD) (tuberculin skin test), blood chemistry profile, and pulmonary function tests. Respiratory or oncology specialists may perform computerized axial tomography (CAT) scans and bronchoscopy among other tests.

#### Interventions

We have a tremendous role to play in the primary prevention of lung cancer in women. At every opportunity, a smoking history should be taken, and women who smoke should be offered support if they desire to quit. School nurses can take an active part in providing educational forums to children of all ages, using their developmental stage to guide the type of educational intervention. Support groups, smoking cessation classes, and behavioral motivation counseling are all ways that we can actively become involved in this issue. In addition, advocating public health and health policy efforts that support women's efforts to protect themselves in their homes, as well as work environments, and supporting community efforts to reduce exposure to second-hand smoke and environmental pollutants are ways that we can intervene to decrease the occurrence of this devastating illness.

## CONDITIONS OF THE BREAST

One of the major reasons that women visit their primary care clinicians is concerns about their breasts. Age-appropriate breast cancer screening guidelines should always be followed for any concerns about breast problems. In addition, any woman who believes she has a breast lump should be evaluated because women of any age can die from breast cancer.

According to Appling (1998) 50% of all women will be seen at some time for a breast disorder, with one third of these having breast biopsies. Concern is stimulated by the well-known statistics showing that 1 in 8 (Hansen and Morrow, 1998) or 1 in 9 (Kuter, 1995; Appling, 1998; Strozzo, 1998) women will have breast cancer during her lifetime. In addition, the significant psychosocial implications, including issues surrounding body image and sexuality, cause women to seek help with questions about normal breast functioning, as well as for breast problems. As members of the health care team, we must each develop the skills necessary to assist women in self-assessment of their breasts. In addition women also need the most up-to-date information about risk factors, early detection, screening, diagnostic testing, and support for surgical and medical interventions for the various conditions that affect their breasts.

The most common concerns expressed by women are breast pain, nipple discharge, breast infection (mastitis), and breast masses. Each of these conditions is discussed further in the following paragraphs, with the exception of mastitis, which usually occurs only in the lactating woman, and therefore is found in the chapters covering postpartum issues.

In addition to these problems, women also have questions regarding size discrepancies between their own breasts and concerns for the overall size of both breasts as compared with other women. Small breast size may bring up concerns about her ability to breastfeed or decrease her sense of sexual attractiveness, especially given the media promotion of larger breast size. Pendulous breasts sometimes create discomfort, especially chronic back pain, and may lead to questions about treatment options. Size discussions are especially common in younger adolescents, as they go through the developmental challenges associated with acceptance of the myriad body changes of puberty. Knowledge about normal breast functioning, self-assessment, and comfort with discussions about sexuality and attractiveness are part of our role in the self-care and advocacy of these patients.

## Breast Pain

Breast pain (mastalgia or mastodynia) is usually associated with cyclic hormonal changes, and although distressing, it rarely indicates a serious problem. Because the levels of circulating hormones are within a normal range in women who have this condition, the exact cause for the pain is unknown. Several theories have been postulated, including increased receptor sensitivity to the normal circulating hormone levels (Ashley, 1998). Two additional classifications of breast pain have also been identified: noncyclic pain and nonbreast pain (Ashley, 1998).

Breast pain is rarely associated with breast cancer (Hansen and Morrow, 1998), but should be taken as a serious symptom, with a thorough history, clinical examination of the breasts, and diagnostic studies as appropriate. Because the history, physical, and diagnostic studies are the same for all breast symptoms, a more thorough discussion appears at the end of this section.

### Cyclic Breast Pain

In the case of cyclic breast pain, once a woman has been assured that there is no cancer, often she will be able to cope with the pain without further therapy. If the pain is such that a woman requires treatment, then the clinician can promote several interventions. Although several studies (Hansen and Morrow, 1998) have not supported a statistically significant therapeutic usefulness of these suggestions, many women report finding some relief, and therefore a trial of the various techniques is worthwhile. These include: dietary changes such as eliminating fat and/or caffeine; increasing the intake of vitamins $B_6$, C, and/or E; increasing intake of high fiber foods; use of evening primrose oil; wearing supportive bras, but avoiding underwire styles and padded bras; wearing athletic bras while exercising; and using over-the-counter (OTC) analgesics such as acetaminophen, aspirin, ibuprofen, naproxen, or other NSAIDs (Miller, 1995; Ashley, 1998; Hansen and Morrow, 1998).

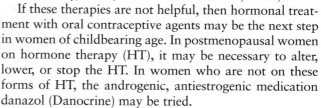

If these therapies are not helpful, then hormonal treatment with oral contraceptive agents may be the next step in women of childbearing age. In postmenopausal women on hormone therapy (HT), it may be necessary to alter, lower, or stop the HT. In women who are not on these forms of HT, the androgenic, antiestrogenic medication danazol (Danocrine) may be tried.

### Noncyclic Breast Pain

In the case of noncyclic breast pain, all of the therapeutic regimens listed above may be tried, with the exception of hormone therapy, which has not been found useful. Some women may opt to try Danocrine, especially if their pain is disabling.

### Nonbreast Pain

Some women experience pain in the breast area that is related to the structural components of their chests rather than to their breasts. For those women with pain that has a nonbreast source, the underlying condition must be treated.

## Nipple Discharge

Nipple discharge is another symptom that greatly worries women, and although it usually has a noncancer-related explanation, it can be a sign of malignancy. There are many causes for nipple discharge, but all of these can fall into one of three categories: (1) physiologic,

(2) galactorrhea, and (3) pathologic (Morrison, 1998). Treatment for the three classifications of nipple discharge varies significantly.

### Physiologic Discharge

**Physiologic discharge** refers to the normal response of the breast to stimulation, such as massage, rubbing from clothing during vigorous exercise, sexual stimulation, and self-stimulation. The discharge is *not* spontaneous, is serous in color, and is bilateral. If all other causes have been ruled out, then an affected woman can be reassured and should adopt a "watch and wait" approach. Explore with her ways to reduce the stimulation to her breasts, and encourage her to report any changes in her discharge.

### Galactorrhea

**Galactorrhea** is breast discharge that is milky white, spontaneous, unrelated to lactation, and often is bilateral. It can be caused by medications, chest wall trauma, breast stimulation, thyroid problems, Cushing's disease, acromegaly, and pituitary tumors known as adenomas, or the discharge can be idiopathic in nature (Morrison, 1998). Treatment depends on the underlying cause.

### Pathologic Nipple Discharge

**Pathologic nipple discharge** includes those cases in which the discharge can be bloody, serous, serosanguinous, watery, or green. It is usually only found in one breast, is spontaneous, intermittent, and persistent. Any woman with this type discharge must be thoroughly examined for the possibility of underlying cancer.

## Fibrocystic Breast Complex

Fibrocystic breast complex refers to a condition of the breast that causes much confusion. In the past, it has been called fibrocystic disease. Two other synonyms for the condition are mammary dysplasia and chronic cystic mastitis (Miller, 1995). When reporting the results of a clinical examination, fibrocystic changes mean that a woman has lumpy breasts that may or may not be painful. She may have cysts that come and go, fluctuating with the menstrual cycle. Biopsies of her breasts might show cysts, hyperplasia, fibrosis, or fibroadenomas, as well as other benign findings. In autopsy reports, up to 90% of women have these benign changes (Bennett and Smith, 1995). Only in a very small percentage of women with biopsy results that show atypical hyperplasia is there an increased risk of breast cancer (NIH, 1998a), and this risk increases if there is a family history of breast cancer (Bennett and Smith, 1995).

According to Bennett and Smith (1995) fibrocystic breast complex is a diagnosis that should be reserved for women in whom recurrent or multiple cysts form and who have localized, persistent nodular tissue or documented atypical hyperplasia. For all other women, the diagnosis is physiologic breast changes, and treatment is symptom-specific.

### Breast Masses

Most breast masses are found by the woman herself. These masses cause a great deal of distress because of the fear of cancer. Because normal breasts can have lumps that vary with the age, menstrual cycle and weight of a woman (Oktay, 1998), it is important that a thorough workup be done when any distinct masses are found. Because physiologic breast changes can cause confusing breast nodularities, it is important to confirm that a distinct mass is identifiable. Once identified, the woman will be provided with further diagnostic testing to distinguish between cysts, fibroadenomas, and carcinomas.

### Cysts

**Cysts** can be identified through the use of ultrasound and/or fine needle aspiration (FNA). Frequently, FNA actually resolves the cyst, and the woman is reassured. Bloody aspirate should be sent to pathology. Abnormal pathology results, and a recurring cyst should be evaluated by a breast surgeon because removal may be indicated (Ziegfield, 1998).

### Fibroadenomas

**Fibroadenomas** are the most common benign tumors of the breast. They can occur at any time, but are found most frequently in women in their 20s and 30s (Deckers and Ricci, 1992). They are usually painless, well-defined, movable, rubbery, round tumors easily distinguished on ultrasound. Management of fibroadenomas depends on a woman's age, her family history, the size of the tumor, and the symptoms the woman is experiencing. For some women, following these benign tumors over time is entirely appropriate. Other women may opt for needle biopsy, or even excision, to be absolutely sure of the diagnosis.

It is important to remember that although the risk of breast cancer spans a woman's lifetime, most cases are identified after the age of 50. According to Hansen and Morrow (1998), "The absolute risk of cancer development between the ages of 35 and 55 is only 2.5% in the absence of other risk factors." In other words, only about 15% of cases occur before the age of 40 (Strozzo, 1998).

Because there is no known primary prevention of breast cancer, it is important to identify women at risk so that cancers are found early and therefore can be treated with more success. One of the techniques for doing this is by careful history taking to identify those women with one or more risk factors. A family history of breast cancer is the most significant risk factor known at this time. A great deal of research is being done on recognition of gene sites that are thought to be the major contributors to this risk. It is the occurrence of mutations at these gene sites that is inherited and leads to a predisposition to develop a type of breast cancer. These gene sites, known as BRCA1 and BRCA2, are associated with cancers that occur in first-degree relatives during the premenopausal years. However, these mutations account for only a small percentage of breast cancer cases (Hansen and Morrow, 1998).

## Risk Factors

Although the risk factors of age, previous diagnosis of breast cancer, atypical hyperplasia, and a first-degree relative with breast cancer are significant, there are also other risk factors; however, their role in cause and effect is difficult to quantify. These include early menarche; late first pregnancy (after 30) or no pregnancies; late menopause; hormone metabolism; density of breast tissue; high-fat diets; obesity; race; alcohol consumption (1 to 2 drinks per day); exposure to high-dose ionizing radiation; exposure to environmental pollutants; smoking, especially as an adolescent; oral contraceptives; and hormone therapy (Kuter, 1995; Appling, 1998; NIH, 1998b; Ziegfield 1998).

## Evaluation of Breasts

### Breast Examination

Regardless of setting, we have a responsibility to teach women how to do breast self-examination (BSE) and to encourage its practice. Regardless of risk profile, all women should perform BSE once per month beginning at age 20. Menstruating women should be reminded to do it at the end of a menses, and postmenopausal women should pick a day once a calendar month. In addition, we should ensure that all women seen for a health care visit have a clinical breast examination (CBE) once every 3 years between the ages of 20 to 40 and yearly after age 40. This frequency clearly should be increased in women with high-risk profiles.

Women between the ages of 35 to 40 should have a first baseline mammogram. Women over the age of 50 should have a mammogram every year. However, there has been some controversy about the cost effectiveness in the scheduling of screening mammography in women ages 40 to 50. In 1997, because of reductions in mortality rates demonstrated in research studies, the American Cancer Society urged women between these ages to have a mammogram every year; previous recommendations were that it be done every 2 years.

### History

A thorough history is an essential tool in helping determine the program of follow-up that a woman receives. The necessary data include the following:

*Family history of breast cancer or ovarian cancer:* age at diagnosis, relationship, sex
*Health history:* age, surgical history of the chest, trauma to the chest, medications
*Gynecologic history:* Menarche, menstrual pattern, last menstrual period (LMP), parity, age(s) when pregnant, contraceptive use and type
*History of breast problems:* type problem, diagnostic studies done, therapies used, woman's understanding of her diagnosis
*Presenting problem at current visit:*
  If discharge: whether spontaneous or not, color, unilateral or bilateral, when it began
  If pain: frequency, relationship to menstrual cycle, location, character, when it began, relieving and exacerbating factors, any associated masses
  If a mass: when discovered, where, consistency, mobility
  In general: changes in the size, color, skin, or shape of the breast or nipple

### Physical Examination

A thorough explanation of how to prepare for a CBE helps reduce a woman's anxiety. She should remove her bra, if she wears one, and put on a shirt or upper body covering. Generally it is designed to open in the front so that one half of the woman's chest may be covered while the other is examined and the time of full exposure is limited. An explanation of the steps of the examination and why they are done also helps her prepare herself mentally for what she may consider to be very intimate touching.

The physical examination for a woman with a problem includes a thorough inspection and palpation of breasts; the nipples; and the cervical, supraclavicular, and axillary nodes. The clinician is looking for nipple discharge, skin changes, retractions, dimpling, or pulling. During palpation, the clinician should note the presence of nodularities, or tenderness. If a discrete mass is palpated, then it should be carefully described, noting size, shape, location, mobility, density, and tenderness.

### Diagnostic Studies

Questionable findings should never be ignored, regardless of the age of the patient. In all cases, proper diagnostic studies should be done. These may include breast ultrasound, needle aspiration, cytology, biopsy, or mammogram. The decision of what tests to order depends on the woman's age, her risk status, her particular clinical findings, and her insurance coverage.

## Breast Cancer

When a woman is diagnosed with breast cancer, several interventions might be offered. Researchers are constantly developing new therapies and comparing cure rates among differing types of surgery, radiation, and chemotherapeutic agents. Depending on the size and type of the lesion, the woman's personal and family history, and the presence or absence of metastases, a woman's breast cancer will be staged from I (small tumor, no metastases) to stage IV (tumor of any size with distant metastases). The oncologist may offer a variety of treatment plans, many using a combination of therapies. The surgical alternatives include lumpectomy, partial (segmental) mastectomy, simple (total) mastectomy, modified radical mastectomy, and radical mastectomy. Radiation therapy is used to treat women with early stage disease. In addition, 50 possible chemotherapeutic agents are used frequently in women with metastatic sites. Autologous bone marrow transplant is also used to treat women with very aggressive cancer or for those with metastases (Branch, 1998).

## Nurse's Role Concerning Breast Health

We have a crucial role to play in promoting breast health for all women. We must educate women about the normal functioning of the human breast, encourage BSE, and perform CBE during all routine screening encounters. We can advocate for women to obtain a mammography, and alert them to programs that offer this service. Some communities offer a breast-screening program free or at a minimal charge.

We must also recognize the enormous impact that breast concerns and problems have on a woman's life and become knowledgeable about the conditions that are relatively benign, so that we can offer reasonable and accurate reassurance. For the woman undergoing diagnostic studies, it is important to be able to describe what will be done, including potential discomfort that might be experienced, and how long it may be uncomfortable. If a woman understands that the better the compression of the breast the better the results of the mammogram, she may have a higher tolerance for the pain she may feel. In addition she may be able to relax more during the procedure and feel less pain.

For the woman with breast cancer, we must be familiar with the various options available; the side effects and risks of the various treatment regimens; and the opportunities for support services, including breast reconstruction. Some communities have programs for women

with breast cancer who are undergoing treatment, a Reach for Recovery program for women who have experienced a mastectomy, and/or a breast cancer survivor's group for those who have had cancer but are now cancer free. Many women find it helpful to be able to talk with other women in the same situation as themselves. Often they are not as comfortable talking about their diagnosis, treatment, and concerns with their friends as they are with women dealing with the same fears and experiences.

### Nursing Diagnoses

Each woman's response to her diagnosis of breast cancer and her treatment plan is unique. Therefore, nursing care plans must be individualized; however, some commonalties in need have been seen and should be considered. The following nursing diagnoses are most prevalent, but not all inclusive:

> Altered role performance
> Anticipatory grieving
> Anxiety
> Body image disturbance
> Fear
> Hopelessness
> Impaired skin integrity
> Ineffective breastfeeding
> Knowledge deficit
> Low self-esteem
> Pain
> Powerlessness
> Sexual dysfunction
> Situational low self-esteem
> Sleep pattern disturbance (Branch, 1998)

After addressing an individual woman's needs as a beginning framework, we can offer the support, expert knowledge, psychologic caring, and physical care needs necessary to help women cope with problems in their breasts.

##  CONDITIONS OF THE PELVIC FLOOR

### Pelvic Floor Relaxation

Usually, the musculature of the pelvic floor supports the pelvic organs. This support positions the organs within the normal pelvic anatomy. The musculature includes muscles, ligaments, and fascia. Any situation that weakens these structures then causes the pelvic organs to lose their support and descend toward the vaginal canal. This is known as **pelvic relaxation syndrome**, and is responsible for prolapses of various organs and some forms of urinary incontinence. This syndrome occurs more frequently as women age; thus, with the aging of the U.S. population, the symptoms caused by this condition are becoming more common.

Pelvic relaxation syndrome can affect the bladder (cystocele), the rectum (rectocele), and the bowel (enterocele). These conditions can be seen in Figure 7-1.

In addition, the uterus can be affected by a condition known as **uterine prolapse**, which occurs when the uterus moves down the vagina. The severity is defined by degrees as shown in Figure 7-2 and as follows:

First degree—prolapse into the vaginal canal
Second degree—prolapse to the level of the hymenal ring
Third degree—protrusion of the uterus beyond the hymenal ring
Fourth degree—the uterus is fully outside the hymenal ring

## Causes

The causes of pelvic relaxation are grouped into three categories: congenital defects, trauma, and aging (Nichols and Brubaker, 1995b). Congenital conditions include lack of connective tissue strength or conditions such as spina bifida. Trauma includes pelvic surgery, childbirth, and sources of increased intraabdominal pressure, such as in heavy lifting, constipation, ascites, obesity, or COPD. Aging is a factor because of the natural reduction in estrogen, which causes atrophy and a weakening in the tissue structure. Furthermore, gravity is also a factor, with the constant downward pulling of organs during the hours when women are upright.

## History

Symptoms include backache, a feeling of fullness in the pelvic region; constipation or painful defecation; urinary incontinence, frequency, and urgency; dyspareunia; discomfort while walking or sitting; or actual protrusion of the uterus from the vaginal introitus. Symptoms may be lessened at night while lying down, but get worse during the day as the woman remains upright. A woman may be too embarrassed to discuss some of these symptoms, especially those involving urinary incontinence. She may also believe that these symptoms are a normal or necessary part of aging and that nothing can be done. We must take the initiative to include questions about incontinence, urgency, constipation, and sexual functioning in our assessments with women.

## Physical Examination

Complete abdominal, pelvic, and rectal examinations need to be done to establish the extent of organ involvement along with the severity of the individual woman's symptoms. A plan of care can then be instituted.

## Interventions

***Nonsurgical Interventions.*** Nonsurgical interventions may be very helpful to those women with first-degree prolapses, as well as those women having occasional problems with urinary incontinence. The pelvic floor elevator exercise (sometimes called the Kegel exercise) can strengthen the muscles of the pelvic floor. (Box 7-5)

Cystocele

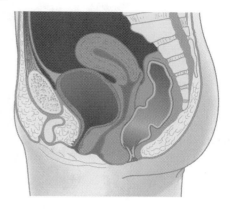

Rectocele

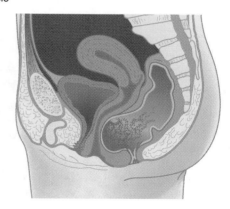

Enterocele

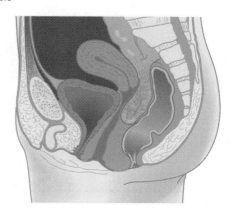

*FIGURE 7-1* • Cystocele, rectocele, and enterocele.

Normal

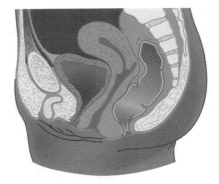

1st Degree

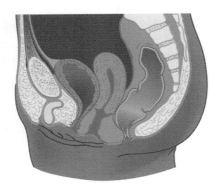

2nd Degree

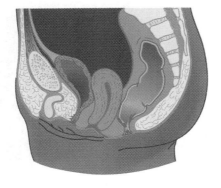

3rd Degree

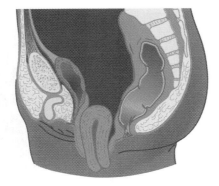

FIGURE 7-2 • Uterine prolapse.

---

### BOX 7-5    Pelvic Floor Elevator Exercise

*To be done six or seven times a day with three repetitions per time.*

1. Empty the bladder.
2. Imagine the pelvic floor as an elevator. It is sitting there at the first floor and by tightening the muscle it is going to be raised several floors.
3. Tighten the muscles to raise it to the first floor . . . second floor . . . third floor . . . fourth floor . . . fifth floor. Hold it there for 5 seconds.
4. Now see if you can go up one more floor. Hold it there for 30 seconds.
5. Now bring the elevator down slowly and steadily, fifth floor . . . fourth floor . . . third floor . . . second floor . . . first floor . . . Hold it.
6. To make vaginal examinations more comfortable or to prepare for childbirth the woman can now "go to the basement" by letting the pelvic floor muscles relax a little and bulge.
7. Repeat back up to the sixth floor and down again two more times.
8. Bring the elevator up to the second floor and leave it there. The muscles of the pelvic floor will be slightly tightened.

---

Other interventions include lifestyle changes, some of which may be more easily achieved than others. Women should be encouraged to attain ideal body weight, avoid or reduce heavy lifting, make changes in the diet to prevent constipation, and practice urination habits that promote bladder emptying. Advanced therapies for pelvic floor strengthening include using biofeedback and electrical stimulation (Maloney and Cafiero, 1999).

Some women strengthen their pelvic floor by using a specially designed product for this purpose. One of a series of progressively heavier weights, approximately the size and shape of a small tampon are placed in the vagina. Starting with the lightest one, the woman inserts the weight into her vagina and then holds it in place during the course of the day, periodically tightening down on it. As her muscles become stronger she moves to the next, heavier weight. By sequentially increasing the weight of the insert she gradually strengthens her pelvic floor muscles.

Pessaries may also be used and are extremely helpful for some women. **Pessaries** are hard rubber or plastic rings of various shapes and sizes that are fitted for each individual woman, much like a diaphragm fitting. It is placed inside the vagina and extends from behind the pubic arch to the posterior fornix. The purpose is to support and maintain the normal position of the uterus. Only health care providers who have experience with these devices should fit a pessary. Women who decide to use a pessary need to learn how to insert and remove it without difficulty. Lubricants are used for insertion. Women also need to know how to care for the device: it can be left in place for a few days at a time, but should be removed about twice a week for cleansing with plain soap and water (Forrest, 1998). The device should not cause discomfort and should not interfere with sexual activity. Possible side effects to pessary use are back pain, UTIs, vaginitis, and cervical erosion. Women should review the symptoms that go along with these complications and report any difficulties to the health care provider (Figures 7-3 to 7-5).

Hormone therapy (HT) may help some women. Both the oral forms, as well as topical cream formulations can be useful. The rationale is that with use of estrogen, the process of atrophy will be halted, and the woman will be less likely to develop pelvic floor relaxation or have it progress.

***Surgical Interventions.*** For women with higher degree prolapses, uterine cystoceles, and rectoceles, surgery may be the intervention of choice. Several pelvic surgeries resuspend the uterus and tighten the support of the musculature. Some women decide that instead of resuspending the uterus they have it removed with a hysterectomy. Regardless of the degree of prolapse, the goal of all the therapies is to restore comfort by reducing as many symptoms as possible.

## Female Genital Mutilation

As the numbers of women immigrating to the United States continues to grow, we must become familiar with cultural practices that effect the health care services provided to immigrant women. **Female genital mutilation (FGM)**, also known as female circumcision, is such a practice (Figure 7-6).

FGM refers to the partial or complete removal of the external genitalia. For purposes of universal monitoring and data collection, WHO (1996) has published the following definition: "Female genital mutilation constitutes all procedures which involve partial or total removal of the external female genitalia or other injury to the female genital organs whether for cultural or any other non-therapeutic reasons."

Although the exact origins of the practice are not known, FGM is known to be an ancient practice. Some researchers hypothesize that the practice started in Egypt and spread to surrounding areas, whereas others think the practice arose in several different regions at the same time (Christiansen, 1996). FGM is practiced in many countries, including the Middle East and Asia, but is most frequently associated with those in Africa. It predates Islam, is not in the Koran, and is practiced by both Muslims and Christians (Momoh, 1999). Prevalence

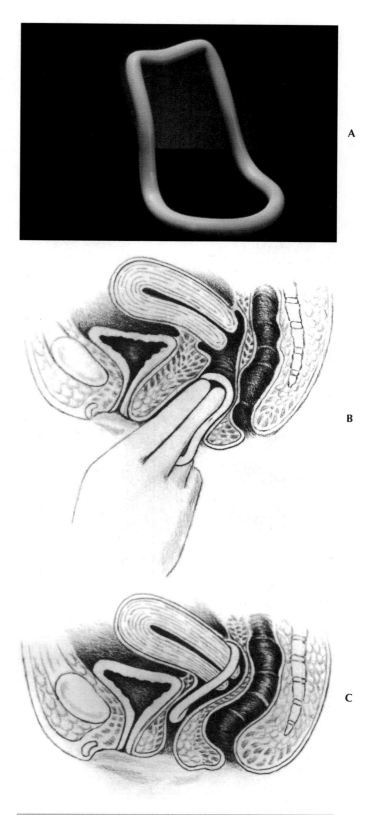

FIGURE 7-3 • **A,** Hodge Pessary recommended for retrodisplacement. **B,** Directing Pessary behind cervix. **C,** Pessary in position. *(Courtesy of Milex Products, Inc., Chicago.)*

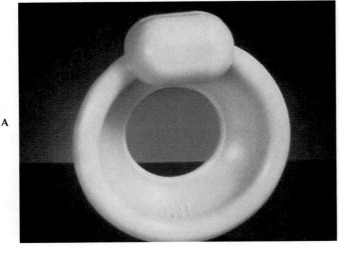

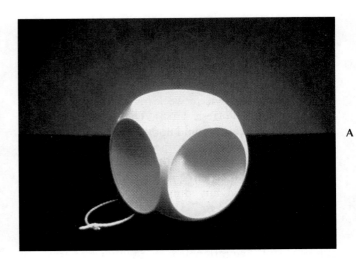

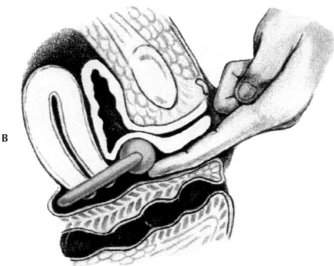

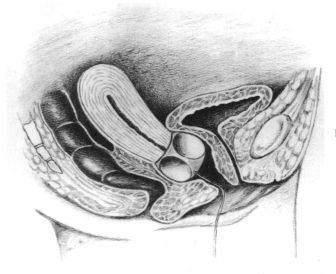

FIGURE 7-4 • **A,** Incontinence disk for stress incontinence with mild prolapse. **B,** Pessary in position. *(Courtesy of Milex Products, Inc., Chicago.)*

FIGURE 7-5 • **A,** Cube athletic support pessary for young women who experience stress urinary incontinence when exercising vigorously. **B,** Pessary in position. *(Courtesy of Milex Products, Inc., Chicago.)*

rates range from 5% in Zaire and Uganda, to 98% in Somalia and Djibouti. It is even known to occur in Europe, Canada, and the United States (Christiansen, 1996).

The procedures vary, but all are meant to exert social and sexual control of women. WHO (1996) has classified the procedures as follows:

> Type I: Excision of the prepuce with or without part or the entire clitoris
> Type II: Excision of the prepuce, clitoris, and partial or total excision of the labia minora
> Type III: Excision of part or all of the external genitalia and stitching/narrowing of the vaginal opening (infibulation)
> Type IV: Unclassified—includes pricking, piercing, stretching, and or incision of the clitoris and/or labia; cauterization/burning of the clitoris and

surrounding tissues; scraping of the vaginal orifice or cutting of the vagina; introduction of corrosive substances or herbs into the vagina to tighten or narrow it; or any other procedure that may be defined according to WHO guidelines.

Type I and II are the most common forms, accounting for 80% of FGM. The age of the female varies from country to country, with some FGM done in infancy, others before puberty, still others at the time of marriage or first pregnancy; average age is 4 to 10 years. The ritual is performed with a variety of implements including knives, scissors, razor blades, and pieces of glass, and is usually done by a local elder woman, assisted by other women. Men are rarely present. Anesthetics or antibiotics generally are not used.

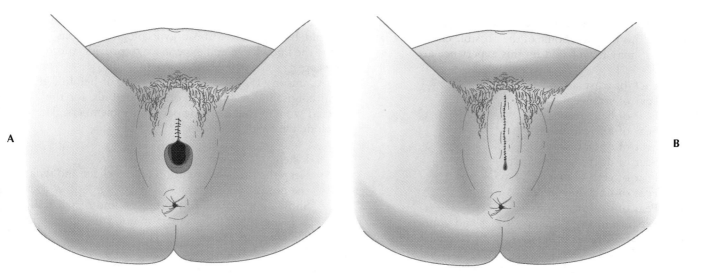

FIGURE 7-6 • Female genital mutilation. **A,** Type II. **B,** Type III.

In some countries to prevent death from blood loss and infection, health care personnel have been trained to perform FGM, using sterilized implements, anesthetics, and antibiotics. However, this practice has been condemned by WHO (1996) as training health care providers to perpetuate a human rights violation.

Complications are many, and include both short- and long-term problems. Short-term complications include hemorrhage, severe pain, infection, urine retention, and injury to adjacent tissues and organs. Any one of these side effects can then lead to shock, sepsis, and death. Long-term consequences include difficulty with urination, frequent UTIs, incontinence, infertility, chronic pelvic pain, chronic pelvic infections, dyspareunia, sexual dysfunction, vulvar abscesses and scar formation, rectovaginal or vesicovaginal fistulas, difficulties with menstruation, depression, anxiety, and complications during pregnancy and childbirth (WHO, 1996; Wright, 1996).

### Understanding the Practice

Various reasons are given for the practice (WHO, 1996; Wright, 1996; Momoh, 1999). These are listed in Box 7-6.

Recognizing the serious nature of this practice, WHO has become the lead organization in the fight to eradicate FGM, offering support and collaboration to any nation's government that requests help. The strategy of WHO is to eradicate the practice, while not condemning or alienating the nations or the cultures involved. Many countries have passed legislation outlawing the practice; the United States did with the passage of "Federal Prohibition of Female Genital Mutilation Act of 1996," Public Law 104-140, 110 Stat. 1327.

Another approach is to replace the traditional imperative with a new and acceptable, but safe cultural practice. Chelala (1998) reports about a new rite in Kenya

---

**BOX 7-6   *Reasons Given for Female Genital Mutilation***

- Custom and tradition
- Religious obligation
- Cleanliness
- Beauty
- Purification
- To enhance fertility
- Increasing matrimonial opportunities
- To enhance a sense of belonging
- To avoid social criticism
- To safeguard virginity
- To cure sexual deviance
- To prevent promiscuity
- To promote family honor
- Increased sexual pleasure for the husband
- Fear of the clitoris as an organ capable of killing newborns

---

and Uganda known as "circumcision through words." Adolescent girls are secluded for a week and "are taught basic concepts of anatomy and physiology, sexual and reproductive health and hygiene, and are counseled on gender issues, respect for adults, self-esteem, and how to deal with peer pressure." These young women are then awarded a certificate, given gifts, and become the center of attention in the community with music, dancing, and feasting. It is hoped that support for such rituals, such as that offered by the Elders Association in Uganda, will spread throughout the countries where FGM is practiced.

### Providing Care to Women

While working to support the organizations that are trying to stop FGM, we must also develop the therapeutic skills necessary to help individual women who have undergone this practice. Some of the possible emotions that a woman may have based on this experience are

- Lack of trust
- Fear of strangers
- Fear of being touched
- Fear of knives, razors
- Fear of operations
- Fear of doctors, midwives
- Fear of getting married, having sex
- Fear of having children
- Fear of new situations
- Separation from friends—older and younger
- Isolation from other family members, including mother and sisters
- It is wrong to cry, shout, or be angry
- There is something wrong with being female
- Being a woman is synonymous with pain (January 18, 2000, http://www.fgm.org/CounsellingGuide.html)

Female students born outside of the United States who seek health care from their college health offices may need a great deal of information. Cultural norms may dictate that these immigrant women not seek help for their health concerns, especially from a Western-based philosophy of health care. In addition to possible health problems, immigrant women may experience a great deal of stress and anxiety adjusting to their new community and living arrangements. History taking and physical examinations may be new experiences and must be done in a respectful, gentle way, without judgment. Women who have experienced FGM must know about the possible risk factors and interventions available for their particular symptom or health problem, and this information should be supplied by a supportive, knowledgeable clinician.

We must offer an understanding of the wide diversity of cultural experiences and a proactive approach to problem solving. For example, although the clitoris is understood to be a major site for sexual pleasure, the loss of the clitoris does not mean that women have to forego sexual pleasure. Kitzinger (1985) describes her conversations with women who have undergone FGM, and who have discovered that the perineal area has become a central area of sexual excitation for them. Stimulation in this area, including anal intercourse can cause orgasm.

### Nursing Role

Within their cultural context, women should be counseled about their bodies and their potential. In particular, women with FGM who are pregnant may come into health care for the first time. They require specialized care, and any presentation of her risks and options must be presented in culturally acceptable ways. Other women

with FGM who wish to pursue surgical repair techniques should be referred to those gynecologic surgeons who have the knowledge and experience to provide appropriate care.

Adamson (1992) outlines a number of helpful, general counseling techniques, of use not only for the affected woman, but also for her family members. These include the following skills:

- Listen.
- Keep the focus of attention on the client and what she needs to talk about.
- Show appreciation of the person and of what she is going through whether or not you agree with the opinions expressed.
- Encourage the woman to express herself, allowing and encouraging verbal and nonverbal forms of emotional release.
- Maintain strict confidentiality.
- Provide information.
- Keep an open mind about traditions and beliefs different from your own.
(January 18, 2000 http://www.fgm.org/CounsellingGuide.html).

If the woman desires, she may need a referral to formal counseling in which she has an opportunity to work in-depth on all aspects of her past and present life that relate to FGM.

We must be supportive of women and their backgrounds by providing culturally competent care that assists each woman in dealing with a personal situation within a family and political arena that they did not ask for and cannot change. Simultaneously, we must strive to increase the awareness of the health complications caused by this unnecessary surgery and support those who wish to establish alternative rituals within their cultures.

 ## CONDITIONS OF THE VULVA AND VAGINA

This region of the body can be the site for five major groups of problems: (1) dermatologic conditions, (2) STIs and vaginitis, (3) benign lesions, (4) carcinomas, and (5) chronic pain syndromes. A discussion of vaginitis follows in another section of this chapter, as does a section devoted to STIs. This first section reviews findings in the four remaining categories.

Symptoms of pain, itching, burning, or finding unusual lesions can all cause significant concern for women. These symptoms can interfere with her comfort, voiding, sexual activity, and exercise. It is important that women obtain a thorough evaluation before any treatments are suggested, so that interventions are focused on the correct cause.

## Dermatologic Conditions

The following dermatologic conditions must be considered when evaluating vulvar problems.

**Tinea cruris** is caused by infection with fungal organisms know as dermatophytes. It causes itching, burning, scaling, erythema, and sometimes fissures. It is usually treated with topical antifungal creams, but occasionally antifungals in pill form are used.

**Seborrheic dermatitis** is a condition that tends to run in families. Typical body areas involved include the ears, scalp, and nasolabial folds, but the vulva can also be affected. The typical appearance is pink to yellow, dull, greasy scaly lesions, which sometimes can be crusty. Mild topical corticosteroids are the treatment of choice.

**Vitiligo** is an autoimmune disorder that interferes with the production of melanin. Affected skin is white, but there are usually no other symptoms. Although topical corticosteroids are sometimes used, their effectiveness is limited. No effective treatment is available for this condition.

**Lichen sclerosus** is thought to be an autoimmune-related condition that causes thinning and hypopigmented changes of the vulva, especially surrounding the introitus. Topical corticosteroids are used to treat this condition.

**Contact dermatitis** refers to the reaction of the skin when in contact with either irritating substances or actual allergens. The skin in the area may be erythematous, itchy, burning, edematous, and/or scaly. Fissures in the skin may also be present. It is important to eliminate the causative agent, if it is identified. Topical corticosteroids are used to alleviate the symptoms.

**Folliculitis** is characterized by small abscesses that form in hair follicles, and therefore can be found on the labia majora, mons pubis, thighs, and buttocks. Topical or systemic antibiotics are used to treat this condition.

**Psoriasis** is a condition that has a genetic component and causes erythema and thickening. Several treatments are available for this condition when it occurs on other body surfaces, but for use on the vulva, topical corticosteroids are usually chosen.

**Lichen planus** is an inflammatory condition that can cause either lacy patterns or erosive changes that can be painful. Although topical corticosteroids can be used, often this condition is treated using intramuscular application of systemic corticosteroids.

All of these conditions can be diagnosed through physical examination alone because their differences may be easily seen. However, if there is doubt about the diagnosis, a biopsy might be done by a dermatology specialist to identify the exact condition.

### Benign Lesions

Benign lesions that may be found on the vulva include normal nevi (moles); epidermal inclusion cysts, which are collections of keratin; and Bartholin's gland cysts, which form when the duct of this gland becomes obstructed. These Bartholin's gland cysts can either be uninfected, or become colonized with bacteria, and infected. The bacterial infection is treated with antibiotics.

### Cancer

Several different types of cancer can be found on the vulva, including melanoma, squamous cell carcinoma, basal carcinoma, and Paget's disease. Definitive diagnoses for these cancers are obtained by having a biopsy of the lesion.

### Vulvar Pain Syndrome

The last category of vulvar conditions is that of vulvar pain syndrome, or vulvodynia. Women who experience this problem have various degrees of pain, burning, stinging, itching, dryness, or irritation (Michlewitz, 1995). Many of the aforementioned conditions can cause vulvodynia, but some women experience the symptoms, although no organic cause can be found. Women who are experiencing the pain without an identified cause are classified as having **essential vulvodynia** (Michlewitz, 1995). A related condition is one known as **vulvar vestibulitis**, which causes exquisite pain with touch or pressure at the vestibule, while the only physical finding is erythema in the area (Kaufman, 1995). When a cause is found, there can be relief of the condition with appropriate treatment. For another subset of women, no known cause can be identified. Relief of the symptoms is the only treatment until the physiologic cause is determined.

Our role in all of these conditions includes educating women about the necessity of having their conditions evaluated thoroughly, making sure that their diagnosis and therapies are understood, and giving women emotional support while they are experiencing symptoms.

### Vaginitis

**Vaginitis** is the inflammation of the vagina. The inflammatory process generally leads to the production of a discharge. According to Moulton and Montgomery (1995), concern about vaginal discharge is one of the 25 most common reasons that women consult their health care providers. Women seek advice and treatment because of lack of knowledge about variation in normal vaginal secretions, discomfort from symptoms, and fear of STIs or even cancer. Other women avoid seeking advice and treatment because of anxiety about pelvic examinations, concerns with sexuality and body image, worry about partner reactions, worry that the provider will not think it is important, the availability of OTC remedies and medications, or cultural norms that discourage gynecologic examinations. Adolescents may avoid care because they believe that the provider will think they are sexually active, or if they are sexually active, they are afraid this information will be disclosed to their parents or guardians. Ignorance of their rights to confidential services may hinder the process of obtaining care.

### Normal Secretions of the Vagina

Normal physiology of the vagina is an important aspect of well-woman education. The vaginal mucosa is a membrane that lines the vagina and produces moisture and mucous, collectively know as secretions. An interesting issue that detracts from women seeking services is one of terminology. Health care providers usually use the term "discharge" to indicate both normal and abnormal secretions from the vagina. It might be more acceptable, for both clients and clinicians, to use the term "secretions" when referring to normal fluids, and "discharge" when referring to abnormal fluids, thus differentiating between the two.

Normal vaginal secretions can be clear, milky, or yellowish if dried. The amount varies depending on timing of the menstrual cycle, menopausal status, sexual arousal, and stress. Normally, the secretions cause no irritation, itching, or inflammation of the vagina or vulva. The normal pH of vaginal secretions is 3.8 to 4.2. Secretions usually contain many different types of bacteria, both anaerobic and aerobic, and small numbers of various species of yeast. The low pH is usually maintained by the production of lactic acid by large numbers of one of these bacteria, the lactobacilli, but other organisms also may contribute (Wakamatsu, 1995). As long as the vagina is in normal homeostasis (a stable balance), pathogenic organisms will not be able to take over the environment of the vagina. But if this homeostasis is subjected to stressors—pregnancy, illness, sexual activity, or other infections, then vaginitis can develop.

### Causes of Discharge

The three most common causes of discharge are BV, *Candida* vaginitis, and *Trichomonas* vaginitis, causing 90% of vaginal infections (Plourd, 1997). Of these three, only trichomoniasis is clearly considered to be an STI because it must be transmitted from one person to the next. However, this condition is discussed here rather than in the section on STIs, because so many of the symptoms are shared, and references and the research often discuss these three conditions together.

***Bacterial Vaginosis.*** Bacterial vaginosis (BV), the most frequent type of vaginal infection, has gone through a number of name changes in the past because of confusion over the causative organism. It is now understood that a mixed group of organisms are responsible for this condition. These bacteria adhere to the squamous epithelial cells of the vagina and give them a fuzzy or irregular appearance. Squamous epithelial cells with these adhering bacteria are called "clue cells" (Figure 7-7).

This condition is called a **vaginosis** instead of a vaginitis because of the minimal amount of inflammation, and therefore limited number of white blood cells (WBCs) seen in the wet prep associated with it. The risk factors for this condition are not clear (Wakamatsu, 1995), and whether or not it is a type of STI is controversial (Secor, 1994; Plourd, 1997). Many clinicians think that it is not an STI because women who have never had intercourse can have the condition, and treatment of male partners does not decrease recurrence rates in affected women (Wakamatsu, 1995; Plourd, 1997).

Affected women may describe an increased discharge that has a fishy odor, especially after intercourse or with menstruation. However, up to 50% of women with BV have no symptoms (Secor, 1994; Migeon, Desnick, and

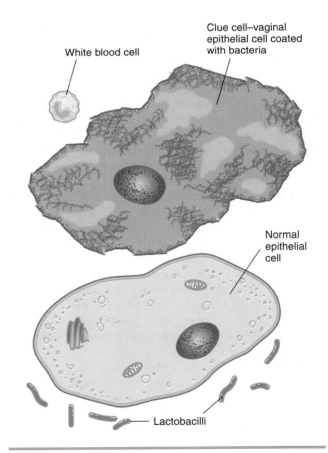

White blood cell

Clue cell–vaginal epithelial cell coated with bacteria

Normal epithelial cell

Lactobacilli

*FIGURE 7-7* • Clue cell found in bacterial vaginosis.

Elmore, 1997; Plourd, 1997). Clinicians' concern about this condition has gone up in the last two decades because of research evidence that links BV with serious outcomes, especially for the pregnant woman. Possible obstetric complications include preterm labor, premature rupture of membranes, preterm delivery, amniotic fluid infection, chorioamniotic infection, and postpartum endometritis. The possible gynecologic complications include PID, postabortion sepsis, and posthysterectomy infections (Secor, 1994; Peipert and others, 1997; Plourd, 1997; Paige and others, 1998; Woodrow and Lamont 1998). In addition, recent studies are beginning to show a link between BV and the acquisition of HIV (Taha, Hoover, and Dalabetta, 1998). It is therefore important for women who are pregnant, for those planning a pregnancy, or for those who will be undergoing gynecologic surgery to have all symptoms of vaginal discharge evaluated, and even if asymptomatic, to undergo examinations to rule out the presence of BV (Carr, Felsenstein, and Friedman, 1998).

**Candida *Vaginitis*.** *Candida* vaginitis occurs when the usual floras are replaced by an overgrowth of candida species (formerly called *monilia*), a type of fungus. The usual organism is *Candida albicans,* but other species are sometimes encountered (Wakamatsu, 1995; Plourd, 1997). On wet prep, hyphae and budding organisms can be seen (Figure 7-8).

In contrast to BV, no serious sequellae are associated with these infections, but the discomfort, frustration, and worry for some women should not be underestimated. Risk factors that increase a woman's chance for developing *Candida* vaginitis have been identified, and include the following: pregnancy, diabetes, recent systemic antibiotic therapy, immunosuppression, and those on immunosuppressive medications such as prednisone

or cyclosporine. Some authors believe that there is also an increased incidence in women taking oral contraceptives (Plourd, 1997), but other studies do not support this relationship (Wakamatsu, 1995).

***Trichomonas Vaginalis.*** **Trichomonas vaginalis** is a flagellated protozoan parasite that is not a part of the normal flora of the vagina (Figure 7-9).

It is easily identified on wet prep because of its movement. The size is slightly larger than that of neighboring WBCs. As mentioned earlier, this organism is transmitted through sexual activity, therefore the partners of women with this infection should also be treated, regardless of whether or not they have symptoms. Both men and women can be asymptomatic despite having this protozoan in either vaginal, urethral or seminal fluid. According to the CDC (1998b), this infection may be associated with premature rupture of membranes and premature delivery, and therefore even asymptomatic women should be treated.

***Other Causes.*** Despite the frequency of these three conditions, it is important to remember that there are also a number of other conditions that can cause the symptoms of vaginitis. These include oral contraceptive use; STIs (see the following section); hypersensitivity or allergic reactions to products such as soaps, pads, medications, or clothing; urinary infections; urinary incontinence; skin diseases such as psoriasis, atopic dermatitis, lichen planus, or lichen sclerosis; post menopausal atrophic vaginitis; cytolytic vaginosis; and foreign bodies. It is therefore of the utmost importance that when a woman describes a vaginal discharge, odor, itching or irritation that she be taken seriously, and a relevant history and physical examination be performed. These symptoms should not be treated over the phone as part of telephone triage, nor should women be encouraged to

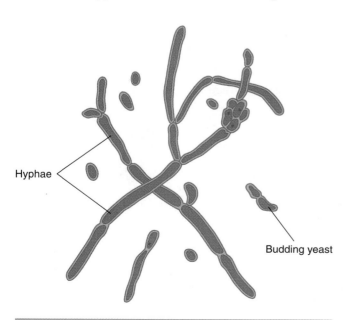

Hyphae

Budding yeast

*FIGURE 7-8* • Candida vaginitis.

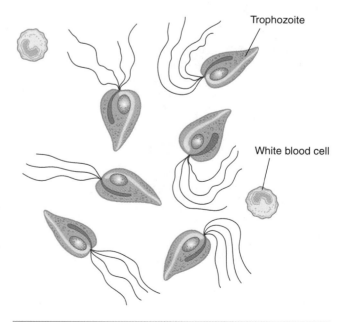

Trophozoite

White blood cell

*FIGURE 7-9* • Trichomonas vaginalis.

self-treat on the basis of her description of the discharge. The only exception is the woman with vulvar itching and discharge who has recently completed a course of antibiotics. (Antibiotics often disturb the homeostasis of the vagina.) In this case, one course of antifungal medications is indicated. If after one course of therapy, her symptoms continue, then she should be evaluated. According to Migeon, Desnick, and Elmore (1999), no prospective studies have found that patient symptoms alone are reliable enough to guide diagnosis and treatment. Missed diagnoses with the potential resultant serious sequellae, unnecessary expense, and medication side effects are all potential problems of women self-treating or clinicians treating by symptoms alone.

*History.* History taking will be the same for women experiencing vaginal symptoms, and for those in whom STIs may be an issue. It should include information in the following areas:

Reason for Visit: description of the discharge, duration, odor, accompanying symptoms such as itching, irritation, pain, problems with urination, symptoms during sexual activity.

Previous Medical History: Previous episodes of vaginitis or STIs, gynecologic surgery, present medical conditions and medications, or abnormal Pap smears.

Menstrual, contraceptive, pregnancy, and complete history of sexual activity.

*Physical Examination.* The physical examination will include an abdominal examination, as well as a pelvic examination. Depending on her symptoms and history, a rectal examination may be indicated.

*Diagnostic Testing.* To differentiate between BV, candidiasis, and trichomoniasis, two laboratory tests must be done. The first of these is to determine the pH of the vagina; the second is a swab of the vaginal secretions or discharge that is then examined on a slide. Both normal saline and potassium hydroxide (KOH) are used to perform this slide test, usually referred to as a "wet prep." These slides are then examined with a microscope. Findings for each of these three conditions, plus treatment options, are listed in Table 7-3.

The "whiff" test refers to the scent of amines, which has a fishlike odor and is released when KOH is added to the slide. These amines are released by anaerobic bacteria, consistent with those found in BV and trichomoniasis.

## Nursing Role

Many women have problems with vaginal discharge and infections, so it is important for us to develop a solid knowledge base concerning normal physiology; the factors that encourage women to seek care and treatment and those that interfere; and information about the causative organisms, symptoms, and necessary examinations; and the available treatments.

Promising new research has shown that collection of vaginal discharge without a speculum insertion is just as valid a method as use of a speculum (Blake and others, 1998). This means that diagnosis and treatment do not require that a woman have a speculum inserted in her vagina, a stressful event for many women. Self-collection

---

**TABLE 7-3** *Vaginitis*

|  | BV | Candidiasis | Trichomoniasis |
|---|---|---|---|
| Discharge type | Homogeneous, thin, adheres to the walls of the vagina, gray or white, often increased | Like cottage cheese, white, sometimes increased | Frothy, yellow or green, increased |
| Patient complaints | Bad odor, more discharge, sometimes worse after sexual activity | Itching, burning, more discharge | More discharge, bad odor, itching, painful urination |
| pH | >4.5 | <4.5 | 5.0-6.0 |
| Whiff test | Positive | Negative | Positive, occasionally |
| Wet prep results | Rare WBCs, clue cells | WBCs, hyphae, budding yeast | Numerous WBCs, motile, flagellated protozoans |
| Treatment | Metronidazole gel<br>Clindamycin cream<br>Metronidazole PO<br>Clindamycin PO | Clotrimazole cream<br>Miconazole cream<br>Butaconazole cream<br>Terconazole cream or suppositories<br>Ketoconazole cream<br>Fluconazole PO<br>Boric acid<br>Vaginal capsules<br>Lactobacillus<br>Yogurt | Metronidazole PO<br>Clotrimazole cream<br>Clotrimazole PO |

of specimens used in the diagnosis of trichomoniasis (specimens are obtained by the woman) were found to be just as valid as those collected by a clinician (Schwebke, Morgan and Pinson, 1997). Understanding and adopting new approaches may make diagnosing these conditions a more acceptable experience for women.

Interpretation of the findings and developing a plan of care acceptable to and fully understood by the woman and her partner is then necessary. Assisting women to make informed decisions about their vaginal secretions is an important role that we play in enhancing their self-confidence and understanding about their bodies.

## Sexually Transmitted Infections

STIs (or sexually transmitted diseases) exact a heavy toll on the lives of women. From the discomfort of symptoms, the difficulty these conditions pose to partner relationships, the possibility that some may be passed vertically to newborns, to the threats to a woman's fertility, sexuality, and life, these infections have become a common issue when discussing the health care needs of women (Soper, 1995; Schafer, 1998).

STIs are a modern day epidemic with an estimated 12 million Americans acquiring an STI every year. (This does not include acquiring the HIV virus.) The infection rates for some of the STIs in the United States are the highest in the industrialized world. According to Felsenstein (1995), 86% of these infections occur in young people between the ages of 15 and 25 years.

More than 25 different infectious organisms can be transmitted through sexual activity, and five of them—chlamydia, gonorrhea, AIDs, syphilis and hepatitis B—are among this country's most frequently reported infections. If detected and treated at an early stage, many STIs are curable. However, others are not. Individuals infected with viral diseases such as genital herpes or HPV are forever at risk of transmitting the disease to their partners. More than 55 million Americans are thought to have these incurable infections (Horton, 1995).

In addition to the toll on an individual's life, there is the enormous burden on the health care system in general as literally billions of dollars are spent on the treatment of these infections and their sequellae (Soper, 1995; Schafer, 1998).

Women are more likely than men to become infected with an STI, but they are less likely to have symptoms, so they generally receive treatment later and suffer more serious sequellae than men. Often the focus of intervention is the treatment of the infection in the individual woman, without simultaneously treating the person that she received the infection from or a person she may have passed it to next. Each infected woman is but a link in the distribution of the organism, and treating only one link does not stop the spread.

### Classification as Communicable Diseases

Because all of the diseases within this category are infectious and are spread from one individual to another through intimate contact, they are classified as communicable diseases. The CDC, located in Atlanta, Georgia, has taken a leading role in collecting and disseminating information about STIs to both health care personnel and the public. This includes collecting statistics about the prevalence and incidence of STIs and providing guidelines for prevention and treatment. Guidelines for treatment of sexually transmitted diseases are available from the CDC, on the web, or through state offices of public health.

Although many of the STIs are reportable to the CDC, not all are, and there is variability from state to state as to which of these diseases is reportable. In addition, not all of these diseases have reliable and affordable diagnostic tests; physicians seeing patients in private offices tend not to report, whereas public sources of health care do report; and not all health care providers are knowledgeable about the reporting guidelines (Horton, 1995). Most resources acknowledge that the rates for many of the diseases discussed here may be actually higher than the statistics indicate.

### Risk Factors

STIs are found in all ages, races, and socioeconomic groups. The most important risk factors are related to the sexual behavior of individuals or their partners. A woman may become infected with one or more organisms from one partner or multiple partners. Because young people tend to experiment more with their sexual behavior, this experimentation is reflected in the higher rates of STIs; and cervical ectopy is a probable factor in the increased rate of infection for young women. Other risk factors include multiple sex partners; history of a previous STI; high rates of partner change; a sex partner who has other sex partners; contact with casual sexual partners; risky sexual practices such as anal intercourse; alcohol and or drug use, which interferes with protective sexual decision-making; and no or limited condom/barrier use.

### Symptoms of STIs

Discussion of STIs can occur using various frameworks. Some authors discuss the conditions according to how frequently they occur in patients, others by the type of organism that causes the disease. The CDC groups STIs according to the major symptom encountered. This framework is used here and is organized as follows:

1. Diseases characterized by genital ulcers
2. Diseases characterized by cervicitis
3. Diseases characterized by vaginal discharge
4. PID
5. HPV
6. Vaccine preventable STIs
7. Ectoparasitic infections

Before beginning the discussion of symptoms, it is important to reemphasize that many women with STIs have no symptoms at all and are unaware that they are infected. This fact increases the challenge for both health care provider and patient. Screening recommendations, therefore, depend not only on symptom profiles, but also on the sexual history information obtained from a woman. Both providers and clients must develop strategies for increasing their comfort levels in both taking and giving a thorough sexual history.

For all of the following problems, there are minimum requirements for the physical examination data that should be obtained and other assessments that may be indicated, depending on symptoms and history. This information is provided in Box 7-7. In addition, several laboratory tests are commonly done. These are listed in Box 7-8. For specific diseases, other tests may be indicated; these are discussed further in the sections that follow.

### Infections Characterized by Genital Ulcers

The diseases included in this category include genital herpes simplex virus (HSV), syphilis, chancroid, granuloma inguinale (Donovanosis), and lymphogranuloma venereum. Of these, this section covers the first two in detail because they are the most commonly encountered. Basic information is provided for the last three diseases.

***Genital Herpes Simplex Virus (HSV).*** Herpes simplex virus is an important entity to discuss because of the large numbers of individuals who have this infection, an estimated 45 million according to the CDC (1998b), and there is no cure. The infection is important to understand because of the morbidity associated with the initial episode, the psychosocial difficulties that affected individuals continue to experience, and the increased risks for other infections, as well as neonatal systemic disease, that exist.

There are two serotypes of the virus: HSV-1 and HSV-2. The **HSV-1 type** is more prevalent in sites other than the genital area, but can also be found in the genital area; **HSV-2** is more commonly known to cause genital lesions. It is important to remember that HSV infections can occur anywhere on the body, with a preference for mucous membranes. The most common area outside the genital area is the nasolabial area of the face, creating what are popularly known as "cold sores." The majority of these infections are from the HSV-1 type virus and are passed on from parent to child during normal affectionate contact and should not be confused with the sexually transmitted form of the disease, nor be a cause for concerns about potential child abuse in the majority of cases. The discussion here is limited to the sexual transmission of HSV.

The virus is passed from one individual to another during intimate contact. Individuals who are infected with the virus may or may not be aware that they have it and therefore are unaware that they are passing it to a partner. For some individuals, the first outbreak of HSV may go completely unrecognized because there are no symptoms or because the symptoms are as nonspecific as a genital itch. For others, the first episode of genital herpes is a severe illness that can cause a great deal of local pain and systemic symptoms such as fever, aches, and other flulike symptoms. In addition, there may be dysuria, abdominal pain, and dyspareunia. The virus causes an eruption of erythematous vesicles on the vulva, the perianal area, or within the vagina. These vesicles rupture, leaving tender ulcerations that eventually heal. Symptoms can last anywhere from a few days to several weeks. Although the involved skin has healed, the virus is still present in a latent state. Recurrent outbreaks can occur whenever the virus is reactivated. Reactivation seems to be related to menstrual cycles; stress; fatigue; ultraviolet light exposure; cannabis use; pregnancy; other infections; trauma or abrasion to the involved area, including intercourse; or any situation that causes immunocompromise or immunosuppression (Wooley, 1998).

There is no cure for HSV disease, although antiviral therapy is available. If begun within the first 48 hours of

---

### BOX 7-7    *Minimum Requirements for a Physical Examination*

**Always includes:**
Vital signs
Abdominal examination including lymph node assessment
External genital examination, including perianal area
Speculum examination
Bimanual examination

**Plus, as indicated:**
Total skin examination
Oropharynx examination
Rectal/Rectovaginal examination

---

### BOX 7-8    *Common Diagnostic Laboratory Tests*

Pregnancy testing
Urinalysis
Wet prep and KOH
Chlamydia
Gonorrhea
Pap smear

the outbreak, these antivirals can reduce the numbers of days, the severity of symptoms, and the extent of involvement. The medications work by interfering with the replication of the HSV virus, and therefore are most helpful when the virus is first coming out of the latency period. Once the outbreak is in full progress, the medications are not as helpful. Often, affected individuals will be aware of an impending outbreak: they might experience local tingling, itching, numbness, and/or pain. They should be encouraged to begin their treatment during this time and not wait for the actual outbreak in the skin. Several medications are in this class, including acyclovir, famciclovir, and valacyclovir, and therapy is generally taken for 5 days.

The number of outbreaks in a year is highly variable for each individual, although the frequency is usually highest in the time that follows the initial infection. Over time, the frequency of outbreaks decreases for most women. For those women who have more than 6 outbreaks in a year, the possibility of taking antiviral therapy on a daily basis is considered. This daily suppressive therapy has been shown to be highly successful in reducing the number of recurrences by 75% or more.

Individuals are most capable of spreading the infection when they have open ulcers, since replication and shedding of the virus are occurring in large numbers. When the infection is in a latency phase, the shedding of the virus is much less, although known to occur in small numbers, and therefore capable of being passed on to partners.

Education and support of women with this condition is a very important component of the treatment program. It is essential for women to understand the nature of the infection, the chronicity, the treatment recommendations, and the concept of viral shedding. It is also important for clinicians and patients to avoid assigning blame to particular partners because the natural history of the infection is so complicated. It is possible for a patient to have been infected by the virus years before, and yet not have a severe outbreak until many months or years have elapsed. Any woman who has had more than one sexual partner cannot determine with certainty which of her partners may have given her the virus. Naturally, there are exceptions, but it is much more important to concentrate on imparting information that can be shared with partners in a nonjudgmental way.

There is some risk of transmitting the virus to the neonate during childbirth. Systemic HSV is life threatening to the neonate. In recent years the risk has been shown to be highest in those women who experience an initial HSV episode during the third trimester of pregnancy. However, any woman who is pregnant or is contemplating pregnancy and who has a history of genital herpes should share this with the health care clinician that is providing prenatal care.

Diagnosis of HSV depends mostly on clinical recognition of the typical ulcerated areas in the genital area. Viral culture can be done and is encouraged, but will only be reliable if there are actual open ulcerations or vesicles, which can be opened and then swabbed. Viral antigen testing is also available.

Care during a severe initial episode revolves around alleviating the pain and discomfort, as well as providing psychologic support and imparting information about the disease. Comfort measures include cool compresses, or Burrow's solution to the ulcerated areas several times a day; gentle spraying of the perineal area with cool water while urinating to decrease the burning experienced from low pH urine; and pain medications such as acetaminophen, ibuprofen, or naproxen. Counseling includes the following information: (1) when and how to take medications; (2) to refrain from sexual activity when outbreaks are present; (3) awareness that the virus can be passed on even during latent periods; (4) to use barrier methods to reduce transmission; (5) awareness that the presence of ulcerated areas can increase the risk of entry of other STIs, especially HIV; (6) discussions of what information partners should be given and advice on how to impart it; (7) referral to supportive services if the client needs assistance to cope with the diagnosis.

***Syphilis.*** **Syphilis** is a systemic illness caused by a bacterium in the spirochete family, *Treponema pallidum*. Transmission occurs through sexual contact, but only when mucocutaneous lesions are present; transplacentally from mother to fetus; and rarely, through blood contact.

There are **three stages of symptomatic syphilis**: primary, secondary, and tertiary. Latent syphilis refers to those individuals who are seropositive, but show no signs of the disease. **Primary syphilis** occurs after exposure to the spirochete and presents as a painless, indurated, solitary ulcer, with yellow-gray exudate. These are known as **chancres**. Usually, there is painless lymphadenopathy in the region. Because chancres are painless, women often are unaware of their presence and are unconcerned about being infectious. While the chancre is present, treponemes are present, and women are infectious.

It takes about 6 weeks for the chancre to heal. If the infection goes untreated, about 50% of those infected will go on to secondary syphilis, the rest will go on to the latent phase. In **secondary syphilis**, the major diagnostic finding is mucocutaneous eruptions, which start out macular in appearance and then progress to a firm, reddish-brown, nonpruritic more papular rash found on the trunk, extremities, and face, but especially on the palms of the hands and soles of the feet. Lesions can also occur on mucous membranes. Secondary syphilis resolves spontaneously, regardless of whether or not the patient is treated.

Latent syphilis occurs in patients who are between the secondary and tertiary phases of the disease. Patients have no symptoms, are not considered to be contagious to sexual partners, but have the spirochetes actively replicating in their systems. About one third of these patients go on to develop **tertiary syphilis,** a condition that causes life-threatening heart disease and bone, liver, skin, or brain damage (neurosyphilis). **Congenital syphilis** refers to those neonates who have had the spirochete transmitted through the placentas of their infected mothers. About 60% of these pregnancies will end in stillbirth or neonatal death; of those that survive, 50% will have a variety of problems, including hepatosplenomegaly, CNS involvement, and skeletal lesions (Schafer, 1998).

Although no culture test is available for syphilis, several diagnostic studies aid in the diagnosis. In primary syphilis the best test result is that of direct microscopic observation of the spirochetes taken from the chancre, using dark field microscopy. A number of serologic tests are also available, which are unreliable during primary syphilis, are very reliable during the secondary stage, and must be used along with the history and clinical picture in tertiary syphilis. No one test gives a complete picture of the stage of the disease, and therefore several different studies are done together.

Fortunately, there is effective treatment available for syphilis, which is penicillin G either by intramuscular or intravenous (required for neurosyphilis) administration. Nonpregnant patients who are allergic to penicillin can by given doxycycline or tetracycline in oral form. Pregnant women with syphilis who are allergic to penicillin will need to be desensitized to it because the two oral medications mentioned cannot be used in pregnancy.

Counseling and education should stress prevention, the necessity of having all lesions in the genital area evaluated, and an understanding of the various stages of the disease and how it is transmitted; the existence of an effective cure; the requirements of partner notification and treatment; the importance of returning for follow-up care; the testing of all pregnant women; and the suggestion that all women with syphilis be tested for HIV.

**Chancroid.** Chancroid is endemic in some areas of the United States. It also occurs in small outbreaks in specific areas. The diagnosis is generally made by assumption. If the person has a painful ulcer and tender inguinal adenopathy, the diagnosis of **chancroid** is suggested. Chancroid is a cofactor in HIV transmission and an estimated 10% of people with chancroid also have HSV. Treatment with antibiotics cures the chancroid infection. A test for the causative organism *H. ducreyi* may be available soon (CDC, 1998b).

**Granuloma Inguinale (Donovanosis).** Granuloma inguinale is rare in the United States, but is endemic in certain tropical and developing areas. The Gram-negative bacterium, *Calymmatobacterium granulomatis* causes painless, highly vascular, progressive ulcerative lesions referred to as **granuloma inguinale.** Treatment requires a minimum of 3 weeks of antibiotic therapy, or until all lesions are healed. A relapse can occur 6 to 18 months later, even after effective initial therapy (CDC, 1998b).

**Lymphogranuloma Venereum.** **Lymphogranuloma venereum** is a rare disease in the United States. It is caused by the invasive serovars L1, L2, or L3 of *C. trachomatis.* The most common manifestation among women is ulcers, then fistulas and strictures in the perirectal or perianal tissues. The infection is cured with an antibiotic, but the tissue damage remains and buboes may need to be aspirated (CDC, 1998b).

### Infections Characterized by Cervicitis

Three conditions considered STIs are included in this category: mucopurulent cervicitis (MPC), chlamydia, and gonorrhea. (*Candida* vaginitis, BV, and trichomoniasis, as previously described, may also cause cervicitis.)

**Cervicitis** refers to an inflamed endocervix, which is characterized by a yellow-white purulent discharge in the endocervical canal, and/or erythema at the cervical os, and/or friability, or easy bleeding of the cervical os. The friability may cause women to experience bleeding after sexual activity or spontaneous intermenstrual bleeding. Other symptoms that may be present with these conditions are pelvic or abdominal pain, dyspareunia, and dysuria. The vaginal discharge of MPC, chlamydia, and gonorrhea may be the symptom that brings a woman to her health care provider.

**Mucopurulent Cervicitis.** Women with MPC can have the previously described symptoms, or they may be asymptomatic. The evidence for MPC, therefore, is only seen when the cervix is observed during an examination with a speculum. All women with MPC should be tested for chlamydia and gonorrhea, have a wet prep and KOH done, and have a Pap done if a smear has not been obtained within the last 12 months. Although chlamydia and gonorrhea are sometimes found when a woman has MPC, in many instances, the causative organism cannot be identified. Some authors equate men's experience with urethritis, caused by *Ureaplasma urealyticum* and *Mycoplasma hominis,* to women's MPC (Schafer, 1998). However, these organisms are frequently found in the vagina without any pathology, and therefore, their role is not at all clear. The antibiotics used in the treatment of chlamydia are also effective against these organisms.

Treatment of MPC is unclear according to the CDC (1998b). Many clinicians may empirically decide to treat a patient with the antibiotic regimens for chlamydia and/or gonorrhea, especially if there is a large incidence rate for these infections in the local community. In particular, antibiotics used for chlamydia seem to be effective in some women with MPC. Use of any other treatment regimens is not recommended. Women should be encouraged to return for follow-up and re-evaluation if her symptoms continue or return. Partner treatment protocols should be followed for any organism that is detected or suspected.

***Chlamydia.*** Chlamydia, one of the most common of the STIs, is found most frequently in adolescents (46% of infections) and young adults (33% of infections) (CDC, 1999b). The organism is found more frequently in women than in men, but this is thought to be a result of the increased screening of women and lack of detection in men (CDC, 1999b). **Chlamydia** is caused by the organism *Chlamydia trachomatis*, which is an obligate intracellular parasite with both bacterial and viral properties. Symptoms can be as previously outlined and may also include cervical motion tenderness (CMT) or adnexal pain. However, many women have no symptoms at all. The sequellae of undetected and untreated chlamydia are serious: PID, infertility, salpingitis, and chronic pelvic pain. Infected mothers can pass the infection on to the neonate during vaginal birth, with the potential for causing conjunctivitis and/or pneumonitis. The CDC (1999b) estimates that the cost of chlamydia and its consequences total more than $2 billion a year, whereas primary care with screening and treatment programs would cost only $175 million. It is imperative for all health care providers and all women to be aware of this infection and when screening and testing should be done.

All sexually active asymptomatic young women should be screened. All women with a change of partner or those whose partners have not been monogamous should be screened. All pregnant women should be screened. Any woman with symptoms should be tested. Several diagnostic tests are available, including culture. Culture is expensive and time consuming, but indicated in cases for which exact diagnosis is required. Several rapid tests are also available; these depend on antigen testing. All of these tests require swabs from the endocervical canal. However, an antigen test using urine as the source material is now available, but currently is not in general use. When available, this test will revolutionize the testing for chlamydia, making collection of the specimen much easier and more economic for both patient and clinician. It is hoped that the frequency of screening and testing will increase as a result.

Several antibiotic treatment regimens are available, including doxycycline and azithromycin; both are very effective. Azithromycin can be given in a one-dose form, which may be preferable in those clients who are less likely to continue with a longer interval of therapy for whatever reason. Doxycycline, however, is less expensive. Alternative treatment medications include erythromycin and ofloxacin.

Patients who are being treated should be encouraged to have partners seen for evaluation and treatment. This is imperative to prevent reinfection. Women should abstain from sexual contact for 7 days after treatment has begun, regardless of the regimen used. Exploring with the woman how to get her partner tested and into treatment and how to explain the prohibition against intercourse to her partner may be helpful. This time without

intercourse should be extended until her partner finishes treatment. If a woman has had several partners in the last 60 days, all partners should be contacted and treated.

It is not necessary to repeat the testing for chlamydia after treatment with doxycycline, azithromycin, or ofloxacin to prove eradication. This procedure is known as "test of cure," and is not indicated with these medications because of their effectiveness. A test of cure may be done after use of erythromycin, which is less effective, or if the patient is still having symptoms.

Reducing the incidence and complications from this infection in women, depends on increasing the use of barrier methods, especially condoms; limiting the number of sexual partners; having all symptoms evaluated in a timely fashion; finishing all medications as prescribed; and referring partners for treatment. For health care providers, it is essential to take the time to obtain complete sexual histories, for screening guidelines to be followed, and to have mechanisms in place for making sure that affected women are treated appropriately, and that all partners are also treated.

***Gonorrhea.*** **Gonorrhea** is caused by the bacteria *Neisseria gonorrhoeae* and has a symptom profile that reflects that of chlamydia. Frequently, dual infection with chlamydia is found. In addition, the risk to the woman of undetected infection is the same for these two organisms. However, there is an additional risk for gonorrhea: disseminated gonococcal infection (DGI), which can lead to pustular skin lesions, arthralgias, and septic arthritis. It can also be passed from mother to newborn, causing conjunctivitis, and possible blindness in the infant. In addition to being found in the endocervix, this organism can be found in the woman's pharynx (rare) and in the rectum (common).

Diagnostic tests include gram-stain slides, culture, and antibody tests. Gram stain of a swab from the endocervical canal will show gram-negative, intracellular diplococci, but they are harder to find in women than in men. The culture is the test of choice, but recent antibody tests have also been shown to be quite reliable.

Several treatment choices are available for gonorrhea, and all of these include treatment of chlamydia at the same time, whether or not this organism is actually tested for or found. The medications for gonorrhea are oral cefixime in a single dose, ceftriaxone in a single intramuscular dose, oral ciprofloxacin in a single dose, or ofloxacin in a single dose. See previous discussion for the medications for chlamydia. DGI requires a different treatment protocol, usually intravenous administration as an inpatient.

As for chlamydia, all sexual partners from the previous 60 days should be referred for evaluation and treatment, and intercourse should be avoided until patient/partners have completed therapy. Education and counseling issues are virtually identical for these infections of gonorrhea and chlamydia. Women should be informed about the risk of developing pelvic inflammatory infection from the organisms *C. trachomatis* or *N. gonorrhoeae*, or both.

### Pelvic Inflammatory Disease

**Pelvic inflammatory disease (PID)** includes a spectrum of infections that have passed through the cervix and caused inflammation in one or more of the pelvic organs—ovaries, tubes (salpingitis), uterus (endometritis), or the peritoneal surfaces (pelvic peritonitis)—and is one of the most serious of the possible sequellae from STIs. Most frequently, it is found to affect the Fallopian tubes, and the causative agent is either *C. trachomatis* or *N. gonorrhoeae*, or both. However, several other organisms have been implicated, including both aerobic and anaerobic types. Most PID is caused by the ascent of microorganisms from the vagina and cervical os into the fallopian tubes. It can cause complications such as infertility, ectopic pregnancy, chronic pelvic or abdominal pain, pelvic abscesses, and pelvic adhesions, and lead to premature hysterectomy. Risk factors include young age, multiple sex partners, a history of STIs or PID, a partner with an STD, recent IUD insertion, and nulliparity. Other risk factors implicated include douching, BV, cigarette smoking, and sex during menses (Forrest, 1998).

*History.* Symptoms vary from the very subtle to the more obvious. Women may complain of abdominal pain or tenderness that can range from minor to severe in intensity. There may be fever, chills, nausea, vomiting, vaginal discharge, symptoms that can be confused with a UTI, dyspareunia, and irregular vaginal bleeding. Women with more subtle symptoms may go undiagnosed, a situation known as "silent PID."

*Physical.* The physical examination requirements are based on the woman's symptoms. A temperature should be taken and thorough abdominal and pelvic examinations should be performed. In addition, a rectal examination may be indicated. Findings may include pain with abdominal palpation, vaginal discharge, cervical friability, CMT, or adnexal pain on bimanual examination. Diagnostic studies include CBC, sedimentation rate, C-reactive protein, urinalysis, wet prep and KOH, chlamydia and gonorrhea, and pregnancy testing (if indicated).

The variety and low severity of findings in some women make clinical diagnosis of PID a challenge. Although positive *Chlamydia*, gonorrhea, *Trichomonas*, or BV findings will certainly aid in the diagnosis, obtaining negative tests does not rule out the condition. Given the seriousness of the sequellae, most clinicians opt to treat women, especially young women, presumptively. In other words, they will treat sexually active women who are experiencing unexplained abdominal or pelvic pain in the hopes of eliminating possible PID. The CDC (1998b) offers the following guidelines: Empiric treatment of PID should be given to women who

are sexually active, and for whom no other cause has been identified, when the following minimum three criteria are present:

1. lower abdominal tenderness
2. adnexal tenderness, and
3. cervical motion tenderness

Additional criteria that support a diagnosis of PID are as follows:

1. oral temperature >101° F (>38.3° C)
2. abnormal cervical or vaginal discharge
3. elevated sedimentation rate
4. elevated C-reactive protein
5. laboratory documentation of chlamydia or gonorrhea.

The only way to definitively diagnose PID is through the procedure endometrial biopsy, transvaginal ultrasonography, or laparoscopic examination.

*Treatment.* Treatment of PID depends on covering the most likely of the etiologic agents, namely chlamydia and gonorrhea, plus a few other groups of bacteria. The CDC (1998b) guidelines should be consulted for a full description of the various treatment regimens. Both oral and intravenous regimens are listed.

One of the most important questions concerning treatment of PID is whether or not the woman should be hospitalized. In the past, all women were admitted; but for various reasons, it is now recommended that hospitalization occur only under the following circumstances (CDC, 1998b):

1. The possibility of appendicitis or other surgical emergencies cannot be ruled out.
2. The patient is pregnant.
3. The patient is immunocompromised.
4. The patient is unable to tolerate oral medication treatment.
5. The patient does not respond to oral medications.
6. The patient is severely ill, with high fever, nausea, and vomiting.
7. The patient has a tuboovarian abscess.

All patients who have been given oral medications must be seen within 72 hours to make sure they are responding to treatment. In addition, they should be encouraged to call if their symptoms are worse, or they are unable to take their medications for whatever reason. Furthermore, it is of the utmost importance for all sexual partners from the last 60 days to be seen, evaluated, and treated empirically. Often they will not have symptoms or will have negative tests, but must be treated anyway to avoid reinfection in the woman with PID. Until all partners have finished therapy, sexual contact should be avoided.

***Follow-Up.*** All women, regardless of treatment regimen, should return for follow-up evaluation. This is an opportunity not only to make sure that a woman's symptoms have resolved, but also to review the information a woman needs to reduce her risk for any further episodes of PID.

Remember that while women are acutely ill, we should limit our counseling to only that information which is absolutely necessary. Once the acute episode is resolved, patients will be able to listen to and retain more information. Education and counseling is the same for PID as for the other reproductive tract infections, with the following addition. It is estimated that fully 50% of ectopic pregnancies occur in women who have had one or more episodes of PID (Soper, 1995). Since undiagnosed ectopic pregnancy is life threatening, women must be made aware of this increased risk in a supportive, nonjudgmental way. They should be encouraged to seek prenatal care as soon as a pregnancy is suspected and should also be advised of the symptoms of ectopic pregnancy.

## HPV Infection

HPV may also be referred to as genital warts. In some women, infection with HPV can actually be visually detected because the virus causes formation of skin lesions. These lesions have three distinct appearances: (1) they can be papular, soft, and grainy (condyloma acuminata); (2) they can be the classic cauliflower-like projections found mostly on moist skin surfaces; or (3) they can have a keratotic form that has a thickened, horny surface and is found on drier skin surfaces (Handsfield, 1997). They can be found singly or in clusters and can grow to be quite large. In women, they are most often found at the posterior portion of the introitus, but they also may be found anywhere on the vulva, rectal area, on the clitoris, in the vagina, or on the cervix. Those seen on the cervix are usually flat-topped. Genital warts are usually flesh-colored, but may be slightly darker in white women, black in black women, and dark brown in Asian women (Fogel, 1995). For the most part, the warts are painless, but they can cause discomfort, especially when large. They can also ulcerate, causing bleeding, or they can cause vaginal discharge and itching, perirectal itching, or dysuria. Although women may be unaware that the warts are present, many women feel the lesions during hygiene procedures, or, if they practice self-examination, may have seen the lesions.

Women who are evaluated and found to have genital warts should be tested for other STIs and also have a Pap smear done, regardless of how recently one has been obtained. Although HPV is an STI, it is often asymptomatic.

Partner evaluation is not required in all cases. Exceptions include the following: (1) male partners with visual lesions, penile discharge, or urinary symptoms; (2) female partners with visible lesions and/or who have not had a Pap test done within the previous year. Also, it may prove useful to have partners evaluated by a health care provider, especially to do a thorough visual examination of the genital area to rule out the presence of observable warts. Furthermore, the visit can be seen as opportunity to discuss the diagnosis of HPV and the risks to the partner. The affected woman may appreciate being able to have this discussion with her partner and provider together.

Although there is no known cure for HPV, counseling and treatment focuses on two issues: techniques to rid the client of the actual warts and evaluation of the Pap smear, since HPV is known to be a risk factor for cervical dysplasia. See the section on cervical dysplasia for a review of Pap smear management.

Several different destructive techniques are used to eliminate the warts. Women should understand the side effects involved, possible inconveniences, and the costs of these therapies. Choice of treatment also depends on the location, number, and size of the warts. Some women may be treated by their primary care clinicians; others will be referred to a specialist in gynecology or dermatology. Common treatment modalities are listed in Box 7-9.

Some of these therapies require multiple visits to the health care provider; others are performed by the client at home; still others require local anesthesia. In some cases, when one technique has been unsuccessful, another treatment modality is then tried.

Women with genital warts should understand the natural history of the virus and the risk of cervical dysplasia. They should be encouraged to have a Pap smear a minimum of once a year and to always tell health care providers their history of HPV.

A woman should also be aware that the virus can be latent for long periods of time (years), and she may have contracted the virus from *any* lifetime partner. Therefore, she should not assume that the present partner is the source of the virus. It is important not to disrupt partner relationships at a time when a woman may be experiencing emotional turmoil because of the diagnosis.

---

### BOX 7-9 *Treatment Modalities for HPV*

Topical trichloroacetic acid
Topical podophyllin
Topical 5-fluorouracil
Topical imiquimod
Cryotherapy
Laser therapy
Simple excision
Electrodessication
Loop electrosurgical excisional procedure (LEEP)
Intralesional interferon therapy

Help her figure out how to inform her partner or partners, perhaps initiating role play as a helpful technique, and as previously mentioned, you may want to offer the patient the opportunity to come in with the partner for discussions in the office.

## Hepatitis A and B

The transmission of hepatitis A and B from an infected to an uninfected person may be stopped by a preexposure immunization. Currently there are licensed vaccines for the hepatitis A virus (HAV) and the hepatitis B virus (HBV). It is recommended that they be given to people as a preexposure prophylaxis. Postexposure prophylaxis is also appropriate in some cases (CDC, 1998b).

## Ectoparasitic Infections

Ectoparasitic infections include infestation of scabies or pubic lice. Since these parasites are easily passed from one person to another during the intimacy of sexual encounters, we assess for their presence when providing care for STIs. Keep in mind that they may also be passed through the sharing of clothing or towels or sleeping in the same bed. The nits of the pubic lice or the lice themselves may be seen on hair shafts and alert the woman to their presence. Treatment is directly to the infested area. Bedding and clothing should be decontaminated. Sex partners and household contacts should be examined and treated (CDC, 1998b).

## Nursing Role

In general, the area of STI prevention, detection, and treatment is a vast area of concern for both health care providers and women. Along with an understanding of each infection process and its risks, there are the overall considerations when counseling women. Carson (1997) discusses the issue of empowerment of women: "Empowerment is a process of helping individuals develop an awareness of the root causes of problems and a readiness to act on this awareness."

In the case of any discussion concerning the issue of STIs, we must also include the discussion of a woman's sexuality—her needs; desires; history of positive, negative, or abusive experiences; and her capacity and strength to shape her own sexual life. Concepts concerning a woman's right to decide whether to engage in sexual activity or not, the exploration and implementation of "outercourse" (sexual activity that does not include the penetration of intercourse), requesting or requiring male partners to use condoms and female partners to use dental dams must be offered as part of our discussions with women. We must go beyond a disease-oriented model and move toward prevention by encouraging an open dialogue of these other issues. The first time you try, a woman may not be interested. However, she will know that if she does seek to pursue such a topic she has a care provider who will be supportive. Each woman's health depends on it.

## Diethylstilbestrol

Diethylstilbestrol (DES) is a potent nonsteroidal estrogen that was given to millions of pregnant women from 1938 until 1971 (NIH, 1995). It was used to treat various pregnancy complications or to prevent complications, including threatened miscarriage; a history of miscarriages, toxemia, in utero fetal death, prematurity, and postmaturity. It was also given to women thought to be at higher risk of complications, including women with diabetes (Lichtman and Smith, 1990). Its use continued through the 1960s and early 1970s, despite placebo-controlled studies, which showed the drug had no therapeutic value (Vieiralves-Wiltgen and Engle, 1988).

In 1970, a higher than expected number of clear cell adenocarcinomas were found in women under the age of 25 years. This was an unusual finding, since this cancer was normally found in women over the age of 50. Further studies revealed the relationship between the development of this cancer and the administration of DES to the affected women's mothers during their gestation. In addition, several anatomic anomalies of the cervix and uterus were also found in women whose mothers had been given DES. In 1971, the FDA withdrew approval for the use of this drug during pregnancy (Lichtman and Smith, 1990).

### Results

Two thirds of the female offspring of women given DES during their pregnancies have suffered congenital anomalies as a result. These women are known as DES daughters. There are approximately 1 to 1.5 million DES daughters in the United States alone (Hill, 1987; Vieiralves-Wiltgen and Engle, 1988). DES daughters have shown a variety of problems because of this intrauterine exposure. These conditions are listed in Box 7-10.

Adenosis is the presence of glandular epithelium on the surface of the vagina. Usually this type of tissue is restricted to the endocervical canal. Although this is normal tissue, and usually regresses over time, it

---

**BOX 7-10** *Problems Experienced by DES Daughters*

- Adenosis
- Anatomic variations of the vagina, cervix, or uterus
- Cervical dysplasia
- Clear cell adenocarcinoma of the cervix or vagina (age <25 years)
- Pregnancy problems—ectopic, miscarriage, premature labor
- Slightly increased risk of infertility

can be accompanied by production of greater levels of vaginal secretions. Anatomic changes include a larger than normal squamocolumnar junction, a hooded or "cockscomb" cervix, a T-shaped uterus, and a narrowing and shortening of the fallopian tubes. DES daughters can have one or more of these problems or experience no problems at all.

### Interventions

DES daughters need to obtain annual gynecologic care from providers who are familiar with their risk profile. Decisions about contraceptive care should be made carefully. IUDs, diaphragms, and cervical caps may not be the methods of choice for those women who have anatomic anomalies. The long-term effects of oral contraception use in DES daughters are unknown, and their use is controversial. Contraceptive jellies may actually aid women with adenosis, by decreasing the usual abundant vaginal secretions that are produced (Vieiralves-Wiltgen and Engle, 1988). All decisions concerning contraception must be made on an individual basis, but with full understanding of the advantages and risks. Furthermore, all DES daughters who become pregnant should make sure that the obstetric health care provider is aware of the history. It is suggested that a high-risk pregnancy team manage their prenatal care.

### Nursing Role

Education and support specific to the condition of the individual woman will be most helpful. Even though a DES daughter has had one or more normal, healthy pregnancies, she is still at risk for problems with subsequent pregnancies. The signs and symptoms of ectopic pregnancy and premature labor should be taught so that they can be easily recognized.

Despite the fact that the cohort of DES daughters has passed through adolescence, and therefore the number of cases of clear cell adenocarcinoma are decreasing, there is still the need for ongoing specialized evaluation of these DES daughters, since the risks for exposure in older women is not known. Research studies are now being done on DES daughters who are postmenopausal to determine if there are problems.

DES daughters should be referred to support groups and to area organizations that specialize in research and education concerning this issue. The National Cancer Institute (800-638-6694) can refer both women and health care providers to their local organizations.

The mothers of the DES daughters should also be provided with supportive care. If a woman feels badly that she "did this" to a daughter she may be reminded that she was carefully following her physicians orders, in an attempt to do what was thought to be best for the child in utero.

##  CONDITIONS OF THE CERVIX

A number of conditions affect the cervix. These include benign lesions, inflammation of the cervix, and precancerous and cancerous lesions. To better appreciate the conditions that affect the cervix, it is important to understand the anatomy of the cervix, in particular the various zones: the endocervix, the squamocolumnar junction, the transformation zone, and the ectocervix (Figure 7-10).

The major cell group found in the endocervical canal is made up of **columnar epithelial cells**, which are one cell layer thick and line the papillae found in the canal. **Squamous cells**, forming multiple layers, are much thicker and resistant and line the ectocervix and the vagina. Imbedded in this layer are mucous-producing cells. The place where these two cell types join is called the **squamocolumnar junction**. Within this **transformation zone**, columnar cells are transformed into squamous cells in a process called **squamous metaplasia**. Before birth, the cervix is lined with columnar cells, but soon after birth, the transformation process begins, and these cells are pushed inside of the cervix and replaced by the squamous cells. At puberty, the process accelerates under the influence of reproductive hormones. The vagina becomes more acidic, the delicate columnar cells are unable to tolerate this low pH, and squamous metaplasia continues so that

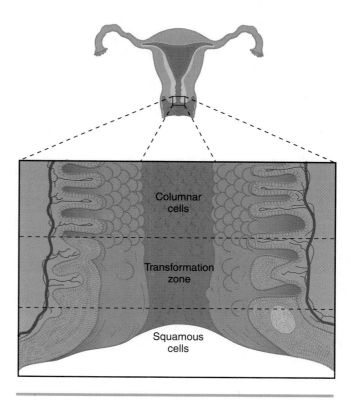

*FIGURE 7-10* • The transformation zone of the cervix.

the more resistant squamous cells mostly cover the cervix, and the columnar cells are in the endocervical canal, where they are protected. It is at the site of the transformation zone that toxic agents can disrupt the cell process of squamous metaplasia, causing dysplasia and leading to cancer, which is discussed later in this section.

## Benign Lesions of the Cervix

Of the benign lesions of the cervix, the two most common are nabothian cysts and polyps. Less frequently, lesions of endometrium may be seen on the cervix (endometriosis). **Nabothian cysts** are found on the ectocervix. They occur when columnar cells become sealed off, and mucous secretions become trapped. These cysts form frequently and usually remain small. When they increase in size, they can be seen during a speculum examination. Most rupture spontaneously and cause no problems. Women who examine their own cervixes may be able to see or feel large nabothian cysts, but the majority of women do not have any symptoms and can be reassured that their presence is not an indication of any problems.

**Polyps** are benign, pedunculated growths that can originate either from the endocervix or ectocervix. They can be single or multiple and are of various sizes. They are usually smooth, reddish or purplish, and can bleed easily when touched. Although the exact cause for polyps is unknown, they are thought to arise from an inflammatory process, but hyperestrogenic states may also contribute (Forrest, 1998). They occur most frequently in women in their 30s and 40s who are multiparous. Many women with polyps have no symptoms. Others may have increased vaginal discharge, bleeding after intercourse, intermenstrual bleeding, or menorrhagia. Polyps should be removed and sent for pathology. Although the vast majority are benign, there is a rare occurrence of malignancy (Star, 1995b). Removal is usually an office procedure, with the major risks being pain during the procedure and bleeding. Women should be encouraged to return for evaluation after 6 months or sooner if they experience any abnormal bleeding.

Lesions of **endometriosis** can form on the cervix and appear as deep purple, red, or chocolate in color. Most are small, but some may form cysts as large as 1 cm. Women may have no symptoms at all or may have abnormal bleeding. Since the lesions may resemble cervical cancer, they should be biopsied to have a definitive diagnosis (Hill, 1987).

## Cervical Dysplasia and Carcinoma

Much is now known about the changes in the cervix that lead to cancer, including the agents that are responsible or that add to the risk. The exact mechanism of how normal cells become cancerous cells is un-

known, but it is thought that agents such as HPV act as carcinogens. Fortunately for women, with the introduction and widespread use of the screening tool known as the Papanicolaou (Pap) smear, which was first described in 1943, the mortality rate for cervical cancer has decreased from being the number one cause of cancer deaths in women, to number eight (Martin, 1997). Despite the fact that fewer women are dying, the rate of abnormalities found on Pap smear has risen dramatically in the last two decades (Muntz, 1995).

The majority of abnormal changes that occur in the cervix are found in the area of squamous metaplasia, or the transformation zone. This area, with the rapidly changing cells, is vulnerable to mutation. The risk factors implicated in these changes are discussed in the following section. In most cases, cervical cancer follows a relatively slow progression of change that begins with low grade (low-grade squamous intraepithelial lesion, LG SIL or LSIL) and progresses to high-grade changes (high-grade squamous intraepithelial lesion, HG SIL or HSIL), then on to carcinoma (Figure 7-11).

The carcinomas are classified as squamous cell, adenocarcinoma, or other malignant neoplasms. Once cervical cancer is invasive, it grows rapidly (Martin, 1997).

### Papanicolaou (Pap) Smear

The purpose of the Pap smear is to discover the changes while in the early, treatable stages. The system of Pap smear classification has changed several times over the past few decades, but the Bethesda System, first developed in 1988, and updated and simplified in 1991, is the preferred system in use today. (Another update is being done in 2000.) It was originally developed to standardize Pap smear results so that research and treatment could be studied and compared.

The Bethesda system includes classifications for Pap smears, as well as information about adequacy of the slide for evaluation, which is very important for the clinician. The cellular changes are described as follows:

Normal—no evidence of atypia, inflammation, or dysplasia found, only normal cells seen
ASCUS—atypical squamous cells of undetermined significance
AGCUS—atypical glandular cells of undetermined significance
LG SIL—low-grade squamous intraepithelial lesion
HG SIL—high-grade squamous intraepithelial lesion

Unfortunately, as a screening tool, Pap smears do have limitations and errors can be made. Both false-positive and false-negative results can occur. Dysplastic cells can be missed (false negative), or essentially normal cells may be evaluated as being abnormal (false positive). Technique errors—errors made by the clinician collecting the specimen—can also occur. Examples include not sampling the entire endocervix, allowing the specimen

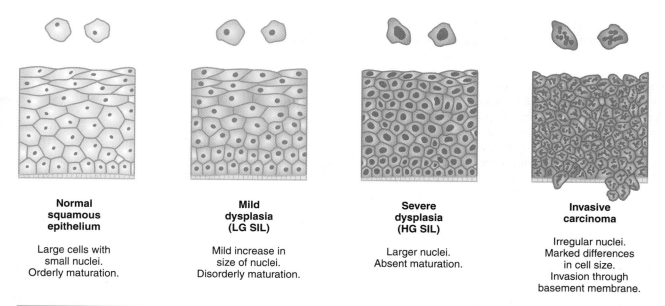

|  |  |  |  |
|---|---|---|---|
| **Normal squamous epithelium** | **Mild dysplasia (LG SIL)** | **Severe dysplasia (HG SIL)** | **Invasive carcinoma** |
| Large cells with small nuclei. Orderly maturation. | Mild increase in size of nuclei. Disorderly maturation. | Larger nuclei. Absent maturation. | Irregular nuclei. Marked differences in cell size. Invasion through basement membrane. |

*FIGURE 7-11* • Cervical dysplasia.

to get dried out, or sampling with too much discharge present, which then obscures the slide. When viewing the slide, cytologists can also make errors of missing dysplastic cells on slides by not studying the whole slide in enough detail or overreading the slide, causing an overestimation of abnormality in the cells. Several new technologies are being developed to attempt to minimize the possibility of errors. These new technologies include automated slide preparations; automated computerized reading devices; cervicography, or enlarged photographs of the cervix (Forrest, 1998); and possible DNA testing to determine the genotype of the HPV present (Shapero, 1991). In the near future, changes may be made in the guidelines for doing Pap smears, which would reflect the statistical studies now being done (McMeekin, McGonigle, and Vasilev, 1997). All of these efforts are an attempt to continue to identify women with early dysplasia while doing so in a cost-effective manner.

### Risk Factors

Several risk factors have been identified with the development of cervical dysplasia (Box 7-11). The most important of these is HPV, with fully 93% of women with cervical cancers having detectable HPV DNA (Koutsky, 1997).

***Human Papillomavirus.*** HPV is a DNA virus responsible for common warts on the skin of any part of the body, including the genital area. There are over 80 different genotypes of HPV (Koutsky, 1997), and of these, over 20 are known to cause genital warts. They are classified according to their association with cervical cancer and are either high, intermediate, or low risk types. Most references agree that types 16 and 18 have the highest oncogenic potential; types 31, 33, 35, 39, 45,

---

**BOX 7-11**  *Risk Factors for Cervical Dysplasia*

Viral exposure—HPV, HSV, HIV
Multiple sex partners
First intercourse before age 17
Partner with multiple partners
History of an STI
Smoking
First pregnancy before age 18
DES exposure
Pregnancy
Poor nutrition
Immunodeficiency
Low socioeconomic status

---

51, 52, 56, and 58 are intermediate in oncogenic potential; and five of the types that commonly cause visible warts—6, 11, 42, 43, and 44—have been determined to be low risk types and rarely associated with cancer.

Genital HPV is considered an STI because it is highly contagious and easily transmitted during mucous membrane contact. It is rarely found in individuals who have never engaged in sexual activity, although the virus can be transmitted from mother to neonate during delivery. This understanding explains why so many of the risk factors associated with cervical cancer are related to sexual activity. In particular, adolescent women under the age of 17 are at higher risk of contracting the virus because of the location of the transformation zone—the area of squamous metaplasia has not fully matured nor has it moved further into the endocervical area, and thus it is more at risk for invasions by HPV. In addition, early sexual activity may actually delay the maturation of the transformation zone, thus allowing more time for the area to come in contact with toxic agents (Carson, 1997).

Smoking is thought to be a cofactor in increasing the risk of cervical dysplasia, although the mechanism is not understood. Another cofactor is poor nutrition, in particular, the lack of vitamins A and C and folic acid. Some sources implicate oral contraceptive use as a risk factor, but the research findings are conflicting (Carson, 1997). Women with herpes simplex virus (HSV) or HIV and transplant patients are thought to be more at risk because of changes in the immune system, which allow for abnormal invasion and changes in the epithelial cells. Low socioeconomic status is thought to increase the risk because of the barriers to obtaining annual health care checks, including screening with Pap smears.

Women may have no symptoms at all in the early stages of dysplasia and may find out only through Pap results. Others might experience vaginal discharge; vaginal or rectal pruritis; or abnormal bleeding, which is the most common symptom. In later stage cervical cancer, the symptoms include back, leg or pelvic pain; abdominal discomfort; edema of the legs; dysuria; urinary frequency; hematuria; and constipation.

### Follow-Up Assessment

If the Pap returns as abnormal because of genital warts, they will be treated. In all other cases of women with abnormal Pap smears, the next choice includes whether to repeat the Pap smear or to do a colposcopy. This technique uses a colposcope, a device that is placed in the vagina for magnifying the cervix, and collection of biopsy specimens. The biopsy may be a punch biopsy alone or also include endocervical curettage (ECC), a scraping of the whole surface of the cervical canal. The results from these specimens help determine the treatment.

### Treatment

Many treatment choices are available, and much depends on the severity of the results and the health history of the individual woman. Therapeutic choices all involve destruction of as many affected cells as possible, and include excision, electrocautery, cryotherapy (a freezing technique using nitrous oxide or carbon dioxide), cone biopsy (removing a cone-shaped section of cervical tissue), laser therapy, loop electrode excision (LEEP), and large loop excision (LLETZ). In some cases a woman may opt for hysterectomy.

The method of treatment of cervical cancer depends on the stage of the disease. Stage I is confined to the cervix. Stage II extends beyond the cervix, but not to the pelvic sidewall or lower third of the vagina. Stage III involves the pelvic sidewall or lower third of the vagina, and Stage IV has spread beyond the pelvis or to the bladder or rectum. In Stage I, hysterectomy may be the

only therapy necessary. In later stages, radical hysterectomy as well as radiation therapies are the usual choices. Chemotherapy is only used in those women who have inoperable or metastatic cancers (Table 7-4).

### Nursing Role

We have a professional responsibility to help women at all three levels of health care intervention: (1) primary or preventive techniques to avoid cervical dysplasia; (2) secondary prevention, or avoidance of more serious sequellae once cervical dysplasia has been found; and (3) tertiary prevention, which includes minimizing disability if a woman is found to have cervical cancer.

#### Primary Prevention

The first stage is in educating women about the risk factors involved with the acquisition of HPV, since it is known to be involved so significantly with cervical dysplasia. Young women should be encouraged to delay sexual intercourse to allow full maturation of the cervical transformation zone. All women should be educated about the risk of having multiple partners and of the necessity of using barrier methods at all times. For all women, it is important to avoid smoking and secondhand smoke, and to eat a balanced diet rich in vitamins.

An essential part of patient education is to make sure that women know the guidelines for having Pap smears done. Women at the age of sexarchy (first sexual intercourse), or at the age of 18 should have a first pelvic examination and Pap smear. According to the American Cancer Society and the American College of Obstetricians and Gynecologists, if three or more annual normal results have been obtained in a woman at low risk, then the Pap may be done less frequently, at the client's and clinician's discretion, but at a minimum of every 3 years. For all other women, Pap smears should be repeated every year.

There are also specific things that women themselves can do to improve the quality of their Pap smears. According to Ginsberg (1991), the best time during the cycle to have cells collected is right before ovulation, when the influence of estrogen causes maturation of the cells. If women keep track of their cycles or can estimate time of ovulation, they can plan their annual examinations accordingly. Pap smears should not be done during menstruation, because the blood cells obscure the reliable reading of the slide. Furthermore, women should refrain from intercourse, douching, use of tampons, vaginal medications, or having anything inside the vagina for 24 to 48 hours before having a Pap done.

#### Secondary Prevention

Once a woman has been found to have dysplasia, the most important counseling involves encouraging women to return for follow-up diagnostic studies in a timely way. Fortunately for many women with dysplasia, these changes can revert to normal without invasive technologies. So even though an abnormal Pap finding may be very frightening, women should be given the necessary support and encouraged to obtain appropriate follow-up. It should be made clear that the earlier intervention is instituted, the more successful it is in protecting women's lives.

In addition if clients are smokers, they should be advised that smoking is a cofactor, and all efforts should be made to provide women with the resources and support to quit. Furthermore, protective measures such as using barrier methods and vitamin supplementation should be encouraged. Mind-body techniques that have been shown to boost the immune system should also be considered, if not already practiced. These include relaxation techniques, yoga, and meditation, among many others. Other protective measures such as getting enough rest and exercise can also be helpful. If not in monogamous relationships, women should consider limiting the number of partners, and barrier protection should be added to a woman's birth control decisions to protect her cervix further. Women should be empowered to institute self-protective mechanisms; often this is difficult to do, especially when there is an impact on her sexual life. Techniques for accomplishing were discussed further under the STD section.

If colposcopy and biopsy are indicated, it is essential for a woman to have a clear understanding of these diagnostic techniques, especially the type of biopsy that will be done. She should know that the biopsy results will take time to be analyzed and should have a supportive network in place to help her through this waiting period.

If the dysplasia is HG SIL, it is essential for a woman to understand her options. She will need to take into account the side effects of treatments and whether or not her potential for childbearing is affected. For example, cone biopsy, because of the amount of tissue that is removed, often is curative because all of the dysplastic cells are removed. However, there is the risk of scarring and stenosis (narrowing) of the cervical canal, which could interfere with fertility. Older women who are done with childbearing and who do not wish, or cannot tolerate a watchful waiting approach, may opt for hysterectomy to eliminate their risk. Each woman should have the information necessary to make the best decision for her self-care needs.

### Tertiary Prevention

When women are diagnosed with cancer, the staging of the cancer has the most significance in determining the treatment plan. The woman should be encouraged to ask questions of her gynecologic oncologist to understand all the options and their probable outcomes.

### TABLE 7-4 Follow-up of Abnormal Pap Smears

| Pap Results | Indicated Follow-Up |
|---|---|
| Negative for dysplastic cells | Follow the guidelines for routine screening. |
| No endocervical cells | Repeat in one month if high risk. Repeat in one year if low risk. |
| ASCUS | Repeat Pap in 6 months. Two ASCUS results: send for colposcopy. |
| LG SIL | Send for colposcopy. Other sources indicate that in women at low risk, the Pap should be repeated every 6 months, and women should be sent for colposcopy only with a second abnormal. After 3 consecutive normals, a woman may return to annual testing. |
| HG SIL | Send for colposcopy. |

*ASCUS,* Atypical squamous cells of undetermined significance; *HSIL,* high-grade squamous intraepithelial lesion; *LSIL,* low-grade squamous intraepithelial lesion.

## The Prevention of Cervical Cancer

The primary goal of nursing, however, is primary and secondary prevention. We should use every available opportunity to share with women how they can lower their risks of HPV, cervical dysplasia, and cervical cancer. The education should start when women are very young (preteens) and continue on as they grow older so that all women understand the risk factors and those who have not had a Pap smear do so. Resources within the community should be researched to find centers where Pap smears can be done for those without health coverage. The optimistic view is that cervical cancer is one type of cancer capable of being eradicated.

## CONDITIONS OF THE UTERUS

Women seek health care advice and evaluation for several problems related to the uterus. The symptoms include pain, abnormal uterine bleeding (AUB), and an inability to become pregnant. The common problems that might cause these difficulties include endometriosis, uterine fibroids, and endometrial cancer.

### Endometriosis

The endometrium refers to the lining of the uterus that increases and decreases in thickness and structure under the influence of reproductive hormones. **Endometriosis** is the presence of small amounts of endometrial tissue, both glands and stroma, in locations outside the uterus. The most common sites are the ovary, the posterior broad ligaments, the cul de sac, uterosacral ligaments, and the posterior uterus. However, this endometrial tissue can be found in any organ of the body (Figure 7-12).

This tissue responds to the circulating hormones by swelling, just as the lining inside the uterus thickens and increases its blood supply over the course of the menstrual cycle. Because it is outside the uterus, the swelling of this tissue causes local pressure and inflammation. This in turn may cause local pain, with eventual formation of adhesions and scar tissue.

### Cause

The cause for endometriosis is not known, although several theories have been offered. Two of these theories are (1) the transplantation theory, or retrograde menstrual flow, which postulates that menstrual flow "backs out" through the fallopian tubes and (2) lymphatic theory, which suggests that endometrial tissue is deposited in distant sites through the lymphatic system. One of the more recent theories proposes that there are immunologic and genetic roles in this process (Forrest, 1998).

Prevalence has been estimated to be between 8% to 15% (Forrest, 1998; Isaacson, 1995; Sutton, Santoro, and Hearns, 1998) in all women of reproductive age. However, these rates increase dramatically in women with pelvic pain and/or infertility and can be as high as 50% (Isaacson, 1995).

### History

As mentioned previously, women will have various symptoms, but most frequently, they may experience chronic pelvic pain, dyspareunia (painful intercourse), secondary dysmenorrhea, and often will have difficulty with infertility (Uphold and Graham, 1998b). Interestingly, the severity of the pain is not related to the number of sites or the amount of endometrial tissue found in external sites. Women with small areas of endometriosis can experience a great deal of pain, while those with larger areas of involved tissue or organs can experience little to no pain. It is not understood why this happens.

### Physical Examination

A pelvic examination of women with endometriosis may be completely normal. For others, there may be palpable nodularities of the fallopian tubes, the uterosacral ligament, fixed retroversion of the uterus, or enlargement of the ovaries, among other findings. Despite these findings, it is not possible to diagnose endometriosis by history and physical alone. A definitive diagnosis can only be made by performing laparoscopy.

### Treatment

Treatment regimens depend on the sites most affected, as well as the symptoms and family planning inten-

tions of the affected woman. In cases of endometriosis found in women who wish to practice contraception, the use of oral contraceptives could help control the amount of menstrual flow, and therefore the pain experienced by some women. Other drug options include GnRH analogs, oral or intramuscular administration of progesterone, and Danazol (a gonadotropin inhibitor). For others, who were diagnosed while the cause of their infertility was being investigated, the options may include surgical ablation, laser ablation, or other interventions that protect and enhance fertility. For those with chronic, unremitting pain in spite of therapy, the choice may be surgical removal of the uterus, a hysterectomy.

### Nursing Role

Our primary role with women dealing with endometriosis is to help them articulate their goals—both family planning and treatment goals, including pain control. In addition, we must ensure that she understands the side effects of the various treatments before choosing a specific intervention. Women may very well need support and counseling for difficulties with the sexuality or depression that may result from their symptoms.

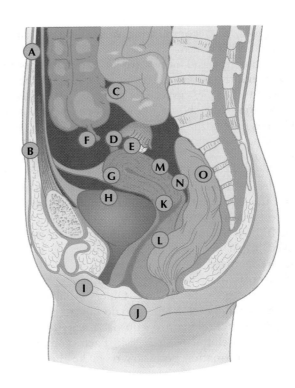

*FIGURE 7-12* ● Sites of endometrial implantation in endometriosis. **A,** Umbilicus. **B,** Scar on abdominal wall. **C,** Ileum. **D,** Fallopian tube. **E,** Ovary. **F,** Appendix. **G,** Uterine wall. **H,** Anterior cul-de-sac and bladder. **I,** Vulva. **J,** Perineum. **K,** Cervix. **L,** Rectovaginal septum. **M,** Posterior surface of uterus and uterosacral ligaments. **N,** Posterior cul-de-sac. **O,** Pelvic colon.

## Uterine Fibroids

Uterine fibroids (leiomyomas, fibromas, myomas, or my-ofibromas) are benign growths of the smooth muscle layer of the uterus. They can occur in the submucous layer, the intramural layer, or in the subserous layer (Figure 7-13). They are estrogen dependent, and therefore mostly affect women during their menstruating years. The most common pelvic tumors in women, fibroids are found in about 40% of women, and more frequently in African-American women than in Caucasians (Friedman, 1995).

### History

Most women with fibroids are asymptomatic; however, depending on their number, size, and location, they can cause chronic pelvic pain, low back pain, bloating, abnormal uterine bleeding (AUB), dysmenorrhea, urinary frequency and/or incontinence, or feelings of heaviness in the pelvic area. Some women with fibroids may experience infertility.

### Physical Examination

During pelvic examination, often the uterus is irregular and enlarged or actual subserous fibroids can be palpated. If there is any possibility of pregnancy, this should first be ruled out. In addition, pelvic ultrasound or MRI should be done to identify and measure the fibromas that are present.

Although it was once thought that the increased levels of estrogen during pregnancy always caused an increase in size of fibromas, this in no longer a hard and fast rule. According to Friedman (1995), serial ultrasounds of pregnant women with fibromas indicate that some grow, usually only during the first trimester; some remain the same size; and some actually regress. Nor do oral contraceptives stimulate growth (Forrest, 1998).

### Treatment

Treatment includes all stages of intervention from conservative to surgical techniques. Watchful waiting (50% of cases), is the treatment of choice for most women, especially if the fibromas are not causing symptoms or cause tolerable symptoms. Most will regress once the woman approaches menopause. If the fibromas are causing AUB, with resultant anemia, NSAIDs can be used to help decrease the amount of bleeding. Medications, which cause a hypoestrogenic state (GnRH analogs), are chosen by some women. Others opt for surgery. Surgery includes myomectomy (i.e., removal of the tumor) but leaves the uterus intact, which is a useful choice for women who wish to become pregnant at some time in the future. Hysterectomy is also an option, especially for women who have symptoms that are severe and interfere with lifestyle. Once again, the choices depend on the severity of symptoms for the affected woman, the side effect profiles of the various interventions, and the woman's desires concerning future childbearing.

## Endometrial Cancer

Endometrial cancer is the most common reproductive tract cancer in the United States (Hubbard and Holcombe, 1990; Horton, 1995; Wertheim, Soto-Wright, and Goodman,1995). Generally, it occurs in women who are postmenopausal, with an average age at diagnosis of 61 years (Wertheim, Soto-Wright, and Goodman, 1995), but younger women can be affected. In the 1970s, the rates of endometrial cancer increased rather dramatically because of the use of unopposed estrogen for hormone therapy (HT). Once this link was understood and progesterone was added to HT, the rates decreased. Thus, the pathophysiology of the disease is related to unopposed estrogen stimulation of the endometrium, and some risk factors are related to this phenomenon. Risk factors are listed in Box 7-12.

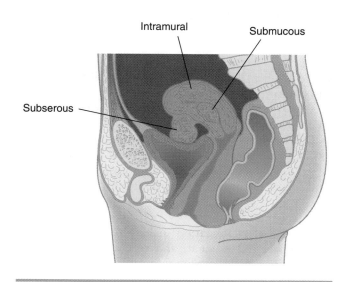

Intramural    Submucous

Subserous

*FIGURE 7-13* • Uterine fibroids.

---

**BOX 7-12**   *Risk Factors for Endometrial Cancer*

Use of unopposed exogenous sources of estrogen
Excessive endogenous estrogen
Obesity
Chronic anovulation
Early menarche
Late menopause
Nulliparity
Liver disease
Diabetes

### History

The most common symptom for women with this type of cancer is AUB. Rarely, do women experience pain with the AUB. If a postmenopausal woman experiences any vaginal bleeding this should be cause for immediate evaluation. Premenopausal women with bleeding patterns that are usually abnormal, with intermenstrual bleeding, spotting after intercourse, or menorrhagia should be evaluated.

Women who pay attention to their cycles and their bleeding patterns, and who are quick to be evaluated for deviations from normal have the advantage. Women with endometrial cancer, who are evaluated early enough, have a very good prognosis. The overall survival rate for endometrial cancer is 85%, a number which increases to 93% when the diagnosis is made early (Horton, 1995).

### Physical Examination

Usually, findings on physical and pelvic examination are normal, although an enlarged uterus and palpable nodes may be found.

### Diagnostic Testing

An endometrial biopsy is currently one of the most common diagnostic studies done to determine the diagnosis. Research is being done to determine the value of the use of transvaginal ultrasound and hysteroscopy in selected populations (Lemcke, Marshall, and Pattison 1995).

### Treatment

Treatment depends on the staging of the disease, and in most cases includes hysterectomy and salpingo-oophorectomy. Women with higher stages of cancer may receive radiation therapy. In some higher stage cancers, however, surgery and radiation are not useful, and treatment depends on systemic agents.

Interestingly, oral contraceptive use has been shown to be protective in the case of both endometrial cancer and ovarian cancer. Women at risk for either of these disorders should be advised of this protective effect. All women should be encouraged to have AUB evaluated thoroughly, immediately. Women who may be obese, diabetic, or who have secondary amenorrhea should be cautioned about their risk and encouraged to pursue options for reducing this risk when possible.

 ## CONDITIONS OF THE OVARIES

The ovaries are the site for more types of tumors, including both benign and malignant types than any other site in the human body (Dambro, 1998). The reason for this has to do with the reproductive capacity of the cells that are found in each ovary and their potential for mutation and change. According to Yon (1995), ovarian cysts and tumors are the fourth most common reason for admissions to the hospital for women in the United States. This section, on conditions of the ovaries, considers benign enlargements of the ovary, meaning those that do not have potential for malignancy; conditions that may be potential precursors to cancer; and ovarian cancer.

## Benign Tumors

Ovarian tumors are common, and fortunately for women of reproductive age, the large majority are benign. Forrest (1998) has classified these benign conditions into the following categories: inflammatory ovarian tumors, metaplastic ovarian tumors, and functional ovarian tumors. The classification of **inflammatory ovarian tumors** refers to inflammation or infection of the ovaries (e.g., PID), which can lead to abscess formation. The classification of **metaplastic ovarian tumors** refers to that form of endometriosis in which the affected sites of endometrial implantation include the ovary. **Functional ovarian tumors** include the following:

> **Follicular cysts** are caused by the failure of the ovarian follicle to rupture at the time of ovulation.
> **Lutein cysts** form when the corpus luteum becomes cystic or hemorrhagic and fails to break down after 14 days.
> **Theca lutein cysts** are associated with polycystic ovary syndrome (PCOS), clomiphene therapy, and others.
> **Polycystic ovary syndrome** (PCOS or Stein-Leventhal syndrome) is associated with androgen excess, anovulation, and secondary amenorrhea; frequently, although not in every case, multiple cysts form within the ovaries.

The majority of benign ovarian tumors in their early stages are asymptomatic. Many are found on routine pelvic examination.

### History

Some women experience mild nonspecific abdominal discomfort, dyspareunia, pelvic pain, and delays in the menstrual cycle or irregular menstrual cycles. In the case of inflammatory conditions such as PID or abscesses, pain is more acute and systemic symptoms such as fever occur. Some cysts may rupture, causing an acute episode of pain. The woman's age, symptoms, degree of pain, and sexual histories are important information.

### Physical Examination

The physical examination includes complete abdominal, pelvic, rectovaginal, and rectal examinations. In the case of a menstruating woman in whom functional cysts are found that are smaller than 8 cm, the clinician may wait one menstrual cycle and then reexamine the client. However, in postmenopausal women, any palpable ovary demands immediate further evaluation, even though benign cysts are now known to occasionally occur in this population (Carlson and Schiff, 1995). PID, abscesses, and endometriosis need treatment specific for these conditions.

### Diagnostic Testing

The woman's age; the size and consistency of the lesion; the accompanying symptoms, plus the degree of pain; and the sexual history all help determine the diagnostic tests to be done. These might include pregnancy testing, screening for an STI, and a pelvic ultrasound.

## Neoplastic Tumors

The second grouping of tumors of the ovary is known as neoplastic. The term **neoplastic** refers to the growth of new, abnormal tissue in an organ. This tissue serves no useful biologic purpose, and usually exists to the detriment of the organ. The neoplastic tissues can be benign (no carcinogenic potential) or malignant. Several ovarian tumors are considered neoplastic, with very low malignancy potential. Included in this group would be dermoid cysts, theca cell tumors, endometriomas, fibromas, mucinous epithelial tumors, and Brenner tumors. Another subset of the neoplastic group is that which has a higher malignant potential. An example of this group would be a granulosa cell tumor (Star, 1995a; MacKay, 1998).

Although primary health care providers may discover an ovarian mass, in all cases except resolving functional cysts, the specialty services of a gynecologist are required. Once an ovarian tumor has been found, it must be classified as (1) functional; (2) neoplastic, but benign; (3) having malignant potential; or (4) malignant (McKay, 1998). Along with the aforementioned diagnostic studies, laparoscopy or laparotomy may be performed to classify the tumor. The woman will need our assistance in coping with her immediate concerns, and then understanding the tests she must undergo for diagnosis and the terminology that is used to describe her tumor.

## Ovarian Cancer

Although ovarian cancer is relatively rare, it is often fatal. It is the leading cause of death among gynecologic cancers. Women with Stage I disease (confined only to the ovaries) have a 5-year survival rate ranging from 66% to 90%. But unfortunately only 25% of the women diagnosed with ovarian cancer have Stage I. For higher stages, those with sites outside of the ovary, the 5-year survival rate ranges only from 28% to 35% (Melnikow and Nuovo, 1997).

**Ovarian cancer** is not just one disease, but many. Many different cell types have been identified. These include epithelial, stromal, and germinal cell cancers, which are then subdivided according to histologic differences (Martin, 1997).

### Risk Factors for Ovarian Cancer

The causes for ovarian cancer are unknown. The only clear risk factor is family history, with the risk increasing as the number of affected family members increases (Yon, 1995). Three different syndromes are included in the familial cancer risk categories: (1) familial ovarian cancer; (2) familial ovarian/breast cancers: and (3) ovarian/breast/endometrial/colon cancers (i.e., the Lynch II syndrome) (Yon, 1995; Thompson, 1998).

Other risk factors are also implicated, however. The most important of these is age: peak incidence occurs between 55 to 59 years of age, with incidence increasing from 15.7 per 100,000 women at age 40 years, to 54 cases per 100,000 at age 75 (Thompson, 1998). In addition, the risk seems to have a hormonal basis of some sort, since women who are nulliparous have an increased risk. Conversely, multiparity seems to be protective: the higher the number of pregnancies, the greater the protection. Furthermore, use of oral contraceptives has repeatedly been shown to be protective (Chi and Hoskins, 1996).

Other risks, including dietary and environmental risks, have been discussed and studied as having an association with ovarian cancer, but none have shown a consistent or substantial effect. These include increased fat in the diet, caffeine intake, exposure to talc or asbestos, menstrual history, infertility, age at first pregnancy, or a history of severe mumps (Yon, 1995; Chi and Hoskins, 1996; Martin, 1997).

### Assessment for Ovarian Cancer

There is no screening program for ovarian cancer, although research is now being done in an attempt to develop such a program (Thompson, 1998). The major stumbling block is that ovarian cancers do not have an identifiable premalignant stage. Complicating the picture even more is the fact that most women with early stage cancer have no symptoms, or very few, vague symptoms. These include bloating, vague GI symptoms, or a change in bowel habits. Currently available tests are not reliable, sensitive, or economic enough to be considered useful screening tests. These include the bimanual portion of the pelvic examination, ultrasound, and measurement of CA-125.

***Bimanual Examination.*** The ability to discern change in the ovary by bimanual examination depends on the skill of the examiner. According to Yon (1995), there is a 30% discrepancy between the findings on bimanual examination, compared with findings on ultrasound. In addition, the group most at risk, postmenopausal women, is the group least likely to continue having pelvic examinations on an annual basis. However, the critical point is that by the time tumors are palpable by an examiner, the disease is usually metastasized and advanced (Thompson, 1998).

***Blood Test.*** CA-125 is a blood test that measures a type of tumor antigen. Eighty percent (80%) of epithelial cell ovarian carcinomas produce this substance, which can then be measured in the bloodstream of affected women. Unfortunately, only one half of patients with Stage I cancer will have elevations of CA-125, and this substance can be elevated in benign conditions such as fibroids, early pregnancy, and endometriosis (Thompson, 1998). Therefore, false-negative and false-positive results are common. This blood test is not useful as a screening tool, although it has been shown to be useful in monitoring therapy for those women with ovarian cancer who are being treated.

***Ultrasound.*** Transabdominal ultrasound does not differentiate early cancers, and therefore, also is not useful as a screening option. Transvaginal ultrasound, however, does show increased specificity over transabdominal ultrasound and may become a part of a screening set of parameters in the future (Thompson, 1998).

Current efforts are focused on early detection of ovarian cancer. Women are divided into two groups—those at high risk and those at low risk. Only women with a history of one of the familial ovarian cancer syndromes as shown by genetic testing or those with two affected first-degree relatives are placed into the high-risk group (Sutton, Santoro, and Hearns, 1998); all others are in the low-risk group. Women at high risk should have a bimanual examination, CA-125 level, and transvaginal ultrasound performed annually. Some women at high risk may be offered a prophylactic oophorectomy. The decision about whether to proceed with the surgery should be made only after careful counseling of the risks and benefits (Thompson, 1998).

All women should be made aware of their risk status and encouraged to seek appropriate evaluation. For those women with low risk, the limitations of the screening examinations and diagnostic studies should be understood. However, all women should be encouraged to have an annual bimanual examination, regardless of whether or not other diagnostic testing, such as Pap smears or STI examinations, is needed. This is especially true of postmenopausal women, a population that may not come for care as frequently.

### Treatment

Treatment of ovarian cancer includes surgical removal of as many tumor sites as possible. Surgical intervention is then followed by combination chemotherapy. Radiotherapy is used only for palliative purposes in women with severe pain, or bleeding from metastases (Martin, 1997).

### Nursing Role

Our role in working with a woman with ovarian cancer is to preserve her quality of life while undergoing treatment for a condition with a high mortality rate, to provide support during therapy, and to place an emphasis on the emotional needs of each woman.

## CONDITIONS OF THE URINARY TRACT

Urinary tract conditions account for a high rate of morbidity in women across the life cycle. These conditions can be classified as either acute or chronic in nature. Although a large number of diagnostic categories are within these two classifications, discussion in this section is limited to UTI as the most common diagnosis from the acute group and interstitial cystitis (IC) from the chronic group.

### Urinary Tract Infection

According to Marchiondo (1998), approximately 20% of women have a UTI each year, compared with a rate of 0.1% in men. Classification of the type of UTI is according to anatomic site: cystitis, referring to infections in the bladder; urethritis, or infection in the urethra; and pyelonephritis, infection in the kidney. In addition, these infections can be classified as acute (symptomatic), asymptomatic, and recurrent, either through relapse or reinfection.

Normally, the urinary tract system is a sterile system. The downward flow of urine prevents bacteria from moving upward and colonizing any of the structures. Furthermore, some physiologic conditions inhibit growth of foreign organisms. These include urine's low pH, high urea concentration, and high osmolarity and the antibacterial properties of the bladder and urethral walls. However, the close proximity of the female urethra, introitus, and rectum, plus the short length of the urethra, increase the risk of organisms being able to overcome these natural defenses. Other risk factors have also been identified and are listed in Box 7-13. It should be noted that this list does NOT include tampon use, nor does it include wiping from back to front after defecation. Although for decades women have been taught that these habits contribute to UTIs, it is now generally recognized that they are not factors (Fang, 1995; Uphold and Graham, 1998a).

### History

The most common symptoms experienced by women with an acute, uncomplicated lower UTI is pain with urination, or dysuria. Other common symptoms are frequent urination; urinary urgency; voiding in small amounts; hematuria; nocturia; and occasionally, lower abdominal pain or heaviness. When systemic symptoms such as fever, chills, nausea, vomiting, and anorexia are also present, then pyelonephritis is a more worrisome part of the differential diagnosis. Along with a symptom analysis, the history should include questions about vaginal discharge, a sexual history, contraceptive history, possibility of pregnancy, risks or history of diabetes or any immunodeficiency condition, and history of previous UTIs.

### Physical Examination

The physical examination includes vital signs; an abdominal examination; a check for costovertebral angle tenderness; and, depending on sexual history, a pelvic examination.

### Diagnostic Testing

The other major focus of the clinical examination is laboratory testing. It is essential for a urinalysis—both dipstick and microscopic examination—to be done, and often on the basis of this test alone, women can receive appropriate treatment. The gold standard of testing is the urine culture, but this test takes 24 hours to grow the responsible organisms in the laboratory, and another 24 hours to determine the sensitivities of this organism to antibiotics. Since 70% to 90% of UTIs are caused by *E.coli* (Komaroff, 1995), and the major classes of antibiotics used for UTIs are very effective, a urine culture is no longer indicated in cases of uncomplicated UTI. For individuals with recurrent UTI or more complicated conditions, however, urine culture and sensitivity are very useful diagnostic tools. Other possible laboratory tests are a CBC for those with systemic symptoms, and when indicated, testing for pregnancy and STIs.

### Treatment

If a lower tract UTI has been established as a diagnosis, treatment depends on the use of appropriate antibiotics. The newer regimens depend on a short course of therapy, usually 3 to 5 days. One-day therapy is also being used, but relapse rates are more common with this therapy (Thompson, 1995; Ryals, Vetroskey, and White, 1997; Marchiondo, 1998). The most commonly used antibiotics include trimethoprim-sulfamethoxazole, trimethoprim, norfloxacin, nitrofurantoin, and ciprofloxacin. Amoxicillin, an antibiotic used frequently in the past, is no longer the drug of choice because of increasing strains of resistant organisms.

In the case of pyelonephritis, often women are managed in the inpatient setting, especially if they are dehydrated, unable to eat, or are debilitated in any way. Under these circumstances, antibiotics are intravenously administered, and women are monitored closely for kidney function.

### Nursing Role

Our role with patients includes sharing information about the risk factors for UTIs and helping women es-

tablish alternate behavioral patterns whenever possible. An example would be to encourage women to pay attention to the urge to void and not delay emptying the bladder; another would be to urinate after sexual activity. Women who use a diaphragm for contraception and who have repeated UTIs may want to change contraceptive method. Recent research has shown that cranberry juice helps reduce the incidence of UTIs through two mechanisms: (1) reducing the pH of urine and (2) interfering with the adherence of bacteria to the bladder wall. Patients should be aware that two to three glasses a day are necessary, and that it takes 4 to 8 weeks for this therapy to be effective; therefore, it should be used as a prophylactic measure, and not be expected to be curative or helpful in the short term (Marchiondo, 1998). While being treated for a UTI, women should be encouraged to finish the entire prescribed antibiotic, to increase fluid intake, and to void every 2 to 4 hours. In some women with extreme discomfort, a prescription for phenazopyridine may be given. Women should know that this medication will turn their urine a deep orange, and that it should be taken for 2 days, after which most pain symptoms subside. Be sure she understands that it is not curative or a replacement for antibiotic therapy. Women should also be encouraged to seek evaluation as soon as they have symptoms and not to wait. Waiting can lead to more serious sequellae such as pyelonephritis.

## Interstitial Cystitis

Of the chronic urinary tract problems that affect women, interstitial cystitis (IC) has caused a great deal of confusion. This disease overwhelmingly affects women, with a ratio of 9:1 women to men. The cause for IC remains unknown, and as a result, it has been difficult to accomplish

---

### BOX 7-13 *Risk Factors for UTI*

Urinary system structural abnormalities
Sexual intercourse
Failure to void after sexual activity
Diaphragm use
Spermicidal jelly use
Spermicidal condom use
Diabetes
Immunocompromised status
Pregnancy
History of UTI or pyelonephritis
Catheterization or other urinary instrumentation
Postponing urination or incomplete voiding
Host genetic susceptibility
Virulence of the colonizing organism

research about the condition and to establish criteria for the diagnosis. The criteria that do exist have been developed by the National Institute of Diabetes and Digestive and Kidney Diseases (NIDDK), and reflect strict conditions that are being used to do research on interstitial cystitis (IC) (NIDDK, 1994).

At present, there are several different theories for the etiology of IC. These include (1) an autoimmune condition; (2) a defect in the bladder wall, which leads to it being "leaky"; (3) an unknown infectious agent; (4) bladder ischemia; and (5) presence of toxic substances in the urine (Pontara, 1997).

### History

The symptoms found in women actually are much broader than the research criteria, and include chronic urinary frequency day and night; decreased bladder capacity; and pelvic, urethral, and/or bladder pain, which is relieved by voiding. But in some women, there is chronic pelvic pain, bladder spasms, urinary urgency, a sense of incomplete voiding, and dyspareunia (NIDDK, 1994; Bavendam and Hart, 1995; Nichols and Brubaker, 1995a). In addition, there are a number of related symptoms such as bloating, nausea, diarrhea, back pain, joint pain, menstrual problems, and certain food intolerances (Webster, 1995). The confusion and variety of symptoms can also lead to a delay in the diagnosis of IC by as much as 5 years (Webster, 1995).

### Diagnostic Testing

Women at midlife are most at risk for the development of IC and usually have undergone diagnostic testing looking for UTIs, STIs, and anatomic defects, which all prove to be normal. At this point it is important that affected women be seen by a urologist who is comfortable and knowledgeable about IC. Since IC is in fact a physical condition, and not an emotional or psychiatric diagnosis, as once thought, it is very important for a woman's concerns to be taken seriously (Webster, 1995). Further testing includes cystoscopy under anesthesia, with distention of the bladder to determine capacity, and biopsy of the bladder wall.

### Treatment

Because the cause is unknown, therapy is directed at controlling the symptoms. A number of medications used are aimed at reducing bladder pain. Some women with chronic debilitating pain may need long-term treatment with narcotic agents. A few antidepressants have been shown to reduce bladder spasms and to decrease inflammation. Pentosan polysulfate sodium is the first drug approved by the FDA specifically for IC. It is not known how it works, but it is hypothesized to repair leaks in the bladder wall (NIDDK, 1994). Other therapies include bladder instillations, use of TENS units, and surgical techniques. Patients are also encouraged to find ways to control their symptoms through quitting smoking, increasing exercise, and practicing bladder training exercises. Although controversial, some patients have found that diet changes have helped. Foods to avoid include caffeine, tomatoes, alcohol, spices, chocolate, and high acid foods (NIDDK, 1994).

### Nursing Role

Interstitial cystitis can have a devastating effect on women's lives, interfering with work, social interactions, family dynamics, and sexual health. In addition, it can have an economic impact, both in regard to lost wages and the cost of diagnostic testing and treatment. Emotional support on the part of family, friends, and especially health care providers is one of the most important interventions for women with IC.

 **SUMMARY**

Due to their anatomy and physiology, women experience unique health problems and threats to their lives. Our role as collaborator in a woman's primary, secondary, and tertiary health care is based on an understanding of her strengths and needs, as well as the options available to her.

---

## Care Plan · The Woman with Endometriosis

**NURSING DIAGNOSIS** **Pain, chronic** related to extrauterine endometrial tissue swelling and inflammation

**GOALS/OUTCOMES** Reported satisfaction with symptom control

**NOC Suggested Outcomes**
- Comfort Level (2100)
- Pain Control (1605)
- Pain: Disruptive Effects (2101)

**NIC Priority Interventions**
- Analgesic Administration (2210)
- Pain Management (1400

## Care Plan · The Woman with Endometriosis—cont'd

**Nursing Activities & Rationale**
- Assess pain location, characteristics, quality, and severity (NIC). *This information is necessary in order to select the most effective pain control method.*
- Ask woman what pain relief measures she prefers; provide information as needed. *This allows her to have control over her pain and use measures she feels will benefit her.*
- Select and implement a variety of pain measures (e.g., pharmacologic, nonpharmologic, interpersonal) to facilitate pain relief, as appropriate (NIC). *Nonpharmologic measures, such as relaxation, are often synergistic with pharmologic measures, providing enhanced pain control.*
- Monitor the effectiveness of pain relief measures. *Depending on the severity of pain and degree of drug effectiveness, different pain control measures may be necessary.*
- Consider cultural influences on pain response. (NIC) *The perception and experience of pain varies between cultures.*
- Monitor for side effects of pharmacologic pain relief measures (e.g., respirations and level of consciousness for narcotics). *Close monitoring is needed in order to achieve a balance between pain relief and dosages that create unwanted or deleterious effects.*

**Evaluation Parameters**
- Verbalizes knowledge of various methods of pain control.
- Reports satisfaction with pain control methods.
- Uses analgesic and nonanalgesic pain relief measures appropriately.
- Reports acceptable comfort level.

NURSING DIAGNOSIS   **Anxiety** related to fear of infertility and/or possibility of need for surgical intervention
GOALS/OUTCOMES   Maintains optimal comfort level *(See the later section on evaluation parameters.)*

**NOC Suggested Outcomes**
- Anxiety Control (1402)
- Fear Control (1404)

**NIC Priority Interventions**
- Anxiety Reduction (5820)
- Coping Enhancement (5320)
- Security Enhancement (5380)

**Nursing Activities & Rationale**
- Encourage verbalization of feelings, fears and concerns. *Verbalization of fear or anxiety can help relieve it.*
- Listen attentively (NIC). *Offers reassurance to the woman that we are focused on her needs. Allows us to understand the woman's needs and concerns.*
- Help woman use coping strategies that have been successful in the past. *It is difficult to learn new strategies when anxious. Previously used strategies that were successful will most likely be successful now.*
- Provide factual information concerning diagnosis, treatment, and prognosis (NIC). *Knowledge reduces fear and anxiety.*
- Monitor for changes in anxiety level. *To detect when further intervention is necessary.*
- Encourage family involvement, as appropriate (NIC). *Emotional support decreases anxiety.*

**Evaluation Parameters**
- Seeks information to reduce fear.
- Maintains control over life.
- Maintains role performance and social relationships.
- Demonstrates ability to focus on new knowledge and skills.

NURSING DIAGNOSIS   **Management of Therapeutic Regimen: Risk for Individual, Ineffective**
GOALS/OUTCOMES   Implementation of prescribed health regimen

**NOC Suggested Outcomes**
- Knowledge: Treatment Regimen (1813)
- Participation: Health Care Decisions (1606)
- Treatment Behavior: Illness or Injury (1609)

**NIC Priority Interventions**
- Behavior Modification (4360)
- Self-Modification Assistance (4470)
- Coping Enhancement (5230)

*Continued*

## Care Plan · The Woman with Endometriosis—cont'd

### Nursing Activities & Rationale

- Determine woman's motivation, social support, and economic ability to maintain therapeutic regimen. *Motivation directs behavior. A highly motivated woman supported by family and friends, and able to meet the economic challenge of the prescribed health regimen, is more likely to succeed in implementing a treatment plan.*
- Reinforce constructive decisions concerning health needs (NIC). *Positive reinforcement increases the occurrence of desired behaviors.*
- Help the woman identify specific goals for following her prescribed treatment regimen. *Self-directed goals provide incentives for changing behavior in a positive manner.*
- Appraise the woman's present knowledge and skill level in regard to following the prescribed therapeutic regimen. *Lack of knowledge or inability to carry out the skills necessary for the treatment plan will result in failure or noncompliance.*
- Encourage woman to identify own strengths and abilities. *This allows her to build on present strengths.*

### Evaluation Parameters

- Describe and follow prescribed health regimen.
- Report symptom control.

---

**NURSING DIAGNOSIS**    **Situational Low Self-Esteem** related to potential inability to conceive secondary to tissue inflammation.

**GOALS/OUTCOMES**    Couple maintains essentially positive self-esteem throughout treatment process

### NOC Suggested Outcomes
- Self Esteem (1205)

### NIC Priority Interventions
- Emotional Support (5270)
- Self-Esteem Enhancement (5400)

### Nursing Activities & Rationale

- Provide emotional support. *Essential for couple while awaiting outcome of treatments.*
- Monitor statements/indicators of self-esteem. *To provide a baseline for and evaluation of interventions.*
- Explore with the couple other areas of competence that they feel good about (e.g., career, relationships). *This promotes self-esteem, focuses on positive instead of "problem" areas.*
- Reinforce statements that reflect positive feelings and attitudes. *Positive reinforcement strengthens self-esteem.*
- Refer to support group for couples as needed. *Provides safe environment for expressing negative feelings.*

### Evaluation Parameters

- Couple demonstrates positive attitudes toward themselves.
- Verbalizes self-acceptance and self-worth.
- Communicates openly.
- Maintains erect posture and eye contact.

## CASE STUDY

Regina has been having a problem with abdominal pain on and off for the past few weeks. She has not noticed any other unusual symptoms, but the discomfort is beginning to bother her, so she decides to come into the urgent care center that is affiliated with her primary care office. She is 26 years old, was divorced 2 years ago, and has never been pregnant. She works full time as a graphic artist. She has been coming to this office for the last few years and is consistent in getting her yearly check-ups; her last pelvic and Pap were 10 months ago. Her history includes an appendectomy at age 17; use of OC for the last 7 years; dysmenorrhea, which is controlled by taking OCs; recent counseling because of issues surrounding her divorce; and a family history (maternal aunt) of ovarian cancer.

- What are the most important things to ask when you begin her history?

## CASE STUDY

- Considering the topics covered in this chapter, list several health conditions that must be included on the differential diagnosis list.
- Which health conditions can be eliminated because of the history she has given so far?
- As you start to gather information from Regina what will be your first question?
- Then what information do you need to learn?

Regina shares with you that she is very worried that the pain may be caused by an STI. She says that the pain is not related to food, urination, or her menstrual cycle. She describes it as a dull ache that comes and goes almost every day, lasting for a few hours. She has no urinary symptoms. She has only taken acetaminophen a few times for the pain, and it has taken the edge off a bit. She has continued to take her oral contraception and has never been late with or missed any pills. Her LMP was 2 weeks ago and was normal for her. Since her divorce, she remained celibate until about 6 months ago, when she began a sexual relationship with a new male partner.

Regina states that during the first few months, she did insist that her partner use condoms, but in the last 3 months, they had stopped. "I know that this was stupid of me, but it seemed like the natural thing to do!" She has had three sexual partners in her lifetime. As far as she is aware, her partner is heterosexual and monogamous with her, although he has had several partners in the past. They have discussed STIs and shared that neither one has ever been diagnosed with any STI. They have vaginal sex, occasionally have oral sex, but never have anal sex. She is experiencing a slight increase in her vaginal secretions, but there is no odor. Occasionally, she has discomfort during intercourse, but not every

time. She states that she has not experienced fever, chills, sweats, a change in appetite, or flulike symptoms.

- With this information, what can you tell her will be done during a physical examination?
- What laboratory tests will probably be collected?

Regina's vital signs, skin, abdominal, pelvic, and rectal examinations are all completely normal. She does not experience any pain during any of the examinations, including no CMT. The wet prep/KOH shows about 10 to 20 WBCs per field, but no yeast, BV, or trichomonads. Results for the DNA tests for gonorrhea and chlamydia are usually available within 24 hours. Before Regina leaves arrangements are made for you to call her the next day with the results. Her results come back positive for chlamydia, but negative for gonorrhea.

- What will you tell Regina when you call her with her results?
- What will you do if you get an answering machine?
- When and where will Regina be taught about her diagnosis?
- What are the important teaching points that must be made?
- What follow-up will be done?
- How should Regina be counseled about her partner's health?
- What other screening test might be offered Regina?
- When will Regina be expected to return to the office?
- What will you do if her insurance will not cover the follow-up visit or travel to the clinic is difficult for her?

# Scenarios

1. Nita, a 24-year-old client at the woman's clinic, tells you that she is there today because she has had "awful itching of her vagina. It itches so bad that I can't stop scratching and now it is bleeding." She tells you that she has never had a vaginal infection before and has not been sexually active in 3 months. She says that she has just finished taking an antibiotic for strep throat and now she feels fine. She has no

symptoms of a UTI although it does burn when the urine touches the excoriated skin. She says that her partner has no symptoms.

- What subjective data do you have about Nita's condition?
- What subjective and objective data do you need?

- What medical condition do you think Nita might be experiencing? Why?
- What nursing diagnoses could apply? How will you validate these?
- What goals might be developed? How will these be prioritized?
- What interventions may you offer?
- How will you evaluate the effectiveness of your interventions?

2. Fatima, born and raised in the Sudan, is a 25-year-old graduate student. She has come to the student health clinic because she has a burning sensation when she urinates. When you are taking her health history, she explains that she has frequent UTIs and a great deal of discomfort when menstruating.

- Based on the information you have learned, what questions must you be sure to include as you continue to take Fatima's history?
- What other subjective and objective data do you need?
- What medical condition might she be experiencing? What led to that assumption?
- What nursing diagnoses could apply? How will you validate these?
- What goals might be developed? How will these be prioritized?
- What interventions may you offer?
- How will you evaluate the effectiveness of your interventions?

3. During a well-woman visit, Rachel, a 28-year-old woman, admits that she does not do BSE. She says, "Is it really necessary? My breasts are so lumpy I don't know what I'm feeling for and when I do feel something it scares me. Why don't I just have you check them for me every year?"

- Based on the information you have learned, what questions must you be sure to include as you continue to take Rachel's history?
- What other subjective and objective data do you need?
- What medical condition might she be experiencing? What led to that assumption?
- What nursing diagnoses could apply? How will you validate these?
- What goals might be developed? How will these be prioritized?

- What interventions may you offer?
- How will you evaluate the effectiveness of your interventions?

4. Sandra, a 39-year-old single woman, is scheduled to be seen periodically because she has fibrocystic breast disease. A CBE reveals palpable nodes in similar areas on both breasts. When you have Sandra feel them she says. "Are these cancer? Can these turn into cancer? Am I going to get breast cancer?"

- Based on the information you have learned, what questions must you be sure to include as you continue to take Sandra's history?
- What other subjective and objective data do you need?
- What medical condition might she be experiencing? What led to that assumption?
- What nursing diagnoses could apply? How will you validate these?
- What goals might be developed? How will these be prioritized?
- What interventions may you offer?
- How will you evaluate the effectiveness of your interventions?

5. Alison, a 30-year-old mother of two preschool children, has come to be seen because she is tired all the time. There are several possible reasons for her feeling this way.

- Based on her chief complaint, what questions must you be sure to include as you continue to take Alison's history?
- What other subjective and objective data do you need?
- What medical conditions might she be experiencing? What led to that assumption?
- What nursing diagnoses could apply? How will you validate these?
- What goals might be developed? How will these be prioritized?
- What interventions may you offer?
- How will you evaluate the effectiveness of your interventions?

6. Jasmine, a 17-year-old college freshman, has come to the health services for oral contraception. When taking her history you learn that she has Type I diabetes.

- Based on the information you have learned, what questions must you be sure to include as you continue to take Jasmine's personal and family history?
- What other subjective and objective data do you need?
- What medical risks does she face?
- What nursing diagnoses could apply? How will you validate these?
- What goals might be developed? How will these be prioritized?
- What interventions may you offer?
- How will you evaluate the effectiveness of your interventions?

---

7. Guerline, a 34-year-old woman in a long-term heterosexual relationship has come into the clinic because she feels like she has the flu. She reports that during the last 12 hours she has experienced abdominal pain, fever, and chills. She took Tylenol but it didn't help. She doesn't remember being near anyone that is sick. She reports no new foods or activities in her life. As she talks she folds her arms across her waist and bends over. She says that she is upset because the weekend is coming and if she is sick her new boyfriend will be mad.

- Based on the information you have learned, what questions must you be sure to include as you continue to take Guerline's personal history and family history?
- What other subjective and objective data do you need?

- What medical conditions might she be experiencing? What led to that assumption?
- What nursing diagnoses could apply? How will you validate these?
- What goals might be developed? How will these be prioritized?
- What interventions may you offer?
- How will you evaluate the effectiveness of your interventions?

---

8. A large pimple-like sore on her vulva has made Ann Marie leave her work as a secretary to come to employee health. She tells you that it started 4 days ago and has just gotten worse and worse. It has been painful when she urinates, but now this afternoon it is too sore for her to sit down. She laughs and says, "My boyfriend had a sore on his mouth that he said hurt when he ate French fries. Now I've got one down there. They're not the same thing are they?"

- Based on the information you have learned, what questions must you be sure to include as you continue to take Ann Marie's personal history?
- What other subjective and objective data do you need?
- What medical conditions might she be experiencing? What led to that assumption?
- What nursing diagnoses could apply? How will you validate these?
- What goals might be developed? How will these be prioritized?
- What interventions may you offer?
- How will you evaluate the effectiveness of your interventions?

## REFERENCES

Adamson F: Female genital mutilation: a counseling guide for professionals, 1992, www.fgm.org/CounsellingGuide.html.

Aguirre A: Recognizing and managing the oral clues that point to Sjogren's syndrome, *Medscape Women's Health* 2(9), 1997, www.medscape.com/Medscape/WomensHealth/journal/02.n09/wh3097.aguirre/wh3097.aguirre.html.

American Diabetes Association: Standards of medical care for patients with diabetes mellitus: position statement, January 1999, *Diabetes Care* 22(suppl):32-41, 1999.

American Heart Association: *1997 Heart and stroke facts statistical update,* Dallas, 1996, American Heart Association.

American Heart Association: Cardiovascular disease in women: a scientific statement from the American Heart Association, *Clin Rev* 8(4):145-147,153-156,159-160,163-165, 1998.

Appling SE: Prevention, early detection, and treatment of breast cancer: a collaborative approach, *Lippincott's Primary Care Practice: A Peer Reviewed Series* 2(2):111-118, 1998.

Ashley B: Mastalgia, *Lippincott's Primary Care Practice: A Peer Reviewed Series* 2(2):189-193, 1998.

Bavendam TG and Hart LJ: Dysuria. In Lemcke DP and others, editors: *Primary care of women,* Norwalk, CT, 1995, Appleton & Lange.

Bennett SE and Smith BL: Benign breast disease and breast implants. In Carlson KJ and others, editors: *Primary care of women,* St Louis, 1995, Mosby.

Berman BM and Swyers J: Establishing a research agenda for investigating alternative medical interventions for chronic pain. In Randall JL and Lazar JS, editors: *Primary care complementary and alternative therapies in primary care* 24(4), 1997.

Blake DR and others: Evaluation of vaginal infections in adolescent women: can it be done without a speculum?, *Pediatrics* 102(4 Pt 1):939-944, 1998.

Boston Women's Health Book Collective: *The new our bodies, ourselves,* New York, 1999, Simon & Schuster, Inc.

Branch LG: Breast health. In Youngkin EQ and Davis MS, editors: *Women's health: a primary care clinical guide.* Norwalk, CT, 1998, Appleton & Lange.

Burdge DR and Money DM: Bridging the gender gap in HIV diagnosis and care, *Medscape Women's Health,* 1(10):www.medscape.com/Medscape/WomensHealth/journal/1996/v01.n10/w83.burdge/w83.burdge.html, 1996.

Carlson KJ and Schiff I: Pelvic masses. In Carlson KJ and Eisenstat SA, editors: *Primary care of women,* St Louis, 1995, Mosby.

Carr PL, Felsenstein D, and Friedman RH: Evaluation and management of vaginitis, *J Gen Int Med* 13(5):335-346, 1998.

Carson S: Human papillomatous virus infection update: impact on women's health, *Nurse Practitioner* 22(4):24,25,28,30,35-37, 1997.

Caufield KA: Controlling fertility. In Youngkin EQ and Davis MS, editors: *Women's health: a primary care clinical guide,* Norwalk, CT, 1998, Appleton & Lange.

Centers for Disease Control and Prevention (CDC): *Critical need to pay attention to HIV prevention for women: minority and young women bear greatest burden,* www.cdc.gov/nchstp/hiv_aids/pubs/facts/women.htm, 1998.

CDC: 1998 Guidelines for treatment of sexually transmitted diseases, *MMWR* 47(No. RR-1):74-75, 1998.

CDC: Diabetes today, *ADVANCE for Nurse Practitioners* 7(4):64-66, 1999.

CDC: *Some facts about chlamydia,* www.cdc.gov/nchstp/dstd/chlamydia_facts.hym, 1999.

CDC Cost-Effectiveness Study Group: The cost-effectiveness of screening for type 2 diabetes, *JAMA* 280(20):1757-1763, 1998.

Chan-Yeung M and Malo JL: Occupational asthma, *New Engl J Med* 333:107-112, 1995.

Chandler MH and others: Premenstrual asthma: the effect of estrogen on symptoms, pulmonary function, and beta 2-receptors, *Pharmacotherapy* 17(2):224-234, 1997.

Chelala C: New rite is alternative to female circumcision, *San Francisco Chronicle,* September 16, 1998.

Chi DS and Hoskins WJ: Ovarian cancer controversy: when and how to use available screening methods, *Medscape Women's Health* 1(11), www.medscape.com/Medscape/WomensHealth/journal/1996/v01.n11/w172.chi/w172.chi.html, 1996.

Chiarmonte CG: Mind-body therapies for primary care physicians. In Randall JL and Lazar JS, editors: *Primary care: complementary and alternative therapies in primary care* 24(4):787-808, 1997.

Christiansen CD: Female circumcision. In McElmurry BJ and Parker RS, editors: *Annual review of women's health, vol. III,* New York, 1996, National League for Nursing.

Conca TJ: Cardiac rehabilitation in women: an innovative approach to increase participation, [unpublished Master's Scholarly Project], 1999.

Dalton CR: Complementary therapies in arthritis treatment, *ADVANCE for Nurse Practitioners,* 33,34,54, November, 1995.

Dambro MR: *Griffith's 5 minutes consult,* Philadelphia, 1998, Williams & Wilkins.

Deckers PJ and Ricci A: Pain and lumps in the female breast, *Hospital Practice* 27(2A):67-73,77-78,87-90,92-94, 1992.

Edelman SV and Henry RR: *Diabetes statistics: diagnosis and management of type II diabetes,* www.medscape.com/PCI/diabetes/diabetes.ch01/pnt-diabetes.ch01.html, 1998.

Elion RA and Cohen C: Complementary medicine and HIV infection. In Randall JL and Lazar JS, editors: *Primary care: clinics in office practice: complementary & alternative therapies in primary care* 24(4):905-919, 1997.

Ernster VL: The epidemiology of lung cancer in women, *Ann Epidemiol* 4(2):102-110, 1994.

Fang and Leslie S-T: Approach to dysuria and urinary tract infection in women. In Goroll AH, May LA, and Mulley AG Jr: *Primary care medicine: office evaluation of the adult patient,* Philadelphia, 1995, Lippincott.

Fantus IG, Delovitch TL, and Dupre J: Prevention of diabetes mellitus: goal for the twenty-first century: part 2, *Can J Diabetes Care* 21(4):14-20, 1997.

Feinerman CE: Pulmonary diseases in women. In *The Medical Clinics of North America: Women's Health Issues, Part II,* 82(2):189-202, 1998.

Felsenstein D: Sexually transmitted disease. In Carlson KJ and Eisenstat SA, editors: *Primary care of women,* St Louis, 1995, Mosby.

Ferrary E and Parker-Falzoi J: Common medical problems: cardiovascular through hematological disorders. In Youngkin EQ and Davis MS, editors: *Women's health: a primary care clinical guide,* Norwalk, CT, 1998, Appleton & Lange.

Ferrel KM: Aquatics for people with arthritis. In Marlowe SM, editor: *Primary care practice: arthritis and related disorders* 2(1):102-104, 1997.

Fogel CI: Sexually transmitted diseases. In Fogel CI and Woods NF, editors: *Women's health care: a comprehensive handbook,* Sage Publications, 1995, Thousand Oaks, CA.

Forrest DE: Common gynecologic pelvic disorders. In Youngkin EQ and Davis MS, editors: *Women's health: a primary care clinical guide,* Norwalk, CT, 1998, Appleton & Lange.

Freund KM and Pastorek II JG: Examining women's health: 1996-1997, *Medscape Women's Health* 2(3), www.medscape.com/Medscape/WomensHealth/journal/97/v02.n03/w3225.freund/w3225.freund.html

Friedman AJ: Uterine fibroids. In Carlson KJ and Eisenstat SA, editors: *Primary care of women,* St Louis, 1995, Mosby.

Gharib SD: Abnormal vaginal bleeding. In Carlson KJ and Eisenstat SA, editors: *Primary care of women,* St Louis, 1995, Mosby.

Gibbons M: Rx for asthma: are providers following the NHLBI strategy?, *ADVANCE for Nurse Practitioners* 4(7):45-48, 1996.

Ginsberg CK: Exfoliative cytologic screening, *J Obstet Gynecol Neonat Nurs* 20(1):39-46, 1991.

Gise LH: Premenstrual syndrome. In Lemcke DP and others, editors: *Primary care of women,* Norwalk, CT, 1995, Appleton & Lange.

Goroll AH, May LA, and Mulley Jr, AG: Evaluation of anemia. In *Primary care medicine: office evaluation of the adult patient,* Philadelphia, 1995, Lippincott.

Goroll AH, May LA, and Mulley Jr AG: Screening for lung cancer. In *Primary care medicine: office evaluation of the adult patient,* Philadelphia, 1995, Lippincott.

Gurevich M: Rethinking the label: who benefits from the PMS construct?, *Women and Health* 23(2):67-98, 1995.

Haan CK: What can be done to prevent coronary heart disease in women?, *Medscape Women's Health* 1(12), www.medscape.com/Medscape/WomensHealth/Journal/1996/v01.n12/w69.haan/w.69.haan.html, 1996.

Handsfield HH: Clinical presentation and natural course of anogenital warts, *Am J Med* 102(5A):16-20, 1997.

Hansen N and Morrow M: Breast disease. In Borum ML and others, editors: *The medical clinics of North America: women's health issues, Part II* 82(2):203-222, 1998.

Harris RE and others: Race and sex differences in lung cancer risk associated with cigarette smoking, *Int Epidemiol* 22(4):592-599, 1993.

Hatcher RA and others: *Contraceptive technology,* New York, 1994, Irving Publishers.

Hill EC: Benign disorders of the uterine cervix. In Pernoll ML and Benson RC, editors: *Current obstetric and gynecologic diagnosis and treatment,* Norwalk, CT, 1987, Appleton & Lange.

Horton JA: *The women's health data book: a profile of women's health in the United States,* ed 2, Washington, D.C., 1995, The Jacobs Institute of Women's Health.

Howes, DG: Cardiovascular disease and women, *Lippincott's Primary Care Practice: A Peer-Reviewed Series* 2(5):514-524, 1998.

Hubbard JL and Holcombe JK: Cancer of the endometrium, *Sem Oncol Nurs* 6(3):206-213, 1990.

Isaacson KB: Endometriosis. In Carlson KJ and Eisenstat SA, editors: *Primary care of women,* St Louis, 1995, Mosby.

Jaffe LS and Seely EW: Diabetes. In Carlson KJ and Eisenstat SA, editors: *Primary care of women,* St Louis, 1995, Mosby.

Janson S: National asthma education and prevention program, expert panel report II: Overview and application to primary care, *Lippincott's Primary Care Practice: A Peer Reviewed Series* 2(6):578-588, 1998.

Johnson D, Silverstein-Currier J, and Sanchez-Keeland J: Building barriers to HIV, *ADVANCE for Nurse Practitioners* 7(5):40-44,46, 1999.

Johnson PA: Hyperlipidemia. In Carlson KJ and Eisenstat SA, editors: *Primary care of women,* St Louis, 1995, Mosby.

Judelson DR: Examining the gender bias in evaluating coronary disease in women, *Medscape Women's Health* 2(2), www.medscape.com/Medscape/WomensHealthJournal97/v02.n02/w28.judelson/w28.judelson.html, 1997.

Kaufman RH: Diseases of the vulva and vagina. In Lemcke DP and others, editors: *Primary care of women,* Norwalk, CT, 1995, Appleton & Lange.

Kazanjian PH, and Eisenstat SA: Human immunodeficiency virus. In Carlson KJ and Eisenstat SA, editors: *Primary care of women,* St Louis, 1995, Mosby.

Kitzinger S: *Education and counseling for childbirth,* New York, 1979, Schocken Books.

Kitzinger S: *Woman's experience of sex,* New York, 1985, Penguin Books.

Klirsfeld D: HIV disease and women. In Borum ML and others, editors: *The Medical Clinics of North America: Women's Health Issues, Part II* 82(2):203-222, 1998.

Komaroff AL: Acute dysuria and urinary tract infections. In Carlson KJ and Eisenstat SA, editors: *Primary care of women,* St Louis, 1995, Mosby.

Koutsky L: Epidemiology of genital human papillomavirus infection, *Am J Med* 102(5A):3-8, 1997.

Kuter I: Breast cancer. In Lemcke DP and others, editors: *Primary care of women,* Norwalk, CT, 1995, Appleton & Lange.

Lammert J: Asthma. In Lemcke DP and others, editors: *Primary care of women,* Norwalk, CT, 1995, Appleton & Lange.

Larkin J and others: HIV in women: recognizing the signs, *Medscape Women's Health,* 1(11) www.medscape.com/Medscape/WomensHealth/journal/1996/v01.n11/w14.larkin/w14.larkin.html, 1996.

Lemcke DP, Marshall LA, and Pattison J: Menopause and hormone replacement therapy. In Lemcke DP and others, editors: *Primary care of women,* Norwalk, CT, 1995, Appleton & Lange.

Lichtman R and Smith SM: Multiorgan disorders. In Lichtman R and Papera S, editors: *Gynecology: Well Woman Care,* Norwalk, CT, 1990, Appleton & Lange.

MacKay HT: Gynecology. In Tierney LM and others, editors: *Current medical diagnosis and treatment 1998,* Stamford, CT, 1998, Appleton & Lange.

Mallory C and Fife BL: Women and the prevention of HIV infection: an integrative review of the literature, *J Ass Nurse AIDS Care* 10(1):51-63, 1999.

Maloney C and Cafiero MR: Urinary incontinence, *ADVANCE for Nurse Practitioners* 7(6):37-42, 1999.

Marchiondo K: A new look at urinary tract infection *Am J Nurs* 98(3):34-38, 1998.

Margolis CG: Hypotic trance: the old and the new. In Randall JL and Lazar JS, editors: *Primary care: complementary and alternative therapies in primary care* 24(4):809-824, 1997.

Martin VR: Gynecologic malignancies. In Varricchio C, editor: *A cancer source book for nurses,* Atlanta, 1997, American Cancer Society, Inc.

McMeekin DS, McGonigle KF, and Vasilev SA: Cervical cancer prevention: toward cost-effective screening, *Medscape Women's Health* 2(12), www.medscape.com/Medscape/WomensHealth/journal/02.n12/wh3023.vasilev/wh3023.vasilev.html, 1997.

Melnikow J and Nuovo J: Cancer prevention and screening in women, *Prim Care Clin Office Pract* 24(1):15-26, 1997.

Merrill JT, Dinu AR, and Lahita RG: Autoimmunity: the female connection, *Medscape Women's Health,* 1(11), www.medscape.com/Medscape/WomensHealth/journal/96/v01.n11/w207.merrill/w207.merrill.html, 1996.

Michlewitz H: Benign vulvar disorders. In Carlson KJ and Eisenstat SA, editors: *Primary care of women,* St Louis, 1995, Mosby.

Midgeon MB, Desnick L, and Elmore JG: Management of vaginal infections, *The Clinical Advisor* May 1999:26-31.

Miller JE: Benign breast disorders. In Lemcke ED and others, editors: *Primary care of women,* Norwalk, CT, 1995, Appleton & Lange.

Minchoff IE and Grandin JA: Syndrome X, *Nurse Practit* 21(6):74,75,79,80,83,84,86, 1996.

Mitchell GJ: Living with diabetes: how understanding expands theory for professional practice, *Can J Diabetes Care* 22(1):30-37, 1998.

Mitus AJ: Blood disorders. In Carlson KJ and Eisenstat SA, editors: *Primary care of women,* St Louis, 1995, Mosby.

Momoh C: Female genital mutilation: the struggle continues, *Pract Nurs* 10(2), www.fgm.org/FGMStruggle.html, 1999.

Morabia A and Wynder EL: Cigarette smoking and lung cancer cell types, *Cancer* 68(9):2074-2078, 1991.

Morrison C: The significance of nipple discharge, *Lippincott's Primary Care Practice: A Peer Reviewed Series* 2(2):129-140, 1998.

Moulton AW and Montgomery KM: Approach to the patient with a vaginal discharge. In Goroll AH, May LA, and Mulley, Jr, AG, editors: *Primary care medicine: office evaluation and management of the adult patient,* Philadelphia, 1995, Lippincott.

Muntz HG: Cervical cancer screening and management of the abnormal Papanicolaou smear. In Lemcke DP and others, editors: *Primary care of women,* Norwalk, CT, 1995, Appleton & Lange.

National Center for Health Statistics: *Health, United States, 1998: with socioeconomic status and health chartbook,* Washington, D.C., 1998, U.S. Government Printing Office.

National Heart, Lung, and Blood Institute, National Asthma Education and Prevention Program: *Guidelines for the Diagnosis and Management of Asthma: Expert Panel Report II,* NIH Pub. No. 97-4051, Bethesda, MD, 1997, The Institute.

Nichols DH and Brubaker L: Chronic bladder disorders and chronic dysuria. In Carlson KJ and Eisenstat SA, editors: *Primary care of women,* St Louis, 1995, Mosby.

Nichols DH and Brubaker L: Incontinence and genital prolapse. In Carlson KJ and Eisenstat SA, editors: *Primary care of women,* St Louis, 1995, Mosby.

NIDDK: *Interstitial cystitis,* NIH publication No. 94-3220, www.niddk.nih.gov/health/urolog/pubs/cystitis/cystitis.htm, 1994.

NIDDK: *Diabetes overview,* NIH publication No. 96-3873, www.niddk.nih.gov/health/diabetes/pubs/dmover/dmover.htm, 1998.

NIH: *DES daughters: women who were born between 1938 and 1971 who were exposed to DES before birth,* Washington, D.C., 1995, Government Printing Office.

NIH: Estimating breast cancer risk, www.cancernet.nci.nih.gov, 1998a.

NIH: *Women of color health data: adolescents to seniors,* NIH Publication No. 98-4247, Washington, D.C., 1998b, U.S. Government Printing Office.

Notelovitz M and Tonnessen D: *The essential heart book for women,* New York, 1997, St. Martin's Press.

Oktay JS: Psychosocial aspects of breast cancer, *Lippincott's Primary Care Practice: A Peer-Reviewed Series* 2(2):149-159, 1998.

Paige DM and others: Bacterial vaginosis and preterm birth: a comprehensive review of the literature, *J Nurse Midwife* 43(2):83-89, 1998.

Parsey K and others: Why the urgency for earlier diagnosis of HIV in women?, *Medscape Women's Health,* 1(8), www.medscape.com/Medscape/WomensHealth/journal/1996/v01.n08/w37.parsey/W37.parsey.html, 1996.

Peipert JF and others: Bacterial vaginosis as a risk factor for upper genital tract infection, *Am J Obstet Gynecol* 177(5):1184-1187, 1997.

Plourd DM: Practical guide to diagnosing and treating vaginitis, *Medscape Women's Health* 2(2) www.medscape.com/Medscape/WomensHealth/journal/1997/v02.n02/w293.plourd/w293.plourd.html, 1997.

Pontara MA: Interstitial cystitis update, *Infectious Urology,* 10(3):75-79,80, 1997.

Redberg RF: Coronary artery disease in women: understanding the diagnostic and management pitfalls, *Medscape Women's Health* 3(5) www.medscape.com/MedscapeWomensHealthJournal/v03.n05.wh3019.redb/pnt-wh3019.redb.html, 1998.

Richman E: Asthma diagnosis and treatment, *Clinician Rev* 7(8):76-78,83,84,86-90,96,97,101,102,107-109,112, 1997.

Rigotti NA and Polivogianus L: Smoking cessation. In Carlson KJ and Eisenstat SA, editors: *Primary care of women,* St Louis, 1995, Mosby.

Ryals JK, Vetroskey D, and White GL: Urinary tract infections, *Lippincott's Primary Care Practice: A Peer Reviewed Series* 1(4):442-445, 1997.

Sarto GE: Controversies in women's health, *Women's Health in Primary Care* 1(10s):5, 1998.

Sawin KJ: Health concerns for women with physical disability and chronic illness. In Youngkin EQ and Davis MS, editors: *Women's health: a primary care clinical guide,* Norwalk, Ct, 1998, Appleton & Lange.

Schafer, SD: Vaginitis and sexually transmitted diseases. In Youngkin EQ and Davis MS, editors: *Women's health: a primary care clinical guide,* Norwalk, CT, 1998, Appleton & Lange.

Schafer SD: Women and HIV. In Youngkin EQ and Davis MS, editors: *Women's health: a primary care clinical guide,* Norwalk, CT, 1998, Appleton & Lange.

Schkade JK and Neville-Smith M: Benefits of occupational therapy for arthritis. In Marlowe SM, editor: *Primary care practice: arthritis and related disorders* 2(1):100-101, 1998.

Schwebke JR, Morgan SC, and Pinson GB: Validity of self-obtained vaginal specimens for diagnosis of trichomoniasis, *J Clin Microbiol* 35(6):1618-1619, 1997.

Secor RM: Bacterial vaginosis: a common infection with serious sequellae, *ADVANCE for Nurse Practitioners* 2(4):11-12,15-16, 1994.

Shapero GH: Screening for cervical intraepithelial neoplasia: two new approaches, *Clinic Rev* I, April, 1991.

Sharp PC and Konen JC: Women's cardiovascular health, *Primary Care: Clinics in Office Practice* 24(1):1-14, 1997.

Skobeloff EM and others: The effect of the menstrual cycle on asthma presentations in the emergency department, *Arch Intern Med* 156(16):1837-1840, 1996.

Skrypzak B: Approach to abnormal vaginal bleeding. In Lemcke DP and others, editors: *Primary care of women,* Norwalk, CT, 1995, Appleton & Lange.

Soper DE: Sexually transmitted diseases and pelvic inflammatory disease. In Lemcke DP and others, editors: *Primary care of women,* Norwalk, CT, 1995, Appleton & Lange.

Star WL: Pelvic masses. In Star WL, Lommel LL, and Shannon MT, editors: *Women's primary health care: protocols for practice,* Washington, D.C., 1995a, American Nurses Publishing.

Star WL: Polyps—endocervical, cervical, and endometrial. In Star WL, Lommel LL, and Shannon MT, editors: *Women's primary health care: protocols for practice,* Washington, D.C., 1995b, American Nurses Publishing.

Strozzo MD: An overview of surgical management of stage I and stage II breast cancer for the primary care provider, *Lippincott's Primary Care Practice: A Peer Reviewed Series* 2(2):160-169, 1998.

Sutton MY, Santoro N, Hearns RM: Gynecologic health and disease. In Borum ML and Hsia JA, editors: *The Medical Clinics of North America: Women's Health Issues,* Part II, 82(2):223-247, 1998.

Taha TE and others: Bacterial vaginosis and disturbances of vaginal flora: association with increased acquisition of HIV, *AIDS* 12:1699-1706, 1998.

Thompson CS: Urinary tract infections. In Lemcke DP and others, editors: *Primary care of women,* Norwalk, CT, 1995, Appleton & Lange.

Thompson SD: Ovarian cancer screening: a primary care guide, *Lippincott's Primary Care Practice: A Peer-Reviewed Series* 2(3):244-250, 1998.

Travis WD, Travis LB, Devesa SS: Lung cancer, *Cancer,* 75(1 Suppl): 191-202, 1995.

Uphold CR and Graham MV: Cystitis and pyelonephritis in adolescents and adults. In *Clinical guidelines in family practice,* Gainesville, FL, 1998a, Barmarrae Books, Inc.

Uphold CR and Graham MV: Dysmenorrhea. In *Clinical guidelines in family practice,* Gainesville, FL, 1998b, Barmarrae Books, Inc.

Uphold CR and Graham MV: Tobacco use and smoking cessation. In *Clinical guidelines in family practice,* Gainesville, FL, 1998c, Barmarrae Books, Inc.

Venn A and others: Questionnaire study of effect of sex and age on the prevalence of wheeze and asthma in adolescence, *Brit Med J* 316:1945-1946, 1998.

Vieiralves-Wiltgen C, and Engle VF: Identification and management of DES-exposed women, *Nurse Practit* 13(11):15,16,19,20,22,27, 1988.

Wakamatsu MM: Vaginitis. In Carlson KJ and Eisenstat SA, editors: *Primary care of women,* St Louis, 1995, Mosby.

Wang CC: Oral contraceptive use linked with increase risk of HIV-1 transmission, *J AIDS* 21:51-58, 1999.

Webster DC: Interstitial cystitis: women at risk for psychiatric misdiagnosis. In Andrist LA, editor: *AWHONN's Clinical Issues in Perinatal and Women's Health Nursing: Women's Issues in Women's Health Care Nursing* 4(2):236-243, 1995.

Wenger NK: The high risk of CHD in women: understanding why prevention is crucial, *Medscape Women's Health* 1(11) www.medscape.com/Medscape/WomensHealthJournal/1996/v01.n11/w60.wenger/w60.wenger.html, 1996.

Wertheim I, Soto-Wright VJ, and Goodman HM: Gynecologic cancers. In Carlson KJ and Eisenstat SA, editors: *Primary care of women,* St Louis, 1995, Mosby.

WHO: Female genital mutilation: information pack, www.who.int/frh-whd/FGM/infopack/English/fgm_infopack.htm, 1996.

Wieker TL: Managing asthma with behavior modification, *Clin Rev* 9(3):65-68,71,72,75,78,79,81,82, 1999.

Wilson DD: *Nurses' guide to understanding laboratory and diagnostic tests,* Philadelphia, 1999, Lippincott.

Woodrow N and Lamont RF: Bacterial vaginosis: its importance in obstetrics, *Hosp Med* 59(6):447-450, 1998.

Wooley P: Update on genital herpes: incidence, treatment, and prevention, *Infect Urol* 11(2):42-46, 1998.

Wright J: Female genital mutilation: an overview, *J Adv Nurs* 24:251-259, 1996.

Yon JL: Evaluation of pelvic masses and screening for ovarian cancer. In Lemcke DP and others, editors: *Primary care of women,* Norwalk, CT, 1995, Appleton & Lange.

Zang EA and Wynder EL: Lung cancer risk elevated in women, *Medscape Women's Health* 1(2) www.medscape.com/Medscape/oncology/journal/1998/v01.n02/wh3275.zang/wh3275.zang.html, 1998.

Zechel MA and Bhagirath S: Vaccination against type I diabetes mellitus by early immunotherapy with autoantigens, *Can J Diabetes Care* 22(s3):S17-19, 1998.

Ziegfield CR: Differential diagnosis of a breast mass, *Lippincott's Primary Care Practice: A Peer Reviewed Series* 2(2):121-128, 1998.

# CHAPTER 8

# Preconception Health Care

*"There is no such thing as making a miracle happen spontaneously. . . You've got to work."*

— MARTINA ARROYO

*What are the components of preconception care?*

*How do we screen for genetic disorders?*

*How do we screen for conditions that make a pregnancy a high-risk condition?*

*What is infertility?*

*What nursing interventions may be necessary to assist with the experience of infertility?*

Some women have the capacity to become pregnant. Others do not. Some women have the desire to become pregnant. Others do not. A woman's desire and ability to become pregnant may change over time because of various personal expectations and physical factors, as well as the desires and expectations of her family and society. To preserve a woman's options, various assessments and interventions are provided as a part of her primary care.

 ## IMPLEMENTING THE PROCESS OF PRECONCEPTION CARE

A woman will have the highest probability of having the best outcome from pregnancy if she is in optimal health before becoming pregnant. Since the majority of pregnancies are unintended, every woman of childbearing age who is sexually active with a male partner should be considered to be at risk for becoming pregnant. Health promotion activities for women of childbearing age are

therefore advised for all women. However, preconception care must be approached in a sensitive manner that does not imply or anticipate that all women want or expect to have babies.

One note of caution should be remembered. A significant number of women of childbearing age are lesbian. It is important not to assume that all women are heterosexual. Avoid any such assumptions when presenting information about pregnancy and childbearing. Some lesbians wish to have children and may elect to have intercourse with a man or obtain sperm and undergo alternative insemination, so assuming that lesbians have no need for preconception health promotion education is inappropriate.

### Understanding Preconception Education

Currently, the concept of preparing for pregnancy is not widespread, and it should be promoted and expanded

313

upon. Preconception health should be addressed at every health promotion visit for women of childbearing age. Achieving and maintaining an optimum level of health becomes a goal of care because of the impact on the woman herself, as well as any child she may conceive, either planned or unplanned. The focus of **preconception** health care is to have every woman who enters pregnancy be in a state of optimal health, thereby increasing the probability of an uneventful pregnancy that ends at term with the birth of a healthy baby. Incorporating preconception health into the well woman health visit can be done in various ways. Teaching materials, such as the example prepared by the March of Dimes (Box 8-1), can be helpful in alerting all women to the concept.

### Unwanted and Unintended Pregnancies

In an ideal world, every pregnancy would be planned and every child would be born into a family that wants that child at that time. It is important to differentiate between an unintended pregnancy and an unwanted pregnancy (Peterson and Moos, 1997). **Unwanted pregnancies** are those that occur to a woman who does not

want to have a child; the woman may be without a partner, she may have had sex with someone other than her long-term partner, she may never want to bear children, or she may already have all the children she wants. Unwanted pregnancies may also occur as the result of nonconsensual sexual activity such as rape or incest. An **unintended pregnancy** is a pregnancy that is mistimed rather than unwanted. The woman wants to have a baby, just not right now. A woman may react very differently to a pregnancy that is unwanted than to a pregnancy that is mistimed.

### Goal of Preconception Care

The goal of preconception counseling is to provide women and their partners with information regarding their health status and to inform them of the potential risks to optimal pregnancy outcome. Women receive information that will be useful to them in reproductive decision making. Some women and their partners may choose to adopt behaviors to alter risk factors; others may choose to delay pregnancy, to postpone pregnancy, or to avoid pregnancy altogether.

---

### BOX 8-1   *Think Ahead*

If you're thinking about having a baby now or in the future, there are things you can do before you conceive to help your baby be born healthy. It's important to keep in mind that you could be pregnant for several weeks before you even realize it. During those early weeks, your baby's vital organs are beginning to form. This is a crucial time so it's important that you be prepared for this possibility in order to give your baby the best chance for a healthy start in life.

If you're trying to become pregnant—or if you could become pregnant unexpectedly—it pays to THINK AHEAD and follow these steps.

Take 400 micrograms of folic acid daily before conception and in early pregnancy. All women of childbearing age should take a daily multivitamin containing folic acid as part of a healthy diet rich in fortified foods (such as fortified breakfast cereals), and in natural sources of folic acid. Natural sources include orange juice, green leafy vegetables, beans, peanuts, broccoli, asparagus, peas, lentils, and enriched grain products.

Have a medical checkup before conceiving so your health care provider can evaluate your health and identify any health risks.

If you're not immune to chicken pox and rubella, check with your health care provider about getting vaccinated

before you conceive.

Now's the time to achieve your ideal weight. Being over- or underweight may cause problems during pregnancy.

Know your family history. If you've had problem pregnancies or birth defects in your family, you should talk to your health care provider and/or a genetic counselor when appropriate.

Adopt a healthy lifestyle; get plenty of exercise; don't drink, smoke, or use drugs. Ask your health care provider if the prescription or over-the-counter drugs you use are safe to take during pregnancy and in the pre-pregnancy period.

Have medical problems like diabetes, epilepsy, and high blood pressure treated and under control before you get pregnant.

Eat a nutritious and balanced diet.

Avoid exposure to toxic substances and chemicals—such as cleaning solvents, lead and mercury, some insecticides, paint thinners and removers, etc.—at home and where you work.

Don't eat undercooked meat or handle cat litter. They can cause toxoplasmosis, which can seriously harm a developing fetus.

March of Dimes website. http://www.modimes.org/HealthLibrary2/healthybaby/think.htm or Toll free # 888-MODIMES

For women who have partners, preconception education involves both members of the dyad. Information about conditions that have genetic components clearly involve both members of the partnership. As we learn more about the environmental influences on pregnancy outcome, it is clear that potentially negative effects are not just related to the mother. For example, several years ago it was noted that nurses who worked in operating rooms had higher-than-expected rates of spontaneous abortions in early pregnancy. The cause was determined to be trace elements of anesthetic gases in the environment, which led to the direct venting of these gases. The female partners of male anesthesiologists also had higher-than-expected rates of spontaneous abortions, so it clearly was important for these couples to include their partners' working conditions in any prenatal education discussion.

## Components of Preconception Education

The most important part of the process of preconception education is gathering data about the woman and her partner, as outlined in Box 8-2. Based on the data information, options can be provided to the woman and her partner so that they can decide whether to alter behavior according to recommendations given, to continue with current behaviors, or to seek advanced counseling because of special circumstances. Preconception education provides clients with information necessary for informed decision making that is systematic, comprehensive, and personalized. This information should be delivered in an appropriate and nonjudgmental manner.

It is important to recognize that different people have different tolerances for risk—what is a negligible risk for one couple may be totally unacceptable for another. Also, it is important to remember that statistics give population-based information. Knowing that you have a 25% risk per pregnancy of having a baby with cystic fibrosis is fine, but to a couple with that risk for a specific pregnancy, the outcome will either be zero or 100%—their child will either have cystic fibrosis or it will not.

The following sections discuss the components of preconception data gathering, with a brief explanation of why each is included in the assessment.

### Personal and Social Information

Personal and social data can elicit valuable information regarding preconception health risks. Maternal age is an important consideration because poor pregnancy outcomes are associated with women at either end of the age spectrum. Certain occupations put women at increased risk of exposure to physical substances or occupational hazards. Women who have intense exercise regimens or who are involved in energy-intense athletic activities may have significantly decreased body fat, which may lead to decreased levels of estrogen and ir-

regular menstrual patterns. Alcohol use has been associated with congenital anomalies, and tobacco use has been associated with increased incidence of low–birth-weight infants. Although many drugs and medications have demonstrated effects on the fetus, other drugs do not. However, for most drugs or drug combinations, the fetal effects are unknown. In the cases of drugs with proven teratogenic effects, it is wise to coordinate medication regimens with pregnancy planning because the most significant drug effects often occur during the first trimester.

Environmental conditions that may affect pregnancy include things such as solvents used in hobbies such as pottery making and furniture refinishing, extremes of heat and cold, exposure to chemicals or radiation, and unsafe living conditions. An assessment of household pets is important because of the potential for infectious diseases such as toxoplasmosis from cat feces and salmonellosis from contact with iguanas.

### Family History

The purpose of the family history is to determine any conditions that may have a genetic component. Although it was originally thought that the genetic component was important for single-gene Mendelian transmission, this is no longer true. As the mapping of the human genome becomes a reality, we are learning more about conditions that are caused by the interaction of more than one gene. This area of knowledge continues to evolve rapidly, and it is important to have a current source of information that is reliable and accurate. The U.S. government provides information on the human genome project at the National Human Genome Research Institute (IVHARI) at www.nhgri.nih.gov/.

Knowing the client's ethnicity and that of the father of her baby allows us to educate the woman about genetic conditions that have increased prevalence in that particular population. For example, Tay-Sachs disease, a progressive, uniformly fatal degenerative neurologic disorder, occurs primarily in people of Ashkenazi Jewish descent. It is also important to question whether the client and the father have any blood relatives in common or whether they have, in their direct lineage, any history of consanguinity, because this would heighten the possibility of expression of any conditions that are transmitted in single-gene Mendelian recessive patterns (Table 8-1).

Other genetic conditions that might be assessed for include disorders such as cystic fibrosis, muscular dystrophy, sickle cell disease, hemophilia, phenylketonuria (PKU), or hereditary hemochromatosis. It is also common to ask about any prior amniocentesis or birth defects that may have occurred in prior pregnancies, since many have a genetic component.

Obtaining a family medical history is important, because many conditions carry increased risk among family members. These conditions include hypertension,

---

## BOX 8-2    *Preconception Data Collection Guide*

**PERSONAL AND SOCIAL HISTORY**
Age
Occupation
Exercise habits
Alcohol use
Tobacco use
Nonprescription drug use
  Over-the-counter medications
  Marijuana, cocaine, and other substances
Occupation
Environmental conditions
Pets in the household

**FAMILY HISTORY**
Ethnicity (patient and partner)
Family medical history
  Diabetes
  Hypertension
  Cancer
  Heart disease
  Seizures
  Mental retardation
  Multiple gestation
History of genetic conditions
  Cystic fibrosis
  Muscular dystrophy
  Tay-Sachs disease
  Sickle cell disease or trait
  Hemophilia
  Hereditary hemochromatosis
  Birth defects
  Down syndrome
  Phenylketonuria (PKU)

**MEDICAL HISTORY**
Allergies
Cancer
Diabetes
Hypertension
Heart disease

Seizures
Previous surgery
Infectious diseases
  Sexually transmitted diseases
  Rubella
  Other childhood infections
Nutrition
  Dietary habits
  Special dietary considerations
    Vegetarianism
    Lactose intolerance
  History of eating disorders
  Use of vitamins, herbs, dietary supplements
  Use of herbal teas, creams, or tinctures
  Unusual food practices or cravings (remember this will
    be usual for the person)

**REPRODUCTIVE HISTORY**
Menarche
Current menstrual pattern
Previous pregnancies
  Age at onset
  Pregnancy outcome
Contraception
  Method(s) used
  Satisfaction
Sexual history
  Partners
    Number
    Male, female, both
  Frequency of sexual activity
  Satisfaction with current practices

**MEDICATION HISTORY**
Prescription medications
Use of nonprescription medications

Is there anything else in your or your partner's personal or family history that you think is important that I haven't asked about?

Adapted from: American College of Obstetricians and Gynecologists: *ACOG guide to planning for pregnancy, birth, and beyond,* Washington, DC, 1990, Author. Cefalo RC and Moos MK: *Preconceptional health care: a practical guide,* ed 2, St Louis, 1994, Mosby. Moos MK: *Preconceptional health promotion,* White Plains, NY, 1994, March of Dimes Birth Defect Foundation.

---

cancer, heart disease, seizure disorders, and mental retardation. Since gestational diabetes is more common among women with family histories of diabetes, it is important to know about any family history of diabetes. Likewise, the spontaneous occurrence of multiple gestations is more common when either parent has a family history of naturally occurring twins, triplets, or higher order multiple births.

### Medical History

The client's personal medical history is relevant because certain chronic illnesses, such as heart disease and dia-

## TABLE 8-1 Increased Risk for Disease Based on Heredity

| Disease | Ethnic group |
|---|---|
| Blood anemias | |
|   Sickle cell anemia | African-American |
|   β-thalassemia | Mediterranean |
| | Middle Eastern |
| | Indian (from India) |
| | Far Eastern |
| | African |
|   α-thalassemia | Southeast Asian |
| | Chinese |
| Endocrine disorder | |
|   Cystic fibrosis | Northern European |
| | Caucasian |
| | Ashkenazi Jewish |
| Neurologic disease | |
|   Tay-Sachs disease | Ashkenazi Jewish |
|   Canavan's disease | Ashkenazi Jewish |

betes, may have an effect on the course and outcome of a pregnancy. Likewise, it is important to know what effect the experience of a pregnancy may have on the course and progression of a chronic illness. For some conditions, such as cancer, there may be an advisable waiting period between the end of treatment and the time at which a pregnancy might be attempted.

Certain infectious diseases have the potential to cause serious damage to a developing fetus. It is advisable, for example, for all women of childbearing age to have a documented titer for rubella; those without documented immunity should be counseled about receiving the rubella vaccine and using a highly effective contraceptive method for 3 to 6 months.

### Nutrition

Pregnancy places significant nutritional demands upon a woman, so it is important that she enter pregnancy in a state of optimal nutrition. When at all possible, a woman who is underweight or overweight should deal with the problem before beginning a pregnancy. An underweight woman may compromise her own health status or that of the fetus if nutrients are not available in sufficient quantity. An overweight woman may mistakenly believe that she can avoid weight gain during pregnancy and use the pregnancy as a mechanism for eventual weight loss. A woman who has special dietary needs, for example those who are lactose intolerant or who follow strict vegetarian diets, may benefit from referral to a nutrition counselor to ensure that her diet contains all of the essential nutrients.

Research has shown that folic acid supplementation is effective in preventing many neural tube defects and may decrease the occurrence of Down syndrome,

leading to a recommendation that all women of childbearing age take 0.4 mg of folic acid per day. In 1995, 52% of the women of childbearing age responding to the March of Dimes Preparing for Pregnancy Survey had heard of folic acid; 5% of the women knew that taking it prevented birth defects, and 28% were taking it daily. When the survey was repeated in 1998, 68% of the women had heard of folic acid (a 28% increase), and 13% knew that it prevented birth defects (this is almost a 300% increase), yet the percentage of women taking folic acid on a daily basis remained relatively the same at 32% (www.modimes.org/HealthLibrary2/factsfigures/folicacid.htm, accessed 4/11/00). These results indicate that even though an increasing number of women have heard about folic acid and its benefit in preventing birth defects, two thirds of them are not benefiting from this knowledge. Educational programs and sources of folic acid must now be developed to enable successful incorporation of folic acid supplementation into the diets of women of childbearing age.

Women who have had pregnancies in which there was a documented neural tube defect may require a higher dose and should be referred for genetic counseling. Recent research indicates that there may be additional health benefits from folic acid, thus suggesting that 0.4 mg of folic acid daily should be continued throughout the woman's life span.

Many women use herbs and other dietary supplements and do not consider these to be medications. It is important to ask about these products when collecting assessment data. Because the Food and Drug Administration (FDA) does not consider these to be medications, they are not subject to the same level of federal oversight and quality control. A referral to a dietician can often be of assistance to a woman as she evaluates these practices.

The craving for substances not normally considered food is called pica. Women have been known to ingest various substances including clay containing dirt, laundry starch, tar, charcoal, and coffee grounds. Pica may interfere with the metabolism of essential nutrients, cause an excessive caloric intake, or cause decreased ingestion of nutritious foods. Women who practice pica may also benefit from referral to a dietician.

Eating disorders, such as anorexia nervosa and bulimia, may make it difficult for women to obtain adequate nutrition to support their own metabolic needs and may constitute health emergencies for the woman. Women who have been successfully treated for eating disorders may have special educational needs regarding preparation for pregnancy and may be referred to a dietician for special education and counseling.

### Reproductive History

A menstrual history includes age at the onset of menses (menarche) and a current menstrual pattern. Women with highly irregular menstrual cycles may have conditions such as polycystic ovarian syndrome that could lead to difficulty conceiving. If women are unaware of these problems and postpone plans for childbearing, they may end up with unwanted infertility. Knowing that there is a possibility of infertility when pregnancy is delayed helps women decide when, and whether, to attempt pregnancy or to seek help from a reproductive endocrinologist.

It is also important to ask about any previous pregnancies, the age at which the pregnancy occurred, and the outcomes of those pregnancies, including spontaneous abortions (miscarriage), induced abortions, stillbirths, live births, and any complications that may have occurred. Make particular note of any incidence of preterm labor or low–birth-weight infants because these are the leading causes of perinatal morbidity and mortality.

Ask about what current contraception, if any, is being used and what methods have been used in the past. Ask if the woman and her partner are satisfied with this means of contraception and whether they have any interest in learning about other methods. Ask as well about present and previous sexual partners, including the number and gender of these partners. Discuss high-risk sexual practices and the need to protect against sexually transmitted diseases as well as pregnancy. Ask whether she is comfortable with her current sexual practices and whether they are satisfactory to her and her partner.

### Medication History

Ask about prescription and nonprescription medication use. Many times medications for chronic conditions, such as seizure disorders or hypertension, can be changed before a pregnancy is attempted so that the woman is stabilized on the medication that is safest for use during pregnancy and also effective in managing the symptoms of the chronic illness.

##  SCREENING FOR GENETIC DISORDERS

One of the purposes of preconception health assessment is to screen for genetic disorders. Some genetic disorders manifest themselves in early childhood and, with our present state of knowledge, have universally poor outcomes. Tay-Sachs disease, for example, occurs primarily in families where both partners are of Ashkenazi Jewish descent. Babies develop symptoms during the first year or two of life and rarely survive beyond the age of 5. Other conditions, such as PKU, manifest themselves in early infancy. Extensive dietary modifications are then required to support the healthy development of the child. Still other genetic conditions, such as Huntington's disease, do not manifest themselves until midlife.

The basis of genetic screening is a family health history that determines the person's age, blood type, occupation, personal health habits and events, as well as the occurrence of these illnesses in close family members. The March of Dimes provides such a form to people interested in collecting the information needed to start the evaluation process (Figure 8-1).

### Genetic Counseling

When a woman and her partner have concerns or unanswered questions about disease traits in family members, they may be assisted by genetic counseling. "A genetic counselor works with a person or family that may be at risk for inherited disease or an abnormal pregnancy outcome, discussing their chances of having children who are affected" (Genetic Counseling, 1994). People should be presented with the option of speaking to a genetic counselor when they have vague or very specific concerns and questions (Box 8-3).

Genetic counseling is complex. As the Human Genome Project continues to teach us more about the genetic basis of certain conditions, it will become even more complex. Genetic nurse specialists, geneticists, and genetic counselors with specialized education in the subject provide information about common genetic conditions and counsel families with complex problems (Williams, 1996).

### Birth Defects

An abnormal gene can cause or contribute to the occurrence of a birth defect. A **birth defect** is an abnormality of structure (e.g., clubfoot), function (e.g., fragile X syndrome, the most common inherited form of mental retardation), or body metabolism (e.g., Tay-Sachs) present at birth that results in physical or mental disability or is fatal.

One out of every 28 babies is born with a birth defect. With more than 4,000 known birth defects, they are the leading cause of death in the first year of life. However, the cause of about 60% of birth defects is unknown. What we do know is that both genetic and environmental factors can cause birth defects.

Every human being has about 100,000 genes, with one half of the genes coming from the 23 unpaired chromosomes in the ovum and one half from the 23 unpaired chromosomes, of the sperm. When the ovum is fertilized by the sperm, a new cell is formed with the combined 46 chromosomes, creating a genetically unique individual. Genes in each pair carry instructions for either dominant or recessive traits. These determine the color of eyes and hair, body build, and the growth and development of every physical and biochemical system.

### Autosomal Dominant Inheritance

Some birth defects are caused by a single abnormal gene from one parent. This is an **autosomal dominant inheritance**. If a parent has the gene for a dominant condition, each child has a 50% chance of having the same condition. Examples of birth defects caused by a single

## Family Health History

Name _____

Date of Birth _____ Blood and Rh type _____

Occupation _____

Please note any serious or chronic diseases you have experienced, with special attention to the following:

- ☐ Alcoholism
- ☐ Allergies
- ☐ Arthritis
- ☐ Asthma
- ☐ Blood diseases (e.g., hemophilia, sickle cell anemia, thalassemia)
- ☐ Cancer (i.e., breast, bowel, colon, ovarian, skin and stomach)
- ☐ Cystic fibrosis

- ☐ Diabetes
- ☐ Epilepsy
- ☐ Familial high blood-cholesterol levels
- ☐ Hearing defects
- ☐ Heart defects
- ☐ Huntington's disease
- ☐ Hypertension (high blood pressure)
- ☐ Learning disabilities (e.g., dyslexia, attention deficit disorder, autism)

- ☐ Liver disease (i.e., particularly hepatitis)
- ☐ Lupus
- ☐ Mental illness (e.g., manic-depressive disorders; schizophrenia)
- ☐ Mental retardation (e.g., Down syndrome, fragile X syndrome, etc.)
- ☐ Migraine headaches
- ☐ Miscarriages or neonatal deaths

- ☐ Multiple sclerosis
- ☐ Muscular dystrophy
- ☐ Myasthenia gravis
- ☐ Obesity
- ☐ Phenylketonuria (PKU)
- ☐ Recurrent or severe infections
- ☐ Respiratory disease (e.g., emphysema, bacterial pnuemonia)
- ☐ Rh disease
- ☐ Skin disorders (particularly psoriasis)

- ☐ Tay-Sachs disease
- ☐ Thyroid disorders
- ☐ Tuberculosis
- ☐ Visual disorders (e.g., dyslexia, glaucoma, retinitis pi osa)
- ☐ Other:

Please note the names of your relatives here, along with indications of any illnesses, such as those above, that affected them. Also make note of lifestyle habits, such as smoking.

Father: _____

Mother: _____

Brothers and sisters: _____

Children of brothers and sisters: _____

If deceased, age and cause: _____

**FIGURE 8-1** • Family health history for genetic screening. *(Adapted from March of Dimes:* Genetic counseling, *White Plains, NY, 1999, March of Dimes.)*

gene are achondroplasia, a type of dwarfism; Marfan syndrome, a connective tissue disease commonly diagnosed when tall athletes collapse and die; familial high cholesterol; Huntington's disease, a progressive nervous system disorder; polycystic kidney disease; some forms of glaucoma; and polydactyly, extra fingers or toes (March of Dimes, 1994) (Figure 8-2).

### Autosomal Recessive Inheritance

More commonly a process of **autosomal recessive inheritance** occurs. Everyone carries a few potentially harmful recessive genes. When the person has one copy of a recessive disorder they are called a carrier. If both parents are carriers of the same recessive gene, this can create birth defects in their children.

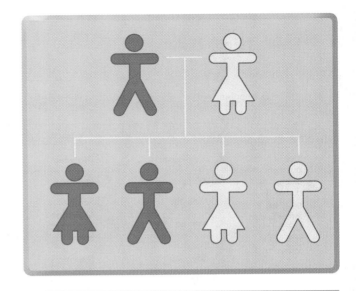

**FIGURE 8-2** • Inheritance of autosomal dominant disorders. *(Adapted from March of Dimes:* Genetic counseling, *White Plains, NY, 1999, March of Dimes.)*

The occurrence of an inherited defect may be a surprise because the parents are healthy. The gene has not manifested itself in their development because they also have a normal gene. If the child receives one gene for the disorder and one normal gene, the development of the condition will also be prevented in the child, but the child will be a carrier. There is a 50% chance of this happening with each pregnancy. Each child also has a 25% chance of being completely unaffected (no recessive gene) and a 25% chance of having the disorder (recessive gene from both parents). Examples of recessive disorders are sickle cell anemia, a painful blood disorder affecting mainly people of African descent; Tay-Sachs disease, a neurologic disease with mental and physical deterioration that occurs mainly in people of Ashkenazi Jewish heritage; cystic fibrosis, a disorder of the lungs and digestion affecting primarily Caucasians; and PKU, a metabolic disorder created by a defective enzyme in mainly Caucasians (March of Dimes, 1994) (Figure 8-3).

### Sex-Linked Recessive Inheritance

Other disorders are passed on by the sex-determining chromosomes, X and Y. Females have two X chromosomes and males have an X and a Y chromosome. If a disorder is passed on by one of the X chromosomes, it is called an X-linked or **sex-linked recessive inheritance**.

A woman who is a carrier of an X-linked abnormal gene will appear normal. However, she has a 50% chance of passing the abnormal gene each time she becomes pregnant, because whether male or female, the fetus receives an X chromosome from the mother. Her sons have a 50% chance of being affected and her daughters have a 50% chance of becoming a carrier.

Examples of X-linked inherited conditions are hemophilia, a blood condition in which there is insufficient substance for clotting; red-green color blindness; and Duchenne's muscular dystrophy, which begins in childhood and causes progressive muscle weakness and death usually by the age of 20 (March of Dimes, 1994) (Figure 8-4).

### Identifying Carriers

When a condition is known to exist in a family, a person may wish to learn if he or she is a carrier. Carrier tests are now available for many genetic traits. Blood tests will reveal that an individual carries hemophilia, beta-thalassemia, sickle cell disease, Tay-Sachs disease, Duchenne's muscular dystrophy, and cystic fibrosis (March of Dimes, 1994).

## Chromosome Disorders

When an egg or sperm is forming, the number of chromosomes may be increased or decreased. This results in an imbalance of genetic material. As the cell division proceeds from fertilization, this may lead to abnormal body structures or functioning. The most common chro-

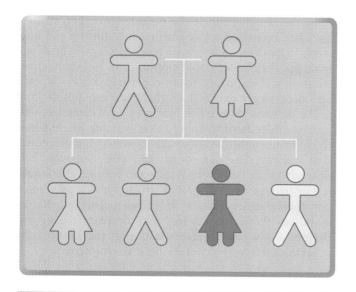

FIGURE 8-3 • Inheritance of autosomal recessive disorders. *(Adapted from March of Dimes: Genetic counseling, White Plains, NY, 1999, March of Dimes.)*

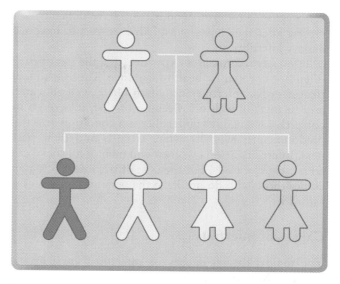

FIGURE 8-4 • Inheritance of X-linked recessive disorders. *(Adapted from March of Dimes: Genetic counseling, White Plains, NY, 1999, March of Dimes.)*

mosomal error of this type is Down syndrome in which affected persons have an extra chromosome, usually number 21 or 22. The result varies from moderate to severe mental retardation with physical abnormalities.

## Multifactoral Inheritance

Less well understood is the development of birth defects when the genes from one or both parents are affected by the environment. Defects that fall into this category are cleft lip and or palate; club foot, deformities of the ankle or foot; spina bifida or open spine, a defect in the walls of the spinal canal; hydrocephalus, accumulation of cerebrospinal fluid within the ventricles of the brain; congenital heart defects; diabetes mellitus; and some forms of cancer (March of Dimes, 1994).

## Ethical Considerations

Ethical considerations are associated with genetic testing. Scientific knowledge is increasing at a rapid rate, and new genetic tests are becoming available constantly. Various ethical issues come with this knowledge. Examples of these concerns are who should be offered testing, what are the long-term effects on the individual when a genetic flaw is detected before it manifests itself, and what possible problems may occur in the future when the individual seeks to obtain health insurance.

In the spring of 1999, the Secretary of Health and Human Services, Donna Shalala, appointed a 13-member committee, the Secretary's Advisory Committee on Genetic Testing (SACGT), to advise her on issues related to genetic testing. The group met for the first time in June, 1999, at which time Dr. David Satcher, the Sur-

geon General, charged them with developing, in consultation with the public, recommendations for federal oversight of genetic testing.

The SACGT made extraordinary efforts to reach out to the public, especially to members of cultural and ethnic minority groups, in an attempt to understand the public's concerns and fears. Committee-approved recommendations for federal oversight were submitted to the Surgeon General (SACGT, 2000). The SACGT recommended additional oversight for tests with complex results and for late-onset conditions for which predisposition can be identified, but no means to prevent the conditions and no definitive treatment are currently available.

 **INFERTILITY**

For many women the dream of having a child is not easily realized. **Infertility** is defined as the inability to achieve pregnancy after a year of unprotected sexual intercourse or the inability to carry a pregnancy to term. It is estimated that somewhere between 10% and 15% of couples experience unwanted infertility (ACOG, 1996). Unwanted infertility can affect self-esteem and result in depression. Furthermore, it can cause stress on the couple's relationship (Bernstein, Lewis, and Seibel, 1994). Although we tend to think of infertility as a problem experienced by married couples, it is important to remember that unmarried heterosexual couples, single women, and lesbians who are partnered may also experience unwanted infertility.

**Primary infertility** is the term used to describe women who have never been able to become pregnant or carry the pregnancy to term. Women who have difficulty conceiving after they have had a baby are said to have **secondary infertility.**

Infertility treatment is expensive, and the treatment is often not covered by health insurance. Those who seek treatment for infertility are often older, well educated, and financially well off. Because of this, it is often incorrectly assumed that infertility is a condition affecting predominantly wealthy white women and their partners. Infertility affects women and men of all social and ethnic backgrounds, but the cost of treatment often excludes those who do not have the personal resources to afford it.

### Causes of Infertility

The major known causes of infertility are listed in Box 8-4. Maternal age is a factor for many reasons. Because more women are choosing to establish themselves professionally before they have children, they delay the onset of childbearing. Fertility peaks during a woman's 20s and then gradually declines until menopause. In addition, women over the age of 35 have an increased risk of a pregnancy with a chromosomal abnormality.

Women who are sexually active with a number of partners have an increased risk of acquiring a sexually transmitted disease. Untreated or chronic pelvic inflammatory disease (PID) can lead to a narrowing or complete blocking of the fallopian tubes, making fertilization difficult or impossible. In some women, the fallopian tubes have wide enough lumena to allow sperm to transverse the tube and fertilize the ovum, but are too narrow for the fertilized egg to pass into the uterus, leading to early miscarriage or ectopic pregnancy.

In the last quarter of the twentieth century, women have had increased employment opportunities and now work in positions previously held only by men. Along with the benefits of equal opportunity in employment comes equal exposure to workplace hazards. Women are increasingly exposed to chemical, ergonomic, and radiation hazards at work that may have deleterious effects on their fertility. In addition, women are exposed to environmental hazards such as water and air pollution and excessive heat from exercise or hot tubs. Fertility also may be adversely affected by cigarette smoking or by ingesting alcohol or drugs. Finally, as women and their partners pursue independent careers, the demands of these dual careers may decrease the opportunities for sexual intercourse during the time of the woman's cycle when conception is most likely.

### Classification of Infertility

Infertility can be classified as female factor; male factor; combined factor; or idiopathic, which means the cause cannot be determined. About 35 percent of couples have female-factor infertility, 30 percent have male-factor infertility, and 20 percent of couples have a combination of male- and female-factor infertility. A cause cannot be identified for about 15% of couples (James, 1998) (Box 8-5).

#### Female Factors

*Hormonal Problems.* Several hormones work in concert during a normal menstrual cycle. Two of these hor-

---

**BOX 8-4    *Major Causes of Infertility***

Age
Sexually transmitted disease
Occupational hazards
   Chemicals
   Noise
   Radiation
Environmental hazards
   Heat
   Smoking
   Alcohol
   Drug abuse
   Environmental toxins
Lifestyle choices
   Delaying pregnancy
   Decreased frequency of coitus

---

**BOX 8-5    *Classification of Infertility***

***Female Factor***
Hormonal problems
Ovulatory problems
Tubal damage
Uterine factors
Cervical problems
Coital problems
Endometriosis
Genetic problems

***Male Factor***
Sperm production problems
Sperm transport problems
Ejaculatory problems
Coital problems
Genetic problems

***Combined Factor***
Sperm antibody problems
Problems with coital technique

mones, follicle-stimulating hormone (FSH) and luteinizing hormone (LH), are secreted by the pituitary gland. In response to the stimulation of FSH, the ovary produces increased estrogen, which stimulates one of the thousands of ovarian follicles to mature and ripen. At the time of ovulation, the LH surge from the pituitary causes the follicle to rupture, expelling the ovum into the peritoneal cavity. After ovulation, and because of the stimulation of LH, the ovary produces progesterone, which works to sustain the ruptured ovarian follicle, now called the corpus luteum, so that, if fertilization does occur, it can maintain the fertilized ovum until after implantation and the development of the placenta. Imbalances in any of these hormones can cause infertility. In addition, elevated prolactin levels, abnormal androgen levels, or decreased thyroid stimulating hormone (TSH) levels can be responsible for infertility.

*Ovulatory Problems.* Women may have problems with ovulation. Some women have **anovulatory** menstrual cycles, cycles in which no egg is produced. Other women may have polycystic ovarian syndrome, also labeled Stein-Leventhal syndrome, in which they experience anovulatory menstrual cycles or infrequent ovulation. Other women have stopped ovulating or experienced an early menopause, have abnormal or absent ovaries, or have the genetic condition of Turner's syndrome. Some women may have ovulatory problems as a result of being treated for cancer.

*Tubal Damage.* Some woman have fallopian tubes that will not allow ovum or sperm to pass through. This tubal damage may be congenital. However, the most common cause of tubal damage is scarring from previous surgery or from PID. Women who have had previous tubal ligation and then **reanastamosis** (surgical repair) of the fallopian tubes may have scarred tubes as well.

*Uterine Problems.* A woman may have an abnormally shaped uterus, or a uterus whose walls contain fibroids, or benign tumors of the muscular layer of the uterus. A woman may have a stenotic opening to the uterine cervix, which may be congenital or due to previous surgery on the cervix. Women whose mothers took diethylstilbestrol (DES) during pregnancy may have congenital abnormalities in their genital tracts.

*Coital Problems.* Some women have thick cervical secretions that are hostile to sperm trying to navigate their way through the cervix into the uterus.

*Endometriosis.* A common cause of female infertility is endometriosis. Endometrial tissue is commonly found only within the uterus. **Endometriosis** is a condition in which endometrial tissue exists outside the uterus.

The endometrium is the innermost layer of the uterus, and it is stimulated by cyclical hormones. During the first half of the menstrual cycle, the endometrium proliferates in anticipation of receiving a fertilized ovum. When pregnancy does not occur, the endometrium degenerates and is sloughed off during menses.

With endometriosis the sloughed off endometrium migrates up and out through the fallopian tubes instead of leaving the body with the menstrual flow. Endometrial implants can exist anywhere in the body; most commonly they are in the abdominal cavity. This tissue continues to proliferate and slough off with every menstrual cycle just as it would if it were in the uterus; the process is quite painful. Abdominal endometrial implants can cause adhesions, and as a result, pelvic structures may not be freely mobile. This can prevent the normal transport of eggs into the fallopian tubes, thus making conception impossible.

### Male Factors

*Sperm-Production Problems.* The production of sperm is an ongoing process. A male may experience hormonal problems in which levels of circulating hormones are insufficient to sustain adequate levels of sperm production, the most common cause of male infertility. The total absence of sperm is called **azoospermia**. Sperm may also be produced in decreased numbers, their motility may be altered, or there may be a high number of abnormally shaped sperm.

*Sperm-Transport Problems.* Sperm mature as they travel through an elaborate system of tubules in the testes. Sperm transport problems may be due to strictures or blockages in these structures. Males who have cystic fibrosis typically have congenital bilateral absence of the vas deferens, rendering them infertile.

*Ejaculation Problems.* Males can also have problems with ejaculation. Some men have premature ejaculation and cannot sustain an erection long enough to complete intercourse and deposit sperm deep in the vagina. Other men have retrograde ejaculation, a condition in which the valve between the bladder and the urethra opens, causing the ejaculate to enter the bladder, rather than travel through the penis to the outside.

### Combined Factor

Combined-factor infertility occurs as a result of individual factors, which alone do not cause difficulty, but when combined cause infertility. One of the more common problems is lack of coital success, in which a couple cannot have successful intercourse. Another type of problem occurs when the woman has antibodies to the man's sperm, causing an antigen-antibody reaction and the immobilization of sperm before they can migrate through the cervix.

## Diagnosis

The decision to undergo the assessment of infertility can be very stressful. Although there is a great deal of joking and innuendo about sex and sexuality in our society, personal intimacy is valued, and many people wish to keep these details private. Having to talk with someone, even a health care professional, about being unable to achieve the most basic of biologic tasks can be a major assault to the self-esteem of either or both partners. Many people postpone seeking professional assistance because they cannot admit to themselves or they fear having to admit to someone else that they need assistance in this area. Others delay because of the need to take time out of work for testing and the possibility that they will have to explain their need for medical care to their colleagues. A summary of diagnostic tests is presented in Box 8-6.

### Assessment of the Male

Although couples often mistakenly believe that infertility is due to a problem with the woman, in fact the problem originates almost equally with partners of either gender. The gynecologist in consultation with the female client may identify the need to begin the diagnostic process, but males are often referred to urologists for this process. Evaluation of the male is easier and less costly. It makes sense to begin the diagnostic workup for a couple by doing the least invasive tests first.

*History.* At the outset it is important to determine whether either member of the couple has ever achieved a pregnancy with a different partner. A comprehensive history looking for factors that may impede fertility is then obtained. This includes exposure to chemicals, radiation, and heat. Since the testes are normally slightly cooler than body temperature, men are asked about whether they wear tight-fitting brief-type underwear or tight pants or restrictive support garments when exercising. Questions are also asked about steam bath or sauna use, hot tub baths, or regular vigorous exercise.

---

**BOX 8-6** *Diagnostic Tests for Couples with Infertility*

**Male**
History
Physical examination
Semen analysis
Blood tests

**Female**
History
Physical examination
Pap smear
Chlamydia test
Basal body temperature chart
Blood tests
Postcoital test
Hysterosalpingogram
Endometrial biopsy
Laparoscopy

---

Past medical history is reviewed, and questions are asked about postpubertal mumps, sexually transmitted diseases, orchitis, or trauma to the external genitalia. Abdominal, inguinal, and reproductive tract surgery is also noted.

Dietary adequacy is also assessed, as is drug, alcohol, and tobacco consumption. A medication history is taken to ensure that the man is not taking any prescribed or over-the-counter medications that could affect sperm production or sexual functioning. An assessment for depression should also be included.

A family history is also important, including asking whether the man's mother took any medications such as DES during the time she was pregnant with him. It was recommended and given as routine prophylaxis by doctors to pregnant women between 1938 and 1971 to prevent abortion, miscarriage, and premature labor.

A family history of cystic fibrosis may suggest that a mutation might be present that does not cause noticeable disease, but may cause congenital bilateral absence of the vas deferens.

*Physical Examination.* A physical examination is performed with special attention to reproductive organs and secondary sex characteristics. It is important to assess for male-pattern hair distribution and structure of the genitalia. Some men have a condition known as hypospadias, in which the urethral opening is on the underside of the penis—a condition that may impair the ability to deliver semen into the vagina. The testes are palpated for any masses or abnormalities, and the scrotum is examined to be certain that the testes are of approximately equal size. A flashlight may be shone on the scrotum to ensure that no hydrocele is present.

*Laboratory Testing.* Blood tests may be done to assess hormonal levels and general well-being. It is important to rule out conditions such as diabetes. The most common laboratory test is a **semen analysis**. The specimen should be collected after 48 to 72 hours of sexual abstinence and is most often obtained by masturbation. For men who have religious or other proscriptions against masturbation, the specimen may be obtained by asking the man to have intercourse wearing a condom. If religious concerns remain, they often can be resolved by having the man poke a minute hole in the condom before applying it. It is important that the condom not contain any lubricants or spermicides. There is often a specified time frame for delivery of the condom with the specimen to the laboratory. If the specimen is obtained at home, the man is often asked to keep the container in a shirt or inner pocket so that it remains close to body temperature.

The semen is analyzed for the number of sperm per milliliter. The shape, or morphology, of the sperm is assessed, as well as their motility, or forward movement. A normal semen analysis includes all three factors. Men who have significantly diminished sperm counts may still be able to have a biologic child through the use of artificial insemination with their sperm, since placement of the sperm directly in the cervix, or directly into the uterine cavity, diminishes significantly the number of sperm needed for a pregnancy to occur.

### Assessment of the Female

*History.* The diagnostic evaluation of the woman likewise begins with a history. A reproductive and menstrual history is taken, with special notice of whether the woman has ever become pregnant.

The menstrual history includes age at menarche, and a comprehensive history of menstrual cycles, including frequency, duration, regularity, discomfort, intermenstrual bleeding, and amount of flow. Women are also asked about symptoms of premenstrual symptom, discomfort at the anticipated time of ovulation, or any other symptoms that are cyclic.

Women are asked about their previous use of contraceptives and their previous sexual patterns, including the number of previous partners and any history of pelvic inflammation or sexually transmitted infections. Diet, medication, alcohol, drug, and smoking information is also gathered. Women are also asked about family history, including maternal DES exposure and any chronic illnesses. Women whose mothers took DES when pregnant with them may have a slightly increased risk for infertility because of some differences in the structure of the pelvic organs in some DES daughters (National Cancer Institute, 1995).

It is also important to ask about a history of physical or sexual abuse, previous surgery or trauma, and depression. Current sexual practices, including frequency and timing of intercourse; positions used for coitus; and the use of any assistive devices, including lubricants, should also be assessed.

*Physical Examination.* The physical examination assesses general health and focuses specifically on the reproductive organs. Body type is examined to assess for the presence of female secondary sex characteristics, including body fat and hair distribution. Excessive facial or body hair may indicate a hormonal imbalance. Severe acne in postadolescent women may also be indicative of a hormonal imbalance.

*Laboratory Tests.* The pelvic examination should include a Pap smear if documented results are not available, and also a culture for chlamydia. Blood tests may be done to assess for hormone levels and to rule out chronic illnesses like anemia or diabetes.

It is important to document rubella immunity, either through having had the disease or having a positive titer following vaccine administration. Women often invest many months and thousands of dollars in infertility treatment, so ensuring rubella immunity before she attempts to become pregnant is important so that the woman will not be faced with the dilemma of delivering

a child damaged by rubella or having an abortion if she contracts the virus. It is also important to ensure that the woman is including a folic acid supplement in her diet during the testing process so that she decreases her risk for having a fetus with a neural tube defect if a pregnancy is achieved.

### Ongoing Assessment

The next steps in testing involve more time and more invasive procedures. The woman especially, and her partner may start to feel like the testing process is defining their lives and absorbing the major focus of their attention. In addition, previously private activities now become public and are shared with health care providers as hormonal cycles are tracked, internal organs are outlined, intercourse is scheduled, and results are recorded and evaluated. Some tests are very uncomfortable and the ones that require general anesthesia present a risk to the woman.

*Monitoring Cycles.* The next diagnostic procedure includes having the woman keep a basal body temperature record for 3 months. A sample chart is shown in Figure 5-13 in Chapter 5.

Using a basal body temperature record to determine when ovulation occurs can either help a woman prevent a pregnancy or enhance her chances of becoming pregnant. Instruct the woman to take her temperature first thing upon awakening in the morning, before she engages in any activity whatsoever. A special basal body thermometer—one that has larger spaces between the lines so that small fluctuations in temperature can be noted more accurately—must be used.

The woman is also instructed to record any medications taken, when she has intercourse, and when she has menses. Some charts include places to note other events such as colds or flulike symptoms that may alter body temperature, headaches, abdominal twinges, cramping, pain, or other events; some providers simply have women note these in the columns.

Several pieces of data can be gleaned from a basal body temperature chart. A biphasic temperature curve, in which the mean temperature for the second half of the cycle is 0.5° F higher than that of the first half, is presumptive evidence of ovulation and adequate hormonal functioning. If the time from the temperature rise to the onset of menses is extraordinarily short, it may mean there is a luteal phase defect. Asking women to note when they have coitus helps determine if intercourse is occurring during the time of the cycle when pregnancy is most likely. Noting the character and duration of menses is also important.

*Postcoital Test.* The next test usually performed is a postcoital test. The test is usually scheduled just before the expected date of ovulation, as determined from the most recent basal body temperature chart. The couple is encouraged to abstain from intercourse for a day or two before the test, and to have intercourse 2 to 12 hours before the appointment. It is important that the couple not use any lubricants for this act of coitus because some lubricants affect sperm motility.

After intercourse the woman is seen in the office and a sample of cervical mucus is obtained and examined under the microscope. It is possible to assess the quality of cervical mucus as well as the characteristics of the sperm. One would expect to see 5 to 10 motile sperm per high power field. An absence of sperm may be due to a low sperm count or to difficulties in coital technique. Immobile sperm may be due to sperm abnormalities or to the presence of antisperm antibodies. If the cervical mucus is not clear and elastic, this may be due to hormonal insufficiency, or it may be too early in the woman's cycle.

***Examination of the Uterus and Fallopian Tubes.*** A hysterosalpingogram is done to determine the shape of the uterine cavity and the patency of the fallopian tubes. The test is scheduled for a time immediately following the completion of menses, so that the woman's risk of being pregnant is minimal. A contrast medium is injected through the cervix, which spreads through the uterine cavity and out the fallopian tubes. X-rays are taken and the shape of the uterine cavity can be determined. Documented evidence of dye flowing out the distal ends of the fallopian tubes into the abdominal cavity is proof of tubal patency.

***Endometrial Biopsy.*** An endometrial biopsy involves the aspiration and microscopic examination of endometrial tissue. This test is done toward the end of the menstrual cycle, shortly before the woman's period is expected to begin. This test is somewhat uncomfortable and often causes cramping that lasts for a short period of time. The results of the test tell whether the lining of the uterus is developing sufficiently to be able to support a pregnancy.

***Laparoscopy.*** A more invasive test is a laparoscopy. After the woman is anesthetized with general anesthesia, a small incision is made, often near the navel. The abdominal cavity is filled with gas, and a slender telescope-like instrument is then inserted through the same small incision. The abdominal contents are then visualized. A dye may be injected into the uterus through the cervix. The presence of the dye in the abdominal cavity documents tubal patency. The surgeon can visualize pelvic structures and see the fallopian tubes and ovaries. The surgeon can also see whether any endometrial implants are present. If minor problems are detected, it may be possible to repair them during the procedure.

### Deciding about Treatment

In most cases, a cause for the infertility is eventually determined. The couple must then decide whether they will seek treatment and, if so, which treatment is most appropriate. These are not easy decisions. Treatment may involve (1) obtaining sperm and then artificial insemination or intrauterine insemination of the woman; (2) procedures in which the woman takes drugs to stimulate egg production, with or without the intention of retrieving eggs; or (3) treatments in which both eggs and sperm are manipulated. This final process is defined by the Centers for Disease Control and Prevention (CDC) as **assisted reproductive technology** (ART). In general, ART includes surgically removing eggs from a woman's ovaries, combining them with sperm in the laboratory, and returning them to the woman's body or donating them to another woman.

Depending on the process required, treatment for infertility may be expensive, costing tens of thousands of dollars, and may require traveling or moving great distances, especially for ART. Three hundred and thirty-five clinics located throughout the United States report offering ART, with the greatest number in the eastern part of the country. Most are located in major cites. There are no reported facilities in Alaska, Idaho, Maine, and Wyoming.

The procedures used to treat infertility are intrusive and may be uncomfortable. The protocols require rigid adherence; many couples comment that they feel like their lives are being put on hold while they follow the demands of a treatment. The medications used have various side effects, and the entire process is extremely stressful for the couple. In the end, success is not guaranteed.

### Stress Management

Couples should have access to psychologic services to help them manage the stress of both the decision-making process and the treatment itself. Starting the process of infertility treatment is often easier than deciding when or if to stop. After investing considerable time and financial resources in trying to become pregnant, it is always tempting to try one more cycle or one more procedure. There are documented cases in which the stress of infertility causes the couple's relationship to end. Others have lost their homes as they spend all their assets on yet one more treatment. Couples need to be reminded that they have the right and obligation to themselves to determine when to stop treatment.

### Success of Treatment

The success of treatment modalities often depends on the individual practice or clinic. Different clinics have different protocols, and the personnel involved have different levels of skill and expertise. Success rates of clinics are reported regularly to the American Society for Reproductive Medicine, and are available to consumers upon request and online from the Centers for Disease Control. It is important to evaluate comparable data when choosing among doctors or clinics. The data can be confusing and difficult to interpret. Since the goal of infertility treatment is achieving a pregnancy that will end in the delivery of a healthy baby, the "take-home baby" statistic is an important one to review. Resolve, an international support group whose purpose is to provide information and support to couples experiencing infertility, is also a good source of information.

## Treatment Procedures

The program of treatment offered to a couple depends on the diagnosis of the problem or problems creating the infertility. It is also determined by the services available to the couples as determined by their access to a treatment facility and their ability to pay for procedures. Some insurance companies are now offering coverage for infertility treatments.

### Alternative or Artificial Insemination

It is possible to increase the probability of pregnancy in women whose partners have low sperm counts by inserting the sperm farther up the woman's reproductive tract, so that more of them reach the distal third of the fallopian tube, where fertilization occurs, than would happen if the couple simply had intercourse. A semen sample is obtained from the male partner, usually by masturbation. Semen may be obtained using alternative means, such as electroejaculation, if the man does not otherwise have the ability to achieve an ejaculation. The sample is allowed to liquefy, and the sperm are washed to remove as much seminal fluid as possible and then suspended in a nutrient medium. This suspension is then deposited near the cervical os or directly into the endometrial cavity of the woman's uterus. The woman is encouraged to remain in a supine position for a short period of time; a cervical cap may be inserted and left in place for several hours; the woman then removes the cap later in the day.

This procedure may also be used with frozen sperm that were banked by the male partner at an earlier time. Many men who are scheduled for surgery or chemotherapy collect semen samples and have them frozen for use at a later date. Frozen sperm from a donor may also be obtained; many single women or lesbians who desire pregnancy use frozen donor sperm in lieu of having coitus with a male, and may prefer to call the procedure alternative insemination, rather than artificial insemination. Donor sperm are frozen and are not released for use until the donor has a negative HIV test 6 months after the donation. Women who have partners who are azoospermic or who have extremely low sperm counts may opt for the use of donor sperm as well.

### Ovulation Induction

Women who do not ovulate, or who ovulate very infrequently, may be candidates for ovulation induction drugs. Medications used include clomiphene citrate, Lupron, Pergonal, and Humegon. It may take several cycles to achieve the desired result, and some medication regimens

carry the risks of ovarian hyperstimulation and the development of a multiple gestation. Women may have intercourse or artificial insemination at the time of ovulation, depending on whether male-factor infertility is also present. Medication regimens may be expensive and may not be covered by insurance plans.

### Assisted Reproductive Technology

If couples are unsuccessful achieving pregnancy using the infertility treatments previously mentioned, they may move to some of the more sophisticated assisted reproductive technologies, including in vitro fertilization (IVF), gamete intrafallopian transfer (GIFT), and zygote intrafallopian transfer (ZIFT). Success rates are affected by many factors, including the quality of the eggs, the quality of the sperm, the general health of the woman, genetic factors, and the skill and competence of the treatment team (National Center for Chronic Disease Prevention and Health Promotion [NCCDPHP], 1999).

In **in vitro fertilization** (IVF) the woman takes ovulation-stimulating drugs in doses sufficient to produce several follicles. The size and development of the follicles are monitored by serial ultrasounds. When the follicles have reached the appropriate size, the woman is given an injection of a drug such as human chorionic gonadotropin and the egg retrieval is scheduled. A sperm sample is obtained, from her partner or from a donor sperm bank, and the oocytes are fertilized in the laboratory. When the fertilized embryos reach the desired size, they are transferred to the woman's uterus through her cervix.

In **gamete intrafallopian transfer** (GIFT) the oocytes are retrieved in a fashion similar to that used in IVF; however, the oocytes and sperm are transferred to the woman's fallopian tubes through a small incision in her abdomen and fertilization is allowed to occur within the woman's body.

**Zygote intrafallopian transfer** (ZIFT) is similar to IVF in that the oocytes are fertilized in the laboratory; however, here the resulting fertilized oocytes are transferred to the fallopian tubes at an earlier stage in their development than in IVF.

In 1997, the number of reported ART cycles was 71,826, using one of the above procedures. Most IVF, GIFT, and ZIFT cycles use fresh, nondonor eggs or embryos. Figure 8-5 shows the percentage of the different types of procedures and the donor and frozen categories.

### Steps of Nondonor ART

The steps for a fresh, nondonor **ART cycle** starts when a woman begins taking medication to stimulate her ovaries to develop eggs or, if no drugs are given, when the woman begins having her ovaries monitored (using ultrasound or blood tests) for natural egg production. If eggs are produced, the cycle then progresses to **egg retrieval**, a surgical procedure during which the eggs are

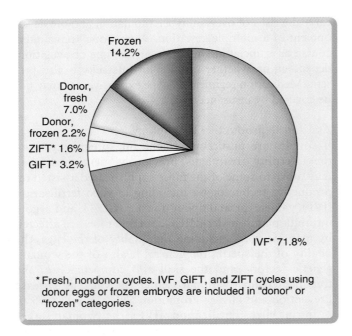

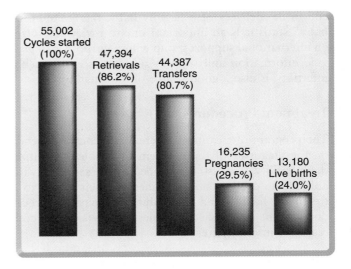

FIGURE 8-5 ● Types of ART procedures—United States 1997 *(From National Center for Chronic Disease Prevention and Health Promotion (NCCDPHP): 1997 Assisted reproductive technology success rates—national summary and fertility clinic reports, Washington DC, 1999, CDC. Page 10 accessed at http://www.cdc.gov/nccdphp/drh/ art.htm.)*

FIGURE 8-6 ● Outcome of fresh, nondonor ART cycles by stage, 1997. *(From National Center for Chronic Disease Prevention and Health Promotion (NCCDPHP): 1997 Assisted reproductive technology success rates—national summary and fertility clinic reports, Washington DC, 1999, CDC. Page 12 accessed at http://www.cdc.gov/nccdphp/ drh/art.htm.)*

collected from the woman's ovaries. Once retrieved, eggs are combined with sperm in the laboratory. If fertilization is successful, one or more of the resulting embryos are selected for **transfer**, most often into a woman's uterus through her cervix (IVF). If one or more of the transferred embryos implants within the woman's uterus, the cycle becomes a clinical **pregnancy**. If one or more live-born infants result it is counted as one **live birth**. An ART cycle may be discontinued at any step for medical reasons or by patient choice (NCCDPHP, 1999).

The most current information about ART outcomes is based on the ART cycles started in 1997. Success rates of procedures can only be calculated and reported 9 months after the year-end when all of the births have occurred. The data collection and analysis must then be performed. The information is then reviewed by agencies with oversight responsibilities and the report is approved (Figure 8-6).

Of the women who used ART in 1997, 78% had not previously given birth. However, 22% had previously delivered children. What the data does not tell is how many had conceived naturally or how many had used ART. It also does not indicate if the need for ART is due to a new partner (NCCDPHP, 1999).

Couples may have one or more causes of their infertility. When there is more than one cause, one is identi-

fied as the primary cause. The primary causes most often reported in those seeking ART are tubal factor, male factor, endometriosis, ovulatory dysfunction, uterine factor, unexplained cause (no cause found in either man or woman), and other causes (i.e., immunologic problems, chromosomal abnormalities, cancer chemotherapy, and serious illness) (NCCDPHP, 1999). The primary diagnoses that led to ART in 1997 are shown in Figure 8-7.

### Success of Nondonor ART Cycles

Several measures are used to assess the success rates of ART. The **pregnancy per cycle** rate refers to the number of cycles that produce a pregnancy. The **live birth per cycle** rate represents the chances of having a live-born infant by ART. It is the percentage of cycles started that result in a live birth. The **live birth per egg retrieval** rate indicates the percentage of cycles in which live births resulted from eggs that were retrieved. It is generally higher than the live birth per cycle rate because those cycles that are canceled before eggs are retrieved are not counted. The **live birth per transfer** rate is even more selective in its statistics so it is generally the highest reported rate of success. It includes only those cycles in which an embryo or egg and sperm were transferred back to the woman. This rate is generally the highest of the four measures because it excludes the attempts in which an egg did not become fertilized, the embryos that formed were abnormal, or other reasons that the transfer could not occur (NCCDPHP, 1999).

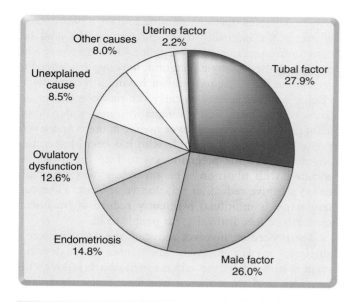

FIGURE 8-7 • Primary diagnoses among couples who had fresh, nondonor ART cycles, 1997. *(From National Center for Chronic Disease Prevention and Health Promotion (NCCDPHP): 1997 Assisted reproductive technology success rates—national summary and fertility clinic reports, Washington DC, 1999, CDC. Page 15 accessed at http://www.cdc.gov/nccdphp/drh/art.htm.)*

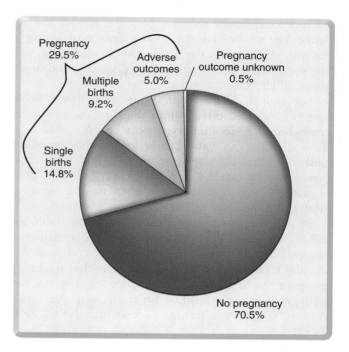

FIGURE 8-8 • Results of fresh, nondonor ART cycles, 1997. *(From National Center for Chronic Disease Prevention and Health Promotion (NCCDPHP): 1997 Assisted reproductive technology success rates—national summary and fertility clinic reports, Washington DC, 1999, CDC. Page 18 accessed at http://www.cdc.gov/nccdphp/drh/art.htm.)*

The actual number of live births varies by the type of ART procedure used. In the data from 1997, GIFT and ZIFT had the highest rates of live births, 29.8% and 28.0%, respectively. IVF had a rate of 27.7%. When a woman learns of her different options, she may not be a candidate for GIFT or ZIFT because of the condition of her fallopian tubes. In addition GIFT and ZIFT are more invasive procedures because they involve surgery (NCCDPHP, 1999).

Most ART cycles *do not* produce a pregnancy. Of all ART cycles reported in 1997, only 29.5% resulted in a pregnancy. Of those pregnancies, 14.8% produced a single live birth; 9.2% resulted in a multiple birth, the majority of which were twins; and 5.0% of the pregnancies had an adverse outcome (ectopic pregnancy, miscarriage, induced abortion, or stillbirth). Information concerning birth defects and newborn deaths is unknown. Also information on multifetal pregnancy reductions is not included (NCCDPHP, 1999) (Figure 8-8).

### Factors Affecting Success of Nondonor ART

Because of the various steps in the ART process, several factors can affect success. Reported factors are the woman's age, whether she has given birth previously, the primary cause of infertility, the number of embryos transferred, the use of intracytoplasmic sperm injection (ICSI), and the number of cycles performed by her treatment facility in the year.

***Woman's Age.*** The most important factor affecting the chance of a live birth when a woman's own eggs are used is her age. In 1997, "among women in their twenties, both pregnancy and live birth rates were relatively stable; however, both rates declined sharply from the mid-thirties onward" (NCCDPHP, 1999).

***Previously Given Birth.*** Whether a woman has had a child naturally or has been assisted through previous ART, her chances of success in having a live birth are greater than if she hasn't given birth before. This is true across all age categories (NCCDPHP, 1999).

***Primary Cause of Infertility.*** The 1997 data demonstrated little variation in success rates among the different primary causes. The success rates ranged from a low of 18.9% for uterine factors to a high of 25.5% for male factors.

***Number of Embryos Transferred.*** The number of embryos transferred during an ART procedure affects the success rate. In 1997, the average number of embryos transferred to a woman younger than 35 ranged from 1.0 to 6.2. In general, transfer of 3 or 4 embryos had the highest success rate, 33.6% and 34.3%, respectively. However, the transfer of multiple embryos not only improved the chance of success, but also raised the risk of a multiple birth. With multiple births comes the concern of additional health risks for both the mother and infants. The mother faces a greater chance of having a surgical delivery and the developing infants are at risk for prematurity, low birth weight, disability, and death (NCCDPHP, 1999).

*Use of ICSI.* ICSI is a procedure in which a single sperm is injected directly into the cytoplasm of a retrieved egg. The resulting zygote can be transferred back as in ZIFT, or the zygote can be kept in the laboratory until it reaches the size of an embryo, and then transferred directly into the uterus as in IVF. This procedure is especially appropriate for use when male factor infertility is the causative factor.

In 1997 approximately 30% of the fresh, nondonor ART cycles used ICSI. When male-factor infertility is the primary diagnosis, success rates per retrieval are slightly higher with ICSI. This indicates that ICSI may improve the chances of fertilization among couples with male-factor infertility. Once the egg was fertilized, ICSI did not affect the success rate (NCCDPHP, 1999).

*Number of Cycles Performed.* In general, the more cycles of procedures a clinic performed, the greater the average success rate. The range of percentage of live births per cycle went from an average low of 20.3% at clinics performing fewer than 50 cycles per year to an average high of 24.5% at clinics performing more than 200 cycles per year (NCCDPHP, 1999).

### Frozen Embryos

Cycles that use frozen embryos are both less expensive and less invasive for a woman. "Approximately 14% of all ART cycles performed in 1997, or 10,181 cycles, used only frozen embryos" (NCCDPHP, 1999). When the percentage of live births was calculated, the frozen embryo succeeded 16.8% per thaw. This is because some embryos do not survive the freezing or thawing process. When they survive the freezing and thawing, they may be used in transfer. Of the frozen embryos transferred, 18.6% resulted in a live birth. This is lower than the comparable result of 29.7% that occurred with fresh embryos (NCCDPHP, 1999).

Couples who undergo ART often obtain more embryos than it is advisable to implant in a single cycle. The surplus embryos may be discarded or they may be frozen for future use. Couples who have frozen embryos they no longer intend to use may donate these embryos for use by other infertile couples. These donor embryos may then be implanted into a woman and the resulting embryo would be genetically unrelated to either member of the couple.

### Multifetal Pregnancy Reduction

One of the most difficult decisions faced by infertile couples is the decision they must make when infertility treatment results in a pregnancy that contains three or more fetuses. Couples start out wanting to have a baby; somewhere in the infertility treatment process the goal becomes reframed to getting pregnant. Once pregnant with a high-number multiple gestation, the couple is forced to reexamine their original goal of having a healthy baby. Higher number gestations carry the risk of preterm delivery of low–birth-weight infants who may suffer significant problems as a result of crowding in utero and severe prematurity. Now the couple who has been desperately seeking to become pregnant has to face the issues associated with abortion. The procedure was originally called selective reduction or selective abortion. The current name is **multifetal pregnancy reduction** because it seems to be less disturbing for people to hear.

The procedure involves reducing the pregnancy to a singleton or twin gestation. The fetuses whose development is stopped are those that are most accessible to the provider, and their tissues are then reabsorbed. This process is similar to what happens when a naturally occurring multiple gestation spontaneously has some fetuses die.

The emotional costs of this procedure can be extraordinary as parents wonder about the fetuses whose development was ended. Parents may need assistance as they grieve their loss. In addition, there is always the risk that the entire pregnancy will be lost as a result of the procedure. The advantage is that if the pregnancy is successfully reduced, the odds of a successful term gestation with normal–birth-weight infants is greatly enhanced. Because of the emotional costs and risks of losing the pregnancy, some parents choose not to have this procedure done.

### The Use of Donors and Surrogates

The use of donor sperm has been routine for many years. A more recent development has been the use of donor eggs, which are fertilized in the laboratory with the male partner's sperm and then implanted in the woman using the most appropriate ART technique. The resulting embryo is genetically related to the male parent, but not to the female parent. In part, the technique was slow to develop because it is technically more difficult to retrieve eggs than it is to harvest sperm. The egg donor must undergo a cycle of ovulation induction and egg retrieval. The time commitment on the part of the donor is significantly increased, and the donor must take medications that have significant side effects (NCCDPHP, 1999).

### Surrogate or Gestational Carrier

A gestational carrier is a woman who carries an embryo that was formed from the egg of another woman and gives birth to a child to whom she has no genetic relationship (NCCDPHP, 1999). A surrogate mother is a woman who is artificially inseminated with the sperm of a woman's male partner and carries the pregnancy to term. After delivery, she surrenders the infant to the couple, who then go through adoption procedures to establish a legal connection. In 1997, there were 600 reported cycles with an overall success rate of 31.2%.

There have been high-profile news stories about gestational carriers who become so attached to the infant that they renege on the agreement to give the child to the infertile couple. In many cases, the infertile couple is successful in finalizing the surrogacy agreement, but these situations do not receive the same degree of media attention.

## The National Report on Assisted Reproductive Technology

Based on the information reported from 335 fertility clinics, a national report is formulated. This presents the overall success rates and shows how rates are influenced by certain patient and treatment characteristics. Because it is based on all reported cases, it presents a good delineation of the average chances of a couple having a child using ART (Table 8-2).

---

**TABLE 8-2**  *1997 National Summary on Assisted Reproductive Technology*

**1997 PROGRAM PROFILE**

| PROGRAM CHARACTERISTICS | | TYPE OF ART* | | ART PATIENT DIAGNOSIS | |
|---|---|---|---|---|---|
| Total clinics | 335 | IVF | 93% | Tubal factor | 27% |
| SART member? | 96% | GIFT | 4% | Endometriosis | 14% |
| Single women? | 76% | ZIFT | 2% | Uterine factor | 2% |
| Gestational carriers? | 37% | Combination† | 1% | Ovulatory dysfunction | 23% |
| Donor egg program? | 78% | | | Male factor | 16% |
| Sharing of donor eggs? | 23% | With ICSI | 35% | Other factors | 10% |
| | | Unstimulated | <1% | Unexplained | 8% |

A comparison of clinic success rates may not be meaningful because patient medical characteristics and treatment approaches vary from clinic to clinic.

**1997 ART PREGNANCY SUCCESS RATES**

| TYPE OF CYCLE | AGE OF WOMAN | | | |
|---|---|---|---|---|
| | <35 | 35-37 | 38-40 | >40 |
| **Fresh Embryos from Nondonor Eggs** | | | | |
| Number of cycles | 24,581 | 12,733 | 10,997 | 6,691 |
| Pregnancies per 100 cycles | 35.7 | 31.3 | 22.8 | 13.2 |
| Live births per 100 cycles‡ | 30.7 | 25.5 | 17.1 | 7.6 |
| Live births per 100 retrievals‡ | 33.8 | 29.6 | 20.9 | 9.9 |
| Live births per 100 transfers‡ | 35.9 | 31.4 | 22.5 | 10.9 |
| Cancellations per 100 cycles | 9.3 | 14.0 | 18.3 | 22.9 |
| Average number embryos transferred | 3.7 | 3.8 | 3.9 | 4.0 |
| Twin gestations per 100 pregnancies | 30.7 | 26.4 | 21.8 | 15.3 |
| Triplet or more gestations per 100 pregnancies | 13.7 | 11.3 | 6.8 | 2.8 |
| Multiple births per 100 live births‡ | 43.0 | 36.8 | 28.4 | 19.0 |
| **Frozen Embryos from Nondonor Eggs** | | | | |
| Number of transfers | 4,862 | 2,144 | 1,385 | 774 |
| Live births per 100 transfers‡ | 21.3 | 18.6 | 14.5 | 10.0 |
| Average number embryos transferred | 3.5 | 3.4 | 3.5 | 3.6 |
| **Donor Eggs** | | | | |
| Number of fresh transfers | 547 | 480 | 846 | 2,625 |
| Live births per 100 fresh transfers‡ | 40.8 | 41.9 | 36.6 | 40.2 |
| Number of frozen transfers | 177 | 134 | 213 | 958 |
| Live births per 100 frozen transfers‡ | 16.4 | 22.4 | 19.3 | 23.6 |
| Average number embryos transferred (fresh and frozen) | 3.5 | 3.6 | 3.7 | 3.7 |

*Includes only fresh, nondonor egg cycles.

†Combination of fresh, nondonor IVF, GIFT, and ZIFT procedures.

‡A multiple birth is counted as one live birth.

From National Center for Chronic Disease Prevention and Health Promotion (NCCDPHP): *1997 Assisted reproductive technology success rates—national summary and fertility clinic reports*, Washington, D.C., 1999, The Center. Accessed at www. edc.gov/nccdphp/drh/art.htm.

## Comparison of Clinic Results

Because of the inconvenience and expense, when a couple decides to undergo fertility treatment, they generally investigate the success rate of the facilities that are available to them. Data are available on the exact number of cycles and success rates of each individual clinic. (For the most current data concerning each facility, go to *www.cdc.gov/nccdphp/drh/art.htm.*) However, comparisons between clinics must be made with caution.

The success of a particular clinic is related to the training and experience of the providers. During the time between the collection of data and the publishing of results the trained personnel and equipment may have changed. The success rates of a clinic may be very changeable from one year to the next when a facility performs a low number of cases. For example, if a clinic performs only one cycle, as some do, the success rate will either be 0 or 100%.

---

### TABLE 8-3   *Sample Clinic Report*

**1997 PROGRAM PROFILE**

| PROGRAM CHARACTERISTICS | | TYPE OF ART* | | ART PATIENT DIAGNOSIS | |
|---|---|---|---|---|---|
| SART member? | Yes | IVF | 72% | Tubal factor | 37% |
| Single women? | Yes | GIFT | 28% | Endometriosis | 18% |
| Gestational carriers? | No | ZIFT | 0% | Uterine factor | 0% |
| Donor egg program? | Yes | Combination† | 0% | Ovulatory dysfunction | 18% |
| Sharing of donor eggs? | No | | | Male factor | 13% |
| | | With ICSI | 16% | Other factors | 13% |
| | | Unstimulated | 1% | Unexplained | 2% |

A comparison of clinic success rates may not be meaningful because patient medical characteristics and treatment approaches vary from clinic to clinic.

**1997 ART PREGNANCY SUCCESS RATES‡**

| TYPE OF CYCLE | AGE OF WOMAN | | | |
|---|---|---|---|---|
| | <35 | 35-37 | 38-40 | >40 |
| **Fresh Embryos from Nondonor Eggs** | | | | |
| Number of cycles | 83 | 41 | 19 | 10 |
| Pregnancies per 100 cycles | 34.9 | 26.8 | 3/19 | 2/10 |
| Live births per 100 cycles§ | 27.7 | 22.0 | 1/19 | 1/10 |
|   (95% confidence interval) | (18.1-37.3) | (9.3-34.6) | | |
| Live births per 100 retrievals§ | 28.4 | 23.1 | 1/15 | 1/8 |
| Live births per 100 transfers§ | 28.8 | 25.0 | 1/14 | 1/8 |
| Cancellations per 100 cycles | 2.4 | 4.9 | 4/19 | 2/10 |
| Average number embryos transferred | 5.2 | 5.6 | 6.8 | 7.5 |
| Twin gestations per 100 pregnancies | 27.6 | 1/11 | 1/3 | 0/2 |
| Triplet or more gestations per 100 pregnancies | 20.7 | 1/11 | 0/3 | 0/2 |
| Multiple births per 100 live births§ | 44.8 | 2/9 | 1/1 | 0/1 |
| **Frozen Embryos from Nondonor Eggs** | | | | |
| Number of transfers | 4 | 3 | 0 | 0 |
| Live births per 100 transfers§ | 1/4 | 0/3 | | |
| Average number embryos transferred | 1.0 | 1.7 | | |
| **Donor Eggs** | | | | |
| Number of fresh transfers | 1 | 0 | 1 | 5 |
| Live births per 100 fresh transfers§ | 0/1 | | 0/1 | 3/5 |
| Number of frozen transfers | 0 | 0 | 0 | 0 |
| Live births per 100 frozen transfers§ | | | | |
| Average number embryos transferred (fresh and frozen) | 5.0 | | 4.0 | 5.6 |

*Includes only fresh, nondonor egg cycles.

†Combination of fresh, nondonor IVF, GIFT, and ZIFT procedures.

‡When fewer than 20 cycles are reported in any one category, rates are shown as fractions.

§A multiple birth is counted as one live birth.

From National Center for Chronic Disease Prevention and Health Promotion (NCCDPHP): *1997 Assisted reproductive technology success rates—national summary and fertility clinic reports,* Washington, D.C., 1999, The Center. Accessed at www. edc.gov/nccdphp/drh/art.htm

The success rate also is related to the patients themselves, with their primary cause diagnoses and age. Some clinics are very selective in who they accept for treatment. Others accept a higher percentage of women with a low probability of success. Some clinics will cancel the treatment of a woman if she produces only a small number of eggs. This lowers the live birth per cycle rate but dramatically increases the live birth per retrieval and live birth per transfer rates.

A sample of a fertility clinic table is found in Table 8-3. For more specific information about a clinic than the report provides, the clinic should be contacted directly. Some clinics are members of the Society of Assisted Reproductive Technology (SART).

## Support During Infertility Treatments

Needless to say, the process of undergoing infertility treatment is emotionally and financially exhausting. Couples may not have shared their treatment plans with friends and relatives because of a desire for privacy, making them feel alone, further adding to the stress. The treatment regimens demand learning new skills, such as administering medication by injection, learning the unpleasant effects of some medications, and becoming attuned to nuances in hormonal and physiologic functioning. Many infertility centers have psychologists or social workers available to assist couples with these stressors. Another valuable resource is Resolve, a national support, education, and advocacy group serving the needs of infertile couples. The organization is headquartered in Massachusetts, but there are local chapters throughout the country.

## New Developments

A new procedure called assisted hatching is being tested. It involves making a hole in the zona pellucida of the egg with a needle, laser, or an acidic solution to enhance the development of the embryo. This procedure is usually reserved for those couples who have had unsuccessful attempts at IVF or for those who are using previously frozen embryos.

## Role of Nursing

Before treatment begins, we are involved in helping couples come to terms with their diagnoses. During the process, we are responsible for patient education, support, and counseling. We are often responsible for teaching the couple what they need to know to make informed decisions about what treatment plans to pursue. Deciding to pursue treatment and then deciding what levels of treatment, and for how long are important. The decision to use ART involves an understanding of the low success rate and the high cost and commitment

of time, effort, money, and emotional energy. With specialized education, we may help couples examine all related financial, psychologic, and medical issues before consenting and beginning treatment.

Once a course is established, we are responsible for coordinating the cycle, teaching about medication, arranging the necessary medical and surgical appointments, and monitoring the woman's progress each day. It is a nurse who often communicates with the patient, instructing her on medication doses and delivering the results of pregnancy tests. The bond formed between the infertility nurse specialist and the couple with the problem of infertility is quite strong; indeed some of those who go on to achieve a pregnancy often describe feeling "lost" when their relationship ends.

A large percentage of couples will fail to achieve a pregnancy. Making the decision to cease infertility treatment can be quite stressful. Couples have described it as the death of their dreams. Some couples elect to adopt and begin another journey as they explore options in this area. There are high-profile news stories in this area as well. Everyone seems to have heard of a couple who, after a long struggle with infertility, adopted a child and then achieved a spontaneous pregnancy. The stories of those who adopt and still do not become pregnant are far more numerous, but these stories do not make the news.

Other couples will choose child-free living. It is an important adjustment for couples come to see this as a choice that they make rather than as a disappointing outcome with which they are stuck. Many couples describe this choice as a step forward, a conscious decision to close the door on a painful time in their lives and a chance to move on to other life experiences. Once resolution is reached, couples often feel positive about this decision and see it as growth-producing experience that frees them to get on with living their lives.

 **SUMMARY**

The goals of preconception education, genetic counseling, and infertility treatment are to provide couples with information and options to maximize their opportunity to have a pregnancy that has a positive outcome. It is important to provide couples with the information necessary to empower them to make decisions that are informed, appropriate for them, and are decisions they feel good about for the long term. We are often the only health care providers who are a continual presence, supporting couples as they make these decisions. It is our compassionate, objective, nonjudgmental counseling and support that are important to give them the confidence to move through the decision-making and possible treatment process in a way that promotes personal growth.

# Care Plan · The Couple Being Treated for Infertility

NURSING DIAGNOSIS **Knowledge Deficit (of human reproduction, tests and treatments, and self-monitoring techniques)** related to no prior experience

GOALS/OUTCOMES Demonstrates knowledge of causes of infertility and of techniques for self-monitoring of fertility cycles

**NOC Suggested Outcomes**
- Knowledge: Fertility Promotion (1816)
- Knowledge: Treatment Procedures (1814)
- Knowledge: Treatment Regimen (1813)

**NIC Priority Interventions**
- Teaching: Disease Process (5602)
- Teaching: Individual (5606)
- Teaching: Procedure/Treatment (5618)

**Nursing Activities and Rationale**
- Assess the couple's level of knowledge related to infertility, self-monitoring, fertility tests, and treatment procedures *to establish database from which to individualize teaching.*
- Provide feedback on any aspects of lifestyle (e.g., nutrition, strenuous exercise) or sexual patterns that may impact fertility *to enhance insight needed to motivate changes in behavior.*
- Correct any misconceptions and provide other information as needed (e.g., preparations for tests and treatments) *to enhance understanding of and adherence to therapeutic measures.*
- Describe rationale for treatment regimens *to promote understanding and informed decision making.*
- Teach procedures for determining when ovulation occurs (i.e., basal body temperature, cervical mucus assessment) *to provides information needed to diagnose cause(s) of infertility and enhance the chances that conception will occur.*

**Evaluation Parameters**
- Describes anatomy of the reproductive system
- Describes normal physiology of the reproductive system
- Describes conditions that can decrease fertility (e.g., hormone levels, sperm count)
- Describes methods for predicting ovulation
- Verbalizes understanding of prescribed tests and treatments
- Reports making any needed lifestyle changes

NURSING DIAGNOSIS **Situational Low Self-Esteem** related to inability to conceive and cultural expectations of fertility

GOALS/OUTCOMES Couple maintains essentially positive self-esteem throughout the course of treatment

**NOC Suggested Outcomes**
- Self-Esteem (1205)

**NIC Priority Interventions**
- Emotional Support (5270)
- Self-Esteem Enhancement (5400)

**Nursing Activities and Rationale**
- Provide emotional support, *which is essential in encouraging the couple to complete the regimen of tests and treatment.*
- Monitor statements/indicators of self-esteem *to provide a baseline for and evaluation of interventions.*
- Explore with the couple other areas of competence that they feel good about (e.g., career, relationships) *to promote self-esteem and focus on positive instead of "problem" aspects.*
- Reinforce statements that reflect positive feelings and attitudes. *Positive reinforcement strengthens self-esteem.*
- Allow adequate time for questions and concerns *to demonstrate regard for the clients.*
- Provide for comfort and privacy during tests and procedures *to decrease embarrassment.*
- Refer to support groups as needed *to provide a safe environment for expressing negative feelings.*

**Evaluation Parameters**
- Couple demonstrates positive attitudes toward themselves
- Verbalizes self-acceptance and self-worth
- Expresses confidence in ability to perform self-care measures
- Communicates openly
- Maintains erect posture and eye contact

## Care Plan · The Couple Being Treated for Infertility—cont'd

NURSING DIAGNOSIS   **Powerlessness** related to complex, long-term regimen of tests and treatments

**NOC Suggested Outcomes**
- Health Beliefs: Perceived Control (1702)
- Health Beliefs: Perceived Resources (1703)
- Participation: Health Care Decisions (1606)

**NIC Priority Interventions**
- Decision-Making Support (5250)
- Emotional Support (5270)
- Self-Esteem Enhancement (5400)
- Values Clarification (5480)

**Nursing Activities and Rationale**
- Explore how clients have coped with stressors in the past *to build on present strengths.*
- Provide information as needed, in language the couple can understand (see Knowledge Deficit). *Knowledge is essential for empowerment.*
- Avoid empty reassurance and false hope, *which invalidates the couple's feelings and interferes with communication.*
- Help the couple establish realistic expectations *to empower by providing hope.*
- Facilitate collaborative decision making (NIC), *which enhances sense of control.*
- Help patient identify the advantages and disadvantages of each option. *Information enhances sense of control.*
- Be accepting and nondirective, *which ensures that choices are the clients' and not a result of caregivers' biases.*
- Refer to support groups to *reduce sense of isolation and enhance coping through sharing of similar experiences.*
- Assist couple to clarify their values *to facilitate effective decision making.*

**Evaluation Parameters**
- Couple verbalizes realistic appraisal of their situation.
- Couple is involved in making decisions about their treatment regimen.

**Other Frequently Encountered Nursing Diagnoses**
- **Altered Sexuality Patterns** related to (1) requirements of tests and treatments and (2) stress of infertility on the relationship
- **Grieving** related to anticipated, perceived, or actual loss of ability for biologic parenting
- **Ineffective Individual Coping** related to inability to conceive and unmet expectations

## CASE STUDY

Maria is a 30-year old woman who has been married to Rosario, age 35, for 8 years. During her annual examination last year Maria stated that she and Rosario were disappointed because they had been trying to get pregnant and it hadn't happened yet. You review when her menses occur and when they have intercourse. You also ask about each of their prior health histories. After her physical examination, during which everything appears normal, the nurse practitioner asks you to set up a referral for Maria to an infertility specialist.

Maria wants to know what the specialist will do. She appears very nervous and says she doesn't know how she should tell Rosario or how he will respond. She looks to you for information and support as she starts to integrate this new information and potential difficulties.

- What immediate response will you provide Maria?

- What are her strengths? Where does she face potential problems?

- What information do you need from Maria to move forward in support of her?

- What nursing diagnoses could apply? How will you validate these?

- What long-term goals might she have for herself? For her family?

- What short-term goals might the two of you develop for Maria? For her family?

- What interventions can you develop and offer?

- How will these interventions be prioritized?

- How will you evaluate the effectiveness of your interventions?

- What note should be put in Maria's chart to prepare providers when she returns for her next annual examination?

# *Scenarios*

1. Ashley, a 31-year-old woman in for her annual examination, tells you that she and her husband have been trying to conceive a child for about 8 months, but every month she keeps getting her period. She asks, "Is there anything we can do to increase our chances of getting pregnant?"

- How will you respond?
- What subjective data do you have about Ashley's condition?
- What subjective and objective data do you need?
- What nursing diagnoses could apply? How will you validate these?
- What goals might be developed? How will these be prioritized?
- What interventions may you offer?
- How will you evaluate the effectiveness of your interventions?

2. Amita and her husband have been using the natural family planning method to prevent pregnancy. They have now decided that they would like a child. Amita asks you to review with her the signs that she may look for to determine when she is fertile (ovulating).

- How will you respond?
- What subjective data do you have?
- What subjective and objective data do you need?
- What nursing diagnoses could apply? How will you validate these?
- What goals might be developed? How will these be prioritized?
- What interventions may you offer?
- How will you evaluate the effectiveness of your interventions?

3. Cheryl, a college senior, spends a great deal of time staying in physical shape and caring for her body. To determine what actions she will take, she reads health magazines. One of the latest articles she read said that "all women of childbearing age should eat foods high in folic acid and take a supplement with folic acid." Cheryl prefers not to take supplements, preferring to get her nutrition from food sources. She says to you, "What's the big deal? Why do I need folic acid anyway? Can't I get enough in food?"

- How will you respond to her?
- What subjective data do you have?
- What subjective and objective data do you need?
- What nursing diagnoses could apply? How will you validate these?
- What goals might be developed? How will these be prioritized?
- What interventions may you offer?
- How will you evaluate the effectiveness of your interventions?

4. Patricia and Michael are both of African-American descent. They are planning on being married next year and starting a family. Patricia confides that she is concerned because both her father and Michael's brother have sickle cell anemia. She and Michael are afraid that their children will have it too.

- How will you respond to her?
- What subjective data do you have?
- What subjective and objective data do you need?
- What nursing diagnoses could apply? How will you validate these?
- What goals might be developed? How will these be prioritized?
- What interventions may you offer?
- How will you evaluate the effectiveness of your interventions?

5. Edna is a 26-year-old woman who has come in for a premarital physical examination and contraception. When giving her family history she reports that her fraternal twin sister Dawn has Down syndrome. Edna says that she and her future husband are concerned about their chances of having a child with Down syndrome.

- How will you respond?
- What subjective data do you have about Edna's condition?
- What subjective and objective data do you need?

- What nursing diagnoses could apply? How will you validate these?
- What goals might be developed? How will these be prioritized?
- What interventions may you offer?
- How will you evaluate the effectiveness of your interventions?

---

6. Jena and Charles are being seen as part of her annual examination for preconception education before she attempts to become pregnant for the first time. They had expressed a desire for genetic assessment and counseling based on family history. The reason they are concerned is that Jena has a sister with cystic fibrosis. Jena has not had any previous pregnancies.

- How will you respond?
- What subjective data do you have about Jena's condition?
- What subjective and objective data do you need?
- What nursing diagnoses could apply? How will you validate these?
- What goals might be developed? How will these be prioritized?
- What interventions may you offer?
- How will you evaluate the effectiveness of your interventions?

---

7. Sean's father has polycystic kidney disease as does Sean. Sean and his wife, Laura, are concerned about the possibility of transmitting the condition to their children. They ask you about how it is inherited.

They also want to know about artificial insemination and if they should consider it.

- How will you respond?
- What subjective data do you have about Sean's condition?
- What subjective and objective data do you need?
- What nursing diagnoses could apply? How will you validate these?
- What goals might be developed? How will these be prioritized?
- What interventions may you offer?
- How will you evaluate the effectiveness of your interventions?

---

8. Katia and her husband, both 38 years old, were diagnosed with infertility problems 2 years ago. Since then they have experienced extensive testing and treatment, with no success. Katia says to you. "We wanted children so much, so that we would be a family. We can't afford any more treatment cycles. We have to stop trying. I am such a failure."

- How will you respond?
- What subjective data do you have about Katia's condition?
- What subjective and objective data do you need?
- What nursing diagnoses could apply? How will you validate these?
- What goals might be developed? How will these be prioritized?
- What interventions may you offer?
- How will you evaluate the effectiveness of your interventions?

## REFERENCES

American College of Obstetricians and Gynecologists (ACOG): *ACOG guide to planning for pregnancy, birth, and beyond*, Washington, DC, 1990, Author.

American College of Obstetricians and Gynecologists (ACOG): *Guidelines for women's health care*, Washington, DC, 1996, Author.

Bernstein J, Lewis J, and Seibel M: Effect of previous infertility on maternal-fetal attachment, coping styles, and self-concept during pregnancy, *J Women Health* 3(2):125-133, 1994.

Cefalo RC and Moos MK: *Preconceptional health care: a practical guide*, ed 2, St Louis, 1994, Mosby.

James CA: Infertility. In Youngkin EQ and Davis MS, editors: *Women's health: a primary care clinical guide*, ed 2, East Norwalk, Conn, 1998, Appleton and Lange.

March of Dimes: *Genetic Counseling*, White Plains, NY, 1994, March of Dimes.

Moos MK: *Preconceptional health promotion* White Plains, NY, 1994, March of Dimes Birth Defect Foundation.

National Cancer Institute (NCI): *DES Daughters*, Washington, DC, 1995, National Institutes of Health.

National Center for Chronic Disease Prevention and Health Promotion (NCCDPHP): *1997 assisted reproductive technology success rates—national summary and fertility clinic report*, Washington, DC, 1999, CDC, *http://www.cdc.gov/nccdphp/drh/art.htm*.

Peterson R and Moos MK: Defining and measuring unintended pregnancy: issues and concerns. *Women's Health Issues* 7(4):234-240, 1997.

Secretary's Advisory Committee on Genetic Testing: *Final report on oversight of genetic testing*, Washington, DC, 2000, The Committee.

Williams JK: *Genetic issues for perinatal nurses*, White Plains, NY, 1996, March of Dimes Birth Defect Foundation.

# CHAPTER 9

# Assessment of a Woman During Pregnancy

*"When women go to practitioners for checkups, they should walk out from every visit feeling 10 feet tall! . . . Every site and style of care, no matter who gives it, ought not only to give surveillance but should educate and empower, should enhance every woman's feeling of her ability to do what she is doing well."*

— A NURSE-MIDWIFE (BOSTON WOMEN'S HEALTH BOOK COLLECTIVE, 1999)

What are the particular needs of pregnant women during their first prenatal visit?

What factors influence the health behaviors of pregnant women?

How can we empower women to make the choices that are right for each of them?

How can we promote wellness for pregnant women and their families?

How do family, culture, and community influence women's pregnancies?

What traditional and complementary health care practices may be safely used in pregnancy?

##  THE PRENATAL PERIOD

The **prenatal** or antepartum period is the time between conception and birth. These months provide an opportunity for a pregnant woman to become more connected with her body and become empowered to care for her health and well-being as she encounters the changes and needs created by pregnancy. It also provides a time when we can assist a woman and her family to prevent health problems from occurring or to reduce negative outcomes (Figure 9-1).

Prenatal care is a program of ambulatory care designed to enhance the health and well-being of both the mother and the fetus while preventing illness and injury. With this as a major focus of professional nursing, we play a pivotal role in increasing the positive outcomes of pregnancy. For many women, participation in prenatal care may be the first time they have received health promotion nursing interventions since they were children.

Pregnancy is an essentially healthy process that can have many normal variations. Each woman enters her pregnancy with unique past experiences that directly affect her ability to cope with the pregnancy and her potential to provide positive parenting (Adams and Kocik, 1997). The way in which a woman defines, perceives, experiences, explains, and maintains her pregnancy depends, in large measure, on past experiences and what she is told by friends, family, neighbors, and members of her community. To be able to participate in her knowledge development, we must convince her that we may also be a resource to her and that we would like to be part of her community of educators and caregivers.

Once accepted, our role is to help the woman identify her strengths and resources and then support her

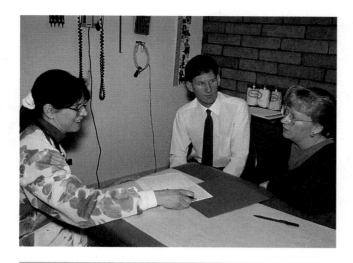

FIGURE 9-1 • Prenatal interview. *(Courtesy of Caroline E. Brown.)*

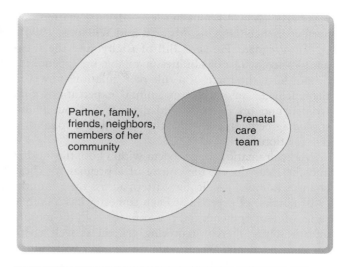

FIGURE 9-2 • Educators and care providers to a pregnant woman.

in making positive life changes and maintaining a healthy lifestyle throughout the pregnancy. The other participants in her care—her partner, family, and friends—should be included as much as the woman desires so that they will understand and be able to support her in her efforts. The closer the two circles of care can work together the better the chances of success (Figure 9-2).

During the initial prenatal visit and throughout the pregnancy, we assess the needs and perceptions of the individual woman and empower her to make appropriate choices for her health and the well-being of her baby. Adaptations will be necessary for women who have serious mental or emotional disorders or who are mentally retarded or brain injured. However, each woman must be respected and involved to the limit of her emotional and cognitive capacities or physical handicap.

Factors that influence the pregnancy include maternal medical conditions, exposure to infectious, occupational hazards, and environmental hazards. Many kinds of prescription and over-the-counter medications also have negative health consequences, as do exposure to violence, tobacco, alcohol, and recreational drugs.

We address some of these risks with the woman directly; other situations, such as the medical conditions of hypertension, diabetes, asthma, and epilepsy, require close collaboration among the woman and her providers, including appropriate specialists. The pregnant woman is not just a partner in this collaboration; she is the key member of the partnership, because it is she who has the most at stake and who is the only one who may create change. Sharing information and resources with the woman empowers her to make positive decisions that can improve her health and her infant's health (Figure 9-3).

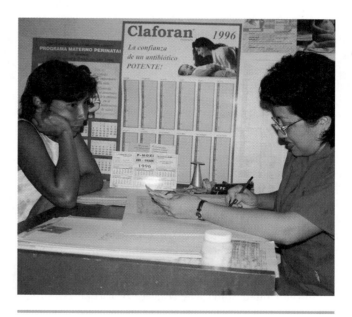

FIGURE 9-3 • Provider with a woman. *(Courtesy of Caroline E. Brown.)*

##  PARTNERING WITH THE WOMAN

The pregnant woman has the right to participate in the decisions involving her well-being and what may or may not be done to her body, unless a clear-cut medical emergency prevents her participation. Some women hesitate to participate in this manner, fearful of making the "experts" angry if she doesn't meet their approval. Others just drop out of care when they feel they are not being heard. A woman's self-esteem and satisfaction with her pregnancy and birth are increased when she makes the choices about her level of participation and her experience (Higgins, Murray, and Williams, 1994).

The **Pregnant Patient's Bill of Rights** and the **Pregnant Patient's Responsibilities** (available in Appendix I) do not have the force of a rule or regulation; however, they provide an outline of mutual expectations that women and providers should discuss. Without philosophic agreement, it is difficult to develop a collaborative relationship.

Many dramatic changes occur within both the mother and the fetus during the course of a pregnancy. These changes follow a predicable pattern across the 9 months (3 trimesters) of pregnancy. Each trimester has a unique series of developments and concerns for both the mother and the fetus, thereby requiring general as well as focused assessments. We provide the woman with anticipatory guidance concerning these changes and explore how to meet her needs.

Collecting baseline information concerning the woman and her pregnancy begins during the first prenatal visit. Knowledge of the components of an initial visit allows for a complete assessment to be obtained and appropriate nursing interventions to be developed with the woman and her family.

## The Development of Prenatal Care

Prenatal care by health care providers is a relatively new phenomenon. For thousands of years, pregnant women were attended by the women in their families or community as they supported and cared for each other. When couples left their communities and moved to urban areas, the women lost the support and guidance of female family members and friends. The women and their families became exposed to poor sanitation, overcrowded living conditions, inadequate nutrition, and poor working conditions. The resulting increase in maternal and infant mortality led to a public health concern (Phillips, 1996).

In the United States, the concept of formalized prenatal care began in 1901 under the influence of social reformer Mrs. Lowell Putman of the Boston Infant Social Service Department. Mrs. Putman established the role of the nurse as a provider of prenatal care, assisting women through their pregnancies. Under Mrs. Putman's supervision, a program of home visits by nurses was instituted. During these visits, information on nutrition was shared and basic maternal physical assessment was performed (Wertz and Wertz, 1989; Thatcher Ulrich, 1991).

The home program was so successful that in 1910, to expand the work, an outpatient clinic was developed for the Boston Lying-in Hospital. By 1914, it was estimated that, with the introduction of this formal prenatal care, the fetal mortality rate within the group of women it served had decreased by 40%. The maternal mortality rates were also significantly reduced through this program (Merkatz, Thompson, and Walsh, 1990).

## Prenatal Care Today

Today, women choose who they wish to collaborate with during their pregnancy and birth experience based on the experience of family or friends, a preference for the place of birth of their baby, their insurance coverage, the ability to access a specific option, convenience, and agreement in philosophy between the client and the practitioner. The health care team may include professional nurses, nurse practitioners, childbirth educators, nurse midwives, and physicians. The prenatal care may be in a private office, a nurse-run clinic, a mobile van, a woman's home, a neighborhood health center, or a clinic within a public facility, such as a church or library. During pregnancy, the woman and her family may prepare to have their baby in a hospital labor, delivery, recovery (LDR) area or room; an alternative birthing center (ABC); a freestanding birthing center; or at home.

### The Prenatal Care Providers

A woman and her family are best served during the prenatal period by a team of providers who collaborate to provide holistic care. Each provider offers a specific expertise to the clients and fulfills an acknowledged role within the overall program of care.

*Professional Nurse.* The professional nurse is often the first health professional that the pregnant woman encounters. Our initial history and basic assessment begins the woman's entry into the prenatal care system. This opening contact sets the tone and expectations for future interactions between the members of the team, the woman, and her support system. Because we are her first contact, the mother often tells us of her concerns and fears, as well as her desires during prenatal care. We often become the woman's initial health educator, with the primary role of counseling and meeting the psychologic needs of the expectant family and performing continuing assessments in these areas during the prenatal period. Integrated within our care are preliminary and ongoing physical assessments.

*Nurse Practitioner.* Nurse practitioners in prenatal care are advanced practice nurses who have education and certification beyond the entry level of professional nurse. They may be certified as a women's health nurse practitioner or a family nurse practitioner. A **Women's Health Nurse Practitioner (WHNP)** has advanced preparation and has passed a certification examination in the promotion of health and prevention of illness in women. A **Family Nurse Practitioner (FNP)** has advanced preparation and has passed a certification examination in the promotion of health and prevention of illness in all persons across the lifespan.

On a prenatal care team, nurse practitioners may take the health and pregnancy histories, perform physical and obstetric examinations, order and interpret diagnostic and laboratory tests, and provide for the continuity of prenatal care for the mother and her family throughout the pregnancy. In some states advanced practice nurses also write prescriptions. Since nurse practitioners do not do deliveries, they work in partnership with nurse midwives and/or physicians.

***Certified Nurse Midwife (CNM).*** The word "midwife" literally means "a woman with . . ." Every culture has had women that were with women as they labored and delivered their babies. In the United States, the first nurse midwifery programs started in the 1920s when the Frontier Nursing Service and the Maternity Center Association started attending to poor women in Appalachia and New York City, respectively. Today a **certified nurse-midwife** (**CNM**) has postgraduate training in the care of normal pregnancy and delivery and then sits for an examination to be certified by the American College of Nurse Midwives (ACNM).

CNMs provide prenatal care in their own private practices, in practices with private physicians, in clinics, health centers, in health departments, and in homes. They assist women with the delivery of their babies in freestanding birthing centers, hospitals, and homes. They always practice in conjunction with physicians, referring women who have problem pregnancies to them. With a focus on assisting women and their families through the pregnancy, nurse-midwives strive to have the addition of a new baby become an unforgettable family event and help ensure a healthy outcome for both mother and child.

During the last decade, as the number of CNMs has increased, so too has the number of women who seek them out for prenatal care and delivery and the number of insurance programs that pay for their services. CNMs are the majority of midwives attending births in hospital settings (98%) and in freestanding birthing centers (67%). They provide 28% of midwife deliveries in nonhospital settings (Horton, 1995).

**Lay midwives** (independent or direct-entry midwives) also offer their services to women and their families. A lay midwife may be as well prepared as a CNM or have very little preparation and experience; only some states have provisions to license lay midwives. Lay midwives sometimes have privileges to deliver in hospital settings or freestanding birthing centers; however, the major focus of their care is helping women in nonhospital locations. When a woman chooses to have a home birth, lay midwives are often the only care providers she can count on for assistance (Phillips, 1996).

***Physicians.*** Both medical doctors (MDs) and doctors of osteopathy (DOs) follow women during their pregnancies and provide care during deliveries. "Physicians attend 96% of all hospital deliveries, 34% of births in freestanding birthing centers, and 20% of all deliveries in residences" (Horton, 1995). Family practice physicians (FPP) and general practitioners (GP) are primary care physicians, skilled in providing care to members of an entire family. Most have experience in obstetrics and some specialize in obstetrics. They generally have a collaborative relationship with an obstetrician for the care of a woman with complications. An obstetrician/gynecologist (OB/GYN) is a physician who has trained primarily to care for high-risk pregnancies and conduct surgical procedures. Although most OB/GYNs are not specialists in normal pregnancies and births, their surgical skills are invaluable in an emergency.

***Other Team Members.*** To meet the needs of women and their families, there may be additional members of the prenatal care team. Home health visitors or aides and lay health workers who are experts in the culture of women and families being served may have positions on the health care team.

## RESPONDING TO THE CONCERNS OF THE WOMAN

When a woman experiences **amenorrhea** (absence of menses) for 1 or more months she may suspect that she is pregnant and seek out a pregnancy test. Test kits that check a woman's urine are available in drug stores and may be done by a woman in her home. A serum pregnancy test that may give results sooner or is used to confirm the findings of a urine test is available in family planning and prenatal care facilities. The desire to confirm a suspected pregnancy often is what brings a woman into a facility and in contact with one or more members of the prenatal health care team.

### Diagnosing a Woman's Pregnancy

Many women first suspect they are pregnant because of amenorrhea. For others, it is the tingling in their breasts. Both of these are presumptive signs of pregnancy that can be caused by other conditions. The **presumptive** or subjective signs of pregnancy are symptoms that the woman experiences. Because they may be caused by conditions other than pregnancy, they are not proof of a pregnancy. The presumptive signs in the first trimester are breast changes, amenorrhea, nausea and vomiting, frequent urination, fatigue, and uterine or abdominal enlargement.

**Probable** or objective signs of pregnancy are signs perceived by an examiner; however, they also may have causes other than pregnancy. A serum pregnancy test, urine pregnancy test, and changes in the woman's vagina and cervix are the probable signs of pregnancy that may be observed during the first trimester of a pregnancy.

**Positive** or diagnostic signs when perceived by an examiner can only be caused by pregnancy. It is not until the examiner can *see* a fetal outline (using ultrasound) or *hear* a fetal heart or *feel* fetal movement that the reality of a viable pregnancy may be confirmed (Box 9-1).

### Pregnancy Tests

Pregnancy tests confirm the presence of the **human chorionic gonadotrophic** hormone (hCG). This hormone is a glycoprotein produced from the day of implantation by the trophoblastic cells of the developing placental tissue. In a normally developing pregnancy, first trimester blood pregnancy levels of hCG double every 48 to 72 hours (Chartier and others, 1979). Distinct from other hormones, the hCG, or β-subunit of the hCG, indicates the presence of hCG in the woman's body and is the basis of the presumption that its presence is being caused by a developing pregnancy. It may be detected in a woman's blood as early as 6 days after conception and in her urine about 20 days later. It is important to note that because hCG is not produced by the fetus, its presence cannot confirm or accurately date a viable pregnancy (Cunningham and others, 1997).

Both women and their providers often place a great deal of importance on the results of urine and blood pregnancy tests, so it is important to have an understanding of their accuracy and the different ways these tests may be interpreted. Pregnancy tests fall into one of four categories of tests: immunoassay, radioreceptor assay, radioimmunoassay, or enzyme-linked immunosorbent assay.

***Immunoassay Tests.*** The **immunoassay** process depends on an antibody reaction between hCG-coated particles and a first morning urine specimen from a woman. If no particle agglutination takes place because of the presence of the hCG in the woman's urine, a woman is generally considered pregnant. The latex agglutination inhibition test (LAI) yields results within 2 minutes and is

accurate 4 to 10 days after a woman's first missed menses. The hemagglutination inhibition (HAI) tests may provide a positive result slightly earlier in the pregnancy, but the test itself takes between 1 and 2 hours (Kochenour, 1994).

***Radioimmunoassay.*** The **radioimmunoassay (RIA)**, which tests a woman's blood for the β-subunit of hCG, is the most sensitive pregnancy test currently available (Pagana and Pagana, 1996). Because of the use of radioactive materials, it is performed in a laboratory and may take from 1 to 5 hours. However, it can provide a positive result earlier at around 6 to 10 days after conception (Varney, 1997).

***Radioreceptor Assay (RRA).*** The **radioreceptor assay (RRA)** test measures the ability of the suspected hCG in the woman's blood sample to inhibit the binding of radio-labeled hCG to receptors. It may be positive at the time of the first missed menses (Pagana and Pagana, 1996). Because the test fails to distinguish between hCG and luteinizing hormone (LH), a woman who is in menopause may receive a false-positive reading (Boston Women's Health Book Collective, 1999).

***Enzyme-linked Immunosorbent Assay.*** The most common test and the basis for most of the over-the-counter (OTC) home pregnancy tests is the **enzyme-linked immunosorbent assay** (ELISA) test. It uses an enzyme to identify the antigen to be measured and may measure hCG amounts as low as 25 mIU/ml. This sensitivity enables it to give a positive reading as early as the time of a missed period. A simple color change indicates a positive reaction that is easily read with the eye or a spectrometer, and results are ready in 5 minutes (Kochenour, 1994).

### Interpretation of Results

The results of a pregnancy test may be **positive, negative, or inconclusive.** Accurate interpretation depends on placing these results within a broader context that considers the type of test used and its degree of specificity and sensitivity; a woman's history of sexual intercourse, her last normal menstrual period, and the usual length of her menstrual cycle; concurrent physical symptoms, her use of medications and recreational drug use, and the techniques used when collecting and handling the specimen.

A **positive pregnancy test** generally indicates that hCG is in the woman's system. A **false-positive result,** although rare, may occur if there is an error in reading the test; the woman has certain drugs in her system (e.g., marijuana, methadone, aspirin, synthetic hormones, or medications that affect the central nervous system); protein or blood is in the urine; the container has soap or other substances on its surface; the woman is experiencing the hormonal changes of menopause; or she has certain tumors or other medical conditions.

A **negative pregnancy test** may indicate that the woman is not pregnant. However, **false-negative** tests are fairly common because the levels of hCG are too low to be detected, the urine is too warm, the urine is not concentrated enough, the woman is on certain medications, the container has other substances in it, there may be problems with the location of the pregnancy, or there is a problem with the testing procedure. Whenever a test result is questionable, repeat testing is required.

Although the presence of hCG is indicative of a possible pregnancy, it does not indicate the potential viability of the fetus or prevent a miscarriage. The presence of hCG may be detected for a period 4 to 6 weeks after miscarriage or abortion or during the postpartum period. However, if the level of a woman's hCG fails to double, it may indicate that she is experiencing an ectopic pregnancy or miscarriage.

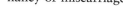

### Estimating the Date of Delivery

Once a pregnancy test is positive, the next question is When will the baby come? The **human gestational period** *averages* 266 days from fertilization or 280 days from the first day of the woman's last true menstrual period. The first day of the **last normal menstrual period** (**LNMP** or **LMP**) is a time that most women are apt to be aware of rather than the time of ovulation. That is one reason why a woman's LMP is the initial point for calculating the length of the pregnancy or gestation. However, when we calculate the length of pregnancy from the LMP we are including the 2 weeks before the time the woman may have ovulated, a time when she was not actually pregnant. Because the length of a woman's cycle, the day of ovulation, and the rate of human growth vary, all calculations to determine a due date add the caveat of plus or minus 2 weeks.

The calculation of fetal age is based on the actual number of weeks of development. **Fetal age** (also referred to as the fertilization age or postconception age) is 2 weeks less than the length of the pregnancy or gestational age in a woman that has regular 28-day menstrual cycles.

#### Estimating Gestational Age

To estimate how far along the pregnancy is and an estimated due date, we must learn the date of the woman's LMP, the length of her normal menstrual cycle, and whether her cycle occurs in a regular pattern. Since ovulation happens 14 days before menses occurs, this is approximately midway through a 28-day cycle.

*Nägele's Rule.* The **estimated date of delivery** (EDD) is often calculated using **Nägele's rule** (LMP − 3 calendar months [90 days] + 7 days = EDD). Gestation age wheels and birth calculators may also be used; however, they are all based on the same formula. The formula may be adjusted to more closely match the possible date of ovulation. If the woman has a longer cycle, add 1 day to the gestational length for every day the menstrual cy-

---

> ### BOX 9-2   *Nägele's Rule**
>
> *First day of LNMP − 3 months + 7 days = EDD*
>
> For example, Nägele's Rule for a 28-day cycle
> Subtract 3 months and add 7 days to obtain EDD
> (e.g., LNMP = 01-01-99
> EDD = 10-08-99)
>
> Adjusted Nägele's for longer or shorter cycles
> (For example, LNMP = 01-01-99 with a 35-day cycle
> EDD = 10-15-99 (35 − 28 = 7, add 14 instead of 7)
> For example, LNMP = 01-01-99 with a 26-day cycle
> EDD = 10-06-99 (28 − 26 = 2, add 5 days instead of 7)
>
> *Nägele's rule can only be applied to a regular menstrual cycle.
> *EDD,* Estimated date of confinement; *LNMP,* last normal menstrual period.

---

cle normally exceeds 28 days. If the client has a shorter cycle, subtract the difference in days (Box 9-2).

Nägele's formula for estimating a date of delivery is based on a belief from the early 1800s. At that time, Franz Carl Nägele declared that pregnancy lasted 10 lunar months (10 × 28 days), counting from the first day of the last menstrual period. More recent research has revealed that patterns of gestation are significantly different. Mittendorf and others (1990) found that healthy, white, private-care women, pregnant for the first time, averaged 288 days, while this same group of women when pregnant again averaged 283 days. These values show a significant difference from Nägele's formula as well as between the groups of women. Mittendorf and others (1990) also reported differences among white, black, and Japanese women, with blacks and Japanese women having a shorter median gestational length of 264 days.

Because of the normal variations in women's fertility cycles, differences in the normal gestational length between ethnic groups, and errors in dating methods, there is *no such thing as a predictable due date.* In general, a birth 2 weeks before or 2 weeks after the EDD is considered within the normal limit (38 to 42 weeks or 266 to 294 days). For that reason, when referring to a woman's EDD we always remind her that it is plus or minus 2 weeks. In fact, since it covers a 4-week period, what we are estimating is a **"due month."** This concept is helpful in allaying fears later in the pregnancy when the EDD arrives and there are no signs of labor.

Sometimes you will see the EDD referred to instead as **"the estimated date of confinement (EDC)."** This term was used in the past to indicate the date that the woman would become "confined," or have her baby.

*Ultrasound.* When a woman has a history of irregular menstrual cycles, is unsure of her LNMP, or has become pregnant before resuming menstruation after a prior pregnancy, ultrasound can be used to assist in estimating the gestational age. Ultrasound measurements can estimate the gestational age of a pregnancy to ± 5 days in the first trimester, to ± 8 days in the second trimester, and ± 22 days in the third trimester (Goer, 1995). However, even the best ultrasound-based estimates result in 80% more errors in dating than following the process of using the LMP (when it is known) plus a confirmatory pelvic examination (Mittendorf and others, 1990).

Ultrasound uses intermittent high-frequency sound waves of 2 to 7 MHz produced by electrical stimulation from a piezoelectric crystal. The sound waves are directed into the body and, by recording their echoes, pictures of the inner organs are created. The procedure may be done either abdominally or vaginally. No harmful effects have been confirmed; however, since we do not know enough about its long-term effects, routine use is not recommended.

Ultrasound can also be used to establish a positive diagnosis of pregnancy with a sonographic outline of the fetus at 5 weeks of pregnancy and reveal the fetal heartbeat at 9 weeks (Reed, 1994).

##  AFTER A PREGNANCY IS CONFIRMED

Learning that her pregnancy test is positive sets off a full array of emotions within a woman. Her response will also depend on her pre-pregnancy health, her emotional status, her past health care, and other events in her life. Helping her adjust to the reality while making plans for her future is a significant task.

### Ambivalence

When we tell a woman that her pregnancy test is positive, she may be simultaneously happy and sad. Such **ambivalence** is a common reaction (Malnory, 1996). Most women need time to explore their feelings about the pregnancy. Initially the joy and excitement of recognizing their fertility may be coupled with fear and doubt about becoming a mother or coping with another child. Even if a pregnancy was actively planned and desired, the reality that it has now occurred can cause mixed emotions. The woman may require a period of time to absorb the information and have it become real.

We may be the first person with whom she feels safe in discussing her ambivalence about the pregnancy. It is important that we let her know that ambivalence during the initial stages of pregnancy is a normal reaction. Assist a woman in exploring her feelings by asking her directly whether she feels ready for this pregnancy (Fischer and others, 1999). Give her time to tell her story and explore her own ambivalence. She may voice concerns about her readiness for motherhood, be unsure of her ability to take on the responsibility of another human being, be anxious about partner support, and fear economic crises (Malnory, 1996). Continue the conversation by asking if there are circumstances that she would wish were different. This provides an opening for the woman to begin to discuss her feelings.

Domestic violence, rape, incest, and assault by a stranger are situations she may not choose to discuss initially, but these are significant factors in the acceptance of the pregnancy. However, asking questions in a supportive and nonjudgmental way may enable her to confide in you later.

### Unintended Pregnancies

It is estimated that 50% to 65% of all pregnancies are **unintended** or unplanned (Henshaw, 1998). As many as 85% of adolescent pregnancies may be unintended (Klima, 1998). A pregnancy may result from contraceptive failure; failure to use contraception; or an unanticipated, undesired event such as rape (Klima, 1998). When we ask a woman if her pregnancy was planned and she responds "no," we cannot assume that because it was unintended it is also unwanted (Rosenfeld and Everett, 1996). Even though most pregnancies are initially unintended, over 90% of pregnant women state that as the pregnancy progresses it becomes a wanted pregnancy. Major factors in adjusting to an unplanned pregnancy are the presence of a supportive partner, the presence of a family support system, and a degree of economic stability (Fischer and others, 1999).

### Unwanted Pregnancies

A woman who states that her pregnancy is unwanted may be looking for help in clarifying her choices (Fischer and others, 1999). We can provide the information she needs to explore her options and act on her decision. When pregnant, she has two options: to terminate the pregnancy (**therapeutic abortion**) or to allow it to continue. When she delivers the infant, she again has two options: she may place it for **adoption** or raise it herself. Some women are unaware of how to act on the options of adoption or abortion; others may not even be aware that the options of abortion and adoption are available to them.

#### Abortion

The rules and regulations concerning therapeutic abortion and the availability of the service vary from state to state. We need to know about the services provided within our state of practice as well as surrounding states. When tax dollars are prohibited from being used to procure an abortion, the options available to poor and uninsured women are limited. Minors also have barriers to this choice, with requirements for parental consent or the necessity of appearing before a judge. If the girl is an **emancipated minor**, is a person less than legal age who is a parent, is in the military, lives away from home, or is self-supporting, and has all the legal rights of an adult, this is not necessary.

Some women find that long distances may have to be traveled to reach a treatment facility, and often there is a 1- or 2-day waiting period once they arrive. For other women, a cultural stigma in obtaining information on an abortion is prevalent. It remains a difficult subject for many people to discuss on a personal level. We should ensure that options are reviewed in a nonjudgmental fashion and that the woman feels supported in whatever choice she makes. If comprehensive counseling is needed, the woman should be referred to appropriate services (Klima, 1998).

### Adoption

Similarly, if the woman wishes to explore the avenue of adoption she may be unaware of the two choices open to her through either agency or private adoption. In **agency adoptions**, the agency selects and performs background screens on the potential adoptive couple. **Private adoption** is usually arranged between the birth mother and adoptive parents. In both cases, the adoptive process can either be closed or open. In a **closed adoption**, full confidentiality on the identity of the birth mother is maintained. This information cannot be accessed, except through legal channels and not before the child is of an age to understand the ramifications involved. In an **open adoption** some relationship between the adoptive family and the birth mother may be maintained. This may consist of simply meeting with one another before or after the birth, or the adoptive parents may give the birth mother regular updates on the child's progress, and in some cases allow visitation. Open adoption is currently being advocated by many professionals in the field, particularly in light of the increasing trend for adoptees to search for their birth mother and vice versa (Rhodes, 1995). Adults often seek to learn about their heritage, not only to discover whom they resemble in appearance or actions, but also to uncover the health history of their biologic family members.

It also may be important to the woman who is considering adoption as an option for her child to choose the adoptive parents or to stipulate characteristics such as the religious or cultural background of the adoptive parents. In the prenatal setting, we should have available various counseling and agency resources to facilitate referral to appropriate resources based on the mother's desires (Fister and Schlomann, 1995).

Once given the requested information, a woman may need time to process and reflect on her options. She may have to deal with feelings of generalized anxiety or guilt about considering options that she may have previously dismissed at other times in her life. She may want to discuss her options with her partner, friend, family member, or spiritual counselor. It is important that she understand how she can access more information, either through care providers in the prenatal setting or by utilizing other resources. We should reiterate support for whatever decision the woman makes and reaffirm that she alone can make the best decision. If she is reluctant to consider further prenatal care at this time, we should develop a plan for further follow-up so that she is not abandoned (Beresford, 1995).

 ## THE INITIAL PRENATAL VISIT

A woman's first prenatal visit may occur at any point within a pregnancy. Some women seek prenatal care when they first suspect they may be pregnant. Others delay seeking care until they feel the need to interact with a health care provider. This may be near the end of the pregnancy or even at the start of labor. The time a woman chooses to seek care is based on her personal and cultural beliefs about pregnancy, her prior relationships with health care providers, her ability to get to the place where care is provided, availability of appointments that she can make, and her ability to pay for the care.

### Nursing Process Overview

Beginning with the initial visit, the process of assessment and education then continues throughout the pregnancy. Because of its vital importance, careful attention to detail is required. As nurses we must practice within the framework of professional standards of the specialty. The *Standards and Guidelines* (Association of Women's Health, Obstetrical, and Neonatal Nurses [AWHONN], 1997) describe the care and professional performance for which all nurses are accountable. They are evidence-based and provide direction on how to meet the needs of patients and their families in ambulatory settings.

### Assessment

Assessment data are collected with interviews, physical examination, and laboratory tests. Because the initial health history is so extensive, data may be collected initially through a questionnaire. This allows the woman to write down information as she waits to see a provider and helps her to begin the process of recalling her pertinent health history. Then as we review the information with the woman during the interview, we can encourage her to expand on the information she has provided and clarify her responses. Assessment and teaching occur simultaneously. Through the interactive interview, a therapeutic relationship is initiated. The woman and her support system will value the prenatal visits and become more active participants in prenatal care if the purpose of all assessments is explained (Box 9-3).

**BOX 9-3**   *Focus of Assessments at First Prenatal Visit*

**HISTORY**
Woman's chief concern
Current pregnancy: gestational age and growth
**Past pregnancies:** history and outcomes
**Gynecologic history:** past problems or surgery on breasts or reproductive organs, sexually transmitted diseases (STDs), pelvic inflammatory disease, Pap smear, use of contraception, risk for STDs
**Family profile:** marital status, father of the baby, current sexual relationship with partner
**Current medical history:** blood type, allergies, hypertension, diabetes, asthma, epilepsy, and other conditions the woman reports
**Past medical history:** childhood diseases, immunizations, surgical procedures, presence of bleeding disorders
**Medical history of the father of the baby:** age, general health, occupation, presence of genetic conditions or diseases, blood type and Rh factor
**Mother's family medical history:** presence of medical conditions, experiences with reproduction
**Cultural/religious expectations:** prescriptive beliefs, restrictive beliefs, and taboos; religious beliefs and expectations
**Occupational history:** screen for working conditions, exposure to toxic substances and diseases
**Personal habits/risks:** seat belt use, exercise, eating habits, caffeine intake, smoking—active and passive, alcohol consumption, use of medications and drugs
**Personal information:** support system, living accommodations, pets in the home, economic resources, personal safety
**Physical Examination:** vital signs, height, weight, complete physical with internal examination
**Laboratory Screening Tests**
**Assessment of well-being of embryo/fetus**

### Nursing Diagnoses

Based on the collected data, nursing diagnoses may be formulated. Examples of diagnoses that may be relevant during an initial prenatal visit include health-seeking behaviors related to exercise during pregnancy, knowledge deficit related to nutritional needs during pregnancy, decisional conflict related to unintended pregnancy, or risk for caregiver role strain related to the care of an aging parent. The woman confirms the correctness of your diagnoses as the interview process continues.

### Establishment of Goals and Implementation of Plans

The time frame of the first prenatal visit must be adequate to learn about the woman's health and possible

needs and also begin to develop a plan to meet those needs. Realistic goals and plans must include those people who are interested in providing support to the pregnant woman as well as the woman herself. Of primary importance is the establishment of a mutual goal that the prenatal visits will continue. The woman must agree with the importance of future prenatal visits and be able to schedule appointments that fit into her life. Unless she can see a value in the prenatal visits for herself and her developing child, she will not have an incentive to come.

### Implementation

A prenatal plan of care will (1) establish a baseline of the woman's current health status, (2) establish the developmental age and baseline status of the fetus, (3) identify possible risks to the woman or the fetus, (4) provide education and resources to the woman and her family, and (5) minimize the impact of these risks on the health of the woman or her fetus. Implementation will be individualized based on the needs of the woman and her support system.

### Evaluation

Evaluation of the care provided during the first prenatal visit should focus on the woman's commitment to a program of collaborative care for the duration of her pregnancy. In addition, she should also be able to respond to concerns or problems specific to her health or the health of her fetus. Examples include the following:

- Woman states that she will return for her next scheduled prenatal visit. Of course stating that she will return is only the beginning. The true evaluation of her acceptance and ability to participate will be when she actually does return.
- Woman states how she will contact the health care provider if she has concerns or experiences cramping or bleeding.

## Conducting the Initial Prenatal Assessment

Although the responsibility for various portions of the initial prenatal visit and the format for obtaining and recording the woman's health history differ from one practice to the next, the type of information deemed as necessary is universal.

### Risk Assessment

Risk is an inherent and integral component of all lived experiences, including pregnancy (Enkin, 1994). Different perceptions of risk can exist between the provider and the pregnant woman and her family. Many women with preexisting medical conditions such as diabetes mellitus, hypertension, and epilepsy consider pregnancy a normal process. They do not perceive that their prior medical conditions place them at greater risk during pregnancy. Conversely, other women who have no "risk factors" for pregnancy and birth may worry a great deal regarding possible risks to their pregnancy. They go through pregnancy with many anxieties after their friends and family members share tales of bad pregnancy and birth outcomes. Based on what they have heard, they cannot perceive that they could possibly go through this process without complications. We cannot arrive at an accurate assessment of a woman's perceived risk without observing how illness and health are linked to the cultural and social context of her identity and community (Spector, 1991).

**Risk factors** are any assessment findings that suggest that the pregnancy may have negative outcomes for either the mother or the fetus. The initial prenatal visit starts the process of identifying the risks the woman perceives as well as her actual risk factors. The major risk factors may be categorized as social-personal, preexisting medical disorders, prior obstetric occurrences, and incidents during the current pregnancy. Through support, education, monitoring, and therapeutic interventions, anxieties can be lowered and the gap between perceptions and reality can be reduced and outcomes improved.

If a woman's condition or her pregnancy is considered to be high risk for negative outcomes, the woman will require more frequent assessment and specific interventions. This nursing care is covered in Chapters 17 and 18.

### Age-Related Adjustments

How we word the questions and the order we follow will be determined in some part by the age and perspective of the pregnant woman. The level of maturity, comfort with her body, and knowledge of the reproductive process vary from one woman to the next, especially if she is an adolescent or an older woman.

To increase the acceptability of teaching materials, be sure that women at both ends of the age and/or educational spectrum can identify with the materials you give them. This necessitates that you have various teaching materials available.

***Pregnant Adolescents.*** A pregnant adolescent more often experiences poor maternal weight gain, premature birth, pregnancy induced hypertension, anemia, and sexually transmitted diseases (STDs). Their incidence of low birth weight is more than double the rate for adults, and the neonatal death rate is almost three times higher (Centers for Disease Control and Prevention [CDC], 1994). When the pregnant girl is younger than 17 years of age, she is at risk for a higher incidence of medical complications for herself and her infant than an adult woman.

Sexual abuse is a common cause of adolescent pregnancy, with up to 66% of pregnant girls reporting a history of abuse (Kenney, Reinholtz, and Angelini, 1997). Sexual abuse is also associated with greater risk-taking behaviors using alcohol and drugs. If a teenager is pregnant, consider that it may be due to sexual abuse and treat her with sensitivity.

***Pregnant Older Women.*** The woman who will be at least 35 years old at the time of her infant's birth is considered to be at an increased risk during the pregnancy. However, many women in their 30s and 40s have developed improved health habits and may be physically and nutritionally much fitter to bear children than they were in their 20s. One risk factor that gradually increases over the life span of the woman is the risk of chromosomal abnormalities that create conditions such as Down syndrome. It is not only the age of the woman, but also the age of the father of the baby, that is a factor. Some women may choose to have genetic testing early in the pregnancy to learn if the fetus has chromosomal abnormalities so that they may consider a therapeutic abortion.

### Learning Style

Early in the interview, ask the woman how she would like you to share information. Is she a visual learner who will feel more comfortable if you show her diagrams and pictures as you answer her questions and provide information? Or does she like to just hear explanations? Or does she prefer a combination of both? Don't assume that the woman can read, comprehend, and retain the information that you provide, at the pace at which you deliver it, or in the language you speak. For the best results in teaching, use various adult learning strategies in your teaching.

### Inclusion of Others

Often her partner, a family member, or a friend will accompany a woman to the prenatal visit. With the woman's permission, they may be encouraged to participate in a portion of the prenatal interview. They are often able to contribute information about the woman's health history or that of her family. In addition, they may use the opportunity to ask questions or express concerns. Inclusion as part of the team will enable them to provide the pregnant woman with more understanding and support within her home. However, there should always be a time during the interview when the woman is alone with you so that she may share private information and concerns.

## Components of the Visit

The health assessment includes a comprehensive review of the woman's current health status and history, screening for risk factors for the woman and the fetus, a physical examination, and laboratory tests (Figure 9-4). The health assessment of a pregnant woman should seek the same information we would obtain when a nonpregnant woman comes in for an annual examination (refer to the well-woman assessment in Chapter 4), plus additional information specific to the pregnancy. Because of the inclusive nature, this visit is lengthy and in more depth than subsequent prenatal visits.

**PRENATAL RECORD**

| Name | | Religion | Date |
|---|---|---|---|
| Address | | | Telephone |
| Occupation | Business address | | Business telephone |
| Husband's name | Business address | | Business telephone |
| Husband's occupation | | Referred by | |

| Age | Gravida | Para | Term | Premature | Abortions | Living |
|---|---|---|---|---|---|---|
| LMP | PMP | | Quickening | | EDD | |

Significant history

Significant findings

| Date | | | | | | | | | | | | | | |
|---|---|---|---|---|---|---|---|---|---|---|---|---|---|---|
| Wt. (   ) | | | | | | | | | | | | | | |
| BP | | | | | | | | | | | | | | |
| Edema | | | | | | | | | | | | | | |
| Ht. of fundus | | | | | | | | | | | | | | |
| Position | | | | | | | | | | | | | | |
| FH | | | | | | | | | | | | | | |
| Urine | Sug / Pro | | | | | | | | | | | | | |
| Gestation | | | | | | | | | | | | | | |
| Movement | | | | | | | | | | | | | | |
| Initials | | | | | | | | | | | | | | |
| RTC | | | | | | | | | | | | | | |

| Blood group | Rh | STS | Hgb. HCT. | Pap | HBsAg |
|---|---|---|---|---|---|
| Rubella | Glucloa | Alpha fetoprotein | | GC | HIV |
| PPD | Chest x-ray | Vitamin supplement | Breast/bottle | Anesthesia preference | Pediatrician |

Problem list

_____

_____

_____

_____

_____

_____

_____

_____

_____

_____

_____

[ ] Family planning information

*Continued*

FIGURE 9-4 • Sample of a prenatal record. *(From Lowdermilk DL, Perry SE, and Bobak IM: Maternity and women's health care, ed 7, St Louis, 2000, Mosby.)*

Name

| **Present Pregnancy** | | | | |
|---|---|---|---|---|
| Nausea: | | Vomiting: | Other symptoms of pregnancy: | |
| Bleeding: | | Cramping: | Pain: | Edema: |
| Pregnancy test | | Date | | |

**Previous Pregnancies**

| No. | Date delivered | Feeding | Sex | Wt. | Wks. preg. | Condition Birth | Condition Now | Duration of labor | Type of delivery | Remarks |
|---|---|---|---|---|---|---|---|---|---|---|
| 1 | | | | | | | | | | |
| 2 | | | | | | | | | | |
| 3 | | | | | | | | | | |
| 4 | | | | | | | | | | |
| 5 | | | | | | | | | | |
| 6 | | | | | | | | | | |

**Past History**

| Menstruation onset | | Frequency | | Duration | | Flow | | Pain | |
|---|---|---|---|---|---|---|---|---|---|
| Usual childhood illnesses | | Rheumatic fever | | Heart disease | | | Pulmonary disease | | |
| Convulsions | | Venereal disease | | Allergies | | | Blood transfusion | | |
| Injuries | | Operations | | Urinary disease | | | | | |
| Alcohol | | Smoking | | Drugs | | | Medication | | |

**Family History**

| Mother | | Father | | Siblings | | Other | |
|---|---|---|---|---|---|---|---|
| Diabetes | | | | Twins | | | |

**Physical Examination**

| General | Ht. | BP | Eyes | Fundi |
|---|---|---|---|---|
| Ears | Mouth | Teeth | Throat | Thyroid |
| Chest | Breasts | Nipples | Heart | Lungs |
| Abdomen | Extremities | | | |
| | | | | |
| | | | | |
| | | | | |

| Ext. genitalia | Perineum | |
|---|---|---|
| Vagina | Cervix | |
| Uterus | | |
| Adnexa | | |
| Bl          cm | DC          cm | Arch |
| Sacrum | | Spines |
| Post. sagittal | SS ligaments | Coccyx |

Signature

FIGURE 9-4, cont'd ● Sample of a prenatal record. (From Lowdermilk DL, Perry SE, and Bobak IM: Maternity and women's health care, ed 7, St Louis, 2000, Mosby.)

The initial assessment is so fundamentally important that some health providers may divide this initial prenatal visit into two, taking the health history, doing a pregnancy test, and providing basic pregnancy information at the first visit, and then performing a physical examination a week or so later. The client may have many initial concerns, so time should be allotted to answer both her questions and those of her partner. This sensitivity to their needs will enhance the growth of the therapeutic relationship and provide for a better collaboration during the pregnancy.

### Initiating the Interview Process

To set a positive tone, the interview should take place in a quiet and private room. Pregnancy is too personal and private an event to have the details discussed where others may overhear. Give the woman your name, tell her how she may address you, and explain your role in her care. Ask her what name she would like you to use when addressing her.

During the interview collect both subjective and objective data. The woman will tell you her appraisal of her health status and the events of her pregnancy—this is the **subjective data**. The **objective data** is what you observe—her affect, posture, body language, skin condition and color, and other physical and emotional indications of her health and well-being. Ask follow-up questions to clarify or enhance the data you collect.

### Chief Concern

Ask the woman directly why she has come for care and record her answer verbatim. This makes all providers aware of the woman's primary concern. Your follow-up question is then, "What prompted you to come today (not last week and not next week)?" This provides an indication of additional factors in her life that influence her ability to seek health care.

Her answer will also lead you to the next area of the interview. If she says that she thinks that she is pregnant based on presumptive signs or a home pregnancy test, ask questions in that area. Ask about the current pregnancy, past pregnancies, and her gynecologic history.

In comparison, if her response refers to her partner, family, or friends, follow her lead and obtained the information about her social history or family profile. Before the interview is complete you will have obtained the necessary information in all areas. However, it flows more easily and is more comprehensive if it follows her train of thought.

### Current Pregnancy

A review of her symptoms and how she has responded to them provides an opportunity for education and the basis of a plan of care. We need to learn:

- The first day of her LNMP (Have a calendar available so that she can figure it out if necessary.)

- Any cramping, spotting, or bleeding since her LNMP?
- The history of her menstrual periods (age at menarche, frequency of cycles, duration of flow, quantity of flow).
- The date when she thinks she conceived and when she thinks she is due.
- Her contraceptive history—method(s), last time used, dates of unprotected intercourse.
- Her feelings about being pregnant—Was it planned? Does she have mixed feelings?
- Any discomforts since her LNMP (e.g., nausea, vomiting, fatigue, frequent urination)?

Ask her if she is experiencing any other symptoms that she is concerned about. Explore their onset and occurrence in relation to the pregnancy.

### Past Pregnancies

Just because a woman is young or unmarried, you cannot assume that this is her first pregnancy. Also you cannot assume that the information she provides to you in front of other people is the most accurate or complete. A woman that has had a prior pregnancy may, for a variety of reasons, not want other people to know. We need to protect her privacy while also allowing her to confide her true history. How and where you record the information she would like to keep private is very important. Be honest with her as to who will have access to it.

The following terms are used to define and record an obstetric history:

- **Gravidity** (G): the number of times that a woman has been pregnant
- **Gravida:** a pregnant woman
- **Primigravida:** a woman pregnant for the first time
- **Multigravida:** a woman who is in her second or a subsequent pregnancy
- **Nulligravida:** a woman who has never conceived a child
- **Parity** (P): the number of pregnancies that reach 20 weeks or viability (500 g birthweight)
- **Para:** a woman who has given birth to an infant weighing at least 500 g after carrying a pregnancy 20 weeks or more, regardless of whether the fetus was born alive or dead
- **Nullipara:** a woman who has never produced a viable infant
- **Primipara:** a woman who has had one birth after 20 weeks of gestation, regardless of whether it was born dead or alive
- **Multipara:** a woman who has carried two or more pregnancies past 20 weeks of gestation or viability
- **Abortion** (AB): a birth that occurs before the end of 20 weeks of gestation. It may be either a **therapeutic abortion (TAB)** or a **spontaneous abortion (SAB)**, often called a miscarriage.

Sometimes the age of viability, generally 24 weeks of gestation or a fetus weighing more than 500 g, is used as the determinant as to whether to label the pregnancy loss as a SAB or as stillborn.

- **Stillborn:** a birth of a dead fetus after 20 weeks of gestation or size of viability.

Document her pregnancies with respect to the number of times she has been pregnant, including the current pregnancy (gravida) and the number of children she has delivered after 20 weeks or age of viability (para). For example, Sara, who is currently pregnant, has previously experienced a TAB and a SAB and the birth of a baby at 40 weeks. Her documentation would be: G 4, P 1, AB 2 or for more specificity G 4, P 1, TAB 1, SAB 1. In contrast, Helen, who is currently pregnant and has previously delivered a full-term live boy and a set of triplet girls at 36 weeks, would be: G 3, P 4. Remember, the terms gravida and para refer to the number of times pregnant, not the number of fetuses carried. Twins, triplets, and more count as one pregnancy and one birth.

If a woman has been pregnant before but does not wish her current partner to know, her status is called a "social" gravida 1. Providers can adjust their assessments and interventions appropriately, but the woman's secret is kept from the partner, family members, or friends.

Some documentation forms require a more detailed approach. In that case the gravida remains the same, but the meaning of the para changes to mean the number of infants born rather than the number of deliveries. The acronym to remember is TPALM with the following meanings:

- **T:** the number of pregnancies ending after 37 weeks of gestation, at term
- **P:** the number of preterm pregnancies ending after 20 weeks or viability but before the completion of 37 weeks
- **A:** the number of pregnancies ending before 20 weeks or viability, either SABs or TABs
- **L:** the number of children currently living
- **M:** the number of multiple pregnancies

Sara, who is currently pregnant, has previously experienced a TAB and a SAB and the birth of a living son at 40 weeks. Her documentation would be G 4, T 1, P 0, A 2, L 1 M 0, or more simply recorded, Gravida 3 Para 10210. Helen, who is currently pregnant and has previously delivered a full-term live boy and a set of triplet girls at 36 weeks, would be G 3, T 1, P3, A 0, L 4, M 1, or Gravida 3 Para 13041.

***Prior Pregnancy Experiences.*** Ask the woman about her experiences with prior pregnancies. Did she experience labor before 38 weeks; a bleeding problem during pregnancy, labor, or delivery; or postpartum depression? Once one of these events has occurred, there is a greater chance that the event will happen again.

If she has experienced either an abortion or miscarriage she may have increased anxiety about this pregnancy. Women who have suffered a prior loss, such as miscarriage, stillbirth, or a previous termination, may need to process and share their experience with a sympathetic provider before participating fully in the current pregnancy. If the woman is still actively grieving, it is important that we have resources available to assist with grief counseling. There are often support groups established within churches and maternal-child health centers that may help (Cote-Arsenault and Mahlangu, 1999).

***Prior Labor and Delivery Experiences.*** Ask about her prior labor and delivery experiences. Was she satisfied with the arrangements? What expectations does she have for this pregnancy and birth? Learning her options and then helping her make the necessary arrangements facilitate her having the experience she wants. Be alert to connections between prior experiences and the current pregnancy. Provide anticipatory guidance and support that help alleviate fear and anxiety. Refer her to specific educational and birth support resources that may assist her.

### Gynecologic History

***Breast and Reproductive Organs.*** Ask about breast problems; infertility problems; gynecologic problems; and past surgeries on the breast or reproductive tract, including the fallopian tubes, uterus, and cervix.

***Sexually Transmitted Diseases.*** Ask if she has been treated for sexually transmitted infections (STIs) or pelvic inflammatory disease (PID). It is important to learn which ones and when. When asking about STIs, be sure to include hepatitis B and HIV.

Also ask the woman if she is currently at risk for acquiring an infection. It is important to identify a potential risk because STIs can cause premature labor, premature births, and problems with the health of the newborn. Most often if the infection is treated during pregnancy, the problem can be prevented.

All women who enter prenatal care should be offered screening for STIs as part of their laboratory work. When an infection is found, the CDC recommends specific treatment guidelines for pregnant women (CDC, 1998). Each woman should also be offered an HIV test. Transmission of the AIDS virus to the newborn can be prevented when detected early and responded to appropriately.

***Papanicolaou Smear.*** Specific information about the date and results of her last Papanicolaou (Pap) smear is important. Also learn if she has ever had a report of an abnormality and, if so, how it was treated. Ask if it might be possible for her to have the records sent from another facility so that her chart will be more complete.

***Contraception.*** Develop a history of her methods of contraception. What method(s) was she using when she became pregnant? What has she used in the past?

What has caused her to change from one method to another? Common reasons are availability, cost, comfort level with the method, partner preference, and comments of members of her family or support system. Determine what factors may lead her to have unprotected intercourse.

This line of questioning will possibly raise the topic of how she became pregnant, the father of the baby, and information about the woman's family. These details are part of her social history or family profile.

## Family Profile

When the woman's family profile is established early in the interview process, a more individualized assessment and series of interventions may be offered. With whom she lives, whom she considers her primary resource, and who provides her social support are all important aspects of her situation. Persons offering social support may include a sister, a girlfriend, her mother, and/or her partner.

*Marital Status.* Asking if she is married may be awkward and only provides information of limited value. Asking instead, "Who else lives with you?" is not only less awkward but also provides the desired information, while giving a more realistic description of her situation. The unmarried woman may respond my partner, or my boyfriend, or my parents and sister. The married woman may respond my husband and my in-laws; or my 3-year-old son and, when he's not on the road, my husband.

*Father of the Baby.* Another potentially awkward question that must be answered if she has a husband or male partner is, "Is your partner the father of the baby?" If the pregnant woman has a female partner the question is, "Do you have access to or know the health history of the man who provided the sperm?" Further questions about the health history of the father of the baby may be found later in the development of this client profile.

*Current Sexual Relationship with Partner.* A woman can remain sexually active during her pregnancy. Whether she chooses to do so and how she chooses to express her sexuality will vary depending on her own feelings, the cultural beliefs she follows, the method by which she became pregnant, the feelings of her partner, the history of prior pregnancies, and the events of this pregnancy.

Ask the woman questions such as, "What have you been told about having sex during pregnancy?" Ask her about her current sexual activity. Is she currently experiencing intercourse with one or more partners? Is this a comfortable experience for her or is she having pain? Is she at risk for being exposed to STIs? Is she using condoms to protect herself and her baby from being infected?

Encourage her to ask questions if she has concerns. Let her know that intercourse during pregnancy is usually considered safe unless she experiences vaginal bleeding or the onset of labor. Also make her aware that during pregnancy not only may her libido, but also the libido of her partner, may vary. Provide the woman with written information or resources so that in private she can learn more about how to be physically and emotionally comfortable. A good resource is the book, *Woman's Experience of Sex* (Kitzinger, 1995).

## Current Medical History

As it becomes more common for women to delay pregnancy, more women enter pregnancy with previously diagnosed medical conditions. Women may present with medical problems such as allergies, hypertension, diabetes, asthma, or epilepsy. The medication or treatment requirements for these conditions may need to be adjusted during the pregnancy. A good baseline assessment followed by close monitoring is essential to ensure the health of the woman and the growing fetus. The following sections discuss some of the pre-pregnancy conditions that can contribute to increased risk during pregnancy.

*Blood Type.* The woman's blood type and Rh factor are determined by the laboratory work. However, if she states that she is Rh negative, we need to learn if she knows if she has ever been pregnant with the child of a man who is Rh positive (even if she had an early spontaneous or therapeutic abortion) or if she has had a blood transfusion.

*Allergies.* Allergies to medications, pollen, environmental sources, or latex should be reviewed. How does her allergic reaction manifest itself? How does she prevent and/or treat the allergic responses? With an increasing number of people developing allergies to latex, it is important to determine if she has a reaction to this substance so that the gloves and equipment we use when working with her do not cause her harm.

*Hypertension.* Hypertension occurs in approximately 10% of pregnancies. Classification of hypertension during pregnancy is divided into four categories: (1) chronic hypertension; (2) preeclampsia and eclampsia, which are medical complications of pregnancy; (3) preeclampsia, superimposed on chronic hypertension; or (4) transient hypertension. Medications for hypertension that are generally considered safe in pregnancy are hydralazine, labetalol, and alpha-methyldopa. Over the past 10 years, studies of children exposed to alpha-methyldopa in utero have not revealed any apparent mental or physical abnormality (The Sixth Report of the Joint National Committee on the Prevention, Detection, Evaluation, and Treatment of High Blood Pressure, 1997).

*Diabetes.* The maintenance of an euglycemic state is of critical importance in pregnant women with diabetes mellitus. Congenital abnormalities such as cardiac defects are associated with maternal hyperglycemia. If a woman is able to adhere to a diet adjusted for the nutritional requirements of pregnancy, participate in regular exercise, and use insulin, she can generally maintain glycemic control. Insulin does not cross the placenta, so its use does not pose a risk to the fetus. It is recommended that the woman's fasting blood sugar levels should be maintained at less than 100 mg/dl, and her postprandial blood sugar levels should be maintained at less than 120 mg/dl before conception and throughout the pregnancy (Report of the Expert Committee on the Diagnoses and Classification of Diabetes Mellitus, 1997).

*Asthma.* Asthma complicates approximately 1% to 4% of pregnancies with variable effects. Therapy for asthma is similar in both the pregnant and nonpregnant state (National Asthma Education Program, 1993). Ask the woman about the triggers for her asthma and explore with her ways that she may be able to minimize her exposure to them. It is important to treat maternal asthma aggressively during pregnancy because the risk of hypoxia to the fetus is greater than the risk of the treatment medications. Information on the medications or alternative remedies she is currently using or has recently discontinued because of the pregnancy should be noted. A woman may have abruptly stopped all use of medication because of concern for her baby. In reality, it may be more beneficial for her to continue her medication or follow a specific tapering regimen, such as that seen with steroid use, than to suddenly stop.

*Epilepsy.* Epilepsy complicates approximately 0.15% of pregnancies. Some anticonvulsants have been found to harm the fetus. It is essential that women with a seizure disorder have an effective medication prescribed to control the seizures while imposing the least risk to the fetus (Kochenour, 1994).

*Other.* Ask her about possible exposure to diethylstilbesterol (DES). Did her mother take DES when she was pregnant with her? Also ask about other health problems such as hypothyroidism; lupus erythematosus; cardiac conditions; anemia; a history of thrombus or coagulation disorders; gall bladder disease; phenylketonuria; tuberculosis; renal disease; mental illness; and previous injuries, especially to the pelvic area or upper leg (Fogel and Woods, 1995). A positive response to any of these conditions should lead to further questions in that area to learn the history and current treatment.

## Past Medical History

*Childhood Diseases.* Ask the woman if she has had the childhood diseases or received the immunizations for chickenpox (varicella), mumps (epidemic parotitis), measles (rubeola), German measles (rubella), or poliomyelitis. Her response will help estimate her risk of contracting one of these diseases while pregnant. If she becomes ill with one of these diseases during the first trimester, it could have harmful effects on the developing fetus. While pregnant, the only immunization for childhood diseases that she may receive is the Salk vaccine for poliomyelitis because the virus is dead. She cannot be immunized against the other childhood diseases while pregnant because they use live virus. She should be instructed to stay away from children as much as possible because they may spread the virus to her before they appear sick themselves.

*Other Immunizations.* Ask her about her history of immunizations. Past immunizations should be documented and the need for additional immunizations determined at this time. If deemed necessary, killed virus or bacteria preparations are probably safe for use during pregnancy. If a woman has multiple sexual partners, uses intravenous drugs or has a partner who does so, or is exposed to blood products at work, it is recommended that she be given the hepatitis B vaccine (CDC, 1997). Tetanus-diphtheria, rabies, and pneumococcal and influenza vaccines are also considered safe to administer, if the woman is at risk during pregnancy. Pneumococcal and influenza vaccines are recommended for pregnant women who have asthma, diabetes, cardiac disease, and renal disease (Friede and others, 1997).

*Surgical Procedures.* Information about past surgeries is important, especially if it was abdominal surgery. Adhesions may affect the expansion of the uterus or cause the mother pain. Asking about surgeries may also remind the woman about other medical events in her history plus give an indication if she has had a negative response to anesthesia.

*Presence of Bleeding Disorders.* The placental site provides an opportunity for bleeding to occur during pregnancy or the birth. Any prior problem with coagulation is important information. Also ask if she has received any blood transfusions and, if so, what year.

## Medical History of the Father of the Baby

The age and general health of the father of the baby must also be learned when considering potential problems with the baby. His health history should include significant health problems and the presence of genetic conditions or diseases. What is his blood type and Rh factor?

Ask about previous or present alcohol intake, drug and/or tobacco use. If the father of the baby uses tobacco products and lives with the mother, where does he smoke? Is she exposed to second-hand smoke? What is his occupation?

The answers to these questions help to determine toxins the woman may be exposed to every day. What level of education has he completed? What is his attitude toward this pregnancy? How involved will he be? What teaching methods would he like used to teach about the changes in the pregnant woman and the developing child? What will be his anticipated role during the delivery?

## Mother's Family Medical History

A family history documents illness that occurs frequently in the woman's family and helps identify potential problems that also may occur in the woman during pregnancy or birth. It is also important to ascertain the ethnicity of both parents, so that screening for conditions such as thalassemia, Tay Sachs disease, and sickle cell disease can be offered when appropriate.

***Presence of Medical Conditions.*** The current presence of an infectious disease, such as tuberculosis or hepatitis B, in a family member requires appropriate testing and counseling. The main reason to ask about past family medical history is to determine the presence of hereditary conditions or diseases. Is there a history of congenital disease or deformities? Learning of the presence of diabetes, cardiovascular disease, or hematologic disease within family members is also important.

***Experiences With Reproduction.*** Ask about the experience of sisters and mothers during pregnancy and birth. A diagnosis of preeclampsia or pregnancy-induced hypertension appears to have a hereditary component and occurs within family groups. Record in the woman's chart if either her mother or a sister had that experience.

Also of importance is how the women in her family viewed their pregnancy and birth. Their experiences provide the cultural basis from which this woman will approach her reproductive experience and will affect not only the way she anticipates events but also how she prepares for the experience. Also learn how they are helping with this woman's pregnancy.

Determine if there is a history of multiple births. If so, were they fraternal or identical multiples? The tendency to ovulate more than one ovum in a cycle and have fraternal multiples can be passed on from a woman to her daughter.

### Cultural/Religious Expectations

To provide prenatal nursing care that is culturally relevant we have to understand cultural needs in the context of the beliefs of the client and her family, and then collaborate in creating strategies that meet those needs. Actions by a woman or her family members during pregnancy may be influenced by either their cultural and/or personal beliefs.

It is important not to make assumptions about a woman's beliefs based on information about her culture. Behavioral norms concerning pregnancy vary within a culture as well as across generations. When the parents of the baby are from two different cultures they may pick and choose the customs to follow, choosing from one or both cultures. Communication patterns, use of conversational space, time orientation, family orientation, male-female roles, religion, health beliefs, nutritional practices, and responses to pain are all factors that have implications during prenatal care. In addition, a woman may be strongly influenced by her culture as to how active a role she is expected or wishes to play in her pregnancy.

All cultures recognize pregnancy as a special transition period, and many have customs and beliefs that dictate the activity and behavior of the woman and sometimes her partner. There are prescriptive beliefs, restrictive beliefs, and taboos. These beliefs affect sexual and lifestyle behaviors during pregnancy, birthing, and the immediate postpartum. These beliefs also influence the nursing care that we provide during pregnancy (Andrews and Boyle, 1995; Purnell and Paulanka, 1998).

***Prescriptive Beliefs.*** **Prescriptive** beliefs are positive statements about what should be done. Prescriptive beliefs may involve wearing special articles of clothing, such as the *muneco* worn by some traditional Hispanic women, to prevent morning sickness and ensure a safe

---

### BOX 9-4 *Cultural Beliefs about Activity and Pregnancy*

**PRESCRIPTIVE BELIEFS**
- Remain active during pregnancy to aid the baby's circulation (Crow Indian).
- Remain happy to bring the baby joy and good fortune (Pueblo and Navajo Indians, Mexican, Japanese).
- Sleep flat on your back to protect the baby (Mexican).
- Keep active during pregnancy to ensure a small baby and an easy delivery (Mexican).
- Continue sexual intercourse to lubricate the birth canal and prevent dry labor (Haitian, Mexican).
- Continue daily baths and frequent shampoos during pregnancy to produce a clean baby (Filipino).

**RESTRICTIVE BELIEFS**
- Avoid cold air during pregnancy (Mexican, Haitian, Asian).
- Do not reach over your head or the cord will wrap around the baby's neck (black, Hispanic, white, Asian).
- Avoid weddings and funerals or you will bring bad fortune to the baby (Vietnamese).

- Do not continue sexual intercourse or harm will come to you and the baby (Vietnamese, Filipino, Samoan).
- Do not tie knots or braid or allow the baby's father to do so because it will cause difficult labor (Navajo Indian).
- Do not sew (Pueblo Indian, Asian).

**TABOOS**
- Avoid lunar eclipses and moonlight or the baby may be born with a deformity (Mexican).
- Don't walk on the streets at noon or five o'clock because this may make the spirits angry (Vietnamese).
- Don't join in traditional ceremonies like Yei or Squaw dances or spirits will harm the baby (Navajo Indian).
- Don't get involved with persons who cast spells or the baby will be eaten in the womb (Haitian).
- Don't say the baby's name before the naming ceremony or harm might come to the baby (Orthodox Jewish).
- Don't have your picture taken because it might cause stillbirth (black).

Purnell LD and Paulanka BJ: *Transcultural health care,* Philadelphia, 1998, FA Davis.

delivery. Or they may involve following certain practices, such as the belief among Polish-American women that they should seek preventive care, eat well, and get adequate rest. Other beliefs involve special rituals, such as the White Shell Woman Way ceremony among traditional Navajos.

***Restrictive Beliefs.*** **Restrictive beliefs** are statements about what the mother can't do if she wants a healthy pregnancy and baby. They cover a wide range of individual activities, including work and sexual, emotional, and environmental constraints. A restrictive belief among the Navajos forbids preparing for the infant before its birth; therefore clothes should not be purchased nor other preparations made during pregnancy. Some families of Latin-American descent believe that if the father sees the mother or baby before they are cleaned up after delivery, it can cause harm to the baby or mother (Andrews and Boyle, 1995; Purnell and Paulanka, 1998).

***Taboos.*** **Taboos** are restrictions that if not obeyed pose the threat of serious negative consequences to the mother or baby. Hispanics believe that an early baby shower will invite bad luck. Orthodox Jews avoid baby showers and divulging the baby's name before the infant's naming ceremony (Andrews and Boyle, 1995; Purnell and Paulanka, 1998). Box 9-4 provides a sampling of various cultural beliefs.

Explore with every woman her views of pregnancy and the practices that she observes, as well as the expectations of her family and her culture. Encourage her to identify for you the prescriptive and restrictive beliefs and taboos that influence her choice in foods, exercise, intercourse, and possible avoidance of weather-related conditions.

When her activity is not harmful, there is no reason to indicate to the woman that she should change. If the activity is potentially harmful, consult and work with someone from her culture to help determine ways to modify the woman's behavior or to find an alternative.

Explore with the woman her plans for the birth. Learn her expectations for the event. What care does she expect for herself? What care does she expect for her baby? What does her partner expect?

Determine whether she wants to have a specific religion specified in her records and what it is. She may want a specific group listed, such as Orthodox Jewish, rather than a general designation such as Jewish. Other general designations are Christian, Muslim or Buddhist. Does she have any religious beliefs or practices that might influence her health care or that of her child? Does she have any prohibitions against receiving blood products? Does she have dietary considerations? Are there special baptism rites, naming rituals, or circumcision rites? When are they performed and who will perform them?

## Occupational History

Questions regarding the client's and her partner's work outside the home and the environments in which she and her family live and work in should be reviewed to screen for possible areas of stress to the woman as well as exposure to toxic substances. **Teratogens** are substances that are known to cause abnormal development in the fetus. Teratogens can be environmental, viral, pharmacologic, or socially induced agents (Stevenson, 1998) (Table 9-1).

Many women have concerns regarding what is safe in pregnancy, especially environmentally. Questions may arise on fumigation of apartments, the safety of painting, and use of hair dyes (Figure 9-5). A Pregnancy Environmental Hotline provides current information on teratogens, as does the March of Dimes.

Learn the number of hours and when during the day the woman works. What type of work does she do?

### TABLE 9-1 *Chemical and Physical Agents that are Reproductive Hazards for Women in the Workplace*

| Agent | Observed effects | Potentially exposed workers |
|---|---|---|
| Cancer treatment drugs (e.g., methotrexate) | Infertility, miscarriage, birth defects, low birth weight | Health care workers, pharmacists |
| Certain ethylene glycol ethers such as 2-ethoxyethanol (2EE) and 2-methoxyethanol (2ME) | Miscarriages | Electronic and semiconductor workers |
| Carbon disulfide ($CS_2$) | Menstrual cycle changes | Viscose rayon workers |
| Lead | Infertility, miscarriage, low birth weight, developmental disorders | Battery makers, solderers, welders, radiator repairers, bridge repainters, firing range workers, home remodelers |
| Ionizing radiation (e.g., X-rays and gamma rays) | Infertility, miscarriage, birth defects, low birth weight, developmental disorders, childhood cancers | Health care workers, dental personnel, atomic workers |
| Strenuous physical labor (e.g., prolonged standing, heavy lifting) | Miscarriage late in pregnancy, premature delivery | Many types of workers |

DHHS (NIOSH): *The effects of workplace hazards on female reproductive health,* Publication No 99-104, 1999.

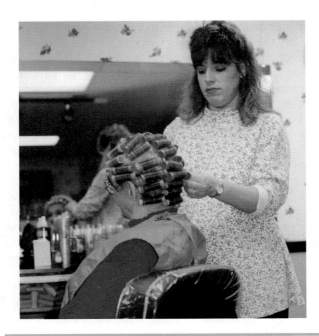

FIGURE 9-5 • A woman exposed to toxic substances at work. *(Courtesy of Caroline E. Brown.)*

Some workplaces may expose women to disease-causing agents that are reproductive hazards (Table 9-2).

Explore if her work involves strenuous activity, such as being a mother to a 2-year-old child or an aerobics teacher, the chronic heavy lifting of a postal worker, or long periods of stationary inactivity. Provide appropriate guidance for her comfort and safety.

Learn about possible restrictions at work that may increase the discomforts of her pregnancy. Are there opportunities in her day for rest? Can she elevate her legs? Can she take bathroom breaks when she needs them? What happens if she is nauseous? Does she have the opportunity for nutritious snacks and lunch? Does she have help at home? Is maternity leave an option? Does she think she will be able to take leave if necessary before the birth?

 ### Personal Habits

In a woman's normal activities of daily living she makes choices concerning her health. Some are advantageous to her health and the developing baby and others are not. The use of caffeine, OTC drugs, cigarettes, and alcohol is sanctioned by society, but is potentially harmful to a developing fetus. When she is unaware of the negative affect on her baby, her use of these choices continues. Research has shown that in the early stages of pregnancy women are very motivated to change their health habits if they know the risks (Fingerhut, Kleinman, and Kendrick, 1990).

When asking about her habits make the questions open-ended. Keep your tone conversational and nonjudgmental. Follow up each response with another ap-

propriate question and develop a dialogue that provides the information you need.

Whenever possible, praise her actions and choices. Almost no woman will be making dangerous decisions in all of the following categories. Complimenting her, as appropriate, helps reinforce positive behavior and encourages further discussion and education. As your relationship continues to develop it can have a positive effect on her personal habits.

*Seat Belt Use.* Seven percent of women sustain trauma during pregnancy, and between 1300 to 3900 annual incidents of fetal demise occur secondary to motor vehicle accidents (MVAs) each year (Pearlman and Phillips, 1996). The mortality rate for persons ejected during an MVA is 33%, whereas, when a person is not ejected, it is 7%. The fetal mortality rate is 47% when a woman does not wear a seat belt and is ejected, and is 11% when a woman remains in the vehicle. It is clear that pregnant women need to be encouraged to use and wear seat belts.

Ask her if she wears a seat belt when in a car. Does she do it every time? She will be more likely to wear a seat belt if she understands the risk and knows how to put the belt on comfortably. She should wear the lap belt under her abdomen and across her upper thighs. The shoulder component should fit snugly between the breasts (Tyroch and others, 1999).

*Exercise.* The physical shape that a woman is in when she starts her pregnancy determines how she will feel during the pregnancy. Learn what she does for physical activity now. Does she follow a regular exercise program? What type? How often does she exercise? How long does she exercise? How does it feel? Does she have any concerns that may lead her to stop?

*Nutrition.* Pregnancy is one of the most nutritionally demanding periods of a woman's life and the nutrition of the mother directly affects the development of the fetus. Because the woman may be particularly receptive to monitoring or changing her eating habits while she is pregnant, nutrition education and support for good eating should be part of every prenatal visit. The basic principles of good nutrition—balance of food groups, variety of foods, and moderation in consumption—should be encouraged during pregnancy and they may become lifelong habits both for herself and her child (ific, 1995).

Ask the pregnant woman to provide a list of all the foods and beverages she has eaten in a 24-hour period. This 24-hour recall is the quickest and simplest method for obtaining a food intake history. Unfortunately it may also be misleading because most individuals are unable to accurately remember everything they consumed the day before. A food diary is much more accurate. Have the woman record all of her food and beverage intake for 3 days, including 1 weekend day. They do not have to be consecutive days. She should then bring that with her to the next visit.

Review the food diary with her and determine where the food was eaten, how much was eaten, and how it

**TABLE 9-2**   *Disease-Causing Agents that are Reproductive Hazards for Women in the Workplace*

| Agent | Observed effects | Potentially exposed workers | Preventive measures |
|---|---|---|---|
| Cytomegalovirus (CMV) | Birth defects, low birth weight, developmental disorders | Health care workers, workers in contact with infants and children | Good hygienic practices such as handwashing |
| Hepatitis B virus | Low birth weight | Health care workers | Vaccination |
| Human immunodeficiency virus (HIV) | Low birth weight, childhood cancer | Health care workers | Practice universal precautions |
| Human parvovirus B19 | Miscarriage | Health care workers, workers in contact with infants and children | Good hygienic practices such as handwashing |
| Rubella (German measles) | Birth defects, low birth weight | Health care workers, workers in contact with infants and children | Vaccination before pregnancy if no prior immunity |
| Toxoplasmosis | Miscarriage, birth defects, developmental disorders | Animal care workers, veterinarians | Good hygiene practices such as handwashing |
| Varicella-zoster virus (chicken pox) | Birth defects, low birth weight | Health care workers, workers in contact with infants and children | Vaccination before pregnancy if no prior immunity |

DHHS (NIOSH): *The effects of workplace hazards on female reproductive health,* Publication No 99-104, 1999.

was prepared (e.g., baked, fried, raw). Are there any foods that she is missing? If she is avoiding certain foods that would be good for her? Explore why that is.

Some cultures prohibit the eating of certain foods during pregnancy. Chinese-American woman avoid eating shellfish during the first trimester because they believe it causes allergies. Following a diet based on "hot" and "cold" foods and "tonic" or "wind" foods, Vietnamese-Americans choose to eat different foods at different times in their pregnancy. During the first trimester the pregnant woman is considered to be weak and cold. She corrects the imbalance by eating "hot" foods such as mangoes, grapes, ginger, peppers, alcohol, and coffee. To provide energy and food for the fetus she eats "tonic" foods, which include a basic diet of steamed rice and pork. "Wind" foods are avoided throughout pregnancy because they are associated with convulsions, allergic reactions, asthma, and other health problems. Leafy green vegetables, fruit, beef, mutton, fowl, fish, and glutinous rice are all part of the "wind" food group (Purnell and Paulanka, 1998). If the woman has strong cultural beliefs, asking her to eat "cold" foods or "wind" foods would probably not be successful.

A woman who eats a vegetarian diet will be following a different pattern of food selection. A **lacto-ovo vegetarian** (a person who eats milk and egg products along with other foods) and a **lacto-vegetarian** (a person who eats milk products but not eggs along with other foods) will be able to meet all of her nutritional needs for proteins. If the woman is a **vegan** (eats no food from animal sources), she should consult with a dietician to ensure that her diet has the adequate amount of pro-

tein and essential vitamins and minerals to support the growth of a baby (ific, 1995).

Recommendations for weight gain are based on a woman's prepregnancy weight and height as well as the number of fetuses she is carrying. On average, the increased demands of pregnancy require an additional 300 kcal per day. Women who are pregnant with twins or a higher number of multiples will need an additional 300 kcal per fetus per day. Weight gain will occur over the course of the pregnancy.

The pregnant woman requires about 1.2 g of calcium and phosphorus every day during pregnancy, and a well-balanced diet generally can satisfy these requirements. Demineralization of the teeth does not occur during pregnancy. Contrary to a popular myth, if a woman loses a tooth, it is related to gingivitis and poor dental hygiene.

Reviewing her dietary intake provides an opportunity to ask if the woman has a history of anorexia or bulimia. If this is acknowledged, address concerns about these issues and refer her to counseling or a nutritionist as needed. Similarly for the overweight client the pregnancy can be a motivating factor to increase activity and change eating patterns.

The routine of weighing a woman at each prenatal visit provides an unwarranted stress for most clients. It may be beneficial to abandon this procedure so that women do not delay or avoid prenatal care, and rely on other, more reliable parameters to assess maternal and fetal well-being.

*Caffeine.* Because of the negative effect on fetal weight gain, a woman often reduces her level of caffeine intake (coffee, tea, cocoa, and colas) during pregnancy. Caffeine should be limited to one to two cups of coffee or caffeinated drinks per day (Hally, 1998). However, the woman should not substitute for these beverages with an increased use of herbal teas. Some of the herbs consumed in teas, capsules, and tinctures contain substances that could affect the developing infant. She should consider the use of these items as self-medication and speak with a health care provider concerning the use of particular teas.

When asking about caffeine intake use nonjudgmental questions such as How many cups of coffee (tea) do you drink a day? Is it regular or decaffeinated? How large are the cups?

*Smoking.* Smoking is a major preventable cause of fetal injury and death. Smoking during pregnancy reduces fetal weight gain and places a constant stress on the fetus because of the reduction of oxygen and nutrients available to the fetus. Women who are exposed to smoke are more likely to have a spontaneous abortion and deliver a low–birth-weight infant (Ward, 1999). The low birth weight of the baby may be due to either premature birth or to intrauterine growth restriction. Even exposure to passive smoking in early pregnancy may increase the risk of a small-for-gestational-age infant (Dejin-Karlson and others, 1998).

Nicotine and carbon monoxide are the major components of tobacco smoke that cause fetal injury. Nicotine causes peripheral and uterine vasoconstriction. Carbon monoxide binds with hemoglobin to produce carboxihemoglobin, which reduces the oxygen-carrying capacity of maternal hemoglobin to fetal tissue (Walsh, 1994). Pregnancy for many women provides an impetus to stop smoking, and 20% to 40% of pregnant smokers stop before their first prenatal visit. Unfortunately, up to 25% of those who stop start again during pregnancy and up to 70% smoke within the first postpartum year (Fingerhut, Kleinman, and Kendrick, 1990).

To determine if a woman is smoking tobacco, ask her directly. How often does she smoke cigarettes? Does she use other tobacco products (this would include chew and cigars)? How many (or how much) does she use per day? How often is she around others who smoke? Is she able to leave the room when others are smoking?

Traditional interventions such as smoking cessation classes have proven ineffective among pregnant women. Women are more successful when counseling sessions that offer coping techniques and skills and educational materials that are specific to pregnant women are combined and offered over the course of the pregnancy (Dolan-Mullen, Ramirez, and Groff, 1994). At each prenatal visit provide continuous supportive counseling to assist women to reduce or stop smoking.

When a woman feels she cannot stop the use of tobacco, encourage reduction of use as gradually as necessary to whatever levels possible. Praising her efforts will bring the best success rather than making her feel guilty because she does not stop altogether. Teaching tools that demonstrate the effect of tobacco on the fetus and prominently displayed posters and literature will help her understand the value of changing this habit. A referral to a smoking cessation group is an important step for her to obtain the assistance she may need to be successful.

*Alcohol Consumption.* Consumption of alcohol during pregnancy can result in lifelong physical and mental impairments for the fetus. Alcohol is now the most common identifiable cause of mental retardation, surpassing Down syndrome and spina bifida (Abel and Sokol, 1986). The ingestion of alcohol disrupts the neural development and brain cell size in a fetus.

Heavy alcohol use (six or more drinks a day or one binge during the first trimester) can lead to **fetal alcohol syndrome (FAS)**, a combination of physical and mental birth defects in the infant. This syndrome includes intellectual impairment, neuromuscular disability, developmental and growth delays, and specific facial deformities. **Fetal alcohol effects (FAE)** is a condition in which some, but not all, of the birth defects associated with FAS occur in the baby.

The most severe damage from alcohol is done during the developmental phase of the first trimester and is not reversible. However, if a mother stops alcohol use, the size of the fetal brain cells will improve. With improved nutrition, decreasing or stopping smoking, and abstinence from alcohol, the fetal brain will continue to grow. Drinking in the latter part of the pregnancy has a greater impact on the birth weight of the baby.

Not all women who drink alcohol during pregnancy give birth to children with FAS. However, there is no safe amount of alcohol for consumption during pregnancy (Bagheri and others, 1998). To determine the consumption of alcohol by the mother, ask her how often she drinks beer, wine, or liquor. How much does she consume? Determine if that amount has recently changed. If there has been a decrease, the woman may be trying to control her use of alcohol.

*Nonprescription Drugs.* OTC drugs should also be used cautiously and only with the approval of the healthcare provider. A list of specific remedies for specific situations with the dosages to take should be given to the woman during this first prenatal visit as a positive teaching tool rather than expecting her to call before taking any OTC medication.

*Acetaminophen* is the pain medication that is often recommended during pregnancy and lactation. Even though a woman may have used *acetylsalicylic acid* (ASA) and *ibuprofen* on a regular basis before the pregnancy, they should now be avoided.

Another area in which to be cautious is the use of megadoses of vitamins. It is generally suggested that women take vitamins during pregnancy. However, more is not better. If a woman has been on a regimen of vitamins before the pregnancy, she should not just add the prenatal vitamin to her intake. Most often the prenatal vitamin will replace all other vitamin use. Too much intake of some vitamins may be toxic to the fetus and/or mother.

Ask the woman, "What OTC medications do you keep in the house? Which ones do you use most often? Which ones have you taken since you have been pregnant? What do you do to help yourself when you get a headache? How many times in a week do you have to do this? What vitamins do you take? How many do you take of each kind? How often do you take them?"

*Prescription Drugs.* No prescription drugs should be taken without consulting the health care provider for the woman and her developing fetus. Not all prescription drugs are safe for a pregnant woman to take. The heath care provider should evaluate each drug to determine whether taking or not taking the drug poses greater possible danger to the embryo or fetus. Sometimes during pregnancy the condition for which the prescription was originally being taken is not currently a problem. For other conditions, a safer, alternative drug may be available to take during pregnancy. Alternatively, the provider may determine that for the health of the mother the same drug is necessary, but the dosage or concurrent medications may be changed.

Ask the woman, "What prescription drugs do you have in the house? Which ones do you take on a regular basis? Have you taken a prescription drug for other than what it was intended? Have you taken someone else's prescriptions?"

*Recreational or Street Drugs.* Marijuana, cocaine, amphetamines, and so on should be avoided for the health and development of the fetus and the health and safety of the mother. These drugs have the potential for causing physiologic and psychologic damage to both the mother and the baby. Cocaine is reported to cause impaired head growth, congenital abnormalities, cerebral infractions, apnea, and is related to a higher rate of sudden infant death (Kenner and D'Apolito, 1997). In addition, a pregnant woman under the influence of mind-altering drugs may make unsafe choices such as drinking, smoking, or having unprotected intercourse. The potential for accidents also increases because she may be involved in a motor vehicle accident or fall, damaging not only herself but also compromising the baby's health (Chasnoff, 1992).

In general, women who are addicted to drugs tend to seek prenatal care later in pregnancy. They often have significantly greater psychologic distress, less parental support, and are more likely to be survivors of sexual or physical abuse. In addition to these problems, there is also a prevalence of post-traumatic stress disorder among these women (Jessup, 1997).

Women do not seek help for their addictions for many reasons—fear that the authorities may take their children away, lack of child care, lack of social support,

violence in the home, and fear of prosecution for fetal endangerment. Residential alcohol and drug treatment programs are especially effective when women can live at a treatment center with their children (NIDA, 1999). However, there are very limited spaces available for pregnant women and women with children.

A nonjudgmental, conversational approach in questioning often works best with this topic. What do you do to help yourself relax? What drugs or medications help you do this? Have you ever used recreational drugs? Which ones? When? How much? Have you used recreational drugs during this pregnancy? When? What? How much? What are your beliefs about using drugs (alcohol; nicotine; and/or OTC, prescription, or recreational drugs) during pregnancy? Be alert for inappropriate behavior or a dazed appearance, tremors, or a poor weight gain. Look for needle or track marks.

Be alert to the fact that women living in situations of domestic violence often self-medicate with tobacco, alcohol, or illicit drugs to cope with the abuse. You may find that her answers lead you to ask about domestic violence next.

## Personal Information

Obtaining some of the basic personal information may be how you start your interview so that the woman may start to relax with you and the environment. Other times she may be so anxious to address her chief concern that you address that issue first. One way or another you will learn her personal information such as age and educational level. Her race and ethnic group also are important to determine a possible need to offer genetic screening or counseling.

*Support System.* A woman's support system may include a partner, family members, friends, community services, and any combination of these. They may provide emotional support as she journeys through her pregnancy and substantive support by helping meet her physical needs. Ask her whom she talks to about the pregnancy. Who cares for her while she is caring for the pregnancy? Who will help her care for the child after it is born?

*Living Accommodations.* Where she is living, the type of housing she currently lives in, where she will live after the birth of the baby, and the stability of these living arrangements are all important. Ask directly about her arrangements. The answers will make a difference in your diagnoses and care if she is living in temporary accommodation such as a shelter, or in a supportive multifamily-housing situation.

*Pets in the Home.* All types of pets are kept in people's homes. Ask if there are pets in the home and if so what they are. Explore where they are allowed to go and where they deposit their waste products. Who cleans up after them?

Many pregnant women are unaware that their cat poses a danger to the developing fetus. Household cats are the greatest source of infection by **toxoplasma gondii**, a protozoan parasite. Toxoplasmosis may also be contracted by eating uncooked meats and vegetables. If a woman develops a primary toxoplasmosis infection during pregnancy it may lead to miscarriage, stillbirth, or premature labor. The earlier in the pregnancy she becomes infected, the higher the fetal morbidity and mortality.

The primary way to prevent toxoplasmosis infection is good handwashing, both before meals and after handling raw meats and vegetables. The woman should also avoid eating raw meat, unwashed fruits and vegetables, gardening without gloves, and changing the cat's litter box. Prevention is the best strategy, and every pregnant woman should be given the information.

If a pregnant woman is at risk, she should be offered a blood test for the toxoplasmosis organism. If that is positive, amniocentesis will be required to determine if the fetus is infected. If that is also positive, drug therapy may be started.

*Economic Resources.* Determining her economic support is important because in some cases her pregnancy may interfere with her ability to work. If she loses her employment, she may lose her insurance coverage. Ask her if she supports herself or if she shares expenses with someone else. Does she anticipate any financial problems because of the pregnancy? Does she anticipate any financial problems after the baby is born?

Provide her with information about programs and services that may be helpful to her. Obtaining the proper food and clothing and the supplies necessary to care for the coming baby can strain household budgets.

*Domestic Violence.* A pregnancy does not always occur under happy circumstances. In addition, when a partner learns of the pregnancy, violence against a woman may start even if there was no prior history. Domestic violence may be a more common problem for pregnant women than preeclampsia, gestational diabetes, and placenta previa—conditions for which women are routinely screened (Gazmararian and others, 1995).

During pregnancy, abuse occurs at rates between 9% and 20% (Gazmararian, Lazorick, and Spitz, 1996). Women who are in an abusive relationship may enter prenatal care late. They are at higher risk for complications of pregnancy, including vaginal bleeding, low weight gain, placental abruption, premature labor, and lower infant birth weight (McFarlane, Parker, and Soeken, 1996). Of pregnant women who come to an emergency room with vaginal bleeding, 33% report physical abuse (Greenberg, McFarlane, and Watson, 1997).

Ask every woman about domestic violence. Women who were interviewed by a nurse are more apt to disclose that they are being abused (29%) than if they are asked to complete a self-report tool (7%) (Parker and McFarlane, 1991). Also observe her for subtle or overt signs of physical, sexual, and emotional abuse.

This part of the interview must take place in a safe and private environment, where the woman's confidentiality is assured. Begin by explaining to her that abuse occurs in one of six pregnancies and that you ask all women about their experiences so you can provide assistance to those who need it. Then proceed with the abuse assessment screening questions (Box 9-5).

If the woman discloses her pain or fear, convey caring and genuine concern. Affirm that no one deserves to be beaten and that being abused is not her fault. Explain to her that although abuse is common, it is also against the law. It happens to all types of women and is rarely a one-time event. Let her know that she is at risk for more severe injuries each time she is attacked. Support her decision to do what she feels is best, either returning to the situation or leaving the situation. "By supporting the woman's independence and autonomy in decision making, you help her to recognize her strengths and resources as a survivor" (Ragozine, 1998).

Help her develop an emergency plan (see Chapter 6). Support and advocacy in a nonjudgmental manner are necessary to prevent further victimization of the woman. Remember that economic constraints prevent many traumatized women from leaving an abusive relationship. Affording a home, finding a job, affording childcare, and raising children alone are barriers to leaving that many women cannot overcome.

## Summarizing Information

In the process of conducting the health assessment, a great deal of information is collected. However, there is also the chance that some vital information is missed. Two techniques may be used to gain an overall picture of the woman—a typical day history and a review of systems.

### Typical Day

Ask the woman to describe one of her typical days. Starting with when and how she wakes up, have her describe her activities and interactions throughout the day. This type of 24-hour recall elicits information that may have been overlooked by the direct questions. It is especially helpful in obtaining data about nutritional intake and patterns of eating outside of normal mealtimes, patterns of elimination, interactions with others, recreation, and rest periods.

### Review of Systems

A review of systems uses a systematic approach to ask about the parts of the woman's body. This method helps her recall diseases or injuries that she may have forgotten earlier. Explain to her that you are going to ask about body parts or systems and any disease that she may have had in them. You may start with her head and work down her body. Use terms that she is familiar with as you name the areas of her body. If she answers yes to any of your questions, ask her to describe the difficulty and when it occurred. The following list includes items you should be sure to ask about:

1. *Head*: Headache? Dizziness? Fainting (syncope)? Seizures? Head injury?
2. *Eyes*: Able to read? Glasses? Double vision? Tearing? Itchiness? Drainage?
3. *Ears*: Hearing loss? Noise in ears? Earache? Infection? Discharge? Sensation of rotation or movement (vertigo)?
4. *Nose*: Allergies? Discharge? Postnasal drainage? Sinus pain? Nose bleeds (epistaxis)?
5. *Mouth and throat*: Teeth or dentures? Toothache? Bleeding from gums? Changes in or loss of voice (hoarseness)? Soreness or difficulty swallowing?
6. *Neck*: Head turns easily? Stiffness? Lumps or masses?
7. *Breasts*: Tingling? Tenderness? Pain? Secretions? Lumps? Breast self-examination done? How often?
8. *Respiratory system*: Asthma? Wheeze? Cough? Shortness of breath? Pain? Tuberculosis? Pneumonia?
9. *Cardiac system*: Blood pressure readings? Anemia? Palpitations? Pain? History of heart murmur? History of heart disease? Has she ever had a blood transfusion?
10. *Gastrointestinal system*: Weight prior to pregnancy? Nausea? Vomiting? Heartburn? Pain? Change in timing or frequency of bowel movements? Diarrhea? Constipation? Hemorrhoids? Rectal itching (pruritus)? Appendicitis? Hepatitis?
11. *Genitourinary system*: Frequency of urination? Pain with urination? Blood in urine (hematuria)? Vaginal discharge? Vaginal bleeding? STDs? Hepatitis B? HIV? PID? Pain in abdomen? Type? When occurs? Contractions?
12. *Arms and Legs*: Any dislocations or fractures? Pain? Stiffness? Swollen joints? Edema? Weakness? Varicose veins?
13. *Skin*: Dry patches? Rashes? Acne? Skin cancer? Recurrent skin disease like psoriasis?

Conclude the interview by asking if there is anything else she wants to add or discuss (Pillitteri, 1999). Tell her that each time she returns she should continue to report changes or concerns and ask questions.

## Physical Examination

The physical examination starts when you first see the woman, inspecting her as you greet her, looking for

---

> **BOX 9-5** *Abuse Assessment*
> *Screening Questions*
>
> 1. Have you ever been emotionally or physically abused by your partner or someone important to you?
> 2. Within the last year, have you been hit, slapped, kicked, or otherwise physically hurt by someone?
> 3. Since you've been pregnant, were you hit, slapped, kicked, or otherwise physically hurt by someone?
> 4. Within the last year, has anyone forced you to have sexual activities?
> 5. Are you afraid of your partner? Are you afraid of someone else that has hurt you?
>
> From Ragozine JE: Abuse during pregnancy, *Contemp Nurse Pract* 3(1):3-10, 1998.

signs of distress or disease. From that point on, use every moment with the woman to observe how she moves, speaks, pays attention to, and relates to others.

### Preparing Woman for the Physical Examination

***Review of the Procedures.*** Explain to the woman what will be done during the complete physical examination. If she has not had an internal examination before, show her the equipment that will be used during the vaginal examination. Explain how it is used and let her handle it if she wishes. Show her the mirror that she will be able to use to see what is happening during the vaginal examination. If she has not yet given a urine specimen have her do so before she undresses. This will ensure that her bladder is empty and she will be more comfortable. The urine specimen is collected by clean catch to rule out asymptomatic bacteriuria.

It may not be necessary for a woman to remove all her clothes for the examination, have her only undress to the degree necessary. Many practices have found creative ways that a woman may retain pieces of her own clothing and her dignity while also allowing providers the necessary access to do the full assessment on one part of her body at a time. Give her directions and then allow her to prepare in privacy.

Many women find the vaginal examination a very stressful part of the physical examination. Putting the client in charge by thoroughly explaining the procedure, including the option to handle and insert the speculum herself, allowing her to choose a support person to be with her, and encouraging her to choose the positioning for the pelvic examination may make the examination less stressful for the woman. Doing the vaginal examination first so that the woman doesn't have to keep anticipating it is also helpful.

Women with physical disabilities may need additional assistance in preparing for the physical examination. Each disability affects the type of preparation needed differently. (See Chapter 7 for details on vaginal examination.)

Women with sexual abuse histories may have difficulty with the idea of a pelvic examination. To help her, give the woman control of the examination (Bohn and Holz, 1996). If she is pregnant as a result of a sexual assault, this may be the first time a provider has inspected her vagina since the attack. Doing the vaginal examination in a position other than the one in which she was assaulted may help reduce her anxiety and pain. Delaying the pelvic examination at the woman's request or having her practice inserting the speculum herself may decrease her anxiety and increase her sense of control over her own body. Ensure that she has a voice in every decision-making process regarding her care. Women who acknowledge a history of sexual or physical abuse also should be referred to a reproductive health counselor or therapist who specializes in this area.

### Vital Signs

The first part of the physical examination consists of the woman's height, current weight, vital signs, temperature, respiration, pulse, and blood pressure. The woman's blood pressure may be checked at each prenatal visit because it may be an important indication of a possible health problem with the pregnancy.

### Weight

A woman's current weight as well has her prepregnancy weight and desired weight should be determined. Some women who view themselves as overweight see pregnancy as a time to lose weight. Others fear pregnancy because of the weight they will gain. The mechanisms of pregnancy (i.e., development of additional tissue such as the placenta, added blood volume, growth of the fetus) that cause a woman to appear to gain weight should be explained.

### The Physical Examination

The physical examination is often the only occasion during the prenatal period that the client is examined from head to toe. The basis behind such a physical examination is to ensure there are no ongoing disease processes and to discuss normal body changes that are occurring with the pregnancy. Generally a nurse practitioner, nurse midwife, or physician conducts this part of the examination. Each practitioner has a pattern in which they progress when doing a complete physical examination; generally it flows from head to toe. The role of the nurse is to be with the woman as she desires, assist the provider doing the physical, and take note of the woman's concerns as the examination progresses. We generally have the advantage of seeing the woman's face when the other provider cannot. Note if she expresses surprise, discomfort, worry, or pain, and follow up appropriately.

The assessment will be a complete physical examination with particular attention being paid to areas affected by pregnancy. It begins with the head and neck, paying close attention to the thyroid. Then her lungs and heart are auscultated and the spine observed for signs of scoliosis or kyphosis. The kidneys are palpated for costovertebral tenderness.

The breasts are observed and palpated with the normal breast changes due to pregnancy reviewed. This is often a good opportunity to review the benefits of performing self-breast examination (SBE) and of breastfeeding. The nipples are observed for inversion or flatness.

The abdomen is palpated, assessing the liver and spleen. If this initial prenatal visit is during the first trimester the uterus will not be palpable abdominally. A fetal heart will usually not be heard with a Doptone until 12 weeks of gestation when the uterus moves into the abdomen.

Throughout the examination, her skin is evaluated regarding general condition, the presence or absence of lesions, bruising, or petechiae. Special attention is given to bruises on the body surfaces that might be used to block an attack on the abdomen/fetus, such as the front of her arms or her thighs. The legs are examined for signs of edema, reflexes are assessed, and the presence of varicosities noted.

The pelvic examination should be performed when the client feels comfortable. The vulva is first inspected, the speculum is inserted, and the cervix visualized. A Pap smear and cultures for STIs may be collected at this point. Many clinicians now include a wet prep to evaluate the vaginal flora for bacterial vaginosis (BV) because BV is thought to be implicated in preterm labor (Johnson and others, 1999).

A bimanual pelvic examination is performed to estimate the size of the uterus. The fallopian tubes and ovaries are palpated to identify inflammation or masses such as a tubal pregnancy or ovarian cyst.

Clinical **pelvimetry** (measurements) may be performed at this point to assess adequacy of the pelvis for labor. It is impossible to predict from the outward appearance of a woman the size of her internal pelvis. Differences in pelvic contours and development occur because of heredity, disease, and injuries (Figure 9-6). Some providers like to take the measurements during this initial visit. Others prefer to wait until later in pregnancy when the pelvic muscles are more relaxed. However, the measurements should be done before the twenty-fourth week. If a routine sonogram is scheduled, those results may be combined with the pelvic pelvimetry to give an estimate. If a woman has given birth vaginally and she has not had an injury to the pelvis since then, the measurements are generally not repeated in later pregnancies.

When the physical assessment is completed, the woman should get dressed and then the prenatal laboratory work is usually drawn.

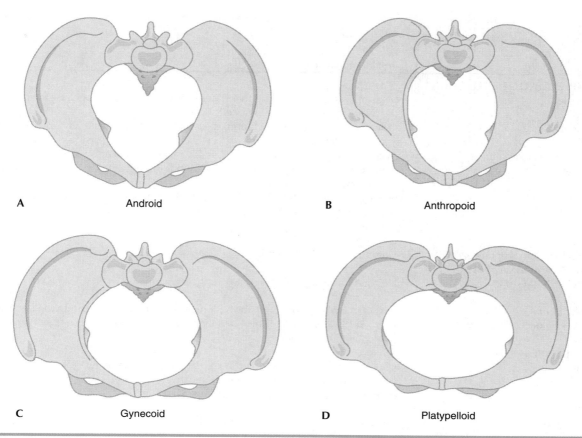

A   Android

B   Anthropoid

C   Gynecoid

D   Platypelloid

FIGURE 9-6 • Types of female pelves.

## Laboratory Screening Tests

Some problems may only be detected by screening tests conducted periodically throughout the pregnancy. A series of tests are generally conducted during the initial prenatal visit so that baseline data may be obtained and possible problems found earlier in the pregnancy process.

Tests that are generally indicated for all pregnant women are urinalysis and blood studies. The urine (collected before the physical examination) is analyzed for albumin, glucose, ketones, and pyuria (pus in the urine). Drawn now, the blood is used to determine blood type (ABO and Rh factor), obtain a complete blood count, screen for antibodies and infection, and measure the alpha-feto protein and glucose levels (Table 9-3).

The need for other studies is determined by a woman's history, physical examination, and health status. When offering the option of screening through more invasive procedures on the mother or fetus, acknowledge that the woman and her partner have a choice and that there is no right or wrong decision in regard to prenatal testing (Kuppermann and others, 1999).

For example, amniocentesis may be offered to determine the chromosomal status of the fetus. Many women who have delayed pregnancy until later in life or who have gone through the invasive procedures associated with infertility treatments may be reluctant to risk losing the pregnancy by having an amniocentesis procedure. At age 35, her risk of having a baby with a chromosomal abnormality is approximately equal to her risk of losing the pregnancy because of miscarriage after the amniocentesis (Pauker, 1994). Women should be supported in the process of weighing the benefits and risk of the procedures offered to them and then making their own decision. If a woman is not going to act on a negative finding and abort the fetus, she may not want to risk losing the child by undergoing a test.

## After the Data Collection

The provider will now review the results of the examination with her. Any risk factors that were found should be discussed and a plan made for follow-up.

* The woman needs to be included in developing a schedule for subsequent visits based on the point she is in her pregnancy and her ability to return for follow-up care.
* She should learn the signs or symptoms of a possible problem and the emergency contact procedures.
* Educational needs should be provided for with written or video materials and other resources.

**TABLE 9-3** *Screening Tests during Pregnancy*

| Test | Results and comments |
| --- | --- |
| **COMPLETE BLOOD CELL COUNT** | |
| Hemoglobin | Measured as g/dl. May drop to 11.5 g/dl later in pregnancy because of increase of plasma in ratio to red blood cells (RBCs). |
| Hematocrit | Volume of RBCs in 100 ml blood, measured in a percentage; 33% is lowest acceptable level. |
| Mean corpuscular volume | Average volume of individual RBC; below average indicates some types of anemia. |
| RBC count | Number of RBCs in each microliter of blood. In pregnancy, hemodilution level may drop to 3.75 million/mm³. |
| WBC count | Neutrophils (50%), lymphocytes (21%-35%), monocytes (4%), basophils (0.3%), eosinophils (2.7%). Total count is 7000-10,000/mm³. Rises to 16,000 by late pregnancy. |
| Platelets | >150,000/mm³ |
| Hemoglobin electrophoresis | Determines sickle cell trait. |
| **MATERNAL SERUM ALPHA-FETO PROTEIN (MSAFP)** | Elevated levels or low levels cause concern. Done between 15-20 weeks. |
| **GLUCOSE** | |
| Hemoglobin A$_{1c}$ | Less than 3.5% is normal; if above, indicates hyperglycemia within the last 6 weeks. |
| 1-hr 50-g glucose load test | Load at 28 weeks; if 1-hr level less than 140, is normal. If above, then glucose tolerance testing is done. |
| **BLOOD TYPE (ABO)** | |
| Rh factor | Check partner's blood type and potential for incompatibility. |
| Coombs' test | Indirect Coomb's test should remain negative. Retested at 28 weeks in Rh-negative woman. |
| **INFECTION*** | |
| Rubella titer | If less than 1:8, immunize after birth. If titer more than 1:128 in early pregnancy, repeat test. |
| Syphilis | Venereal Disease Research Laboratory (VDRL) or fluorescent treponemal antibody absorption (FTA-ABS) test; repeat at 32 weeks for high risk. |
| Vaginal and cervical smear Gonorrhea | Gram stain or enzyme-linked immunosorbent assay (ELISA) test; repeat at 28 weeks. |
| Chlamydia | Direct examination of smear on slide. |
| Gram-positive *Streptococcus* | Direct slide examination. |
| Hepatitis B surface antigen | Vaccination advised. |
| Tuberculosis | Screen for tuberculosis. Skin tests: tine, Mantoux. Radiographic examination after positive finding. |
| **URINE** | |
| Glucose, ketones, albumin | Dip-stick test each visit. |
| Cells: leukocyte, RBCs, bacteria casts | Urinalysis performed first visit and as necessary. Catch clean, midstream specimen for culture if cells present. |
| Specific gravity | |

*Some physicians also check all women for toxoplasmosis.

 **SUPPORTIVE PRENATAL PROGRAMS**

## Centering Pregnancy Program

An alternative approach to traditional prenatal care is the Centering Pregnancy Program that promotes prenatal care in a group setting rather than on an individual basis. Groups consisting of 8 to 12 women are formed based on age and a similar EDD. They meet for ten 90-minute prenatal visits. Women are encouraged to actively participate in their own care by determining gestational age, weighing themselves, checking blood pressure, and making appropriate chart entries. Each woman has individual time with the provider to address any personal concerns and to assess fetal growth and fetal heart tones. The provider acts as facilitator for group discussion. The range of discussion varies from the normal physical changes associated with pregnancy to family and social issues that are of interest to the group. The social support and networking opportunities provided by group interaction assist women in normalizing their responses to pregnancy (Schindler Rising, 1998). This type of program works especially well with women who feel they are outside the norm of other women in the waiting room, such as the pregnant adolescent or the older woman (Figure 9-7).

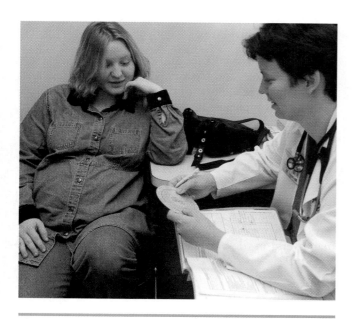

FIGURE 9-7 • Care provider with a pregnant teen. *(Courtesy of Caroline E. Brown.)*

## Teenage Mothers Grandmothers Program

Teenagers often respond well to a program that facilitates open communication and support. Such a program is the Teenage Mothers Grandmothers Program.

Family communication frequently breaks down when a teen becomes pregnant, yet this is just when the teen needs the most support. Up to 85% of teen mothers reside with their own mothers during pregnancy and after the delivery of the baby (Brooks-Gunn and Chase-Lansdale, 1995). That makes it important for health care providers to develop strategies that help grandmothers confront and cope with their own feelings of disappointment and anger so that they can then help their daughters.

This program is structured to provide prenatal care and prenatal classes to the teen. In addition, individual counseling is provided to the teen and her mother during the first two sessions; then in the third session a social worker assists them in discussing their individual feelings regarding the pregnancy and what they will do after the birth. During the fourth session the social worker meets with the grandmother alone, to discuss issues. Two additional sessions are scheduled at the first and second well-baby visit to assess the family's adjustment to the newborn (Roye and Balk, 1996).

## Early Pregnancy Classes

Early pregnancy classes provide a complementary addition to the individual care a woman receives, with additional discussions concerning fetal development, nutrition, and adjustment to pregnancy. Educating the pregnant woman, and giving her the support she needs to make informed decisions regarding pregnancy and childbirth empower her to be an active participant in her care, no matter her age.

Education provides reassurance and assists with adjustment to the new reality of becoming a parent. Most health insurance companies do not cover prenatal classes despite their obvious benefits. Therefore, many women who would benefit from the information and support provided by attending classes are excluded.

## COMPLEMENTARY THERAPIES USED DURING PREGNANCY

Pregnancy is often a time when women seek out traditional, folklore, and culturally based practices to handle the discomforts of pregnancy or to ensure a healthy pregnancy and baby. Some cultures have identified alternative healers within their community, who the woman first turns to for advice. Other clients may be seeing various care practitioners and combining multiple techniques and therapies. Many of the remedies and practices that the client incorporates may benefit and nourish her during the pregnancy, while a few practices should be avoided and may cause harm. It is important to learn what therapies the woman may be using.

Simple questions such as, "What have you tried or has been suggested that you try to deal with the discomforts of pregnancy?" may elicit some practices that can then be discussed. Encourage the woman to inform any care provider that she consults that she is pregnant (Houston and Valentine, 1998).

### Acupuncture, Acupressure, and Shiatsu

Acupuncture, acupressure, and shiatsu have been shown to be beneficial in the treatment of morning sickness and hyperemesis (Murphy, 1998). They are also used to assist in the turning of breech babies at term, in starting labor if the pregnancy has gone past 42 weeks of gestation, and for the reduction of pain in labor. Another value of acupuncture during pregnancy is to assist in smoking cessation. Because these interventions theoretically risk stimulating labor before term, it is advised that only trained providers perform the techniques (Beal, 1992a; Beal, 1999).

### Aromatherapy

Aromatherapy stimulates the limbic system of the brain by the olfactory route. Small quantities of essential oils are used for specific ailments and to restore balance. Aromatherapy is considered safe for pregnancy in the quantities prescribed for its use. The oils can either be used with a safe heating device to scent the room, in massage, or when bathing. If they are used in direct contact with the skin, then care should be taken to use appropriate portions to prevent excess absorption of oil. Some oils used in aromatherapy during pregnancy are rosewood for massage, lavender for varicose veins and muscle aches, and sandalwood and orange for relaxation (Kane, 1997a).

## Art Therapy

Art and music therapy are used to aid in the expressions of grief and anger and to promote healing (Watkins, 1997). Art therapy may help a pregnant woman adjust to her pregnancy and work through feelings of anger and pain (Roller, 1992).

## Ayurveda

Ayurvedic therapies focus on the individual, combining lifestyle changes along with meditation and herbal remedies. Clients usually receive their care through an Ayurvedic practitioner (National Women's Health Resource Center, 1998).

## Biofeedback and Hypnosis

Biofeedback and hypnosis are especially useful in promoting relaxation and aid in addiction treatment and smoking cessation. There are no contraindications to their use in pregnancy.

## Chiropractic

Treatment is useful for neck and shoulder pain, headaches, and back pain. Chiropractic care is considered safe for pregnancy so long as a position is used during the adjustment that prevents supine hypotension (National Institute of Alternative Medicine, 1999).

## Herbalism

Many cultural groups use herbal therapies, and they are generally considered safe, particularly if the plant is used rather than the essential oil, which may be more toxic (Kane, 1997b). However, some herbs are used as abortifacients and can cause premature labor and abruptio placentae (Stapleton, 1995). Other herbs, such as sage, may decrease milk in a lactating woman (Youngkin, 1996). All herbal use should be reviewed in light of the woman's pregnancy. Some herbs that should not be self-administered in pregnancy unless under supervision are listed in Box 9-6 (Beal, 1998).

## Homeopathy

A small amount of a substance similar to the client's ailment is prescribed stimulating the body's own defense mechanisms to respond and heal. Because very dilute potencies are used, homeopathy is considered safe for pregnancy (Lockie and Geddes, 1995).

## Meditation and Yoga

Yoga is meant to balance and connect the mind, body, and spirit (Roth and Creaser, 1997). During pregnancy it encourages relaxation of the mind and promotes flexibility and suppleness in the body (Collins, 1998).

## Prayer and Spirituality

A woman may derive strength, gain peace and acceptance, and develop strategies for coping with her pregnancy and changing life through prayer and spiritual support. A church group may also provide physical support with meals and assistance throughout the pregnancy and in the postpartum period (Corrine and others, 1992).

## Reflexology

The manual massage of the bottoms of a woman's feet can relieve stress and muscle tension and produce relaxation. It may also be helpful in the treatment of diarrhea, constipation, migraines, and anxiety (Nurse's Handbook of Alternative and Complementary Therapies, 1999).

## Therapeutic Touch, Energy Healing, and Reiki.

Therapeutic touch, energy healing, and Reiki restore an individual's normal life energy patterns. They are considered safe and beneficial for pregnancy (Ryburn-Starn, 1998).

---

### BOX 9-6 *Herbs That Require Supervision in Pregnancy*

| | |
|---|---|
| Angelica | Marjoram |
| Arbor vitae | Meadow saffron |
| Barberry | Motherwort |
| Beth/birth root | Mugwort |
| Black cohosh | Pennyroyal |
| Blue cohosh | Poke root |
| Cascara sagrada | Rue |
| Cichona | Sage sqaw vine |
| Cotton root bark | Sqaw vine |
| Goldenseal | Tansy |
| Greater celandine | Wormwood |
| Juniper | |

Some of these herbs may be used appropriately in pregnancy to induce labor or separate a stubborn placenta, but, if not used under supervision, they may cause such problems as miscarriage or preterm labor (Beal, 1998).

# SUMMARY

There are many factors to consider when a woman presents for the first time for prenatal care. However, not every aspect and risk of pregnancy can or must be addressed at the first prenatal visit. The focus of assessment and interventions must be prioritized based on the concerns of the woman and the findings of the providers. What is vital is that the woman and provider establish a therapeutic partnership that will lead to future visits. This partnership will continue to develop with each return visit as the woman progresses through her pregnancy.

The woman should leave this visit believing in the uniqueness of her pregnancy, feeling a beginning level of security with her providers, and having faith that she is respected and will be making choices concerning her care in the coming months. Every woman should leave feeling that she has found a safe place to return to as her pregnancy develops.

## Care Plan · The Woman with an Unwanted Pregnancy

**NURSING DIAGNOSIS** **Decisional Conflict** related to unwanted pregnancy *(as manifested by client statements, "We simply can't afford a baby. . . I'm just beginning to get my business going; this will make it go under, for sure. . . I'm not sure I ever wanted to be a mother anyway. . . I don't know what to do. Could I deal with an abortion?")*

**GOALS/OUTCOMES** By the end of this visit, the client discusses the situation openly and demonstrates reduced anxiety; by the end of the next visit, the client and partner begin to resolve their emotional conflict and begin active problem solving for resolution of decisional conflict *(see "Evaluation Parameters" for indicators of goal achievement)*

### NOC Suggested Outcomes
- Decision Making (0906)
- Information Processing (0907)
- Participation: Health Care Decisions (1606)

### NIC Priority Interventions
- Decision-Making Support (5250)
- Family Planning: Unplanned Pregnancy (6788)

### Nursing Activities and Rationale
- Evaluate carefully whether the woman is experiencing true decisional conflict. *The nurse cannot assume that everyone faced with a difficult decision is experiencing conflict. Data could also represent the normal ambivalence that is present in first trimester.*
- Assess the woman's level of tension or distress *to offer support or, in extreme cases, make a referral.*
- Assess the partner's and family's feelings about the pregnancy and their effect on the client. *Decisions will affect the entire family, and family members might be a source of support.*
- Clarify (nurse's) own values regarding the available options. *Self-awareness helps prevent the nurse from being judgmental about client choices or from influencing the client.*
- Acknowledge client's feelings about the pregnancy. *This shows support and caring, which builds rapport.*
- (If this is the first prenatal visit), briefly present the options of abortion and adoption, but do not elaborate. Encourage the woman to take some time to think about her alternatives and to telephone or return if she wishes to discuss the options further. *She needs time to take in the new situation. Her feelings may change. Presenting too much information about alternatives at the first visit might imply that the nurse favors abortion or adoption. It is important to remain neutral until the client comes to her own decision. If this is a later visit and the choice has definitely been made, then more information should be given.*
- Provide information requested by the client (e.g., names of adoption agencies in the community). *Lack of knowledge contributes to decisional conflict.*
- As soon as appropriate, help patient/partner identify advantages and disadvantages of each alternative, *which supports the decision-making process.*
- Assess level of conflict and status of decision making at the next prenatal visit. *If the decision is not made by the end of the first trimester, the client will have one less option (abortion) available to her.*

*Continued*

## Care Plan  ·  The Woman with an Unwanted Pregnancy—cont'd

### Evaluation Parameters

By the end of this visit, client:
- reports and demonstrates decreased anxiety and tension.
- verbalizes awareness that she has options for coping with the pregnancy.
- verbalizes intent to discuss her feelings with appropriate family members and contact the health care professional as needed.

By the next prenatal visit, client:
- reports having arrived at a decision about continuing or terminating the pregnancy, or freely discusses options with health professionals.
- identifies her feelings as normal ambivalence of pregnancy, or verbalizes intent to pursue other options.
- verbalizes understanding of the choices available.
- evaluates available choices (i.e., abortion, adoption, becoming a parent) in relation to personal values.
- uses problem solving to work toward achieving the chosen outcome (i.e., abortion, adoption, becoming a parent).

**NURSING DIAGNOSIS**  **Risk for Altered Development** related to unplanned or unwanted pregnancy (NOTE: This diagnosis is most useful if the client's decision is to continue with the pregnancy.)

**GOALS/OUTCOMES**  Achieves normal developmental tasks of pregnancy; demonstrates conditions and behaviors indicative of maternal and fetal well-being; engages in behaviors to promote maternal and fetal health *(see "Evaluation Parameters" for indicators of goal achievement)*

### NOC Suggested Outcomes
- Maternal Status: Antepartum (2509)
- Prenatal Health Behavior (1607)
- Risk Detection (1908)

### NIC Priority Interventions
- Anticipatory Guidance (5210)
- Attachment Promotion (6710)
- Support System Enhancement (5440)

### Nursing Activities and Rationale
- Assess emotional attachment to fetus and level of acceptance of the pregnancy (see "Evaluation Parameters"). *If the client chooses to continue the pregnancy, one of the developmental tasks is to resolve her initial ambivalent feelings and develop emotional attachment to the fetus.*
- Provide opportunity to hear fetal heart tones (FHTs) and see ultrasound image of fetus as soon as possible; observe and discuss parental reactions, which *helps make the pregnancy real and promotes attachment; identifies lack of attachment.*
- Encourage parents to note fetal movement; discuss their reaction. *Promotes attachment and helps make the pregnancy a reality.*
- Instruct about developmental tasks of pregnancy. *Knowledge of normal responses reassures the woman that her own feelings are "OK" and helps her to evaluate her own progress.*
- Help identify available resources and options for action (e.g., options for childcare, hiring someone to help with her business, LaLeche League for breastfeeding support). *Information is essential to good problem solving and also relieves anxiety.*
- Suggest books and literature about pregnancy and psychosocial adjustments, as needed. *Reinforces teaching done at prenatal visits.*
- Provide a phone number to call for assistance, if necessary. *The initial conflict may not be completely resolved. If so, the client can be expected to experience more of the normal discomforts of pregnancy and find role adjustments more difficult. Continued support is reassuring.*
- Assess the amount of emotional and financial support provided by the client's partner. *An adequate support system facilitates developmental tasks and adaptation; if partner support is not adequate, nurse can make other recommendations. Information about financial support is important if the client initially expressed concern about money.*
- Involve partner and other family members (as client desires) in care planning. *Strengthens family ties, provides support for client. Helps family members view the pregnancy and baby as a cooperative effort.*

### Evaluation Parameters
- Demonstrates emotional attachment to fetus (e.g., chooses name for baby, asks questions about sonogram, smiles or makes positive comments when hearing fetal heart tones)
- Demonstrates acceptance of pregnancy (e.g., expresses happiness and pleasure)
- Develops a fantasy image of her unborn child

## Care Plan · The Woman with an Unwanted Pregnancy—cont'd

- Copes well with normal discomforts of pregnancy
- Maintains healthy preconceptual state (e.g., keeps appointments for prenatal care; practices good nutrition; avoids nicotine and alcohol)
- Attends childbirth preparation classes
- Recognizes "danger signs" of complications of pregnancy; reports to health professional as needed
- Uses health care services (e.g., prenatal classes) congruent with needs

**NURSING DIAGNOSIS**   **Risk for Altered Family Processes** related to situational crisis created by unwanted pregnancy

**GOALS/OUTCOMES**   The couple acts together to manage stressors, demonstrates healthy family internal environment, and indicates that their needs are satisfactorily met during the pregnancy; the family demonstrates adjustment to pregnancy and life changes; client and partner maintain adequate role performance *(see "Evaluation Parameters" for indicators of goal achievement)*

### NOC Suggested Outcomes
- Family Coping (2600)
- Family Environment: Internal (2601)
- Family Functioning (2602)
- Family Normalization (2604)
- Parenting (2211)
- Psychosocial Adjustment: Life Change (1305)
- Role Performance (1501)

### NIC Priority Interventions
- Family Integrity Promotion: Childbearing Family (7104)
- Family Process Maintenance (7130)
- Normalization Promotion (7200)

### Nursing Activities and Rationale
- Convey an attitude of acceptance and establish a trusting relationship with parents. *Because this is a potential problem rather than an actual problem, nursing activities focus on assessment and data gathering. Clients must trust the nurse to share personal information and feelings.*
- Evaluate the relationship between the parents; observe their interaction when they are together at prenatal visits; observe their expression of feelings and their ability to comfort one another to *provide data about family functioning.*
- Ask for information about family functioning (e.g., "Have you talked about who will get up when the baby cries at night?" "How much help are you getting from your husband at home now?"), *which provides data for early detection of Altered Family Processes, should the problem actually develop.*
- Note any reports of fatigue or inability to manage at work or home, *which may signal a lack of support from partner.*
- Assess parents' self-esteem and self-perceptions. *Low self-esteem may hinder goal achievement, for example, by inhibiting expression of true feelings.*
- Assess degree of financial burden of the pregnancy and the implications for lifestyle changes *to provide data to identify needs and begin a plan.*
- Identify and discuss existing social supports (e.g., extended family, church members, friends, financial aid) *to help the family manage stressors and meet their needs, if necessary. Adequate support helps foster growth of individual family members and reduces the stress of role changes.*
- Assess for indications of negative behaviors (e.g., not eating properly, using alcohol or tobacco, reluctance to give information and discuss concerns, not keeping appointments). *These may be cues that the family is not meeting an individual's needs.*
- Involve the couple in decisions about the pregnancy and birth as much as possible. *Provides some control and empowerment. Fosters confidence in ability to decide and problem solve.*
- Provide anticipatory guidance *to allow time for adaptation.*

### Evaluation Parameters
- Reports incidents of role flexibility (e.g., partner assumes some household chores)
- Reports making joint decisions with partner (e.g., about role expectations after the baby is born)
- Client and partner express feelings freely with each other
- The couple maintains financial stability
- Reports participating in activities, recreation, and so on with partner.
- Reports working together to solve problems and meet goals.
- Expresses realistic expectations of parental role
- Expresses optimism about ability to manage new roles and responsibilities after birth of the baby

*Continued*

## Care Plan · The Woman with an Unwanted Pregnancy—cont'd

**Other Nursing Diagnoses That Might Apply**

- Health Seeking Behaviors (Subsequent Prenatal Visits) related to desire for a healthy pregnancy
- Possible Knowledge Deficit (personal habits necessary for a healthy pregnancy; for example, nutrition, caffeine use, exercise) related to lack of prior experience
- Risk for Injury (during prenatal period) to Mother and/or Fetus related to preexisting medical conditions or obstetric developments during pregnancy
- Risk for Noncompliance (e.g., with dietary instructions) related to lack of commitment to the pregnancy outcome and reluctance to alter lifestyle to accommodate the pregnancy
- Risk for Altered Parenting related to unwanted pregnancy

## CASE STUDY

Tina, a 27-year-old secretary at a large insurance company, has come to see her primary provider because she thinks she has the flu. She is tired and nauseous. As you do her intake interview she tells you that for the last few weeks, she has not wanted to be around food. When she does try to eat, she feels like throwing up. She also says that she is having trouble getting up in the morning for work even though she is going to bed by 9 PM.

When you ask about her personal habits you learn that she smokes socially when out with friends, about five cigarettes a week. She says she prefers to drink bottled water rather than alcohol so that she doesn't get the calories. She says that her nutrition is good. She doesn't eat breakfast. Her favorite lunch is a salad. For dinner she usually grabs a frozen dinner.

Tina lives with her mother, who is divorced, and her brother, a senior at the local college. Her support system consists of her friends from high school, who are also single and employed.

As you continue the interview she tells you that she has been sexually active for about 2 years but has never been pregnant. She leaves the process of contraception up to her male partner. She doesn't remember the date of her last menstrual period (LMP) but says it has been awhile. When you ask if she thinks she is pregnant she says she doesn't know, but she hopes not. She says, "If I am pregnant, I will have the baby."

Tina is 5'4" and weighs 100 pounds. Her vital signs are within normal limits. Her urine specimen comes back positive for pregnancy.

- What immediate reponse will you provide Tina?
- What are her strengths? Where does she face potential problems?
- What information do you need from Tina?
- What nursing diagnoses could apply? How will you validate these?
- What long-term goals might she have for herself?
- What short-term goals might the two of you develop for Tina?
- What interventions may you offer?
- How will these interventions be prioritized?
- How will you evaluate the effectiveness of your interventions?

## Scenarios

**1.** Maggie, a 35-year-old G3 P3, has missed a menstrual period and has come to the office requesting a pregnancy test. Her 2-year-old son James has accompanied her. She appears nervous while waiting for results of the urine pregnancy test. You bring Maggie into a private room and tell her the test is positive. It is apparent to you that she is in severe emotional distress and needs time to regain control.

Once Maggie is calm you ask about her response to the positive pregnancy test. She tells you that her husband is not happy with her, and she is afraid the pregnancy will upset him. This is one more thing she has to deal with now. You ask Maggie about her safety and the safety of the children. She says that her husband is verbally abusive, but she doesn't think he would ever hit her or her children.

- Before you can provide further care to Maggie, what subjective and objective data do you need?
- What do you think Maggie might be experiencing? Why?
- What nursing diagnoses could apply? How will you validate these with Maggie?
- What goals might be developed? How will these be prioritized?
- What interventions may you offer?
- What crucial information should Maggie have today before she leaves the office?
- How will you evaluate the effectiveness of your interventions?

---

2. Fatima is a 30-year-old G5 P4 who has recently arrived from Saudi Arabia. She has come into the clinic in the third trimester of her pregnancy. Her mother and sister accompany her. Her sister acts as intrepreter and explains that Fatima is a Muslim and that her beliefs forbid a male to provide her care. They are all very concerned and want reassurance that a woman will provide her prenatal care and be at the birth.

- What subjective data do you have about Fatima's condition?
- What subjective and objective data do you need?
- What possible resources will provide the information you need?
- What possible nursing diagnoses might apply?
- How will you validate these diagnoses with Fatima?
- What interventions will you need to be prepared to discuss with Fatima?
- How will you evaluate the effectiveness of your care?

---

3. Susan, a 16-year-old young woman, G1 P0, has come to your OB/GYN clinic accompanied by her mother. During the assessment interview, Susan explains that she is currently living in a supportive environment with her boyfriend and his mother.

Susan's mother explains that she has come with her daughter to ask you to persuade her daughter to terminate her pregnancy for the good of all the family. Susan's mother states, "This baby will ruin my daughter's life. My husband will not let her back into the house unless she has an abortion." Susan's mother reveals that she and her husband were teen parents also. She explained that they had received little support from family and friends and that "it has taken years to get to where we are today."

- What subjective data do you have about Susan's condition?
- What subjective and objective data do you need?
- How will you separate Susan from her mother so you may speak with Susan alone?
- What nursing diagnoses could apply? How will you validate these?
- What goals might be developed? How will these be prioritized?
- What interventions may you offer?
- How will you evaluate the effectiveness of your interventions?

---

4. Sherine is a 32-year-old woman with a G2 P0 obstetric history of an ectopic pregnancy and spontaneous abortion (SAB). She has been married for 5 years. Having missed her last two menstrual cycles, she performed a home pregnancy test yesterday, and the results were positive. She tells you that she is scared. When she had her miscarriage, her provider told her not to think about it; it was nothing. She has not had anyone to talk with about what happened, and she wonders why it happened and what her baby was like. She also wonders if it will happen again. You reassure her that her anxiety is normal under the circumstances.

- What subjective data do you have about Sherine's condition?
- What subjective and objective data do you need?
- What do you think Sherine might be experiencing? Why?
- What nursing diagnoses could apply? How will you validate these?
- What goals might be developed? How will these be prioritized?
- What interventions may you offer? How can you ensure that her needs are met? What about the needs of her husband?
- How will you evaluate the effectiveness of your interventions?

5. Jean is a 41-year-old woman, G1 P0, who comes to the office newly pregnant. She has many concerns regarding her age and the pregnancy. The father of the baby is 56 years old, and they are both in good health and are nonsmokers. Both of their health and family histories are negative for any problems. They express concern about their age and pregnancy risks. She is already taking folic acid 1 mg daily. You reassure Jean regarding the normalcy of her feelings.

- What subjective data do you have about Jean's condition?
- What subjective and objective data do you need?
- What do you think Jean might be experiencing? Why?
- What nursing diagnoses could apply? How will you validate these?
- What goals might be developed? How will these be prioritized?
- What interventions may you offer?
- How can you ensure that Jean's needs are met? What about the needs of the father of the baby?
- How will you evaluate the effectiveness of your care?

6. Fay is a 24-year-old woman, G1 P0, who is 9-weeks pregnant through artificial insemination. You are seeing her for her first prenatal visit, and she has a severe migraine headache. She says she has had a history of migraines since age 16. She has stopped taking her regular medication for the migraines on the advice of her care provider. She does not want to hurt the baby by taking any medications while she is pregnant, but her migraine is intolerable. She is also anxious that the migraines will keep recurring during the pregnancy and that she will not be able to work. To begin to calm her anxieties, you inform Fay that frequently during the second trimester of pregnancy, migraines decrease.

- What subjective data do you have about Fay's condition?
- What subjective and objective data do you need?
- What do you think Fay might be experiencing? Why?
- What nursing diagnoses could apply? How will you validate these?
- What goals might be developed? How will these be prioritized?

- What interventions may you offer that ensure Fay's needs are met? What about the needs of her partner?
- How will you evaluate the effectiveness of your interventions?

7. Kathy is a 38-year-old woman with a G9 P7 obstetric history. She had a positive pregnancy test at home 1 week ago. She has come to the clinic with a history of scant vaginal bleeding. The bleeding began after she had intercourse last night. She does not have any pain. She is worried that she may be miscarrying. You reassure Kathy about the normality of her concerns and tell her she did the right thing to come in.

- What subjective data do you have about Kathy's condition?
- What subjective and objective data do you need?
- What do you think Kathy might be experiencing? Why?
- What nursing diagnoses could apply? How will you validate these?
- What goals might be developed? How will these be prioritized?
- What interventions may you offer?
- What crucial information should Kathy have today before she leaves the office?
- How will you evaluate the effectiveness of your interventions?

8. Susan has come to the nurse's office in her high school because she is worried. Her last menstrual period was only one day long, and instead of needing to use 6 tampons during 24 hours, she only needed three. She is concerned about all the "blood and stuff" that is still in her. She says, "I'm glad I got my period because that means I'm not pregnant. But why did my period change?"

- What subjective data do you have about Susan's condition?
- What subjective and objective data do you need?
- What nursing diagnoses could apply? How will you validate these?
- What goals might be developed? How will these be prioritized?
- What interventions may you offer?
- How will you evaluate the effectiveness of your interventions?

# REFERENCES

Abel EL and Sokol RJ: Fetal alcohol syndrome is now the leading cause of mental retardation, *Lancet* 2:1222-1228, 1986.

Adams D and Kocik SM: Perinatal social work with childbearing adolescents, *Soc Work Health Care* 24(3/4):85-97, 1997.

American College of Obstetricians and Gynecologists (ACOG): *Ultrasound in pregnancy,* ACOG Tech Bull No 187, 1993.

Andrews MM and Boyle JS: *Transcultural concepts in nursing care,* ed 2, Phildelphia, 1995, Lippincott.

Association of Women's Health, Obstetrical and Neonatal Nurses (AWHONN). *Standards and guidelines,* ed 5, Washington, DC, 1997, Author.

Bagheri MM and others: Fetal alcohol syndrome: maternal and neonatal characteristics, *J Perinatal Med* 26:263-269, 1998.

Beal MW: Acupuncture and related treatment modalities, *J Nurse Midwifery* 37(4):254-259, 1992a.

Beal MW: Women's use of complementary and alternative therapies in reproductive health care, *J Nurse Midwifery* 43(3):224-233, 1998.

Beal MW: Acupuncture and accupressure: applications to women's reproductive health care, *J Nurse Midwifery* 44(3): 217–230, 1999.

Beresford T: Intervention for the unintended pregnancy. In Carr PL, Freund KM, and Somani S, editors: *The medical care of women,* Philadelphia, 1995, Saunders.

Bohn DK and Holz KA: Sequelae of abuse. Health effects for childhood sexual abuse, domestic battering, and rape, *J Nurse Midwifery* 41:442-456, 1996.

Boston Women's Health Book Collective: *Our bodies, ourselves,* New York, 1999, Touchstone.

Brooks-Gunn G and Chase-Lansdale C: Adolescent parenthood. In Bornstein MH, editor: *Handbook on parenting,* Mahwah, NJ, 1995, Lawrence Erlbaum Associates.

Centers for Disease Control and Prevention (CDC): *1998 Guidelines for treatment of sexually transmitted diseases,* Jan 23, 1998. Retrieved June 4, 1999 from *http://www.cdc.gov/wonder/prevguid.*

Centers for Disease Control and Prevention (CDC): *Pregnancy, sexually transmitted diseases, and related risk behavior among U.S. adolescents* [Brochure]. Atlanta, 1994, Author.

Centers for Disease Control and Prevention (CDC): Prevention and control of influenza: recommendations of the Advisory Committee on Immunization Practices (ACIP), *MMWR Morbid Mortal Wkly Rep* 46:1-17, 1997.

Chartier M and others: Measurement of human chorionic gonadotrophin (hCG) and CG activities in the late luteal phase: evidence of spontaneous abortion in infertile women, *Fertil Steril* 31:134, 1979.

Chasnoff IJ: Cocaine, pregnancy, and the growing child, *Curr Probl Pediatr* 22:302-318, 1992.

Collins C: Yoga: intuition, preventive medicine, and treatment, *J Obstet Gynecol Neonatal Nurs* 27(5):563-568, 1998.

Corrine L and others: Spiritual interventions in maternal-child health, *Matern Child Nurs J* 17(3):141-145, 1992.

Cote-Arsenault D and Mahlangu N: Impact of perinatal loss on the subsequent pregnancy and self: women's experiences, *J Obstet Gynecol Neonatal Nurs* 28(3):274-290, 1999.

Cunningham F and others: *Williams obstetrics,* ed 20, Norwalk, Conn, 1997, Appelton & Lange.

Dejin-Karlson E and others: Does passive smoking in early pregnancy increase the risk of small for gestational age infants? *Am J Public Health* 88:1523-1527, 1998.

Dolan-Mullen P, Ramirez G, and Groff JY: A meta-analysis of randomized trials of prenatal smoking cessation interventions, *Obstet Gynecol* 171:1328-1334, 1994.

Enkin MW: Risk in pregnancy: the reality, the perception, and the concept, *Birth* 21(3):131-134, 1994.

Fingerhut LA, Kleinman MC, and Kendrick JS: Smoking before, during, and after pregnancy, *Am J Public Health* 80:541-544, 1990.

Fischer RC and others: Exploring the concepts of intended, planned, and wanted pregnancy, *J Fam Pract* 48(2):117-122, 1999.

Fister S and Schlomann P: The role of the perinatal nurse in open adoption, *Matern Child Nurse* 20:9-13, 1995.

Fogel C and Woods NF: *Women's health care,* Thousand Oaks, Calif, 1995, Sage.

Friede A and others, editors: *Centers for disease control and prevention. General recommendations on immunizations: a guide to action,* Baltimore, 1997, Williams & Wilkins.

Gazmararian JA and others: The relationship between intendedness and physical violence in mothers of newborns, *Obstet Gynecol* 85:131-138, 1995.

Gazmararian JA, Lazorick S, Spitz AM: Prevalence of violence against pregnant women, *JAMA* 275:1915-1920, 1996.

Goer H: *Obstetric myths versus research realities,* Westport, Conn, 1995, Bergin and Garvey.

Greenberg EM, McFarlane J, and Watson MG: Vaginal bleeding and abuse: assessing pregnant women in the emergency department, *Matern Child Nurs* 22:182-186, 1997.

Hally S: Nutrition and reproductive health, *J Nurse Midwifery* 43(6): 459-470, 1998.

Henshaw SK: Unintended pregnancy in the United States, *Fam Plann Perspect* 30(46):24-29, 1998.

Higgins P, Murray M, and Williams E: Self-esteem, social support, and satisfaction differences in women with adequate and inadequate prenatal care, *Birth* 21:26-33, 1994.

Horton JA: *The women's health data book,* Washington, DC, 1995, Elsevier.

Houston RF and Valentine WA: Complementary and alternative therapies in perinatal populations: a selected review of the current literature, *J Perinatal Neonatal Nurs* 12(3): 1-15, Dec 1998.

ific: Healthy eating during pregnancy, 1995. Retrieved Nov 11, 1999 from http://ificinfor.health.org/brochure/eatpreg.htm.

Jessup M: Addiction in women: prevalence, profiles, and meaning, 1997, *J Obstet Gynecol Neonatal Nurs* (26):449-458, 1997.

Johnson R and others: Advances in screening and management of infections in pregnancy, *The Female Patient* 24:50-57, 1999.

Kane A: Childbirth and aromatherapy, *Int J Childbirth Educ* 12(1): 14-15, 1997a.

Kane A: Herbal medicine and childbirth, do they mix? *Int J Childbirth Educ* 12(1):22-24, 1997b.

Kenner C and D'Apolito K: Outcomes for children exposed to drugs in utero, *J Obstet Gynecol Neonatal Nurs* (26):595-603, 1997.

Kenney JW, Reinholtz C, and Angelini PJ: Ethnic differences in childhood and adolescent sexual abuse and teenage pregnancy, *J Adolesc Health* 21:3-10, 1997.

Kitzinger S: *Woman's Experience of Sex,* New York, NY, 1995, Penguin.

Klima CS: Unintended pregnancy, *J Nurse Midwifery* 43(6):483-491, 1998.

Kochenour NK: Normal pregnancy and prenatal care. In Scott, JR and others, editors: *Danforth's obstetrics and gynecology,* ed 7, Philadelphia, 1994, Lippincott.

Kuppermann M and others: Who should be offered prenatal diagnosis? The 35 year old question, *Am J Public Health* 89:160-163, 1999.

Lockie A and Geddes A: *The complete guide to homeopathy,* London, UK, 1995, Dorling Kindersley Ltd.

Malnory ME: Developmental care of the pregnant couple, *J Obstet Gynecol Neonatal Nurs* 25(6):525-532, 1996.

McFarlane J, Parker B, and Soeken K: Abuse during pregnancy: associations with maternal health and infant birth weight, *Nurs Res* 45:37-42, 1996.

Merkatz IR, Thompson JE, and Walsh LV: History of prenatal care. In Merkatz IR and Thompson JE, editors: *New perspectives on prenatal care,* New York, 1990, Elsevier.

Mittendorf R and others: The length of uncomplicated human gestation, *Obstet Gynecol* 75(6):929-932, 1990.

Murphy PA: Alternative therapies for nausea and vomiting of pregnancy. *Obstet Gynecol* 91:149-155, 1998.

National Asthma Education Program. *Report of the Working Group on Asthma and Pregnancy. Management of asthma during pregnancy,* National Institutes of Health Publication No 93-3279A, Washington, DC, 1993, Government Printing Office.

National Institute of Alternative Medicine: Chiropractic health care, May 1999. Retrieved May 22,1999 from http://nccam.nih.gov.

National Institute on Drug Abuse (NIDA): About women, drug abuse and AIDS, Jan 1999. Retrieved June 6, 1999 from the World Wide Web: http://www.nida.nih.gov/notes/

National Women's Health Resource Center: Alternative therapies and women's health, *National Women's Health Report* 17(3):1-5, 1998.

Nurse's Handbook of Alternative and Complementary Therapies: Springhouse, Penn, 1999, Springhouse.

Pagana K and Pagana T: *Mosby's diagnostic and laboratory test reference,* ed 3, St Louis, 1996, Mosby.

Parker B. and McFarlane J: Identifying and helping battered pregnant women, *Matern Child Nurs* 16:141-164, 1991.

Pauker S: Prenatal diagnosis: Why is 35 a magic number? *N Engl J Med* 330:1151-1152, 1994.

Pearlman MD and Phillips ME: Safety belt use in pregnancy, *Obstet Gynecol* 88:1026-1029, 1996.

Phillips CR: *Family-centered maternity and newborn care,* ed 4, St Louis, 1996, Mosby.

Pillitteri A: *Maternal and child health nursing,* ed 3, Philadelphia, 1999, Lippincott.

Purnell LD and Paulanka BJ: *Transcultural health care,* Philadelphia, 1998, FA Davis.

Ragozine JE: Abuse during pregnancy, *Contemp Nurse Pract* 3(1):3-10, 1998.

Reed K: Ultrasound during pregnancy. In Scott JR, editors: *Danforth's obstetrics and gynecology,* ed 7, Philadelphia, 1994, Lippincott.

Report of the Expert Committee on the Diagnoses and Classification of Diabetes Mellitus: *Diabetes Care* 326:1183, 1997.

Rhodes A: Adoption: an overview, *Matern Child Nurse* 20:7, 1995.

Roller CG: Drawing out young mothers, *J Matern Child Nursing* (17):254-255, 1992.

Rosenfeld JA and Everett KD: Factors related to planned and unplanned pregnancies, *J Fam Pract* 43:161-166, 1996.

Roth B and Creaser T: Mindfulness meditation and stress reduction: experience with a bilingual inner city program, *Nurse Practitioner* 22(3):150-176, 1997.

Roye CF and Balk SJ: Evaluation of an intergenerational program for pregnant and parenting, *J Matern Child Nurs* 24:32-40, 1996.

Ryburn-Starn, J: Energy healing with women and children. *J Obstet Gynecol Neonatal Nurs* 27(5):576-584, 1998.

Schindler Rising S: Centering pregnancy: an interdisciplinary model of empowerment, *J Nurse Midwifery* 43(1):46-54, 1998.

Spector RE: *Cultural diversity in health and illness,* ed 3, Norwalk, Conn, 1991, Appelton and Lange.

Stapleton H: Women as midwives and herbalists. In Tiran D and Mack S, editors: *Complementary therapies for pregnancy and childbirth,* ed 2, London,UK, 1995, Bailliere Tindall.

Stevenson AM: Teratogens, Nov 1998. Retrieved May 06, 1999 from http://www.Irp-mcn.com.

Thatcher Ulrich L: *A midwife's tale: the life of Martha Ballard, based on her diary, 1785-1812.* J. Laslocky, editor, New York, 1991, Vintage.

The Sixth Report on the Joint National Committee on the prevention, detection, evaluation, and treatment of high blood pressure, *Arch Intern Med* 157:2413-2420, 1997.

Tyroch A and others: Pregnant women and car restraints: beliefs and practices, *J Trauma Injury* 42(2):241-245, 1999.

Varney H: *Varney's midwifery,* ed 3, St Louis, 1997, Mosby.

Walsh RA: Effects of maternal smoking on adverse pregnancy outcomes: examination of the criteria of causation. *Hum Biol* 66: 1059-1092, 1994.

Ward S: Addressing nicotine addiction in women, *J Nurse Midwifery* 44(1):3-18, 1999.

Watkins GA: Music therapy: proposed physiological mechanisms, *Clinical Nurse Specialist* 11(2):43-50, 1997.

Wertz R and Wertz D: *Lying in: a history of childbirth in America,* New Haven, Conn, 1989, Yale University Press.

Youngkin EQ: A review and critique of common herbal alternative therapies, *Nurse Pract* 21(10):39-62, 1996.

# CHAPTER 10

## Nursing Care During the First Trimester (Weeks 1-13 of pregnancy)

*"At the beginning of pregnancy, whether it is your first or your fifth, your feelings can shift from delirious joy to deep sadness, with a whole range of possibilities in between."*
— Boston Women's Health Book Collective, 1998

What signs and symptoms may lead a woman to think she is pregnant?

Describe a woman's initial response to the reality of pregnancy.

Describe the physical changes that take place in a woman's body during the first trimester.

Describe the changes taking place in the embryo/fetus during this trimester.

What cognitive changes will a woman experience during this trimester?

What other factors influence the woman and her support system during this trimester?

What assessments are necessary during this trimester?

What anticipatory guidance is required during this trimester?

What is the therapeutic response if the woman loses this pregnancy during this trimester?

A healthy woman is pregnant for an average of 6,384 hours. During that time, she will spend only 13 or 14 hours consulting with health care providers. The woman herself will make the day-to-day determinations that affect her health and the baby during pregnancy. She is the actual provider of her own prenatal care, often assisted by her partner, family members, and friends.

Pregnancy is a dynamic state that changes the woman's entire body to meet the demands of the developing fetus. During the pregnancy, health care providers meet periodically with a woman to support the care of her health and well-being and assess the growth and development of the fetus. We answer her questions and monitor the dramatic

changes as part of the normal care of pregnancy and help her maintain her mental and physiologic comfort. Each prenatal visit requires a multifaceted response to the woman's concerns based on her individual needs and the gestational period she is experiencing. To be culturally relevant and appropriate for our diverse clients, the care we provide must be individualized. We can learn from each woman and her family about their needs.

When a woman learns she is pregnant, she experiences a variety of emotions from wonder, excitement, awe, and reverence to ambivalence, anxiety, and fear. How she responds is influenced by how she views herself in the role of motherhood, as well as what she has been told by others. The period of transition into this new identity is a time of much uncertainty. The woman may react by seeking information and help from a number of sources. The assistance we provide can have long-term effects for both her and her child (Mercer, 1995). By listening and exploring with the woman, we can learn what thoughts and concerns she is bringing to this pregnancy and birth experience, because what one believes to be true is often as important as what is true. We can carefully and sensitively provide her with a broader knowledge base from which to make her choices.

## MATERNAL PHYSIOLOGIC CHANGES DURING THE FIRST TRIMESTER

The female human body is an amazing, adaptable being. The changes that occur during pregnancy are extraordinary. All changes are for nurturing the developing fetus while maintaining the health of the mother and preparing her to give birth to a new human being.

Changes occur in most systems of the body and often a change in one system relates to a change in another system. It is important that the pregnant woman understand these changes. Knowing what is going on in her body and why, helps to promote the normalcy of the process. This knowledge also helps the woman to cope with the associated discomforts. As we describe the physiologic adaptations, we will also explain the effects on her.

### Physiologic Changes in the Woman's Reproductive System

All aspects of a woman's reproductive system change to support the health and well-being of pregnancy. There are both structural and functional changes in the reproductive organs, but they will revert to their prepregnant or near prepregnant state after birth.

*Breasts.* Breast tenderness is one of the earliest signs of pregnancy. A woman may notice that her breasts may be full, tingle, and have increased sensitivity as early as 4 weeks of gestation. Estrogen and progesterone are the primary hormones that are responsible for breast changes. The increased estrogen enhances fat storage, as well as development of the mammary ducts, alveoli, and nipples. Progesterone promotes the growth of glandular tissue and the lobular alveoli (Davis, 1996). After 2 months, the breasts will begin to enlarge and the vascular circulation will expand, with veins becoming more visible under the skin. The nipples will become larger and more erect. Both the nipples and the surrounding areola will become deeply pigmented. **Montgomery's glands,** sebaceous glands located in the areola, will also become more prominent.

*Uterus.* When fertilization occurs, ovulation stops and most women experience **amenorrhea** (absence of a menstruation). A "missed period" is one of the first indications to a woman that she might be pregnant. Only 20% of women who are pregnant have slight spotting during the first trimester. If this slight bleeding occurs, it may be related to low progesterone levels or implantation. Implantation is when the fertilized ovum becomes embedded in the uterine mucosa about 6 days after fertilization.

Before pregnancy, the uterus is a small pear-shaped organ, weighing about 60 to 70 g with an internal capacity of 10 ml or less. As the pregnancy develops, the uterus changes from a pear shape to a more globular shape. By the end of the pregnancy, the uterus will have increased from about 2 oz (60 g) to 2 lb (1000 g) (Cunningham and others, 1997).

During the first few months of pregnancy, estrogen and possibly progesterone stimulate uterine growth. Growth is the result of increased vascularity and dilation of the blood vessels, hyperplasia (the formation and growth of new cells) and hypertrophy (enlargement of existing cells), and the development of the endometrium (decidua) of pregnancy. Similar uterine growth is seen with ectopic pregnancies, in which there is no developing embryo within the uterine cavity (Cunningham and others, 1997). Throughout pregnancy, the uterus remains globular and ovoid in shape. By 10 weeks, it is the size of an orange, and by 12 weeks it is the size of a grapefruit (Lowdermilk, Perry, and Bobak, 1997).

Physical findings during the first trimester include a positive **Hegar's sign,** which is a softening of the lower uterine segment, the isthmus. This finding is present as early as 8 weeks of pregnancy. By 14 weeks, the uterus may be palpated as the fundus (top of the uterus) is at or slightly above the symphysis pubis.

When the pregnant woman's abdomen is auscultated, three distinct sounds may be heard over the uterus. A **uterine soufflé** (or bruit) is a soft blowing sound that is caused by the increased uterine blood flow through the arteries of the uterus and occurs at the same rate at the maternal pulse. A **funic soufflé** is a soft blowing sound caused by the blood moving through the umbilical cord that occurs at the same rate as the fetal heart rate. The **fetal heart rate (FHR)** is the actual heartbeat of the fetus.

*Ovaries and Fallopian Tubes.* Ovulation ceases during pregnancy because the elevated levels of estrogen and progesterone suppress the secretion of the follicle-stimulating hormone (FSH) and luteinizing hormone (LH) by the anterior pituitary. The ovaries become active in hormone production in support of the pregnancy. The corpus luteum secretes progesterone until 10 to 12 weeks, when the placenta becomes fully functional. The ovaries are usually not palpable after the uterus fills the uterine cavity at 12 to 14 weeks. The fallopian tubes remain relatively unchanged, demonstrating only slight hypertrophy.

*Cervix.* At 8 weeks of pregnancy, the cervix may feel soft, which is referred to as **Goodell's sign,** a change created by the hormones of pregnancy. Increased vascularization of the cervix causes **Chadwick's sign** (the blue/violet coloring of the vaginal mucosa and cer-

vix) to occur about the same time. Estrogen also stimulates the glandular tissue of the cervix, causing an increase in the normal mucus production during pregnancy (Cunningham and others, 1997). The endocervical glands secrete thick tenacious mucus that forms a **mucous plug** (operculum) that prevents bacteria and other substances from entering the cervix during pregnancy.

The increased vascularization of the cervix creates cervical friability in that the cervix bleeds easily when scraped or touched and releases small amounts of blood. Contact with the penis during intercourse can lead to spotting during pregnancy.

***Vagina and Vulva.*** An increase in a whitish vaginal discharge, called **leukorrhea,** occurs during pregnancy. The fluid is whitish because it contains exfoliated vaginal epithelial cells. An increase in vascularity occurs within the vagina, causing a sensation of increased pelvic congestion. The vaginal secretions become more acidic, white, and thick. The increased acidity of the secretions (pH 3.5 to 6.0) helps to prevent infection but also makes the vagina more susceptible to the overgrowth of *Candida albicans,* leading to monilial vaginitis (Cunningham and others, 1997).

## Hormonal Changes with Pregnancy

### Human Chorionic Gonadotropin (hCG)

The **trophoblast** (the peripheral cells of the blastocyst that attach the fertilized ovum to the uterine wall) secretes human chorionic gonadotropin (hCG) in early pregnancy. This stimulates progesterone and estrogen production by the corpus luteum until the developing placenta assumes this role. If a woman is pregnant with multiple embryos, the hCG levels will be more than twice as high than with a single pregnancy (Simpson and Creehan, 1996). The presence of hCG in a woman's blood may be detected as early as 24 to 48 hours after implantation and reaches a measurable level 7 to 9 days after conception. A urine pregnancy test may detect hCG as early as the first missed menses. The levels continue to increase, peaking between the sixtieth and eightieth day of fetal gestation and then decline and are barely detectable at the end of the pregnancy.

### Human Placental Lactogen (hPL)

The **syncytiotrophoblast** (the outer syncytial layer of the trophoblast) of the placenta produces a hormone called human placental lactogen (hPL), which is also known as human chorionic somatomammotropin. The serum levels of hPL rise with placental growth.

### Estrogen

In early pregnancy, the ovaries secrete estrogens. By 7 weeks of gestation, the placenta secretes more than half of the estrogen. The primary estrogen produced by the placenta is estriol.

### Progesterone

First the corpus luteum and then the placenta produce progesterone, which is crucial to maintaining the pregnancy. Progesterone maintains the endometrium, inhibits uterine contractility, and assists in the development of the acini and lobules of the breasts for lactation.

### Relaxin

Relaxin is primarily secreted by the corpus luteum and in small amounts by the placenta and endometrium or decidua lining the uterus. Relaxin is detectable by the first missed menstrual period and affects the pregnancy by inhibiting uterine activity, diminishing the strength of the uterine contractions, and softening the cervix. Relaxin may also relax the woman's intravertebral joints as the pregnancy progresses.

### Prostaglandins

Prostaglandins are complex lipid compounds synthesized by many cells in the body. They are found in high concentrations in the woman's reproductive tract and endometrium during pregnancy. Although their exact function during pregnancy is unknown, prostaglandins affect smooth muscle contractility, and some are also potent vasodilators. Prostaglandins play an important role in the mechanism of labor.

### Prolactin

Prolactin is released from the anterior pituitary and is responsible for initial lactation. Serum prolactin concentrations begin to rise in the first trimester and at term are 10 times their nonpregnant concentration.

## Physiologic Changes in the Woman's Other Physiologic Systems

### Cardiovascular System

The most profound changes are in the cardiovascular system. The woman's normal functions continue while her body adapts to meet the demands of the pregnancy. Changes in the cardiovascular system affect all of the other organ systems.

***Heart.*** The woman's heart enlarges slightly because of increased blood volume and cardiac output (Harvey, 1991) and returns to its normal size after childbirth.

***Blood Volume.*** The woman's blood volume starts to increase during the tenth to twelfth week and continues through the thirty-second to thirty-fourth week of pregnancy. A 30% to 50% increase in blood volume is needed during pregnancy to provide sufficient blood flow to the uterus, fetus, and maternal tissues, as well as to protect the mother and the fetus from impaired venous return when sitting or standing (Mattson and Smith, 2000). One sixth of the total blood volume is within the vascular system of the uterus (Cunningham and others, 1997). Because of this shift, bleeding in the uterus at anytime during the pregnancy presents a risk to both the mother and the developing fetus.

Systemic vascular resistance (SVR) decreases during pregnancy because of dilatation of peripheral blood vessels and the large placental vascular system. Progesterone, which relaxes smooth muscles, decreases the vascular tone, causing the vessels to dilate, increasing their capacity. This decrease in SVR facilitates the flow of the increased blood volume.

*Cardiac Output.* Cardiac output is the product of heart rate times stroke volume. During pregnancy, cardiac output begins to increase during the first trimester, mostly due to increase in stroke volume. By the end of the second trimester, cardiac output will have increased by 30% (Mattson and Smith, 2000). The majority of the increased output is distributed to the uterus, kidney, breasts, and skin (Harvey, 1991).

*Blood Pressure.* Blood pressure (BP) is one of the screening tools used to monitor the health of the mother and fetus. Many factors can affect a woman's arterial blood pressure. Age, activity level, concurrent health problems, and anxiety can all increase a pregnant woman's blood pressure. If a woman's readings are elevated when you take a reading, give her time to rest and then repeat the measurement.

A woman's blood pressure may be influenced by her assumption of a particular position. It is generally found to be highest when she is sitting, intermediate when she is in the supine position, and lowest when she is in the lateral recumbent position (Simpson and Creehan, 1996). To enable comparisons between visits, we should take her blood pressure in the same arm and with her in the same position. These specifics should be noted along with the reading in her chart.

Diastolic blood pressure tends to gradually decrease approximately 5 to 10 mm Hg because of peripheral dilation. **Pulse pressure** (the difference between systolic and diastolic pressure) widens slightly during the first trimester (Simpson and Creehan, 1996).

*Hematologic Changes.* In response to the increased need for oxygen, the red blood cell (RBC) volume increases by 18% to 30%. The percentage of the increase depends on the amount of iron available. As the plasma volume increases more than the RBC volume, the woman's hematocrit may decrease by approximately 7%, resulting in a condition called **physiologic anemia**. The normal hematocrit values for pregnancy are 37% to 47% (Cunningham and others, 1997). Hemoglobin levels also tend to be slightly lower (e.g., 12 to 16 g/dl of blood). A value less than 11.0 g/dl, however, is considered abnormal and is usually due to iron deficiency rather than to hypervolemia (Cunningham and others, 1997).

Over the course of the pregnancy, iron requirements increase to about 1000 mg/day in contrast to the 300 mg needed by healthy nonpregnant young women. Actual iron demands are minimal, however, during the first trimester (Cunningham and others, 1997).

Coagulation and fibrinogenic systems also change during pregnancy. Several coagulation factors (fibrinogen, factors V, VII, VIII, IX, and X) increase. Prothrombin time remains unchanged or increases only slightly. The number of platelets and the clotting time remain unchanged. The clotting factors XI and XIII decrease slightly. All of these changes help to support the pregnancy and accommodate the bleeding that occurs when the placenta separates from the uterus during the delivery process. These coagulation changes and the potential for venostasis during pregnancy place the pregnant woman at risk for venous thrombosis.

Women with normal cardiovascular function are able to adjust to the major cardiovascular changes that occur during the pregnancy. However, the alterations in the blood volume and cardiac output do place women with previous cardiovascular disease at risk.

### Respiratory System

Changes in the respiratory system are essential to support maternal and fetal well-being. The woman's oxygen requirements increase to accommodate her increased metabolism. Adjustments are also needed to facilitate the oxygen–carbon dioxide exchange to the fetus.

*Structural Changes.* Over the course of the pregnancy, the length of space available to accommodate the woman's lungs decreases as the diaphragm shifts upward 4 cm. To compensate for this decrease in length, the transverse and the anteroposterior diameters of the rib cage enlarge by 2 cm. The thoracic cage increases 5 to 7 cm, and the lower ribs flare out. Although it seems logical that these structural changes are caused by the enlarging uterus, the changes seem to occur prior to uterine enlargement and are in response to the hormones of pregnancy (Harvey, 1991). As a result of these changes, the woman's breathing becomes more diaphragmatic than abdominal.

*Functional Changes.* Vital capacity does not significantly change in normal pregnancy. A slight increase of 2 breaths per minute in the respiratory rate may occur. A progressive increase of the tidal volume begins in the first trimester.

*Oxygenation.* A gradual increase in oxygen consumption occurs during pregnancy, which leads to increased alveolar and arterial $PO_2$ levels. Circulating hemoglobin will also gradually increase. The maternal hemoglobin has a decreased affinity for oxygen, and the fetal hemoglobin has an increased affinity.

### Renal/Urinary System

Changes in the renal system help to accommodate to the cardiovascular changes of pregnancy. The kidneys must handle the increased metabolic and circulatory requirements of pregnancy in addition to excreting both maternal and fetal waste. The kidneys are responsible for maintaining homeostasis (i.e., electrolyte balance, acid-base balance, maternal-fetal waste management, extracellular fluid volume regulation, and conservation of essential nutrients). Approximately 1000 to 2000 ml of blood flow through each kidney per minute (Harvey, 1991).

***Structural Changes.*** Anatomically, the kidneys enlarge somewhat during pregnancy, most likely due to the increased vascular and interstitial volume (Cunningham and others, 1997). As early as the tenth week, the renal pelvis, calyces, and ureters dilate. Progesterone is thought to cause this dilation because of its relaxing effect on smooth muscle. Estrogen causes increased bladder vascularity, predisposing the mucosa to injury and bleeding more easily.

Early in pregnancy—beginning at approximately 5 weeks, many women report bladder irritability, nocturia, urinary frequency, and an urgency to void. During the first trimester, this usually results from an increased sensitivity of the bladder and the pressure on the bladder from the growing uterus. The discomfort resolves when the expanding uterus lifts up and out of the pelvis during the second trimester.

***Functional Changes.*** Changes in renal function occur due to the hormones of pregnancy; the increase in blood volume; and the woman's posture, physical activity, and nutritional intake. The renal plasma flow (RPF), which is the volume of blood flowing through the kidneys every minute, increases. As the blood flow increases, so does the glomerular filtration rate (GFR). The GFR is the amount of plasma filtered by the glomeruli of both kidneys per minute. The pregnancy causes a change from 100 to 125 ml/min to 140 to 170 ml/min. Both the GFR and the RPF rise after the twelfth week and increase up to 50% at term (Barkauskas and others, 1998).

The renal changes are thought to result from the growth hormone effects of placental lactogen. The increased blood volume, increased cardiac output, and lowered peripheral resistance in the kidneys are related factors (Simpson and Creehan, 1996). Because of the increased GFR and RPF, renal clearance of amino acids, glucose, proteins, electrolytes, and vitamins is more rapid, lowering their circulating levels. The increased GFR also causes the serum urea and creatinine levels to decline (Simpson and Creehan, 1996).

Renal function is most efficient when the woman lies in a lateral recumbent position. This position should be encouraged throughout the pregnancy because as the renal perfusion increases, urinary output increases and edema decreases.

### Fluid and Electrolyte Balance

Sodium maintains the increased intravascular and extracellular fluid volumes and the normal isotonic state. Sodium regulation is difficult during pregnancy because there is a tendency toward sodium depletion. As blood volume increases, however, sodium retention also occurs due to an increase in tubular reabsorption. Therefore additional sodium does not need to be added to the woman's diet, but her sodium intake should not be restricted either. The implementation of sodium restriction and/or diuretics was once a common practice, but newer research has led to the discontinuation of that practice (Harvey, 1991).

***Glycosuria.*** Glycosuria is a common finding during pregnancy because the renal tubules cannot absorb the increased glucose filtered by the glomeruli. Many factors, including anxiety, may increase it to a 1+ level. When this occurs, the possibility of diabetes mellitus or gestational diabetes should be assessed. When diabetes mellitus is present, serum glucose—instead of urine glucose—must be measured (Simpson and Creehan, 1996).

***Proteinuria.*** Proteinuria does not occur during a normal pregnancy except during labor or delivery, but small amounts of protein may be detected in the woman's urine when the level of amino acids in her system exceed the capacity of the renal tubes to absorb it. Values of 1+ protein on a dipstick are generally considered acceptable during pregnancy, but if a woman also experiences hypertension or greater proteinuria she requires further evaluation.

### Gastrointestinal System

Pregnancy increases a woman's nutritional requirements. In response to pregnancy, changes occur in her gastrointestinal system with the alimentary tract altered both anatomically and physiologically. While the woman's appetite increases, her intestinal secretions are reduced, liver function is altered, and the absorption of nutrients is enhanced.

***Stomach.*** Progesterone relaxes the smooth muscles of the stomach, decreasing the gastrointestinal tone and motility of the stomach. Many women (50% to 89%) experience nausea and vomiting (morning sickness) during the first trimester of pregnancy, which may start as early as her first missed period. Excessive morning sickness (10% of cases) may require medical intervention (Mattson and Smith, 2000).

Other common discomforts of pregnancy related to the gastrointestinal system include a sensitivity to the taste of some foods and beverages or the odor of foods, personal care products, and/or environmental pollutants. Some women experience an increase in the production of saliva (**ptyalism**), which may become excessive. Hyperemia and softening of the gums may cause them to bleed easily, so the woman should take care when she brushes her teeth or flosses.

***Liver.*** The liver does not change in size or structure during pregnancy, although liver function is altered. If liver function tests were to be performed on a pregnant woman, the results would be suggestive of hepatic disease even though it is not present. These results occur because the serum concentration of many of the proteins produced by the liver increases during pregnancy in response to the increased estrogen levels.

***Gallbladder.*** The gallbladder is affected by the elevated progesterone levels, causing it to become hypotonic and distended. The function is altered because smooth muscle contraction is impaired, which possibly leads to a stopped or diminished flow (stasis) of bile and an increased risk for developing gallstones. Emptying time is especially reduced after 12 weeks of gestation.

## Endocrine System

Changes in the endocrine system facilitate the metabolic functions that maintain the health of the mother and the fetus throughout the pregnancy.

***Thyroid Gland.*** Due to increased vascularity and hyperplasia, the thyroid increases in both size and activity during pregnancy. Increases in the production of thyroid hormones, particularly T3 and T4, increase the woman's basal metabolic rate (BMR), cardiac output, vasodilation, heart rate, and heat tolerance. Hyperthyroidism during pregnancy is rare, but when it occurs, poor metabolic control can cause preterm labor, fetal loss, or thyroid crisis. Hypothyroidism has been associated with spontaneous abortion.

***Parathyroid Glands.*** The size of the parathyroid gland and the concentration of the parathyroid hormone (parathormone) increases during pregnancy. Parathormone regulates the metabolism of calcium and phosphorus in the body. Because regulation of calcium is interrelated with magnesium, phosphate, vitamin D, calcitonin, and parathormone, an alteration in the amount of one substance is likely to alter homeostasis.

***Adrenal Glands.*** Few structural changes occur in the adrenal glands, but the corticocosteroids secreted by the cortex of the adrenal glands serve several functions. Cortisol regulates the woman's carbohydrate and protein metabolism, and aldosterone accommodates increased sodium excretion. Androgens and small amounts of progesterone and estrogen are also present in adrenal secretions.

***Pituitary Gland.*** The anterior pituitary enlarges during pregnancy, but there is no significant change in the posterior lobe. The anterior lobe produces the follicle-stimulating hormone (FSH) that stimulates ovum growth and the luteinizing hormone (LH) that influences ovulation, secretion of estrogen by the cells of the ovary, and formation of the corpus luteum. The anterior lobe also produces thyrotropin (thyroid-stimulating hormone) and adrenotropin (adrenal-stimulating hormone) to stimulate the thyroid and adrenal glands in support of pregnancy. Prolactin, which is also secreted by the anterior pituitary, facilitates lactation after delivery.

The posterior pituitary secretes oxytocin, which stimulates uterine contractions in pregnancy and the "let down" of milk from the breasts after delivery of the baby. Vasopressin increases blood pressure by causing vasoconstriction, as well as maintains water balance with its antidiuretic abilities.

## Neurologic System

In general, there are no changes in the nervous system during pregnancy, but it is common for a woman to experience headaches during pregnancy. Possible causes of the headaches during the first trimester include hormonal changes, sinusitis, fatigue, lowered blood glucose, emotional tension, noxious fumes, allergens, and increased tension or stress. Treatment for the headaches is limited to relieving the symptoms with comfort measures, rest, light massage, and—with the care provider's direction—an analgesic.

To reduce the occurrence of headaches, pregnant women should be counseled to avoid skipping meals, eliminate the use of caffeine and tobacco, and avoid strong odors. Stress-reduction techniques, periods of resting their eyes, and using a natural tear replacement if their eyes are dry may also help. Healthy habits such as taking walks in the fresh air, taking warm baths, meditating, and performing conscious relaxation (i.e., a process of consciously releasing tension) are beneficial (Davis, 1996).

## Integumentary System

Changes in the integumentary system are primarily caused by hormonal factors and the growth of the breasts and abdomen. General changes include increases in skin thickness and subdermal fat, hyperpigmentation, increased hair and nail growth, accelerated sweat and sebaceous gland activity, and increased circulation and vasomotor activity.

Alterations in skin pigmentation begin early in pregnancy. Under the influence of estrogen and progesterone, ACTH, and the melanocyte-stimulating hormone, melanocytes in all portions of the skin become active. Pigmentation becomes darker over the nipples and areola of the breasts. The dark line that extends from the umbilicus to the mons pubis is called the **linea nigra**. **Melasma** (previously referred to as chloasma), or "the mask of pregnancy," is a darkening of the skin on the cheekbones, forehead, and around the eyes. It disappears after pregnancy but may reappear with excessive sun exposure or oral contraceptive use. The axillae, the anal area, the vulva, and the inner thighs may also have increased pigmentation.

Estrogen also contributes to the development of pregnancy-specific vascular changes and markings. Blood flow to the skin increases to 3 or 4 times the prepregnant levels. Skin changes include feelings of warmth, vascular spider nevi, palmar erythema, and increased nail and/or hair growth. **Spider nevi** are tiny, bright, red angiomas that appear mostly on the face, neck, chest, arms, and legs during the second to fifth month of pregnancy, usually disappearing after the birth of the baby. Sixty-five percent of white women and 10% of black women experience them. **Palmar erythema,** which is experienced by 60% of white women and 35% of black women, is a well-delineated pink area on the palmar surface of the hands. Some women notice accelerated nail growth or a softening or thinning of their nails by the sixth week. Acne may become more pronounced or clear up completely. Hair growth, of fine and/or coarse hair, may occur. For some women, the hair on their head becomes fuller as the number of hairs in the growth phase remains stable. After delivery, the fine hair will usually disappear, but the coarse hair may remain. Women experience an increase in hair loss 2 to 4 months after delivery because the proportion of hairs entering the resting phase doubles after delivery (Simpson and Creehan, 1996).

### Musculoskeletal System

Anatomic changes in the musculoskeletal system result from the influence of hormones, growth of the fetus, and maternal weight gain. Early in pregnancy, the ligaments of the woman soften from the effects of progesterone and relaxin. To facilitate delivery, the sacroiliac, sacrococcygeal, and pubic joints of the pelvis also soften.

A woman's posture and body mechanics may cause backaches as early as the first trimester. We should provide information and educational materials to help the woman minimize these problems as she moves about and carries items (Figure 10-1). If she has to stand for long periods of time, placing one foot slightly higher on a stool helps. She should also wear supportive shoes with heels less than 1 inch high. Daily exercise (e.g., walking, swimming, or stretching) will tone muscles and decrease back weariness. An evaluation by a chiropractor may determine that her spine needs to be realigned.

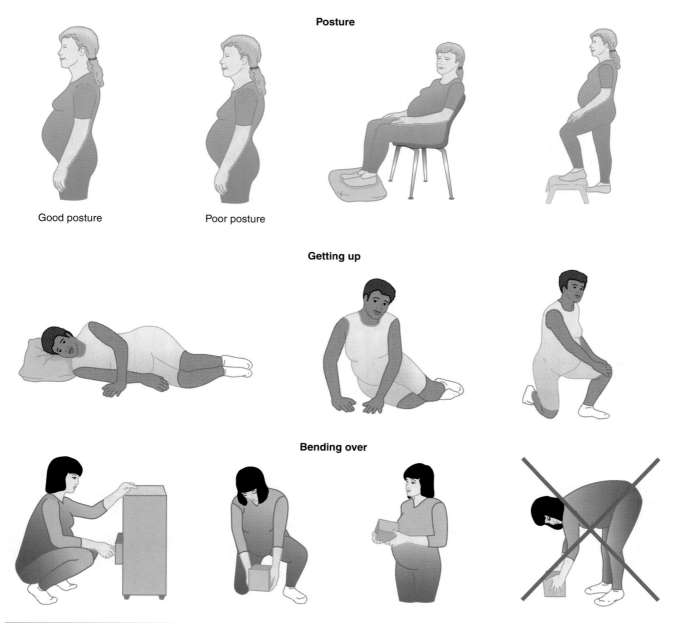

**Posture**

Good posture     Poor posture

**Getting up**

**Bending over**

*FIGURE 10-1* • Body mechanics in pregnancy.

### Metabolic Changes

In normal pregnancies, complex metabolic changes occur to provide for the development and growth of the fetus. Fats stored in the early months of pregnancy are more completely absorbed later in the pregnancy, as the demand for carbohydrates increases.

*Pancreas.* In early pregnancy, insulin production increases in response to the rise in serum levels of estrogen, progesterone, and other hormones. In addition, the mother's body tissues develop an increased sensitivity to insulin, thus decreasing the mother's need and resulting in a build-up of insulin during the first half of pregnancy.

## EMBRYO AND FETAL DEVELOPMENT DURING THE FIRST TRIMESTER

During the 266 days (38 weeks) after conception, amazing growth and development takes place. That the process works and works well so often is extraordinary in itself. **Growth** is the increase in the number and size of the cells of an organism as it gains weight and length. **Development** refers to the way primitive cells differentiate into tissues that perform specific functions. Both must occur in a certain sequence for the outcome to be successful. When parents ask about the formation, growth, and development of their infant, how we answer their questions helps them to relate to the developing baby and provides them with the necessary information to foster the health of their child.

### Preembryonic Stage (First 2 Weeks, Beginning with Fertilization)

Human development follows three stages, all of which occur during the first trimester. The first 14 days of development, starting the day the ovum is fertilized, are called the **preembryonic stage.** Fertilization is only possible if the sperm and the ovum are mature and the sperm can reach the ovum and penetrate it (Table 10-1).

### Week 1 of Development

**Conception,** the union of an ovum and sperm, generally occurs in the outer third of the fallopian tube. From this fertilized ovum, the infant and all the support structures necessary for development (e.g., the placenta, the fetal membranes, the amniotic fluid, and the umbilical cord) are formed (Pillitteri, 1999).

With fertilization, the genetic foundation—including the sex—for the growth and development of an infant is determined. All ova contain X-chromosomes. Sperm may contain an X or a Y chromosome, so the male partner determines the sex of the baby. In 1959, scientists determined that embryos carrying the Y-chromosomes develop as males.

The **zygote** (fertilized ovum) then generally travels down the fallopian tube, entering the uterus approximately 3 to 4 days after fertilization. During this time, the cells are rapidly multiplying and differentiating and the embryonic membranes and the primary fetal germ layers, from which all body systems are formed, are being established.

The amnion and chorion are the fetal membranes that protect and support the embryo as it grows and develops. First the **chorion** forms from the trophoblast and encloses the amnion, embryo, and yolk sac. The **amnion,** a thin protective membrane, forms from the ectoderm and surrounds the embryo and yolk sac and then fills with amniotic fluid. The space between the amnion and the embryo is the amniotic cavity, which fills with amniotic fluid that cushions the fetus, keeps it at an even temperature, equalizes pressures, and allows the fetus to move freely without adhering to the amnion. As the embryo grows, the amnion expands until it comes in contact with and adheres to the chorion. Together, the amnion and chorion are known as the amniotic sac or **bag of waters (BOW).**

### Week 2 of Development

Approximately 7 days after fertilization and 3 or 4 days after entering the uterus, the floating zygote attaches to the surface of the endometrium and settles into the tissue, becoming implanted in the lining of the uterus. Implantation is a vital step to a successful pregnancy, but it is estimated that 50% of zygotes never achieve it. Failure to implant causes the pregnancy to end as early as 8 to 10 days after conception, so the woman may never know that pregnancy has occurred because she did not miss a menstrual period.

Once implanted, the zygote is called an **embryo.** By the eleventh or twelfth day, when implantation is successfully achieved, the chorionic villi (projections on the chorion) reach out into the endometrium. The chorionic villi under the embryo make up the fetal side of the placenta. The growing embryo, no longer able to survive only on nutrients from its own yolk sac, begins to obtain nourishment through the **placenta** and its membranes, which are fully functional by the twelfth week (Sadler, 1995) (Table 10-2).

| TABLE 10-1 | *Terms Used to Label Fetal Growth* |
|---|---|

| Name | Time period in fetal development |
|---|---|
| Ovum | From ovulation to conception (fertilization) |
| Zygote | From conception (fertilization) to implantation |
| Embryo | From implantation to 8 weeks after conception |
| Fetus | From 8 weeks after conception until term |

## TABLE 10-2  Milestones in Human Development before Birth since LMP

| 4 Weeks | 8 Weeks | 12 Weeks |
|---------|---------|----------|
| **EXTERNAL APPEARANCE** | | |
| Body flexed, C-shaped; arm and leg buds present; head at right angles to body | Body fairly well formed; nose flat, eyes far apart; digits well formed; head elevating; tail almost disappeared; eyes, ears, nose, and mouth recognizable | Nails appearing, resembling a human, head erect but disproportionately large, skin pink, delicate |
|  |  | |
| **CROWN-TO-RUMP MEASUREMENT, WEIGHT** | | |
| 0.4 to 0.5 cm, 0.4 g | 2.5 to 3 cm, 2 g | 6 to 9 cm, 19 g |
| **GASTROINTESTINAL SYSTEM** | | |
| Stomach at midline and fusiform, conspicuous liver, esophagus short, intestine a short tube | Intestinal villi developing, small intestines coiling within umbilical cord; palatal folds present, liver very large | Bile secreted, palatal fusion complete, intestines withdrawn from cord and assuming characteristic positions |
| **MUSCULOSKELETAL SYSTEM** | | |
| All somites present | First indication of ossification—occiput, mandible, and humerus; embryo capable of some movement, definitive muscles of trunk, limbs, and head well represented | Some bones well outlined, ossification spreading; upper cervical to lower sacral arches and bodies ossifying; smooth muscle layers indicated in hollow viscera |
| **CIRCULATORY SYSTEM** | | |
| Heart developing; double chambers visible, beginning to beat; aortic arch and major veins completed | Main blood vessels assuming final plan, enucleated red cells predominate in blood | Blood forming in marrow |
| **RESPIRATORY SYSTEM** | | |
| Primary lung buds appearing | Pleural and pericardial cavities forming, branching bronchioles, nostrils closed by epithelial plugs | Lungs acquiring definite shape, vocal cords appearing |
| **RENAL SYSTEM** | | |
| Rudimentary ureteral buds appearing | Earliest secretory tubules differentiating, bladder-urethra separation from rectum | Kidney able to secrete urine, bladder expanding as a sac |
| **NERVOUS SYSTEM** | | |
| Well-marked midbrain flexure, no hindbrain or cervical flexures, neural groove closed | Cerebral cortex beginning to acquire typical cells; differentiation of cerebral cortex, meninges, ventricular foramens, cerebrospinal fluid circulation; spinal cord extending entire length of spine | Brain structural configuration roughly complete, cord showing cervical and lumbar enlargements, fourth ventricle foramens developed, sucking present |
| **SENSORY ORGANS** | | |
| Eye and ear appearing as optic vessel and otocyst | Primordial choroid plexuses developing, ventricles large relative to cortex, development progressing, eyes converging rapidly, internal ear developing | Earliest taste buds indicated, characteristic organization of eye attained |
| **GENITAL SYSTEM** | | |
| Genital ridge appearing (fifth week) | Testes and ovaries distinguishable, external genitals sexless but beginning to differentiate | Sex recognizable, internal and external sex organs specific |

Modified from Wong DL: *Whaley and Wong's nursing care of infants and children*, ed 5, St Louis, 1995, Mosby.

## The First Month of Pregnancy (2 Weeks of Development)

The end of the first 2 weeks of development that resulted in an embryo is also dated as the end of 4 weeks of pregnancy for the woman. The embryo is a rapidly growing mass of cells but does not yet resemble a human being. It is .75- to 1-cm long and weighs about 400 mg. The spinal cord is formed and is fused at the midpoint. The tissues that will form the body are folded forward and fused at the midline. The head is prominent and makes up about one third of the length. The embryo is in the shape of a C, so that the head and the tail are almost touching. The heart is starting to form on the anterior surface. The buds that will develop into arms and legs are present. As they start to form, the location of the eyes, ears, and nose can be seen.

## Embryonic Stage

The embryonic stage begins on day 15 (the third week after conception) and continues until approximately the eighth gestational week of development, or until the embryo reaches a crown-to-rump (C-R) length of 3 cm (1.2 in) about 56 days after fertilization. During this time, the woman may start to suspect that she is pregnant because she has missed one or possibly two menses.

During the embryonic stage, the tissues differentiate into essential organs and the main external features develop. Development of the embryo is **cephalocaudal,** proceeding from the head to the tail. Because this is a time of basic development, the embryo is now most vulnerable to **tetratogens** (i.e., nongenetic factors that can produce malformations of the embryo/fetus). The embryo is susceptible to radiation exposure, maternal infection, drugs and chemicals, and maternal conditions.

Although there is no direct mingling of fetal and maternal blood, virtually everything that a woman puts in her body has the potential to cross the placenta and enter the fetus through the umbilical cord. The umbilical cord, which is formed from the amnion and chorion, connects the developing embryo and the placenta. There are originally four cord vessels, but one atrophies, leaving one large umbilical vein and two smaller umbilical arteries. The cord vessels are surrounded and stabilized by a substance called **Wharton's jelly.** The umbilical vein carries blood with oxygen and nutrients from the placenta to the fetus. The umbilical arteries return the deoxygenated blood to the placenta. Approximately 400 ml of blood flow through the cord per minute.

The development and circulation of the placenta occurs during the third week. The placenta functions as the fetal lungs, kidneys, and gastrointestinal tract, as well as as a separate endocrine organ throughout pregnancy. The placenta secretes progesterone and the estrogen, estriol— hormones essential for maintaining the pregnancy. It also secretes human placental lactogen (hPL), a hormone that prepares the mother's body for lactation.

By the end of 4 weeks of development (28 days after conception), the fetal heart begins to beat. The brain is forming. There are the beginnings of eyes, ears, and nose; and small buds will eventually grow into arms and legs.

During the next 4 weeks (days 29 through 56 after conception), the embryo grows to be about 1 ⅛ inches long. Because of the cephalocaudal pattern of development and the rapid development of the brain, the head is very large compared with the other parts of the embryo. External genitalia appear, but the sex is not discernable. The beginnings of all essential external and internal structures are present, and the embryo clearly resembles a human being. By 8 weeks, all body organs are formed. The remainder of the pregnancy is devoted to the fetus's growth and maturation. The embryo is now developed enough to be called a **fetus.**

---

### BOX 10-1  *Documentation of Ongoing Prenatal Care*

In general, follow-up prenatal visits are made to measure the growth of the fetus, assess the effect of the pregnancy process on the mother's health and well-being, and provide for educational needs.

**MATERNAL HEALTH**
- Updated history
- Physical assessment
- Laboratory testing as indicated
- Assessment of actual or potential risk factors
- Woman's adaptation to the idea of pregnancy

**FETAL HEALTH**
- Fetal growth
- Fetal well-being (activity level is indicated)

**FACTORS WITH POTENTIAL TO INFLUENCE MOTHER OR FETUS**
- Cultural customs
- Socioeconomic stressors
- Environmental stressors

**FACTORS TO CONSIDER FOR WOMAN AND FAMILY**
- Strengths and resources
- Educational needs

## Fetal Stage

By the ninth week of development, the fetus is 5-cm (2-in) long and weighs about 14 g. The head is large, making up almost half of the fetus's entire length. Between weeks 8 and 12, fetal heart tones can be heard with an ultrasound fetoscope. By the tenth week, the eyelids are fused shut. The body begins to grow faster and longer.

### At the End of the First Trimester of Pregnancy (11 Weeks of Fetal Development)

The fetus is now 7- to 9-cm long (the primitive tail is regressing) and weighs 45 g. Spontaneous movements are possible but are too faint for the mother to feel. The heartbeat—at a rate of 120 to 160 beats/min— is audible with an ultrasound fetoscope device. Bone ossification centers are apparent in most bones, and the tooth buds for the first teeth are present under the gums. Nail beds are beginning to form on fingers and toes. Some reflexes, such as the Babinski reflex, are present. The kidneys have begun to secrete urine. All organ systems are formed and simply require maturation. Documentation of the assessment of the physical changes of the woman and her fetus is vital (Box 10-1).

## THE COGNITIVE CHANGES OF PREGNANCY

Pregnancy produces a period of transition between a woman's self-image as an unpregnant woman and as a pregnant woman, as well as a transition between the accompanying lifestyle changes. "The transition to parenthood is a psychological process of unfolding that keeps pace with and complements the physical development of the fetus inside—a transition that carries with it variable amounts of resistance and progress" (Lederman, 1996).

Rubin (1984) referred to pregnancy as "a period of gestation of a child and of the maternal persona." The pregnant woman thinks about and strives to come to terms with the reality of her pregnancy, her potential role as a birth mother, and her feelings of uncertainty and vulnerability as the stability and continuity of her personal domain are disrupted. From the moment a woman first suspects that she is pregnant, she begins to think about what this means to her. If she continues with the pregnancy, she may have concerns about bodily harm and permanent physical change, as well as about her ability to survive childbirth intact and with dignity.

As the pregnancy progresses, a woman moves through a series of four cognitive maternal tasks that lead her to take on the maternal identity (Mercer, 1995). The woman's maternal identity develops as she affirms her maternal role and receives feedback from her partner, mother, family members, and friends. The four themes of maternal tasks during pregnancy, as identified by Rubin (1984), focus on the woman herself, the woman and child subsystem, and the woman and her family. These themes are as follows:

1. *Seeking safe passage through pregnancy, labor, and childbirth.* The woman expresses a desire to implement a plan that fosters her ability to adjust to the variables in her life and pass through pregnancy, labor, and childbirth safely.
2. *Seeking social acceptance for herself as a mother and for her child.* The woman's identity of herself as a mother is facilitated when her partner accepts the expected child, acknowledges the woman's personal sacrifice to carry a pregnancy, and willingly makes supportive changes. The pregnant woman also seeks acknowledgement that her mother and any earlier born child or children accept the pregnancy.
3. *Attaching and committing herself to the new role and to her unborn child.* The woman starts to become attached to the child during pregnancy, which provides motivation to assume the maternal role, as well as initial satisfaction in the role (Mercer, 1995).
4. *Giving of self on behalf of the child.* "Whether the transition to the maternal role is viewed from a purely physical basis, in terms of gains and losses in a career or educational trajectory, or in social and psychological costs, the mother is unequivocally the parent who gives and sacrifices the most in creating, bearing, and rearing a child" (Mercer, 1995). The woman develops the ability to delay self-gratification or deny her own needs as she attempts to place the needs of her baby before her own needs.

Pregnancy provides the time for major developmental changes in a woman, as well as in her family and friends. All persons involved must adapt in their own way to the anticipated role changes and the idea of an the addition of a family member in their own way.

### Adapting to Pregnancy during the First Trimester

The woman and her partner, family, and friends will each have different thoughts and feelings as they learn of the possible or actual pregnancy. How they respond individually and collectively has implications for the development of the woman-child dyad, the family, and their future place within their community (Box 10-2).

The woman and her partner experience a period of disruption and radical change during the first trimester. From their identification of conception until the twelfth

## BOX 10-2    Reactions to Pregnancy in the First Trimester

People's reactions to pregnancy are as individualized as the people themselves. There are several common responses, however, that may occur in a pregnant woman and her partner.

### MOTHER'S REACTION
- Differs according to culture, view of role, age, and relationship to father of baby
- Feels ambivalent toward reality of pregnancy
- May tell partner
- Anxious about process of labor and prospect of caring for child
- Becomes aware of physical changes in body
- Worries about miscarriage
- May think of her relationship with her mother with new interest, now with a common experience of motherhood

### PARTNER'S REACTION
- Differs according to culture, view of role, age, and relationship to pregnant woman
- Accepts pregnancy and pregnant woman, or rejects woman and pregnancy and breaks off communication
- May develop more or less sexual interest
- May develop new interest or hobby outside of partnership as a way of distancing self

Compiled from Lederman RP: *Psychosocial adaptation in pregnancy,* ed 2, New York, 1996, Springer; Mercer RT: *On becoming a mother,* New York, 1995, Springer; Rubin R: *Maternal identity and the maternal experience,* New York, 1984, Springer.

week of the pregnancy, they must identify and consider many physical and psychosocial processes.

### The Woman

Am I really pregnant? What does it mean to be pregnant? What is happening to my baby and me? What status will pregnancy bring me (Mercer, 1995)? A woman asks these questions of herself as she comes to terms with a positive pregnancy test.

As a woman's health care provider, we explore with her the meaning of the pregnancy and the positive, negative, and ambivalent feelings she may be experiencing. How does she feel about pregnancy in general? How does she feel about this pregnancy with this partner in particular? What is she anxious about? What are her economic concerns? Who is her support system? Helping her to validate the pregnancy and her needs is essential to her well-being.

***Mood Swings.*** The many changes—both physical and hormonal—in a woman's body contribute to the emotional lability she may experience. The woman may initially experience the physical discomforts of pregnancy

while contemplating who she is and her new role. Externally, she may have other stressors such as an unsupportive partner or financial or professional concerns.

Helping a woman and her family understand that  mood swings are common is the first step to decreasing her concern about what is happening to her. Assistance in dealing with the physical discomforts also helps her become more comfortable with her body. Encouraging her to "brain storm" with family and friends for solutions to the external problems, as well as offering our own positive reinforcement for her decisions also helps. If the mood swings appear to be from alcohol use, drug use, or a personal crisis, referral to social services for counseling and care may be necessary.

***From Ambivalence to Acceptance.*** Acceptance of a positive pregnancy test is one of the first tasks of pregnancy. As many as 50% of pregnancies are unintended, unwanted, or mistimed. To some extent, every pregnancy is a surprise, because either it was unplanned or the woman is surprised that the process worked. Even after a positive pregnancy test, a woman will look for confirming signs within her body that she really is pregnant. Until she is able to verify the pregnancy in some way, there is room for denial or disbelief. Hearing the fetus's heartbeat, seeing an ultrasound image, and later feeling the sensations of movement cause the child to become more of a reality in the parents' minds.

A woman may be motivated to have a child and become a mother for a variety of reasons. Learning about her motives, and if she intended pregnancy to happen now or later, help us respond to her expectations, hopes, values, dreams, fears, and fantasies about pregnancy and childbirth. Motivations for motherhood and childbearing may include "confirmation of femininity, a fondness for children, a wish to reproduce a happy family life, fulfillment of a motherhood wish, and the desire to have someone to nurture for whom love, affection, and tenderness can be expressed" (Lederman, 1996). Other women may want a child so that someone loves them.

Ambivalence, the simultaneous feeling of conflicting feelings, is a common response even when a desired pregnancy is first confirmed. Planning and striving for a pregnancy are very different from accepting a pregnancy. Ambivalence is a normal response of most women. As excited as a woman may be about the pregnancy, she knows that her life is now forever changed. As the pregnancy becomes a reality and the woman comes to terms with the changes in her body, however, she starts to integrate the idea of mothering into her self-image (Rubin, 1984). To evaluate ambivalence, Lederman (1996) believes it is important to assess the following factors:

"1. How honestly ambivalence is expressed;
2. The reason for ambivalence;
3. The intensity of the ambivalence;
4. How sustained the ambivalence is."

The woman's motivation and eagerness for pregnancy, as well her life situation, will affect the extent of her ambivalence and her movement toward accepting the pregnancy. For a first-time mother, pregnancy moves her self-image from girl to woman and from childless woman to expectant mother. Some women grieve the loss of an image or a lifestyle. Others may feel that they are not ready or are inadequate to become mothers. If a woman already has a child, she may not feel capable of caring for another child. If she is pregnant as the result of a sexual assault or if the relationship with the father of the baby has disintegrated, the woman may be angry about her current condition. If she is young, single, or in a difficult relationship, she may unconsciously ignore the existence of a pregnancy for months.

To evaluate a woman's acceptance of her pregnancy it is necessary to assess the extent to which she exhibits the following characteristics:

1. She consciously planned and desired this pregnancy.
2. She is predominantly happy (vs. being depressed).
3. When she has discomfort during the pregnancy, she addresses that discomfort.
4. She accepts the changes in her body instead of rejecting them.
5. Her ambivalence and conflict are resolved as she nears the end of the pregnancy (Lederman, 1996).

If a woman accepts the pregnancy, she will have simultaneous positive and negative responses, but the feelings of well-being will prevail (Brown, 1988). By the end of the first trimester, she may seek information from experts or role models that she can imitate. She will start to confront and resolve issues about the type of mothering she has received and the type of mother she envisions she will be. She may attend early pregnancy or parenting classes, watch friends and relatives with children, or rehearse the mothering role by babysitting for a friend's baby. These activities provide the woman with a sense of certainty at a time when she is feeling very uncertain. Multiparas tend to do less role playing during later pregnancies and use themselves as models (Mercer, 1995).

*A Woman's Concerns.* During the first trimester, a woman is normally more concerned about herself, the physical changes that come with pregnancy, and her feelings about the pregnancy. As she tries to gauge how normal she is and if she should worry, our assessment and interventions should focus on the customary changes at this time in pregnancy (e.g., breast fullness, urinary frequency, nausea and vomiting, and fatigue). The woman may wonder about the need to adopt lifestyle changes (e.g., giving up tobacco or alcohol, changing exercise routines or eating habits, or using a seat belt when in a car).

The relationship with her partner may also concern her. If this is an unexpected pregnancy, she may be fearful of her partner's negative response to the prospect of a child or to the continuation of their partnership. She may also wonder how the pregnancy will affect their sexual relationship.

A woman and her partner may have specific expectations for care during the pregnancy, birth, and postpartum experience, and these should be explored. We should explain the individuals or team that is available to them, as well as the pattern and purpose of planned prenatal visits and how to get assistance between visits. The procedures the woman should follow if something unexpected or disturbing occurs are also important.

*Indications of Difficulty in Acceptance.* Because pregnancy presents enormous implications to a woman's life, all women have the potential for maladaptive behavior during pregnancy. We must work with them and their families to develop interventions directed toward reducing the effect of the situations that lead to maladjustment.

The task of accepting a pregnancy permeates a pregnant woman's behavior. She may exhibit exaggerated discomforts such as nausea and vomiting, sleeplessness, or fatigue. She may be angry with her partner or fear new patterns of behavior he may be exhibiting. In some relationships, incidents of domestic violence start after the woman becomes pregnant.

In general, a low degree of acceptance—evidenced by greater conflicts and fears, more physical discomforts, and depression—is associated with an unplanned pregnancy. If a woman does not accept the pregnancy, she will tend to despair, be depressed, and feel overwhelmed by the possibility of the physical and emotional disruption in her life.

Listening to her concerns and encouraging her to talk with her partner or supportive family members or friends can be helpful. If the woman appears to be suffering from depression, we should assess the onset, severity, and duration of the symptoms. We should observe the effects and listen for other related symptoms (e.g., headaches). We should be positive and nonjudgmental, establishing a comfortable climate that will facilitate communication. Just telling her one genuine, valid reason why we like her as a person and a patient will help her feel less isolated and alone.

Mild depression can usually be treated with encouragement, positive reinforcement, and therapy. Give the woman time to express her fears and apprehensions. We should provide clear, concise verbal and written instructions because her condition will make it difficult for her to retain what we tell her. Referring the woman to a provider who can provide cognitive therapy may be helpful. If finances or health insurance is a concern, we should connect her with a service that is subsidized, free, or low-cost.

Depression is an increased risk during a pregnancy when the physical and psychologic adjustments are added to an existing situation of unresolved conflicts, emotional turmoil, poor coping skills, and genetic predisposition. About 15% to 20% of all pregnant women may require referral for mental health considerations. This percentage includes the women who have been sexually assaulted and are pregnant due to incest or rape. Coerced or forced intercourse by someone she trusted (e.g., a family member, husband, boyfriend, or date) can be especially devastating, and a mental health facility can provide the most appropriate treatment. Major depressive disorders usually require therapy and, in some cases, pharmocologic treatment to prevent the woman from harming herself (Davis, 1996). Pharmacologic treatment for the mother's benefit must be balanced against the potential risk to the fetus's development.

### The Partner

Within much of the white, middle class culture of the United States, it has become expected that the partner will be actively involved in the pregnancy process, labor experience, and parenting role after delivery. This is not universally accepted across ethnic and social groups, however, so we should not make any assumptions and assess the situation of each pregnant woman individually. When her partner learns about the pregnancy, he may view himself anywhere on a continuum from being just the "sperm donor" to this process or as an active participant and supporter as the woman "grows" their child.

The role of partners has often been minimized in the childbearing process, as they have been dismissed as unimportant contributors or influences on a pregnancy or to the woman's health. We now know, however, that how the father of the baby and/or the woman's partner views the pregnancy has a direct effect on the pregnant woman's health and adaptation to pregnancy (Mercer, 1995). The encouragement and support that the partner gives the woman as she tries to take on the role of mother is important to her development.

When a partner is told of a pregnancy, it means accepting not only the pregnancy but also the idea that the changes in the woman (e.g., fatigue and nausea) are related to the fact that she is pregnant. At first, this is often difficult to do. As the pregnancy progresses, hearing a heartbeat, feeling the baby kick, or seeing the fetus on ultrasound makes the pregnancy more real.

Like the mother-to-be, partners may also experience feelings of ambivalence, fluctuating between being proud and happy and being concerned. The extent of the ambivalence depends on the partner's relationship with the woman, previous experiences with pregnancy, age and economic stability, and if the pregnancy was planned. Whether the couple is married or not, most states will hold a male partner responsible for the financial support of the child.

Just as the pregnant woman does, the partner will seek recognition as a parent from her family, friends, coworkers, and society—and then from the baby. Parenting partners may prepare by reading and planning, fantasizing and thinking about the baby and the subsequent changes in their lifestyle, attending classes, and talking to other fathers. The factors that are important to first-time fathers' readiness for parenthood are as follows: a prior intention to become a father at some point in his life; his perception of the stability of the couple's relationship; the couple's relative financial security; and his sense of having completed the childless period of his life (Lederman, 1996).

Some partner's experience a series of health symptoms and complaints similar to what the mother is experiencing, which is termed **couvade.** Couvade behaviors vary in different cultures but end with the birth of the child. Symptoms occur for which there is no apparent physiologic cause. Intestinal gas pains, nausea, hunger and weight gain, restlessness, sleeping difficulties, and bad dreams about the child or birth have all been reported. It is thought that couvade indicates that the partner has a positive level of identification with the pregnant woman and the developing child. Men who report symptoms of couvade score higher on scales measuring paternal role preparation than men who report no symptoms (Longobucco and Preston, 1989).

### The Couple

If the couple views it as "our pregnancy" and "our infant," both partners become participants. This joint view of the pregnancy may help to prevent the jealousy that some partners develop for the baby during the first trimester when the woman spends time focusing on the baby.

A young and/or unwed father may have a great deal of difficulty accepting a pregnancy, negotiating his role within the childbearing process, and working with the mother to consider his role or possible involvement with the child in the future. If the woman decides to abort the pregnancy, he may attempt to stop her legally, have a deep sense of loss if an abortion does occur and yet, having no one to turn to for understanding, must suffer the loss alone.

Pregnancy generally causes a couple to look at the long-term potential of their relationship. Within an ongoing relationship, an assessment of the effect of a pregnancy is difficult because neither partner may be comfortable in disclosing concerns or problems to a new provider. Areas to evaluate are as follow:

1. *The partner's concern for the woman's needs as an expectant mother.* Is empathy, cooperativeness, availability, and trustworthiness demonstrated?
2. *The woman's concern for her partner's needs as an expectant partner.* Does she demonstrate empathy and understanding about how this new role will affect the partner? Does

she include the partner in the pregnancy process?

3. *The effect of the pregnancy on the relationship bond.* Do they maintain the same level of closeness as before the pregnancy? Has the pregnancy created conflict? The anticipation of a newborn, as well as the actual presence of a fetus, adds a new dimension to the way couples relate to one another. Pregnancy and parenthood do not help to resolve conflicts and relationship problems.

4. *The partner's adjustment to the parenting role.* Has the partner established a role for himself and accepted that role with relatively little ambivalence and conflict? Fathers who are most successful accept children, are eager to nurture a child, and have confidence in their ability to do so (Lederman, 1996).

## Other Children

Once one or both partners in a relationship has a child, the response of that child or children must be considered with the news of a new pregnancy. The effect of a new baby on the current family structure, as well as previous children's acceptance of a parent or parents taking on additional responsibility, are concerns. For the woman especially, the anticipated response of older children will affect her view towards this pregnancy. As providers, we can encourage siblings to be involved in aspects of the pregnancy and prenatal care. During this trimester, older children who have a good sense of time and understand how long a pregnancy continues may be included in aspects of the woman's prenatal visits and listen to the fetus's heartbeat. Inclusion of younger children occurs later in the pregnancy.

## Grandparents

Grandparents, or at least the pregnant woman's mother, are often the first people told about a pregnancy. The pregnant woman will turn to her mother or a mother figure "for information about childbearing, child rearing, and the validation of her ability to mother" (Mercer, 1995).

During the daughter's first pregnancy, the mother-daughter relationship may be strengthened as the daughter develops a sense of autonomy and differentiation from her mother while sharing a common experience. This permits the daughter and mother to assume more of a peer relationship, as they are now both mothers. Any previous mother-daughter conflicts may be resolved during the daughter's pregnancy.

The response of the grandparents as a unit is determined by events in their own lives, their current identities, and their view of what being grandparents means. Family cohesiveness is promoted by frank discussions between the two generations.

## Social Support System

Friends' and co-workers' responses to the pregnancy are also important to the way the pregnant woman and her partner feel about the pregnancy. Unsure of their own feelings, each partner may test the response of others by telling trusted friends and observing their responses. The parents usually will not make a general announcement until they have come to terms with their ambivalence and have passed the first trimester of development so that the risk for miscarriage has decreased.

When a woman thinks that her employment might be jeopardized or her job might be changed if her employer learns that she is pregnant, she may choose to keep the news private until the pregnancy becomes apparent. It is illegal for a woman to be discriminated against because she is pregnant, but there are methods employers have used to remove pregnant women from positions. Such action—if proven to be illegal, however—takes time and money to pursue.

## Community

The immediate and broader community within which the couple lives may or may not be supportive of couples having children. Possible restrictions on children within a residential building, as well as the location of prenatal providers, child care services, and playgrounds and schools will demonstrate the values of the community. Couples must consider these factors as they come to terms with the idea of pregnancy.

## OTHER INFLUENCES ON THE FIRST TRIMESTER OF PREGNANCY

We must understand the factors that influence this stage of a woman's pregnancy in order to provide care that will make a woman feel comfortable and that she will accept.

## Cultural Expectations

Women in many American cultures perceive pregnancy as a normal physiologic process and see themselves as healthy and not in need of health care services. However, the expectation of the health care community is that women should enter care as soon as pregnancy is suspected. A woman may come to prenatal care during the first trimester to validate the pregnancy and address concerns about the changes in her body and the discomforts of pregnancy. Other women handle these issues themselves and often choose to delay prenatal care until they have a more severe problem or delivery is eminent. Rather than making a woman feel guilty if she delays prenatal services, she should be welcomed when she does seek prenatal care. If a woman benefits from the visit, she will be more apt to come in earlier during her next pregnancy and encourage other women to do so, as well.

## Myths

Prenatal care provides the opportunity for health care providers to learn the woman's perspective on the information she hears from others. There are many myths surrounding pregnancy and childbirth, some of which center on the needs of the women during pregnancy and others of which focus on the unborn child. We must explore a woman's attitudes and beliefs about pregnancy and birth with her so that we can connect her beliefs and practices with our expectations for her prenatal care.

One myth often repeated is that "a woman loses a tooth with every pregnancy." This statement is based on the erroneous belief that the fetus draws its calcium for bone growth from its mother, which is untrue because the fetus acquires its calcium from the maternal blood supply (Worthington-Roberts and Williams, 1993). When a woman loses a tooth or teeth during pregnancy, the loss is actually related to the condition of her gums or her general need for dental care.

Preventing harm to the developing fetus is the focus of some myths. Women are cautioned not to "reach over their head or the umbilical cord will strangle the baby." Once the anatomy of pregnancy is explained to a woman, she will see that there is no relationship between her arms being over her head and the placement or tension of the umbilical cord.

Determining the baby's sex before birth is often desired. There are "tests" with household chemicals or a needle suspended by a thread, as well as determinations based on the fetal heart rate. None of these, however, are accurate assessment tools. A fetal heart rate above or below 140 does not indicate the sex of the fetus. Neither does the way an abdomen protrudes, although pregnant women often hear, "If you carry the baby low, it is a boy" or "If you stick out in front, it is a girl." Others will predict, "She [the mother] looks beautiful, so she is carrying a girl." Because each person guessing the sex of the baby has a 50% chance of being right, these myths continue.

Other myths equate the physical symptoms a mother may be experiencing with characteristics of the expected baby. For example, if the woman frequently has heartburn, "the baby has curly hair"; or if the baby is active, he will be a poor sleeper after he is born. Again, these are not actual predictors of the baby's characteristics.

The last category of myths relates to the woman's upcoming birth experience and ability to breast feed if she chooses. A woman may hear that she will duplicate the experience her mother had when she delivered her. Some women are told by their mothers, "I almost died having you (or another sibling)." The labor and childbirth experience of a woman is not determined by the experience of her mother but by the physical and emotional factors that the woman brings to the experience, her preparation for the experience, and the fetus that she is carrying. A woman's ability to breast feed her infant is also unrelated to her mother's experience.

## Spiritual Beliefs

Individuals, couples, and families may attach a spiritual meaning to the pregnancy and its development. Spirituality has been defined in a variety of ways within the profession of nursing and is defined individually by each client. A person may have spiritual beliefs without being religious and attending services.

Spirituality has been described as having two dimensions. The vertical dimension is a person's relationship to a higher being, a trust relationship with or in a transcendent being that provides a basis for meaning and hope in her life experiences. A client's spiritual beliefs related to a supreme being greatly influence how she views life and copes with the change and stress (both good and bad) that these beliefs bring. A client's beliefs determine how she responds to life's crises of illness, suffering, and loss.

The horizontal dimension of a person's spirituality reflects her relationship with a supreme being through her beliefs, values, lifestyle, quality of life, and interactions with others and with her environment. The horizontal dimension is the core of her being; it is what she is and is becoming. This dimension is concerned with bringing meaning and purpose to the woman's existence; that is, what or who she ought to live for (Carson, 1989).

When a woman learns she is pregnant, her spirituality affects how she views the condition and responds to the news. Her spiritual beliefs have implications for the services that she seeks, when she seeks them, and the adjustments she makes in her life to support the well-being of the fetus. Her spirituality also affects how she responds to a threatened or actual loss of the pregnancy.

## Maturity

The needs of a woman during her pregnancy depend upon her level of maturity. Maturity often corresponds with—but is not totally dependent upon—a person's chronologic age. During pregnancy, a woman grows from caring for herself to include caring for another. Some adolescents are capable of doing this, and some older women are not.

### Pregnant Adolescents

Most adolescent pregnancies are unintended. Middle class adolescents get pregnant, but poor teens more often have the babies, do not finish school or get married, and do not get good jobs (Musick, 1993). Pregnant girls should be encouraged to remain in school. The opportunity for peer interaction and possible peer support is greater in school than if the girl isolates herself at home.

By virtue of her own developmental level, when an adolescent girl becomes pregnant, she is generally unable to care adequately for herself, not to mention to ensure the adequate development of her child. Pregnant adolescents face physical, psychologic, and sociocultural risks associated with pregnancy (Moore, 1996).

Over 90% of the adolescents that carry the pregnancy to term keep and raise the infant (Steinberg, 1998). Some of these adolescents may make that choice to meet their needs for belonging, love, and self-esteem; and fulfill cultural expectations. However, many teens do not have access to information about the process of adoption, so they are unable to make that choice. We should raise the option of placing the child for adoption at some time during early pregnancy and provide appropriate information.

Most adolescent females are impregnated by adult men—not adolescent males, as is often assumed. Faced with physical or sexual abuse, neglect, and even abandonment, these often emotionally needy girls retain a preoccupation to please the fathers of their children in order to gain and retain their support (Musick, 1995). In such a relationship, a pregnant adolescent may be compelled to remain single rather than marry the father of her child, although her life may continue to focus on an overwhelming need to please this or other men. Once pregnant, other girls, however, want nothing to do with men—not even the father of their child.

The two common qualities within this otherwise diverse group of pregnant adolescents are poverty and the tendency to define themselves through motherhood. Poverty forces them to live in more dangerous neighborhoods, where they have access to fewer support services and have fewer opportunities for employment. In addition, each girl often does not have one of the two pathways for getting out of poverty: a family that instills high expectations and a community environment that provides a vision of a productive future beyond mothering (Musick, 1995).

Pregnant adolescents are less likely to seek early, regular prenatal care but are apt to come to care in middle-to-late pregnancy. They tend to deny to themselves the signs and symptoms of pregnancy that they are experiencing. Others feel embarrassed that they were assaulted or did not use contraception or that they believed their partner when he said he was either sterile or "taking care of it."

When an adolescent girl seeks services during the first trimester, she should be welcomed in a nonjudgmental way and provided care at a pace that makes her comfortable. The age and development of the girl determines how we approach her and which concerns are most important to her. If she is under the age of 15, she may be a concrete thinker, so we will have to be specific and directive in providing her with prenatal education. She will probably not be fully capable of making plans for the future. Before the age of 15, most girls have not even decided how they will prepare for an occupation in adulthood much less how they will be a mother to an infant. Her locus of control is generally outside of herself, so she may be very eager to take direction. She is probably also under the control of another adult (e.g., the father of the baby or a parent or guardian). Pregnant adolescents should be encouraged to involve a trusted adult in their pregnancy and prenatal care.

If the girl is between the age of 15 and 17, she may be more of a risk-taker, feel invulnerable, rebel against conformity, and use alcohol and drugs. Her support group is important, providing her with social experiences, information, and advice. This peer group offers a symbiotic relationship, helping her to develop toward independence. Now that she is pregnant, she may be forced to partially withdraw from her group and become more dependent upon her parents, which may cause her to be angry about her situation and act out against her parents. Older adolescents are generally capable of abstract thinking and future planning but may have difficulty anticipating the long-term implications of their actions. Health teaching can occur within a dialogue that respects them as individuals while also giving guidance about their choices and assistance with problem solving.

If the girl is between the ages of 17 and 19, we may generally relate to her as an adult. She is developing individuality, can picture herself in control, and is making decisions based on her judgements. Thinking abstractly and anticipating consequences, she is generally capable of identifying and solving problems.

During the assessment process, we can learn from her about her self-image, expectations for her future and the future of her child, and resources to care for herself and her child. What does she envision? To what level can she—or does she want to—make her own decisions about prenatal care? How may we help her achieve her goals while maintaining the health and well-being of her and her fetus?

The physical care of an adolescent during the first trimester is the same as for an adult woman with the additional evaluation of her physical maturity. If she is a young adolescent, her bone growth may be incomplete and the increased levels of estrogen during pregnancy may lead to the early closure of the epiphysis, arresting her bone growth. She is most at risk for this to occur in the first 4 years after menarche. In addition, her pelvic bones have not yet reached adult dimensions, increasing the risk for a **cephalopelvic disproportion** and the need for a surgical delivery (**cesarean birth**).

Regular monitoring of her blood pressure is necessary to assess for the development of **pregnancy-induced hypertension (PIH),** which is the most prevalent medical complication in pregnant young adolescents. The increased risk for PIH may be caused by less-than-optimal development of the vascular system of the placenta or the lack of adequate nutrition for the adolescent (Mattson and Smith, 2000).

Other common problems experienced by adolescents are eating disorders, substance abuse, or depression. An evaluation of these risk factors should be accomplished as early as possible. Poverty, as well as the typical eating habits of teenagers, may mean that her diet is inadequate. Because of the increased need for adequate nutrition for her own growth and maintenance, as well as for that of her child, diet counseling is required. If the adolescent is comfortable meeting another person, referral to a dietician is helpful. If she prefers to stay with us, we should start by finding out what foods she likes and can access. We should determine who does the shopping and cooking in her household. Starting with what she likes and gradually modifying her diet will provide a greater chance of success. We should encourage a balanced selection of foods from the food pyramid and limit nonnutritional food and snacks. Healthy pregnant adolescents should eat nutrient-dense foods and gain about 35 pounds in a gradual increase over the course of their pregnancy (Worthington-Roberts and Williams, 1997).

It also helps to have an adult caretaker be involved in the educational session, the purchasing and cooking meals. Careful periodic assessment and positive reinforcement are necessary. If the adolescent came into the pregnancy with an eating disorder, counseling may be needed along with the nutritional guidance.

## Delayed Pregnancy

Women over the age of 35 years also become pregnant—some with their first child. Some of these women have purposely delayed childbearing until they found a suitable partner with whom to raise the child. Others are intent on remaining single while raising the child. Mature women are generally well-educated and financially secure but may be anxious about the realities of having and raising a child. Although the pregnancy may have been planned and desired, the woman may be ambivalent and concerned about how motherhood will affect her. Accomplished in her personal and possibly professional life, the woman returns to the level of novice in the area of pregnancy and birth. In other cases she may be surprised that she is pregnant, and the child is an unplanned pregnancy. If she is newly married, she may worry about the effect on her relationship. If pregnancy has been delayed due to an infertility problem, she may fear losing this fetus and never becoming pregnant again. The life situation and feelings of the woman must be assessed.

There has been an ongoing debate in the literature about the safety of pregnancy after age 40. The concerns have generally been based on an increased risk for chromosomal abnormalities in the fertilized egg and simultaneously managing preexisting medical conditions with the pregnancy. The sharpest rise in maternal mortality occurs after age 40 when a woman is more likely to experience prenatal complications, as well as difficulties with her medical conditions. A thorough medical history is vital.

The two areas of care to address during the first trimester are the woman's concerns about the well-being of the fetus and about having the energy to care for a new baby. Gentle questioning about her feelings, reassurance about the health of the fetus, and offering her the option to be involved as much as she desires in her own care will help the woman adapt to the situation.

Be sensitive to the fact that some of the literature about women who are over 35 and pregnant with their first child may refer to them as elderly primigravidas. The use of the term "elderly" may have a negative connotation for many women, and most prefer the terminology of "mature primigravida."

The ongoing assessment of a woman whose pregnancy occurs later in life is the same as for other maternity clients. Pay particular attention to her nutritional status, history of disease, and immunization status, as well as her reproductive, medical, social, and occupational history and her use of medications and drugs. Explore her concerns about the possible risks due to her age. If she is interested, offer information about genetic risk counseling and testing.

Physical assessment should include an evaluation of the presence of uterine fibroids, which are more common in older women, while the embryo/fetus is still relatively small. Detected early in the pregnancy, this information will help to explain possible discrepancies in estimating gestational age and the size of the uterus later in pregnancy. Fibroids may also cause other complications during pregnancy and labor.

There is also an increased risk for multiple gestation in women over 35 and those who have received fertility treatments. Because women with delayed pregnancies may fall into one or both categories, a careful assessment should be done to determine how many fetuses are developing. These findings will have implications for the nutritional needs of the woman.

The incidence of vaginal bleeding also increases in women over 35 years, so they must know when and how to contact their healthcare providers. Bleeding during this trimester may be due to a spontaneous miscarriage, an ectopic pregnancy, or trophoblastic disease (a molar pregnancy). These conditions require immediate assessment and intervention to maintain the health and safety of the woman.

## Resources

The resources to be considered during a woman's pregnancy are both material and relational. Material resources (e.g., housing, clothing, food, transportation, and access to services) become even more important when the woman is also experiencing the first 3 months of pregnancy. The discomforts of early pregnancy (e.g., frequent urination, fatigue, nausea and vomiting) are harder for the woman to respond to when she is unable to leave the assembly line, when she does not have enough money to buy a variety of foods to see which ones she may tolerate, or when she is unable to take naps or rest periods during the day.

Relational resources are developed with friends, family, and organizations designed to respond to needs. The support system that a woman develops depends upon if she believes that she needs support, if she is able to accept care and emotional assistance from others, and if she has people around her that care about her and are willing to help. Family members, friends, neighbors, coworkers, members of her church, and human service agencies are general resources for social support.

During the first trimester, a woman may seek someone to talk to about her pregnancy and her body's response to it, her fears and apprehensions of how it will affect her and her life, and how she will provide for herself and her child. Single or partnered, young or old, most women seek out others beside the father of their baby. A woman's culture may determine where she seeks out and finds social support.

Keeping in mind that there are always individual differences within cultures, there are some concepts that are common in certain cultures. Young, pregnant, Native American women have a strong belief that their family or "people" will take care of them. African-American teenagers believe that their families will help them meet all of their needs during pregnancy, and this is generally true. White adolescent mothers actually receive little or no familial or social support except from boyfriends and worry most about meeting basic needs such as food and shelter (Andrews and Boyle, 1995).

## ASSESSMENT OF CHANGE DURING THE FIRST TRIMESTER

### Signs and Symptoms of Pregnancy

Many women first suspect that they are pregnant because of amenorrhea (i.e., absence of menses). Others experience tingling in their breast. Both of these are presumptive or subjective signs of pregnancy, however, because they may be caused by other conditions. Other presumptive signs of pregnancy in the first trimester are breast changes, amenorrhea, nausea and vomiting, frequent urination, fatigue, and uterine or abdominal enlargement.

**Probable** or objective signs of pregnancy are the changes perceived by an examiner, although these may also be due to causes other than pregnancy. A positive serum pregnancy test, a positive urine pregnancy test, Goodell's sign, Chadwick's sign, and Hegar's sign are the probable signs of pregnancy that may be found during the first trimester of a pregnancy.

A **positive** or diagnostic sign of pregnancy as perceived by an examiner can only be caused by pregnancy. The two positive signs that may be found during the first trimester are when the fetus can be seen (i.e., sonographic evidence of fetal outline) or heard (i.e., fetal heart is audible). A third positive sign, feeling the fetus, does not occur until the second trimester when the fetal movement may be palpated (Table 10-3).

### Ongoing Assessment of the Woman and Fetus

After it is determined that a woman is pregnant, she will be scheduled to be seen on a regular basis (Figure 10-2). The purpose of these visits is to monitor the woman's well-being—including to check her emotional adjustment, screen for maternal disease or problems caused by the pregnancy, and evaluate the growth and well-being of the fetus. These visits also provide time to address concerns and health promotion with the members of the woman's support system. Explaining the changes she is experiencing and the methods for assisting with her comfort are especially important for first-time mothers.

These periodic revisits are more focused than the initial visit described in Chapter 9, so they generally require less time. The agenda is determined by the gestational age of the pregnancy, the summary of events since the last visit by the mother, and the assessment and evaluation of the maternal and fetal status. In some health care practices, the woman conducts part of her own prenatal assessment by taking her own weight and blood pressure, testing her own urine for glucose and protein, and reporting or charting the results when she meets with the provider. In other practices, nurses aides or nurses conduct this part of the evaluation.

#### Schedule of Visits

The intervals for return visits have traditionally occurred every 4 weeks throughout the first and second trimester. This pattern of visits is not based on research. Other scheduling patterns that decrease the total number of visits for healthy women and differentiate between the needs of nulliparas and multiparas have been suggested but have not yet come into common use (Fogel and Woods, 1995).

#### Nursing Care of the Mother

Assessment of a pregnant woman entails searching for risk factors based on her past health and on the physical and psychosocial developments of this pregnancy. We should individualize our approach with a woman by following up on the questions and concerns she raised during her previous visit, as well as asking her how she is feeling and about any changes or new symptoms she may have experienced since the last visit.

Be alert for subtle or overt signs of physical, sexual, and emotional abuse. Ask her specifically, "Since your last visit, have you been emotionally or physically abused or slapped by your partner or someone important to you? Are you afraid of your partner or someone else in your home?" This assessment should occur at each visit because it allows the woman to discuss the

**TABLE 10-3**  *Signs of Pregnancy in the First Trimester*

| Approximate time in pregnancy | Presumptive signs | Probable signs | Positive signs | Description | Reason not definitive/ other possible causes |
|---|---|---|---|---|---|
| 3 | | Serum laboratory test | | Blood work reveals presence of human chorionic gonadotropin (HCG) | Have a 95% to 98% accuracy; hydatiform mole; choriocarcinoma |
| 4 | Breast changes | | | Breasts feel tender, full, or tingly; enlargement and darkening of areola | Premenstrual symptoms; oral contraception; other hormonal changes; pseudocyesis |
| 4 | Amenorrhea | | | Absence of menses | Hormonal imbalance; emotional disturbance; disease; environmental changes; excessive exercise |
| 4 | | Urine pregnancy test | | Test of urine reveals HCG | 97% accurate; pelvic infection; tumors; hydatiform mole |
| 4 | Nausea and vomiting | | | Nausea and vomiting when arising in morning | Gastrointestinal illness; acute infections; food poisoning; emotional disorder |
| 5 | Frequent urination | | | Need to void frequently | Urinary tract infection; diabetes; pressure from pelvic tumor; congestive heart failure; emotional tension or stress |
| 6 | | | Sonographic view of fetal outline | Fetal outline can be seen and measured | No other causes |
| 8 | | Goodell's sign | | Softening of the cervix | Pelvic congestion; estrogen-progestin oral contraceptives |
| 8 | | Chadwick's sign | | Color of vagina changes from pink to blue/violet | Pelvic congestion; vulvar, vaginal, cervical hyperemia |
| 8 | | Hegar's sign | | Softening of the lower uterine segment | Pelvic congestion, excessively soft walls of nonpregnant uterus |
| 12 | | | Fetal heart audible | Doppler ultrasound reveals heartbeat | No other causes |
| 14 | Fatigue | | | General feeling of fatigue | Stress, illness |
| 14 | Uterine/ abdominal enlargement | | | Uterus can be palpated over symphysis pubis | Uterine tumor; pelvic tumors; ascites; ovarian cyst |

subject when she chooses and also encourages her to disclose her situation. Research shows that only 7.3% of women report abuse on their own initiative. That number jumps to 29.3% when women are asked specifically about it during an assessment (McFarlane and others, 1991).

Assess her progress—physically and psychosocially— in adapting to the pregnancy. Determine with whom she has shared the news of her pregnancy. How have they responded? How has that made her feel? What are her personal and family strengths that support her? What are her educational needs? What are the educational needs of her support system? Does she need a referral to obtain goods or services that would help her?

Ask about the physical changes and discomforts usually experienced at her stage of pregnancy. If she has ex-

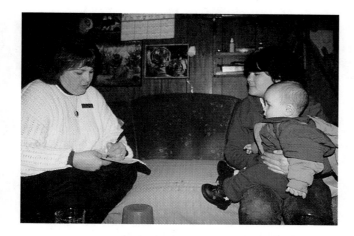

FIGURE 10-2 • Home visit with expectant mother. *(Courtesy of Caroline E. Brown.)*

**TABLE 10-4   *Signs and Symptoms of Potential Complications***

| Signs/symptoms | Possible causes |
| --- | --- |
| Severe vomiting | Gastrointestinal infection; "morning sickness" |
| Abdominal cramping and/or vaginal bleeding | Spontaneous abortion |
| Severe abdominal pain | Ectopic pregnancy |
| Chills, fever over 101°F | Infection |
| Diarrhea | Gastrointestinal infection |
| Burning on urination | Urinary tract infection |

perienced discomfort, encourage her to describe how she has responded. Using appropriate teaching tools, explain to her the changes in her body that are causing the discomfort. Cultures have developed different ways to address the discomforts of pregnancy. Learn the prescriptive and possibly restrictive ideas that she has followed to increase her comfort.

Provide anticipatory guidance appropriate for her stage of the pregnancy and individual needs. Answer any questions she may have or obtain someone more knowledgeable to provide her with the information.

During the first trimester, the woman should immediately report any cramping, vaginal bleeding, or severe and prolonged vomiting. Review this information with her and ask if she has experienced any of these. Also go over with her what she should do if she becomes concerned about the baby or experiences any signs of potential complications (Table 10-4). Some women intuitively know that something is wrong before they are fully aware of a danger sign. Encourage her to call with any questions or concerns.

At each visit, we will evaluate the effect of the pregnancy on the woman's body by checking her vital signs, blood pressure, and weight. Her urine may be tested for protein and glucose, and she will be assessed for edema, especially of the hands and face. A complete blood count (CBC) with differential smear, hemoglobin (Hbg), and hematocrit (Hct) is obtained, and screening for sexually transmitted infections is done as indicated.

The nurse-midwife, nurse practitioner, or physician may repeat some or all of the prior assessment, review the history and findings, and complete the examination, which includes the following:

- Review of the woman's history and current findings
- Assessment of deep tendon reflexes
- Assessment of the status of the fetus

### Assessment of the Fetus

Toward the end of the first trimester, the fundus of the uterus may be felt and the fetal heartbeat can be heard with an ultrasound fetoscope or ultrasound stethoscope. The nurse midwife, nurse practitioner, or physician listens to the fetal heart tones as part of the fetal assessment. If culturally acceptable, the pregnant woman and those with her may also be relieved to hear the child's heartbeat. If possible, the mother is helped to feel the top of the uterus as a way of making the fetus seem real to her.

### Additional Assessment Measures

During the course of a pregnancy, additional assessment tools may be used. These tools are selected based on availability, provider preference, the need for evaluating the mother or fetus, the expense, and if the data that might be obtained will make a difference in the course of the pregnancy.

***Laboratory Testing.*** Based on the woman's and the father of the baby's family history, genetic screening may be indicated to identify babies with possible inherited or acquired defects. "Approximately 50% of spontaneous abortions and 5% to 7% of intrauterine fetal deaths are caused by chromosomal abnormalities." Clients with potential risks should receive further education and counseling, so they may then choose whether to do nothing and proceed with the pregnancy—often because they see it as "a gift from God"—or to choose only noninvasive assessment procedures so that they do not put the pregnancy at risk. Others may choose to undergo further testing and evaluation, often with the thought of aborting the fetus if abnormalities are found.

Between weeks 12 and 16 of the pregnancy, genetic testing may be done using either amniocentesis or α-fetoprotein serum. Another option is sampling the chorionic villi (CVS) after 10 weeks to evaluate the chromosomal, enzymatic, and DNA status of the fetus. A CVS provides less accurate data and provides more risk to the successful continuation of the pregnancy than amniocentesis.

Testing the father of the baby may also occur. He may be screened for blood type and Rh factor and sickle cell disease or other genetic risk if indicated.

***Ultrasound.*** Ultrasound may be used for a number of screening and diagnostic tests during the first trimester. Five to six weeks after the woman's last menstrual period, an endovaginal ultrasound can confirm the presence of a pregnancy by estimating the gestational sac volume. If the date of conception is unknown and of concern, the crown-rump length of the embryo can be measured when visualized by ultrasound between weeks 6 and 10. More measurements (i.e., of the biparietal diameter, femur length, and abdominal circumference of the fetus) may be taken during the thirteenth week. To appraise problems with fetus growth, ultrasound can be used to ascertain a ratio of the size of the head to the size of the abdomen after 13 weeks. If a CVS is desired, ultrasound is used to see the chorionic villi.

Ultrasound is also used to identify actual or potential problems for the mother. An ectopic pregnancy or a multiple gestation may both be detected by ultrasound. Other maternal conditions (e.g., a bicornate uterus, ovarian cysts, and fibroids), as well as placental abnormalities, may be seen.

### Close of the Visit

Before the woman leaves each prenatal visit, address any further questions and concerns, provide appropriate anticipatory guidance, review the expected changes that will occur before her next visit, and praise her positive health behaviors. Review the signs and symptoms of possible problems and be sure she knows when and where to contact a provider. Confirm the date and time of her next appointment.

During the first trimester, visits are generally 4 weeks apart, which may be a long time for a woman or family member to carry a concern or remember a question. Encourage the woman to call with major concerns and write down the questions that she wants to have answered at the next visit.

Some providers do not encourage a woman to call with questions because of the non-billable time they take. The connection that is offered to a woman when she knows she can call, however, will help to keep her anxiety level lower and include her as a collaborator in the prenatal health care process. The reality is, if she has a question she will ask someone. Her continuity of health care will be improved when she is able to ask a health care provider rather than a friend or acquaintance, who may have a more limited knowledge base.

### Anticipatory Guidance during the First Trimester

During the monthly prenatal visits, a woman or her partner may ask many questions. Based on research and our experience, we can anticipate what these areas of concern may be and be prepared to raise the issues ourselves and then, in dialogue, offer anticipatory guidance (Figure 10-3). During the first trimester, areas of concern are sexual activity, hygiene, nutritional needs, safety, drug use, and the discomforts of pregnancy.

### Sexual Activity

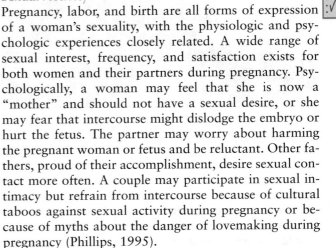

Pregnancy, labor, and birth are all forms of expression of a woman's sexuality, with the physiologic and psychologic experiences closely related. A wide range of sexual interest, frequency, and satisfaction exists for both women and their partners during pregnancy. Psychologically, a woman may feel that she is now a "mother" and should not have a sexual desire, or she may fear that intercourse might dislodge the embryo or hurt the fetus. The partner may worry about harming the pregnant woman or fetus and be reluctant. Other fathers, proud of their accomplishment, desire sexual contact more often. A couple may participate in sexual intimacy but refrain from intercourse because of cultural taboos against sexual activity during pregnancy or because of myths about the danger of lovemaking during pregnancy (Phillips, 1995).

Because childbirth is a sexual experience, we must have a basic understanding of a couple's personal and cultural attitudes about pregnancy and birth, as well as of their attitudes toward expressing love, sex, and intimate relations during pregnancy. To incorporate sexuality into the assessment and subsequent teaching plan, we must ask about their personal and cultural beliefs and expectations; present the wide range of normal behavior; and allow them to integrate the practices that meet their needs (Phillips, 1995).

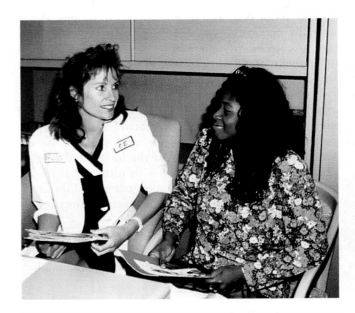

*FIGURE 10-3* • Expectant mother and nurse discuss prenatal care concerns. *(From Dickason:* Maternal-infant nursing care, *ed 3, St Louis, 1998, Mosby.)*

A woman's physiologic sexual responses during pregnancy are similar to her nonpregnant responses. What may change during the course of the pregnancy is her desire. During the first trimester, most women experience a decrease in sexual desire and, consequently, in their desired frequency of intercourse. Sensations of fatigue, nausea, vomiting, breast tenderness, or anxieties about miscarriage are factors that may decrease desire.

Fatigue—even exhaustion—is often experienced by women during this trimester because they may require more sleep. A woman who desires sexual intercourse but is feeling fatigued may persuade her partner to participate in lovemaking earlier in the day or evening, helping her to relax before she falls asleep.

Nausea and vomiting may be a sexual turnoff. The woman may feel uneasy and be preoccupied with maintaining control of this discomfort, rather than enjoying sex at this time. "'I felt really awful,' one woman said. 'Drained of all vitality, smelly, with a tinny taste in my mouth. I wondered where this much-vaunted pregnancy radiance was. I felt ghastly! And sex was out of the question'"(Kitzinger, 1985). By the end of the first trimester, the nausea and vomiting usually subside. At this point, the couple may become more sexually active.

Early pregnancy brings many changes to a woman's breasts; they grow in size and, in some cases, become extremely sensitive. These physical changes and the need for some women to sleep with a bra on for comfort, often begin to shift the significance of the breasts from erotic objects to the means by which to feed a baby. If a woman is comfortable with allowing her breasts to be caressed and experience nipple stimulation, it must be gentle because pummeling, biting, or energetic sucking will hurt and bruise her. During sexual arousal, the breasts swell by as much as 25% so the already enlarged breasts become more engorged. Nipple stimulation should begin with a touch as light as a feather and become firmer only as it feels good to her. Gentleness becomes the norm for sex to be pleasurable to pregnant women (Kitzinger, 1985).

The experience of a miscarriage with a previous pregnancy or the threat of a miscarriage with the current pregnancy may cause the mother or both partners to feel very apprehensive and see sex as a direct threat to the baby. The couple may be so fearful that they even avoid cuddling or caressing each other because they fear sexual arousal. Prohibitions against lovemaking, which are so often given when a woman has bleeding during early pregnancy, have not been shown to help avoid miscarriage. In addition, when couples do "break the rules" and not only touch each other but experience intercourse, they generally will not tell us. With respect and support for a couple's desire for caution during this trimester, however, we can teach and encourage other ways that they may demonstrate mutual love and caring without penetrating the woman's vagina (Kitzinger, 1985). Encouraging them to meet each other's sexual needs without intercourse may be a new concept so teaching materials and diagrams may be helpful. A loving touch, hugs, kissing, stroking of the breasts and/or clitoris, and oral stimulation of the breasts or clitoris are ways that a partner may "make love" to a woman without having intercourse. A man may wish to have his partner perform oral sex. Oral/genital sex on either partner should only be done if it is known that infection is not present.

Providers may tell a woman to avoid sexual intercourse during this trimester if she has a partner with a sexually transmitted infection, a history of miscarriage or a possibility of threatened miscarriage (even though research does not support this), or undiagnosed vaginal bleeding. Once these difficulties are overcome during the first trimester, many women enjoy consensual sex more than ever before.

### General Hygiene

A woman may take both regular tub baths and showers throughout her pregnancy as she experiences oilier skin, increased perspiration, and increased vaginal discharge. Douching is not necessary at any time but is definitely not allowed during pregnancy. Hot tubs should not be used during pregnancy because they create a danger of hyperthermia and the risk for fetal abnormalities.

### Nutritional Needs

Patterns of weight gain are as important to monitor as the woman's total weight gain for the pregnancy. Know the goals that were set with the woman at the beginning of the pregnancy, and support her progress. It is more important that the woman eats in a nutritionally sound pattern every day rather than be tempted to diet just before a visit so that she will not be "overweight" for the provider. It is only when the woman has persistent and extreme deviations from expected patterns that reassessment of weight-gain goals and other factors in her life become signals for intervention. Weight maintenance or a slight weight loss during pregnancy is normal during the first trimester (ific, 1999).

The cause of nausea and vomiting during the first trimester is unknown. A combination of hormonal, psychologic, and neuralgic factors, as well as general fatigue may have a causal effect (Davis, 1996). In pregnancies where chorionic gonadatropins are elevated, women generally experience more frequent and severe nausea and vomiting (Simpson and Creehan, 1996).

Because of the nausea and vomiting, the woman may restrict her diet to foods that she can tolerate (e.g., toast, crackers, cereal). Fluids are often better tolerated between meals rather than with them. Some women will not even be able to stand the thought of food and tolerate only "flat" soft drinks—especially ginger ale or cola; popsicles; or hard candy. These substances will supply fluid and a few calories (ific, 1999). The woman should not take supplemental iron until her nausea and vomiting improve.

A woman may experience nausea and vomiting at any time of the day. Assessment includes onset, frequency, time, and duration of symptoms, as well as the gestational age of the pregnancy. The woman may also report ptyalism (i.e., excessive, bitter salivation). Identifying and avoiding foods or food smells that trigger nausea is the first step. Keeping something in her stomach by eating smaller meals more frequently (i.e., every 2 or 3 hours) and/or by snacking on bland crackers or cookies or hard candy between the frequent meals also helps. Preferred foods are low-fat protein foods and carbohydrates that are easily digested. Small amounts of non-carbonated liquids consumed between meals help to prevent gastric distention.

We should assess the woman for dehydration by observing pallor, poor skin turgor, or dryness of skin and mucous membranes. Vital signs, weight changes, the presence of ketones in her urine, and positive bowel sounds should also be noted (Davis, 1996). Review with each woman possible ways to maintain an appropriate level of fluid and nutritional intake during this time. There is no evidence that supplementing a woman's diet with large doses of vitamin $B_6$ will effectively treat morning sickness (ific, 1999).

A woman may experience nausea and vomiting when she gets up in the morning. Eating toast, a few saltines, or graham crackers before lifting her head off the pillow may help reduce the sensations. Many women do not like the blandness of saltines, however, and prefer a different food. Interestingly, a nutrient analysis of saltine crackers and ginger ale vs. baked potato chips and lemonade determined that a better nutrient value was obtained with the potato chips and lemonade. The potato chips provide potassium, which is lost during vomiting, and more folic acid and vitamin C than the saltines. Potato chips also help to settle the stomach and increase thirst. The lemonade reduces the amount of saliva, making it more palatable to women experiencing the excess saliva associated with nausea and vomiting (Davis, 1996).

Different cultures have remedies for nausea and vomiting. For example, Cuban-American women believe that eating coffee grounds will cure it (Pernell and Paulanka, 1998). Acupressure helps some women because it triggers sensory and neurologic impulses that control vomiting. Acupressure wristbands are available at businesses that provide remedies for motion sickness (e.g., boating stores and travel clubs). A sensory afferent stimulating unit that delivers electrical stimulation to the volar aspect of the wrist has also been useful to some women (Davis, 1996).

### Promotion of Safety

Seat belts must be worn at all times during pregnancy. There is greater risk to the developing fetus if the mother is injured in an auto accident than to the fetus itself from the seat belt.

The home and other workplaces expose women to a variety of dangerous substances and hazards. Harmful substances may enter a woman's body by inhalation, skin contact, or swallowing (ingestion) and may cause a great deal of damage during the first trimester when the embryo and/or fetus is developing. Reproductive hazards do not affect every woman or every pregnancy. Whether a woman and her fetus are harmed depends on *how much* of the hazard they are exposed to, *when* they are exposed, *how long* they are exposed, and *how* they are exposed.

In her home the woman should avoid exposure to cleaning supplies, paint supplies, pesticides, etc. If there is a cat, she should not be changing the litter box because of the risk for toxoplasmosis from the feces of the cat. Other adults living in the home may unknowingly carry contaminants home on their work clothes. To prevent home contamination, these adults should change out of the contaminated clothes and into street clothes that have been stored in a safe area of the workplace, as well as wash-up with soap and water before going home. Ideally, the work clothes should be washed at work. If this is not possible they should be transported home in a sealed plastic bag and washed separately from the rest of the family's clothes by someone other than the pregnant woman.

The harmful effects of a few agents found in the workplace have been known for many years. For example, more than 100 years ago lead was discovered to cause miscarriages, stillbirths, and infertility in female pottery workers. Exposure to fumes and chemical agents that are toxic, radiation, and the strain of heavy lifting may lead to miscarriage or abnormalities in fetal development. Table 9-1 lists some of the chemical and physical reproductive hazards for women in their places of work. The list is not complete and is constantly being revised. Do not assume that a substance is safe because it is not on the list.

Some workers are also exposed to disease-causing agents that are reproductive hazards. Table 9-2 lists viruses and other disease-causing (infectious) agents that are found in some workplaces and that have harmful reproductive effects in pregnant women. Women with immunity through vaccinations or earlier exposures are generally not at risk from diseases such as hepatitis B, human parvovirus B19, German measles (Rubella), or chicken pox (varicella-zoster virus). Pregnant workers without prior immunity, however, should avoid contact with infected children or adults—especially during the first trimester.

Women should also use good hygienic practices (e.g., frequent hand washing) to prevent the spread of infectious diseases among workers in elementary schools, nursery schools, and daycare centers. They should also use universal precautions (e.g., wear gloves and safely dispose of needles) to protect against disease-causing agents found in blood.

Women should be alert to possible exposure both in and outside the home. Employers are responsible for training and protecting their workers. Employees are responsible for learning about the hazards, using personal protective equipment, and following proper protective practices. Because much is unknown about hazards, however, a woman can increase her safety by doing the following:

- Storing chemicals in a sealed container when not in use.
- Washing hands after contact with hazardous substances and before eating and drinking.
- Avoiding skin contact with chemicals.
- Washing skin contacted by chemicals as directed by the material safety data sheet accompanying all hazardous materials. Home cleaning supplies have this information on the side of the container. For jobs outside the home, employers are required to have this information available to workers.
- Participating in all safety and health education, training, and monitoring programs offered by her employer.
- Learning about proper work practices and engineering controls (e.g., proper ventilation).
- Using personal protective equipment (e.g., gloves, respirators, and protective clothing) to reduce her exposure.
- Preventing home contamination by other adults living in the same home (National Institute for Occupational Safety and Health, 1999).

If a woman is concerned about a possible hazard in the workplace, she should consult her health care provider. We can educate the woman, her family, and employers about how she can continue to function without the risk of exposure. We should be aware, however, that many women will not mention their concerns to their employers for fear of losing their job and—with it—their health insurance.

### Drug Consumption

There are many times in a woman's normal activities of daily living when she makes choices concerning her health. The use of caffeine, herbal teas, over-the counter drugs, cigarettes, and alcohol are all activities sanctioned by society yet potentially harmful to a developing fetus. Asking about her use and providing clear explanations about the effects of these drugs, as well as assisting her in making changes in her personal habits, can have a positive effect. Continue to assess her choices in the use of drugs throughout her pregnancy.

***Caffeine.*** No association between caffeine consumption and birth defects has been found. Moderate con-

sumption of caffeine does not increase the risk for spontaneous abortion or preterm delivery, although some studies suggest that drinking more than 2 or 3 cups of coffee daily (i.e., 8 cups of tea or 9 cans of carbonated soft drinks) increases the chances of a low–birth-weight baby. This may be because caffeine curbs the appetite, increases gastrointestinal motility—decreasing absorption of nutrients with negative affect on fetal weight gain, and increases production of hydrochloric acid. A reasonable guideline for daily caffeine intake is around 300 mg. Caffeine content varies in food and beverages, but if the woman understands caffeine levels she may make wise choices (Table 10-5).

Pregnant women should not substitute herbal teas, however, for these beverages. Many of the herbs consumed in teas, capsules, and tinctures contain substances that could affect the developing infant. Remind the woman to ask about the possible effects of an herb before using it.

Continue to assess the woman's beverage habits throughout pregnancy. Appropriate questions are, "How many cups of coffee do you drink a day now? Is it caffeinated or decaffeinated? How large are the cups? What herbal teas are you drinking?"

***Smoking.*** Smoking during pregnancy reduces fetal weight gain and places a constant stress on the fetus because of the reduction of oxygen and nutrients available

### TABLE 10-5 *Caffeine Content of Food and Beverages*

| Item | Average milligrams | Caffeine range* |
|---|---|---|
| Coffee (5 oz cup) | | |
| Brewed, drip method | 85 | 65-120 |
| Instant | 65 | 30-120 |
| Decaffeinated | 3 | 2-4 |
| Espresso (1 oz cup) | 40 | 30-50 |
| Tea (8 oz cup) | | |
| Brewed, major U.S. brands | 40 | 20-90 |
| Brewed, imported brands | 60 | 25-110 |
| Instant | 28 | 24-31 |
| Iced (8 oz glass) | 25 | 9-50 |
| Some soft drinks (8 oz) | 24 | 20-40 |
| Cocoa beverages ( 8 oz) | 6 | 3-32 |
| Chocolate milk beverages (8 oz) | 5 | 2-7 |
| Milk chocolate (1 oz) | 6 | 1-15 |
| Dark chocolate semisweet (1 oz) | 20 | 5-35 |
| Baker's chocolate (1 oz) | 26 | 26 |
| Chocolate-flavored syrup (1 oz) | 4 | 4 |

*The amount of caffeine varies according to the brewing method, the variety of plant that is used, the concentration of the brand, etc.

From the U. S. Food and Drug Administration and National Soft Drink Association. Printed in *Healthy Eating During Pregnancy,* http://ificingo.health.org/brochure/eatpreg.htm

to the fetus. In addition, women who smoke are more likely to use caffeine and/or alcohol. Each of these substances has an addictive effect, making it difficult for some women to stop use totally.

With each visit, ask about the woman's exposure to tobacco products. If she was a smoker before pregnancy and has continued to smoke ask the following questions, "How often do you smoke cigarettes? Are you using other tobacco products (i.e., chew and cigars)? How many (or how much) per day?" If the woman is a non-smoker, ask about her exposure to passive smoke. For example, "Does anyone in your home (or place of work) smoke around you?"

If the woman cannot stop using tobacco but is trying to cut back, encourage her efforts and sympathize with her about how difficult it is. Praise, rather than guilt, will help to bring about a higher level of success. Teaching tools that demonstrate the effect of tobacco on the fetus and prominently displayed posters and literature will reinforce our teaching. Offer to refer her to a smoking-cessation group.

Exposure to secondhand smoke also has a negative affect on the fetus. Ask about her exposure to other smokers. Help her figure out ways to reduce her exposure.

***Alcohol Consumption.*** The ingestion of alcohol disrupts the neural development and brain-cell size of a fetus. The most severe damage is done during the developmental phase of the first trimester and the limitation in the number of cells developed is not reversible. If a mother is able to stop using alcohol later in the first trimester, however, the size of the existing fetal brain cells will improve. With improved nutrition, decreased or stopping of smoking, and abstinence from alcohol, the fetal brain cells will continue to grow as the pregnancy continues.

Ask the mother the following: "How often have you had beer, wine, or liquor? How much did you consume? How has that amount changed?"

***Nonprescription Drugs.*** Rather than expecting the woman to call before taking any over-the-counter medication during the first trimester, we should provide her with a list of remedies for specific situations with proper dosages as a positive teaching tool. Remind the woman that although she may have taken either *acetylsalicylic acid* (ASA) or *ibuprofen* on a regular basis before the pregnancy, they should now be avoided. *Acetaminophen* is the pain medication that is often recommended during pregnancy and lactation.

The fatigue of pregnancy may cause the woman to consider increasing her use of herbs and vitamin supplements. Encourage her to start taking prenatal vitamins when they are prescribed, but remind her that more is not better. Too much of some vitamins may be toxic to the fetus and/or mother.

Ask the woman the following: "What over-the-counter medications have you used? What do you do to

help yourself when you get a headache? How many times per week do you have to do this? What vitamins do you take? How many of each kind do you take? How often do you take them?"

***Prescription Drugs.*** No prescription drugs should be taken without being evaluated by a heath care provider for the possible danger to the embryo or fetus.

Ask the woman the following: "Have you needed to take a prescription drug recently? Have you taken a prescription drug for other than what it was intended? Have you taken someone else's prescriptions?"

***Recreational or Street Drugs.*** Marijuana, cocaine, and amphetamines continue to be a threat to the well-being of the woman and her fetus. The use of these drugs crosses all economic classes and ethnic groups. Continue to screen every woman. During the physical examination, look for fresh needle or track marks.

Ask the woman the following: "What are you doing to help yourself relax? What drugs or medications help you do this? Are you using recreational drugs? Which ones? When? How much? What recreational drugs have you used during this pregnancy? When? What? How much?"

We should keep the questions open-ended and in our own words and the tone conversational and nonjudgmental. Each response should be followed up with other questions and dialogue as appropriate to obtain the information we need. We should praise her actions as appropriate. Almost no woman will be using substances from all these categories so complimenting her as possible helps to keep the door open for further discussion and education. As we develop a relationship of trust with her, she will be more open to sharing information.

### Discomforts of Pregnancy

During the course of a pregnancy, women experience a variety of discomforts related to the physical changes occurring in her body. We may see these discomforts as minor, but they are not experienced as such by the pregnant woman. If she does not expect them or understand their cause, she may become unduly anxious.

Fatigue in early pregnancy is common, although the physiologic basis is unknown. A variety of physiologic factors (e.g., poor nutrition, anemia, and slowed circulation), however, are thought to influence it. Excessive fatigue may indicate that the woman is depressed or experiencing other psychologic or physiologic causes. Poor nutrition may also contribute to fatigue when the woman is experiencing nausea and possibly vomiting. Maintaining a mild to moderate level of exercise (i.e., with walking, swimming, or stretching) can have a positive influence on a number of body systems, improve circulation, and provide the woman with a greater sense of vitality.

If the woman is fatigued, investigate ways that she may rest during the day and activities that will enhance her ability to sleep at night. If she finds that she is hav-

## TABLE 10-6   *Relief of the Common Discomforts of the First Trimester*

| Condition | Helpful interventions |
|---|---|
| Nausea and vomiting | Avoid odors or factors that trigger nausea |
| | Eat dry toast or crackers before getting up in morning |
| | Eat small but frequent meals without drinking fluids, and drink fluids between meals |
| | Avoid greasy or highly seasoned foods |
| | Drink ginger ale or other carbonated beverages or herbal teas (e.g., ginger, peppermint, chamomile, or spearmint) |
| | Consider the use of acupressure wrist bands or the self-care practice of acupressure to appropriate pressure points |
| Ptyalism (excessive secretion of saliva) | Use an astringent mouthwash |
| | Chew gum |
| | Suck on hard candy (different flavors may have different effects) |
| Breast tenderness | Wear a well-fitting, supportive bra during the day |
| | Sleep in a bra at night |
| Leukorrhea (increased vaginal discharge) | Bathe daily |
| | Wear cotton underpants |
| | Avoid the use of nylon panties and pantyhose |
| | Do not douche |
| Urinary frequency | Drink most of daily fluid allowance in the morning |
| | Void when the urge is present |
| | Know that pressure on bladder will gradually be relieved with the growth of fetus |
| Nasal stuffiness and epitaxis | Maintain fluid intake |
| | Use nasal moisture sprays |
| | Avoid nasal sprays for congestion and/or "cold" symptoms |
| | Avoid decongestants |

From Davis DC: The discomforts of pregnancy, *J Obstet Gynecol Neonat Nurs* 25(1):73-81, 1996; *Nurses handbook of alternative and complementary therapies*, Springhouse, PA, 1998, Springhouse; Snyder and Lindquist: Complementary and alternative therapies in nursing, ed 3, New York, 1998, Springer).

ing difficulty staying asleep, explore with her what is waking her (i.e., environmental noise or temperature, the need to urinate, dreams, muscle cramping), and solve the problem together.

Women assume the general responsibility for identifying and treating their discomforts within each trimester of pregnancy. They will base their interventions on information from family, friends, and health care providers. Giving the woman anticipatory guidance and teaching materials are the best way to lessen or prevent the discomforts (Table 10-6). Take-home information is important because the woman will only remember about 20% of what she hears you say. The materials also serve to inform the others in her support network. A multifaceted approach has the best chance of being successful.

How a woman responds to the discomforts of pregnancy depends on her personal knowledge and the experiences of her friends. She may welcome the discomforts of the first trimester as confirmation that she is pregnant; think that they are a right of passage to be endured; or be very upset with the experiences of nausea and vomiting, ptyalism, fatigue, frequency of urination, breast tenderness, increased vaginal discharge, nasal stuffiness, or epitaxis. The knowledge that these discomforts generally only occur for a limited time often helps the woman to cope.

## PREGNANCY LOSS—POTENTIAL AND ACTUAL

Bleeding at any time during a pregnancy indicates a physical and emotional crisis that may lead to the death of the embryo/fetus and endanger the life of the mother. When bleeding occurs in the first trimester, the most common causes are spontaneous abortion, ectopic pregnancy, and gestational trophoblastic disease (GTD). The woman will most often call her regular prenatal provider when she is worried. We respond by providing immediate care, as well as preparing her for the possibility of admission to an inpatient facility (see Chapter 18 for in-hospital prenatal nursing care).

### Spontaneous Abortion

A spontaneous abortion (i.e., miscarriage) is the ending of a pregnancy before the point of fetal viability. The period of gestation will not be more than 20 weeks, and the conceptus will not weigh more than 500 g or be longer than 16.5 cm (crown to rump).

It is unknown how many pregnancies end in spontaneous abortion, but estimates vary from 12% to 15%. A woman may assume that her "period" was late, so she is now having a heavy menstrual period, when she actually may be having an early abortion.

Spontaneous abortions have several classifications depending on the process the woman is experiencing. A **threatened abortion** causes cramping, backache, and vaginal bleeding early in the pregnancy that may persist for several days and possibly lead to pregnancy loss, although the pregnancy may continue. The uterine size remains compatible with dates, the os remains closed, and no products of conception are passed. The long-term prognosis is unpredictable; the pregnancy may continue without further problems or an abortion may eventually occur. An **imminent or inevitable abortion** is a pregnancy that cannot be saved. The bleeding and cramping increase, the internal os dilates, and the membranes may rupture, but the products of conception have not yet been passed. A **complete abortion** is when all of this occurs *and* all of the products of conception are expelled. If moderate to severe uterine cramping and heavy bleeding occur and the cervix dilates while some of the products of conception—usually the placenta—are retained, the process is labeled an **incomplete abortion.** A **missed abortion** occurs when an early fetal intrauterine death occurs, but the fetus is not expelled. Uterine growth stops, breasts return to their nonpregnant state, and pregnancy tests are negative. Bleeding may initially be absent, but then a brownish discharge or spotting of blood may occur and then a heavier flow. If the fetus is retained beyond 6 weeks, the breakdown in fetal tissues may result in the release of thromboplastin, and disseminated intravascular coagulation (DIC) may occur, placing the woman's life at risk. A woman experiences **habitual abortions** if she has three consecutive pregnancies that end in spontaneous abortion.

The exact cause of spontaneous abortions is unknown, but they may result from fetal, placental, or maternal factors that influence development and implantation during the first trimester. Fetal factors include defective development of the embryo, faulty implantation of the embryo, or rejection of the embryo by the endometrium. Chromosomal defects account for most of the first trimester spontaneous abortions. Placental factors include an abnormally functioning placenta and abnormal platelet function. Maternal factors include infection, drug injection, and trauma.

### Assessment

When a woman reports vaginal bleeding, she should be seen and evaluated as soon as possible. Other signs and symptoms of a spontaneous abortion during the first half of pregnancy include cramping in lower abdomen; symptoms of infection (e.g., fever or malaise); dry skin or mucous membranes; thirst; nausea; or anorexia. An ultrasound scan may be useful in determining the cause of bleeding. Other possible causes of bleeding that must be ruled out are as follows: polyps, a ruptured cervical blood vessel, cervical erosion, cervicitis, ectopic pregnancy, or gestational trophoblastic disease (GTD).

Nursing assessment includes the woman's vital signs, amount and color of bleeding, current level of comfort, as well as assessment of cramping and/or contractions and overall physical health. The level of understanding and response of the woman and her family to this potential loss must also be assessed. The woman and her family may exhibit a variety of responses. Their behaviors will be influenced by the value of the pregnancy to the woman and her support system; their desire for the pregnancy; the length of gestation; the history of other pregnancy outcomes; the relationship of the woman and her partner; their social support network; their spiritual, religious, and ethnic beliefs; and their coping mechanisms.

### Nursing Plan

Both the physical and the emotional well-being of the woman and her family must be provided. An explanation about the cramping that is occurring, the tests that may be ordered, and ways to increase her physical comfort is necessary. When a woman is experiencing a miscarriage, the contractions often feel very strong—not only because she is experiencing the process of labor but also because she is either consciously or unconsciously tightening up her lower abdomen trying to hold onto the fetus. Conscious relaxation and breathing techniques, analgesics for pain, and the presence of a caring person (i.e., either a family member, friend, or provider) are of great help.

Objective data are collected by the nurse practitioner or midwife or the physician to determine the actual diagnosis. Such data may include palpation of the uterus for sizing, auscultation for fetal heart tones, observation of the cervix, the use of transvaginal or transabdominal ultrasound to see the embryonic sac, or measurement of progesterone or serial measurement of $\beta$-hCG in the woman's blood. We should prepare the woman and her partner for the assessment process and answer their questions.

Emotional support for the threatened or actual loss of pregnancy is important because the woman started to become attached to the fetus when the pregnancy was first diagnosed. With the cramps and or bleeding, she may now feel shocked or exhibit disbelief. As the reality becomes more apparent, she may begin to feel guilty that it is happening because she was ambivalent about being pregnant or did not take care of herself or that this is a punishment for wrongdoing.

Explaining the natural processes that can lead to spontaneous abortion can decrease a woman's feelings of guilt. Encourage the woman and her partner to talk about their fears and feelings both for this pregnancy, as well as for future possibilities, and give them the privacy to grieve together. We should be available, however, as the outcome of this crisis unfolds.

Inevitable and incomplete abortions are treated with a dilation and curettage or suction evacuation to remove the products of conception as soon as a definitive diagnosis is made. If the woman has experienced a missed abortion, a wait-and-see approach may be taken as the provider waits for the woman's body to start labor spontaneously. For many women, this is emotionally difficult because they know their fetus is dead and the thought of carrying it around waiting for labor to start is hard. Other women welcome the delay because it gives them time to become accustomed to their circumstances. In the first trimester, some providers may offer a suction curettage to remove the tissues of conception rather than delay the process. If the woman is Rh negative and not sensitized, anti-D Rh immune globulin will be given within 72 hours.

The grieving period for a couple after a spontaneous abortion may last from 6 to 24 months, which may surprise family and friends as they expect the couple to quickly "get over it." Each person involved will grieve differently and come to resolution and acceptance in a different way. Understanding the unique response of each individual will help partners support each other. Providers often neglect the needs of the partner after a spontaneous abortion because the mother is the focus of care and the partner is also involved in caring for the mother. Be sure to leave time to provide individual attention and support to the partner. Many couples are helped in their grieving process by attending support groups for parents who have experienced a miscarriage.

## Ectopic Pregnancy

An **ectopic pregnancy** is the implantation of a fertilized ovum outside of the uterine cavity. In the United States, an ectopic pregnancy occurs in approximately 1 in 50 pregnancies—and this rate is increasing. An ectopic pregnancy is a potentially life threatening condition for the mother that may require the decision to end the pregnancy to save her life.

Most ectopic pregnancies attach in a fallopian tube but may also occur in the cervix or migrate out the fallopian tube and attach on an ovary or in the abdominal cavity. As the pregnancy continues, the normal signs and symptoms of pregnancy occur.

When the embryo grows in the fallopian tube, the tube stretches and ruptures, causing bleeding into the abdominal cavity. The blood irritates the peritoneal tissue, causing a sharp, one-sided pain; syncope (fainting); and sometimes pain in the shoulder. The woman may also see irregular vaginal bleeding. It is the sharp pain that most often makes a woman seek care, although the risk of hemorrhage, shock, and peritonitis are what place her life at risk.

### Assessment
Where the embryo implants determines the symptoms that occur. The woman may experience vague or less than acute symptoms (e.g., gastrointestinal disturbances, malaise, dizziness) or signs of shock. Later signs are hypotension and tacycardia. An ectopic pregnancy should be considered when any woman of childbearing age, whether using contraception or not, reports mild or severe abdominal symptoms. The severity of the symptoms does not indicate the severity of the health risk.

Physical examinations by the nurse practitioner or midwife or the physician may reveal adnexal tenderness and sometimes an adnexal mass. When there is bleeding, the abdomen may become rigid and very tender. The cervix and vagina may also be tender. For diagnosis, blood work to measure hemoglobin and hematocrit levels, rising leukocyte levels, and $\beta$-hCG levels and visualization with ultrasound, culdocentesis (i.e., withdrawal of fluid from the abdomen through the vaginal wall) to detect blood, and laparoscopy or laparotomy may be necessary.

### Nursing Plan

Teach the woman about the procedures and support her as the diagnosis and treatment options are determined. Some procedures will require her to be hospitalized. We must clearly state information about the possible procedures and treatment plan to the woman and her partner, family member, or friend. We must also answer questions and offer appropriate reassurance, as well as explain that if the woman is Rh negative and not sensitized, anti-D Rh immune globulin will be given to her within 72 hours.

The gestational age and placement of the fetus determines the medical treatment. If the woman is not hemorrhaging and the mass measures less than 4 cm (as measured by ultrasound) and is unruptured, she is a candidate for drug therapy. Methotrexate, which inhibits cell division, can be used to stop the developing pregnancy. This drug is administered via muscular injection, local infiltration, or orally and clears the trophoblastic tissue, reducing the need for a laparotomy (Youngkin and Davis, 1997).

Surgery is required for treatment in some cases. Depending on the situation, the surgery may remove the products of conception or the tissue around it—including a piece or all of the fallopian tube, if that is where it is located. If rupture has occurred with infection, the uterus, tubes, and ovaries may be removed. The goal of treatment is to save the woman's life. In the process, she loses the pregnancy and, depending on the medical treatment required, might lose a fallopian tube or ovary or, in extreme cases, the ability to have a future pregnancy.

We must provide emotional support as the woman grieves the loss of her baby and comes to terms with the medical complications of the situation. Following surgical procedures, the woman will also need information on how to care for herself, prevent infection, what symptoms to watch for and report, and when to have a follow-up visit.

## Gestational Trophoblastic Disease

**Gestational trophoblastic disease** describes a spectrum of neoplastic disorders that have common clinical findings (e.g., abnormal proliferative tissues) and abnormally high chorionic gonadatropin (HCG) levels. These disorders are hydatiform mole, invasive mole, and choriocarcinoma. The **hydatiform mole** may be classified as a **complete molar pregnancy** (i.e., no fetus or amnion present) or **partial molar pregnancy** (i.e., a fetus or evidence of an amniotic sac is present). The progression of the disease creates what looks like clusters of grapes, and the trophoblastic tissue proliferates. The **invasive mole** (i.e., chorioadenoma destruens) is more severe than a hydatiform mole because it is usually locally invasive. The myometrium of the uterus is invaded as the trophoblastic tissue grows. **Choriocarcinoma** is a rare chorionic malignancy that may occur years after any type of pregnancy. About one half of the choriocarcinomas occur after a complete hydatiform mole (Mattson and Smith, 2000).

### Nursing Assessment

The first signs of this disease usually appear like a spontaneous abortion at about 12 weeks of pregnancy. Women may report spotting, bleeding, nausea and vomiting, cramping, and sometimes the passing of "a grape." Vital signs and blood pressure are usually stable, and no medical emergency seems to exist. We must monitor the amount of bleeding, and draw blood as required. Blood work will reveal high levels of $\beta$-hCG that continue to rise 100 days after the last menstrual period.

A physical examination by the nurse practitioner or midwife or the physician reveals an abdomen that is soft and a uterus that may be "large for date" and feels doughy rather than firm. No fetal heart tones or activity is detected. Ultrasound reveals the characteristics of a molar pregnancy.

Medical treatment begins with dilatation and curettage of the uterus to remove the mole and all fragments of the placenta. If the woman wants no further pregnancies or there is excessive bleeding, a hysterectomy (i.e., removal of the uterus) may be performed to reduce the woman's chances of developing choriocarcinoma later in life. While the woman is hospitalized, a chest radiograph is done to establish a baseline for later comparisons if there is a question of invasive choriocarcinoma. The lungs are the site of metastases 75% of the time.

In addition, the woman is followed for a year with serial $\beta$-hCG levels. These are drawn weekly for the first 3 weeks, then monthly for 6 months, and then every 2 months for 6 months. Measuring the $\beta$-hCG levels determines if hCG is present, which indicates that residual trophoblastic tissue is present. Because pregnancy also elevates hCG levels and a pregnancy test cannot differentiate normal early pregnancy from beginning invasive disease, a woman is placed on a highly effective method of contraception for a year.

If hCG levels become nondetectable and remain normal for a year, no further treatment is necessary and the woman may attempt to become pregnant again. If hCG levels remain or rise, however, dilatation and curettage are performed and the tissue examined for malignant cells. If cancer cells are found, chemotherapy is initiated.

### Nursing Plan

Just as with an abortion or ectopic pregnancy, we must provide the couple with the opportunity to grieve the loss of their pregnancy. The couple must also deal with the possibility of cancer development in the woman and wait a year to see if this occurs. Arrangements must be made for the weekly and then monthly blood draws to check for the woman's hCG levels. The provider must accommodate transportation difficulties or a conflict with a woman's work schedule. The risk for pregnancy during that time must be explained to the couple. We must discuss and select with them a contraceptive option that complies with their individual needs and religious and ethnic beliefs, and that they can afford. Encourage the couple to verbalize their concerns. Understanding that the risk of the woman developing choriocarcinoma is low may decrease their anxiety. We must reiterate the importance of the follow-up care to increase her chances of survival and provide them with information about resources for support and additional understanding.

## Assisting in the Grief Process

When a woman experiences a spontaneous abortion, ectopic pregnancy, or gestational trophoblastic disease, she endures the loss of a baby. This is a time of bewilderment, disappointment, and grief. The couple will have questions about what happened, why it happened, and if it will happen again. They may also want to know what has happened to the remains of their baby. We must answer the questions as truthfully and completely as possible, although some of the questions will have no definitive answers. With careful investigation, however, other answers may be found. If the couple is offered testing to see if a cause can be found, we should encourage them to participate.

Unfortunately, the woman or the couple may have to endure their grief alone because others cannot relate to the extent of the loss. If it is early in the pregnancy, family members and friends may not even know about the expected child. As health care providers, we can empathize with the couple, help them understand the normalcy of their individualized responses, and guide them on how to move through the grief process.

Helping a grieving woman and her family is not a comfortable intervention. Fear of saying or doing the wrong things prevents some people from offering support and assistance. We should feel free to say, "I'm so sorry. I would like to help, can I _____ [give suggestions] for you?"

Alternatively, be more open by disclosing, "I don't fully understand what you are going through, but I care and would like to help." We should be aware of our own feelings as we work with the parents. This work may cause us to relive some of our own losses. We might consider sharing some of these feelings and tears because they show our humanness. However, we must not overwhelm the couple with our own emotions and needs.

We should try to be sensitive to the family's grieving style and the needs of each individual by giving them the freedom to be themselves. We should help the parents to understand the normal process of grief and the physical symptoms to expect (e.g., insomnia, achiness, depression, anger, and self-blame). We should also explain that they will not be "over this" in a few months, but that things will gradually get better. It will take time and effort for them to integrate this loss into their lives. They are forever changed, and each of them will find a "new normal." The woman is no longer considered as never before pregnant, but she will not have a child to share with the world. Her view of herself is forever different.

Help the couple prepare themselves for what others might say and how they might react. Family and friends might avoid conversations about the pregnancy or the baby or give advice that is not helpful. Be careful not to assume that the couple can or will have another baby because sometimes it is not possible. Sometimes the parents find the pain too great to risk having another pregnancy. Besides, another pregnancy would produce a new child—not a replacement for this one.

Help the couple determine who and where they will find a support system. It may be their clergy, family members, friends, coworker, or a local grief-support program. Help them figure out how they can ask for help. Offer as many resources as you can find and let them choose which they will use. Just because they appear to be doing "fine," do not assume they will not need the resources. After the immediacy of the situation has passed, the couple will be left alone to deal with the event, and then the resource list will be most helpful.

Box 10-3 provides some *dos* and *don't*s for providing nursing care to a family grieving a pregnancy loss during the first half of the pregnancy.

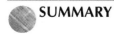

## SUMMARY

Pregnancy changes a woman's entire body to meet the demands of the developing infant. We help a woman by caring for her health and well-being, answering her questions, monitoring the dramatic changes as part of

---

### BOX 10-3  How to Help a Grieving Family with an Early Pregnancy Loss

Let your concern and care show.
(Don't avoid them.)

Reach out, through your uncomfortableness, and be available to listen.
(Don't talk, listen. Be comfortable with silence.)

Say you are sorry about what has happened
(Don't say "I know how you feel." Even if you have had the same loss, you don't know how they feel.)

Allow them to express as much grief as they are feeling, to cry.
(Don't say "You'll feel better soon," or "Why don't you stop crying.")

Reassure them that this is not their fault.
(There are so many unknown reasons for early pregnancy loss.)

Encourage them to be patient with themselves. It takes time to grieve the loss of another person.
(Don't say, "Get over it and get on with your life.")

Allow them to express their feelings, anxieties, and worries about possible future pregnancies.
(Don't say, "You can always have another child.")

Provide supportive care to other children and the grandparents.
(Don't exclude the others in the family. Each one of them will be grieving in his or her own way. They can only help each other if someone has been of help to them.)

---

the normal care of pregnancy, and helping her maintain her mental and physiologic comfort. To be culturally relevant and appropriate in our care for diverse clients, we must provide individualized care. We can learn from each woman and her family about their needs.

When a woman learns she is pregnant, she experiences a variety of emotions—from wonder, excitement, awe, and reverence to ambivalence, anxiety, and fear. How a woman responds to the news of her pregnancy and the changes that occur in her body during the first trimester is influenced by the circumstances of the impregnation, how she views herself in the role of motherhood, as well as what she has been told by others. The period of transition into this new identity occurs during the first trimester. By listening and exploring with the woman, we can learn what ideas she is bringing to this pregnancy and then carefully and sensitively provide her with a broader knowledge base from which to make her self-care choices.

## Care Plan · The Woman with a Threatened Abortion

**NURSING DIAGNOSIS**    **Fear** related to possible loss of pregnancy

**GOALS/OUTCOMES**    Experiences reduction of fearful feelings; copes successfully with situation (*see "Evaluation Parameters" for indicators of goal achievement*)

**NOC Suggested Outcomes**
- Fear Control (1404)

**NOC Additional Outcomes**
- Coping (1302)

**NIC Priority Interventions**
- Anxiety Reduction (5820)
- Emotional Support (5270)
- Coping Enhancement (5230)
- Presence (5340)
- Security Enhancement (5380)

**Nursing Activities and Rationale**
- Assess responses of client and family, especially their coping mechanisms and ability to comfort each other. *To determine the nature and amount of support needed from professionals.*
- Observe for nonverbal signs of fear: hyperalertness; wide-eyed look; increased pulse, respirations, and blood pressure. *Sympathetic response to fear.*
- Assess understanding of spontaneous abortion. *Provides appropriate information.*
- Provide information in a calm, simple, direct manner. *Removes the fear of the unknown, so that the client has only to cope with fear of the known (possible fetal loss); provides a sense of control.*
- Encourage client and family to verbalize feelings and fears. Listen sympathetically to their concerns about this and future pregnancies. *Relieves tension produced by the fear; communicates caring and support.*
- Express empathy for the client's experience. *Promotes a trusting relationship.*
- Encourage participation in treatment decisions. *Restores sense of control.*
- Explain all medical and nursing interventions, including sensations the client can expect during the procedure. *Promotes a sense of control; prevents fear progressing to powerlessness.*
- Stay with the client. *To promote safety and reduce fear.*
- Use physical touch to express concern. *Provides nonverbal reassurance.*

**Evaluation Parameters**
- Reports feeling less fearful
- Verbalizes a sense of control
- Able to concentrate and focus on information given
- Pulse and blood pressure within normal limits for client
- No signs of physical arousal (e.g., hyperalertness, wide-eyed look)
- Verbalizes feelings openly
- Participates in treatment decisions, requests information

---

**NURSING DIAGNOSIS**    **Risk for Situational Low Self-Esteem** related to feelings of guilt and responsibility for "causing" the abortion

**GOALS/OUTCOMES**    Demonstrates essentially positive self-esteem (*see "Evaluation Parameters" for indicators of goal achievement*)

**NOC Suggested Outcomes**
- Decision Making (0906)
- Self Esteem (1205)

**NIC Priority Interventions**
- Self-Esteem Enhancement (5400)

**Nursing Activities and Rationale**
(NOTE: Emotional assessment and support interventions for the nursing diagnosis, Fear, will also promote self-esteem and are not repeated here.)

- Monitor all evaluation parameters. *To evaluate goal achievement.*
- Observe interactions of client and partner for expressions of guilt or blaming (of self or each other). *Early in pregnancy, most women are ambivalent about being pregnant. They may then see the threatened abortion as punishment or as something they caused; guilt is a common reaction, as is anger toward self and/or partner.*

## Care Plan  •  The Woman with a Threatened Abortion—cont'd

- Observe for comments such as, "I probably shouldn't have played tennis," or "Do you think it was because I drank a beer?" *The woman often expresses guilt in terms of wondering whether she should have done something differently.*
- Use open-ended questions and active listening. *To encourage expression of feelings and initiate emotional healing.*
- Provide information about the various causes of spontaneous abortion. *To increase understanding that she was not the cause; the client should know that a direct cause cannot always be determined.*
- Express confidence in the client and family's ability to handle the situation. *Promotes autonomy and increases positive self-evaluation.*
- Help the client and family identify significant cultural and religious factors that influence their feelings of guilt and responsibility. *To assist them in gaining insight into their feelings.*
- Administer sedatives if ordered. Sometimes these are needed for extreme emotional upset.

### Evaluation Parameters
- After initial expression of feelings, verbalizations of guilt and/or blaming decrease
- Communicates freely and accepts factual information and explanations
- Participates in decisions about therapeutic regimen

NURSING DIAGNOSIS    **Risk for Injury (to Fetus)** related to birth before age of viability

GOALS/OUTCOMES    Threatened abortion will not progress to inevitable abortion; pregnancy is maintained

### NOC Suggested Outcomes
- Risk Control (1902)
- Symptom Control (1608)

### NIC Priority Interventions
- Electronic Fetal Monitoring: Antepartum (6771)
- High-Risk Pregnancy Care (6800)
- Home Maintenance Assistance (7180)
- Surveillance (6650)

### Nursing Activities and Rationale
- Assess for presence of uterine contractions. *To establish diagnosis of threatened abortion and determine prognosis.*
- Determine date of last menstrual period. *To confirm and date the pregnancy and age of the fetus.*
- Assess fetal heart rate (if gestational age >10 to 12 weeks). *To establish fetal viability.*
- Ask patient to describe the bleeding she experienced at home; ask specifically if she passed any tissue. *To rule out bleeding from other causes and determine if the client can be treated at home or in the hospital.*
- Ask the patient to describe other symptoms (e.g., cramping, backache). *To rule out bleeding from other causes.*
- Prepare client for ultrasonography, if ordered. *To determine placental integrity, stage of abortion, and fetal viability, as well as to rule out ectopic pregnancy.*
- Prepare client for speculum vaginal exam. *To determine if there is any cervical dilation, and to rule out polyps. A Pap smear may also be done to rule out cervical cancer. If cervix is closed, treatment is a matter of watchful waiting; if cervix is dilated, the prognosis for the pregnancy is poor.*
- Withhold fluids until medical work-up is completed. *Food and fluids are usually withheld because of the possibility that surgery will be needed if threatened abortion progresses to complete.*
- If being treated at home, be sure that the client and family understand the medical regimen (e.g., limited activity, no douching, no cathartics, and probably bedrest until cramping and spotting cease). *To assure compliance with regimen intended to maintain the pregnancy.*
- If the client is being treated at home, discuss the need to refrain from sexual activity. Teach about alternative methods of sexual gratification and intimacy. *Prostaglandins in semen may stimulate uterine contractions. For threatened abortion, it may still be possible to continue the pregnancy, so usual activities are limited. Most couples appreciate this information, but will not introduce the topic themselves, so we must initiate.*
- If the client is being treated at home, inform her and her family to notify physician if bleeding persists or becomes heavier, or cramping becomes more severe. *Indications that*

*Continued*

## Care Plan · The Woman with a Threatened Abortion—cont'd

*situation is progressing to inevitable abortion. Bedrest and abstinence are the only effective treatments for threatened abortion. If symptoms worsen, the woman may be advised to resume normal activities in an attempt to hasten the inevitable abortion; hospitalization may be necessary.*

- Provide written instructions for the treatment regimen and calling the physician. *Reinforces verbal instructions.*
- If the client is being treated at home, help her identify family, friends, and other personal support persons who can help during her period of limited activity; involve the client and partner in a plan for managing work and home responsibilities. *Supports compliance with treatment regimen: if others are doing the work, the woman will be less likely to feel she must do it herself.*

### Evaluation Parameters
- Uterine contractions not detectable on monitor; cramping and backache cease
- Fetal heart detectable at 120 to 160 bpm (if gestational age >10 to 12 weeks)
- No cervical dilation
- Verbalizes understanding and intent to follow treatment regimen
- Identifies personal support systems and begins to plan for managing activity limitations
- Verbalizes symptoms for which she will notify the physician

NURSING DIAGNOSIS **Risk for Injury (maternal)** related to complications of spontaneous abortion: (1) Infection, (2) Hemorrhage

GOALS/OUTCOMES Infection will not occur; hemorrhage will not occur *(see "Evaluation Parameters" for indicators of goal achievement)*

### NOC Suggested Outcomes
- Risk Control (1902)
- Symptom Control (1608)

### NIC Priority Interventions
- High-Risk Pregnancy Care (6800)
- Surveillance (6650)

### Nursing Activities and Rationale
- Assess pulse and blood pressure (BP). *When hemorrhage occurs, pulse increases and BP drops (compensatory mechanism). For threatened abortion, normal vital signs allow for hope that pregnancy can be maintained.*
- Monitor urine output. *Adequate output is an indicator of adequate circulating volume and helps confirm diagnosis that abortion is only "threatened," not "inevitable."*
- Monitor bleeding; count or weigh vaginal pads if more than just spotting. *For early recognition of developing problems (e.g., disseminated intravascular coagulation, progression to complete abortion, hemorrhage); confirms diagnosis of threatened rather than inevitable abortion.*
- Assess maternal and paternal blood types. *To evaluate need for RhoGAM if fetal loss occurs. Also for possible blood replacement if hemorrhage occurs.*
- Monitor temperature. *A temperature above 100.4°F is a sign of intrauterine infection (a white blood cell count of >16,000 is another indicator).*
- Assess odor of lochia; general malaise; elevated white blood cell count; and constant lower back, pelvic, or abdominal pain. *Signs of intrauterine infection.*
- If the client is being treated at home, instruct her to call physician if any of the signs and symptoms of infection or hemorrhage occur; provide written instructions. *To receive early treatment and avoid progression to a more serious condition. Written instructions reinforce verbal teaching.*

### Evaluation Parameters
- Pulse and BP within the woman's normal limits
- Urine output at least 30 cc/hr and appropriate for intake
- Bleeding remains only spotting and gradually stops
- Temperature <100.4°F
- No low back, pelvic, or abdominal pain
- Lochia essentially odor free
- Reports her usual energy level
- Verbalizes knowledge of symptoms of infection and hemorrhage and intent to notify physician if they appear

## Care Plan · *The Woman with a Threatened Abortion—cont'd*

**NURSING DIAGNOSIS**   **Pain** related to uterine cramping secondary to threatened abortion

**GOALS/OUTCOMES**   Absence of pain or satisfactory pain relief *(see "Evaluation Parameters" for indicators of goal achievement)*

### NOC Suggested Outcomes
- Comfort Level (2100)
- Pain Control (1605)
- Pain: Disruptive Effects (2101)
- Pain Level (2102)

### NIC Priority Interventions
- Analgesic Administration (2210)
- Anxiety Reduction (5820)
- Environmental Management: Comfort (6482)
- Medication Administration (2300)
- Pain Management: (1400)

### Nursing Activities and Rationale
- Ask client to rate pain as 1 to 10, with 1 meaning no pain and 10 representing the worst pain imaginable. *To plan appropriate pain-relief measures.*
- Assess severity, location, frequency, and quality of pain. *Comprehensive assessment aids in differential diagnosis and is essential to effectively treat the pain. Pain may reflect progression of abortion or intrauterine infection.*
- Observe for nonverbal expressions of pain. *Some clients do not express pain verbally.*
- Consider cultural influences on expression of pain. *People are unique in their perception and expression of pain.*
- Assess pulse, BP, and respirations. *Increases reflect sympathetic response to pain.*
- Perform comfort measures (e.g., position changes, back rub, breathing/relaxation techniques). *To promote relaxation, which decreases pain perception.*
- Manipulate environment to promote comfort (e.g., adjust lighting and room temperature, provide blankets, limit noise). *To limit pain by decreasing tension.*
- Explain the cause of the pain. *Understanding removes fear of the unknown.*
- *Administer analgesics if ordered. Pain of threatened abortion is usually mild; if abortion progresses, it may worsen.*
- Use a calm, supportive approach. *Promotes relaxation and decreases pain perception*

### Evaluation Parameters
- Rates pain as less than 2 on a 1 to 10 scale
- Expresses satisfaction with pain-control measures
- Nonverbal expressions of pain absent (i.e., no grimacing, muscle tension, or guarding)
- Vital signs within normal limits for client

### Other Nursing Diagnoses that Might Apply
- **Impaired Home Maintenance Management** related to prescribed bedrest or limited physical activity
- **Powerlessness** related to inability to change the outcome or prevent the loss
- **Spiritual Distress** related to blaming self or God for the possible loss

## CASE STUDY

Genevieve is a 21-year-old who has come for continuing prenatal care at 12 weeks. She is gravida 3, para 0, TAB 2. Both terminations occurred at approximately 9 weeks for social reasons. Genevieve used oral contraception after the first termination but had stopped after 4 years because of weight gain. The couple then used male condoms for contraception. The second pregnancy occurred when the condom broke. Shortly after the second termination, they married and the current pregnancy was planned.

Menarche was at age 11 years, and menstruation occurs every 28 days and lasts for 4 to 5 days.

Personal habits include smoking 2 cigarettes a day. When she conceived, she was swimming daily at the

## CASE STUDY—cont'd

local YWCA and restricting herself to 1000 calories per day. She says she has tried to keep this up so that she doesn't "get too fat" during the pregnancy.

Past medical history includes an episode of cystitis that responded well to medication. Genevieve's vital signs are within normal limits. Her weight has not increased since her prior visit. The nurse midwife indicates that Genevieve's physical examination confirms that her uterine size is compatable with a 12 week gestation. There are no abnormalities of her genitalia or discharge present.

- What immediate reponse will you provide Genevieve?

- What are her strengths? Where does she face potential problems?

- What information do you need from Genevieve?

- What nursing diagnoses could apply? How will you validate these?

- What long-term goals might she have for herself and for her family?

- What short-term goals might the two of you develop for Genevieve and for her family?

- What interventions may you be able to develop and offer?

- How will these interventions be prioritized?

- How will you evaluate the effectiveness of your interventions?

- When will Genevieve return for further care?

# Scenarios

1. Kristin is gravida 1, para 1 and is being seen for her first prenatal examination. She asks you the following, "What is going to happen to me during this visit?", "What are you testing and measuring and why?", and "Is this visit different from the rest of the visits?"

- What subjective data do you have about Kristin's condition?

- What subjective and objective data do you need?

- What do you think Kristin might be experiencing? Why?

- What nursing diagnoses could apply? How will you validate these?

- What goals might be developed? How will these be prioritized?

- What interventions may you offer?

- How will you evaluate the effectiveness of your interventions?

2. Kerry, G1 P0, is 12 weeks pregnant when she comes for her second prenatal visit. She tells you that her main problem is fatigue. She states, "Sometimes I'm so tired by the end of the day that I can hardly

make it home to cook dinner. I can't tell you how many meals Larry has cooked lately because I don't have the energy to do it. Is something wrong with me?" You check Kerry's blood work and find a hemoglobin level of 12.9 g/dL, a hematocrit level of 39%, and a white blood cell count of 4600.

- What subjective data do you have about Kerry's condition?

- What subjective and objective data do you need?

- What do you think Kerry might be experiencing? Why?

- What nursing diagnoses could apply? How will you validate these?

- What goals might be developed? How will these be prioritized?

- What interventions may you offer?

- How will you evaluate the effectiveness of your interventions?

3. Meghan has come to the Women's Center because she feels nauseated all the time. She is 8 weeks pregnant and knows that this is normal, but she is tired of it. She wants to know what she can do to feel better.

- What subjective data do you have about Meghan's condition?
- What subjective and objective data do you need?
- What nursing diagnoses could apply? How will you validate these?
- What goals might be developed? How will these be prioritized?
- What interventions may you offer?
- How will you evaluate the effectiveness of your interventions?

---

4. Lana is a 25-year-old married woman of Hispanic decent. She is seeing you during a prenatal visit; she is 12 weeks pregnant with her first child. She is of normal weight and says, "I don't want to gain too much weight with this pregnancy but my mother keeps telling me I have to eat. What do I really have to do so my baby is okay?"

- What subjective data do you have about Lana's condition?
- What subjective and objective data do you need?
- What do you think Lana might be experiencing? Why?
- What nursing diagnoses could apply? How will you validate these?
- What goals might be developed? How will these be prioritized?
- What interventions may you offer?
- How will you evaluate the effectiveness of your interventions?

---

5. Kathryn has come to the Women's Center for her first prenatal visit. She detected that she was pregnant after missing a period and then performing a home pregnancy test. Her LMP was 6 weeks ago, starting on April 23rd, and it was a normal period in duration and flow. She wants to know when her baby is going to be born and whether it is a boy or a girl.

- What will be your first response to Kathryn?
- What subjective data do you have about Kathryn's condition?
- What subjective and objective data do you need?
- What nursing diagnoses could apply? How will you validate these?
- What goals might be developed? How will these be prioritized?

---

- What interventions may you offer?
- How will you evaluate the effectiveness of your interventions?

---

6. Tamar is 14 years old and has been brought to the clinic by her mother, Julie, because she seems to be gaining weight. Julie says that Tamar is a good student with lots of friends who has been lying around the house and gaining weight. She wants her to see a nutritionist. You explain to Julie that Tamar will also need a physical and ask her to step out into the hall for a few minutes while Tamar gets ready.

- What will be your first statements and questions for Tamar?
- What subjective data do you have about Tamar's condition?
- What subjective and objective data do you need?
- What nursing diagnoses could apply? How will you validate these?
- What might be Tamar's medical diagnosis?
- What goals might be developed? How will these be prioritized?
- What interventions may you offer?
- How will you evaluate the effectiveness of your interventions?

---

7. Tyanna is 38 years old, single, and pregnant for the first time with a planned pregnancy after artificial insemination. She is a branch manager at a bank and has a master's degree. She lives alone, but her mother lives in the same town. Tyanna's last menstrual period was 6 weeks ago. She is a life-long vegetarian and has an uneventful medical history. After having a positive pregnancy test last week, she has returned to start prenatal care.

- What subjective data do you have about Tyanna's condition?
- What subjective and objective data do you need?
- What nursing diagnoses could apply? How will you validate these?
- What goals might be developed? How will these be prioritized?
- What interventions may you offer?
- How will you evaluate the effectiveness of your interventions?

8. Lydia is 13 weeks pregnant and is feeling great. She and her partner Pamela are very excited about the pregnancy and attend all prenatal appointments together. Pamela is expressing concern because she is not sure that Lydia is eating correctly or getting enough exercise. Her favorite meal is steak with macaroni and cheese. Lydia doesn't like vegetables so she eats a lot of lettuce and cucumber salads. In regard to exercise, Lydia says, "It's difficult to walk because as soon as I leave the house it seems that I have to use the bathroom."

- What subjective data do you have about Lydia's condition?
- What subjective and objective data do you need?
- What nursing diagnoses could apply? How will you validate these?
- What goals might be developed? How will these be prioritized?
- What interventions may you offer?
- How will you evaluate the effectiveness of your interventions?

## REFERENCES

Andrews MM and Boyle JS: *Transcultural concepts in nursing care*, ed 2, Phildelphia, 1995, J.B. Lippincott.

Barkauskas V and others: Health and physical assessment, St Louis, 1998, Mosby.

Beckman CR and others: *Obstetrical and gynecology*, ed 3, Baltimore, 1998, Williams & Wilkins.

Brown M: A comparison of health responses in expectant mothers and fathers, *West J Nurs Res* 10(5):527-549, 1988.

Carson VB: *Spiritual dimensions of nursing practice*, Philadelphia, 1989, Saunders.

Cunningham FG and others: *Williams obstetrics*, ed 20, Stamford, CT, 1997, Appleton and Lange.

Davis DC: The discomforts of pregnancy, *J Obstet Gynecol Neonat Nurs* 25(1):73-81, 1996.

Fogel C and Woods N: *Women's health care*, Thousand Oaks, CA, 1995, Sage.

Gloger-Tippelt G: A process model of the pregnancy course, *Hum Devel* 26:134-148, 1983.

Harvey MG: Physiologic changes of pregnancy. In Harvey CJ, editor: *Critical care obstetrical nursing*, Gaithersburg, MD, 1991, Aspen.

ific: Healthy eating during pregnancy, *http://ificinfor.health.org/brochure/eatpreg.htm*, 1999.

Kitzinger S: *Woman's experience of sex*, New York, 1985, Penguin Books.

Lederman RP: *Psychococial adaptation in pregnancy*, ed 2, New York, 1996, Springer.

Longobucco DC and Preston MS: Relation of somatic symptoms to degree of paternal role preparation, *J Obstet Gynecol Neonat Nurs* 18(6):482, 1989.

Lowdermilk DL, Perry SE, and Bobak IM: *Maternity and women's health care*, ed 6, St Louis, 1997, Mosby.

Mattson S and Smith J: *Core curriculum for maternal-newborn nursing*, ed 2, Philadelphia, 2000, Saunders.

McFarlane J and others: Assessing for abuse: self-report versus nurse interview, *Pub Health Nurs* 8(4):245-250, 1991.

Mercer RT: *On becoming a mother*, New York, 1995, Springer.

Moore R: Overview of developmental and physical milestones and psychosocial issues, *Curr Pract Issue Adolesc Gynecol*, Fair Lawn, NJ, 1996, MPE Communications.

Musick JS: *Young, poor, and pregnant—the psychology of teenage motherhood*, New Haven, CT, 1995, Yale University Press.

National Institute for Occupational Safety and Health: *The effects of workplace hazards on female reproductive health*, DHHS (NIOSH) Publication No. 99-104, Washington, DC, 1999, US Department of Health and Human Services.

*Nurses handbook of alternative and complementary therapies*, Springhouse, PA, 1998, Springhouse.

Pernell L and Paulanka BJ: *Transcultural health care*, Philadelphia, 1998, F.A. Davis.

Phillips CR: *Family-centered maternity and newborn care*, St Louis, 1995, Mosby.

Pillitteri A: *Maternal and child health nursing*, ed 3, Philadelphia, 1999, Lippincott.

Rubin R: *Maternal identity and the maternal experience*, New York, 1984, Springer.

Sadler T: *Langman's medical embryology*, ed 7, Baltimore, 1995, Williams & Wilkins.

Simpson KR and Creehan PA: *AWHONN perinatal nursing*, Philadelphia, 1996, Lippincott.

Snyder M and Lindquist R: *Complementary/alternative therapies in nursing*, ed 3, New York, 1998, Springer.

Steinberg L: *Adolescence*, New York, 1998, McGraw-Hill.

Worthington-Roberts BS and Williams SR: *Nutrition in pregnancy and lactation*, ed 6, Boston, 1993, McGraw-Hill.

Youngkin EQ and Davis MS, editors: *Women's health: a primary care clinical guide*, Stamford, CT, 1997, Appleton & Lange.

# CHAPTER 11

# Nursing Care During the Second Trimester (14 to 26 Weeks)

*"I was lying on my stomach and felt something, like someone lightly touching my deep insides. Then I just sat very still and for an alive moment felt the hugeness of having something living growing in me."*

— (BOSTON WOMEN'S HEALTH
BOOK COLLECTIVE, 1998)

*Describe the physical changes that take place in a woman's body during the second trimester.*

*Describe the changes taking place in the fetus during the second trimester.*

*What cognitive changes does a woman experience during the second trimester?*

*What other factors influence the woman and her support system during the second trimester?*

*What assessments are necessary during the second trimester?*

*What anticipatory guidance is required during the second trimester?*

*What is the therapeutic response if the woman miscarries during the second trimester?*

The second trimester of pregnancy is often a time of well-being for the woman. The fatigue of the first trimester is gone, morning sickness has usually stopped, and the risk of miscarriage is decreased. "The middle months of pregnancy are a time when many women feel happy with their bodies and glow with a kind of pregnancy radiance" (Kitzinger, 1985). If the woman has come to terms with the pregnancy and feels well physically, she will often now share the news of the pregnancy with friends and relatives. If things are going well for the couple, her desire for sexual encounters generally increases (Phillips, 1995).

 **MATERNAL PHYSIOLOGIC CHANGES
DURING THE SECOND TRIMESTER**

The woman's various body systems continue to change both to sustain the pregnancy and to prepare gradually for the more strenuous third trimester and the birth process (Table 11-1).

## Physiologic Changes in the Woman's Reproductive System

### Breasts and Reproductive System

**Breasts.** As the woman's breasts enlarge, striae (stretch marks) may start to develop. Breast enlargement is created by growth of the mammary glands and is completed by 20 weeks of gestation. Palpation of the breasts reveals a generalized coarse nodularity because of the proliferation of the lactiferous ducts and lobule-alveolar tissue. The high levels of estrogen and progesterone inhibit lactation until after birth by inhibiting the release of prolactin, a hormone that stimulates and sustains lactation.

**413**

**TABLE 11-1** *Signs of Pregnancy in the Second Trimester*

| Approximate time in pregnancy (weeks) | Presumptive signs | Probable signs | Positive signs | Description | Reason not definitive/ other possible causes |
|---|---|---|---|---|---|
| 16-18 | Quickening | | | Fetal movement felt by mother | Flatus (gas) Peristalsis Abdominal muscle contractions Shifting of abdominal contents |
| 16-20 | | Ballottement | | When the lower part of the uterus is tapped during a bimanual examination, the fetus can rise to be felt through the abdomen | Uterine tumors, cervical polyps, ascites |
| 18 | | Braxton-Hicks | | Periodic uterine tightening | Myomas, other tumors |
| 20 | | Fetal outline felt by examiner | | Fetal outline palpated through abdomen | Uterine myomas |
| 20 | | | Fetal movement felt by examiner | Fetal movement can be palpated through abdomen | No other cause |

As the breasts enlarge, a supportive bra becomes even more necessary for the woman's comfort. The cups must be structurally firm to hold the breasts up and away from the chest. The area underneath the breast and the nipples should be kept dry to prevent the growth of *Candida*.

 During this trimester, colostrum starts to develop. **Colostrum,** rich in antibodies, is the thick yellowish fluid that is the precursor to breast milk. It may be secreted or expressed from the nipples as early as 16 weeks of gestation. Some women rub it on the nipple area. No other nipple preparation is necessary at this time unless the nipples are inverted. Exercises to evert the nipples are seldom successful. If the woman wishes to breastfeed, the inverted nipples may be treated with breast shells—vented domes worn over the nipples that allow the nipples to evert. The cups of a well-fitting bra hold the shells in place (Davis, 1996) (Figure 11-1).

*Uterus.* By the fourth month of pregnancy the globular uterus may be palpated above the symphysis pubis. The uterus continues to become larger and heavier while the muscular walls become somewhat thinner. The growth of the uterus occurs with the stretching and marked hypertrophy of the existing cells, with some distention related to fetal development. The size and number of blood vessels and the lymphatics also increase. The increase in the uterus's weight is attributable, in large part, to the increasing blood volume associated with its vascular system (Simpson and Creehan, 1996).

A nulliparous woman may notice fetal movements, (**quickening**) at about 18 weeks of pregnancy or later. Multiparous women may recognize these sensations as early as 16 to 18 weeks. The fetus's first movements are generally light and fluttering, like "butterfly flutterings" and are felt only by the mother. As they become stronger, others can feel them through the abdomen. Fetal movements gradually become more intense and frequent as the pregnancy continues.

By 16 weeks, the fundus of the uterus is midway between the symphysis and the umbilicus, and by 20 weeks, the fundus is at the umbilicus. Uterine enlargement occurs in a linear fashion, with growth occurring at the rate of about 1 cm per week after the twentieth week. After this time, the cells' hypertrophy ends and the muscular wall thins, allowing palpation of the fetus by the fifth month.

The uterus is a muscle that contracts intermittently. At  about 4 months of pregnancy (approximately 18 weeks) some women can feel oxytocin-induced uterine contractions as uterine firmness through the abdominal wall, or the contractions may be visible as they push the uterus forward. These are called **Braxton-Hicks** (or false labor) contractions. They are light, regular or irregular contractions that may be felt every 10 to 20 minutes. Most women do not find them painful, but some do find them annoying. The contractions promote placental perfusion, enhancing the delivery of oxygen to the fetus.

The enlarging uterus also may stretch the ligaments that support it. Some women report a sharp, stabbing, "knifelike" pain that surprises them and takes their breath away. The pain, which immediately comes and then goes, may occur when ligaments holding the uterus in position are strained. When a woman reports such a pain, further assessment is needed to rule out other possible causes. Assessment includes location, frequency, and nature of the pain and any accompanying symptoms; relationship to changing position or other activities; presence or absence of fever; and palpation for masses or tenderness. Reviewing good body mechanics with the woman may help her minimize the pain's occurrence. As the uterus grows, some women reduce the strain on the ligaments by actually holding the uterus as they stand up and move about. Repeated spasms may cause local tenderness that may be helped by fingertip massage. If at any time the pain is prolonged or associated with other symptoms, the woman should call her provider (Davis, 1996).

***Ovaries.*** The ovaries are usually not palpable after the uterus fills the uterine cavity at 12 to 14 weeks of gestation (Bailey, 1998).

***Cervix.*** The mucous plug continues to seal the cervix. Production of mucus continues to increase.

Between the sixteenth and twentieth week of pregnancy, while doing a vaginal/cervical examination, the examiner may palpate the fetus by pushing up on the cervix with two fingers. This causes the fetus to rise or bounce up in the amniotic fluid before it sinks, creating the sensation of a gentle tap that may be felt by the examiner's finger. This procedure is called **ballottement.** If ballottement is done during a bimanual examination, the fetus may be felt twice: first as it taps against the examiner's hand on the woman's abdomen, and then again when it sinks down and touches the examiner's hand in the woman's vagina.

***Vagina and Vulva.*** The external structures of the perineum enlarge because of increased blood supply, skin and muscle hypertrophy, and new fat deposits. The hypertrophy and increased vascularity that cause the vagina to enlarge and take on a bluish tinge also affect the vulva. The vaginal introitus, clitoris, labia minora, and labia majora enlarge and become bluish. With the increasing vascularity, pelvic congestion and sensitivity also are increased. For some women this leads to greater sexual interest as increased pelvic engorgement contributes to easier and more frequent sexual arousal. As the abdomen stretches and the pregnancy starts to show, a partner who was having trouble relating to the fact of a pregnancy now sees the reality. He may feel very warm, loving, and protective of his mate and their child. The second trimester can be a time of loving caresses, expressions of appreciation for each other, and a fulfilling sex life. With no need for contraception, sexual spontaneity may increase (Phillips, 1995).

With the increased congestion, the walls of blood vessels relax, and the growing uterus places more pressure on the tissues of the vagina and vulva: the vulva may become edematous and varicose veins may develop in the vulva and perineum. They create an aching feeling and sense of heaviness. By resting in a supine position with her legs and one hip elevated to relieve the pressure on the pelvis without compressing the vena cava, a woman may increase her comfort. If she must be

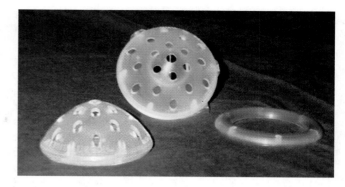

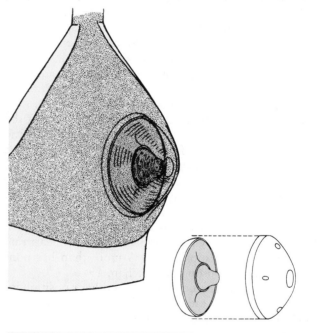

**FIGURE 11-1 •** Breast shell. *(Modified from Lawrence RA: Breastfeeding: a guide for the medical profession, ed 4, St Louis, 1994, Mosby.)*

in an upright position, she can support her vulva by wearing two sanitary pads within her underpants. The varicosities should resolve after the delivery of the baby.

## Physiologic Changes in Other Body Systems

### Cardiovascular System

Physical symptoms may start to become more apparent in response to cardiovascular changes. Some women report palpitations, light-headedness, and a decreased tolerance for standing quickly or excessive activity. Dependent edema may also be present and worsen as the pregnancy continues.

***Heart.*** As the uterus enlarges, it elevates the diaphragm, displacing the heart upward and to the left. This displacement also results in a slight anterior rotation of the heart. The apical impulse, a point of maximum intensity (PMI) on the chest where the impulse of the left ventricle is felt most strongly, is shifted upward and laterally about 1 to 1.5 cm (1/2 inch). The extent of these changes depends on the size and the position of the uterus, the strength of the abdominal muscles, and the configuration of the abdomen and the thorax (Cunningham and others, 1997).

Alterations in the heart sounds are common during normal pregnancy and may be most easily heard after 20 weeks of gestation. The second heart sound remains normal, but there is an exaggerated splitting of the first heart sound and the presence of a third sound. Systolic murmurs, found in 90% of pregnant women, are benign and disappear after birth. The murmur is usually heard during inspiration. No significant changes occur in the electrocardiogram (ECG).

***Blood Volume.*** The woman's blood volume is increasing rapidly, now reaching a maximum of a 50% increase over her prepregnant level. If there are multiple fetuses, the blood volume increase is in proportion to the number of fetuses (Mattson and Smith, 2000).

***Cardiac Output.*** The cardiac output peaks during the second trimester at 30% and remains stable until the end of the pregnancy. The increase in cardiac output changes from being mostly due to an increase in stroke volume to now also being caused by an increase in the heart rate. Between 14 and 20 weeks the pulse increases about 10 to 15 beats per minute and maintains that rate until delivery. Women also may experience palpitations. If the woman is carrying multiple fetuses, the heart rate may increase even more to 40% more than her nonpregnant rate (Simpson and Creehan, 1996).

As the uterine size increases, the mother's position influences her cardiac output. The lateral recumbent position promotes the greatest cardiac output, the sitting position produces an intermediate decrease in cardiac output, and the supine position results in a cardiac output that is less than that of a nonpregnant woman. Because the lateral recumbent position promotes the greatest cardiac output, it is the preferred resting position.

***Blood Pressure.*** The woman's diastolic blood pressure has been decreasing gradually as a result of peripheral dilation, and now in the second trimester reaches its lowest levels—as much as 20 to 25 mm Hg below prepregnancy state. Systolic pressures are not significantly changed because they only decrease about 10 to 15 mm Hg; as a result, her pulse pressure continues to widen (Mattson and Smith, 1993; Simpson and Creehan, 1996).

As the uterus enlarges, be aware of supine hypotensive syndrome (also identified as vena cava syndrome). If the woman lies on her back, the enlarging uterus can occlude venous return, causing a decrease in cardiac output and thus a drop in systolic blood pressure of more than 30 mm Hg. After 4 or 5 minutes a reflex bradycardia occurs, and cardiac output is reduced by half. When this occurs the woman may experience dizziness, nausea, light-headedness, or diaphoresis. The woman should be assisted to turn on her side to restore circulation. Encourage the woman to never lie on her back. If she must, she should place a folded towel or blanket underneath her right hip. This displaces the uterus as she rolls slightly to the left, preventing pressure on the large blood vessels.

Just telling a woman not to lie on her back may not be enough. In some cultures, such as the Mexican-American community, women may sleep on their backs because they believe it protects the baby from harm (Purnell and Paulanka, 1998). Slight adjustments, such as using a pillow under the hip, may be acceptable.

***Hematologic Changes.*** Even with an increased production of red blood cell (RBC) volume, hemoglobin values decrease ( 12 to 16 g/dl blood) and hematocrit values decrease (37% to 47%) during pregnancy. This decrease in hemoglobin and hematocrit values is most obvious in the second trimester (Simpson and Creehan, 1996).

The simultaneously rapid increase in plasma volume creates a condition called **hemodilution**. This is sometimes called the "physiologic anemia of pregnancy" because proportionately fewer RBCs are in the blood plasma, which in a nonpregnant state would indicate a possible anemic condition (Drummond, 1992). However, this is not an actual pathologic state. The woman is not considered anemic until the hemoglobin drops below 11 g/dl or the hematocrit value drops to 35% or less.

The total white blood cell (WBC) count starts to increase during the second trimester and continues on through the third trimester. The primary increase is in the number of granulocytes (range moves from 55% to 70% to 60% to 85% of circulating leukocytes), while the lymphocyte count remains consistent throughout pregnancy (20% to 35% of circulating leukocytes). A person's WBC count can vary at different times of the day, so note the time the blood sample is taken (Tilkian, Conover, and Tilkian, 1995).

### Respiratory System

As the pregnancy advances it becomes less possible for the diaphragm to descend with inspiration. Women may state they feel short of breath. They may sleep more easily if their head and shoulders are elevated with several pillows.

***Functional Changes.*** The tidal volume (volume of air exhaled or inhaled during quiet breathing) continues to increase which, in turn, causes an increase in respiratory minute ventilation (volume of air expired over 1 minute) (Barkauskas and others, 1998). The woman's $PaCO_2$ levels range from 27 to 32 mm Hg in the second half of pregnancy, as compared to the nonpregnant level of 40 mm Hg. This lower level of $PaCO_2$ in the mother allows the transfer of $CO_2$ from the fetus to the mother. The process is aided by an increased renal excretion of bicarbonate, causing a slight increase in pH and facilitating the removal of fetal carbon dioxide. Oxygen consumption increases as pregnancy advances and is greater in multiple gestations.

***Basal Metabolic Rate.*** By the fourth month of the pregnancy a woman's basal metabolic rate has usually started to rise. This reflects the increased demand for oxygen created by the uterine-placental-fetal unit and the increased oxygen needs for maternal cardiac work.

### Renal/Urinary System

***Structural Changes.*** As the pregnancy progresses, the enlarging uterus lifts up and off the bladder so urinary frequency is less common during the second trimester. After 4 months of pregnancy, the hyperemia of the pelvic organs and hyperplasia of all the muscles and connective tissue push the bladder forward and upward, causing the urethra to lengthen to 7.5 cm (3 inches). During this process the bladder's shape changes from convex to concave, reducing its capacity to retain urine.

***Functional Changes.*** Both the glomerular filtration rate (GFR) and the renal plasma flow (RPF) continue to rise until term. Because of the increased GFR and RPF, renal clearance of many substances is increased, lowering the serum levels. The increase in the GFR causes an increase in protein excretion, but it is not abnormal until the values have reached greater than 250 mg/dl. Higher levels are found with pregnancy-induced hypertension (PIH), renal disease, and urinary tract infections (Simpson and Creehan, 1996).

***Fluid and Electrolyte Balance.*** Calcium and phosphorus are excreted, creating an increased requirement for calcium during pregnancy. The amount recommended varies around the world. In the United States, the recommended daily allowance (RDA) for calcium during pregnancy is 1200 mg daily, 400 mg more than for a woman over age 24 who is not pregnant. Research has demonstrated that a satisfactory calcium intake provides protection against hypertensive disorders in pregnancy (Worthington-Roberts and Williams, 1997).

The RDA for phosphorus is also 1200 mg daily. The U.S. diet is high in phosphorus and, in fact, may be too high. At high levels, phosphorus binds to calcium and inhibits its absorption, so a woman should be cautioned against eating large amounts of processed meats, snack foods, and carbonated beverages (Worthington-Roberts and Williams, 1997).

A well-balanced diet can satisfy a woman's nutritional requirements for calcium and phosphorus. Supplementation is not required during routine prenatal care (Worthington-Roberts and Williams, 1997).

### Gastrointestinal System

The general nausea and vomiting of pregnancy usually improve about the sixteenth gestational week. If nausea and vomiting continue during the second trimester, the self-care interventions mentioned in Chapter 10 should be continued. In addition, a homeopathic evaluation and treatment for the nausea and vomiting may be helpful.

A complete evaluation and possible inpatient medical treatment may be needed if the nausea and vomiting are severe. **Hyperemesis gravidarum** is a less common but more pronounced form of nausea and vomiting usually occurring after 16 gestational weeks. It can produce weight loss, starvation acidosis, hypokalemia, alkalosis (loss of hydrochloric acid), and dehydration. Hospitalization may be needed for fluid and electrolyte replacement through intravenous therapy. In addition, the woman must be evaluated to determine if she has an illness causing this condition rather than the pregnancy.

***Stomach.*** As the size of the uterus increases it moves the stomach upward. Relaxation of the esophageal sphincter, caused by the higher levels of progesterone, permits reflux of gastric contents into the esophagus causing "heart burn" (**pyrosis**). If a woman eats smaller meals, reduces the spiciness of her food, and remains in an upright position for at least an hour after eating, the occurrence of this may be reduced.

***Gallbladder.*** In the second and third trimesters, fasting and residual volumes are twice as great as in a nonpregnant woman, and the rate the gall bladder empties continues to slow. When bile is retained, the woman is more at risk for developing excess cholesterol in the blood (hypercholesterolemia) or gallstone formation.

### Endocrine System

***Parathyroid Glands.*** Between 15 to 35 weeks, the slight increase in the size of the parathyroid gland and the amount of parathyroid hormone it produces peaks. It remains at this level until birth, controlling the metabolism of calcium and magnesium and enhancing the growth of the fetal skeleton.

***Placental Hormones.*** During the second trimester the levels of estrogen, progesterone, and human placental lactogen (hPL), or human chorionic somatomammotropin, continue at the levels achieved during the first trimester.

### Neurologic System

Mild frontal headaches related to hormonal changes or caused by tension may continue to occur in the second trimester. Severe headaches, especially after 20 weeks of gestation, may be associated with PIH. This type of headache is the result of edema from vasoconstriction. The ongoing monitoring of the woman's blood pressure helps screen for PIH.

Assessment of the headaches includes patient's headache history with onset and duration, location and radiation, and associated symptoms; relationship to events or activities; and relief therapy used and its effectiveness. A brief neurologic examination and inspection of the nasal and oral cavities with palpation and percussion of the sinus area help rule out possible causes of the pain. The woman should be told that if she experiences blurred vision and is seeing spots, both symptoms associated with hypertension, she should call her provider immediately (Davis, 1996).

### Integumentary System

The increase in pigmentation that started in the first trimester continues until delivery. In addition, the skin on the breasts, hips, upper thighs, and abdomen begins to stretch during the second trimester. Straie gravidarum, or stretch marks, result from the normal stretching of the skin and softening and separating of the underlying collagenous and elastic tissues of the skin. They become much more noticeable during the third trimester. From 50% to 90% of pregnant women develop at least one. Even though products are sold to prevent stretch marks, none of them have been demonstrated to work, and there is no known way to prevent them. Whether a woman develops them or not seems to depend in large part on her heredity.

Hypertrophy of the gums also may occur. Around the third month of pregnancy, a woman may develop an **epulis**—a red, raised nodule on her gums that bleeds easily. It may continue to enlarge as the pregnancy progresses and then regress after the birth of the baby. Using a soft toothbrush minimizes trauma to the lesion and the rest of the gum area.

### Musculoskeletal System

As the pregnancy advances, the growing uterus tilts the pelvis forward, increasing the lumbosacral curve and creating a gradual lordosis. The woman's enlarging breasts may pull her shoulders forward, and she may assume a stoop-shouldered stance. Mild muscle spasms, back tenderness, or back strain usually respond well to gentle stretching exercises, localized cold or heat, rest, and administration of analgesics. A nonelastic sacroiliac belt can offer relief for posterior back pain but not posterior pelvic pain.

If a woman reports periodic backaches she should be evaluated for preterm labor, which may manifest as lower back pain. Immediate and aggressive treatment may be necessary if it is preterm labor.

### Metabolic Changes

During the second half of this trimester (from 16 to 32 weeks of pregnancy) plasma lipids increase, with an increase in the ratio of low-density proteins (LDL) to high-density proteins (HDL). This increase in the plasma remains stable until after birth. Because serum lipids are affected by pregnancy, tests taken at this time may not provide valid results (Barkauskas and others, 1998).

*Pancreas.* During the first half of pregnancy, the mother's increased production of insulin combined with her decreased need leads to a buildup of insulin. This ensures that the fetus has an adequate supply of glucose. During the second half of pregnancy, maternal hormones cause an increased resistance to insulin, resulting in a breakdown of insulin stores when the mother experiences periods of fasting.

Gestational diabetes mellitus occurs as a result of disruption in this delicate homeostatic balance. Pregnant women may be screened for gestational diabetes between 24 and 28 weeks of gestation. A fasting glucose of greater than or equal to 135 mg/dl is considered a positive screen for gestational diabetes.

### Nervous System

Some women experience backaches that occur during the night. As the pregnancy progresses and the uterus grows in size and weight, venous stasis and overdistention of venous blood vessels may exert pressure on the nerve fibers innervating the lower back and create backache.

##  FETAL GROWTH AND DEVELOPMENT DURING THE SECOND TRIMESTER

### End of 14 Weeks of Fetal Development (16 Weeks of Pregnancy)

The fetus is growing in length and is now 10 to 17 cm long and weighs 55 to 120 g. A fine downy hair, called **lanugo,** covers the body and keeps oil on the skin. Fetal heart sounds may be audible with a regular stethoscope. The liver and pancreas are functioning. The fetus can suck and swallow amniotic fluid.

### End of 16 Weeks of Fetal Development (18 Weeks of Pregnancy)

The external sex organs of the fetus can be seen. Although thin, the fetus is beginning to look like a baby.

### End of 18 Weeks of Fetal Development (20 Weeks of Pregnancy)

The fetus has grown considerably and is now approximately 25 cm long and weighs about 223 g. The mother can now feel it as it moves around, stretches, and extends its arms and legs. The hair on the head and the eyebrows is forming. Meconium (a thin, dark green to black sterile substance) begins to form in the upper intestine. The fetus's biorhythms create definite and distinguishable sleep and activity patterns.

Several protective mechanisms for the well-being of the fetus are also developing. **Vernix caseosa,** a cream-cheese-like substance produced by the sebaceous glands, begins to form. It coats and protects the skin during the remainder of the pregnancy. Brown fat, a special fat that aids in temperature regulation at birth, begins to form behind the kidneys, sternum, and posterior neck (Mattson and Smith, 2000).

## End of 22 Weeks of Fetal Development (24 Weeks of Pregnancy)

After 22 weeks of development, the fetus is now 28 to 36 cm long and weighs about 550 g. The fetus's eyebrows and eyelashes are well defined, and the eyes begin to open and close. The pupils are capable of reacting to light. **Vernix caseosa** covers the entire body. Meconium is now present as far down as the rectum. In preparation for life outside the uterus, active production of **lung surfactant** begins. This substance reduces the surface tension of the pulmonary fluids and thus prevents the alveoli from collapsing when the infant breathes after birth. As early as 18 weeks, but definitely by 22 weeks of development, the fetus receives a passive antibody transfer from its mother. Because the infant has no naturally developing immunities, this transfer of antibodies protects the infant until its own stores of immunoglobulins can be built up (Mattson and Smith, 2000).

If the fetus is delivered at 22 weeks of fetal development, 24 weeks of pregnancy, or with a weight of 601 g, it is at the low-end of viability and must be cared for in an intensive care facility (Table 11-2).

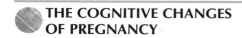

## THE COGNITIVE CHANGES OF PREGNANCY

Parents do most of the psychologic work of pregnancy during the first 4 months of gestation. (Hees-Stauthamer, 1985). By the second trimester, the woman is dealing with her ambivalence regarding the pregnancy and is starting to adjust to the changes in her body. Because her partner has not had the same physical sensations and experiences that she has had, he may not be at the same developmental level in associating with the pregnancy.

A major change in how the woman and her partner view the pregnancy occurs when movement is felt. The parents begin to think of the fetus as separate from themselves. Being able to feel fetal movement initiates a period of new attitudes and behaviors very different from the first or third trimester.

The responses of other family members, friends, and community members continue to influence, negatively or positively, the couple's adaptation to new roles. Select members of their support system may be invited to share in feeling the baby kick and hearing the parents' reports as the trimester progresses.

## Adapting to Pregnancy During the Second Trimester

### The Woman

During the second trimester, continue to assess the woman's adaptation to the pregnancy and the physical changes she is experiencing. Explain the growth and development of the fetus and provide pictures so that she can more easily imagine the developing fetus within her. Explain how her own body is adapting both physically and emotionally to support the development of the child. She will seek reassurance that she is doing the right things to help her baby and that it is okay. She may be convinced to eat and take care of herself to help the baby grow. Now that she is feeling better, this is the time to plan ahead. Help her investigate childbirth education options and enroll in a class that matches her philosophy on preparation for and involvement in the childbirth process.

***Self-Image.*** How a woman describes herself during pregnancy may be indicative of how she feels about herself as a person. Seeing herself as a pregnant woman is a change in body image. Women with positive views of themselves during pregnancy have better coping skills, are happier and more content with the pregnancy, and more frequently practice healthy behaviors (Davis, 1996). As an ongoing process, evaluate whether the woman is concerned about the changes in her body. Observe her appearance and how she is presenting herself. Ask how her family and/or friends are supporting her during the pregnancy. Ask about her activities.

Early in the second trimester, women may have increased sexual interest and experience arousal easily. Near the end of this trimester, physical changes and concern for the baby's well-being may cause concern that alters her desire for intercourse. Explore her concerns and correct any misinformation. Explain any specific restrictions she may have been given and the reason for them. Explore options for her sexual expression that both address her concerns and meet her needs.

***Acceptance of Pregnancy.*** The point at which a woman loses her ambivalence and definitely knows she wants the child can vary from when she first learns she is pregnant until now. One way to measure the level of a woman's acceptance is to determine how well she follows your prenatal advice. Until she thinks of the fetus inside her as a person separate from herself, she may be unable to to act in the child's best interests. Of course, a woman may not follow prenatal instructions because she does not understand them, the instructions are in conflict with her cultural beliefs, she cannot implement the directions, or her partner prevents her from doing so.

***Separating Self from Fetus.*** During a physical examination, the woman may first become aware of the separate person within her by simultaneously listening to her own heartbeat, which is relatively slow, and the faster heartbeat of the fetus. This is a first step toward differentiating between herself and the fetus. With quickening, the woman becomes even more aware that although the fetus is within her, it is a separate entity. Each time it moves, the fetus reminds her of its presence and health. This process of **fetal differentiation** is normally complete by the end of the second trimester. If an ultrasound

**TABLE 11-2**   *Milestones in Human Development Before Birth Since LMP*

| 16 Weeks | 20 Weeks | 24 Weeks |
|---|---|---|
| **EXTERNAL APPEARANCE** | | |
| Head still dominant; face looking human; eyes, ears, and nose approaching typical appearance on gross examination; arm-leg ratio proportionate; scalp hair appearing | Vernix caseosa and lanugo appearing, legs lengthening considerably, sebaceous glands appearing | Body lean but fairly well proportioned, skin red and wrinkled, vernix caseosa present, sweat gland forming |
| **CROWN-TO-RUMP MEASUREMENT, WEIGHT** | | |
| 11.5-13.5 cm, 100 g | 16-18.5 cm, 300 g | 23 cm, 600 g |
| **GASTROINTESTINAL SYSTEM** | | |
| Meconium in bowel, some enzyme secretion, anus open | Enamel and dentine depositing, ascending colon recognizable | |
| **MUSCULOSKELETAL SYSTEM** | | |
| Most bones distinctly indicated throughout body, joint cavities appearing, muscular movements detectable | Sternum ossification, fetal movements strong enough for mother to feel | |
| **CIRCULATORY SYSTEM** | | |
| Heart muscle well-developed, blood formation active in spleen | | Blood formation increasing in bone marrow and decreasing in liver |
| **RESPIRATORY SYSTEM** | | |
| Elastic fibers appearing in lungs, terminal and respiratory bronchioles appearing | Nostrils reopening, primitive respiratory-like movements beginning | Alveolar ducts and sacs present, lecithin beginning to appear in amniotic fluid (weeks 26 to 27) |
| **RENAL SYSTEM** | | |
| Kidney in position and attaining typical shape and plan | | |
| **NERVOUS SYSTEM** | | |
| Cerebral lobes delineated, cerebellum assuming some prominence | Brain grossly formed, cord myelination beginning, cord ending at level S-1 | Cerebral cortex layered typically, neuronal proliferation in cerebral cortex ending |
| **SENSORY ORGANS** | | |
| General sense organs differentiated | Nose and ears ossifying | Ability to hear |
| **GENITAL SYSTEM** | | |
| Testes in position for descent into scrotum, vagina open | | Testes at inguinal ring in descent to scrotum |

**TABLE 11-3**  *Signs and Symptoms of Potential Complications*

| Signs and symptoms | Possible causes |
| --- | --- |
| Abdominal pain or cramping | Spontaneous abortion, placenta previa, placental separation |
| Vaginal bleeding | Placenta previa, placental separation |
| Nausea and vomiting | Hyperemesis gravidarum |
| Burning or painful urination | Infection |
| Fever | Infection |
| Reduction in fetal movements after quickening | Problems with fetus |
| Absence of fetal movements | Fetal death |

has to be performed for medical reasons, "seeing" the child for the first time and receiving an ultrasound "picture" is also helpful. The picture can be shared with family and friends as part of the process of making the pregnancy real.

With the fetus's movement, the woman starts to visualize the child and become aware of periods of sleep and activity, as well as what disturbs or soothes the fetus. Some begin to play with the fetus, poking it and provoking activity as well as "rocking and soothing it to sleep." The mother may start to daydream about caring for the child, teaching it a nursery rhyme, or how to play ball. Others experience dreams at night that reveal fears and concerns for the fetus's well-being and safety. These dreams also are signs that she has differentiated the child from herself.

As she thinks about her child, the woman may become increasingly introspective, distancing herself from her partner and others. If her emotional lability persists, her partner may feel left out of the process and withdraw. She may then feel emotionally deserted when she is in need of love and affection. The mother's intense preoccupation with the unborn infant generally occurs between 21 and 24 weeks of pregnancy, creating a vulnerable period for relationships (Hess-Stauthamer, 1985).

Some women refer to the developing fetus as "it," whereas others give it a name such as "pumpkin," or if a given name has been selected for the child, they may start to use it. Certain cultures believe that referring to the child in a specific way will bring bad luck or disappointment.

***Caring for the Fetus.*** To reinforce her interest in the growth of the fetus, a chart or informational handout on the growth and development of the fetus is useful. In addition she will want to know the measurements obtained at each prenatal visit. With an increased focus on the infant, the mother will ask about her diet and whether it is meeting the needs of the baby. She will seek answers about what she can and cannot do regarding clothing, work, exercise, and travel. This concern for the baby easily leads into reviewing with her the warning signs of possible problems during this trimester. She should feel comfortable in knowing when and whom to call if she experiences a physical change that disturbs her (Table 11-3).

***Indications of Difficulty in Acceptance.*** If the woman appears angry or depressed or focuses on her needs rather than the needs of the baby, it may indicate that she is continuing to have difficulty with accepting the pregnancy. If she does not follow through with prenatal care or suggested activities that support the development of the fetus, further assessment is necessary.

If the mother has not completed her own development and cannot view herself as an individual (as is true for some adolescents), she will have difficulty viewing the fetus as different from herself. It will surprise and upset her that the infant has reactions different from her own.

Pregnancy is a difficult time, and now that the reality of another life is clear to her, she may be overwhelmed, lose the support of her partner, or find that her cultural beliefs and values are incongruent with her own beliefs (Box 11-1).

### The Partner

Although the partner's role in the second trimester is still vague, reality will increase when fetal movement is felt and the heartbeat is heard during a prenatal visit. The pregnant woman plays a critical role in making the partner feel as though he or she is integral to the pregnancy experience by including the partner in her physical sensations and emotional experiences.

The expectant father continues to confront and resolve issues around the type of fathering he has received and the type of father he envisions he can be. He also examines other relationships and may start to seek interactions with men who are parenting their children.

The growing change in his partner's appearance may either increase or decrease his desire for sexual intimacy. If he has concerns about harming the baby or his partner, he may not act on his desires even if he is interested. If a father is attending the prenatal visits with the mother or is attending pregnancy classes, he may raise the issue. In other cases, it may be the woman that raises the issue with the provider. Information and illustrations can help with this situation.

The partner and the pregnant woman may now reach the point at which they start to look toward the end of the pregnancy and the childbirth experience. The parents will discuss their expectations for each of their roles. Each partner's level of anxiety is reduced when they agree on the role each will play. If a partner sees himself or herself exclusively as a financial supporter and caretaker of the family while the mother expects an active comrade with her in childbirth and in subsequent childcare, compromise decisions need to be made. Resolution should be reached before the birth, or future occurrence of unmet expectations may lead to conflict within the family.

### Other Children

With the onset of detectable fetal movement through the abdomen, older children living within the household are usually now told about the pregnancy. The children's individual responses may vary based on their age, development, and current interests, as well as how they think having a new baby will affect their lives.

With about 4 and a half months before the birth of the baby, parents have the opportunity to address older children's issues and to prepare them appropriately for the addition to the family. Some children like age- and situation-appropriate books about families that are having babies. Others like to hear stories about when their mother was pregnant with them.

Because of their impatience with the passage of time, telling younger children should be delayed until they ask or it is closer to the delivery date. They can then participate in hearing stories, "reading" books, attending classes, role playing with their dolls, and in making household preparations for the baby.

### Grandparents and Social Support System

During the second trimester grandparents may be involved to varying degrees, depending on how much input the pregnant couple desires and how much the grandparents are willing and able to provide in emotional support. In African-American families, the family support network, especially the grandmother and maternal relatives, are often the primary advisors to a pregnant woman (Purnell and Paulanka, 1998).

Friends serve as role models and resources for information and services, teach new skills, and offer the opportunity to talk about our concerns. As the parents start to make choices based on the well-being of the fetus, friends are useful in supporting those choices.

### Community

The community may support the development of the parents and the expanding family in several ways. It may offer resources for information and stress reduction, programs and facilities that allow new parents to meet other parents or role models, and partnerships with people and facilities that help them plan the process of preparing for and then caring for their child.

Some communities have rituals in which they offer support to the mother. The Navajo Indians have a pregnancy recognition ceremony in which the extended family and community recognize the pregnancy as a reality (Purnell and Paulanka, 1998).

## OTHER INFLUENCES ON THE SECOND TRIMESTER OF PREGNANCY

### Cultural Expectations

Pregnancy is a time when Filipino-American women can demand attention and pampering from their husbands and families. Families come together in anticipation of the new baby. The woman is protected from sudden fright or stress because these might harm the baby. The pregnant woman's mother has a great deal of influence during this period, and the mother and daughter generally become very close. The pregnant woman will be asked "personal" questions, receive advice, and hear stories from many Filipino-American women (Purnell and Paulanka, 1998).

Prescriptive, restrictive, and taboo practices continue to affect the behaviors of the woman during this trimester. Mexican-Americans believe that hot and cold foods influence a woman's health and pregnancy. During pregnancy a woman is more likely to choose hot foods because they are believed to provide warmth for the baby and enable it to be born into a warm and loving environment. Cold foods are thought to have a negative effect on the pregnancy (Purnell and Paulanka, 1998).

Although some families may begin to prepare for the arrival of the baby at this stage of the pregnancy, others do not. "A restrictive belief among the Navajo is that clothes should not be purchased for the infant before birth because preparing for the infant is forbidden by Indian tradition. When an expectant woman does not prepare for the birth of her baby, it does not mean that she does not care about herself or her baby." (Purnell and Paulanka, 1998).

## Maturity

### Pregnant Adolescents

Adolescents generally enter prenatal care during or after this trimester of pregnancy. Once seen and having had their pregnancy confirmed, their visits may be sporadic. To encourage adolescents to come back on a more regular basis it sometimes helps to have programs in the neighborhood specifically for pregnant adolescents. They sometimes feel more comfortable when they can be seen in a more casual environment (such as their school) and are not surrounded by pregnant adults. Other facilities set aside certain clinic sessions for just adolescents. Whether an adolescent who is 17 to 19 years of age will be more comfortable in the adolescent or adult clinic time is a matter of judgment.

Thorough evaluations and teaching should be done whenever possible. Some teaching is more accepted when done in a group. Prenatal classes for adolescents include all the information provided to adults, but it is tailored to their learning needs. It includes child development, providing for child safety, age-appropriate discipline, and planning for child-care arrangements. The goal is to prevent unintentional child abuse or neglect through lack of knowledge. Learning and practicing appropriate techniques for stress reduction and anger management prevent future child abuse. In some areas, mentoring programs are available in which an experienced mother, who may be slightly older than the teen, is partnered with the new mother to provide role mod-

eling. Other programs assign a parent-aide to make weekly visits, monitor the health and well-being of the mother and child, teach the mother new skills as the infant grows and develops, and provide positive feedback.

Realistic short-term and long-term goal setting should be included. Will she return to school or continue her education through a GED program? What are her career or life plans to support herself and her child? How will she coordinate caring for her child while maintaining social relationships with her peers?

Continue to assess how her parents and others significant to her are adjusting to her pregnancy. Learn how the father of the baby is treating her. Is he still involved with her? Is he interested in the pregnancy?

Continue to assess the growth and development of the girl and her fetus. Be positive and reaffirming about any changes she has made in her diet. She may be restricting her caloric intake to prevent protrusion of her abdomen. An alternative may be that she is overeating, especially on high-calorie foods to mask the bodily changes of pregnancy.

Continue to collaborate on improving her nutritional choices. If finances are a problem, she may be helped with government assistance programs such as the food voucher program of WIC (Women, Infants, and Children). Other support programs at both the state and federal level are in an almost constant state of flux and vary from one state to another. Be aware of what area services adolescent mothers may be eligible for and how to make the referral.

As the second trimester progresses and the pregnancy becomes more evident, the adolescent may decide to quit school, leave school and take advantage of a home tutoring option, or transfer to a school for pregnant adolescents. Support any interest she demonstrates for continuing her education and looking toward her future.

### Delayed Pregnancy

The physical relief the second trimester offers to younger pregnant women may not occur as readily with women who are 35 and older. Her body is dealing not only with the stress of pregnancy, but also with the effects of more years of living. As a result of more years to engage in poor health habits, she may not have entered this pregnancy in good physical shape and she may feel more aches and pains and a continuing level of fatigue. Because of her life experiences, she is more likely to have developed chronic diseases (i.e., arthritis, hypertension, or diabetes) that need concurrent treatment with the prenatal care.

The second trimester may bring the older woman an increasing level of confidence that her pregnancy will be successful. Knowing that at her age her "biological clock is ticking," she may feel the pressure of not knowing if she will have another opportunity for pregnancy. Psychologically she may now feel more at ease, having successfully completed the first trimester with its higher risk for spontaneous miscarriage. In addition, she may have chosen to proceed with genetic testing during the first trimester and has received good reports.

With the pregnancy now more of a reality, she may express increasing ambivalence about the role change or role addition she has taken on. If she is involved in a career, she may wonder about balancing her career and the psychologic demands of first pregnancy and then motherhood.

Because of the increased risk for gestational diabetes, hypertension, and vaginal bleeding due to advanced maternal age, vigilant monitoring is maintained throughout the last two trimesters. Blood glucose screening for gestational diabetes, if not done as part of routine screening for all pregnant women, is usually offered to pregnant women over the age of 35 years between the twenty-fourth and twenty-eighth week of pregnancy.

The incidence of PIH is higher in women over the age of 35. In addition, women with chronic hypertension have an increased incidence of superimposed PIH. Screening and ongoing monitoring for this pathology is required. Education of the client and her family about the importance of monitoring and treatment is essential.

The incidence of vaginal bleeding also increases in women over 35 years of age. During the second and third trimester, it may be due to abruptio placentae or placenta previa. Both conditions require immediate assessment and intervention. The treatment options for each of these conditions are explained in Chapters 17 and 18.

## Resources

During the second trimester the pregnant woman and her partner will consider the resources they may need to adjust to the addition of a baby to their lives. They may seek information through enrolling in classes or individualized reading.

Relational resources continue to develop, and the parents may seek out new friends who are also pregnant or new parents. A social support system generally becomes more extensive as the pregnancy becomes more obvious. The cultural background of a woman may limit where she seeks support.

 ## ASSESSMENT OF CHANGE DURING THE SECOND TRIMESTER

During the second trimester, the prenatal visits remain 4 weeks apart unless a problem is detected in either the mother's health or the growth of the fetus.

### Ongoing Assessment of the Woman

#### Care of the Mother

During this trimester, the mother generally feels well and possibly is more energetic than in the first trimester.

As her abdomen grows, the pregnancy now becomes more obvious to others. Virtual strangers will offer advice on pregnancy, tell stories about labor and delivery, and question her about how she will feed her baby. Ask her if she has started to get advice from others and what she has heard. Help her determine what she needs to consider and what she can forget. Remind her that each person and each pregnancy are different.

Ask the mother how she is doing and how she feels the pregnancy is going. Determine if she has felt quickening yet (if appropriate by gestational age) and explain to her what that may feel like. Encourage the woman and her partner or other support person to enroll in prenatal classes for the third trimester. Prenatal classes vary in purpose, content, the number of participants, and cost. Given time to investigate several different programs provides the couple an opportunity to find a class that meets their needs and expectations.

Assess for subtle or overt signs of physical, sexual, and emotional abuse. Ask her specifically, "Since your last visit, have you been emotionally or physically abused or slapped by your partner or someone important to you? Are you afraid of your partner or someone else in your home?"

The results of any prior laboratory testing are reviewed with her. If the mother is Rh-negative, the antibody screen titer that was obtained earlier will be reevaluated to determine if she is a candidate for RhoGam. RhoGam is the trademark name for an immune globulin that prevents the formation of antibodies after an abortion or delivery of an Rh-positive baby from an Rh-negative mother. However, if the Rh-negative woman has already formed antibodies during a prior pregnancy, the RhoGam is ineffective and will not be given.

During the second trimester, the woman should immediately report if she experiences abdominal pain or  cramping, vaginal bleeding, nausea and vomiting, burning or painful urination, fever, or reduction in or absence of fetal movements. Review this information with her and ask if she has experienced any of these. Review with her what she is to do if she becomes concerned about the baby or experiences any signs of potential complications. Some women know intuitively that something is wrong before they become fully aware of a danger sign. Encourage her to call with any questions or concerns.

Preterm labor is the presence of regular uterine contractions that cause the effacement and dilation of the cervix after 20 weeks but before 38 weeks of gestation. The cause of preterm labor is generally unknown. The occurrence of preterm labor and delivery may be decreased by early identification of risk factors, explaining the condition to the couple, and providing them with appropriate guidance (such as the woman refraining from experiencing an orgasm). In addition, if she is experiencing contractions, frequent assessment of the cervix may be done to assess for changes in the position, consistency, length, and possible dilation of the cervix. Treatment is limited to interventions that reduce controllable factors. (For further information on diagnosis and treatment see Chapter 17.)

### Assessment of Fetus

The growth and assumed health of the fetus is determined by measuring fundal height and comparing it to the prior measurement and by assessing fetal heart tones. The positive aspects of the fetal examination, normal heart tones and good growth, are shared with the mother. This serves to include her as a partner in the process of prenatal care and supplies her with positive reinforcement to continue to care for herself and her child.

Most healthy babies move at least 10 times in 4 hours. Once the mother can feel the fetus move about the womb on a daily basis, teach her how to count and record the number of times she feels her baby kick, twist, or turn. Kick counts should be done during the baby's most active time of the day and at approximately the same time every day. The activity of the baby may be generated or increased by the mother palpating her abdomen, eating and/or drinking, or walking. To do the count, the woman records the time she starts to count the kicks, twists, and turns. After the fetus has moved 10 times she writes down the time again. If it has taken the baby more than 4 hours to move 10 times, she should call the nurse midwife or doctor right away (Box 11-2).

### Additional Assessment Measures

*Laboratory Testing.* Blood may be drawn for a remeasurement of hemoglobin and hematocrit. A glucose screening to detect gestational diabetes may be done.

*Ultrasound.* During the second trimester ultrasound may be used to confirm viability and estimate how advanced the pregnancy is by measuring the biparietal diameter, femur length, and abdominal circumference, and estimating fetal weight. It can allow for visualization of the placement of the fetus for test procedures and possible observation of some congenital abnormalities and problems.

Ultrasound is also helpful in measuring the amount of amniotic fluid present and detecting abnormalities such as polyhydramnios, oligohydramnios, congenital abnormalities, and intrauterine growth retardation (IUGR).

### Close of the Visit

Before the woman leaves each prenatal visit, address any further questions and concerns, provide appropriate anticipatory guidance, review the expected changes that will occur before her next visit, and praise her positive health behaviors. Review the signs and symptoms of possible problems with the pregnancy and be sure she knows when and where to contact a provider.

Remind her about being "fair game for every horror story" there is. Reaffirm that every person's circumstances and pregnancy are different and that her expec-

---

**BOX 11-2** *Recording Kick Counts*

Date _____

Start time:
First kick
Second kick
Third kick
Fourth kick
Fifth kick
Sixth kick
Seventh kick
Eighth kick
Ninth kick
Tenth kick
End time:

Call your midwife or doctor if it is longer than 4 hours between the "start time" and the "end time."

If you have any concerns about the movement of your baby, call your provider immediately.

---

tations and decisions are her own. Ask her to call if any questions arise based on what she hears or learns. Finally, confirm the date and time of her next appointment (Figure 11-2).

## ANTICIPATORY GUIDANCE DURING THE SECOND TRIMESTER

### Sexual Activity

By the beginning of the second trimester the tissues of a woman's vagina and labia have become slightly engorged and will remain that way until delivery. Increased blood supply puts the woman in a state of permanent gentle sexual arousal. With the increased vaginal secretions she is also more moist. The pressure on the genital organs from about the fourth month is so great for some women that they are easily aroused (Kitzinger, 1985). These sensations may lead a woman to seek more sexual activity with her partner or self-pleasuring with masturbation.

The woman's partner may be reluctant to have intercourse for fear of breaking the bag of waters, starting labor, or damaging the baby. Review the anatomy and physiology with the couple and suggest a gentle form of intercourse. Provide information about positions they might try, such as side-lying or with the man entering from behind (Kitzinger, 1985). Be aware that many cultures have taboos against intercourse with a pregnant woman (Figure 11-3).

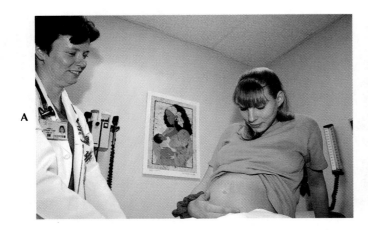
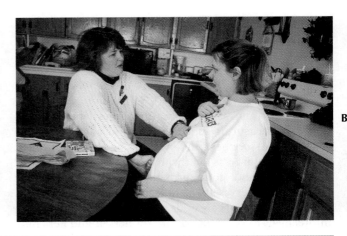

A

B

FIGURE 11-2 • **A,** Prenatal visit. **B,** Prenatal evaluation during home visit. *(Courtesy of Caroline E. Brown.)*

 The following contraindications most often preclude sexual intercourse during this trimester: undiagnosed vaginal bleeding; a history of premature dilation of the cervix, without cerclage; severe vulvar varicosities; premature rupture of the membranes; or premature labor. If premature labor is a concern, caution the couple about the woman experiencing orgasm from nipple stimulation or masturbation, even without vaginal penetration.

## Oral Hygiene

Gentle tooth brushing and flossing should continue on a regular basis. A soft tooth brush should be used to prevent injury to gums that are more tender during pregnancy. During the second trimester many women schedule appointments for their teeth to be cleaned and to check for needed repairs. Waiting until after "morning sickness" has passed makes it more comfortable and yet allows the time for scheduling of any work that may need to be done before the arrival of the baby.

## Nutritional Needs

During the second trimester, continue to review with the woman her eating habits and preferences for food and beverage. Show her how she is doing compared to the Food Guide Pyramid. If the woman started the pregnancy at a healthy weight, and she is pregnant with only one fetus, she will be gaining an average of 1 pound per week during the second and third trimesters. If she was initially underweight, she should gain more than 1 pound per week. If she was initially overweight, she should eat amounts of food and maintain an activity level that help her gain at the slower rate of 2/3 a pound per week. Her weight gain should be evaluated by look-

ing at the total picture, not just her weight. Consider the nutritional status and weight at which she started the pregnancy, her activity level, and the selections of foods she is consuming.

Although it is possible to meet the nutritional requirements of pregnancy through a balanced diet, most women are encouraged to take a daily prenatal vitamin supplement starting by the second trimester. These generally include iron (30 mg), folic acid (400 $\mu$g), calcium (250 mg), vitamin C (50 mg), vitamin $B_{12}$ (2 $\mu$g), vitamin D (5 $\mu$g) copper (2 mg), zinc (15 mg) and vitamin $B_6$ (2 mg). If a woman is a vegan, the amount of vitamin D should be increased to 20 $\mu$g and vitamin $B_{12}$ should be increased to 4 $\mu$g. Because excessive amounts of vitamin A can be toxic, supplementation during pregnancy is not recommended. It is strongly recommended that all women who either are vegetarians, smoke tobacco, drink alcoholic beverages, use illicit drugs, or are pregnant with more than one fetus take prenatal vitamins (ific, 1995).

A woman's culture may influence the way she follows your diet and vitamin supplementation recommendations. Many Cuban women eat for two during pregnancy and gain excessive amounts of weight. Some believe that eating more fruit ensures a baby with a smooth complexion (Brewer, 1995). During the second trimester, the pregnant Vietnamese-American woman may add cold foods to her diet. She will continue to eat animal protein, fat, sugar, and carbohydrates that are generally hot and sweet. Chinese-American women may refuse iron supplementation, often started in the second trimester, because they believe it will make the delivery more difficult. Filipino-American women may refuse to take vitamins because they avoid medications for fear of harming the fetus (Purnell and Paulanka, 1998).

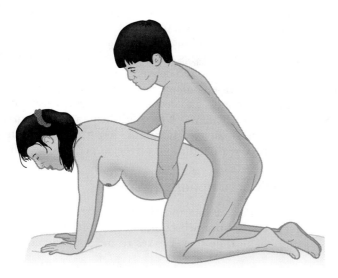

Hands and knees take the weight of
the uterus and baby off the woman's back

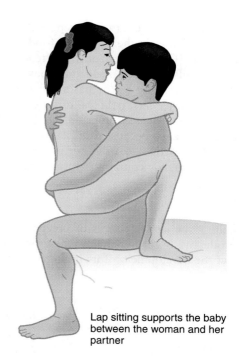

Lap sitting supports the baby
between the woman and her
partner

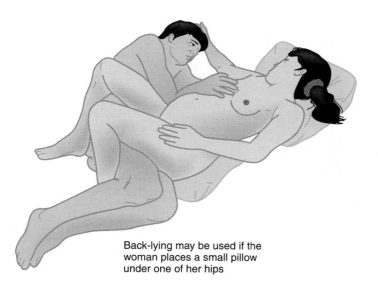

Back-lying may be used if the
woman places a small pillow
under one of her hips

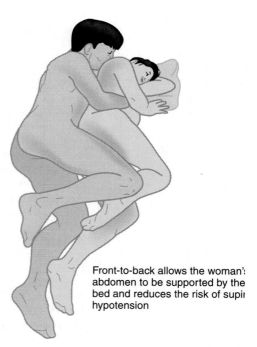

Front-to-back allows the woman':
abdomen to be supported by the
bed and reduces the risk of supir
hypotension

FIGURE 11-3 • Positions for intercourse during second trimester.

Constipation, a problem sometimes exacerbated by the intake of iron supplements, becomes more of a problem when intestinal motility gradually decreases during the second and third trimesters. Fruits and vegetables, whole grain breads, and cereals are not only good for their nutrients, but also they provide the fiber needed to help alleviate constipation. A regular pattern of walking or other forms of exercise and 64 ounces of fluid a day can also be helpful (ific, 1995).

**Pica,** the craving for nonnutritive substances, occurs in women of all cultures. The etiology of pica has been speculated to be cultural, psychologic, or a response to a physiologic need such as anemia. None of these hypotheses universally are supported.

Initially the woman may report that she has experienced a change in the way some food or beverages smell and taste. Commonly reported offenders are coffee, tobacco, milk, and red meats. She may then mention that she has a craving for or has started to ingest nonfood items such as clay, pebbles, dirt, starch, ice, and other substances. The consumption of nonfood items should be discouraged because it displaces nutritious foods and interferes with adequate nutrient intake. In addition, these items may contain harmful substances (ific, 1995).

### Safety

During the last 6 months of pregnancy, exposure to reproductive hazards can slow the growth of the fetus, affect the development of its brain, or cause premature labor. The workplace hazards of most concern during this trimester include infectious agents, demanding labor, and less-than-ideal working conditions. "Physically intensive employment increases the likelihood of low birth weight and preterm labor and delivery. Standing for long periods of time; increased pulling, pushing, or lifting of more than 10 to 25 pounds; and decreased rest periods also increase these risks" (Bailey, 1998). With help, a woman may be able to negotiate two 10-minute rest periods and a nutrition break with bathroom privileges per 8-hour shift.

### Drug Consumption

During the second and third trimester, restricting caffeine consumption becomes even more important. The amount of time that it takes to metabolize and excrete

| TABLE 11-4 | *Relief of the Common Discomforts of the Second Trimester* |
|---|---|
| **Condition** | **Helpful interventions** |
| Constipation | Herbal therapy |
| | High-fiber diet |
| | Drink 48 ounces of water per day |
| | Walk |
| | Maintain time in day for regular bowel movements |
| | Accupressure |
| | Homeopathy |
| | Yoga |
| Feeling faint or fainting | Change positions slowly |
| | Assist circulation with moderate level of exercise, deep breathing, leg exercises, wearing elastic hose |
| | Stay cool and warm; avoid crowded areas |
| | Provide body with a consistent supply of food throughout the day |
| | Avoid becoming hungry or hypoglycemic. |
| Flatulence | Avid gas-producing foods |
| | Chew food slowly to avoid swallowing air |
| | Maintain regular bowel habits |
| Food cravings | Respond to them as long as the substances eaten are not harmful or interfere with a nutritious diet |
| Headaches | Ice pack or bag of frozen vegetables to area |
| | Conscious relaxation |
| | Meditation |
| | Accupressure |
| | Biofeedback |
| | Chiropractic manipulation |
| | Diet changes to remove common triggers such as chocolate, aged cheeses, citrus fruits, processed meats containing sodium nitrates or MSG, and red wine |
| | Herbal therapy |
| | Homeopathy |
| | Sound therapy |
| | Tai chi chuan |
| | Yoga |
| | Call care provider if sudden onset or severe |
| Heartburn | Eat small meals; adjust diet to avoid food high in fats and oils, tomatoes, citrus fruits, garlic, onions, chocolate, coffee, alcohol, and peppermint |
| | Accupressure |
| | Herbal tea made from ginger, chamomile, or slippery elm |

caffeine takes longer—up to 18 hours. So there is a cumulative effect when regular consumption continues within a 12- to 18-hour period.

Exposure to a smoky environment, as well as smoking herself, affects the growth of the fetus. Smoking during pregnancy reduces a mother's appetite and creates vascular changes in the placental tissue. It doubles the risk of having a low–birth-weight baby. If a mother can stop smoking before the third trimester, some of the negative changes may be reversed, and the weight of the baby may improve.

## Discomforts of Pregnancy

During the second trimester, women are generally the most comfortable of their pregnancy. The morning sickness, frequent urination, and fatigue have generally passed. They may be replaced with discomforts, but these generally don't interfere with their daily activities as much.

Women treat the discomforts of pregnancy based on information from family, friends, and their health care providers. Anticipatory guidance and teaching materials to take home are the best ways to prevent or lessen the discomforts (Table 11-4).

## PREGNANCY LOSS

Once a pregnancy enters the second trimester, most couples relax their concern about losing the fetus. With the pregnancy firmly established continuing processes

---

**TABLE 11-4**  *Relief of the Common Discomforts of the Second Trimester—cont'd*

| Condition | Helpful interventions |
|---|---|
| Heartburn—cont'd | Homeopathic remedies |
| | Hydrotherapy of placing an ice pack over your stomach for 5 to 10 minutes before eating |
| | Note: Milk is not a remedy for heartburn; it may soothe at first but fat, calcium, and protein cause increased acid secretion |
| Hemorrhoids | Prevent constipation and forceful bearing down when moving bowels |
| | Relieve swelling and pain with witch hazel compresses, sitz baths |
| Itchiness of skin (pruritus) | Find a distraction or use meditation |
| | Reduce sensations with herbal therapy, homeopathy, oatmeal or corn starch baths, Keri baths |
| | Apply petroleum jelly or other lotions or oils that help retain moisture |
| | Use mild soap or replace use of soap with lotion-based body cleaners |
| | Wear loose clothing |
| | Ask health care provider about a mild sedation |
| Joint pain | Conscious relaxation |
| | Maintain good posture and body mechanics |
| | Sleep on firm mattress |
| | Wear shoes with heels as low as are comfortable |
| | Do pelvic rock |
| | Use abdominal support |
| | Acupressure or acupuncture |
| | Body work such as Alexander technique and the Feldenkrais method |
| | Chiropractic |
| | Herbal therapies that cause muscle relaxation |
| | Yoga |
| Leukorrhea (increased vaginal discharge) | Bathe daily |
| | Wear cotton underpants |
| | Avoid the use of nylon panties and pantyhose |
| | Do not douche |
| Periodic numbness/finger tingling | Maintain good posture and body mechanics |
| | Wear supportive bra |
| Supine hypotension | Use side-lying or semiupright sitting position |
| Varicose veins | Avoid crossing legs, lengthy periods of standing still, socks or stockings that constrict the leg at specific points such as the calf or the thigh |
| | Walking, resting with legs above hips, wearing support stockings may help |

(Compiled from Davis DC: The discomforts of pregnancy, *J Obstet Gynecol Neonatal Nurs* 25(1):73-81, 1996; *Nurses handbook of alternative and complementary therapies*, Springhouse, PA, 1998, Springhouse; Snyder M and Lindquist R: *Complementary/alternative therapies in nursing*, ed 3, New York, 1998, Springer.)

now support the growth of the baby. Even though they happen less often, spontaneous abortion, ectopic pregnancy, and gestational trophoblastic disease (GTD) may be diagnosed in this trimester. The photo essay depicted in Figure 11-4 takes you on a visual journey with a mother meeting her infant son, who was stillborn at 19 weeks of gestation. The process of becoming acquainted is clearly visible in this new mother's gentle exploration of her son.

## Spontaneous Abortion

A spontaneous abortion can, by definition, occur through 20 weeks of gestation. Because the woman's abdomen has increased in size, it is now considered a more established pregnancy. The parents may have told friends and relatives about their news. The couple also may feel more attached to the baby as an individual, and the mother has become aware of the movements of the fetus. A loss at this time may be more difficult for her and her family.

The categories of miscarriage are the same as are the assessment and planning processes that are required. A missed abortion may be resolved in the second trimester with a dilation and curettage or admission to a hospital where labor may be induced. Because the couple has not yet attended childbirth preparation education, they must be prepared now for the labor process.

**Laminaria** (a type of seaweed) may be placed in the os of the cervix the night before to start the dilation before the procedure. The laminaria swells as it absorbs the moisture in the cervix, gradually and nontraumatically opening the os. The labor may be started with an intravaginal prostaglandin $E_2$ ($PGE_2$) suppository and then intravenous administration of oxytocin (Pitocin) (Youngkin and Davis, 1998). The woman has the full experience of labor while knowing that she will deliver a dead baby. She may be medicated for the pain.

The mother or both parents may wish to see their child. If the woman experiences a spontaneous abortion at home, she may have retrieved the tissue she expelled and brought it in with her. Depending on the gestational

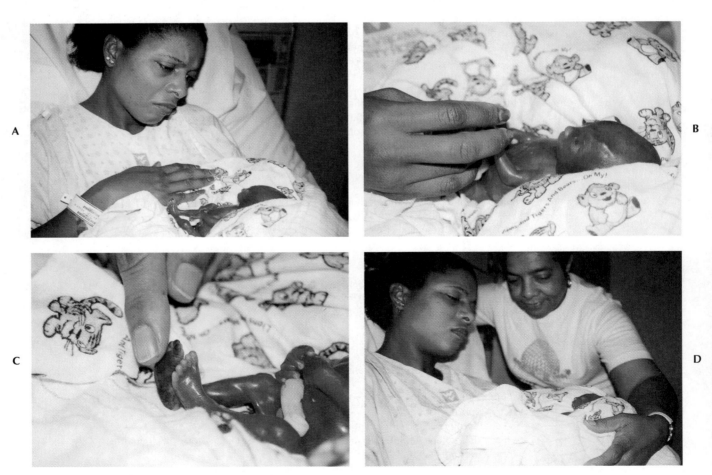

*FIGURE 11-4* • **A,** Early in the contact, maternal contact centered around visual inspection. **B,** Gentle touch beginning with fingertip exploration of the extremities. **C,** Progressive touch using more of the fingers to delicately explore the infant's face and then body. **D,** Quiet time supported by the family. *(Courtesy of Caroline E. Brown.)*

age and condition of the fetus, we can generally clean and wrap it so that it looks like a sleeping infant. Be cautious about denying parents their right to see their child. What they imagine it looks like is generally much worse than the reality. Seeing, touching, and holding even the tiniest fetus helps them in their grief process.

## Ectopic Pregnancy

An ectopic pregnancy may survive into the second trimester when attached in a place other than the fallopian tube (Figure 11-5). If the woman reports that it just does not feel right or if bleeding or pain is present, further investigation and a definitive diagnosis are needed. The assessment and interventions remain the same as during the first trimester. With the confirmation of an ectopic pregnancy, the woman must be prepared for the loss of her baby and the prospect of surgery.

## Gestational Trophoblastic Disease (GTD)

Women experiencing severe nausea and vomiting in the second trimester may be treated for hyperemesis gravidarum. Others exhibit the fluid retention and swelling edema at 24 weeks that are generally associated with PIH later in pregnancy. Both symptoms are indications of a possible molar pregnancy and warrant investigation (Youngkin and Davis, 1998). A molar pregnancy may be expelled through the cervix or lead to the rupture of the uterus (Figure 11-6). A partial mole may not be noticed until after a spontaneous abortion occurs.

The nursing assessment and treatment are the same as during the first trimester. The family will experience grief over the loss of the baby they thought they were having and concern for the future health of the mother, as well as uncertainty as to how to explain this to their friends.

## Stillborn

If at any time after 20 weeks the fetus stops developing and dies in utero, it is called a stillborn. A woman may come in for a regular prenatal visit and report that the baby has not moved in the last few days or week. A fetal heart cannot be found and ultrasound reveals no heartbeat.

### Nursing Care

The woman and her partner need information to understand what has happened and time to assimilate the loss of their child. The woman must be prepared for a hospital admission and dealing with the process of labor. Labor will start spontaneously or be induced. The assessment and grief work provided to the woman and her family are similar to when they experience a miscarriage.

## Bleeding in the Second Trimester

Placenta previa is the abnormal implantation of the placenta in the lower uterine segment, near or over the os. The condition causes painless bleeding primarily in the third trimester; however, it may occur in the second trimester at about 24 weeks of gestation, and even as early as 20 weeks.

Abruptio placentae is the partial or complete detachment of a normally implanted placenta before delivery of an infant. Detachment and bleeding occur more often during the third trimester, but may occur anytime after 20 weeks of gestation. Both of these events are described in more detail in Chapter 12.

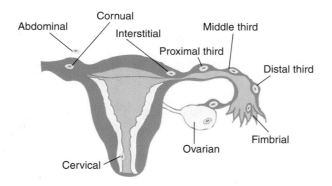

FIGURE 11-5 • Ectopic sites of implantation. *(From Dickason and others: Maternal-infant nursing care, ed 3, St Louis, 1998, Mosby.)*

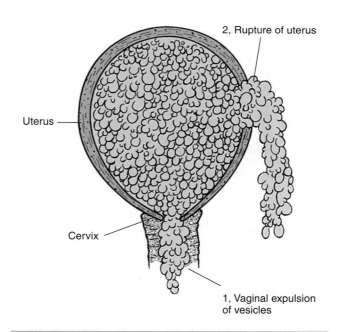

FIGURE 11-6 • Molar pregnancy. *(From Lowdermilk DL: Maternity and women's health care, ed 7, St Louis, 2000, Mosby.)*

**SUMMARY**

The second trimester of pregnancy is often a time of well-being for the woman and she glows with a kind of pregnancy radiance. The woman's body continues the process of change in various systems both to sustain the pregnancy and to gradually prepare for the more strenuous third trimester and the birth process. The fetus continues to grow and move actively within the uterus. The second trimester is an opportune time for the woman and her partner to engage in education programs and prepare their home for the addition of the infant.

---

## Care Plan · Promoting Wellness During the Second Trimester

**NURSING DIAGNOSIS** **Potential for Enhanced Physical Growth and Development** (Fetal)(NOTE: Because this is a wellness diagnosis, no etiology is needed.)

**GOALS/OUTCOMES** Fetus grows and develops normally throughout second trimester; client practices behaviors that foster fetal development and avoids behaviors that are hazardous to the fetus *(See "Evaluation Parameters" for indicators of goal achievement.)*

**NOC Suggested Outcomes**
- Fetal Status: Antepartum (0111)
- Health Seeking Behavior (1603)
- Prenatal Health Behavior (1607)

**NIC Priority Interventions**
- Anticipatory Guidance (5210)
- Electronic Fetal Monitoring: Antepartum (6771)
- Prenatal Care (6960)

**Nursing Activities and Rationale**
- Measure fundal height (with a tape measure, in centimeters) and compare with gestational age. *Accurate measurement data can be used to evaluate adequacy of fetal growth.*
- Monitor fetal heart rate and pattern. *Normal rate and pattern reflect fetal well-being and intact fetal nervous system.*
- Instruct client to monitor fetal activity at home and to contact health professionals if less than 10 movements in 4 hours, no movement in 24 hours, or a decrease in the usual activity. *Decreased movement may indicate fetal distress. Involving client promotes self-care, which is appropriate when viewing pregnancy as a normal state.*
- Provide anticipatory guidance about expected physiologic changes (e.g., fetal movement) to *enable the client to be prepared for changes and to detect any variation from normal.*
- Teach about fetal growth and development to *help the client understand body changes and promote attachment.*
- Instruct about harmful effects of smoking, alcohol, and drugs (including over-the-counter medications) on the fetus. *Social support by the nurse encourages positive health practices.*
- Encourage the client to attend prenatal classes; provide a referral if needed. *This provides information needed for healthy behaviors and choices. A referral facilitates client's choices.*
- Teach and support healthy behaviors (e.g., nutrition, exercise). See *"Effective Individual Management of Therapeutic Regimen."*
- Suggest books and literature to read *to reinforce personal teaching done by nurse.*

**Evaluation Parameters**
- Fetal heart rate is 120 to 160 beats/minute.
- FHR pattern shows good variability and accelerations with fetal movement.
- Mother reports that fetal movements occur approximately 10 times in a 4-hour period (varies).
- Fundal height corresponds to gestation in weeks, using McDonald's method.
- Ultrasound imaging reveals normal fetal development.
- Maternal alpha-fetoprotein screening is normal level for gestational age.
- Client reports practices to promote optimal wellness (see *"Potential for Enhanced Maternal Physical Development"* and *"Effective Individual Management of Therapeutic Regimen"*).
- When asked, client describes appearance of fetus during second trimester.

## Care Plan · Promoting Wellness During the Second Trimester—cont'd

**NURSING DIAGNOSIS** **Potential for Enhanced Physical Development (Maternal)** (NOTE: Because this is a wellness diagnosis, no etiology is needed.)

**GOALS/OUTCOMES** Experiences physiologic growth and development expected during second trimester *(See "Evaluation Parameters" for indicators of goal achievement.)*

**NOC Suggested Outcomes**
- Maternal Status: Antepartum (2509)
- Risk Detection (1908)

**NIC Priority Interventions**
- Anticipatory Guidance (5210)
- Health Education (5510)
- Prenatal Care (6960)
- Risk Identification (6610)

**Nursing Activities and Rationale**
- Monitor vital signs at prenatal visits *to discriminate between normal discomforts of pregnancy and beginning complications (high-risk conditions). For example, increased BP is a symptom of pregnancy-induced hypertension (PIH); increased temperature may indicate an infection.*
- Provide anticipatory guidance regarding physiologic changes to expect during second trimester. *Client needs information to recognize and adjust to normal changes.*
- Monitor for edema and sudden weight gain *to differentiate between normal, dependent type and that associated with preeclampsia.*
- Test urine for glucose, protein, and nitrites. *Proteinuria of +1 or more is associated with PIH. Elevated glucose may indicate gestational diabetes. Nitrites may indicate infection.*
- Assess sleep and rest patterns *to provide baseline data and serve as an indicator of healthy behaviors.*
- Assess for urinary tract infection. Teach signs and symptoms to report (urinary frequency, urgency, dysuria, hematuria). *UTI is common in pregnancy because of urinary stasis that results from loss of smooth muscle tone in kidneys, ureters, and bladder under the influence of elevated progesterone levels.*
- Teach to not postpone voiding, wipe from front to back after elimination, and wash hands after voiding *to minimize urinary stasis and contamination by* Escherichia coli.
- Teach danger signs that should be reported immediately to health professionals: vaginal bleeding, abdominal pain, rupture of membranes, edema of hands/fingers, severe/persistent headache, visual disturbances, persistent emesis, fever, chills, and dyspnea *to begin immediate treatment and prevent serious complications.*
- Assess nutritional status and eating habits *to determine if calories and nutrients are adequate for pregnancy.*
- Teach nutritional requirements for pregnancy, using the food guide pyramid *to provide knowledge for selecting healthful foods. Good nutrition is essential for the health of both mother and fetus.*

**Evaluation Parameters**
- Vital signs within normal limits for client.
- Gains recommended amount of weight (*see "Potential for Enhanced Nutritional Status"*).
- Recognizes signs and symptoms of high-risk conditions.
- Exhibits symptoms of high-risk conditions (e.g., no headache, edema, or blood pressure increase; no vaginal bleeding or infection; no premature labor or premature rupture of membranes).

**NURSING DIAGNOSIS** **Effective Individual Management of Therapeutic Regimen** (NOTE: Because this is a wellness diagnosis, no etiology is needed.)

**GOALS/OUTCOMES** Client practices behaviors that foster maternal health and avoids behaviors that are hazardous to maternal health *(See "Evaluation Parameters" for indicators of goal achievement.)*

**NOC Suggested Outcomes**
- Health Beliefs (1700)
- Health Seeking Behavior (1603)
- Participation: Health Care Decisions(1606)
- Prenatal Health Behavior (1607)

**NIC Priority Interventions**
- Exercise Promotion (0200)
- Health Education (5510)
- Health System Guidance (7400)

**NOC Additional Outcomes**
- Knowledge: Health Behaviors (1805)

*Continued*

## Care Plan • Promoting Wellness During the Second Trimester—cont'd

### Nursing Activities and Rationale
- Teach methods for managing common discomforts of pregnancy (e.g., morning sickness, heartburn, breast tenderness, leg cramps, shortness of breath, constipation) *to provide information the woman needs to manage self-care during this normal developmental event.*
- Teach about increased need for rest: 8 hours sleep plus one nap; schedule a rest period at work *to minimize the normal fatigue that occurs with pregnancy.*
- Instruct client about the benefits of exercise *to motivate the client.*
- Teach appropriate exercises, including tailor sitting, Kegel exercises, pelvic lifting and rocking, and modified sit-ups. Explain that usual exercise routines can be maintained (as a rule), but to introduce new exercises gradually. *This safely promotes muscle tone for childbirth and return to prepregnant state.*
- Advise resting or sleeping on left side *to reduce vena caval compression and facilitate uteroplacental circulation.*
- Provide written instructions (e.g., for exercises, for return visits) *to reinforce oral instructions.*
- Inform client/family about different types of health care facilities (e.g., hospital, clinic, birthing center) as appropriate *to promote participation in health care decisions and provide choices.*
- Assess for barriers to healthy behaviors (e.g., transportation to clinic appointments) *to evaluate the kind and amount of support needed. Client may not volunteer such information.*

### Evaluation Parameters
- Describes and uses strategies to manage normal discomforts of pregnancy.
- Contacts health professionals when indicated (e.g., by unusual symptoms).
- Reports exercising regularly.
- Reports she is getting 8 hours of sleep at night, plus a nap during the day.
- Reports eating a balanced diet with adequate calories.
- Uses correct body mechanics.
- Attends childbirth preparation classes.
- Keeps appointments for prenatal visits.
- Consults with health provider before using over-the-counter medications.

| | |
|---|---|
| NURSING DIAGNOSIS | **Potential for Enhanced Psychological Development (Maternal)** (NOTE: Because this is a wellness diagnosis, no etiology is needed.) |
| GOALS/OUTCOMES | Adapts to physical changes of pregnancy: maintains positive self-esteem; completes psychologic developmental tasks of pregnancy *(See "Evaluation Parameters" for indicators of goal achievement.)* |

### NOC Suggested Outcomes
- Health Seeking Behavior (1603)
- Prenatal Health Behavior (1607)
- Maternal Status: Antepartum (2509)
- Self-Esteem (1205)

### NIC Priority Interventions
- Attachment Promotion (6710)
- Family Integrity Promotion: Childbearing Family (7104)
- Prenatal Care (6960)
- Self-Esteem Enhancement (5400)
- Teaching, Sexuality (5624)

### Nursing Activities and Rationale
- Assess for anger, depression, and focusing on her own needs to the exclusion of the baby, *which may indicate difficulty accepting the pregnancy.*
- Assess for past negative experiences with pregnancy or birth, *which is a risk factor for difficult psychologic adaptation in this pregnancy.*
- Assess for persistent and many physical complaints, *which may indicate psychologic failure to adapt.*
- Assess amount of support from partner, parents, and other family members. *Lack of family support systems makes it difficult to achieve psychologic tasks.*
- Provide opportunity to listen to fetal heart tones and give parent(s) the ultrasound "picture." Discuss parents' reactions. *This supports the process of fetal differentiation and parent-fetus attachment.*
- Discuss parent(s) reaction to fetal movement, *which supports the processes of fetal differentiation and attachment.*
- Assess extent to which client is following prenatal advice; if not following advice, assess reasons (e.g., lack of understanding, conflict with cultural beliefs) *to provide an indication of acceptance of the pregnancy.*

## Care Plan · Promoting Wellness During the Second Trimester—cont'd

- Explore concerns about sexuality; provide information about alternative positions for intercourse; correct any misinformation; teach contraindications to intercourse (e.g., vaginal bleeding, previous premature dilation of cervix, severe vulvar varicosities, premature rupture of membranes, or concern about premature labor). *Many women are more sexually active in second trimester. Explanations and information support the sexual relationship and strengthen bonds between the partners.*
- Give client a chart showing the growth and development of the fetus. Share the measurements obtained at each prenatal visit, *which supports fetal differentiation and attachment to fetus.*
- Facilitate discussion with partner of their expectations for each of their future roles. *Each partner's level of anxiety is reduced when they agree on the role each will play.*
- Explore client's body image; be alert for negative comments (e.g., "I'm a fat pig."). *During the second trimester the woman's body image changes because of her enlarging abdomen, normal weight gain, and other changes. If she perceives these changes as negative, it can damage her self-esteem.*
- Praise client's positive behaviors and normal body changes (e.g., "Great! You've gained just the right amount of weight for your baby") to *enhance self-esteem.*
- Explain to partner and family the importance of positive comments and reassurance. *The woman looks to important others for reassurance during this time.*

**Evaluation Parameters**
- Loses ambivalence about the pregnancy and definitely knows that she wants the child.
- Begins to recognize fetus as a separate being. Completes fetal differentiation by end of second trimester.
- Describes fetal activity patterns as well as what disturbs or soothes the fetus.
- Dreams or daydreams about caring for the baby.
- Refers to fetus as "it"; by a pet name; or by given name, if one has been selected.
- Client and partner openly discuss their feelings about the pregnancy and the baby, their fantasies, and role expectations.

## CASE STUDY

Raeanne is a 21-year-old single, college student who was first seen for prenatal care approximately 6 weeks ago accompanied by the father of the baby, also a student.

At her first visit, Raeanne, who is 5 feet tall, weighs 105 pounds. Her blood pressure is 120/70 mm Hg. Her hemoglobin level is 13.5 g/ml. VDRL is negative, and the rubella antibody titre indicated that she is immune. Her blood type is A, Rh+.

Raeanne is unsure of the date of her last menstrual period. Physical examination determines that the size of her uterus is consistent with a 14-week gestation. When explained to Raeanne, she agrees that this is probably right, based on missed menses. A fetal heart is easily heard with a portable Doppler. An ultrasound scan shows a gestation by crown-rump length of approximately 13 weeks.

When she returns for her next prenatal visit 4 weeks later, she has not gained weight, but she generally feels well with no nausea or tiredness. The fetal heart is again heard with the Doppler. Measurement of the uterus seems to be about 16 weeks. A repeat ultrasound scan determines that amniotic fluid is diminished. Another ultrasound is scheduled in 2 weeks when she would be at 20 weeks of gestation.

Raeanne has returned today, at 19.5 weeks of gestation, worried that she has not felt any fetal movements for the last 2 days. A fetal heart could not be heard with the Doppler and an ultrasound confirmed there is no fetal heartbeat.

- What immediate response will you provide Raeanne?
- What are her strengths? Where does she face potential problems?
- What information do you need from Raeanne to move forward in support of her?
- What nursing diagnoses could apply? How will you validate these?
- What long-term goals might she have for herself? For her partner?

- What short-term goals might the two of you develop for Raeanne? For her partner?
- What interventions may you be able to develop and offer?
- How will these interventions be prioritized?

- How will you evaluate the effectiveness of your interventions?
- What note should be put in Raeanne's chart to prepare providers when she returns for her next annual examination?

# Scenarios

1. Joanne is G 1, P O and is naturally concerned about her pregnancy. She asks, "Are there different signs and symptoms of possible problems that I should watch for?"

- What subjective data do you have about Joanne's condition?
- What subjective and objective data do you need?
- What nursing diagnoses could apply? How will you validate these?
- What goals might be developed? How will these be prioritized?
- What interventions may you offer?
- How will you evaluate the effectiveness of your interventions?

2. Aisha is 24 years old and 16 weeks pregnant. This is her second pregnancy, the first one having ended with a spontaneous abortion at 14 weeks. She has been very nervous about the status of this fetus as it grows. She asks you, "How can I tell that my baby is healthy? I am just so worried something is going to happen. My friend told me that she did kick counts when she was pregnant. What is that and will it help?"

- What subjective data do you have about Aisha's condition?
- What subjective and objective data do you need?
- What nursing diagnoses could apply? How will you validate these?
- What goals might be developed? How will these be prioritized?
- What interventions may you offer?

- How will you evaluate the effectiveness of your interventions?

3. You are providing Anne, a woman of Chinese descent, with nutritional counseling. When you tell her that she should take iron supplementation she becomes quiet and seems to disengage from the conversation. You become aware that you have lost her interest and try to identify why that might have happened.

- What subjective data do you have about Anne's situation?
- What subjective and objective data do you need?
- What nursing diagnoses could apply? How will you validate these?
- What goals might be developed? How will these be prioritized?
- What interventions may you offer?
- How will you evaluate the effectiveness of your interventions?

4. Christine, age 26 years old, is 20 weeks pregnant. During her prenatal visit she confides to you that she and her husband haven't had sex for the last 6 weeks. Christine states, "I don't know why this has happened, although I haven't been interested for awhile. But now I am." She continues, "It's funny. Greg seems rather timid and nervous about touching me. That's not like him. In the past he has always been interested in being sexually intimate."

- What subjective data do you have about Christine's condition?

- What subjective and objective data do you need?
- What nursing diagnoses could apply? How will you validate these?
- What goals might be developed? How will these be prioritized?
- What interventions may you offer?
- How will you evaluate the effectiveness of your interventions?

---

5. Ellen is a 16-year-old who is in her second trimester of pregnancy. She has come to the clinic for her first prenatal visit. She is by herself. She learned she was pregnant using a home pregnancy test after missing two menstrual cycles. She was excused from track and field practice by her high school coach so that she might "have her annual examination." She has not told her coach or her family that she had a positive home pregnancy test.

- What subjective data do you have about Ellen's condition?
- What subjective and objective data do you need?
- What nursing diagnoses could apply? How will you validate these?
- What goals might be developed? How will these be prioritized?
- What interventions may you offer?
- How will you evaluate the effectiveness of your interventions?

---

6. Heather and Nathan, both 34 years old, have been married for 4 years, and this is a planned pregnancy. Now that she is in her second trimester, Heather is no longer experiencing nausea and vomiting. As she feels the baby move she begins to plan for its arrival. Heather says that Nathan is becoming more and more involved in fishing with his friends. When he is home he doesn't want to talk about the things she wants to buy for the baby.

- What subjective data do you have about Heather and Nathan's situation?
- What subjective and objective data do you need?
- What nursing diagnoses could apply? How will you validate these?
- What goals might be developed? How will these be prioritized?

- What interventions may you offer?
- How will you evaluate the effectiveness of your interventions?

---

7. Monica is 20 weeks pregnant with her first child. She has been paying close attention to the physical changes that have been occurring in her body. Today she says, "My face is a mess. I can't stand the blotchy color. And now my nipples are dark brown and I have this line going down from my belly button. What's going on? What else is going to happen to me?"

- What subjective data do you have about Monica's condition?
- What subjective and objective data do you need?
- What nursing diagnoses could apply? How will you validate these?
- What goals might be developed? How will these be prioritized?
- What interventions may you offer?
- How will you evaluate the effectiveness of your interventions?

---

8. Phyllis is 33 years old and lives in the women's shelter two doors down from the clinic. She moved to the shelter to escape her abusive husband and may stay there for 6 months. She has come to the clinic today because she thinks she might be pregnant. Her history and examination reveal that she is right. She appears to be about 22 weeks along. Taking her vital signs you find that her blood pressure is 122/72, pulse 52 per minute, respirations 34 per minute. Her height is 5'10" and her weight is 120 pounds.

- What subjective data do you have about Phyllis's condition?
- What subjective and objective data do you need?
- What nursing diagnoses could apply? How will you validate these?
- What goals might be developed? How will these be prioritized?
- What interventions may you offer?
- How will you evaluate the effectiveness of your interventions?

## REFERENCES

Bailey CW: Assessing health during pregnancy. In Youngkin EQ and Davis MS, editors. *Women's health: a primary care clinical guide,* Stamford, Conn, 1998, Appleton & Lange.

Barkauskas V and others: *Health and physical assessment,* ed 2, St Louis, 1998, Mosby.

Brewer S: *Conception, pregnancy and childbirth rituals, taboos, and beliefs within the Filipino and Cuban cultures,* Miami, Florida International University. Unpublished manuscript, 1995.

Cunningham FG and others: *Williams obstetrics,* ed 20, Stamford, Conn, 1997, Appleton & Lange.

Davis DC: The discomforts of pregnancy, *J Obstet Gynecol Neonatal Nurs* 25(1):73-81, 1996.

Drummond SB: Cardiac disease in pregnancy: Intrapartum considerations, *Crit Care Nurs Clin North Am* 4(4):659-665,1992.

Harvey MG: Physiologic changes of pregnancy. In Harvey CJ, editor: *Critical care obstetrical nursing,* Gaithersburg, Md, 1991, Aspen.

Hees-Stauthamer JC: *The first pregnancy: an integrating principle in female psychology,* Ann Arbor, Mich, 1985, UMI Research Press.

ific: *Healthy eating during pregnancy,* 1995. *http://ificinfor.health.org/ brochure/*eatpreg.htm (11/18/1999).

Kitzinger S: *Woman's experience of sex,* New York, 1985, Penguin Books.

Lee W and Cotton D: Cardiorespiratory changes during pregnancy. In Clark S and others, editors: *Critical care obstetrics,* Boston, 1991, Blackwell Scientific Publications.

Mattson S and Smith J: *Core curriculum for maternal-newborn nursing,* Philadelphia, 1993, W.B. Saunders.

Mattson S and Smith J: *Core curriculum for maternal-newborn nursing,* ed 2, Philadelphia, 2000, W.B. Saunders.

*Nurses Handbook of Alternative and Complementary Therapies,* Springhouse, Penn, 1998, Springhouse.

Purnell L and Paulanka BJ: *Transcultural health care,* Philadelphia, 1998, F.A. Davis.

Phillips CR: *Family-centered maternity and newborn care,* St Louis, 1995, Mosby.

Simpson KR and Creehan PA: *AWHONN perinatal nursing,* Philadelphia, 1996, Lippincott.

Snyder M and Lindquist R: *Complementary/alternative therapies in nursing,* ed 3, New York, 1998, Springer.

Tilkian SM, Conover MB, and Tilkian AG: *Clinical and nursing implications of laboratory tests,* ed 5, St Louis, 1995, Mosby.

Worthington-Roberts B and Williams AR: *Nutrition in pregnancy and lactation,* ed 6, Boston, 1997, WCB McGraw-Hill.

Youngkin EQ and Davis MS, editors: *Women's health: a primary care clinical guide,* Stamford, Conn, 1998, Appleton & Lange.

# CHAPTER 12

# Nursing Care During the Third Trimester (Weeks 27 to 40)

*"My kid is dancing under my heart."*
— (Boston Women's Health Book Collective, 1998)

*Describe the physical changes that take place in a woman's body during this trimester.*

*Describe the changes taking place in the fetus during this trimester.*

*What cognitive changes will a woman experience during this trimester?*

*What other factors influence the woman and her support system during this trimester?*

*What assessments are necessary during this trimester?*

*What anticipatory guidance is required during this trimester?*

*What is the therapeutic response if the woman loses this pregnancy during this trimester?*

During the third trimester, the developing fetus becomes more obvious and the effect of nurturing and carrying the fetus becomes more evident in the woman's day-to-day life. The mother's fatigue level increases as the fetus grows, and carrying the expanding uterus becomes more strenuous. Fatigue levels may also increase from sleep disturbances due to increased urinary frequency, leg cramps, breathing difficulties, and other problems during this trimester. When the baby moves, the mother focuses on the fetus and continues to mentally prepare herself for motherhood.

## MATERNAL PHYSIOLOGIC CHANGES DURING THE THIRD TRIMESTER

A number of the woman's body systems continue the process of change to maintain her health, sustain the pregnancy, and gradually prepare for the strenuous birth process.

## Physiologic Changes in the Woman's Reproductive System

### Breasts and Reproductive System

**Breasts.** In about 50% of women, the enlarged breasts may continue to develop striae. During this trimester, women may experience periodic leaking of colostrum from the breasts.

**Uterus.** The uterus is becoming a relatively thin-walled muscular organ that accommodates the fetus, placenta, and amniotic fluid. The thin wall of the uterus allows parts of the fetus to be palpated, but the uterus still maintains a globular and ovoid shape. At term, the uterine size is approximately 20 times that of its nonpregnant size—32-cm (12.5-in) long, 24-cm (9.5-in) wide, and 22-cm (8.5-in) deep. The uterus weighs approximately 1000 to 1200 g (2.5 lbs) and has 500 to 1000 times the capacity of the nonpregnant uterus. Its volume increases from about 10 ml to 5000 ml during pregnancy (Cunningham and others, 1997).

A large portion of the increase in the organ's weight can be accounted for by the increase in blood volume because about one sixth of the total maternal blood volume is within the vascular system of the uterus. The rate of blood flow from the uterine and ovarian arteries to the uterus is approximately 500 ml/minute, with 80% going to the placental bed (Simpson and Creehan, 1996).

Uterine enlargement continues in a consistent, linear fashion with growth occurring at the rate of about 1 cm per week until 36 weeks. Between 38 and 40 weeks, the fetus moves down into the pelvis and the fundal height decreases gradually.

 During this last trimester, **Braxton-Hicks** contractions gradually increase in intensity and frequency and may be confused with prodromal labor contractions. They are differentiated from labor contractions in that the pattern of contractions rarely becomes closer than 5 minutes apart and, on vaginal examination, cervical dilation is not occurring. These contractions may be painful but manageable. Generally, if the woman changes what she is doing, they will stop (e.g., if she is walking, she should sit or lie down and rest; if she is resting, she should get up and walk).

*Vagina and Vulva.* The increase in vascularity and secretions prepares for the distention of the vagina and vulva during the birth process, but the woman may now become uncomfortable due to increased pelvic congestion.

Loosening of the connective tissue and hypertrophy of the smooth muscle cells also occur (Cunningham and others, 1997). By the end of the pregnancy, the vaginal—as well as the perineal—walls are relaxed enough to allow for the stretching needed to accommodate the birth of the infant.

*Cervix.* As with the vagina, there has been increased vascularization in addition to edema, softening, and dilation. Estrogen stimulates the glandular tissue, causing hypertrophy and hyperplasia of the cervical glands (Cunningham and others, 1997). The **mucous plug,** created by secretion from the endocervical glands, remains in the cervical os. Some women observe the passing of the mucous plug—often tinged with blood, which is an indication that the cervical os has started to dilate.

## Physiologic Changes in the Woman's Other Bodily Systems

### Cardiovascular System

*Heart.* The woman's cardiac volume is 10% to 20%, or approximately 75 ml above her nonpregnant state and her heart rate 10 to 15 beats per minute above her nonpregnant rate. If she is pregnant with multiple fetuses, it may be as much as 40% above her nonpregnant rate.

*Blood Volume.* Blood volume is 25% to 45% greater than in her nonpregnant state. This increase will peak at about 34 weeks and then decrease slightly at the 40th week and return to normal 2 to 3 weeks postpartum. The blood volume increase is created by a plasma volume increase of 45% and a red cell mass increase of 20% to 30% by term. This increase will offset the normal loss at birth.

During this last trimester of pregnancy, the increased volume serves to protect the mother and the fetus from impaired venous return when sitting or standing. Despite the increase in blood volume, blood pressure remains normal due to peripheral vasodilation (Cunningham and others, 1997). The increase in volume in a multifetal pregnancy is greater than for a single fetal pregnancy (Fuschino, 1992).

*Cardiac Output.* Cardiac output remains stable after increasing 30% to 50% during the second trimester. Maternal position remains important to the cardiac output as uterine size increases during the third trimester. In the supine position, pressure exerted on the inferior vena cava from the gravid uterus decreases venous return, resulting in decreased cardiac output. Cardiac output can change 25% to 30% when the woman rolls the fetus off the inferior vena cava by moving from a supine position to a lateral position. Cardiac output will increase with exertion.

At term, most of the additional blood volume is flowing through the uterus (33%) and the kidneys (30%). **Hyperemia** is evident in the cervix and vagina, as well as the breasts, where glandular growth, distended veins, and engorgement reflect the increased blood flow. Blood flow to the skin also increases, which helps to lower the body temperature of the mother.

*Blood Pressure.* Blood pressure rises toward prepregnant levels in the third trimester. The pulse pressure returns to prepregnant values at term. When recording the woman's blood pressure, we must be sure to note both the mother's body position and on which arm it was taken.

As the fetus grows, the risk for supine hypotensive syndrome increases. In addition, compression of the  iliac veins and inferior vena cava by the uterus contributes to the development of dependent edema, vericose veins in the legs and vulva, and hemorrhoids during this trimester. We should continue to encourage the woman to lie on her side whenever she rests or sleeps.

*Hematologic Changes.* The greatest need for an increase in iron for hemoglobin production is evident during the last half of the pregnancy. The amount of iron from diet, together with that mobilized from maternal iron stores, may be insufficient to meet the demands imposed from pregnancy. Therefore supplemental iron is often recommended. It is important to note that hemoglobin production in the fetus will not be impaired even if the mother has severe iron-deficiency anemia. The placenta will obtain sufficient iron from the mother to establish normal fetal hemoglobin levels (Cunningham and others, 1997).

The total white blood cell count that started increasing during the second trimester peaks during the third trimester. An average white cell count in the third trimester is 5,000 to 12,000 per cubic millimeter (Cruikshank and Hays, 1991).

The coagulation and fibrinolytic changes continue to help support the pregnancy and will accommodate the bleeding that occurs when the placenta separates from the uterus during the delivery process. As the growing uterus increases, the potential for venostasis and the clotting factors increase, and the woman is at increased risk for venous thrombosis. At term, the fibrin in the blood has increased by 40%. With delivery, the platelets and fibrinogen levels decrease as the fibrin forms clots at the placental site. If copious bleeding takes place and an insufficiency of platelets and fibrinogen occurs, the woman may experience the DIC syndrome (disseminated intravascular coagulation).

### Respiratory System

***Structural Changes.*** Even though the size of the rib cage has expanded, the increasing uterine size generally prevents women from taking deep breaths. Sleeping in a reclining position may become difficult, even with several pillows under the head. As the pregnancy progresses, some women—especially those carrying multiple fetuses—find it most comfortable to sleep semi-upright in a comfortable chair.

The increased estrogen levels make the upper respiratory tract more vascular. The tissues of the nose, pharynx, larynx, trachea, and bronchi become engorged, and edema and hyperemia develop. As a result, a woman may experience nasal stuffiness, epistaxis (nose bleeds), changes in her voice, and a seemingly out of proportion inflammatory response to even a mild upper respiratory tract infection. She may have a sense of fullness in her ears, impaired hearing, or earaches.

***Functional Changes.*** There is little change in respiratory rate during pregnancy, but a woman's tidal volume continues to increase so that by the end of the pregnancy, it has increased from 500 to 700 ml—an increase of 30% to 40%. This increase in tidal volume causes an increase in respiratory minute ventilation, which is the amount of air inspired in 1 minute. By late pregnancy, the respiratory minute ventilation has increased 40% and reaches 6.5 to 10 L/min by term. These alterations create an increased risk for hyperventilation in the mother.

Although hyperventilation normally causes alkalosis, in this instance it does not because of the compensatory increase in the renal excretion of bicarbonate. The hyperventilation is caused by progesterone's direct effect on the respiratory center. The decreased level of $PaCO_2$ (as a result of hyperventilation) facilitates the removal of carbon dioxide from the fetal to the maternal system (Harvey, 1991).

***Basal Metabolic Rate.*** The increase in thyroid hormones may cause a woman's basal metabolic rate (BMR) to be 30% above average by term. By the end of the third trimester, 50% of the oxygen is distributed to the reproductive tissues and the fetus, which increases to an even greater level during labor. The BMR returns to nonpregnant levels 5 to 6 days after delivery (Sims and others, 1995).

### Renal/Urinary System

***Structural Changes.*** Dilation of the ureters continues and is greater on the right side than on the left. With the increasing weight of the uterus on the bladder, nocturia, urinary frequency, and an urgency to void are again common. The increasing pressure on the renal system can impair drainage of blood and lymph, increasing the risk for infection and trauma.

The structural changes also cause a larger volume of urine to be held within the renal pelvis and the ureters. The resulting urinary stasis or stagnation makes pregnant women more susceptible to urinary tract infections. A urinary tract infection may first be identified as flank pain (Mattson and Smith, 2000). If the urine culture is positive, antibiotic therapy is given and the woman is encouraged to drink eight glasses of water a day, which is often a difficult task because of the already increased frequency of urination due to the pressure on the uterus. If the woman's symptoms become worse or her temperature becomes greater than 101° F, she is instructed to contact her health care provider.

***Functional Changes.*** Both the glomerular filtration rate (GFR) and the renal plasma flow (RPF) continue to rise until term. The increase in the GFR causes an increase in protein excretion but is not abnormal until the values are above 250 mg/dl. Higher levels may be an indication of pregnancy-induced hypertension, renal disease, and urinary tract infections (Simpson and Creehan, 1996). Blood urea nitrogen and uric acid, which declined during the first 2 trimesters, now increase.

**Edema** can occur at any point during a pregnancy and is the result of several hormonal, structural, and functional mechanisms. Each time a woman is seen, we must assess her for venous distention; facial puffiness; and pitting edema of the hands, legs, and ankles. Any weight gain since the previous visit, her blood pressure, and the presence or absence of proteinuria should also be determined. It is important to differentiate between the normal edema of pregnancy and the pathologic edema that indicates there is a medical problem.

If the woman has edema, ask when she first noticed the "puffiness," as well as about her activities, diet, and the severity now when compared with when it started. Also learn what she has done to try to decrease the swelling and what the results were. If the edema is systemic or her face is puffy, she should receive further medical evaluation. Dependent edema is a more common situation created by pregnancy.

 **Dependent edema** (swelling of the lower body parts) can be reduced if the woman lays on her side instead of her back, elevates her feet and legs, reduces the amount of time she stands, and does not constrict the flow of fluids through her leg tissues with tight clothes or knee-high stockings. The woman may be more comfortable wearing support hose or elastic stockings. She should also walk or swim to increase the blood flow to the lower body and increase her water consumption. Diuretics, however, should not be used. A woman with edema must be closely monitored in case it is the manifestation of pregnancy-induced hypertension (Davis, 1996).

*Glycosuria.* Glycosuria is a common finding during pregnancy. The renal tubules cannot absorb the increased glucose filtered by the glomeruli. The glycosuria is usually not pathogenic. Therefore evaluation of a pregnant woman with diabetes requires the measurement of serum/capillary glucose and not urine glucose (Simpson and Creehan, 1996).

### Gastrointestinal System

*Stomach.* Gastric motility and emptying time are reduced due to hormonal changes and the mechanical pressures of the uterus pressing on the gastrointestinal system. Gastric reflux is most common during this trimester due to displacement of the stomach, relaxation of the esophageal sphincter due to the hormones of pregnancy, and delayed gastric emptying time.

As the size of the uterus continues to increase, the stomach is displaced farther upward. In 15% to 20% of pregnant women, a **hiatal hernia** (i.e., herniation of the upper portion of the stomach through the esophogeal hiatus of the diaphragm) occurs after the seventh or eight month of pregnancy. Multiparas and older or obese women are more prone to develop such a hernia, which increases a woman's experience with "heartburn."

*Small and Large Intestines.* The intestines are also pushed upward and laterally by the expanding uterus. Progesterone relaxes the muscles of the gastrointestinal tract, decreasing intestinal motility and allowing increased absorption from the colon. Increased water absorption causes the feces to become harder and drier, making the woman more prone to constipation. If she strains during bowel movements, pressure on the blood vessels below the uterus is increased and hemorrhoids may develop or worsen.

If a woman reports being constipated, ask her to describe her stools (firmness and color); the frequency of the movements; the time of defecation; and any feelings of bloating, gassiness, or cramping. Ask about her diet and fluid intake, iron supplements, and her physical activities. Learn what she has already done to treat the condition and how well these remedies worked. Auscultation should reveal bowel sounds in all four quadrants. Palpation should not reveal abdominal tenderness.

Increased fluid intake; setting aside the same time each day for a bowel movement; and consuming dietary fiber daily with fruits and vegetables (5 servings per day), whole grain cereals, and breads can help prevent constipation. A stool softener or mild laxative may be given if preventive measures are unsuccessful. Prevention and treatment of constipation will help prevent formation of hemorrhoids or assist to not worsen their status.

**Hemorrhoids** are created when veins in the rectal and anal mucosa are dilated and venous return is impeded. Contributory causes are the pressure of the uterus, straining due to constipation, and standing still for long periods. A woman may describe a feeling of rectal fullness, pain, itching, or bleeding after defecation. These symptoms occur when the veins bulge through the anal opening and bleed when irritated by bowel movements.

Relief can be provided by warm sitz baths, warm and then cold compresses, and application of a witch hazel solution or a topical lubricant. Kegel exercises help to prevent the development of hemorrhoids by toning the rectal/anal sphincters (Davis, 1996).

*Gallbladder.* In the third trimester, fasting and residual volumes remain twice as great as in a nonpregnant woman and the rate the gall bladder empties continues to slow. Women are at increased risk for an excess of cholesterol in the blood (hypercholesterolemia) or gallstone formation.

### Endocrine System

*Parathyroid Glands.* The size of the parathyroid gland and the concentration of the hormone peak between 15 to 35 weeks and then return to normal after birth. Other hormones remain at pregnancy-sustaining levels until the birth process starts.

### Neurologic System

The size and placement of the uterus may create some concerns during the third trimester. Dizziness and lightheadedness may be associated with supine hypotensive syndrome (i.e., vena cava syndrome), vasomotor instability, and postural hypotension—especially after prolonged periods of sitting or standing. **Postural hypotension** may result from a transient deficiency in the volume of blood (oligemia). **Meralgia paresthetica** (i.e., pain, numbness, and a prickly or tingling feeling in the thigh) may be caused by the pressure of the uterus on the lateral femoral cutaneous nerve. **Carpel tunnel syndrome** may create burning, tingling, and pain in the hand (i.e., usually in the thumb and the first three fingers). The pain may shoot through the wrist, up the forearm, and sometimes to the shoulder, neck and chest. This syndrome is a repetitive stress injury to the wrist that causes inflammation and constriction of the median nerve that runs through the carpal tunnel.

**Leg cramps** are sudden, intense gripping contractions of the calf muscle that may occur when a woman rests or awakens from sleep. These cramps are caused by a lowered serum ionized calcium and increased phosphates, or inadequate intake of calcium (Sims and others, 1995; Davis, 1996). When they occur, the woman should flex or bend the foot in the opposite direction or stand on the leg. There is some thought that stretching exercises before going to bed and keeping the bed covers untucked may prevent the occurrence. An evaluation of the woman's calcium intake and consumption of phosphate-containing edibles (e.g., soft drinks and processed foods) may find an imbalance that if corrected will help. A woman should be instructed to not massage the leg because the pain may also be from a thrombophlebitis.

## Integumentary System

**Straie gravidarum,** or stretch marks, develop in response to weight gain and growth of the expanding uterus. Although they may start during the second trimester, straie gravidarum become much more noticeable during the third trimester. In light-skinned women, they are pinkish-red, slightly concave streaks that may appear over the abdomen, breasts, and sometimes the buttocks and thighs. In dark-skinned women, the straie appear lighter than the surrounding skin. In women who have been pregnant before, silver lines (in light-skinned women) or dark purple lines (in dark-skinned women) may appear. Reassure women that after delivery many of these lines fade. The striae will become silvery white or dark purple.

Melasma, the linea nigra, and the vascular marking that began in the first trimester will fade in the weeks after pregnancy. The increased pigmentation of the nipples and areola, however, may remain after the pregnancy.

## Musculoskeletal System

The framework provided by the musculoskeletal system faces a challenge during the third trimester. Abdominal distention causes the pelvis to tilt forward. The growing uterus may cause the **rectus abdominis muscles** to separate, allowing the abdomen to protrude. The weight of the uterus and breasts, along with the relaxation of the pelvic joints, changes the woman's center of gravity, stance, and gait. Movement of the **symphysis pubis** and lumbosacral joints and relaxation of the pelvic ligaments may cause general soreness and discomfort for many women. A woman's shoe size, especially the width, may increase permanently.

Because of the increasing **lumbosacral curve,** back tiredness or backaches are a common occurrence—particularly for women who do a lot of standing. It is estimated that 48% to 56% of all pregnant women report having back pain. The reports are more prevalent, however, in adolescents, older women, women with a history of back pain before pregnancy, and women who have had previous pregnancies. There are fewer reports from women who are tall and/or thin or were physically fit before becoming pregnant (Davis, 1996).

In normal pregnancy, there is no loss of maternal bone density because the increased parathyroid hormone levels enhance gastrointestinal absorption and decrease renal excretion of calcium. Calcium intake should be increased to 1.5 g/day in this last trimester and during lactation.

**Prodromal labor** (i.e., early labor) sometimes starts with a mild backache that comes and goes. The woman may find herself rubbing her back for relief for a minute and then not need to for 5 or 6 minutes and then the backache returns in a short time. This discomfort should respond to basic comfort measures. If it is a sharp pain, the woman should report it immediately because she must be evaluated for the possibility of preterm labor.

## Metabolic Changes

The fats stored in the first trimester are now mobilized in correlation with the fetus's increased use of glucose and amino acids. The ratio of low-density lipoproteins (LDLs) to high-density lipoproteins (HDLs) continues to increase until birth.

### Weight Gain

The weight gain by the end of pregnancy includes much more than the weight of the fetus. For a pregnancy with one fetus, the weight gain is distributed as follows:

Fetus—7.0 to 8.0 lbs
Placenta—1.5 to 2.0 lbs
Amniotic fluid—2.0 to 3.5 lbs
Increased uterine size—2.5 to 3.0 lbs
Increased blood volume—3.0 to 4.5 lbs
Increased breast size—1.0 to 1.5 lbs
Increased extracellular fluid—4.0 to 6.0 lbs
Fat deposits—4.0 to 6.5 lbs
TOTAL—25.0 to 35.0 lbs (Phillips, 1995)

### Pancreas

All women are generally screened for gestational diabetes by 28 weeks of gestation. A fasting glucose of 135 mg/dl or above is considered a positive screen for gestational diabetes. If a woman develops gestational diabetes mellitus, the treatment goal focuses on achieving and maintaining a normal level of glucose in the blood (euglycemia) and avoiding hypoglycemia.

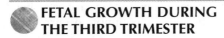

# FETAL GROWTH DURING THE THIRD TRIMESTER

### End of 26 Weeks of Fetal Development (28 Weeks of Pregnancy)

The fetus is 35 to 38 cm long, and its weight has almost doubled (i.e., to approximately 1200 g). It is about two thirds of its final size, but it still appears generally long and thin. The lung alveoli have begun to mature, and surfactant may be found in the amniotic fluid. If the fetus is a male, the testes begin to descend into the scrotum from the lower abdominal cavity.

### End of 30 Weeks of Fetal Development (32 Weeks of Pregnancy)

The length of the fetus generally ranges from 38 to 43 cm, with a weight of 1600 g. The fingernails are now to the end of the fingertips. The fetus is starting to look less wrinkled, red, and "stringy" as subcutaneous fat is deposited. The lecithin continues to increase, creating a lecithin/sphengomyelin (L/S) ratio of 1.2:1. Iron stores start developing and will provide iron for the infant during the time it will only ingest milk. An active Moro reflex is present. The fetus is aware of and may react to sounds not only inside but also outside the mother's body. Within its increasingly tight quarters, the fetus may assume a delivery position—either **vertex** (head-down) or breech, although this position may change again before delivery.

### End of 34 Weeks of Fetal Development (36 Weeks of Pregnancy)

The fetus is 42 to 49 cm and weighs 1900 to 2700 g (5 to 6 lbs). The soles of its feet have begun to develop creases and have one or two crisscrosses. By the time the fetus is full-term, there will be a full pattern of crisscrosses. Preparing for life after birth, body stores of glycogen, iron, carbohydrate, and calcium, as well as additional stores of subcutaneous fat, develop. The L/S ratio is now equal to or greater than 2:1. The **lanugo** that covered the fetus, now starts to diminish. If not already positioned, most fetuses turn into a vertex position during this period in preparation for labor.

### End of 38 Weeks of Fetal Development (40 Weeks of Pregnancy)

The average length of a fetus at this time is 48 to 52 cm, with the distance between the crown and the rump ranging from 35 to 37 cm. The average fetal weight is 3000 g (i.e., 7 to 7.5 lbs). At this point, the fetus may kick often and hard enough to make the mother very uncomfortable. The vernix caseosa is only apparent in the creases and folds of the skin, and lanugo only remains on the upper arms and shoulders. The fingernails extend over the fingertips, and at least two thirds of the soles of the feet are covered by creases. These details are some of the measures used to determine the developmental age of a newborn. Fetal hemoglobin also starts being converted to adult hemoglobin. At birth, in approximately 2 weeks, about 20% of the hemoglobin will be adult in character.

## Transition from Fetus to Neonate

With delivery, the fetus becomes a **neonate**—an infant between birth and 28 days old (Table 12-1).

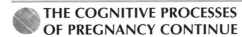

# THE COGNITIVE PROCESSES OF PREGNANCY CONTINUE

During the third trimester, the work of adapting to the role of parent continues. The parents focus on the developing child, prepare a place for the child within their home (i.e., nesting), and plan for the birth phase of their experience (Gloger-Tippelt, 1983). Family members, friends, and community may support the couple as they prepare for their new roles (Box 12-1).

## Psychologic Challenges During the Third Trimester

### The Woman

By the third trimester of pregnancy, the woman becomes more interested in meeting the baby's needs, as well as her own. She anticipates the approaching labor and birth and begins to prepare for it. As she reaches the end of pregnancy, we should determine if the woman feels ready for the birth process, as well as to assume the care of the infant afterwards. It is normal for her to simultaneously feel prepared and anxious. We should explore her expectations about labor, birth, and the newborn. Her dependency on others may peak during this trimester as she deals with her fears of motherhood, concerns about the pain of labor, loss of control, and perceived potential for harm to herself or the fetus. We should encourage her support system and suggest ways they may meet her needs.

Anxiety tends to increase during this trimester. Vague fears that occurred earlier in the pregnancy now become larger. The woman now faces the unknown of a labor and delivery, which even if she has gone through it before, is an unknown. She is concerned about safe passage for both herself and her infant and fears she may not do well during labor and birth. She may be concerned about pain or anxious about losing control or having a surgical delivery.

Assessment of anxiety is difficult because the woman may feel it is inappropriate for her to experience it and try to hide her feelings. Be alert to apprehension, restlessness, irritability, nervousness, impatience, or fearfulness. Bring up the subject with, "Many women become

**TABLE 12-1   *Milestones in Human Development before Birth since LMP***

| 28 Weeks | 30-31 Weeks | 36 Weeks | 40 Weeks |
|---|---|---|---|
| **EXTERNAL APPEARANCE** | | | |
| Lean body, less wrinkled and red; nails appearing | Subcutaneous fat beginning to collect, more rounded appearance, skin pink and smooth, assumption of birth position | Skin pink, body rounded, general lanugo disappearing, body usually plump | Skin smooth and pink, scant vernix caseosa, moderate to profuse hair, lanugo on shoulders and upper body only, nasal and alar cartilage apparent |
| **CROWN-TO-RUMP MEASUREMENT, WEIGHT** | | | |
| 27 cm, 1100 g | 31 cm, 1800-2100 g | 35 cm, 2200-2900 g | 40 cm, ≥3200 g |
| **GASTROINTESTINAL SYSTEM** | | | |
| **MUSCULOSKELETAL SYSTEM** | | | |
| Astragalus (talus, ankle bone) ossification; weak, fleeting movements; minimum tone | Middle fourth phalanxes ossification, permanent teeth primordia visible, able to turn head to side | Distal femoral ossification centers present; sustained, definite movements; fair tone; able to turn and elevate head | Active, sustained movement; good tone |
| **CIRCULATORY SYSTEM** | | | |
| **RESPIRATORY SYSTEM** | | | |
| Lecithin forming on alveolar surfaces | L/S ratio = 1.2:1 | L/S ratio ≥ 2:1 | Pulmonary branching only two-thirds complete |
| **RENAL SYSTEM** | | | |
| | | Formation of new nephrons ceasing | |
| **NERVOUS SYSTEM** | | | |
| Appearance of cerebral fissures, convolutions fast appearing; indefinite sleepwave cycle; cry weak or absent, weak suck reflex | | Ending of spinal cord at level (L-3), definite sleep-wake cycle | Myelination of brain beginning, patterned sleep-wake cycle, strong suck reflex |
| **SENSORY ORGANS** | | | |
| Eyelids reopening; retinal layers completed, light receptive; pupils able to react to light | Sense of taste present, awareness of sounds outside mother's body | | |
| **GENITAL SYSTEM** | | | |
| | Testes descending to scrotum | | Testes in scrotum, labia majora well-developed |

anxious as their pregnancy nears the end. What concerns do you have?" Without being too positive or negative, we should provide sound, basic explanations that are realistic and refer the woman to counseling if her anxiety is related to issues beyond the scope of a normal pregnancy.

The woman's anxiety may increase if she experiences sleep deprivation during this time. Relaxation and breathing exercises, meditation, and massage can be used not only to prepare for the birth experience but also to decrease stress, promote a sense of well-being, and help the woman to relax for sleep now. Planning quiet, relaxed activities before bed and developing a pattern of high fluid intake early in the day and decreased intake in the hours before bed may reduce problems of falling asleep and nocturnal awakenings (Davis, 1996). Eating small amounts of food throughout the day and continuing mild to moderate exercise should also facilitate the woman's ability to rest.

***Preparing for Fetal Separation.*** As the woman prepares for the end of pregnancy and the birth of her infant she may again feel ambivalent. As the fetus has grown, it has made her physically uncomfortable, so she anticipates the freedom of not having to carry the fetus with her at all times. She looks forward to seeing it and welcoming it into her arms, but she must prepare for letting go of the fetus and the sense of unity she has developed with it. She is dealing with the process of **fetal separation.**

***Determining Roles.*** The mother and her partner must reach a decision about the roles they will play during the labor and delivery experience. Couples who are planning on going through childbirth together will seek out expert advice and attend childbirth-preparation classes. They establish their roles and learn to work through the experience of birth together. The woman will be especially interested in how to relieve the discomforts, and her partner will want to know how to assist her. Both the imagery and relaxation techniques taught in the classes help to enhance a woman's sense of control. The parents also learn the roles of the providers they have chosen for assistance and determine who else they might want to have present.

Classes tailored for groups with specific needs (e.g., women who have had a cesarean section [CS] and now want to attempt a vaginal birth after cesarean section [VBAC] or adolescents who are pregnant) fill a critical need. In addition, the woman and her support person are encouraged to attend classes to assist with parenting and infant safety and massage, which are critical to parental development.

The Pregnant Patient's Bill of Rights and The Pregnant Patient's Responsibilities, shared with the woman during her first prenatal visit, should be reviewed (see Appendix I). The birth plan, which started being developed during the initial prenatal visit (see Chapter 9) and evolved through subsequent educational sessions, is now finalized. A **birth plan** outlines the desires and expectations of the woman and her partner during the labor and delivery experience based on their philosophy of birth (see Chapter 13 for more information).

***A Woman's Concerns.*** A woman in the third trimester of pregnancy expresses some universal needs. She focuses on the well-being of the infant, the process of labor, and the changes she is experiencing both in her body and her emotional status. Between the 27th and the 32nd weeks, as the size of the baby continues to increase, the woman has increasing concerns about the adequacy and integrity of her body (Richardson, 1990).

The mother will seek reassurance about the health of her baby and wonder about how it will tolerate labor and be affected by medication and anesthesia, as well as if any birth defects are suspected. As the reality of providing for another family member becomes closer, the woman may reach a higher level of concern about how expenses will be met.

Braxton-Hicks contractions will remind the woman of the impending labor process. Her fears of physical inadequacy and the possible intensity of pain, as well as her misconceptions about the labor process will all come to the forefront. We must reassure her as to whom and when she should call if she has concerns and, if she is going to a birthing center or hospital for delivery, when she should go. If she has other children, she will be concerned about how to arrange childcare for an unpredictable event such as birth. She will wonder about who will care for the children, how will she contact them, and where will the children go.

The woman has known her expected date of delivery (EDD) since her first prenatal visit. Even though cautioned from the beginning that the delivery date is actually a delivery month because it can occur any time from 2 weeks before to 2 weeks after that date, she and her family have probably fixed on that as "the" date. Remind her that less than 5% of pregnancies end exactly 280 days from the first day of the mother's last menstrual period. In fact, fewer than 50% of births are within 1 week of the 280th day. Help the woman to think of ways to handle the comments, such as "You haven't delivered yet?" without becoming disappointed herself.

***The Final Preparations.*** The last 2 months generally find the mother "nesting" (i.e., creating a place for the infant) and preparing for the birth. These activities may be accompanied by feelings of disorientation, poor coordination, and heightened vulnerability. As the woman grows closer to term, her dependency needs continue to increase. She must be nurtured as she moves toward the role of nurturer. Information about the postpartum recovery and self-care and infant care should be presented at this time.

Because she is about to give birth, the mother will come to the strong realization that there is no going back. She is to become the provider of care for this child and can never return to her previous life. She also must now learn to deal with comments and possible criticism from others as they evaluate how she "measures up" in her new role. She is differentiating herself from others to become the kind of mother she wants to be (Rubin, 1984).

***Emotional Discomfort.*** If a woman is still experiencing a high level of anxiety after the 33rd week of pregnancy, she may need help determining what is making her anxious. Once the cause or causes are identified, we may guide her in developing solutions. If she neglects to prepare for the coming infant, it may indicate that there are cultural taboos against it or she is not yet able to adjust to the approaching birth, which may be caused by high levels of stress in her life. If the woman demonstrates the inability to plan for the birth in a way that she finds acceptable both for herself and within her culture, she will need increased assistance through counseling and increased visits. Helping a woman to achieve personal satisfaction with the birthing process—however she conceives it to be—is the first step to developing her confidence as a new mother.

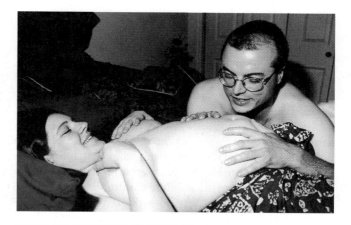

**FIGURE 12-1** • Partner becoming more focused on child. *(Courtesy of Caroline E. Brown.)*

### The Partner

During the third trimester, the partner also becomes more focused on the birth and the needs the infant will have when they bring it home. Participating in the preparation of a room or purchase of equipment and supplies may be the first time the partner actually feels included in providing for the child (Figure 12-1).

As the end of pregnancy approaches, the partner's anxiety increases and finances may become a concern. There may be concerns about the well-being of the mother and the health of the child. The partner may wonder about fulfilling his partner's expectations and being capable of caring for the child—especially if it is their first child. Just as the mother requires more nurturing, so does the partner. The partner may also begin to grieve the loss of a previous lifestyle and wonder about the life that is to come.

### Other Children

It is best to tell young children about the coming baby during the last trimester of pregnancy. For very young children, the time between being told and the time the baby arrives can seem like forever. For school-age children, however, classes may be available to teach them about new babies, provide them with the opportunity to ask questions, and let them learn how they may help as the family takes in this new member. Such classes also allow them to observe that they are not the only child experiencing this change in their lives. Just as the parents experienced earlier, children are often ambivalent about a new baby and wonder about how it will affect their current relationship with the adults in the family. Including children in prenatal visits allows them to hear the baby's heartbeat and feel like a part of the process.

### Grandparents

Clarifying the roles of the grandparents during the labor and delivery process, as well as in the early postpartum period, is important and must be done with frank discussion. If there are other children to be cared for that may be the job of one or more grandparents. The pregnant couple may want to have the woman's mother present for the labor and delivery. In that situation, the role expectation must be discussed so that the new parenting unit is supported in the way it desires.

Effective communication between the new grandparents and parents is important so that all are clear on what is expected. Grandparenting classes may be available in the community to teach grandparents about the options and choices their adult children are making so that the grandparents can be supportive of their decisions. These classes can also offer suggestions about ways that grandparents may support the child-bearing couple.

### Social Support System

During the last few weeks of pregnancy, family members and friends can step forward and take on some of the nurturing requirements of both the mother and her partner. They can also help with care of other children as the woman may find it increasingly difficult to move. Family members and friends may participate in the preparation for the birth experience and plan to be there. In some cultures, members beyond the extended family become active participants in supporting the new family and developing or performing welcoming rituals for the new infant.

### Community

A family may perceive their community as valuing and supporting the development of their family by the services they receive. Some communities demonstrate their concern during pregnancy by planning for and informing the family that they will provide a new baby visit after the birth of the baby. Parents feel reassured that a health care provider will come to their home and assess the needs of the infant and the family, as well as offer referrals and support to help the family during this stressful time.

## OTHER INFLUENCES ON THE THIRD TRIMESTER OF PREGNANCY

### Cultural Expectations

There are few new cultural considerations during the third trimester. Cuban-American women have a restriction against wearing necklaces during pregnancy because they fear it will cause the umbilical cord to wrap around the baby's neck (Brewer, 1995). Navajo Indian communities perform rituals during pregnancy to prepare for the birth of the child. "During the pre-cradleboard phase (before birth), a hogan is designated for the birth and a religious practitioner ties a red sash for a girl and a buckskin rope for a boy. These are used

to give the mother support during delivery" (Purnell and Paulanka, 1998).

### Maturity

#### Pregnant Adolescents

By the third trimester, the pregnancy has generally become an undeniable fact to all adolescents. Some enter prenatal care at this point. With the level of assessment and teaching that is necessary because there has been no prior prenatal care, prenatal visits may be scheduled weekly or twice a week. Explanations about what is happening in her body may not be as important to the girl as addressing her concerns about how she is going to get "It" out. Individual or group prenatal and child-birth education should start immediately with the girl  and whoever will go through labor with her. Premature labor occurs more frequently in adolescents. Be sure she understands the signs and symptoms of labor and the signs of possible danger to her and her baby, as well as how to respond. Written instructions at the level of her reading and comprehension and in her language should also be given to her and her support person.

An adolescent will occasionally present in an office, clinic, or emergency room for treatment of abdominal pain. She may actually be pregnant—or close to full term in some cases—and in labor. Responding to her immediate needs, the needs of her baby, and the needs of her support system takes an efficient and caring team of health care providers. A calm, blameless atmosphere must prevail in order to keep the anxiety level of the adolescent within appropriate levels. Depending on the speed of the labor, all that may be possible to do is deal with the immediate physical and psychosocial needs of the moment. After the delivery, a special effort must be made to help the girl understand what has happened to her and answer her questions.

#### Delayed Pregnancy

Vigilant monitoring for gestational diabetes, hypertension, and vaginal bleeding continues during the third trimester. In some practices, prenatal visits of older mothers become more frequent during this trimester, while in other practices the mothers are expected to monitor for signs and symptoms and call the office with concerns. The nursing care and medical treatment of a woman with gestational diabetes, hypertension, and vaginal bleeding are covered in Chapters 17 and 18 because these conditions place the woman's health and the pregnancy at risk.

### Resources

Depending on the couple's culture, "nesting" may become a dominant theme in their lives. The place where the baby will sleep and live may be prepared. Clothing and supplies may be gathered as friends pass on items their own children have outgrown, gifts are given, or the couple purchases supplies. Participation in childbirth preparation classes offers not only information about choices in childbirth but also the opportunity for relationships with others with similar experiences and needs.

Prenatal care providers are often asked about the needs of an infant. Ask the parents what they think they will need, then clarify and support their views. Have additional information available that the couple may follow to help them prepare adequately for the infant without excessive cost. Many products are sold that are overpriced or of minimal use, but new parents wanting to provide for their child may be unable to discern what is actually needed and can be managed on their income. What the parents ultimately provide for their infant is determined by their culture, values and beliefs, financial status, and the availability of products.

## ASSESSMENT OF CHANGE DURING THE THIRD TRIMESTER

After 28 weeks of gestation, the prenatal visits are generally scheduled every 2 weeks until 36 weeks of gestation. Then they are every week until childbirth or 40 weeks of gestation. If the pregnancy goes past 40 weeks, the appointments may become twice a week.

### Ongoing Assessment of the Woman

#### Care of the Mother

Ask the woman how she is feeling and how the pregnancy seems to be going. Also assess her for subtle or overt signs of physical, sexual, and emotional abuse. Ask her specifically, "Since your last visit, have you been emotionally or physically abused or slapped by your partner or someone important to you? Are you afraid of your partner or someone else in your home?"

Learn from the woman the frequency and duration of any Braxton-Hicks contractions she may be experiencing. Review with her what to do if she experiences a gush of fluid from her vagina.

Also review with the woman the signs and symptoms of labor. Remind her that the timing of a periodic backache (i.e., as it comes and goes) may indicate that she is in early labor. Provide her with a handout detailing, in a language and at a literacy level that she can read, how to respond as labor approaches and begins. This handout should include comfort measures, timing of contractions, and when and how to contact her care provider.

Other assessments during this trimester include the mother's vital signs, weight gain, a complete blood count (CBC) with differential smear, hemoglobin (Hbg), hematocrit (Hct), the Rh antibody screen and a blood glucose screen at 24 to 28 weeks, and tests for sexually transmitted diseases as indicated. Review the results of any prior laboratory testing.

Ask about visual disturbances, headache, a swollen face (facial edema), fever, abdominal pain, uterine contractions, vaginal bleeding, nausea and vomiting, a gush of fluid from the vagina (premature rupture of membranes), or a decline or lack of fetal movements. Review with the woman what to do if she experiences any of these (e.g., call immediately, present for further evaluations by the nurse practitioner or midwife or the physician) (Table 12-2).

Review her expectations for her labor experience and her preparations. Is her birth plan complete? Does she understand the policies that affect the providers and the facility where she is planning to deliver? Answer any questions she may have in order to facilitate her preparation process.

Help the woman plan for a health care provider for her infant. If the woman is seeing a family nurse practitioner or family physician for her prenatal care, either of those providers may also provide care for the infant. The woman and/or prenatal care provider, however, may need to choose a pediatrician for delivery.

## TABLE 12-2   *Signs and Symptoms of Potential Complications*

| Signs/Symptoms | Possible causes |
| --- | --- |
| Visual disturbances: blurring, double vision, or spots | Hypertension; pregnancy-induced hypertension |
| Headache: severe, frequent or continuous | Hypertension; pregnancy-induced hypertension |
| Facial edema or swelling of fingers or skin over sacrum | Hypertension; pregnancy-induced hypertension |
| Fever | Infection |
| Uterine contractions or pressure and cramping | Preterm labor |
| Abdominal pain | Appendicitis; placenta previa; abruptio placenta |
| Severe backache or flank pain | Kidney infection; kidney stone; labor |
| Vaginal bleeding | Placenta previa; abruptio placenta |
| Nausea and vomiting | Hyperemesis gravidarum |
| Fluid from the vagina | Premature rupture of membranes |
| Decline in fetal movements | Fetal distress |
| Lack of fetal movements | Fetal death |

Looking beyond labor, review with the woman her preferences and options for postpartum contraception. Some methods may be started immediately after delivery, before there is any chance of pregnancy. Other women may choose sterilization, however, and arrangements will need to be made at the facility.

If the baby is not born at home and the family will be transporting it by car, an infant car seat will be necessary to move it from where it is born to its home. If the couple cannot afford to purchase a car seat before the baby is born, assist them in locating a program that will provide a seat at a reduced rate or loan them a seat.

## Assessment of Fetus

The nurse practitioner or midwife or the physician will evaluate the growth of the fetus by measuring uterine size and fundal height (Figures 12-2 and 12-3). The fetal heartbeat will be auscultated, and Leopold's maneuver will be used to estimate the approximate size and current position of the fetus. Women are very aware of daily movement as the fetus grows. Explain the position of the fetus to her so that she may see the location of el-

bows, feet, etc. Encourage her to stop periodically during the day and focus on the movement of the fetus. Have her continue to record daily kick counts.

The position and presentation of the fetus will be assessed between 36 and 40 weeks. An internal examination to assess the cervix may be repeated during the last weeks of the pregnancy. During this examination, the cervix will be evaluated for effacement and dilation.

After 40 weeks of gestation, fetal surveillance will include ultrasound for viability, measurement of amniotic fluid volume (AFV), nonstress tests—and possibly a stress test, and biweekly office visits.

## Additional Assessment Measures

### Laboratory Testing

A vaginal/anorectal culture for group beta strep (GBS) may be obtained at between 34 and 36 weeks. Depending on the protocol of the setting, weekly cultures for active herpes simplex virus (HSV) may be done in women with a history of this infection. Women who were infected with chlamydia and gonorrhea earlier in pregnancy may be retested.

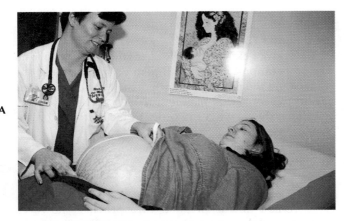

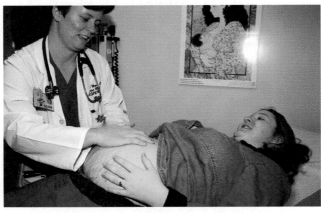

FIGURE 12-2 • **A,** Measuring fundus to evaluate growth of the fetus. **B,** Palpating uterus to determine position of fetus. (*Courtesy of Caroline E. Brown.*)

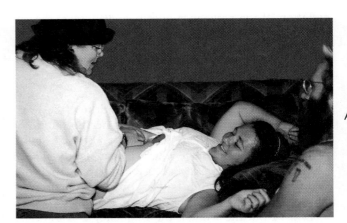

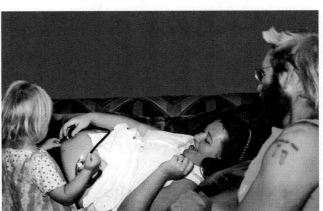

FIGURE 12-3 • **A,** Prenatal evaluation during home visit. **B,** Expectant mother surrounded by supportive family. (*Courtesy of Caroline E. Brown.*)

## Ultrasonography

Possible uses of ultrasound are estimating the gestational age of the pregnancy, comparatively measuring the growth of the fetus, detecting congenital abnormalities, and confirming fetal viability. Ultrasound can also be used to localize the position of the placenta for amniocentesis and determine the cause of bleeding (e.g., placenta previa or abruptio placenta). Ultrasonography helps in the assessment of fetal status during a biophysical profile, a nonstress test, or a contraction stress test. Fetal echocardiography may diagnose cardiac problems. An ultrasound will obtain more information about a breech presentation as labor approaches and during an external version of the fetus, ultrasound is used for visualization of the necessary maneuvers.

## Electronic Fetal Heart Monitoring (EFHM)

Not every woman requires electronic fetal monitoring during the prenatal period, so it is only performed when there is concern about the well-being of the fetus. Concerns may be raised because of the health of the mother (e.g., diabetes) or the length of the pregnancy, or when a mother reports decreased fetal movement.

The EFHM procedures demonstrate the response of the fetal heart to activity, sounds or vibrations, or spontaneous or induced uterine contractions. The most common EFHM methods are the non-stress test (NST), the fetal acoustic stimulation and vibroacoustic stimulation tests (FAST/VST), and the contraction stress test (CST). EFHM, in the form of an NST is also a component of the biophysical profile used to confirm a healthy fetus and identify a fetus that might be at risk.

The heart rate of a healthy fetus will increase in response to 90% of its movements. A **non-stress test (NST)** monitors the responses of the fetal heart to movement over a 30 to 40 minute period. The test is said to be negative or reactive (indicating a healthy response) if the following occur: (1) the baseline of the FHR is between 120 and 160 beats per minute, (2) there are two FHR accelerations within a 10-minute period, with each acceleration increasing the heart rate by at least 15 beats per minute and lasting at least 15 seconds, and (3) the overall tracing shows a long-term variability amplitude of 10 or more beats per minute. If the NST does not meet these three criteria, it is considered abnormal or nonreactive and requires further evaluation that day (Figure 12-4).

The advantages of the NST are that it is noninvasive and can be performed in an office or clinic, is relatively inexpensive, and has no known contraindications. The disadvantage of the NST is that it has a high rate of false-positive results caused by nonactivity of the fetus due to fetal sleep, medications, or fetal immaturity. The NST is less sensitive a measure than the contraction stress test (CST) or the biophysical profile (BPP).

Two adjuncts to the NST are the **fetal acoustic stimulation test (FAST)** and the **vibroacoustic stimulation test**

**(VST)**. In this case, the FHR is monitored for 5 minutes to obtain a baseline reading. A device is placed on the woman's abdomen over the head of the fetus, and a low-frequency vibration (LFV) and a buzzing tone (FAST) are generated for up to 5 seconds. (It is not known if the fetus responds more to the sound or the vibration.) If FHR accelerations do not occur after the first stimulus, the procedure is repeated at 1-minute intervals for a maximum of three times. The monitoring continues for 5 minutes after the last stimulation. A reactive test is when there are two FHR accelerations of at least 15 bpm for at least 15 seconds within 10 minutes. Advantages of the FAST and VST are that they are noninvasive techniques, the tests are easy to perform, and the results are obtained more quickly than with the NST.

Contractions stress the fetus by decreasing blood flow through the placenta. In a fetus already having difficulty due to complications with the umbilical cord, disease, or other factors, contractions may alter the heart rate that is detected during EFHM. During a **contraction stress test (CST)**, the FHR is monitored during spontaneous or created uterine contractions. Contractions may be started by breast stimulation. Either manipulation of the nipples or application of moist heat to the breasts will cause the release of oxytocin and the start of contractions. Alternately, a low dose of oxytocin is infused piggyback through an intravenous line. If Pitocin—a synthetic oxytocin—is given to the woman to cause contractions, it is called an **oxytocin challenge test (OCT)**. EFHM records the activity of the fetal heart as

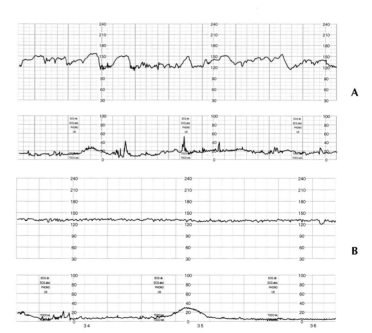

**FIGURE 12-4 ● A,** NST reactive (FHR acceleration with fetal movement). **B,** NST nonreactive (no FHR acceleration with fetal movement). *(From Tucker SM: Pocket guide to fetal monitoring, ed 4, St Louis, 2000, Mosby.)*

the fetus experiences three contractions within 10 minutes, each lasting 40 to 60 seconds. If the fetal heart displays a normal heart rate pattern with no decelerations, the test is considered negative, meaning that no problems are anticipated in the FHR during the next week (Figure 12-5).

The advantage of the CST is that by stressing the fetus it provides an earlier warning of the potential for fetal compromise than the NST. With the CST, there are also fewer false-positive results.

The disadvantages of the CST are that the initiation of contractions to perform the test may continue on into the labor process. If exogenous oxytocin is necessary, it introduces the need for an invasive procedure. It is also more expensive and time-consuming than the NST.

The **biophysical profile** (BPP) of a fetus is based on an assessment of five variables. The following four are obtained through the use of ultrasound: (1) fetal breathing movement, (2) fetal body or limb movements, (3) fetal tone as the fetus extends and flexes arms and legs, (4) and amniotic fluid volume around the fetus. The fifth measurement is a negative NST. Scoring is on a scale of 0 to 10 (0 or 2 points for each test). Scores of 8 (with a normal pocket of amniotic fluid) and 10 indicate a normal fetus (Table 12-3).

Most women and their fetuses will not undergo these evaluations, although many women may ask about them because they have heard about the testing undergone by other pregnant women. Providing a brief overview of each of the assessment tests and the reassurance that the current health of her fetus does not indicate the need for further assessment should ease her mind. If the need to use one of these tools does arise, provide a more in-depth explanation of the procedure and what it is measuring. Also explore with her any concern she may be experiencing about the health of her baby.

### Close of the Visit

The prenatal visits are now closer together, so our contact with the woman will occur more often. The health status of the maternal-fetal unit can change rapidly, however, so we should continue to offer a chance for her to ask questions and review directions she has been given. Continue to praise her positive health behaviors. Review the signs and symptoms of possible problems with the pregnancy and be sure she knows when and where to contact a provider. Confirm the date and time of her next appointment.

Between 36 and 40 weeks of pregnancy, a copy of the client's prenatal records detailing the events of the pregnancy for both the woman and the fetus will be made available to the agency where she expects to deliver the baby. Some women are also provided a copy of this

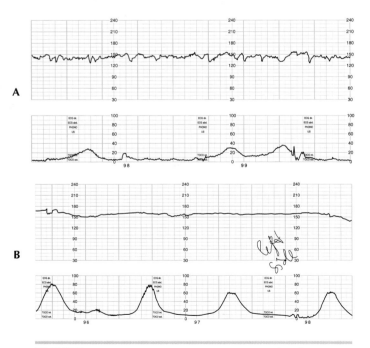

FIGURE 12-5 • **A,** CST negative (no FHR decelerations). **B,** CST positive (late decelerations of FHR with contractions). *(From Tucker SM: Pocket guide to fetal monitoring, ed 4, St Louis, 2000, Mosby.)*

| TABLE 12-3 *Biophysical Profile* | |
|---|---|
| **Criteria** | **Scoring*** |
| Reactive NST | _____ |
| Fetal breathing movements (one or more episodes of 30 seconds or more within 30 minutes) | _____ |
| Fetal movements (three or more discrete body or limb movements in 30 minutes) | _____ |
| Fetal tone (one or more episodes of extension with return to flexion) | _____ |
| Amniotic fluid (one or more pockets of fluid measuring at least 2 cm in two perpendicular planes) | _____ |
| TOTAL | _____ |

| **Interpretation** | |
|---|---|
| 10 | Normal, delivery not indicated |
| 8 (with a normal amniotic fluid measurement) | Normal, delivery not indicated |
| 6 | Equivocal, consider delivery of fetus |
| ≤4 | Abnormal, deliver fetus if gestation is longer than 26 weeks |

*If present, 2 points; if absent, 0 points.

From Mattson S and Smith J: *Core curriculum for maternal-newborn nursing,* Philadelphia, 2000, Saunders; Manning F: Fetal biophysical assessment by ultrasound. In Creasy R and Resnick R, editors: *Maternal-fetal medicine,* ed 3, Philadelphia, 1994, Saunders.

record to carry with them. With a complete record of the events of pregnancy, the woman and fetus are able to receive continuity of care no matter where and when a prenatal emergency or labor and delivery occur.

##  ANTICIPATORY GUIDANCE DURING THE THIRD TRIMESTER

### Sexual Activity

The expression of sexual intimacy and intercourse, when comfortable, are possible throughout the third trimester. However, couples often decrease their sexual activity.

The pregnant woman may experience indigestion and heartburn if she reclines. She may have backaches and other physical discomforts, increasing uterine irritability or Braxton-Hicks contractions, excessive pelvic congestion, or vulvar or femoral vericosities that make her reluctant to experience intercourse. This does not necessarily mean that her desire for physical intimacy has subsided. She may crave physical closeness and caressing in order to feel safe and secure. If she desires intercourse, the couple may have to experiment to see what is comfortable and pleasurable. She may prefer to be sitting or lying on her side. When the baby's head is low in the uterus, however, even these positions are uncomfortable for some women and they decline to participate in vaginal penetration.

Fathers may hesitate to initiate sexual interest for fear of hurting the now very evident fetus. Some couples sometimes hesitate because they do not know how to position themselves in a way that does not put pressure on the fetus. Others are reluctant because the fetus may kick and squirm during physical intimacy.

During the last few weeks of pregnancy, the baseline levels of oxytocin will increase; when the mother is sexually aroused, it will be released into her bloodstream. When a baby is due to be born but labor has not yet started, a couple may assist the process through passionate lovemaking. Prostaglandins supplied by the semen deposited in the vagina will soften the cervix and the release of oxytocin will initiate contractions that may start labor (Kitzinger, 1985).

When a couple is advised to refrain from intercourse, it is based on an appraisal of the couple's individual needs, desires, and circumstances. Couples are most likely to implement this advice if both partners hear the advice from the providers and are given a clear explanation as to the reasons for the advice. A chance to ask questions and learn about acceptable ways to experience physical closeness also increases the likelihood that a couple will comply.

 The contraindications to sexual penetration during this trimester are vaginal infection; undiagnosed vaginal bleeding; premature dilation of the cervix, without cerclage; severe vulvar varicosities; premature rupture of the membranes; premature labor; or placenta previa.

### General Hygiene

The general hygiene activities of prepregnancy and prior trimesters continue. With the increased production of oil and perspiration of pregnancy, many women feel dirty and clammy. During the third trimester, the woman may find it awkward to move in and out of a bathtub, so showers may be preferable. Be sure to cover safety issues with the woman so that the possibility of her slipping and falling in the shower is reduced.

### Nutritional Needs

Women's nutritional needs remain the same during the third trimester. She may have a problem eating all that she needs without developing heartburn. Most of her food intake should occur in the morning, giving her more time to digest it before she lies down. The total amount of food that she requires may have to be divided into small amounts that are eaten more frequently. This practice is called "grazing" and often occurs even when women are not pregnant: some oatmeal at 7:00 AM, half a banana at 8:00 AM, a half-glass of orange juice at 9:00 AM, a handful of raisins at 10:00 AM, celery sticks at 11:00 AM, a whole wheat pita at noon, pieces of cooked chicken at 1:00 PM, etc.

Cultural prescriptive and restrictive practices related to foods continue through the third trimester. Women nearing the end of pregnancy often feel hot and experience indigestion and constipation. Cultural responses to these experiences vary. For example, Vietnamese-American women eat "cold" foods, including mung beans, green coconut, spinach, and melon. Tonic foods (e.g., animal proteins, fat, sugar, and carbohydrates) eaten in the first 2 trimesters to increase the baby's weight are now limited (Purnell and Paulanka, 1998).

### Safety

As the abdomen protrudes more, some women find it uncomfortable to wear seatbelts. Others are afraid they will hurt the baby. Encourage the woman to wear a seatbelt at all times when in a car. The lap strap should be placed under the abdomen.

On the job, the woman may experience edema in her legs if she is required to sit or stand for long periods of time. Sleep, which is already difficult due to the pregnancy, may become more so if the woman is working a rotating shift. Increasing fatigue also makes her more vulnerable to accidents. Heavy lifting and physical labor may become impossible. As the size of her abdomen increases, the woman will not be able to work in places where a good sense of balance is required.

Because of the changes in her body and the potential risks, a woman may seek either a reassignment to another position (which may bring a lower salary) or find it necessary to leave her job temporarily. Some women find that when they want to return to their position after delivery, however, it is no longer available. This may make other pregnant woman hesitant to make such a decision. The Family Leave Act was passed in an attempt to prevent this from happening but only applies to companies with a large number of employees. Even companies to which it applies may find ways to circumvent the system. When this occurs, the woman may not have the financial resources to litigate against her former employer.

## Drug Consumption

At the end of a pregnancy, the amount of caffeine consumed becomes more important because the half-life of the drug in a newborn is 4 days. Some fetal heart arrhythmias have been attributed to maternal coffee consumption just before labor. With high caffeine levels at birth, the newborn may experience caffeine withdrawal after delivery (Dickason, Silverman, and Kaplan, 1998).

The results of active or passive smoking during pregnancy may reduce fetal birth weight by 150 to 300 g. The risk for premature delivery is also increased. After delivery, fetuses that were exposed to smoke are at increased risk for sudden infant death syndrome and asthma.

Use of all kinds of drugs (i.e., over the counter, prescription, and recreational or street drugs) continues to have implications for the fetus. The drugs in the fetus's system will affect its response to labor and ability to survive after delivery.

## Discomforts of Pregnancy

As the size of the uterus increases during the third trimester, the woman may feel like the fetus has taken over her body. She may feel miserable, but the daily, sometimes constant, activity of the fetus provides a reminder of why this is happening to her. (This is unlike the first trimester when she may have felt miserable but had no interaction with the fetus.) Knowing that the end of pregnancy is near may help her withstand the discomforts. As health care providers, we can offer support and empathy, praise her efforts, and help her brainstorm about what she might do to be comfortable.

We must simultaneously encourage her to maintain her intake of water at appropriate levels (which will increase her need to urinate and interfere with periods of rest and sleep) and maintain an adequate level of nutrition (which may give her increased heartburn). By drinking most fluids in the morning and eating small amounts almost constantly, her discomforts may be minimized. The woman may also have solutions as to how to be successful in her intake while remaining relatively comfortable. Functioning as a collaborator, she will be empowered to be successful (Table 12-4).

One of the major concerns of a mother during the third trimester is being able to know the difference between Braxton-Hicks contractions and labor contractions. Braxton-Hicks contractions occur on and off for hours, days, or even weeks before true labor begins. Most of the time they are felt only in the front of the abdomen and do not increase in intensity. These contractions are usually not regular or rhythmic and can often be relieved or even stopped by walking or taking a warm shower or bath.

True labor contractions may feel different from  Braxton-Hicks contractions. The contractions generally become gradually more uncomfortable and occur at regular intervals that become closer and closer over time. In contrast to Braxton-Hicks contractions, true labor contractions usually become stronger when the woman walks around.

Review with the woman how to time contractions. Review relaxation breathing techniques with her so she can stay comfortable. Advise her to call if her contractions become stronger or different from previous contractions; if there is bleeding, leaking, or rupture of membranes; or if there is increased vaginal discharge so that she may be evaluated for cervical dilation (Youngkin and Davis, 1998).

 ## PREGNANCY RISK AND LOSS

The woman may find the survival of her fetus at risk due to bleeding from placenta previa or abruptio placenta. These may occur as early as 20 weeks of gestation, but the greater risk is more often during the third trimester. The woman may experience preterm labor (i.e., labor before the end of the gestational period), placing her fetus at risk for not surviving life outside the uterus. (See Chapter 18 for nursing care of the woman in preterm labor.) A woman may also complete the full gestational period and then deliver a stillborn child, one who dies before taking a breath.

### Placenta Previa

Placenta previa occurs when the placenta becomes attached to the lower segment of the uterus. When the cervix begins to soften and efface, the placenta is pulled away from the endometrium and bleeding can occur. The life of the fetus is at risk from hypoxia if the bleeding is profuse or a preterm delivery occurs. Any significant bleeding that leads to hemorrhage also endangers the mother.

#### Classification of Previa
The degree that the internal cervical os is covered by the placenta determines the classification of the condition. The placenta previa may be total, partial, or low-lying. When the placenta completely covers the internal os,

TABLE 12-4   *Relief from Common Discomforts of the Third Trimester*

| Condition | Helpful interventions |
|---|---|
| Ankle edema | Rest with legs elevated above hips.<br>Walk and do ankle exercises.<br>Do not cross legs.<br>Maintain fluid intake.<br>Maintain balanced nutrition.<br>Put on support stockings before edema occurs. |
| Braxton-Hicks contractions | Change position or activity when they start (e.g., if resting, walk; if walking, rest).<br>Practice breathing techniques.<br>Use the massage of effleurage. |
| Gingivitis | Use a soft toothbrush and brush gently.<br>Use mouthwashes (e.g., baking soda and hydrogen peroxide, bayberry and prickly ash).<br>Gently massage gums to improve circulation.<br>Massage cashew oil, vitamin E oil, or poultices of goldseal or myrrh into the gums to protect against infection.<br>Maintain a well-balanced diet.<br>Have teeth cleaned. |
| Insomnia | Reduce stimuli before going to bed.<br>Keep bedroom quiet and dark, using earplugs if necessary.<br>Maintain a scheduled pattern of sleep.<br>Exercise earlier in the day.<br>Use aromatherapy and/or biofeedback.<br>Use herbal therapy (e.g., chamomile, lime blossom, or passion flower tea), relaxation therapy and massage, and meditation or yoga.<br>Avoid sweets and fruit juices in the evening. |
| Leg cramps | Stand with foot flat on floor or pull toes back toward knee.<br>Increase calcium and decrease phosphorus intake.<br>If pain continues, see health care provider. |
| Mood swings | Talk with a supportive person.<br>Seek information about factors that are causing anxiety.<br>Talk with health care provider.<br>Remain active.<br>Relax and understand that this is normal. |
| Perineal pressure | Good posture with back straight and pelvis rocked up so uterus is resting within pelvis.<br>If standing, place one foot on a stool.<br>Rest with feet and hips raised. |
| Shortness of breath | Maintain good posture with back straight and shoulders back to provide lungs with maximum space.<br>Eat small meals.<br>Sleep with pillows under head and shoulders or reclining in a chair. |
| Urinary frequency | Empty bladder on a regular basis even when the urge is not present.<br>Do Kegel exercises to maintain or increase control of flow.<br>Drink most of the necessary fluids earlier in the day and minimize intake 4 hours before bedtime. |

Compiled from Davis DC: The discomforts of pregnancy, *J Obstet Gynecol Neonat Nurs* 25(1):73-81, 1996; *Nurses handbook of alternative and complementary therapies*, Springhouse, PA, 1998, Springhouse; Snyder M and Lindquist R: *Complementary/alternative therapies in nursing*, ed 3, New York, 1998, Springer.

it is classified as a **total (or complete) previa.** A **partial (or incomplete) previa** describes the condition when the placenta covers part of the os. When the edge of the placenta is at the os but does not obstruct it, it is classified as a **low (or marginal) previa** (Mattson and Smith, 2000; Youngkin and Davis, 1998) (Figure 12-6).

### Etiology

The etiology of placenta previa is unknown. The incidence is 1 in 200 deliveries, with a range from 1/1500 nulliparas and 1/20 grand multiparas. Placenta previa occurs more frequently in the following women: (1) Those who have had a prior placenta previa; the incidence is

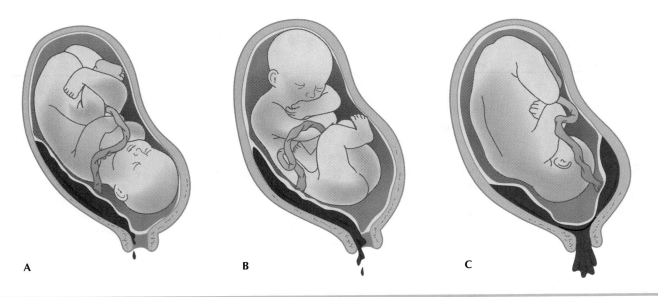

**A**          **B**          **C**

*FIGURE 12-6* • Classifications of placenta previa. **A,** Low; **B,** Partial; **C,** Total.

12 times greater. (2) Those who are older; women over 35 years of age account for 33% of the cases. (3) Those who have had other children; 80% of affected women are multiparous. (4) Those who have experienced uterine surgery. (5) Those carrying multiple gestations. A lack of sufficient uteroplacental surface area is involved in most risk factors (Hilton, 1992; Mattson and Smith, 2000; Youngkin and Davis, 1998).

### Clinical Manifestations

Bleeding from previa may occur as early as 20 weeks. If a woman reports intermittent, painless, vaginal bleeding of bright red blood after 24 weeks, previa is suspected. The first episode of bleeding is usually self-limiting, stopping as clots form and requiring no further treatment. If the bleeding continues, however, the woman may be admitted to the hospital, stabilized, and discharged within 48 hours of the last bleeding episode.

As the pregnancy progresses, the previa is resolved in 88% to 98% of the partial or low implantation cases. This occurs because as the pregnancy progresses, the lower segment of the uterus stretches and the area where the low lying placenta is attached moves away from the os.

### Nursing Care

Obtain a description of the bleeding, including when it started, how much has been lost, what the woman thinks might have caused it, and if there is cramping. Explain the possible causes of bleeding at this time in pregnancy and prepare the woman for further evaluation by abdominal ultrasound. Monitor her vital signs and the fetal heart rate. Prepare the woman for possible admission to a hospital if the bleeding does not stop. If the woman is sent home, work with her family members and employer so that she will be able to follow the in-structions for bed rest or limited activity. Review with her the self-care instructions (e.g., rest, nothing in her vagina) and what to do immediately if she has another episode of bleeding.

### Abruptio Placentae

**Abruptio placentae** is the partial or complete detachment of a normally implanted placenta prior to the delivery of an infant. Detachment occurs more often during the third trimester, but may occur anytime after 20 weeks of gestation. The risk of hypoxia or death exists for the fetus. The mother may also die from hemorrhagic shock (Mattson and Smith, 2000; Youngkin and Davis, 1998).

### Classification

An abruptio placenta may be classified as one of three types: (1) **marginal separation** with apparent bleeding, (2) **partial separation** with concealed bleeding, or (3) **complete separation** with concealed bleeding. The marginal separation is the least risky because the occurrence of the separation leads to visible bleeding and provides an earlier indication that there is a problem. With a partial separation, the bleeding is trapped under the placenta. The abdominal area may become tender. This "silent" abruption may continue with more of the placenta becoming detached. A complete separation will cause massive vaginal bleeding and hypoxia for the fetus (Phillips, 1996; Youngkin and Davis, 1998) (Figure 12-7).

### Etiology

The etiology of abruptio placentae is unknown. It occurs in 1 in 120 births (i.e., in about 1% of deliveries) and leads to 15% of all perinatal deaths. A woman is at

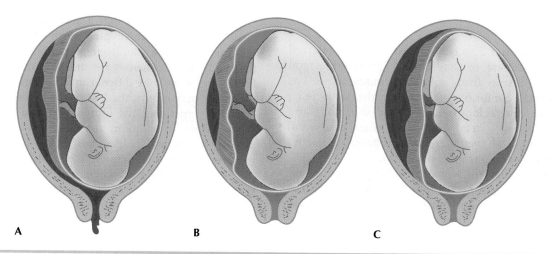

FIGURE 12-7 • Types of abruptio placenta. **A,** Marginal; **B,** Partial; **C,** Complete.

TABLE 12-5   *Comparison of Placenta Previa and Abruptio Placentae*

| Placenta previa | Abruptio placentae |
|---|---|
| No underlying chronic disease | Associated with hypertension, diabetes, and kidney diseases |
| Warning signs of spotting hemorrhage always externally visible | Usually no warning signs |
| No pain | Hemorrhage may be internal or externally visible |
| Occurs rarely during labor but is unrelated to labor | Pain may be present in varying degrees |
| FHTs and movement usually present and unaffected | Usually occurs in labor |
| Placenta in lower uterine segment | FHTs reflecting uteroplacental insufficiency |
| Soft uterus | Placental attachment in normal locations |
| | Uterus tender to woodlike |

*FHTs,* Fetal heart tones.

Adapted from Dickason E and others: *Maternal-infant nursing care,* ed 3, St Louis, 1998, Mosby

more risk for having a premature separation of the placenta if she has had one before (recurrence risk is 10% to 30%); smokes cigarettes or uses cocaine; experiences trauma to the abdomen from a domestic violence dispute, automobile accident, or a fall; or has a chorioamnionitis, poor nutrition, or hypertension (Mattson and Smith, 2000; Youngkin and Davis, 1998).

### Clinical Manifestations

The symptoms a woman reports will vary depending on the extent and the location of the separation (Table 12-5). In the case of a mild separation, there may be no symptoms, so it will not be known until the placenta is inspected after delivery. In other cases, the woman may report bleeding; a small amount of dark, old blood; or a profuse amount of bright, red blood. She may report labor pains with a constant tenderness that does not go away or a sharp, knifelike pain. Her uterus may feel as hard as a board, with a severe constant pain. If the mother has lost a great deal of blood from circulation (it may be hidden behind the placenta), she may experience symptoms of shock (e.g., falling blood pressure, nausea,

vomiting, dizziness, or fainting) (Hilton, 1992; Mattson and Smith, 2000; Youngkin and Davis, 1998).

### Nursing Care

When a woman reports a combination of abdominal pain and bleeding, she must be seen immediately for diagnosis, stabilization, and treatment. The woman and her family must be informed about the impending diagnostic tests and the possibility of hospitalization. If a woman calls with these symptoms, instruct her to go to the nearest emergency facility for further evaluation. Be sure that she can arrange for the care of her other children, as well as for transportation. Further evaluation will focus on the fetal heart rate, the presence or absence of vaginal bleeding and abdominal pain, and maternal symptoms. An ultrasound examination may be used to locate a retroplacental clot. Intravenous fluids and oxygen will be used to stabilize the woman's condition. The woman should not be left alone, and all procedures should be explained to her. Fetal viability and the maternal condition will determine if and how delivery will occur (Dickason, Silverman, and Kaplan, 1998).

## Fetal Death

If the fetus dies after 20 weeks of gestation, it is referred to as a fetal demise or "stillbirth." Intrauterine fetal death (IUFD) results from unknown causes, as well as from maternal conditions that affect the fetus (e.g., preeclampsia and eclampsia, diabetes, infection, and isoimmune disease), fetal conditions (e.g., congenital abnormalities), and events created by pregnancy (e.g., placenta previa and abruptio placenta).

When a fetus dies, the woman and her partner are left wondering what happened as they confront the death of hope. When a woman and her partner reach the second half of pregnancy, they have generally resolved any ambivalent feelings they might have had and begin to fantasize about the baby. The growing fetus represents not only an addition to their family but also evidence of their fertility and the embodiment of their immortality.

It is to be expected that a woman whose baby has died—whether before or after birth—will want to cry, talk about the baby, and reminisce about her time with the child. Because men and women grieve differently, the father's response may differ from the mother's. Although the father may mourn the loss of the fantasized child, he does not experience the humiliation and guilt that the woman does. In addition, insensitive handling by health care providers and inadequate family and community recognition of the loss may make it difficult for the couple to resolve their grief. The couple's other children, the grandparents, and others involved in the pregnancy are often forgotten in the facilitation of their grieving process.

### Nursing Care

Women who have had a stillborn child still require a postpartum examination. If they return to the person who cared for them during pregnancy, it presents an opportu-

---

### BOX 12-2 *How to Help a Grieving Family with a Fetal Death*

Let your concern and care show.
(Don't avoid them.)

Reach out, through your uncomfortableness, and be available to listen.
(Don't talk, listen. Be comfortable with silence.)

Say you are sorry about what has happened to their child: "I am sorry your baby died."
(Don't say, "I know how you feel." Even if you have had a baby, you don't know how they feel.)

Allow them to talk about the child as much and as often as they want.
(Don't change the subject.)

Ask them if they named the child. If so, call it by name.
(Calling the child by name legitimizes that it was an individual.)

Talk about the special qualities of the child they have lost.
(Commenting on the child's beautiful hair, cute face, etc. may lead to tears but is helpful.)

Allow them to be angry that their baby died, to cry, and to withdraw from others.
(Don't' say, "You can't be angry" or "That's enough crying now. Be strong.")

Reassure them that this is not their fault, that they did everything they could.
(There are many unknown causes of problems in utero and of fetal death.)

Encourage them to be patient with themselves. It takes time to grieve the loss of another person.
(Don't say, "Get it all out now before you go home.")

Explain that everyone grieves differently. They should try to be patient with each other as each will work through this in his or her own way.
(Without this understanding, the loss of a child is more apt to drive a couple apart.)

Allow them to express their feelings, anxieties, and worries about possible future pregnancies.
(Don't say, "Go home and have fun making another one.")

Provide supportive care to the other children and grandparents.
(Don't exclude the others in the family. Each will be grieving in his or her own way. They can only help each other if someone has been of help to them.)

Remember the anniversary of the child's birth and death. The parents will remember and appreciate that you also care enough to.
(Their friends and relatives may never mention the child again.)

If the woman has lost a child and then has another pregnancy, provide frequent opportunities for the family to check on the health status of the developing fetus.

nity for them to bring the cycle to a conclusion. Women will want to talk about the infant they became attached to in utero. If the woman had the opportunity to look at and hold the baby after delivery, she will want to share what she observed. If she has keepsakes (e.g., a lock of hair, a picture, the blanket the baby was wrapped in, the hat on the baby's head), she may want to share them.

Grieving the loss of a fetus is a process that may take a year or longer. Health care providers, uncomfortable with a less than optimal outcome, often retreat from the couple and offer them only the most obligatory contact.

Parents find comfort when we allow our compassion to surface and display the sadness we feel about what has occurred. Box 12-2 provides some *dos* and *don'ts* when providing care to a family grieving the loss of a baby during the second half of pregnancy.

## SUMMARY

During the third trimester of pregnancy, the developing fetus grows, becoming more obvious and expanding the woman's uterus and abdomen. The effect of nurturing and carrying the enlarging fetus becomes more evident in the comfort level, physical abilities, and activities of the woman. As the onset of labor approaches, the mother should understand what is happening to her body, feel that she is empowered to participate as desired in the birth experience she has prepared for, and continue to mentally prepare herself for the act of giving birth. Our assessments and interventions during the third trimester support her desires and empower her to plan for the experience she desires.

---

## Care Plan · The Woman with Normal Discomforts of Third Trimester Pregnancy

NURSING DIAGNOSIS   **Risk for Injury** related to inability to recognize signs and symptoms of complications of pregnancy
GOALS/OUTCOMES   Complications will be recognized and treated immediately if they occur

**NOC Suggested Outcomes**
- Knowledge: Pregnancy (1810)
- Health Seeking Behavior (1603)
- Risk Control (1902)

**NIC Priority Interventions**
- Prenatal Care (6960)
- Surveillance: Late Pregnancy (6656)

**Nursing Activities & Rationale**
- Instruct client to call the appropriate health professional if she experiences any of the following: (1) visual disturbances, severe headache, finger or facial edema (*pregnancy-induced hypertension*); (2) fever (*infection*); (3) uterine contractions, pressure, or cramping (*preterm labor*); (4) abdominal pain (*appendicitis, placenta previa or abruptio*); (5) severe back or flank pain (*kidney infection, labor*); (6) vaginal bleeding (*placenta previa or abruptio*); (7) nausea and vomiting (*hyperemesis gravidarum*); (8) fluid leaking from the vagina (*premature rupture of membranes*); (9) reduced or lack of fetal movements (*fetal distress, fetal death*).
- Monitor for potential problems at routine prenatal visits. *To compare current status with previous status and identify problems before they become severe.*

**Evaluation Parameters**
- Lists signs and symptoms that indicate the need to notify health professional.
- Notifies health care professional immediately if symptoms occur.
- Vital signs within normal limits for this client.
- If complications occur, they are detected and treated before they become severe.

---

NURSING DIAGNOSIS   **Altered Comfort** related to edema of lower extremities
GOALS/OUTCOMES   Reports satisfactory relief of discomfort from pedal and ankle edema

**NOC Suggested Outcomes**
- Comfort Level (2100)
- Knowledge: Pregnancy (1810)
- Symptom Severity (2103)

**NIC Priority Interventions**
- Prenatal Care (6960)
- Surveillance: Late Pregnancy (6656)
- Teaching: Disease Process (5602)

**Nursing Activities & Rationale**
- Instruct to rest often with legs elevated above the hips. *Gravity facilitates venous return from legs.*
- Instruct not to cross legs when sitting (*blocks venous return from lower legs*).

*Continued*

## Care Plan · The Woman with Normal Discomforts of Third Trimester Pregnancy—cont'd

- Instruct not to sit or stand for long periods; alternate with walking about and/or ankle exercises. *When walking, "muscle pump" facilitates venous return against gravity.*
- Instruct to limit added table salt and avoid high-sodium foods and beverages. *High-sodium intake contributes to water retention; however, adequate sodium intake is important to prevent dehydration.*
- Monitor blood pressure, reflexes, and weight; assess for visual disturbances, headache, epigastric pain; assess for edema in hands and face. *Mild edema is common in third trimester but could also represent the beginning of pregnancy-induced hypertension.*

### Evaluation Parameters
- Reports compliance with instructions (e.g., walking, support stockings).
- Pedal edema 1+ or less.
- Reports that discomfort does not interfere with usual functioning or sleep.

---

**NURSING DIAGNOSIS**   **Altered Comfort** related to Braxton-Hicks contractions

**GOALS/OUTCOMES**   Reports coping satisfactorily with Braxton-Hicks contractions

### NOC Suggested Outcomes
- Comfort Level (2100)
- Knowledge: Pregnancy (1810)
- Symptom Severity (2103)

### NIC Priority Interventions
- Prenatal Care (6960)
- Surveillance: Late Pregnancy (6656)
- Teaching: Disease Process (5602)

### Nursing Activities & Rationale
- Teach to differentiate Braxton-Hicks (B-H) contractions from true labor. *True contractions are regular and increase in intensity. Knowledge may help relieve anxiety and, therefore, minimize pain perception.*
- Teach to change position or activity when contractions start. *B-H contractions can often be relieved by walking.*
- Teach to take a warm shower or bath when contractions start (*often relieves B-H contractions*).
- Advise to practice effleurage and/or breathing techniques (*for relaxation and distraction from abdominal sensations*).
- At prenatal visits, palpate and electronically monitor uterine contractions (*to validate client's verbal reports*).

### Evaluation Parameters
- Correctly verbalizes differences between B-H and labor contractions.
- Reports use of techniques for managing B-H contractions.
- Verbalizes obtaining satisfactory relief from techniques used.

---

**NURSING DIAGNOSIS**   **Altered Comfort** related to shortness of breath

**GOALS/OUTCOMES**   Reports satisfactory management of shortness of breath

### NOC Suggested Outcomes
- Comfort Level (2100)
- Knowledge: Pregnancy (1810)
- Symptom Severity (2103)

### NIC Priority Interventions
- Prenatal Care (6960)
- Surveillance: Late Pregnancy (6656)
- Teaching: Disease Process (5602)

### Nursing Activities & Rationale
- Teach the relationship between posture and ease of breathing. *Keeping back straight and shoulders back provides maximum space for lung expansion.*
- Instruct to eat small frequent meals. *Prevents full stomach from encroaching on space for lung expansion.*
- Advise to sleep with head and shoulders elevated on pillows, or in a reclining chair. *Relieves pressure of enlarged uterus on diaphragm.*
- Assess for symptoms of cardiac problems. *Shortness of breath is a normal finding in third trimester, but cardiac problems must be ruled out.*

### Evaluation Parameters
- Reports compliance with instructions (e.g., eating small meals).
- Reports that shortness of breath does not interfere with usual functioning or sleep.

## Care Plan · The Woman with Normal Discomforts of Third Trimester Pregnancy—cont'd

**NURSING DIAGNOSIS**    **Altered Comfort** related to heartburn

**GOALS/OUTCOMES**    Expresses satisfaction with symptom control; maintains adequate intake of nutrients and calories

**NOC Suggested Outcomes**
- Comfort Level (2100)
- Knowledge: Pregnancy (1810)
- Symptom Severity (2103)

**NIC Priority Interventions**
- Prenatal Care (6960)
- Surveillance: Late Pregnancy (6656)
- Teaching: Disease Process (5602)

**Nursing Activities & Rationale**
- Instruct to eat frequently in small amounts, *to accommodate the decreased size of the stomach in pregnancy. Increased progesterone in pregnancy contributes to decreased gastrointestinal motility and relaxation of the cardiac sphincter, allowing for regurgitation of acidic gastric contents.*
- Teach and give rationale for good posture. *Allows more room for the stomach to function.*
- Teach to avoid fatty and fried foods. *These aggravate heartburn.*
- Teach to not lie down soon after eating. *Horizontal position increases regurgitation of stomach contents.*
- Assess client's food intake; have her keep a food diary if necessary. *Despite the discomfort that eating may create, good nutrition is essential for the developing fetus.*
- Warn not to self-medicate with baking soda or Alka-Seltzer. *May cause electrolyte imbalance.*

**Evaluation Parameters**
- Reports compliance with instructions (e.g., avoiding fried foods).
- Reports self-care interventions provide effective relief from heartburn.
- Reports eating a well-balanced diet.

**NURSING DIAGNOSIS**    **Sleep deprivation** related to physical discomfort and insomnia

**GOALS/OUTCOMES**    Reports receiving adequate amount and quality of sleep

**NOC Suggested Outcomes**
- Comfort Level (2100)
- Knowledge: Pregnancy (1810)
- Symptom Severity (2103)

**NIC Priority Interventions**
- Prenatal Care (6960)
- Surveillance: Late Pregnancy (6656)
- Teaching: Disease Process (5602)

**Nursing Activities & Rationale**
- Instruct to drink most fluids in the morning hours. *This decreases the amount of circulating fluid to be eliminated during sleeping hours, so that she will not need to get out of bed to urinate.*
- Teach to avoid caffeinated drinks and stimulating activity at bedtime (*to promote relaxation*).
- Keep bedroom quiet and dark; use earplugs if needed (*to decrease stimuli*).
- Use aromatherapy, biofeedback, meditation, rexalation therapy, and/or massage (*to promote relaxation*).
- Teach to use pillows to support back, legs, and arm when lying on side. *The enlarged uterus makes it difficult to find a comfortable position for sleep.*
- Avoid sweets and fruit juices in the evening (*to avoid stimulating fetal activity*).
- Suggest drinking a warm beverage (e.g., chamomile, lime blossom, or passion flower tea) at bedtime (*to promote relaxation*).

**Evaluation Parameters**
- Reports compliance with instructions (avoiding caffeine at bedtime).
- Reports that she is sleeping 8 hours a day or that lack of sleep does not interfere with her usual functions.

**NURSING DIAGNOSIS**    **Pain** related to leg cramps

**GOALS/OUTCOMES**    Reports ability to relieve leg cramps when they occur

**NOC Suggested Outcomes**
- Comfort Level (2100)
- Knowledge: Pregnancy (1810)
- Symptom Severity (2103)

**NIC Priority Interventions**
- Prenatal Care (6960)
- Surveillance: Late Pregnancy (6656)
- Teaching: Disease Process (5602)

*Continued*

## Care Plan · The Woman with Normal Discomforts of Third Trimester Pregnancy—cont'd

### Nursing Activities & Rationale

- Teach to stand with foot flat on floor or pull toes back towards knee (for cramps in calves). *Stretching the muscle relievs the spasm.*
- Teach to do stretching exercises before bedtime (*prevents leg cramps*).
- Encourage to rest during the day; assess for sleep deprivation. *Fatigue increases the likelihood of leg cramps.*
- Instruct to consult primary care provider if pain continues. *The care provider may recommend limiting milk intake and taking calcium carbonate or aluminum hydroxide gel to absorb the phosphorus (one theory is that cramps may be caused by an imbalance in the calcium/phosphorus ratio).*

### Evaluation Parameters

- Reports compliance with instructions (e.g., stretching before bedtime).
- Reports obtaining adequate rest.
- Reports that self-care interventions provide effective relief from leg cramps.

NURSING DIAGNOSIS   **Pain** related to hemorrhoids

GOALS/OUTCOMES    Reports relief from hemorrhoids; able to perform usual functions of living

### NOC Suggested Outcomes

- Comfort Level (2100)
- Knowledge: Pregnancy (1810)
- Symptom Severity (2103)

### NIC Priority Interventions

- Prenatal Care (6960)
- Surveillance: Late Pregnancy (6656)
- Teaching: Disease Process (5602)

### Nursing Activities & Rationale

- Teach to notify health care provider if hemorrhoids become hardened or very tender to touch or if rectal bleeding after a bowel movement is more than spotting (*to detect and provide early treatment for thrombosis*).
- Teach to reinsert hemorrhoids digitally and assume a side-lying (Sims') position (at bedtime or at a daily rest period). *Reinsertion provides some relief; lying down relieves some of the pressure by removing the effects of gravity and promoting venous return to the heart.*
- Teach to include adequate fluids and fiber in the diet (*to prevent constipation and straining at stool; to prevent or relieve the discomfort*).
- Teach to use ice packs and topical ointments. *Provides local anesthesia.*
- Teach to use warm soak (in sitz pan or shallow water in bathtub). *Increases circulation locally, allowing for swelling to subside.*

### Evaluation Parameters

- Notifies health care provider as appropriate.
- Has daily, soft bowel movement.
- Reports adequate relief from self-care interventions.
- Reports ability to continue.

## CASE STUDY

Kim is 15 years old, pregnant with her first child, and due to deliver in 3 weeks. She has been participating in prenatal care since she first realized she was pregnant at 20 weeks of gestation. She has kept all of her appointments and seems to have followed all directions. Prenatal growth is progressing satisfactorily, with Kim demonstrating appropriate weight gain. Fundal growth and fetal activity have been within normal limits. Kim has not experienced significant changes in her vital signs or laboratory values.

Kim lives with her mother, Lorraine, and her 17-year-old sister in a small town. Her parents divorced when

## CASE STUDY

she was 12. Lorraine works at a department store and is away from home from 8:00 AM to 6:00 PM. Kim's sister is a senior in high school, preparing to leave for college. Lorraine is very supportive of Kim and attends childbirth classes with her. Lorraine is planning to be Kim's labor support person. Lorraine loves to shop and plan for the new baby. Kim is quiet and spends little time outside their home because all of her friends are in school. She has nothing to do except watch television. The father of the baby is in college and is no longer interested in Kim. His family does not know about the pregnancy.

Kim is here for her weekly prenatal visit. She plans to keep the baby but is demonstrating little enthusiasm for the future.

- What immediate response will you provide Kim?

- What are her strengths? Where does she face potential problems?

- What information do you need from Kim to move forward in support of her?

- What nursing diagnoses could apply? How will you validate these?

- What long-term goals might she have for herself and for her family?

- What short-term goals might the two of you develop for her and for her family?

- What interventions may you be able to develop and offer?

- How will these interventions be prioritized?

- How will you evaluate the effectiveness of your interventions?

# Scenarios

**1.** Courtney is in her third trimester of pregnancy. She feels well and continues to work full-time. You have just told her that her prenatal visits will now be every week. She responds, "Every week!! Why? Is there something wrong? I can't miss that much time from work. What do you have to do that is so important?"

- What will be your initial response?
- What nursing diagnoses could apply? How will you validate these?
- What goals might be developed? How will these be prioritized?
- What interventions may you offer?
- How will you evaluate the effectiveness of your interventions?

---

**2.** Melissa is 33 weeks pregnant with her first child. She tells you that she and her partner, Steve, are still having sexual intercourse. In order to be more comfortable, they are positioning themselves so that Melissa is in the superior position or they are both lying on their sides. Melissa asks, "Is this normal? Can we keep having intercourse until the baby is born? Can anything happen to the baby?"

- What subjective data do you have about Melissa's condition?
- What subjective and objective data do you need?
- What do you think Melissa might be experiencing? Why?
- What nursing diagnoses could apply? How will you validate these?
- What goals might be developed? How will these be prioritized?
- What interventions may you offer?
- How will you evaluate the effectiveness of your interventions?

---

**3.** Annalyn and her husband are at the clinic early this morning because they are worried. Last night after having intercourse, there was some bright red bleeding from Annalyn's vagina. She has continued to feel the baby kick this morning but the bleeding has her concerned.

- What subjective data do you have about Annalyn's condition?
- What subjective and objective data do you need?
- What nursing diagnoses could apply? How will you validate these?
- What goals might be developed? How will these be prioritized?
- What interventions may you offer?
- How will you evaluate the effectiveness of your interventions?

---

4. Susan, now at 32 weeks of gestation, has had a comfortable pregnancy. She calls the clinic today because she is having "terrible heartburn." She says, "I can't eat meals anymore. What am I going to do? I have to feed this baby so it will grow strong."

- What subjective data do you have about Susan's condition?
- What subjective and objective data do you need?
- What nursing diagnoses could apply? How will you validate these?
- What goals might be developed? How will these be prioritized?
- What interventions may you offer?
- How will you evaluate the effectiveness of your interventions?

---

5. Kelli, age 34 and a G5 P3, is experiencing pain in her legs and vulva due to varicose veins. She says, "What can I do to get comfortable? I have the three kids to take care of: two are in school and the baby naps during the afternoon."

- What subjective data do you have about Kelli's condition?
- What subjective and objective data do you need?
- What nursing diagnoses could apply? How will you validate these?
- What goals might be developed? How will these be prioritized?
- What interventions may you offer?
- How will you evaluate the effectiveness of your interventions?

---

6. Juanita is a 30-year-old school teacher who is married to Roberto and pregnant with their first child.

She has a due date of June 1, which is 2 weeks from now. At this prenatal visit she says, "I am really concerned. Roberto is the manager of a bank 45 minutes away from the birthing center, and I work 30 minutes away. I am afraid he won't be able to make it in time for the baby's birth. How will I know when labor starts so that I can call him?"

- What subjective data do you have about Juanita's situation?
- What subjective and objective data do you need?
- What nursing diagnoses could apply? How will you validate these?
- What goals might be developed? How will these be prioritized?
- What interventions may you offer?
- How will you evaluate the effectiveness of your interventions?

---

7. Inga, at 30 weeks of gestation, has called the clinic to report that she has increased vaginal discharge and pelvic pressure. She wants to know what she should do. When you ask if she can come to the clinic she asks, "Why do I need to come in? What do you think is going on?"

- How would you respond to her? Why?
- What subjective data do you have about Inga's condition?
- What subjective and objective data do you need?
- What nursing diagnoses could apply? How will you validate these?
- What medical diagnosis could apply? What test will be done to determine this?
- What goals might be developed? How will these be prioritized?
- What interventions may you offer?
- How will you evaluate the effectiveness of your interventions?

---

8. Katia, at 36 weeks of gestation, is at the clinic for her weekly prenatal visit. It is 4:00 PM, and she has come from her job as a bank teller. When taking her vital signs, you determine that her blood pressure is 122/80. Looking back in her chart, her prepregnant blood pressure ranged from 110/75 to 120/80. You examine her hands and face for puffiness and find nothing unusual. Her ankles are slightly swollen, with a +1 edema.

- What subjective data do you have about Katia's condition?
- What subjective and objective data do you need?
- What nursing diagnoses could apply? How will you validate these?
- What medical diagnosis could apply? What test will be done to determine this?

- What goals might be developed? How will these be prioritized?
- What interventions may you offer?
- How will you evaluate the effectiveness of your interventions?

## REFERENCES

Brewer S: *Conception, pregnancy and childbirth rituals, taboos, and beliefs within the Filipino and Curban cultures,* Unpublished manuscript, Miami, 1995, Florida International University.

Cruikshank D and Hays P: Maternal physiology in pregnancy. In Gabbe S, Nieyl J, and Simpson J, editors: *Obstetrics: normal and problem pregnancies,* ed 2, New York, 1991, Churchill Livingstone.

Cunningham FG and others: *Williams obstetrics,* ed 20, Stamford, CT, 1997, Appleton & Lange.

Davis DC: The discomforts of pregnancy, *J Obstetr Gynecol Neonat Nurs* 25(1):73-81, 1996.

Dickason EJ, Silverman BL, and Kaplan JA: *Maternal-infant nursing care,* ed 3, St. Louis, 1998, Mosby.

Fuschino W: Physiologic changes of pregnancy: impact on critical care, *Crit Care Nurs Clin North Am* 4(4):691-701, 1992.

Gloger-Tippelt G: A process model of the pregnancy course, *Hum Devel* 26:134-148, 1983.

Harvey MG: Physiologic changes of pregnancy. In Harvey CJ, editor: *Critical care obstetrical nursing,* Gaithersburg, MD, 1991, Aspen.

Hilton D, editor: *Maternal-newborn nursing,* New York, 1992, Lippincott.

Kitzinger S: *Woman's experience of sex,* New York, 1985, Penguin Books.

Manning F: Fetal biophysical assessment by ultrasound. In Creasy R and Resnick R, editors: Maternal-fetal medicine, ed 3, Philadelphia, 1994, Saunders.

Mattson S and Smith J: *Core curriculum for maternal-newborn nursing,* ed 2, Philadelphia, 2000, Saunders.

*Nurses Handbook of Alternative & Complementary Therapies,* Springhouse, PA, 1998, Springhouse.

Purnell L and Paulanka BJ: *Transcultural health care,* Philadelphia, 1998, F.A. Davis.

Phillips CR: *Family-centered maternity and newborn care,* St Louis, 1996, Mosby.

Richardson P: Women's experiences of body change during normal pregnancy, *Mat Child Nurs J* 19:93-111, 1990.

Rubin R: *Maternal identity and the maternal experience,* New York, 1984, Springer.

Simpson KR and Creehan PA: *AWHONN perinatal nursing,* Philadelphia, 1996, Lippincott.

Sims LK and others: *Health assessment in nursing,* Redwood, CA, 1995, Addison-Wesley.

Snyder M and Lindquist R: *Complementary/alternative therapies in nursing,* ed 3, New York, 1998, Springer.

Youngkin EQ and Davis MS, editors: *Women's health: a primary care clinical guide,* Stamford, CT, 1998, Appleton & Lange.

# CHAPTER 13

# Childbirth Preparation

"We all came to welcome you, we all
came to your birth.
We all came to welcome you, to
welcome you to earth."

— A SONG OF THE BLESSINGWAY
CEREMONY OF THE NAVAJOS
(STARCK, 1993)

What factors have influenced women's childbirth options during the last century?

In what ways may a woman become involved in the birth of her baby?

Explain the two divergent philosophies of formal childbirth education programs.

What difference does social support make to a woman in labor?

What must be considered when designing and developing childbirth preparation classes?

What content is included in childbirth preparation classes?

How can the empowerment of women and their partners also assist them in parenting?

For millennia, women have given birth to the next generation. The majority of births in the world today occur in the home with experienced women caring for women. Women possess an innate capacity to experience childbirth, supported by women and unassisted by chemical or mechanical intervention. Traditionally, women have learned about birth and the nurturing of babies as they grew up observing their extended families and learning from tribal or cultural lore and information passed on by close female relatives. The educational process was completed once a woman became pregnant and received support and specific care from a midwife during the pregnancy, birth, and postpartum period.

"The removal of birth from the seclusion and protection of the home and family and its placement in the mysterious, clinical and unfamiliar territory of the hospital has completely disrupted the natural educational process. . . . Pregnant women now find themselves facing birth with little idea of what will happen and few social supports within a health care system that is more focused on its own needs rather than on the needs of the woman herself and her family" (Robertson, 1994). Health care professionals must prepare women for birth in a manner that empowers them to choose the level of self-determination and active participation they desire. By providing accurate and complete information to the expectant woman and her support network during pregnancy, we may empower them to make informed decisions about their birth experiences.

## THE HISTORY OF CHILDBIRTH IN THE UNITED STATES

To understand our current expectations and procedures surrounding birth, an overview of the developments during the last 100 years is in order. In the United States before the twentieth century, births occurred in homes attended by midwives, relatives, and friends. The natural process and tempo of labor and birth was allowed to occur with limited intervention (Jordan, 1987; Wertz and Wertz, 1989; Rooks, 1997). By the 1940s, radical changes had occurred related to where and how women gave birth. Culturally approved birth moved from the home to the hospital, changing the percentage from less than 5% of women giving birth in the hospital in the early 1900s to as many as 75% of women giving birth in the hospital by 1940 (Wertz and Wertz, 1989; Rooks, 1997).

The underlying assumption was that the doctors in the hospital could offer optimal safety during the birth process (Wertz and Wertz, 1989). The acceptance of physician dominance over birth created an environment of sterility, precision, and control over the birthing process (Wertz and Wertz, 1989; Rothman, 1991).

By the 1950s, hospital birth had become a routine depersonalized procedure aided by technology. Many women were brought to the hospital and left by family members. The women were then cared for by strangers, medicated or anesthetized, and delivered of their babies. The father of the baby and other family members were then called to come back to the hospital. After the anesthesia wore off, women were introduced to their infants.

This trend in hospital birth steadily increased and peaked in the early 1960s, at which time greater than 95% of all births occurred in hospitals (Wertz and Wertz, 1989). Since that time, the number of women choosing to have their babies born at home or in birthing centers has gradually increased.

### Factors that Influenced Change

This change in the type and place of care during labor and childbirth occurred because of several factors and underlying assumptions, discussed in the following sections.

#### Medical Sanctions against Midwives

In the early 1900s physicians began to move into the business of childbirth and promoted themselves as the sole authorities. Beginning in 1920, medical organizations pressured state after state to restrict the practice of obstetrics to physicians. This occurred even though a study in 1912 indicated that most American doctors were less competent handling the majority of pregnancies and deliveries than were midwives (Ehrenreich and English, 1973). The physicians campaigned against the midwives by pressing the idea that pregnancy and birth were to be feared; therefore, only highly educated physicians were qualified providers.

Believing this campaign, women started to enter hospitals for births. Since hospitals were places that you went to if you were sick and dying, birth gradually came to be seen as an unhealthy event instead of a healthy event, a process that women needed physicians to help them endure. Planting the seeds of doubt, physicians denied women their competence to give birth, and began the process of restricting who could provide them with care.

The attempt to limit midwifery practice continues today in the United States. Certified nurse midwives are now licensed in all states; however, where they may practice their profession is sometimes restricted. The ability of direct entry midwives and lay midwives to practice without fear of prosecution varies from one state to the next.

Consumers continue to work with midwives to push for legislation that protects their right to provide care. They do so because "midwifery care differs from obstetric care in philosophy, style, and practices. It promotes the normal, speaks to psychological care as well as the physical care, is woman rather than doctor centered, empowers women, and looks to simple, noninterventionist remedies before resorting to technology" (Goer, 1995).

#### Women's Social Roles

Women's social roles were evolving during the nineteen hundreds. As middle class women became increasingly employed outside the home they were no longer solely defined by the activities of childbearing and child rearing. By the early 1960's most notions of **confinement** (forced retirement from employment and/or home seclusion) during pregnancy were abandoned (Rooks, 1997; Wertz and Wertz, 1989).

#### Medical Developments

New medical developments created changes in childbearing practices (Oakley, 1984; Wertz and Wertz, 1989). A desire for painless birth led to the introduction of a German anesthetic technique labeled "twilight sleep," which involved hospitalization of the woman early in her labor followed by the administration of the analgesic, morphine and the amnesiac, scopolamine. When "twilight sleep" was introduced in the 1920s even women who could afford private doctors at home decided to go to the hospital. This combination of drugs offered to create a painless birth. However, with the administration of the drugs, the necessity for other interventions occurred. Women were unable to control themselves during labor and delivery, and the drugs sometimes made them vomit so they could have no food or drink. Often forceps were necessary to pull the baby out because the drugged women could not push effectively. To be able to apply the forceps the vagina had to be enlarged by cutting an episiotomy. With increased medications, the need for cesarean deliveries increased. The drugs given to the mother during labor remained in the baby's system after delivery, increasing the risk of respiratory distress and leading to further interventions. Because of the administration of scopolamine, a hallucinogen, most women were left with no memory of their labor or birth; however, some experienced nightmares and flashbacks (Wertz and Wertz, 1989; Boston Women's Health Book Collective, 1998).

Initially, a strong women's rights movement educated women to view "twilight sleep" as the modern way to give birth, and it supported the physicians' efforts to make the technique available to American women. During the 1940s as the effect of the drugs on the respiratory efforts of infants became more apparent, it gradually dropped out of favor so that by the 1970s the use of "twilight sleep" was rare (Wertz and Wertz, 1989). However, the use of analgesic and anesthetics in combinations with other medications and in various patterns during hospitalized labor continues. Women delivering at home because of personal desires, cultural beliefs, or lack of ability to pay for hospital care continued to handle their birth experiences in a traditional manner.

### Personal and Professional Control

By the 1960s, as women gained increasing control over their personal and professional lives some also expressed an increasing desire to regain control of their birthing experiences. Women-centered childbirth, both in and outside the hospital environment, challenged an assumed physician dominance over birth. Yet, many of the health care providers within institutions stood firm and were not receptive to change (Wertz and Wertz, 1989).

### Competition for Clients

As the total number of births started to decline in the 1970s, competition among doctors and hospitals led to the offering of childbirth options that would attract pregnant couples to a facility. There was an increase in classes for prepared childbirth; birthing rooms within hospitals and birth centers outside of hospitals; and inclusion of maternal support systems and family-centered care before, during, and after the birth experience.

### Expectation of Perfection

During the 1980s and 1990s increasing numbers of middle-class couples planned on having a few children within a specific time frame. These expectations led women to once again turn their birth process over to health care providers and submit to being measured and monitored, being given drugs to speed labor and to control pain, and other interventions as their physicians deemed appropriate.

Other women relinquished control to a physician so they could plan on the delivery date. A scheduled labor induction or surgical delivery allowed them to plan what day their child would be delivered. Within these expectations and care environment, growing numbers of women become passive recipients in their birthing process (Wertz and Wertz, 1989; Rothman, 1989, 1991; Davis-Floyd, 1992).

Our social values continue to shape practices surrounding birth. Along with our culture's fascination with technology is the belief that perfection is possible in the process and outcome of birth. Technology is thought to be the operational link to achieving this perfection.

Childbirth is a rite of passage within our culture. A woman's ultimate perception of her birth experience as positive or negative, empowering or victimizing, depends on the degree to which her experience confirms or undermines her desires and expectations for the experience.

### Infant Outcomes

Looking at the total birth outcomes for women in the United States and comparing it to other countries, reveals that the selection of a medical model of care for birth does not guarantee the successful birth of an infant. In 1997, the U.S. infant mortality rate was 7.2 infant deaths per 1000 live births. This placed us at about eighteenth among the world's nations.

A disparity in outcomes also exists within our country. Mortality rates were lowest for infants born to Asian and Pacific Islander mothers (5.0%), followed by white (6.0%), American-Indian (8.7%), and African-American (13.7%) mothers (CDC, 1998, 1999).

In the United States, we spend more per capita on medical care than any other country. Why does our infant mortality rank higher than countries expending less money yet experiencing better outcomes? Some argue that reliance on a medical system of care that responds after a situation has developed (i.e., dehydration, immobility, and/or fear during labor), rather than preventive care has created more problems than benefits (Tew, 1990; Rothman, 1991; Consumer Reports, 1991, 1992; Goer, 1995). These considerations now challenge us to educate women about their bodies and the birth process, to be with them and their family as they journey through birth, and to assist them to become as actively involved in their birth process as they desire.

## WOMEN'S INVOLVEMENT IN CHILDBIRTH

In this brief history of childbirth practices, socialization emerges as a major factor influencing women's patterns of involvement in the process of pregnancy and childbirth (Davis-Floyd, 1992; Davis-Floyd and Sargent, 1997). **Socialization** is the transfer of socially condoned norms formed by the dominant group to the members of that group (Davis-Floyd, 1992).

Women are socialized to be dependent on medical care throughout their reproductive health cycle (Miles, 1991; Sherwin, 1992). From menarche on, the medical community views a woman's reproductive organs as possible problem areas (Sherwin, 1992). The medical community maintains power and authority over the domain of a woman's health and illness and thus comprises the dominant force in socialization (Miles, 1991; Sherwin, 1992). Women repeatedly select obstetricians and gynecologists (trained surgeons) as their primary health care provider, reflecting the extent to which this has become the cultural belief.

In addition, medical and institutional practices, rules, and regulations have evolved into socially sanctioned rituals that have created an environment whereby women believe they need technologic interventions to proceed through or survive the birth experience (Rothman, 1981, 1991; Shaw, 1974; Romalis, 1981; Oakley, 1984; Eakins, 1986; Wertz and Wertz, 1989; Davis-Floyd, 1992).

Davis-Floyd (1992) examined American birth practices in an ethnographic study. The sample consisted of 100 middle-class women and focused on their first pregnancy. Seventy percent of the women she studied ascribed to the current technologic model of birth. The women's narrative stories revealed that women might not have actually desired a technologic birth, yet they accepted the experience. Of the remaining 30%, 15% desired and were able to achieve a natural birth within the confines of the hospital, and 9% desired but were unable to achieve a natural birth within the hospital setting. The remaining 6% pursued home births.

## Women's Patterns of Involvement

Women and their providers bring various expectations and concerns to the labor and birth experience. Women's expectations of being involved, control of self, control of situation, and satisfaction with birth experience vary from client to client and over time.

### Being Involved

The sense of being involved reflects a woman's desire to participate in decision making related to her care. Some women voice satisfaction in their level of involvement when they are informed of decisions made by the health care providers, thus feeling that they are cared for and correct decisions are being made. Other women need to actually participate in the decision-making process (Davis-Floyd, 1992). Being involved is an individualized concept, representative of differing desires for involvement in decision making, ranging from control over decision making to believing in the correctness of the decisions made (Green, Coupland, and Kitzinger, 1990; Simkin, Whalley, and Keppler, 1991; Davis-Floyd, 1992).

### Control of Self

The sense of being in control relates to a woman's concern with maintaining self-control during the birth process (Mackey, 1990; Simkin, Whalley, and Keppler, 1991; Davis-Floyd, 1992). Women fear that loss of self-control will lead to personal embarrassment and negative feedback from health care providers. Women describe loss of self-control as crying, screaming, and general feelings of helplessness during labor and birth (Mackey, 1990; Davis-Floyd, 1992).

Women identify negative feedback from health care providers as a source of low self-esteem following birth (Simkin, Whalley, and Keppler, 1991). Women have a pervasive desire to "do it right," and want to behave in a socially acceptable manner (Bromberg, 1981).

Mackey (1990) found that women describe "being in control" as having control over their behavior during labor and delivery and behaving in a socially sanctioned manner through labor. "Managing well" was defined as proper application of Lamaze techniques, whereas, "managing poorly" indicated use of negative behaviors such as screaming. Fifty-nine percent of the women felt confident in their ability to manage well, while the remaining 41% were uncertain about their ability to perform in an acceptable manner.

### Control of Situation

Women's desire for control of their situation leads them down varying pathways. Women may verbalize a strong need to maintain control, yet select different ways to gain control. Some women employ medical technology to its fullest, while others seek nurse midwifery care and actively participate in the birth process (Davis-Floyd, 1992).

Women who select nurse-midwives have a different locus of control compared with those who select physicians. Women selecting midwifery care expect to be an active participant and score higher on internal locus of control. Women selecting physician providers do not expect to be as involved and score higher on "powerful others" locus of control (Aaronson, 1987; Littlefield and Adams, 1987; Rothman, 1989, 1991; Davis-Floyd, 1992).

Some women may think their desire for control is an unattainable ideal. Instead they speak of feelings of helplessness, powerlessness, and vulnerability. Feelings of helplessness emerge when the needs of a minority group (pregnant women) are subsumed within the beliefs of the dominant group (medical community). The uncontrollable nature of childbirth and the societal valuing of technology serve to reinforce women's perceived inadequacies to proceed autonomously through the process of birth, creating a dependence on medical control of birth.

## Satisfaction with Involvement

A woman's satisfaction with her birth process is a multidimensional construct. It is related to congruence between the women's belief system and the reality of her birth experience (Davis-Floyd, 1992). A woman's perception of her control over her behavior and the events occurring during the birth process is positively associated her satisfaction with the birth experience. Involvement in decision making, rather than having the sole responsibility for decision making is a key factor in a woman's perception of personal control (Sequin and others, 1989; Green, Coupland, and Kitzinger, 1990; Davis-Floyd, 1992).

## THE DEVELOPMENT OF CHILDBIRTH EDUCATION

Preparation for childbirth dates back to 1908 when the Red Cross incorporated maternal and infant concerns into a course on home health and hygiene (Sasmor, 1979). Prepared childbirth as a movement for social change later evolved from dissatisfaction with existing obstetric care practices.

As society drifted away from thinking of birth as a natural woman's event, several obstetricians, nurses, and activists organized to maintain a women-centered perspective. A series of publications furthered this work. In 1957, the *Ladies Home Journal* published a letter written by an obstetric nurse who described the cruel conditions in an obstetric department. It described the dehumanization of women experiencing childbirth in the hospital (Eakins, 1986; Wertz and Wertz, 1989). Sheila Kitzinger, an anthropologist, and Suzanne Arms, a journalist, researched and wrote consumer-oriented books that explored current childbirth practices and proposed alternative approaches (Arms, 1975). And in 1975, a French doctor addressed the adaptation process of the infant in his book, *A Birth Without Violence* (Leboyer, 1975).

### Initial Programs

#### Natural Childbirth

Birth, as conceptualized by British obstetrician Dr. Grantly Dick-Read, is an instinctive natural process controlled by the woman. He was one of the first physicians to speak out about the medicalization of the birth process (Robertson, 1994). Dick-Read's (1933) publication, *Childbirth Without Fear*, introduced the concept of **natural childbirth**, of which preparation was a key component (Enkin, 1982). Dick-Read presented the concept of the fear-pain-tension cyclic response. His philosophy was that knowledge about childbirth reduces fear, breaking the fear-tension-pain cycle and allowing childbirth to occur naturally. He promoted exercise and the use of two levels of breathing to promote relaxation during labor.

Whether attending a home or hospital birth, he did not consider pain and trauma an inherent aspect of the birth process. Social support was seen as primary to minimize pain and negate the need for anesthesia (Rothman, 1991;

Davis-Floyd, 1992). Natural childbirth classes consist of basic pregnancy and birth information, progressive breathing, and physical and relaxation exercises.

Women who agreed with the philosophy of natural childbirth and desired a natural or unmedicated birth within a hospital often met resistance because of the expectations of the providers within the institution (Rothman, 1991). To most easily achieve a natural birth, women either avoided delivery within institutions or carefully selected providers and attendants who believed in the birth process as a natural function and encouraged and assisted them to maintain control during a birth in a facility (Rothman, 1991; Davis-Floyd, 1992).

#### Bradley Method

In the 1940s, Dr. Robert Bradley developed the **Bradley Method**, which supported the notions of natural birth espoused by Dick-Read. Bradley, also an obstetrician, initiated humanistic changes in birthing routines by making the hospital environment soothing and safe and helping a woman know how to relax during labor. He was the first physician to endorse the active role of the father during the birth process (Davis-Floyd, 1992). The American Academy of Husband Coached Childbirth, founded in 1970, trained childbirth educators in this method. Preparation in the Bradley method, also known as **husband-coached childbirth,** involves transmitting information that enables participants to approach childbirth with a proactive stance. Bradley strongly advocated for woman-controlled childbirth, and his practice supported his beliefs, with a cesarean delivery rate of 3% and a medication rate of 3% (Davis-Floyd, 1993).

The Bradley method, based on a philosophy of holistic care, did not gain wide acceptance by providers within institutional settings for the same reason that natural childbirth was resisted. The childbearing couple was encouraged to remain in charge and the process of birth was allowed to unfold as required by the woman's body and the response of the infant.

#### Lamaze Method

The **psychoprophylactic** (or Lamaze) method originated in 1945 with Russian scientist Nicolaiev (Beck, Geden, and Brouder, 1979). This method is founded upon the tenets of Pavlovian classical conditioning. These concepts were translated to the West in 1952 by Lamaze and Vellay, French obstetricians (Cherok, 1967). Marjorie Karmel and Elizabeth Bing popularized the **Lamaze method** of psychoprophylaxis in the United States (Enkin, 1982) about the same time as interest in the Bradley method was growing.

Dr. Lamaze presented his alternative in *Painless Childbirth: The Lamaze Method,* published in 1956. Lamaze proponents theorize that the painful stimulus of uterine contractions can be blocked by a conditioned response. If the mind is busy concentrating on another activity, the woman would not have as strong a perception of discomfort or pain from her contractions. These classes provide basic anatomy, physiology, and obstetric information; exercises; patterned breathing; and relaxation techniques. Emphasis is placed on distraction techniques to remove or minimize the actual perception of pain.

The Lamaze techniques are based on the technocratic model of birth rather than helping women learn how to trust their instincts (Robertson, 1994). Members of the medical community more readily accepted this technique because it supported the medical model of birth. As stated in the American Society for Psychoprophylaxis training manual, "In all cases the woman should be encouraged to respect her own doctor's word as final. . . . It is most important that his job and hers are completely separate. He is responsible for her physical well-being and that of her baby. She is responsible for controlling herself and her behavior" (Bing and Karmel, 1961). These are the divergent beginnings from which the philosophy of childbirth education has evolved, one branch supporting a holistic model of birth and the other supporting the technocratic model.

## Development of Organizations

With the education of both the providers and the public, interest in childbirth options grew. The **International Childbirth Education Association** (ICEA) emerged in the 1960s to join professionals and consumers together in bringing about change in childbirth practices. The organization advocated "freedom of choice through knowledge of alternatives" and trains childbirth educators who provide information and support to pregnant women and their families.

The **American Society for Psychoprophylaxis (ASPO)** emerged in the early 1970s (Davis-Floyd, 1992). ASPO advocates "prepared-childbirth" and is actively involved in childbirth educator training and consumer education. With a focus that remains within the medical system, women are prepared for the hospital experience of birth and provided with specific techniques to handle labor (Davis-Floyd, 1992).

## Continuing Changes in Childbirth Preparation

During the 1970s prepared childbirth classes were taught both within doctor's offices and hospitals and independently by community groups. Most classes focused on training a woman for birth and taught a prescribed method of dealing with labor and birth. Some of them chose to present information and techniques from the natural childbirth, Bradley, and Lamaze methods so that women could choose to follow the prescribed techniques that met their individual needs. No matter what their emphasis or scope of informa-

tion, all provided information to women on the birthing process and how to cope with labor.

### Overview of Information

In general, information on basic obstetric principles continues to be conveyed. Physical conditioning, relaxation techniques, and patterned breathing remain an integral aspect of preparation programs. Beyond that, the specific content varies with the discretion of each instructor and the perceived needs of their employer, whether physician, institution, or couple.

Although methods vary, some similarities exist. The idea of fear strengthening the perception of pain continues to provide the rationale for the inclusion of information concerning anatomy and physiology and the physical process of birth. The belief that tension increases pain perception provides the rationale for teaching the principles of relaxation. The inclusion of patterned breathing is closely linked to the relaxation process and consistently surfaces in preparation programs.

### Expanded Options

The educated couples pressured hospitals to open up the labor and delivery area to partners and even other members of the family. As couples became more informed about their options for family-centered care, they lobbied increasingly for full participation and more options for birth. Some birthing facilities adopted a more woman-centered perspective in which women are informed and actively engaged in decision making throughout the childbearing and childbirth experience.

In 1975 in his book, *Birth Without Violence,* Dr. Frederick Leboyer promoted the philosophy that the external environment surrounding the birth is important to neonatal adaptation. Following his directives, parents began to push for using soft lights, gentle music, and a warm, comforting environment to ease the infant's transition into life outside the womb. Birth attendants or partners became involved in placing the newborn into a warm water bath immediately following birth.

### New Philosophy

In the early 1980s a philosophy based on women's innate abilities slowly reemerged. Based on observations of women who gave birth in familiar and protective atmospheres, most often their homes, it encouraged and supported each woman in following her natural and personal responses to labor. Rather than learn a specific method of breathing and relaxation, women were increasingly encouraged to learn about and then trust their bodies. During labor they used various innate behaviors, born of instinct and hormonal physiology, to successfully manage their labors (Robertson, 1994).

Sheila Kitzinger (1972, 1979, 1985), an anthropologist and childbirth educator, delineated a psychosexual method of responding to birth. The woman focuses on internal sensory experiences so that she can respond to the signals her body gives her. Being aware of her body enhances the sensuality of childbirth, which some women experience as similar to orgasm. A woman increases her comfort by relaxing through imagery and an inward focus. Her breathing pattern is not predetermined but is the relaxed response to her contractions. She doesn't push until she feels the urge to do so.

Elizabeth Noble, a physical therapist and childbirth educator, also supported the normalcy of birth and encouraging a woman to be aware of her feelings and rely on her ability to respond to labor. She popularized the technique of "gentle pushing" in *Essential Exercises for the Childbearing Year* (1982) and *Childbirth with Insight* (1983).

Dr. Michel Odent, an obstetrician, reinforced the focus on childbirth as a sexual experience and the interaction between members of the new family in *Birth Reborn* (1984). He believed that women could be self-reliant during childbirth because they have an instinct for and innate knowledge of the natural process. He supported women in experiencing childbirth with spontaneity and freedom. In his practice, he used pools of warm water, music, and dim lights to help the woman relax during labor. She was encouraged to assume any position that was comfortable for her during labor and birth. After the birth of the baby, contact between the mother, her family, and the baby was immediate. In some instances the baby was put into a warm bath to relax.

## Current Choices for Childbirth

Now a woman may follow either a natural or technical pathway within a woman-centered perspective; the emphasis is on informed decision making. A woman may choose (1) birth at home, (2) birth in a freestanding birthing center, (3) birth in a birthing center attached to a hospital, (4) birth within a birthing suite in a hospital,

---

### BOX 13-1   *An Empowered Woman*

For a woman to feel empowered within our maternity care system, the following principles must be in place:

- She is fully aware of her rights and responsibilities.
- She is able to exercise her rights and make decisions about care affecting herself and her baby.
- She has the necessary social supports to ensure her physical and emotional well-being.
- She is not discriminated against because of her age, sex, or state of pregnancy.
- Her ability to grow, produce, and nurture her baby is respected and accepted within the framework of birth as a normal bodily function.

---

or (5) birth within a labor and delivery room. However, her choice is still limited by her knowledge of the birth process and what options are available in her area; what is covered by her insurance, if she has insurance; and her personal and cultural beliefs about her body and the birth process.

## Benefit of Childbirth Preparation

The efficacy of childbirth education has been explored in the research literature. Huttel and coworkers (1972) demonstrated a significant relationship between preparation for childbirth using the Lamaze psychoprophylaxis method and decreased use of analgesia in labor. Timm (1979) compared women's choices in labor after participating either in a childbirth preparation class, a knitting class (the placebo), or no class (the control). The study found that the women who attended the childbirth preparation used significantly less amounts of analgesia when compared to the control and placebo groups. No studies have determined that participation in a childbirth preparation session has a negative effect.

## Evolving Curricula

Curricula of childbirth preparation programs continue to vary. Some are designed to give information and ensure compliance with the woman's chosen provider and facility. Others engage and support the woman in making her own choices and participating to the level she desires in advocating for her own needs. The most recent variation is a new philosophic approach to birth, termed "active birth." Here the woman is empowered to give birth using her own resources and abilities (Robertson, 1994) (Box 13-1). The prenatal class helps the parents develop the skills needed to obtain the kind of birth they desire. Didactic lectures of information and advice are replaced with a flexible teaching approach based on the individual parent's goals, practical problem solving, and the development of communication and negotiating skills they will need. Birth is viewed, not as an end point, but rather as a step in becoming a parent (Robertson, 1994).

Having various education and preparation options from which to choose is necessary because women's personal and cultural beliefs vary. Appropriate and responsive classes to prepare for childbirth result in a woman's increased satisfaction with the birth (Mackey, 1990; Strychar and others, 1990).

## SOCIAL SUPPORT DURING THE CHILDBEARING YEAR

Positive outcomes are associated with social support networks for pregnant women during the childbearing year (the 9 months of pregnancy plus the first 3 months postpartum). During pregnancy social support enables a woman to share her joys and concerns with others and receive both information and validation. Family members, friends, coworkers, and providers can provide this support.

During labor and birth, social support has been associated with decreased length of labor, decreased use of epidural and other analgesic drugs, a reduction in oxytocin use, a reduction in surgical deliveries, increased feelings of maternal satisfaction with the birth experience, and increased interactions with the newborn. Information sharing, advocacy, tangible assistance including physical comfort measures, and emotional support are dimensions of support generally included under the broader concept of social support (Sosa and others, 1980; Bloom, 1990; Kennel and others, 1991; Gagnon, Waghorn, and Covell, 1997).

## Support from Family and Friends

To provide assistance and support during the labor and delivery process, one or more people may attend childbirth classes with the pregnant woman. It is through this process that they become aware of the woman's wishes for her birth experience and learn how to support her desires. Included in the childbirth preparation may be the woman's partner, and/or other female friends.

The woman's partner may or may not decide to take an active role in providing care to the woman during labor, but just his or her presence may offer her support through the process. Others may choose not to or cannot attend classes with the woman. The comfort level and desires of both partners are to be considered. Some cultures prohibit males from being present at births and rely on women to provide support through the labor and birth.

## Support from Specialists

During the perinatal period, a woman and her family may receive support from several providers, each having a different expertise. Each provider may offer different philosophies of care and depth of knowledge in specific areas, so the woman and her family can select the support and care that meets their unique requirements.

### Support During Pregnancy

During her pregnancy the woman may receive care from a childbirth educator to learn about pregnancy and her needs during pregnancy and to start to prepare for the birth. If she decides to breastfeed her baby, she may seek the services of a lactation consultant. Prenatal assessments of the health status of the woman and her baby may be provided by a nurse practitioner, either specializing in women's health or family, a certified nurse midwife or a direct entry midwife, or a physician.

### Selecting a Provider for Childbirth

Care providers attend labors and deliveries in hospitals, birthing centers, and homes. The team of providers that supports a woman during pregnancy, labor, and birth strives to empower the mother to take responsibility for herself, her baby, and her birth. Providers that empower women:

* Believe childbearing to be a fundamentally healthy and normal part of a woman's psychosocial life
* Treat women holistically, taking their thoughts, feelings, concerns, and priorities into consideration
* Respect the woman's right to make informed decisions for herself and her baby
* Respect labor as an experience with its own lessons and rewards
* Offer supportive care rather than intervening with their own desires
* Assess individually and do not treat by rules and regulations
* Start small when intervention becomes necessary
* Keep abreast of the research (Goer, 1995).

### Support During Childbirth

Where a woman chooses to deliver her baby determines the providers available to her. Some women choose the provider they want and then make plans to deliver where he or she provides care. Others select where they want to give birth and then seek a provider. Attendants during labor may be a doula or monitrice hired to provide support to the childbearing woman, nurses who specialize in assessing women in labor, a certified nurse midwife, or a direct entry midwife. A certified nurse midwife, direct entry midwife, family practice physician, or an obstetrician may provide care during the birth itself.

The term **doula** is of Greek origin and means "woman servant." Doulas are becoming a familiar part of the birthing woman's support system for home, birth center, and hospital births. They provide information, emotional support, physical comfort measures, and advocacy during the pregnancy, birth, and postpartum period. A doula does not replace the woman's partner, but she assists the partner as desired and provides care to both the woman and the partner. A doula may be educated and certified for this role as a member of the labor support team by one of two organizations, the Doulas of North America (DoNA) or the International Childbirth Education Association (ICEA). Some certified childbirth educators are also certified doulas. Families that desire this help contract with and pay the doula for these services.

A **monitrice**, the term is of French origin, may be present instead of a doula to provide labor support. A monitrice has the clinical skills to provide both nursing care

## BOX 13-2 *Options for Care Providers*

Health care providers differ in the services and level of care they provide. Women commonly choose a network of providers that includes a combination of the following:

**Obstetrician:** A physician/surgeon who specializes in the care of women during pregnancy, labor, and the postpartum.

**Pediatrician:** A physician who specializes in infants and children.

**Family doctor:** A physician who cares for the whole family; some provide care during pregnancy, labor, and the postpartum.

**Certified nurse midwife:** A licensed registered nurse with additional education who specializes in providing women with care throughout the life cycle, including during pregnancy, birth, and postpartum of low-risk mothers and babies.

**Direct-entry midwife:** A provider trained in the care of a woman during pregnancy, birth, and the postpartum who has passed an examination and received a license from the state to provide this care.

**Women's health nurse practitioner:** A licensed registered nurse with advanced education who specializes in providing women with care throughout a woman's life cycle—including pregnancy and the postpartum, but not during the birth process.

**Family nurse practitioner:** A licensed registered nurse with advanced education in family health care, providing care throughout the family's life cycle, not including the birth.

**Childbirth educators:** A person, who may or may not be certified, who provides information about pregnancy, childbirth, and the postpartum and assists pregnant woman and their support network to make the decisions they need to have the experience they desire. Preparation avenues for being a childbirth educator vary.

**Lactation consultant:** A person with specialized education to assist women and their babies with breastfeeding who has passed a credentialing examination and maintains requirements for being a lactation consultant.

**Breastfeeding specialist:** A person with a special interest and knowledge in breastfeeding.

**Doula:** A person with specialized education and experience in assisting women and their families during the pregnancy, birth, and postnatal period. They may achieve certification and maintain their level of expertise through a specialty organization.

**Monitrice:** A nurse who has the clinical skills and experience to provide both nursing care and labor support on an individual basis to a childbearing woman.

If a woman or her baby is at risk, the following providers might also become part of the team:

**Perinatologist:** A physician who specializes in high-risk pregnancy and birth.

**Neonatologist:** A physician who specializes in premature and sick babies.

---

and labor support. Nurses often feel that they need to be doing something to be helpful, but the monitrice's role is different. When assisting women journeying through labor the most important thing a monitrice can offer the clients is patience and calm. Patience prevents the monitrice from interfering when nothing is really helpful except time and a belief in the natural process.

Nurses, nurse midwives, and physicians may also provide continuous or periodic support during the labor and delivery process. However, because of other role expectations, this is not their primary role unless they are specifically hired by the couple to do so. A normal labor can extend well beyond 14 hours, covering more time than would normally be considered a shift or the amount of time that a nurse, nurse midwife, or physician could devote solely to one client (Box 13-2).

### PLANNING PREPARED CHILDBIRTH CLASSES

**Preparation for childbirth** has been defined as a program of instruction based on a theoretic framework, with specific objectives and structured content (Cogan,

1981; Hassid, 1984). An integrated, flexible approach to preparing women for childbirth is necessary to meet diverse needs. Incorporating various options does not pose an insurmountable task, nor does it incur significant costs (Figure 13-1).

Formal childbirth class offerings should be tailored to the needs of a particular community. Originally childbirth classes were offered once a week for 6 or 8 weeks, with individual class sessions lasting 2 to 2½ hours. Today a wide variety of class format options are offered. Childbirth classes may range from 12 weeks with the Bradley format to a two-session hospital-based class. Another format is the weekend session format in which class is held for two 4-hour periods over 2 weekend days.

Class size is an important consideration. Small groups of 10 or fewer women and their labor supporter tend to be more interactive and facilitate learning. Large class size can inhibit group participation, reduce the ability for individualization and discussion, and reduce the effectiveness of practice sessions. A program schedule with options daytime, evening, and weekend sessions offers the best opportunity for many women and their partners to be able to participate.

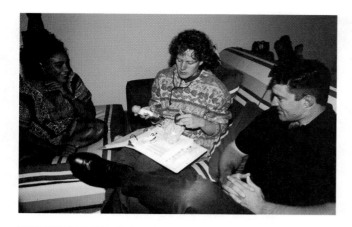

FIGURE 13-1 • Home visit instruction for upcoming parents. *(Courtesy of Caroline E. Brown.)*

It is optimal if class participants share somewhat similar age and educational levels, interests, cultural backgrounds, and expectations of the experience. When a class is randomly grouped with a wide variation in age or language, the groups dynamic are altered and the educational process is impaired.

## Content

Childbirth instructors typically feel the need to teach participants all there is to know about pregnancy, nutrition, labor and delivery, postpartum care, and newborn care. The appropriateness of this has been disputed, and the current trend is to focus on the needs of the woman herself and her understanding of the labor and birth process, with minimal information on postpartum and newborn care.

Content guidelines for childbirth preparation programs have been established to correlate with the four maternal tasks of pregnancy identified by Rubin (1984). Most commonly childbirth preparation itself occurs during the third trimester, however the educational process may begin with introductory classes earlier in pregnancy.

### Classes in the First Trimester

During the first trimester, the woman focuses on herself and ambivalence to pregnancy. When early pregnancy classes are designed, the content generally includes nutritional information, physiologic changes to the mother, dental care needs, maternal and fetal risk factors, and anticipated psychologic changes (Box 13-3).

### Classes in the Second Trimester

The maternal focus shifts during the second trimester, focusing more on the pregnancy as the infant becomes a reality. The mother begins to show interest in learning and to prepare for her new role. Classes during this period of time are uncommon. If desired, they would in-

---

### BOX 13-3   *Possible Content in Early Pregnancy Classes*

Although the actual content may vary depending on the specific needs of attendees, potential topics for an early pregnancy class include the following:

- Normal physiology of pregnancy
- Fetal growth and development
- Physical and emotional adaptation to pregnancy
- Prenatal testing and care
- Nutritional considerations
- Lifestyle considerations
- Common discomforts and relief measures
- Warning signs and how to respond
- Rights and responsibilities as a care consumer
- Choices in birth attendants and birth place
- Role of health care providers
- Possible roles of family members and friends

---

clude content on fetal growth and development, proper body mechanics, comfort measures, considerations for intimacy, and evolving roles.

### Classes in the Third Trimester

The maternal focus during the third trimester is the closure of pregnancy, her concern about and preparation for labor, and completing preparations for the infant. Childbirth preparation classes are generally conducted during this time. Content includes maternal and fetal risk factors, psychologic and physiologic changes, danger signs and how to respond, feelings about labor and the developing infant, signs of onset of labor, responding to labor and delivery, comfort measures during labor, support during delivery, the situation of cesarean birth, and establishment of family-centered care (Box 13-4).

### Classes in the Postpartum

Once the class members have gone through preparation classes together, they generally develop a bond and often desire to continue meeting as they take on their new parenting roles. Postpartum classes are conducted during the fourth trimester or postpartum phase and focus on the completion of the birth process and a shifting of concern to the infant. Content during this phase may include infant caretaking skills, parenting, family planning, role transition, and intimacy (Box 13-5).

## The Learning Climate

To be able to receive the information you are sharing, participants must feel physically and emotionally comfortable. Physical barriers to paying attention and learning are the comfort of the seat, the quality of the air, the

---

**BOX 13-4** *Possible Content in Late Pregnancy Classes*

Although the actual content may vary depending on the specific needs of attendees, potential topics for a late pregnancy class include the applicable information that may be provided in early pregnancy classes, plus the following:

- Normal physiology of late pregnancy
- Common discomforts and relief measures
- Birth process
  - Signs
  - Stages and physiology
  - Variations of normal
- Management of labor
  - Comfort measures
  - Relaxation skills
  - Breathing techniques
- Positions to facilitate birth process
- Role of labor supporters
- Role of health care providers
- Options for place of birth and expected routines (home, birthing center, hospital)
- Preparation/participation of sibling(s) of baby
- Guidelines for birth and birth options
- Analgesia and anesthesia
- Medical procedures with benefits, risks, alternatives
  - Induction of labor
  - "Nothing by mouth" directive
  - Intravenous fluids
  - Electronic fetal monitoring
  - Episiotomy
  - Forceps or vacuum extraction

- Preparation for unexpected occurrences
- Cesarean delivery
  - Indications
  - Surgical procedure
  - Anesthesia options
  - Role of labor supporter
  - Postoperative course
  - Implications for future pregnancies
- Postpartum considerations
  - Immediate reaction to birth
  - Postpartum assessment and care: explanation of routines and options
  - Physical and emotional changes
  - Integration of the family in the home
  - Exercises to regain comfort and strength
- Care of the newborn
  - Immediate assessment and care
  - Needs and characteristics
  - Initiation of infant feeding
  - Initiation of parental care
  - Providing for the health and safety of the newborn
- Parenting
  - Expectations of self and others
  - Emotional adjustments
  - Resumption of sexual relationship and social relationships
  - Understanding of community resources

---

ease of access to a bathroom, and the temperature of the room. Before deciding where to hold a class, evaluate the possible space to see how it will meet the needs of pregnant women. Encouraging couples to bring extra pillows and wear comfortable clothing can increase their physical comfort.

Emotional and psychologic comfort are also important. Pregnancy can bring a wide range of emotional reactions and heightened psychologic needs. Couples may be puzzled about the childbearing process, combined with curiosity, anxiety, excitement, fear, concern, and confusion over the process. When these feeling are shared with a class, a collegial atmosphere can develop. "Anxieties and worries may be reduced if they are acknowledged, and it may be possible to eliminate some altogether if solutions can be found for problems, or questions can be answered with factual information" (Robertson, 1994).

Be warm, friendly, relaxed, and hospitable. Create a permissive atmosphere so that people can talk about deep feelings in a safe, nonjudgmental atmosphere, without fear of recrimination or adverse reaction from others. Maintain confidentiality when you learn things that the participant has not shared with the group as a whole.

Make no assumptions about the participants because this disempowers them. The only assumption we can safely make about another woman is that she is an individual, with needs, reactions, feelings and responses that are uniquely hers. To be supportive and empowering, we must accept our clients as they are, stay open to their individual uniqueness, and help them explore choices.

## Methodology

### Adults as Learners

Adults bring a wide range of life experiences with them to a learning encounter. They generally have a vision of themselves and seek out specific information when they perceive a need. This means that they present with a readiness to learn and a desire to apply that knowledge in a practical manner within a real life orientation. Factors that may have a positive influence on their learning are linkage of new information with past information and experiences, an opportunity for active participation and immediate feedback when applying new knowledge or skills, continuing reinforcement of learning, and an acknowledgement of their emotional response to the material to be learned.

### Adult Education Techniques

Adult teaching methods are used during childbirth preparation programs to present information ranging from anatomy and physiology to initial parenting concerns. The use of imagery, flexible breathing patterns, and relaxation techniques are integrated into the class format (Kitzinger, 1977).

A primary assumption when teaching adults is that the learner and the instructor are involved in an interactive, educational process. Adults are problem-focused learners with a need to immediately apply information. They are self-directed, have past experiences to draw from, and a readiness to learn based on their need for the information (Renner, 1994). These factors must be considered when designing classes.

***Multiple Types of Presentations.*** Lecture, discussion, and demonstration are commonly used within childbirth preparation classes. Using short lectures geared to the educational level of the learners is an effective means of providing information in a uniform and timely way. The lecture format can be augmented with visual aids to facilitate identification and highlight important aspects of the lecture. The disadvantage of a lecture format is that communication is unilateral, reducing group participation. The addition of discussion to the educational session encourages the sharing of past experiences and enhances active participation and problem solving (Rorden, 1987).

Demonstrations are used to present psychomotor skills such as the stretching exercises, relaxation and breathing patterns, positions for labor and birth, techniques for breastfeeding, and so on. Return demonstrations are a means to evaluate a participant's understanding of skill-based learning content.

Audiovisual tools are an integral aspect of childbirth preparation. Audiovisual aids reinforce learning and en-

gage another sense in the learning process. Posters and models are useful adjuncts to enhance the effectiveness of lecture. Videotapes of labor and birth are a common part of childbirth education classes. It is important to allow time for discussion of reactions to the videotape shown.

***Participation and Rehearsal.*** The use of role play and rehearsal immediately facilitate use of learned information, encourage group participation, and allow participants to engage in problem solving in a safe environment. Role-play techniques can be facilitated with the use of simple teaching aides. One example is the use of 5 x 7 inch index cards each illustrating a different physical position, the benefits of the position, and when to use the position in labor and birth (Brown and Shocker, 1995). The cards are distributed to class participants with instructions to try out the position on their card. After a time of practice the participants are asked to share with the group the information on the card, describe how the position felt in practice, and how it could be used in childbirth.

The use of rehearsal techniques, such as responding to simulated contractions with relaxation and breathing techniques also assists in the learning and evaluation processes. Cognitive rehearsal facilitates a person's ability to rehearse specific aspects of the event, thus decreasing anxiety with a resultant increase in pain tolerance.

## TEACHING PREPARATION FOR CHILDBIRTH

Comprehensive childbirth education realistically prepares the woman for the labor and birth process; therefore, it must be more than instructions about what to do and procedures to follow in labor. It should be based on a holistic philosophy that birth is a biologic, psychologic, and social event and that women and their partners have inner strengths and resources they may use during labor and delivery. Part of the goal of educational preparation is to help them become aware of these inner strengths (Perez, 1997).

### Becoming a Childbirth Educator

Teaching preparation for childbirth classes requires a set of specialized skills and knowledge. These may be obtained through informal or formal mechanisms. Quality assurance is maintained through certification programs and ongoing professional development.

### Certification

Various organizations provide a process for certifying childbirth educators. Certification indicates to potential students that a given set of competencies about childbearing and childbirth have been achieved and maintained. The particular route an individual chooses for certification depends on individual preferences, time, convenience, and cost. The American Society for Psychoprophylaxis and the ICEA are examples of organizations offering options for childbirth certification.

## Education for Childbirth Education

Each certifying body has its own individual educational pathway established. Knowledge of educational techniques as well as knowledge of childbearing, childbirth, and early child care are common competencies required for the childbirth educator. Familiarity with adult learning principles, instructional design, teaching strategies, and evaluation of learner needs and the efficacy of the program is necessary. Some programs accept professionals already educated in one area and provide in-depth instruction in the other. For example, experienced teachers learn the aspects of birth, or nurses learn the role and activities of teachers. Some programs conduct formal classes, while others arrange for distance learning or modular home study. There are various ways for committed individuals to become certified childbirth educators.

## Roles of the Childbirth Educator

Advocacy, support, and informational exchange are the three focal areas of the childbirth educator. **Advocacy** is the process of informing and supporting a woman so that she may actively participate in the decision related to her health care. **Support** encompasses both emotional buttressing and reassurance. **Informational exchange** is your most obvious role as a childbirth educator. Class information incorporates content focusing on childbearing as well as community resources.

The childbirth educator functions as a part of the pregnant woman's health care network, along with other health care providers, labor support assistants,

and with the pregnant woman's support network of family members and friends. As a childbirth educator, you may also collaborate with individuals, groups, or others within the community at large to advocate for a broad scope of childbirth options.

## Professional Development

Professional development begins with the initial learning process of becoming a childbirth educator. However, this process is only the beginning of a career-long commitment of personal growth and development in both educational techniques and the expanding research-based pool of knowledge concerning pregnancy, childbirth, and the adaptation to parenthood.

## The Language of Empowerment

The words we use in the health care system can dehumanize the participants, create barriers to understanding, and project a negative image on the woman (Kahn, 1995; Davis-Floyd and Sargent, 1997). In addition to the words, how we say them, our nonverbal behavior, and the connotations given to them by the listener all affect how the listener perceives what we say.

Many words commonly used to discuss the process of labor and birth are derived from medical usage and therefore have the connotation of describing a problem rather than a healthy, normal situation. Some very simple changes in our selection of words can make a difference in how class attendees relate to the topic (Table 13-1).

Unless we carefully select our words, the pregnant women are coerced into adopting a medical view of labor and birth each time we use a medical term to describe a process. Given the insidious and pervasive nature of the masculine view, and the medical, problem-oriented

| TABLE 13-1 *The Use of Normalizing Terms* | |
|---|---|
| **Commonly used** | **Try instead** |
| Fetus | Baby |
| Contractions (of the uterus) | Expansions (of the cervix) |
| Cesarean section | Cesarean birth |
| Labor | Birth process, birth journey (as appropriate) |
| Delivery | Birth |
| Antenatal | Prenatal |
| Class | Group, session, discussion |
| Coping (with labor, pain, etc.) | Managing (labor, pain, etc.) |
| Birth plan | Guidelines for birth |

Robertson A: *Empowering women—teaching active birth in the 90s,* Camperdown, Australia, 1994, ACE Graphics.

| TABLE 13-2 *The Use of Positive Terms* | |
|---|---|
| **Commonly used** | **Try instead** |
| Adequate pelvis | Capable pelvis |
| Failure to progress | Pause in labor |
| Expected date of confinement | Approximate birth date |
| Incompetent cervix | Elastic cervix |
| Girls, ladies | Women |
| Trial of labor | Vaginal birth after previous cesarean birth |
| Class | Group, session, discussion |
| Control (of anything) during labor | Eliminate from use—birth is uncontrollable |
| Losing (lost) a baby | The baby died |

Robertson A: *Empowering women—teaching active birth in the 90s,* Camperdown, Australia, 1994, ACE Graphics.

language often used today in midwifery and obstetrics, it will be hard for women to feel empowered and confident (Robertson, 1994).

Some words can inadvertently convey negative messages to women about the natural process of birth and their ability to be successful. Replace negative phrases and terms with terms that reflect a more feminine and positive approach to the events of labor and birth, supporting the woman's ability to give birth (Table 13-2).

## Learning Needs

The perceived needs of the learner are an important consideration when engaging someone in a learning activity. Women who have prior experiences with childbearing and childbirth will have different learning needs than women experiencing a first pregnancy. As educators we must strike a balance between the information we determine to be important and the information the learner desires to learn. We need to be flexible to accommodate both the learner who brings ideas about what they are interested in learning and the learner who has limited experience and is interested in being guided through the learning experience.

## Designing Educational Sessions

"The traditional teacher-student power imbalance is familiar to everyone who as attended school at any level. The teacher has the power to . . . offer opinions and judgements, and to speak. The student is . . . defined as a receiver of the teacher's opinions and judgements, and

the listener. Overcoming these expectations for roles and behavior is not easy" (Wheeler and Chinn, 1991) but must be accomplished to develop educational sessions that truly meet the needs of the attendees. "Two values . . . consistently welcomed by classroom participants are empowerment for all and demystification of content and processes" (Wheeler and Chinn, 1991). It may be helpful as you develop a series of informational and practice sessions to consider the type of power you are assuming as the convener of the group (Table 13-3).

When developing a teaching plan, it helps to take a broad view of the purpose, which is to work with people making the transition to parenthood. This process becomes easier when the parents have "specific skills, such as:

- the ability to solve problems and make decisions,
- knowledge of resources and how they may be used,
- stress management techniques,
- flexibility in their approach and thinking,
- confidence in their competence as parents, and
- an ability to recognize their limitations" (Robertson, 1994).

Most adults have some or all of these skills because of their life experiences. They just may need to become aware of the transferability of prior learning and experiences to the role of parenting. Pregnant adolescents are less likely to have developed these skills and may need more time and attention (Figure 13-2).

Attendees may come to class with different agendas from you, the convener, and each other. "As an educator,

## TABLE 13-3  *Shifting the Power in the Learning Process*

| Replace the power of . . . | With the power of . . . |
|---|---|
| Results | Process |
| Prescription | Letting self-knowledge and cooperation emerge |
| Division created by the hoarding of knowledge and skills | The whole to encourage the flow of new ideas, images, and energy from all |
| Force for or against another | Collectivity that values the personal power of each individual |
| Hierarchy and a linear chain of command | Unity and shared responsibility for decision making and actions |
| Command in which others are made passive | Sharing that encourages leadership to shift |
| Opposites that polarize issues and lead to value judgments | Integration, which views situations without value judgments |
| Use of resources and people | Nurturing life and experiences |
| Accumulation of things | Distribution of resources |
| Causality through technology without regard to the consequences | Intuition and self-knowledge |
| Expediency | Consciousness of long-range outcomes and ethical behaviors |
| Xenophobia (the fear of strangers) | Diversity to encourage creativity, alternative views, and flexibility |
| Secrets and mystification of the process | Responsibility and demystification of the process |

Adapted from Wheeler C and Chinn P: *Peace and power*, ed 3, New York, 1991, NLN.

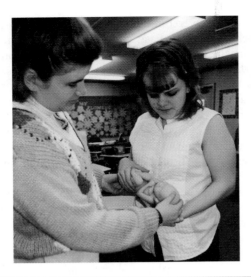

FIGURE 13-2 • School-board childbirth and parenting classes for pregnant adolescent girls.

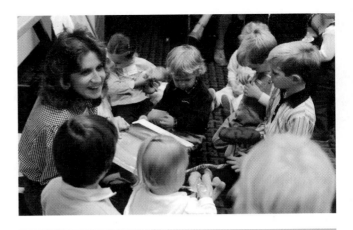

FIGURE 13-3 • Sibling classes.

you have a responsibility to meet not only your own aims and objectives, but also those of your client or group, enabling them to meet . . . their own goals" (Robertson, 1994). It is not always easy to determine the expectations and needs of your clients. They may be unsure about what they need to know or uncertain about what is appropriate for them to ask. As they begin to participate in the sessions and you arouse their curiosity, inspiring them to seek further information and take responsibility for their own learning, they will express new needs. As these needs become apparent, incorporate them into the objectives of the sessions.

### Classes for Family and Friends

Reaching out to family support networks is another important consideration for educators helping to prepare families for childbirth and a new baby. Specialty classes may be designed for grandparents, fathers, siblings, and members of the labor support network. By educating interested family members and friends, the childbearing couple gains support for their desires and endeavors, making this transitional process much smoother (Figure 13-3).

 ### Addressing Different Learning Styles

We primarily take in information through our eyes and ears, supplemented by the rest of our senses. By the time we are adults we have a preference for learning through one or more modes. The members of each learning group will have different preferences, so when devising ways to present information and developing learning activities, various methods must be used so that everyone receives the desired information.

**Visual learners** like pictures, demonstrations, models, videos, and written handouts. Try to present as much information as possible using one of these formats. They also appreciate being able to takes notes, using questionnaires and worksheets, and having written references or reading materials to take home. They use their eyes to take in information, so face them when you talk, use examples and statistics, and allow time for them to visualize situations.

**Auditory learners** use their sense of hearing as their primary way of taking in information. They like to talk things over, debate issues, and participate in discussions, as well as hear the experiences of others and listen to stories. They are especially attune to the music and words spoken on the videos. Sometimes they will look down or close their eyes when someone is speaking so that they may listen more intently. Present information using a story format, provide opportunities for discussion, and make audiotapes available for their use outside the classroom.

**Kinesthetic learners** prefer experiences that engage all of their senses. They learn most readily through practice sessions, physical movement, role playing, tours of facilities, and demonstrations. Your teaching methods should include exercise sessions; practice of techniques and positions; handling models; and role playing, with the participants being as physically involved as possible.

Even though an adult may have a preferred learning style, each tends to take in information in more than one way. Because any group of learners will have a mixture of learning styles, it is important to include various methods that will appeal to everyone. Plan to present your material in at least three different ways so that each person in the class receives your message. At the same time, be sensitive to individual preferences regarding participation. Some may wish to talk, while others prefer just to listen; some may wish to be involved in games and activities, while others prefer to sit and watch. Structuring situations so that attendees may comfortably choose their own level of participation helps accommodate individual preferences (Table 13-4).

**TABLE 13-4   Responsibilities of the Educator and the Client**

| Educator responsibilities | Client responsibilities |
|---|---|
| Set up the group | Attend the group |
| Serve as a resource | Use the resources |
| Devise a program appropriate to client needs | Make use of the information provided |
| Take into account the differing learning styles within the group | Learn |
| Empower clients to make decisions | Make decisions |
| Be aware of own needs | Be aware of own needs |
| Be open, nonjudgmental, and flexible | Deal with emotional baggage |
| Provide what the group wants to get the job done | Cooperate to the get the best from what is offered |
| Be resourceful | Be resourceful |

Adapted from Robertson A: *Empowering women—teaching active birth in the 90s,* Camperdown, Australia, 1994, ACE Graphics.

## Evaluation of Benefit of Sessions

Evaluation is a continuous and systematic process that incorporates various outcome criteria. The goals and objectives of the educational program as well as the activities, exercises, and discussions planned for the sessions should all fit the broad agenda of obtaining these desired knowledge and skills. A **summative evaluation** of the success of the program is based on the degree to which participants feel satisfied at the end of the sessions with the information and skills they have acquired. It should not be based on things over which you have no control, such as birth outcomes and parenting behaviors because these are influenced by many factors beyond your control.

If at the end of the series the attendees have the knowledge they desire, feel comfortable making decisions, can better manage stress, can remain flexible in their approach and thinking, and have confidence in their competence while being aware of their strengths and limitations, they can better handle the process of birth and parenting. The summative feedback serves as a reference for ongoing revision of the program.

The evaluation process also includes formative components. **Formative evaluation** is incorporated throughout the educational process beginning with an informal needs assessment during the first class and followed with ongoing feedback and discussion. This feedback serves to guide the focus of the specific class and subsequent classes within the series.

Evaluation data are collected using both formal and informal methods. A formal evaluation may be completed during the final class of a series. The focus may be on attainment of objectives, effectiveness of the methodology used, and an overall impression of the course and suggestions for additional content or approaches for teaching.

The postpartum or reunion class may be held after all the babies are born. This class is generally designed to be a celebration of birth and provides an ample time for participants to recount their experience and elaborate on the components of the class they found most applicable.

## CONTENT INCLUDED IN THE PREPARATION PROCESS

Not all members of the health care team are, or need to be, capable of teaching childbirth preparation sessions. However, all members of the team need to be aware of the scope of what is covered so they will understand how women are prepared. The following sections give an overview of the information presented in childbirth preparation classes and some of the rationale for doing so. The amount and focus of information and the way it is presented vary, based on the teacher's knowledge and skills and attendees' needs, desires, and learning styles.

### The Pregnant Patient's Bill of Rights and Responsibilities

With knowledge and the right to make choices also comes the assumption of responsibility. *The Pregnant Patient's Bill of Rights and Responsibilities* by the ICEA (see Appendix I) provides clients with a basis from which to start to think about and plan for their childbirth experience. Participation in preparation classes may help couples determine how they will participate in their pregnancy, their desires for the birth experience, and the choices they will make as they assume the parenting role. Their choices and sense of empowerment will lead to the choice of a location for birth and the selection of the providers who will collaborate with them to meet their needs.

### Selecting Birth Preferences

Birth preference lists, sometimes called birth plans, are a written communication tool highlighting a woman's preferences, desires, and beliefs for her pregnancy, the birth, and her newly born infant. They are not so much a script or a legal contract, but rather a tool to learn about birth options and an aid to demystify labor and the birthing experience. Developing a personalized list can help a woman and her partner think through their options together and then communicate these preferences to a potential health care team. Learning their options and establishing what they envision for their birth are outcomes of attending childbirth preparation sessions.

Common formats for organizing and sharing this information include a narrative description, a checklist, or a summary outlining important points. The length and readability of the document is an important consideration. However, it can include anything the woman feels is an import consideration for her care (Table 13-5).

Common points addressed include who is to be present at the birth, the birth environment, the roles of the attendants during the process of labor and birth, and expected care of the mother and infant following the birth. Choices regarding the birth environment include issues such as privacy, desire and preference for music and/or aroma therapy, desire to wear personal clothing, and provisions for a gentle birth with low light and water available in a bath. The discussion about labor and birth can incorporate preferences for eating and drinking, movement and positioning, if and how the baby's heart rate will be monitored, process of deciding about an amniotomy, comfort and pain management strategies, and the desire for an episiotomy. The infant and maternal care section can address where the initial evaluation of the infant will take place, desire for skin-to-skin contact for infant thermoregulation, timing of the

---

**TABLE 13-5** *Example of a Birth Preference List*

Developing a birth preference list is important to determine what factors are important to the woman and what options are available. The following list is not all-inclusive but gives an idea of some of the choices a pregnant woman may make. If she chooses to not make a decision, she is by default making a decision.

| Choice | I would like to have | | Available | |
|---|---|---|---|---|
| **Care provider:** | | | | |
| Certified nurse-midwife | yes | no | yes | no |
| Direct entry midwife | yes | no | yes | no |
| Family physician | yes | no | yes | no |
| Obstetrician | yes | no | yes | no |
| **Birth setting:** | | | | |
| Birth center | yes | no | yes | no |
| Hospital | yes | no | yes | no |
| Birthing room | yes | no | yes | no |
| Labor/delivery room | yes | no | yes | no |
| Home | yes | no | yes | no |
| **Environment:** | | | | |
| Dimmed lights | yes | no | yes | no |
| Voices respectfully lowered | yes | no | yes | no |
| **Partner present:** | | | | |
| During labor | yes | no | yes | no |
| During birth | yes | no | yes | no |
| During cesarean delivery | yes | no | yes | no |
| During the immediate postpartum | yes | no | yes | no |
| **During labor I wish to:** | | | | |
| Ambulate as desired | yes | no | yes | no |
| Shower if desired | yes | no | yes | no |
| Wear own clothes | yes | no | yes | no |
| Use hot tub | yes | no | yes | no |
| Use a rocking chair | yes | no | yes | no |
| Have fluid or ice as desired | yes | no | yes | no |
| Have food as desired | yes | no | yes | no |
| Have music during labor and birth | yes | no | yes | no |
| **With regard to medical interventions:** | | | | |
| Internal exams at a minimum | yes | no | yes | no |
| Membranes | yes | no | yes | no |
| Rupture naturally | yes | no | yes | no |
| Amniotomy if needed | yes | no | yes | no |

first bath, timing of the eye prophylaxis, maternal care following birth, and teaching and support.

Many resources for learning about birthing options are available. Some interactive personalized birth plans are available on the Internet. Once the couple has determined what is important to them, they seek out providers who have a philosophy and practice that matches their own. Ultimately the agreed-upon wishes will be shared in writing with the providers, the birthplace staff, and the birth partner.

### Body Mechanics and Prenatal Exercises

As a woman's body gradually changes during pregnancy, attention must be paid to maintaining balance and good posture, not only for comfort but also for safety reasons. Body mechanics and various prenatal strengthening and conditioning exercises are taught to women to increase their comfort level during the last trimester of pregnancy and their flexibility and comfort during labor. Other prenatal exercises focus on specific areas of the body and are intended for use both before and after the baby is born.

### Body Mechanics

During pregnancy a woman will be more comfortable if she maintains good posture. Good posture means not only standing and walking so that the baby is cradled in the pelvis, but also performing everyday movements in a way that avoids unnecessary strain. To achieve good posture, she needs to improve the tone of her muscles and learn how to use only those muscles that are necessary as she moves through her daily activities (Figure 13-4).

The human backbone is curved. Because of this, the increasing size of the abdomen may put a strain on the

| TABLE 13-5 *Example of a Birth Preference List—cont'd* | | | | |
|---|---|---|---|---|
| **Choice** | **I would like to have** | | **Available** | |
| Labor stimulation, if needed | yes | no | yes | no |
| Intermittent fetal monitoring | yes | no | yes | no |
| Fetoscope | yes | no | yes | no |
| Doppler | yes | no | yes | no |
| Electronic monitoring | yes | no | yes | no |
| Continuous fetal monitoring | yes | no | yes | no |
| Medication | yes | no | yes | no |
| Type _____ | yes | no | yes | no |
| Episiotomy | yes | no | yes | no |
| **Position during second stage:** | | | | |
| Squatting | yes | no | yes | no |
| Hands and knees | yes | no | yes | no |
| Kneeling | yes | no | yes | no |
| Water birth | yes | no | yes | no |
| Birthing bed | yes | no | yes | no |
| Birthing chair | yes | no | yes | no |
| On side | yes | no | yes | no |
| **Family friend participation:** | | | | |
| Family members present | yes | no | yes | no |
| Filming of birth | yes | no | yes | no |
| Partner to cut umbilical cord | yes | no | yes | no |
| **Choices during third stage:** | | | | |
| Hold baby immediately after birth | yes | no | yes | no |
| Breastfeed immediately after birth | yes | no | yes | no |
| Keep baby with me | yes | no | yes | no |
| Save the placenta | yes | no | yes | no |
| **Newborn care:** | | | | |
| Delay propholaxis eye treatment | yes | no | yes | no |
| Vitamin K injection | yes | no | yes | no |
| Breastfeeding | yes | no | yes | no |
| Formula feeding | yes | no | yes | no |
| Circumcision | yes | no | yes | no |
| **Postpartum care:** | | | | |
| Rooming-in | yes | no | yes | no |
| Infant care classes | yes | no | yes | no |
| **Other considerations:** | | | | |

## POSTURE AND BALANCE

Good posture is essential to your physical well-being during pregnancy. This means not only learning to stand and walk in the best way, so that your baby is cradled in the pelvis in a position that is comfortable for both of you, but also performing other everyday movements, such as getting out of bed, in a way calculated to avoid unnecessary strain. To achieve good posture, you need to improve the tone of your muscles and learn how to use only those muscles necessary for whatever you are doing. If you are looking good and walking with a spring in your step, you will probably also feel much better.

### MAINTAINING GOOD POSTURE

Make a point of tucking in your buttock muscles, and feel your abdominal muscles working to straighten out your spine. Keep your shoulders dropped. Now imagine a string is pulling your head straight up, and notice the back of your neck lengthening.

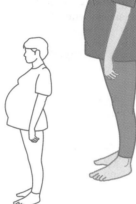

### WRONG

If the weight of your uterus makes you stand back on your heels, with your bottom stuck out and your shoulders flung back, your spine becomes hollowed and you get low backache.

### TAILOR SITTING

Tailor sitting is an ideal way of rounding out the lower back. As long as you take care not to slouch over, it can be one of the most comfortable positions for sitting during pregnancy.

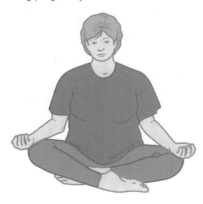

### BRIDGING

In late pregnancy, your abdominal muscles can feel so stretched that it might be difficult to exercise them consciously. If this is the case, it helps to tighten your buttock muscles, since this means that you pull in your abdominal muscles too. Bridging improves the tone of your buttock muscles and helps the circulation in your legs.

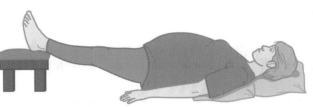

1. Lie on the floor with your heels raised on a low table or stool.

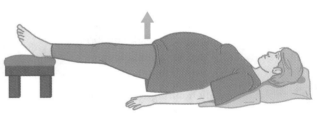

2. Tighten your buttock and abdominal muscles and lift your bottom up off the floor, keeping your back straight.

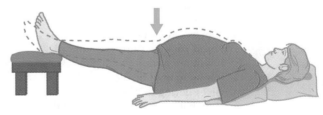

3. Hold this position for several seconds, then slowly lower your hips.

---

FIGURE 13-4 • Posture and balance. *(Redrawn from Kitzinger S:* The complete book of pregnancy and childbirth, *London, 1990, Knopf.)*

## THE ROCKING-CHAIR EXERCISE

This exercise encourages good posture by allowing you to press out the small of your back while keeping the rest of your body aligned. You become the rocking chair that rocks to and fro, and you need a partner to set you in motion and provide the firm surface against which you press your lower back. Avoid hollowing your back at any time.

## GETTING UP FROM LYING DOWN

If you sit up suddenly after you have been lying on your back, you put great pressure on your stomach muscles, especially in advanced pregnancy. The method below is a way of avoiding undue strain on these muscles, and, since it involves changing from a horizontal to an upright position in gentle stages, it is also good for the circulation.

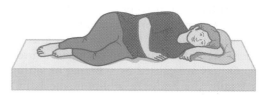

1. Roll over to one side, swinging your shoulders round and drawing up your knees.

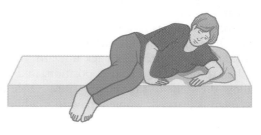

2. Push yourself up with your upper arm while swiveling your legs from the hips over to the edge of the bed.

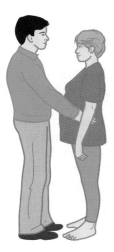 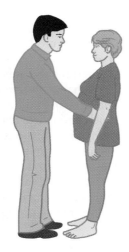

1. Your partner stands in front of you with his hands on your hips.

2. You rock your pelvis gently backwards and forwards between his hands several times.

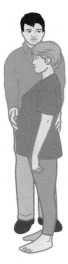 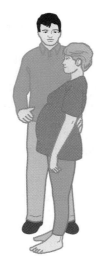

3. Now he stands at your side and puts one hand on the small of your back and the other hand over your lower abdomen.

4. You continue the rocking movement, pushing against his hand with the small of your back and then moving away from it.

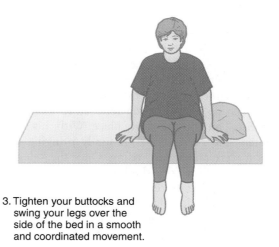

3. Tighten your buttocks and swing your legs over the side of the bed in a smooth and coordinated movement.

FIGURE 13-4, *cont'd* ● Posture and balance.

spine, especially in the small of her back. When this occurs the woman's upper back must compensate, and this can lead to back strain and back pain. Girdles do not help much because they can only partially compensate for the work the muscles should be doing. The best girdle is composed of the woman's own abdominal and buttocks muscles, and both need to be in tone to provide the necessary support. Exercises such as pelvic rocking and leg sliding can be very helpful (Figure 13-5).

As the pregnancy progresses and the woman carries more weight, she may feel more aches and pains. Some of these are natural and will occur no matter what she does. Others are caused by standing or sitting in a way that strains the body. In addition, the baby's position can cause the woman sharp shooting pains when it presses against a nerve. Exercises that bring the body back into realignment, increase circulation to tissues, or move the baby can increase comfort.

*Pelvic Rock or Tilt.* The pelvic tilt or rock is useful in pregnancy to alleviate back pain. One common way to teach this exercise is referred to as "the angry cat" position. Once on her hands and knees, the women is instructed to slowly arch her back upward, like an angry cat, then to return to a resting position, taking care not to allow the spine to sag (Figure 13-6). Once the pelvic movement is learned, women may do it while sitting or standing.

### Preparing for Labor

*The Kegel—a Pelvic Floor Exercise.* Pelvic floor exercise is an essential exercise for women's gynecologic health. Help the woman learn how to control the pelvic floor so that she may relax it during labor and then tone the muscle after delivery. This reduces the occurrence of problems with bladder control in the early postnatal period and later in life. One of the easiest ways to teach the woman to identify the muscle is to have her stop the flow of urine when on the toilet. Once identified she may then do what is often referred to as the "elevator exercise," any time and any place. With this exercise she tightens the pelvic floor gradually bringing it up, just as if it were an elevator rising. Once the "elevator" has reached the fifth floor she holds it there for 30 seconds and then gradually relaxes it floor by floor. Before delivery, she should relax the muscles so much it is as if they go to the "basement." After delivery she no longer goes to the "basement," she just tightens and releases it gradually. Some women find it helpful to remember to do this exercise by associating it with an event that occurs often, such as every time she talks on the phone or while stopped at a red light. A way to measure the strength of the muscles is to tighten around a penis during intercourse.

*Tailor Sitting.* Tailor sitting helps gently stretch the muscles in the thighs. It involves sitting on a firm surface, back upright, soles of feet touching with knees

gently fallen open. This position is incorporated into many activities during educational sessions as well as many of the activities a woman may do at home such as watching television or playing with a child.

*Squatting.* The squatting position can reduce back pain during pregnancy. It is also excellent for the second stage of labor. However, it is not a position that many women in our culture are comfortable assuming, so it must be practiced. Many variations of squat positions can be used. There are also other positions a woman may assume in labor (Figure 13-7). These may also be practiced.

*Touch and Massage.* A woman's preference for touch and massage is highly individual, and the woman's preferences can change during pregnancy as well as during labor. The woman and her birth partner can learn how to use touch and massage techniques to facilitate relaxation during class sessions. They can then practice between sessions so the partner can learn how to use the techniques in a way that enhances the woman's ability to relax and cope. Tension and pain in her back, hips, thighs, and legs are common during labor, but they respond well to massage (Figure 13-8).

## Understanding Labor and Birth

Teaching about the process of birth begins with a broad introduction about the unique nature of labor and birth for each woman. The physical, emotional, and spiritual dimensions of the birthing process are addressed. The physical aspects of birth incorporate the physiology and change process of labor and birth. The emotional dimension of birth is explored through discussions of "letting go" and working with the body during labor. The spiritual nature of birth focuses on each woman's sense of self in this process and her feeling of birth energy.

### When Delivery Will Occur

One of the first and then ongoing questions of pregnant women is, "When will by baby come?" In presenting information about the onset of labor, it is important to address the tentative nature of the **estimated date of delivery** (EDD) or estimated date of confinement (EDC). Once an EDD has been established, the mother and her partner or their family and friends often consider it a specific end point to the pregnancy. It can be helpful to conceptualize the EDD with a more flexible perspective. It is, in fact, a midpoint around which the baby may be born; a birth 2 weeks before or 2 weeks after the EDD is still on time. Many providers, instead of giving a specific date, speak of a due "month," which places the EDD in the middle of that month.

### Factors that Influence Process

When teaching about the process of labor and birth, critical factors that influence the process are presented. These factors—the power, passenger, passage, and the

**KEEPING FIT DURING PREGNANCY**

While you are pregnant, it is easy to allow muscles that were previously firm and elastic to sag. You are putting on weight, your figure is changing, and you may assume that sagging muscles are an inevitable accompaniment to these changes. However, gentle, toning exercises, aimed at firming up your abdominal muscles and avoiding back strain, can do you and your baby nothing but good.

PELVIC ROCKING

Lie on a flat surface, your head and shoulders supported by pillows and your knees bent with the feet flat. Experiment with pressing the small of your back against the floor or bed and then releasing it so that you produce a gentle, rhythmic, rocking movement. Then roll your hips round in a very slow, circular, hula-hoop movement.

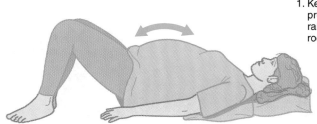

1. Keeping your upper back pressed firmly down, slightly raise your hips and buttocks and rock them gently to and fro.

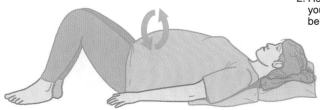

2. Roll your pelvis around—as if you were doing a slow languorous belly dance while lying down.

WRONG

Although double-leg raising and sit-ups are exercises often recommended for pregnant women, they do not in fact strengthen the abdominal muscles. These muscles do not work to lift the legs but to stabilize the lower back. If they are not strong to start with, they cannot cope with the effort involved when the legs or trunk are raised, and the result is back strain or torn abdominal muscles.

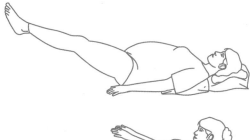

Double-leg raising is rarely effective in toning abdominal muscles and should never be done in pregnancy or in the 4 weeks following birth.

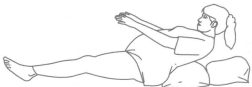

Sit-ups can cause harm in pregnancy. They should never be done with the knees and back held straight if you are pregnant or in the first 6 weeks after childbirth.

FIGURE 13-5 ● Avoiding back strain. *(Redrawn from Kitzinger S:* The complete book of pregnancy and childbirth, *London, 1980, Knopf.)*

*Continued*

## LEG SLIDING

Leg sliding is a gentle exercise that allows you to tone up your abdominal muscles efficiently without straining them. Do it five or six times at first and gradually build up until you can do it comfortably 10 or 15 times. If at any point you feel your back aching, stop. Leg sliding is best done lying on your back on a firm surface with a pillow under your head and shoulders.

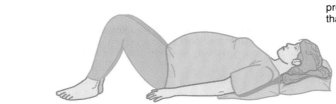

1. Keeping the small of your back pressed down, bend your knees so that your feet are flat on the floor.

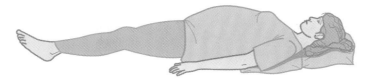

2. Slowly extend both legs until they are straight.

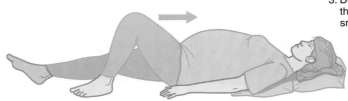

3. Draw one knee back up, then the other, without lifting the small of your back off the floor.

## TESTING FOR SEPARATION OF THE RECTUS MUSCLE

If you are starting exercises in the last three months of pregnancy, find out whether you have already damaged your rectus muscle. You will need to be careful when doing exercises for toning up your abdomen if this muscle has separated.

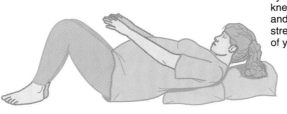

1. Lying on your back with your knees bent, slowly raise your head and shoulders about 8 in (20 cm), stretching your arms out in front of you.

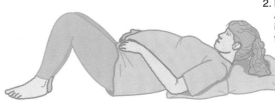

2. Place your hands on your abdomen. A small soft bulge like a marshmallow in the middle below your navel means the rectus muscle has probably separated.

*FIGURE 13-5—cont'd* • Avoiding back strain.

## ACHES AND PAINS

In late pregnancy, you are carrying more weight that—instead of being evenly distributed—is centered in one area and so affects your balance. This extra weight alone can cause aches and pains by straining muscles and causing you to adopt an unnatural stance, leading to further strain. The way the baby is lying can also cause discomfort and occasionally sharp shooting pain when the baby is pressing against a nerve.

## FOOT EXERCISES

Foot exercises discourage varicose veins in the legs by simulating the blood flow back to the heart. When you are sitting down or having a rest, practice drawing the letters of the alphabet with your feet, one foot at a time, keeping your legs still. You will find that you can easily read or do some work at the same time.

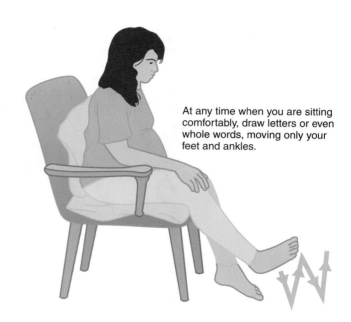

At any time when you are sitting comfortably, draw letters or even whole words, moving only your feet and ankles.

## THE ANGRY CAT

However many exercises you do with your back well supported, it feels good to get the weight of the baby off your spine occasionally. You can do this by going on to all fours and rocking your pelvis, an exercise sometimes known as "the angry cat." This is a kind of pelvic rocking reversed.

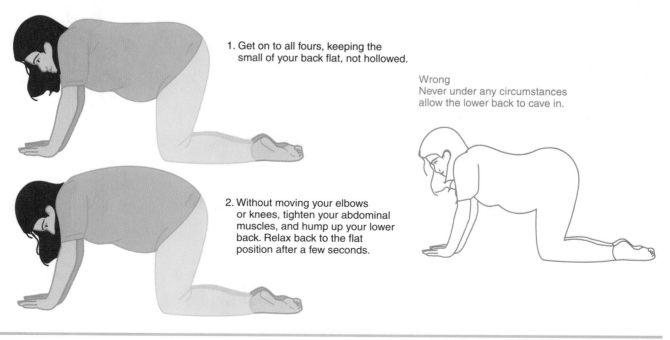

1. Get on to all fours, keeping the small of your back flat, not hollowed.

2. Without moving your elbows or knees, tighten your abdominal muscles, and hump up your lower back. Relax back to the flat position after a few seconds.

Wrong
Never under any circumstances allow the lower back to cave in.

FIGURE 13-6 • Overcoming aches and pains. *(Redrawn from Kitzinger S:* The complete book of pregnancy and childbirth, *London, 1980, Knopf.)*

*Continued*

**THE WHEELBARROW**
Towards the end of pregnancy many women
have pain in the groin. This usually occurs
as a result of pressure from the baby on the
joints of the pelvis. To relieve the discomfort,
try this exercise, your partner kneeling very
close to you.

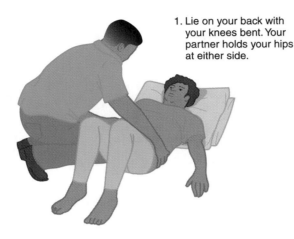

1. Lie on your back with
your knees bent. Your
partner holds your hips
at either side.

2. Your partner slowly
lifts your hips, holding
them up for a moment,
then gently lowering them.

**WALL STRETCHING**
A good way to lift your ribs off your expanding uterus is simply
to stretch high with first one arm than the other, until you
are comfortable. A similar exercise may be done by sitting with
your back pressed against a wall to help alignment.

**THE SHOULDER ROLL**
Upper backache, which is caused
by poor posture or heavy breasts,
can be relieved by doing the
shoulder-roll exercise

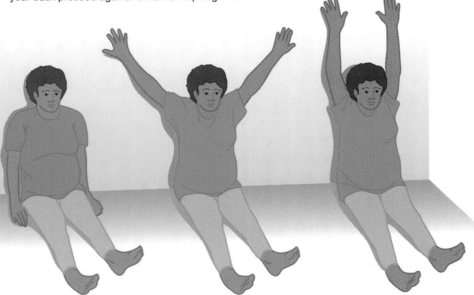

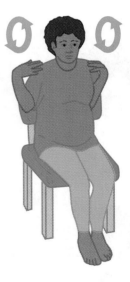

1. Sit with your back
pressed against a wall and
your legs stretched out in
front of you.

2. Swing your arms out to
the sides at shoulder level
and, with your hands
pressed against the wall,
walk your fingers up it.

3. Turn your palms
outward when your hands
have reached as high as
they can go.

Rest your fingertips on your
shoulders and rotate your
elbows back.

*FIGURE 13-6—cont'd* ● Overcoming aches and pains.

## MOVEMENT AND POSITIONS FOR LABOR

Descriptions: Moving about freely during labor allows you to find the most comfortable positions. Restriction to bed often adds to your discomfort. Beyond the freedom to move, it helps to know specific movements and positions that can help with painful or challenging situations.

In general:
- Upright movements and positions (walking, swaying; slow dancing with your partner; leaning against the wall, on your partner, or over a raised bed) give you a gravity advantage that may enhance comfort and labor progress.

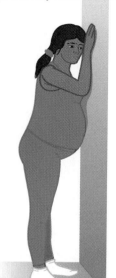

- A knee chest position for a half hour or more may help reposition a posterior baby or reduce swelling of the cervix. Ask your caregiver for advice and assistance.

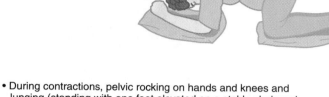

- During contractions, pelvic rocking on hands and knees and lunging (standing with one foot elevated on a stable chair and leaning sideways toward the elevated foot) may help rotate an occiput posterior baby or speed a slow labor. Lunge in the direction that feels best or in the direction toward which your baby's occiput is pointed, if you or your caregiver knows.

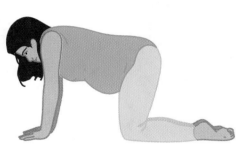

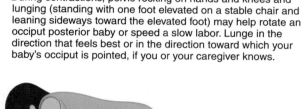

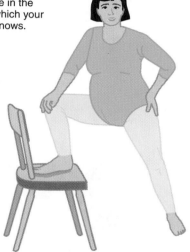

- Positions in which you kneel and lean forward ease back pain.

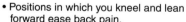

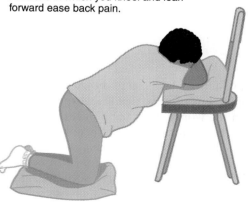

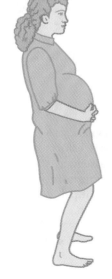

- Gently lifting your abdomen during contractions with your hands placed below your uterus sometimes relieves back pain and speeds labor, especially if you are standing up. Bend your knees as you lift your abdomen.

---

**FIGURE 13-7** ● Position changes in labor. *(Redrawn from Simkin P: Simkin's ratings of comfort measures for childbirth, Minnetonka, MN, 1985, Meadowbrook Press.)*

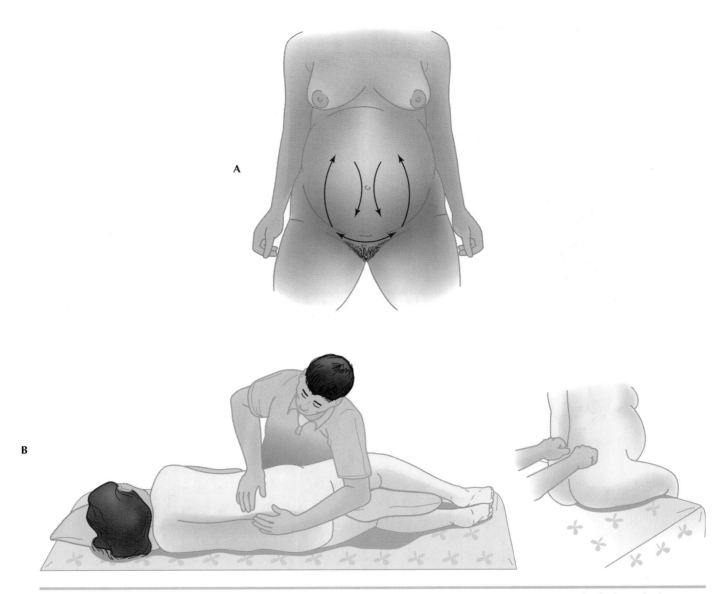

FIGURE 13-8 • Massage techniques. **A,** Effleurage; **B,** Back. *(Redrawn from Whitley N: A manual of clinical obstetrics, Philadelphia, 1985, Lippincott.)*

psyche—vary within the woman from one pregnancy to the next. Contractions that create the expulsive efforts of labor and birth provide the **power**. The **passenger** is the infant, with its size, position, and presentation influencing the process. The **passage** is the maternal pelvis and soft tissue that the baby must pass through. The **psyche** considers the energy, anxieties, and fears the woman brings to the event as well as the support she perceives from the network that surrounds her.

### The Birthing Environment

The birthing environment influences the process of labor and birth. Some women choose to give birth in their homes or an alternate birth center because they want to be in a familiar, safe place so that their experience is personal. When the woman is in her home, the birth environment is familiar with the smell, people, and sounds that she is accustomed to experiencing.

Other women choose a hospital for birth because in the United States it has become the socially condoned place for birth to occur. Yet others choose a birthing center where they can experience many of the comforts of home but have more space and options available.

When the woman is planning a birth away from home she will prepare by taking a tour of the facility. Tours are most effective when they are conducted in

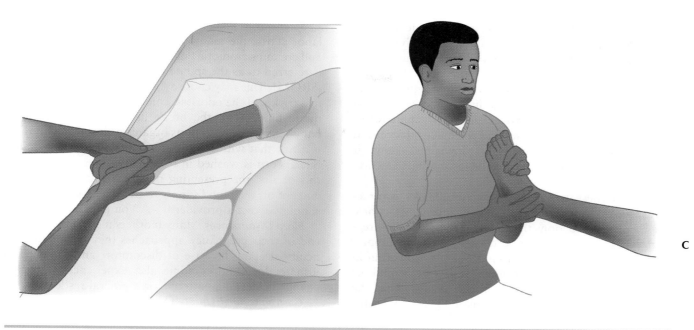

C

FIGURE 13-8—*cont'd* • Massage techniques. **C,** Extremities.

small groups and involve the staff in the birthing area. On the tour she can become familiar with the setting and start to determine how she will make the setting more culturally appropriate and comfortable for herself. The hospital setting contains sights, smells, and sounds that can distract and influence the mother's degree of relaxation and her birthing process. A woman can help reduce some of these distractions by bringing things from home to counterbalance distraction.

A woman may choose to wear her own clothing rather than the clothing provided. Taped music can soften the existing sounds of the environment and provide a sense of the familiar for the woman. This is especially true if the woman brings music she listened to as she practiced her relaxation and breathing at home during the pregnancy. Pictures of family members, friends, or favorite places also provide the woman with a connection outside the facility. Aroma therapy can be used to help the woman relax and soften the "smells" of the hospital.

No matter where a woman chooses to give birth, positive energy is vital. Supporting the woman's personal sense of confidence and having positive and supportive people around her create positive energy. Some educators have women and their partners create a birthing poster with peaceful and positive images of pregnancy, birth, and the newborn. The woman may place the poster where she can see it as she moves about in her labor. It will provide a visual reminder of the positive images she enjoys.

## Self-Assessment Techniques

During pregnancy women are responsible for monitoring the activities and changes within their body and determining when they should contact a health care provider. Childbirth preparation classes help them understand and become more proficient in the process of self-assessment.

### Signs and Symptoms of Impending Labor

Predictable changes may or may not be noticed by the woman as her body transitions from carrying a baby to preparing for the experience of labor and delivery. Referred to as **premonitory signs,** they are not indications that a woman is in labor but that her body is preparing for labor. They include lightening, increased vaginal discharge, Braxton Hicks contractions, show, rupture of amniotic sac, sleep disturbances, gastrointestinal upset, burst of energy, and weight loss.

*Lightening.* **Lightening** is when the uterus and presenting part of the baby move down into the pelvis. On average it occurs 10 days before the onset of labor in a woman having her first baby (primigravida). In women pregnant with their second or succeeding baby (multigravidas), it may not happen until closer to the start of labor.

As a result of the change in position, a woman may now be able to breathe more easily as the baby has moved away from her diaphragm. However, she may experience more urinary frequency, backache, and leg pain; increased vaginal discharge; and dependent edema because of the pressure of the baby in her pelvis. Confirmation of lightening is achieved by abdominal and pelvic evaluation by a provider.

***Increased Vaginal Discharge.*** During pregnancy the woman normally experiences an increase in vaginal discharge, **physiologic leukorrhea.** As labor approaches, mucous production increases and the mucus thickens in consistency. As the mucus moves down the vagina, it helps reduce the occurrence of an ascending infection during this time.

***Braxton Hicks Contractions.*** Braxton Hicks contractions, sometimes referred to as false labor contractions, are uterine contractions that occur throughout the pregnancy but may not be noticed until the ninth month. They may be random or rhythmic in nature and occur in a short sequence or last for hours. It may be helpful for the mother to think of them as practice contractions. She can practice her relaxation and breathing as they occur.

***Mucous Plug.*** During pregnancy the os of the cervix is filled with a thick mucus called the **mucous plug.** The passing of the mucous plug indicates that the cervix is softening and the os is opening. Because the cervix is friable, the mucous plug sometimes has red blood attached to it or may be brownish in color. This has led to the term, "bloody show."

***Spontaneous Rupture of Amniotic Sac.*** Sometimes before labor starts, the amniotic sac that surrounds the baby and contains amniotic fluid, ruptures spontaneously; this is referred to as the **spontaneous rupture of membranes (SROM).** This may cause a "gush" of fluid or may result in a trickle of the odorless, colorless, clear or cloudy amniotic fluid. With the break in the amniotic sac, the baby's barrier to infectious organisms is gone. Also there is a risk that with the rupture of the sac the baby's umbilical cord is washed in front of the presenting part. If this occurs, the presenting part may press on the cord and cut off the blood supply to the baby (see "A woman should contact a provider if . . ." on page 496).

***Sleep Disturbances.*** Many mothers mention that as the end of their pregnancy approaches they have more difficulty sleeping because of discomfort and the need to urinate. In addition, some also experience dreams, a change in sleeping patterns, or a general restlessness.

***Gastrointestinal Upset.*** The hormonal changes at the end of pregnancy sometimes cause women to experience "flulike" symptoms for a few days. In addition some may experience indigestion, diarrhea, nausea, and vomiting. If caused by hormonal changes, these symptoms generally pass before labor starts.

***Burst of Energy.*** A burst of energy in the mother often occurs 24 to 48 hours before the onset of labor.

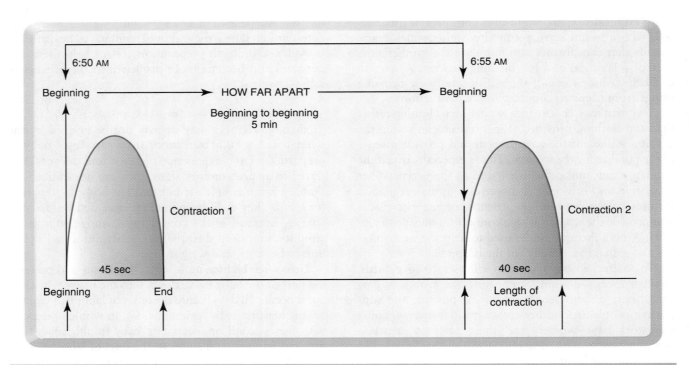

FIGURE 13-9 • How to time contractions. *How far apart are the contractions?* Contractions are timed from the beginning of one to the beginning of the next—usually minutes. *How long are the contractions?* Contractions are timed from beginning to end—usually seconds.

An increase in the amount of released epinephrine is caused by a decrease in the release of progesterone as the hormones shift to initiate labor. Because some women take advantage of this time to finish final preparations for the baby, it is sometimes referred to as "nesting." Women should be cautioned to relax and enjoy their newly found energy, saving it for the birth experience, rather than running around in preparation activities.

***Weight Loss.*** Women may experience a 1- to 3-pound weight loss 24 to 48 hours before the onset of labor. This is the beginning of the shift to her prepregnancy status.

If a woman experiences one or more of these events and is eager to finally deliver her baby, she may wish to be seen for an evaluation. Physical assessment may be able to measure a weight loss and observe the descent of the uterus. An internal examination may determine that the cervix has moved from a posterior position to an anterior position and softened. **Effacement** (thinning of the cervix) and **dilation** (opening of the cervix) may be in process. The fluids within the vagina can be tested to determine if there is amniotic fluid present. If the amniotic sac ruptured, the fetal heart should be monitored to ensure that the presenting part of the baby is not pressing on the umbilical cord.

Because these signs indicate approaching labor and not labor itself, the woman will be reassured and sent home to rest. Labor contractions will generally start within the next few days. The only concern will be if the SROM has left the umbilical cord in front of the presenting part of the baby. This becomes a medical emergency requiring immediate attention.

## Timing of Contractions

Contractions are the regular tightening of the uterine muscles as they thin and open the cervix and then push the baby out through the vagina. By learning to recognize and time contractions, women can determine when active labor starts (Figure 13-9).

As a contraction starts, the uterus gradually becomes hard. After reaching a peak, it will gradually relax again. To determine when the uterus is contracting, a hand is placed on the top of the uterus.

Contractions are timed from the beginning of one contraction to the beginning of the next, generally a length of time measured in minutes. Contractions last from when the uterus tightens until it relaxes, usually measured in seconds.

## Differentiating between Prelabor and Labor Contractions

The only definitive way to determine between prelabor contractions and labor contractions is that labor contractions produce a baby. Some signs may help a woman in the self-assessment process; however, remind women that each of them may experience prelabor and labor differently. Some women are only aware of one contraction before they deliver their babies. Others have Braxton Hicks contractions in a regular pattern, for a period of time every day for 6 months before their babies are born. The woman herself, rather than the type and pattern of contractions, is the best judge of whether she is experiencing labor (Table 13-6).

When a woman notifies her provider that her contractions are 3 to 5 minutes apart (if a primipara) or 5 to 8 minutes apart (if a multipara) with the characteristics of true labor, the woman will be directed go to the birth center or hospital. However these directions will vary based on the woman's pregnancy history, prior birth experiences, mode of transportation, and distance to the facility. If a woman is planning a home birth, she probably will have alerted her provider when her contractions started.

Although the mother or her support system may worry or hope that the baby will soon arrive, that generally is not the case. Most women will have hours to settle into their environment as they accomplish the work of childbirth.

## Signs and Symptoms of Potential Problems

Some signs and symptoms may indicate a potentially serious problem for either the mother or the baby. If a mother experiences one or more of these she should call her health care provider or go to an emergency room for an immediate evaluation.

**TABLE 13-6** *Self-Assessment of Prelabor and Labor*

| Factor | Prelabor | Labor |
| --- | --- | --- |
| Contraction | May be irregular; no shortening of interval between | Regular rhythm, a wavelike shape lasting 40 sec or more |
| Discomfort | Abdomen | Moves from back to front of lower abdomen/cervix area |
| If woman changes position or activity | Contractions decrease | No change or contractions increase |

A woman should contact a provider if:

* Vaginal bleeding
* Puffiness of the face, eyes or fingers, especially if it is of sudden onset
* Severe, continuous headache
* Dimness or blurring of vision
* Severe abdominal pain or cramping, especially if constant
* Persistent vomiting and diarrhea, lasting more than 24 hours
* Chills and fever over 100° F
* Pain or burning when urinating, or only producing a scant amount of urine
* A sudden gush of fluid from the vagina
* The baby moves fewer than 10 times in 4 hours

Women should be alert to the possible occurrence of any of these symptoms, without being fearful. Their occurrence doesn't always mean that a serious problem has developed because some of them may have multiple causes, and many of the causes can be treated before a harmful result occurs.

## Explaining Options for Childbirth

The process of childbirth encompasses four stages. The **first stage** of labor is when uterus contractions cause the baby to press on the cervix, creating the process of effacement and dilation. This is the longest stage of labor. It encompasses both the gentle contractions of early labor and the strongest and longest contractions, those of transition. The contractions build in strength and duration during first stage, and once established come in a very predictable manner. Between contractions the woman generally feels "normal" and can move about and converse freely. Many women see first stage as the time to remain relaxed, breathe comfortably, and experience in awe the process as they just let their bodies do the work as intended.

The **second stage** is when the baby is pushed down and out of the vagina. The uterine contractions during this stage are generally farther apart and shorter in time than they were in transition. This allows both the mother and baby time to become reoxygenated and to rest between contractions. With second-stage contractions, women experience an urge to push. Women may welcome this as an opportunity to now work with their bodies to bring their babies into the world.

**Third stage**, the delivery of the placenta, may occur without the woman paying much attention as she focuses on her baby and her support system. After the baby is born, the uterus collapses down into the woman's pelvis and the placenta becomes detached. With a concentrated push or two, the placenta is gently delivered. The **fourth stage** of childbirth is the immediate postpartum, during

which the woman and baby become acquainted and her body starts the process of returning to a nonpregnant state.

In preparation for childbirth, each stage is explained and discussed with regards to maternal physical and emotional response, the role of the support team, comfort techniques that may be used, and the various choices available to the mother. Woven throughout these topics are the conceptual threads concerning the natural process and each woman's innate capacity to give birth, the role of the support people and health care providers, and active coping strategies the woman can achieve independently or with her labor support team.

### Understanding Anatomy and Physiology

Pregnant women and their partners are curious about what is going on inside her abdomen and, if given the opportunity, will ask many questions. During the sessions, just as understanding of the developing infant increases, so too is the realization of the unique personhood of the yet unborn child.

Because women are born with innate instinct and knowledge on how to reproduce, we do not need to teach them *how* to give birth. What is helpful is to teach about the anatomy and physiology of birth (Figure 13-10), while also helping the woman get in touch with her personal insights and instincts (Robertson, 1994).

*Pelvis.* The female pelvis is the bony cradle in which the baby rests. It is an elasticized system of bones and ligaments that only open to their full capacity during actual labor. Any measurements of pelvis before labor will not show the true capacity of the labor. The only true way of exploring the "fit" between the mother and baby is during the labor and birth process. During labor a woman may increase the opening of the pelvis through body movement.

*Posture and Gravity.* A woman's labor is shorter during the first stage if she is upright because gravity helps bring the baby's head down against the cervix. The contractions are also less painful if the weight of the baby and uterus are pressing downward on the pelvic floor muscles rather than on other abdominal muscles, tissues, and organs when she lies down.

During second stage, when the woman is pushing, assisting her in an upright position enhances the uterine action and speeds the process. The woman finds that the need to provide the primary force for pushing the baby out is reduced as gravity assists her. This is not true if the woman is lying on her side, since gravity has no helpful effect, or lying on her back when the baby must be forced first horizontally and then vertically upwards (Robertson, 1994).

Based on anatomy and physiology, some positions are much more helpful than others. In addition, some positions allow the mother to move about and change position much more freely in labor. Because movement enhances the labor process, this is encouraged.

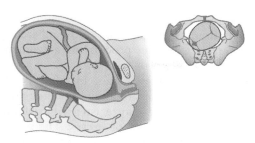

1. Head floating, before engagement

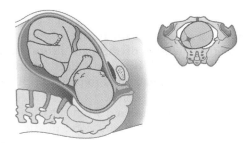

2. Engagement, flexion, descent

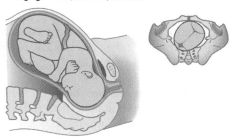

3. Further descent, internal rotation

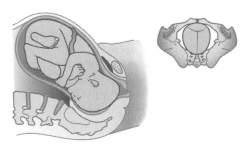

4. Complete rotation, beginning extension

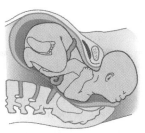

5. Complete extension

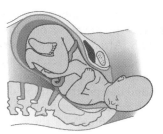

6. Restitution, external rotation

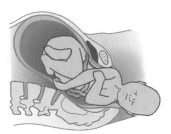

7. Delivery of anterior shoulder

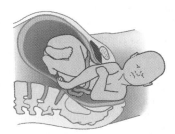

8. Delivery of posterior shoulder

FIGURE 13-10 • Mechanisms of birth.

**Role of Hormones.** Hormones are involved in every facet of reproduction from ovulation through lactation in the postpartum period. Three major hormones are central and essential elements of a woman's normal labor and delivery: oxytocin, endorphin, and catecholamines (adrenaline).

**Oxytocin** is released from the posterior pituitary gland and, among other activities, is responsible for causing uterine contractions and the let-down of milk when an infant sucks at the breast. Once labor has begun, oxytocin shapes the pattern of the contractions.

"The hormone is released as a result of pressure from the presenting part of the baby's head against the cervix. If the head becomes well applied, the contractions become regular and consistent" (Robertson, 1994) and the cervix effaces and dilates efficiently. Once through the cervix, with the beginning of the second stage of labor, the baby presses on the pelvic floor muscles and causes the ongoing release of oxytocin until shortly after the birth of the baby.

**Endorphins** are natural substances similar to opiates in both structure and effect. Produced in the brain stem, nerve endings, and placenta, endorphins are released whenever the body is stressed beyond its normal limits. They work to modify pain, create a sense of well-being, and alter perception of time and place. Women enter labor with moderately high levels of endorphins already circulating. When labor begins, the levels continue to rise and help the woman manage her labor. "Her behavior indicates that this process is occurring: she becomes withdrawn, more sedentary, rests between contractions, closes her eyes, and appears "spaced out." These signs are all proof that her endorphin levels are adequate for her needs and that the labor is progressing normally" (Robertson, 1994). During second stage, endorphin levels remain high. After the baby is born they contribute to her elation, sense of achievement, and positive state. Following birth, the endorphin level falls dramatically and by the second day postpartum is almost at a prepregnancy level. This precipitous change may contribute to the mother feeling "blue" on the third postpartum day.

**Catecholamines (adrenaline)** are made in the brain, in the adrenal glands, in the nerve endings, as well as other location in the body and are responsible for the "fight or flight" behaviors of survival. If a woman in labor experiences a real or perceived threat while in labor, adrenaline is released. Caregivers will notice that the woman becomes agitated and restless, her breathing becomes more rapid. She makes direct eye contact and her pupils may dilate. She may start to shiver or become cold and her blood pressure may rise and her pulse may increase. The adrenaline she releases will cause her level of oxytocin to fall, and her labor contractions will slow or stop. In addition, the circular fibers in the lower third of the uterus contract, halting the process of effacement and dilation. The blood supply is diverted away from the uterus, so that she has the capacity to respond to the threat. If the muscles of the uterus become hypoxic, they will be more painful when they contract. The endorphin levels also fall in response to the adrenaline. It will only rise again when the source of the threat is removed. It may take a woman an hour of more after the threat is removed for her level of adrenaline to sufficiently drop and the productive level of endorphins and oxytocin to resume.

## Pain in Childbirth

The main symptoms of labor are contractions of the uterus and a sensation of some degree of pain. There are probably two main reasons for the experience of pain during the birth process. The physical reason is so that a woman will be aware that the baby is about to be delivered and can judge the progress. This gives her the time to get herself into a safe and supportive environment. Women who experience painless or precipitous births often find them frightening events. The psychologic advantage of experiencing pain in labor "offers women unique opportunities for self-discovery and

growth through mastery of this powerfully life threatening situation. . . . weathering of the inherent pain of labor is an empowering process for a woman. . . ." (Robertson, 1994).

The primary source of pain in labor is from the stretching of the cervix. Abdominal organs and tissues around the uterus may also register pain from pressure and compression of bones or nerves. The pain is most intense at the end of first stage, when the woman enters transition. This is because the contractions are longer with the shortest periods of rest in between, and the greatest tension is being placed on the cervix to open and let the head of the baby through. Once the baby is through, the intensity of the pain drops because the cervix is no longer being stretched. However, the mother now feels pain related to pressure on the tissues of the vagina or pelvic bones.

The amount of pain that a woman experiences in labor is related to several factors, some physical and some psychologic. Her perception of sensations of pain is increased if she is frightened or anxious. Being in certain positions alters the amount of physical pain she feels. If her baby is malpositioned (which may cause the pain of back labor) or if some other mechanical problem, such as having a full bowel or bladder, is present, her pain may be increased.

*Relationship between Fear and Pain.* Explaining the interaction of fear and pain has been a traditional aspect of childbirth education programs (Dick-Read, 1933). Knowledge of the physiologic interaction between pain and fear and its possible effect on the woman during the labor process is important to understand because the perception of pain is influenced by several factors as discussed in the following sections.

*Influences on Perceptions of Pain.* A woman's physical state can influence her perception of pain. If she is fatigued, sick, or otherwise physically challenged she will respond differently to pain than if she is in an optimal physical state. Increased anxiety, cultural expectations, knowledge about the process, expectations of the process, self-esteem, and past experience with pain all have the potential for increasing or decreasing a woman's perception of pain.

The duration and predictability of the painful stimulus also impact her overall perception of pain. If the increase and decrease of pain is predictable and has a rhythm to it, as much of the pain of labor does, it is easier to handle. Stress and anxiety-reduction techniques such as patterned breathing, relaxation, and distraction; role modeling how to respond; and conditioning activities may alter perceptions of pain. Childbirth preparation classes use various principles to assist women and their support system in preparing for responding to the birth process.

When preparing for childbirth, women may learn of the cause and value of pain in labor and explore a full range of ways to manage their pain. Particular options vary with labor attendant preferences and practices, as well as with regional and institutional preferences and practices.

## Nonpharmacologic Pain Management

Relaxation and conscious breathing techniques offer assistance in reducing fear, anxiety, stress, and discomfort not only during labor, but throughout the parenting experience and life. A variety of methods are taught and practiced.

***Relaxation Techniques.*** **Relaxation techniques** are critical elements in birthing preparation because tense muscles lead to fatigue and increased pain. Relaxation works by increasing the descending inhibitory activity in the higher brain centers while it lowers heart rate, respiratory rate, blood pressure, and level of blood lactates (Perez, 1997).

The physical environment, the woman's breathing pattern, and the position she assumes are all elements of the relaxation process. The environment a woman chooses should enhance her positive emotions and physical state; it should be comfortable and familiar to her. Sounds and smells are part of an environment, and some of these may be transferred from the woman's home to wherever she chooses to give birth, if it is not in her home. Breathing should be maternally directed and based on physiologic need.

The position in which a woman chooses to practice relaxation techniques should vary according to her desire and comfort, as long as it promotes uteroplacental blood flow. Walking, sitting, squatting, and any other position in which she is upright and supported should be encouraged. Generally, the supine position should be avoided. Comfort, both physical and emotional, is essential to achieving relaxation. Pillows are wonderful tools to increase comfort as the woman assumes a succession of different positions.

There are many different approaches to achieving relaxation. Because the woman may be able to implement one more easily than another, several approaches may be presented in a preparation series. **Progressive relaxation** is a systematic process of actively tensing then relaxing a muscle group. The process begins at the head with the facial muscles and moves progressively down the central body, out the arms to the hands, and finally out the legs ending with the feet. Deep breathing is used to release tension as the tensing and releasing process unfolds.

**Tension relaxation** is active relaxation in response to a noxious stimulus. The stimulus that a woman responds to can be identified as a tense muscle group, pressure on her thigh mimicking a contraction, or a cold source such as ice applied to an area of her body. The concept is that the stimulus mimics the duration and pattern of the contracting uterus during labor and

the woman practices responding with relaxation. The stimuli can be applied with no coping techniques, then tried again with the use of relaxation and breathing awareness.

Another relaxation technique, **touch relaxation,** combines massage and touch with breathing awareness and active relaxation. With touch relaxation a partner provides a firm but gentle touch to an area to facilitate the release of tension.

**Meditation** encourages dwelling on an object by repeating a sound or gazing at an object while clearing the mind of all other thoughts and distractions (Perez, 1997).

***Visualization Techniques.*** **Visualization** and imagery used in combination with relaxation can be helpful throughout pregnancy and the birthing process. When the woman feels stress or is uncomfortable, she can picture herself in a peaceful setting or her favorite relaxing environment, perhaps on a deserted beach or under a tree. Women can visualize positive birthing scenarios as they progress through labor. They can focus on opening up to let the baby emerge or center on picturing the baby as it moves down the birth canal.

Exercises that assist women in developing their skills in relaxation and visualization can be conducted during class. Before a session of guided imagery starts the woman should get in a comfortable, well-supported position and then close her eyes. When you guide a visualization experience it is important to let the woman pick the place she wants her mind to go. By not being specific in describing the scenario, you don't force the woman to confront unwanted memories or associations.

Practice time at home for relaxation, breathing awareness, and exercises is critical to successful application of these techniques during the labor and birth process. Couples will appreciate hints about ways in which these strategies can be incorporated into the context of daily activities, thus increasing the probability that participants will practice outside class times.

***Affirmations.*** Every woman has intuitive knowledge related to her body, but sometimes we need to remind her of that strength. We tend to create our own reality, and it helps if we create a positive one. Affirmations can do that. **Affirmations** are positive statements that can be used as support tools throughout labor. They may be based on religious statements or scripture or just be a simple statement that a woman finds affirming. Examples are "Be strong and of good courage. Fear not" (1 Chronicles 22:13); "My body will show me how to give birth," "I can do this," or "Come on, baby, we can do this."

It is important that those supporting and caring for the mother also use affirmations. Being verbally positive will reinforce to the mother her beliefs about herself and her abilities. It will also remind caregivers about the mother's strengths and abilities.

***Breathing Techniques.*** The breathing techniques for labor have changed in nature from the early prepared childbirth movement and the use of the highly structured patterns of the Lamaze techniques. With educators and labor support assistants currently presenting a more physiologic and natural approach to women's use of breathing techniques in labor, the current emphasis is on breathing awareness. Most techniques include starting and finishing with the traditional cleansing breath. The **cleansing breath,** is a deep and deliberate inhalation and exhalation that gives the mother a boost of oxygen, while indicating the beginning and completion of a contraction. It is also referred to as a welcoming breath or a greeting breath (Figure 13-11).

Between the beginning and ending cleansing breaths, the woman breathes in a pattern that makes her comfortable. The woman can best determine the depth and rate of breathing. Sometimes a woman may inadvertently hyperventilate and need to slow her pattern of breathing. Hyperventilation can leave a woman nauseated and dizzy, but simple remedies can help. The woman can cup her hands over her mouth and nose and rebreathe her air for a few contractions. As an alternative, the woman may be given a small paper bag to breathe into for several contractions.

Breathing patterns for second stage may be in one of two patterns: breathing lightly to reduce the tendency to bear down before her cervix is fully dilated or breathing in a long, slow exhale as the baby is pushed down and out. To help the woman focus, the partner or birth attendant can breathe along with the woman or provide short and clear verbal directions.

The most common breathing techniques for light breathing are rapid panting or blowing patterns. A "candle blowing" pattern uses breaths that are shallow and rapid—repetitive breaths similar to that of lightly playing with a candle flame. Another pattern is light like a panting puppy.

Breathing patterns for pushing the baby down and out involve nonphysiologic and physiologic patterns. Nonphysiologic breathing involves extended breath holding, in essence creating a Valsalva maneuver. This is not as productive in moving the baby down the birth canal as physiologic breathing. With physiologic breathing, the woman creates a pattern of breathing in which she slowly releases her breath, with or without vocalization. This second pattern is less stressful to the woman, is more efficient in moving the baby forward because of the secondary involvement of her abdominal muscles, and facilitates a better supply of oxygen to the mother and baby.

*Hypnosis.* Some women have found that hypnosis before labor is useful. They are awake and aware during the labor and delivery process; however, with the process of posthypnotic suggestion, they are comfortable.

***Motion and Position.*** Freedom of positional choice is important through both first and second stage labor. A woman will feel freer to move in labor if she has practiced various positions while pregnant. Freedom of movement is a critical component for the woman to maintain physiologic comfort. Supporting a woman's choice to move and select positions during labor enhances her feelings of control and comfort.

Upright positions and movement are also helpful as the infant fits through the maternal pelvis. The supine position should continue to be avoided during labor and birth because it precipitates supine hypotension and reduces uteroplacental blood flow.

Positions or movements are limited only by the imagination of the birthing women, her partner, and birth attendants (see Figure 13-7). Upright positions commonly assumed for labor include standing, leaning, and walking. The benefits include increased contraction effectiveness, improved alignment for the infant entering the maternal pelvis, and reduction of back pain. When resting during contractions, she may lean on a raised countertop or bedside table, cushioned with pillows.

When the woman wants a rest, positive sitting positions include being upright on the bed; semisitting, such as leaning back against partner; sitting in a rocker or recliner; and sitting on the toilet or bedside commode.

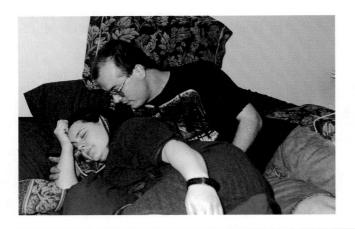 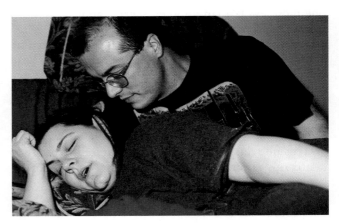

*FIGURE 13-11* • Partner learning relaxation and breathing. *(Courtesy of Caroline E. Brown.)*

A woman can change the baby's position in several ways, including being on all fours. Other postures such as just resting on hands and knees, doing the pelvic rock from the hands and knee position, and kneeling and leaning forward on a large exercise ball or chair seat also help to change the baby's position. These positions are particularly useful when the woman is experiencing back pain during labor, and assuming this position may facilitate rotation of an infant from a posterior to an anterior position. They can also reduce pressure on hemorrhoids.

Lateral positions, lying on either her left or right side, are particularly useful at night or when the woman needs a rest period or a backrub. However, the woman should maintain motion by alternating from one side to the other every hour.

Squatting positions include squatting without support, squatting with the support of a labor attendant, use of a squatting stool, squatting while hanging on to a bar for stabilization, and squatting by sitting on the toilet or bedside commode. The squat position may open the diameter of the pelvis by 2 cm. It also increases intra-abdominal pressure, which helps move the infant into the maternal pelvis. For these two reasons, it is not only useful during the first stage of labor, but also is the optimal position for second stage.

***Heat and Cold.*** Heat and cold may both be used during the process of labor. What the woman wants will change from one time to another. Teach the partner to cover the area with a towel or cloth to reduce the risk of thermal injury when applying heat or cold.

Local application of heat can reduce a woman's perception of pain and enhance her relaxation response. Heat can be provided with a heating pad or with moist warm towels or wash cloths. Fabric-covered bags filled with rice can be warmed in the microwave to provide a source of heat as well.

Local application of cold can reduce edema as well as muscular and skeletal pain. Ice pack can be made from vinyl gloves filled with ice, traditional ice packs, or cold cloths.

***Counter Pressure.*** Firm counter pressure is most commonly applied to a woman's lower back if she experiences back contractions or pain during labor. Tennis balls or the heels of her partner's or the birth attendant's hands may be pressed into her lower back (see Figure 13-8).

***Reflexology and Acupressure.*** Reflexology and acupressure are complementary therapies that use the technique of applying pressure at certain points to help the woman feel more comfortable. "**Reflexology** is a widely practiced form of manual therapy that involves the application of pressure to specific parts of the body, usually the soles of the feet (but sometimes the palms of the hand). It is based on the theory that these parts of the feet (or hands) correspond to, and can therapeutically affect, various organs and glands of the body" (Nurse's

Handbook of Alternative and Complementary Therapies, 1998). In use for more than 3,000 years, it is believed that these points follow the same meridians as those used in acupressure and acupuncture.

When using **acupressure,** also known as Chinese massage, the practitioner applies deep finger pressure to acupoints. Acupoints are the locations on the body that when stimulated by needles or pressure, "balance, release, or enhance the flow of *qi* (the vital life force) and thus relieve pain or restore health" (Nurse's Handbook of Alternative and Complementary Therapies, 1998). Application of these techniques requires additional knowledge of these specialty practices.

***Hydrotherapy.*** **Hydrotherapy,** being in a pool of warm water, can enhance relaxation, normalize blood pressure, and reduce a woman's perception of pain. Getting into a bath tub or a pool with water 89° to 100° F provides the optimal results. If this option is not available, a shower may be used as an alternative. Water can be used at any point throughout the birthing process and may be the preferred choice for the birth of the baby as well.

Used around the world, hydrotherapy was first promoted in the United States by Dr. Michel Odent during the 1980s. It is now more commonly offered as an option. Most women feel relaxed and find great comfort in warm water. When a woman in labor relaxes in a warm tub, free from gravity's pull on her body, with sensory stimulation reduced, her body is less likely to produce adrenaline and more able to produce endorphins. Another benefit is that the water makes the tissues of the perineum more elastic, reducing the incidence of tearing or the use of an episiotomy.

When the baby is born while under water it continues to receive oxygen through the umbilical cord and placenta just as it did in utero. It is not until the newborn makes contact with the cooler air that the complex physiologic process of breathing begins. During the first few seconds after birth, while underwater, the newborn makes the gentle transition to life outside the womb.

***Intradermal Water Injections.*** Intradermal sterile water injections are used in many European countries to assist with pain management during the first stage of labor. The technique is slowly becoming more common in the United States as certified nurse midwives offer it as an option. The technique involves injecting 0.1 ml of sterile water intradermally with a 25 gauge needle at four points in the lower back (Simpkin, 1986). The technique is especially effective for back discomfort.

***Transcutaneous Electrical Nerve Stimulation.*** Some birth facilities provide the woman with the option of using a transcutaneous electrical nerve stimulation (TENS) unit to reduce her sensations of pain. The TENS device is commonly used in physical therapy for pain management. The technique involves placement of the TENS electrodes on either side of the lower spine during the first stage of labor. During contractions the woman creates electrical stimulation with the unit. This stimulation provides an alternate sensation for her thereby decreasing her perception of pain from the contractions. The technique works most effectively if the woman has a chance to practice before active labor.

### Pharmacologic Pain Management

Information about the pharmacologic agents and techniques available during birth are also explained during childbirth preparation classes. Women need to have this information in advance of the labor process so that they have a chance to further explore and think about the options they have. If medication techniques and the effect of the individual drugs are not discussed during the prenatal period, the woman will be vulnerable to agreeing to something she doesn't fully understand while she is in labor.

General considerations to include in giving women information include purpose of the drug; how it is administered; when it is administered; how often it may be repeated; how it works to reduce pain; and the effects on the mother, the baby, and the partner. The possible cascade effects of a drug or medication technique should be explained. The **cascade** effect explains the possible outcomes of the use of the intervention beyond the intended effect. It involves more than side effects because it explains how one response might then require another response. (This is discussed further on page 504.)

*Analgesia.* The goal of analgesia during labor is to provide the highest level of pain relief with least amount

---

**TABLE 13-7** *Analgesia or Anesthesia in First Stage of Labor*

| Systemic Medications | Effect |
|---|---|
| **Sedatives (barbiturates) (infrequently used)** pentobarbital (Nembutal) secobarbitol (Seconal) | • Provide sedation or sleep<br>• Reduce tension and fear<br>• Used to help woman rest |
| **Tranquilizers (infrequently used)** hydroxyzine (Vistaril) promethazine (Phenergan) | • Reduce anxiety<br>• Provide muscle relaxation<br>• Decrease nausea and vomiting<br>• Thought to potentate narcotics, but there is no objective evidence |
| **Opioid analgesic (agonist)*** meperidine (Demerol) morphine | • Raise woman's threshold for pain<br>• May increase or decrease uterine contractions<br>• May cause drowsiness<br>• Used when antagonist or mixed antagonist will precipitate withdrawal in drug-dependent individuals and should not be given |
| **Opioid analgesic (Mixed agonist/antagonists)** butorphanol (Stadol) nalbuphine (Nubain) | • Provide same anesthesia as narcotics without causing respiratory depression in the mother or neonate |

| Regional Anesthesia | Effect |
|---|---|
| **Epidural or caudal†** local anesthetic injected into the epidural space | • Cause sensory blockage by acting on nerve fibers as they cross the epidural space<br>• Affect entire pelvis and lower extremities so woman can sense touch but not pain<br>• May cause maternal hypotension, which will decrease the uterine blood flow, leading to potential fetal distress<br>• Adding a narcotic decreases the amount of local anesthetic needed, speeds the onset of action, improves the quality of pain relief, and increases the duration of action<br>• Labor may be lengthened |
| **Intrathecal narcotic** narcotic injected into subarachnoid space | • Provides pain relief but woman is able to maintain mobility and sensation; sometimes referred to as a "walking epidural"<br>• May cause pruritis, nausea and vomiting, and urinary retention |

*Before giving a narcotic, be sure that a narcotic antagonist (e.g., naloxone hydrochloride [Narcan]) is available.

†May be given in diluted concentration combined with narcotics (e.g., fentanyl or sufentanil) via continuous infusion pump.

Adapted from Mattson S and Smith J, editors: *Core curriculum for maternal-newborn nursing*, ed 2, Philadelphia, 2000, W.B. Saunders; Simpson K and Creehan P: *Perinatal nursing*, Philadelphia, 1996, Lippincott.

of risk for the woman and baby. Analgesic agents are selected based on the expected effects on the woman, the baby, and the progress of the labor. All systemic drugs given for pain relief cross the placenta. High doses remain active in the fetal circulation longer than in the mother's circulation.

To reduce the chance that the analgesia will slow the labor contractions it is generally not given to the woman until labor is clearly established, and the woman's cervix has dilated at least 3 to 5 centimeters. The birth attendant generally decides when the woman can receive the medication. If it is given too early it will slow her labor. If it is given too late the woman will not get the effect she desires and the infant may be born with a sufficient amount of medication in its system to cause respiratory distress. Within hospitals, the labor nurse generally decides when to give the woman the systemic medications prescribed as needed (PRN) by the physician, nurse-midwife, or nurse anesthetist (Table 13-7).

Because of the pressure the baby places on the tissues as it descends the birth canal and pushes up against the perineum, every woman experiences a numbing of these tissues. Some women select to have additional anesthesia for delivery. Options are determined by what providers are available because only an anesthesiologist or nurse anesthetist can provide some of the selections. Birth attendants also determine options after assessing the status of the baby, the woman, and the birth process.

*Anesthesia.* Some women may have the caudal or epidural anesthesia started during the first stage of labor, and it continues throughout the second stage (Figure 13-12). Alternative anesthesia options available in the second stage of labor are a pudendal block, a saddle block, or local infiltration (Table 13-8). Regional anesthesia related to the spinal cord is given by a nurse anesthetist or anesthesiologist.

## Unexpected Situations in Pregnancy and Birth

Although pregnancy and birth proceed in an uneventful manner most of the time, the possibility of experiencing unexpected outcomes still exists for some women. Pregnant couples will hear many childbirth stories by well-meaning family members, friends, and even complete strangers. Some of them will be disconcerting, and others will be frightening. Couples come to sessions with this information and wonder what options and control they have. Being able to ask questions and receive accurate information helps control their anxiety and boost their confidence.

The educational discussion always begins with a presentation of the typical and expected process of birth. As the various topics are raised, situations that may fall outside the normal experience are addressed. For example, one of the typical discussion points is the length of labor. Discussion begins by presenting the average length, but then proceeds to preparing for both a longer and a shorter time frame.

Because every condition occurs on a continuum, the discussion of possible situations that might unfold and the role the mother and her labor support person may be gently presented. As educator, you can introduce the woman's options and choices in the context of each unexpected intervention.

### Medical Management of Birth
The medical management approach to childbirth views birth as a potential emergency. However, many of the

---

## TABLE 13-8  *Anesthesia in the Second Stage of Labor*

| Regional Anesthesia | Effect |
|---|---|
| **Pudental block**<br>Anesthestic is injected through the lateral vaginal walls near the ischial spines | • Anesthetizes the lower vagina, vulva, and perineum<br>• Because it is given close to birth, it has little or no effect on baby |
| **Saddle block**<br>Local anesthetic introduced into the subarachnoid space of the spine | • Motor and sensory nerves of lower part of body are blocked<br>• Woman may not be able to feel the sensations and continue to push the baby out<br>• Decreased blood flow to fetus with maternal hypotension secondary to peripheral vasodilation |
| **Local infiltration**<br>Anesthetic injected into the perineum and posterior vagina | • Performed just before delivery; if an episiotomy is to be cut, it is done before that<br>• Has no effect on fetus<br>• Provides anesthesia for the repair of the episiotomy |

Adapted from Mattson S and Smith J, editors: *Core curriculum for maternal-newborn nursing,* ed 2, Philadelphia, 2000, W.B. Saunders; Simpson K and Creehan P: *Perinatal nursing,* Philadelphia, 1996, Lippincott.

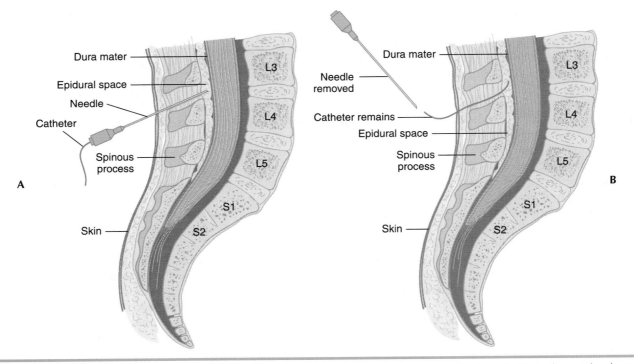

FIGURE 13-12 • Epidural. **A,** A needle is inserted into the epidural space; **B,** A catheter is threaded into the epidural space, then the needle is removed. The catheter allows medication to be administered intermittently or continuously to relieve pain during labor and childbirth.

prevailing practices and beliefs are based on false, out-moded, or unverified assumptions. "The myths concerning childbirth include commonly used obstetrical practices that are unnecessary and that actually interfere with the normal physiology of the birth process" (Harper, 1994) (Box 13-6).

The appropriateness of the broad use of routine interventions for births in the United States remains in question. Routine electronic fetal monitoring, restricted movement, amniotomy, oxytocin use, extensive use of analgesia and anesthesia, cesarean delivery, episiotomy, vacuum extraction, and forceps delivery are potentially useful in select high-risk pregnancies. However, their value in low-risk pregnancies has not been demonstrated.

In some cases these interventions create problems in otherwise normal labors and deliveries. Comprehensive reviews of technologic practices in obstetrics have caused some providers to critically reflect on interventions that have become routine. In many instances the use of one medical intervention necessitates the use of others. This can be considered a cascade effect.

### Exploring the Cascade Effect

During preparation classes, exploring the cascade effect is a strategy that engages participants in exploring various dimensions of an intervention. First the intervention is described in a factual manner, discussing the advantages and benefits of an intervention. Then the ripple effect of the intervention is considered.

This strategy can be used to explore various interventions that are options during childbirth. In addition to providing information, it makes clear that there are no right or wrong decisions, but various options that may be contemplated based on a woman's needs. It also demonstrates how an intervention selected for one reason may lead to other conditions. Having followed this line of thinking in class, women are prepared to do it again when presented with options in childbirth. This practice allows faster dissemination of information and facilitates the ability of the woman to participate in decision making more quickly.

Developing flow charts helps clarify the ramifications of a given issue. With a growing knowledge base and little bit of encouragement, class participants can soon participate in the construction on the flow sheets. Examples of cascade flow sheets for amniotomy, Pitocin use, and supine position follow. These and other like them may be constructed during educational sessions in response to attendees' questions (Figures 13-13 to 13-15).

## PREPARING FOR THE JOURNEY TO BIRTH

The most important decisions prospective parents will make, in terms of the outcome of the birth and the potential future health of their child, concerns their choices for their pregnancy, labor, and birth experience. Women are more satisfied with their care when they have been considered as individuals, supported in their journey to parenthood. One aspect of this support

## BOX 13-6 *Medical Myths Surrounding Childbirth*

**Myth #1:** *The hospital is the safest place to have a baby.*
**Reality:** The countries with the lowest mortality and morbidity rates are those where home birth is a common practice.

**Myth #2:** *Maternity care should be managed only by a physician.*
**Reality:** Research has demonstrated that qualified midwives offer competent maternity care for women seeking normal, natural, gentle births.

**Myth #3:** *Family and friends interfere during birth.*
**Reality:** Never leaving a woman alone in labor and providing her with strong emotional support have been shown to decrease the length of labor and reduce stress in the infant.

**Myth #4:** *Labors progress in a predictable manner for a predictable length of time.*
**Reality:** Each woman's labor may be different both from other women as well as from her prior experiences.

**Myth #5:** *Once in labor, a woman should stay in bed.*
**Reality:** Mobility improves contraction quality and improves the labor progress.

**Myth #6:** *Artificial rupture of the membranes (amniotomy) will speed labor.*
**Reality:** Amniotomy may have little or no effect on labor length or have an effect only in some subgroups.

**Myth #7:** *It is better not to eat or drink during labor.*
**Reality:** The practice of withholding foods or liquids increases the risk of dehydration and negative nitrogen balance in the laboring woman. In addition, fasting does not guarantee an empty stomach.

**Myth #8:** *Drugs for pain relief won't hurt the baby.*
**Reality:** There is little research on the effects of drugs on the baby during childbirth and later as the child grows.

**Myth #9:** *The electronic fetal monitor will save babies.*
**Reality:** At best, electronic fetal monitoring can only detect whether an infant is doing fine. It has not demonstrated the ability to predict or prevent neurologic morbidity.

**Myth #10:** *When a baby is in a breech presentation, it must be delivered by a cesarean.*
**Reality:** External version, near term can safely increase the number of babies in vertex position and decrease the need for cesarean deliveries.

**Myth #11:** *An episiotomy heals better than a tear.*
**Reality:** Episiotomies do not heal better than tears nor are they less painful than tears.

**Myth #12:** *Birth needs to be sterile.*
**Reality:** Birth cannot possibly be sterile because when the baby emerges it is coated with a film of the mother's vaginal bacteria.

**Myth #13:** *Once a cesarean always a cesarean.*
**Reality:** Most women who are supported in a vaginal birth after a prior cesarean delivery will succeed.

**Myth #14:** *The baby must go to the newborn nursery for observation.*
**Reality:** For the normal, unmedicated mother and newborn, separation interferes with the initial process of getting to know each other during the maternal sensitive period.

**Myth #15:** *Baby boys need to be circumcised*
**Reality:** In 1975, the American Academy of Pediatrics announced that there is no absolute medical indication for routine circumcision.

From Goer H: *Obstetric myths and research realities,* Westport, Conn, 1995, Bergin & Garvey; and Harper B: *Gentle birth choices,* Rochester, Vt, 1994, Healing Arts Press.

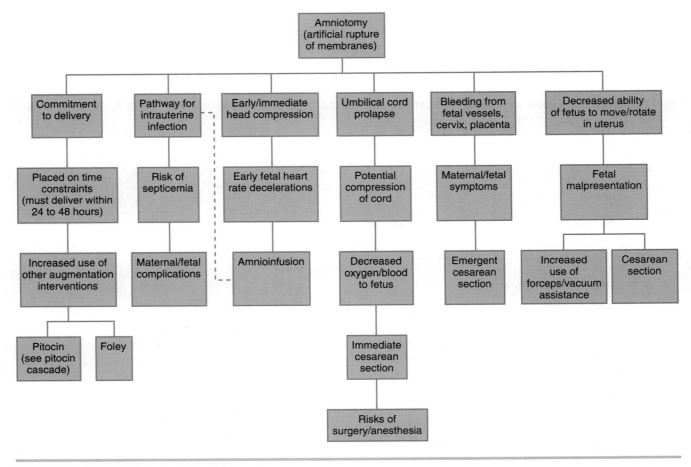

FIGURE 13-13 • Possible cascade with amniotomy.

is providing information from which they may make their choices. An informed choice is one in which:

- Accurate information, based on the most up-to-date research, is provided
- The specific areas where choice is available are detailed and outlined
- The advantages and disadvantages of the various options are given
- Enough time is given for consideration of the physical and psychologic implications of each choice
- Information included about any potential risks, flowing from specific decisions, is presented in a sensitive, nonthreatening manner
- Crisis decisions, based on information that is unavailable to the parents(s), are delegated to the medical attendants
- Emotional support is available, regardless of the decisions made
- Evaluation is made to ensure that the information that is given is understood (Robertson, 1994).

Participation in childbirth preparation can be empowering and may be pivotal in helping women, and their partners, achieve the birth experience of their choice.

 **SUMMARY**

The process of giving birth is a powerful experience in a woman's life. During these hours, she can expect to work harder than ever imagined while simultaneously experiencing a wider variety of sensations than she has at any other time in her life.

Because each experience is unique for each woman, participation is essential. Understanding how her body is designed for the process, learning how she may work with her body, and the birthing options available to her empower the woman to assume the level of participation she desires.

Birth involves more than the mother and the fetus. Preparation must also be offered to the woman's partner and/or the person or persons who will provide her labor support to ensure the desired birth experience.

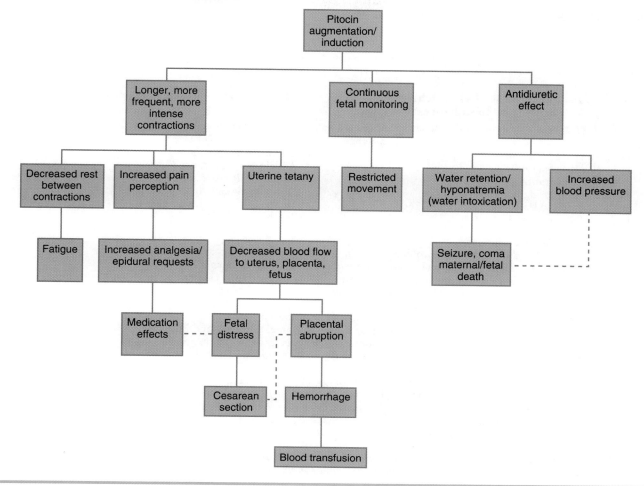

FIGURE 13-14 • Possible cascade with pitocin.

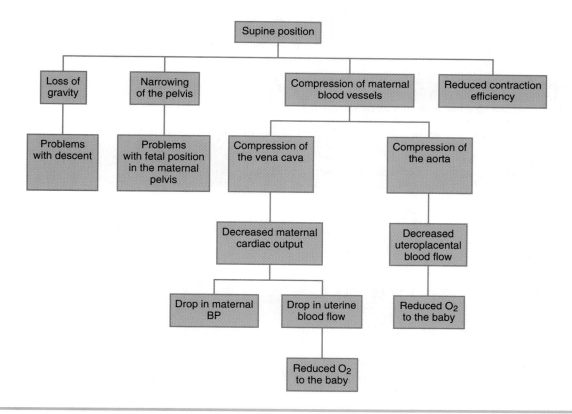

FIGURE 13-15 • Possible cascade with supine position.

## Care Plan · The Couple Preparing for Childbirth

NURSING DIAGNOSIS **Health-Seeking Behaviors (Childbirth Preparation)** related to desire for making informed decisions about birth experiences

GOALS/OUTCOMES Chooses and experiences the desired level of self-determination and active participation in childbirth

**NOC Suggested Outcomes**
- Health Beliefs (1700)
- Health Orientation (1705)
- Health Promoting Behavior (1602)
- Participation: Health Care Decisions (1606)
- Social Support (1504)

**NIC Priority Interventions**
- Anticipatory Guidance (5210)
- Childbirth Preparation (6760)
- Decision-Making Support (5250)
- Health System Guidance (7400)
- Teaching: Individual (5606)

**Nursing Activities and Rationale**
- Assess woman's and partner's desire to participate in decision making related to her care. *People vary in their desire for control in decision making about their health care.*
- Assess woman's concern about maintaining self-control during the birth process *because it influences choices such as type of pain relief measures.*
- Assess amount of control over situation and events desired by woman and partner *because it influences choice of care provider (e.g., midwife or physician).*
- Explore options for childbirth: type of provider, setting (e.g., home, hospital), and birth philosophies (e.g., Leboyer, Odent, Noble methods), *which provides information needed for informed choice. Waving various options is important because women's beliefs and wishes vary.*
- Provide a list of childbirth preparation programs available in the community that most closely meet the needs expressed by the couple, *which supports self-determination. Appropriate, responsive classes result in increased satisfaction with the birth.*
- Assess social support network (e.g., family, friends, specialists, care providers for the birth). *Social support is associated with positive labor outcomes and increased satisfaction with the birth experience.*
- Assist woman/partner in developing a birth plan *to help demystify the birthing experience and help the couple think through their options and communicate preferences to the health care team.*
- Explain options for pharmacologic and nonpharmacologic pain management during the birth process *to reinforce explanations given in childbirth preparation class.*
- Correct myths about the medical management of childbirth *to provide balanced information to empower the woman/partner to make informed decisions about their birth process.*
- Use the "cascade effect" to discuss advantages and benefits of an intervention *which makes clear that there are no right or wrong decisions, but various options; advance practice facilitates the ability of the woman to participate in decision making during the birth process.*

**Evaluation Parameters**
- Freely discusses options for birth.
- Expresses preferences for decision-making involvement.
- Expresses concerns about maintaining self-control.
- Chooses type of provider, setting, and childbirth preparation program; verbalizes comfort with choice.
- Completes a birth plan.
- Decides in advance on the type of pain relief desired during the birth process.
- Discusses the pros and cons of medical interventions such as oxytocin administration and episiotomy.
- Expresses satisfaction with the birth experience

## CASE STUDY

Emily, a 23-year-old woman of Irish descent, is 30 weeks pregnant. She has called you, a certified childbirth educator, in response to a flyer her nurse-midwife gave her. She explains that her midwife encouraged her to call about the childbirth preparation classes, saying that they would be helpful to her. She asks, "Why should I come to class when I can read and practice everything I need to know at home?"

## CASE STUDY

- What other information would you like to have before you offer an answer?

- What would you say that would explain the value of the series to her?

Emily then says, "What do I do if both my mother and the father of the baby want to come too? How should I handle this?"

- What other information do you need before you explore this situation with Emily?

- In general, how will you answer her?

Emily thanks you for your time and information and then says, "I'm still not sure. I don't know what I will get out of the class. I am legally blind and everything I read has to be in Braille. How am I going to be able to get anything out of these classes?"

- With this new information revealed, how will you alter your assessment of how the classes will be helpful?

- What adaptations might you have to make so that Emily will obtain full benefit from the program?

# Scenarios

**1.** Melissa and her partner Linda come to the clinic for their first prenatal visit. At the conclusion of the visit, you tell them that you offer early pregnancy classes every Wednesday night and you would like to invite them to come. Melissa asks, "What is covered in the classes? Why couldn't we just read a book? What would be the value of our coming?"

- What subjective and objective data do you need before you answer?

- What nursing diagnoses could apply? How will you validate these?

- What goals might be developed? How will these be prioritized?

- What interventions may you offer?

- How will you evaluate the effectiveness of your interventions?

**2.** Sophy, a 22-year-old primigravida, is 14 weeks pregnant and attending your early pregnancy class. When the topic of fetal development comes up she asks, "When will my baby look like a baby? How long is it and how much does it weigh? When will I feel my baby move?"

- What subjective and objective data do you need before you answer?

- What nursing diagnoses could apply? How will you validate these?

- What goals might be developed? How will these be prioritized?

- What interventions may you offer?

- How will you evaluate the effectiveness of your interventions?

**3.** Katia is an 18-year-old woman, pregnant with her first child. She is attending early pregnancy classes with her partner, Luke. Katia says to you, "My friend had a baby last month and she is still upset about the things that were done to her. I'm scared! What can we do that will keep that from happening to us?"

- What subjective and objective data do you need before you answer?

- What nursing diagnoses could apply? How will you validate these?

- What goals might be developed? How will these be prioritized?

- What interventions may you offer?

- How will you evaluate the effectiveness of your interventions?

**4.** During childbirth classes Jim helps his partner Liz with the relaxation and breathing exercises by massaging her shoulders and breathing with her through the simulated contractions. During a break in the class, he shares with you that he has gained weight since Liz became pregnant, that he has had some nausea and vomiting, and now he is experiencing heartburn.

- What subjective data do you have about Jim's condition?
- What subjective and objective data do you need before you answer?
- What nursing diagnoses could apply? How will you validate these?
- What goals might be developed? How will these be prioritized?
- What interventions may you offer?
- How will you evaluate the effectiveness of your interventions?

5. Ted also attends the childbirth education classes and remains at his wife Susan's side during all the exercises. However, Ted does not touch Susan or offer any visible support to her during class.

- What objective data do you have about Ted's activities?
- What subjective and objective data do you need?
- What nursing diagnoses could apply? How will you validate these?
- What goals might be developed? How will these be prioritized?
- What interventions may you offer?
- How will you evaluate the effectiveness of your interventions?

6. Inga and Peter are practicing their relaxation techniques in class. As Inga sits cross-legged on the floor and Peter massages her shoulders and back, Inga starts to gradually relax and her breathing becomes deeper. Then you notice that she starts shifting her body around, raising her head and turning it from side to side. Finally she raises her head and says, "It's no use, I can't concentrate. I'll never be able to do this in labor!"

- What subjective and objective data do you have?
- What additional data do you need before you answer?
- What nursing diagnoses could apply? How will you validate these?

- What goals might be developed? How will these be prioritized?
- What interventions may you offer?
- How will you evaluate the effectiveness of your interventions?

7. Roberta, a 27-year-old woman of Haitian descent, tells you that she wants to attend classes to learn how to have a baby in the United States, but her husband is hesitant to come with her.

- What subjective data do you have?
- What subjective and objective data do you need before you answer?
- What nursing diagnoses could apply? How will you validate these?
- What goals might be developed? How will these be prioritized?
- What interventions may you offer?
- How will you evaluate the effectiveness of your interventions?

8. Doreen and her best friend Donna are attending childbirth preparation classes together. Donna will be present during the labor and is preparing to be Doreen's primary labor support person. This is Doreen's first child but Donna is older and already has three children, the oldest being 15 years old. Donna went to prepared childbirth classes during her first pregnancy.

During class Doreen and Donna are practicing together in response to a labor simulation exercise that you are conducting. As Doreen relaxes and breathes deeper and deeper, you hear Donna say to her, "This is never going to work. You have to breathe quicker, when the contractions are this long. It has to be more structured; do 'pant blow'!"

- What subjective and objective data do you need before you answer?
- What nursing diagnoses could apply? How will you validate these?
- What goals might be developed? How will these be prioritized?
- What interventions may you offer?
- How will you evaluate the effectiveness of your interventions?

# REFERENCES

Aaronson L: Nurse-midwives and obstetricians: alternative models of care and client "fit," *Res Nurs Health* 10:217-226, 1987.

Arms S: *A new look at women and childbirth: immaculate deception,* Toronto, 1975, Bantam Books.

Arms S: *Immaculate deception II: a fresh look at childbirth,* Berkley, 1994, Celestial Arts.

Beck N, Geden E, and Brouder G: Preparation for labor; a historical perspective, *Psychosom Med* 41(3):243-258, 1979.

Bing E and Karmel M: *A practical training course for the psychoprophylactic method of childbirth,* New York, 1961, American Society for Psychoprophylaxis in Obstetrics.

Bloom JR: The relationship of social support and health, *Soc Sci Med* 30(5):635-637, 1990.

Boston Women's Health Book Collective. *Our bodies, ourselves.* New York, 1998, Touchstone.

Bromberg J: Having a baby: a story essay. In Romalis S, editor. *Childbirth alternatives to medical control,* Austin, 1981, University of Texas Press.

Brown C and Shocker B: Preparing women for nontraditional positional approaches for labor and birth: a childbirth education strategy, *Midwifery Today* 33:22, 1995.

Centers for Disease Control and Prevention (CDC): Report of final mortality statistics, 1996. Vol. 47, No. 9. pp. (PHS) 99-1120, 1998. Available at *http://www.cdc.gov/nchswww/releses/98facts/98sheets/finmort.htm.*

Centers for Disease Control and Prevention (CDC): Infant Mortality Statistics from the 1997 Period Linked Birth/Infant Death Data Set. Vol. 47, No. 23. pp. (PHS) 99-1120, 1999. Available at *http://www.cdc.gov/nchswww/releses/99facts/99sheets/infmort.htm.*

Chute G: Expectation and experience in alternative and conventional birth, *J Obstet Gynecol Neonatal Nurs* 14(1):61-67, 1985.

Cogan R: Effects of childbirth preparation, *Clin Obstet Gynecol* 23(1):1-14, 1981.

Consumer Reports: Too many cesareans, *Consumer Rep* (Feb):1-6, 1991.

Consumer Reports: Wasted health care dollars, *Consumer Rep* (July): 435-449, 1992.

Davis-Floyd R: *Birth as an American rite of passage,* Berkley, 1992, University of California University Press.

Davis-Floyd R: Hospital birth as a technocratic rite of passage, *Mothering Magazine* (67):69-75, 1993.

Davis-Floyd R and Sargent C: *Childbirth and authoritative knowledge,* Berkley, 1997, University of California Press.

Dick-Read G: *Childbirth without fear,* New York, 1933, Harper and Row.

Eakins P: *The American way of birth,* Philadelphia, 1986, Temple University Press.

Ehrenreich B and English D: *Complaints and disorders: the sexual politics of sickness,* New York, 1973, Feminist press.

Enkin M: Antenatal classes. In Enkin M and others, editors. *Effectiveness and satisfaction in antenatal care,* Philadelphia, 1982, Lippincott.

Gagnon AJ, Waghorn K, Covell C: A randomized trial of one-to-one nurse support of women in labor, *Birth* 24:71-77, 1997.

Goer H: *Obstetric myths versus research realities,* Westport, Conn, 1995, Bergin and Garvey.

Green J, Coupland V, and Kitzinger J: Expectation, experiences, and psychological outcomes of childbirth: a prospective study of 825 women, *Birth J* 17(1):15-24, 1990.

Harper B: *Gentle birth choices,* Rochester, Vt, 1994, Healing Arts Press.

Hassid P: *Textbook for childbirth educators,* Philadelphia, 1984, Lippincott.

Huttel C and others: A quantitative evaluation of psychoprophylaxis in childbirth, *J Psychomatic Res* 16:81-93, 1972.

Jordan B: The hut and the hospital: information, power, and symbolism in the artifacts of birth, *Birth* 14(1):36-40, 1987.

Kahn R: *Bearing meaning.* Urbana, 1995, University of Illinois Press.

Kennell J and others: Continuous emotional support during labor in a U.S. hospital, *JAMA* 265(17):2197-2201, 1991.

Kitzinger S: *The experience of childbirth,* ed 3, Baltimore, 1972, Penguin.

Kitzinger S: *Education for counseling and childbirth,* New York, 1977, Schoeken.

Kitzinger S: *Birth at home,* New York, 1979, Penguin Books.

Kitzinger S: *Women's experience of sex,* New York, 1985, Penguin.

Kitzinger S: Episiotomy, *Mothering Magazine* June(55):62-67, 1990.

Kitzinger S: Birth plans, *Birth: Issues in Perinatal Care* 19(1):36-37, 1992.

Lamaze F: *Painless childbirth: the Lamaze method.* New York, 1956, Pocket.

Leboyer F: *Birth without violence,* New York, 1975, Knopf.

Littlefield V and Adams B: Patient participation in alternate perinatal care: impact on satisfaction and health locus of control, *Res Nurs Health* 10:139-148, 1987.

Mackey M: Women's preparation for the childbirth experience, *Matern Child Nurs J* 19(2):143-173, 1990.

Mattson S and Smith J, editors: *Core curriculum for maternal-newborn nursing,* ed 2, Philadelphia, 2000, W.B. Saunders.

Miles A: *Women, health, and medicine,* Philadelphia, 1991, Open University Press.

Noble E: *Essential exercises for the childbearing year,* ed 2, Boston, 1982, Houghton-Mifflin.

Noble E: *Childbirth with insight,* Boston 1983, Houghton-Mifflin.

Noble E: Essential exercise for the childbearing year, ed 4, Harwich, 1995, New Life Images.

*Nurses handbook of alternative and complementary therapies*: Springhouse, Penn, 1998, Springhouse.

Oakley A: *The captured womb,* Oxford, 1984, Basil Blackwell Published Ltd.

Odent M: *Birth reborn,* New York, 1984, Patheon Books.

Perez P: *The nurturing touch at birth: a labor support handbook,* Katy, Tx, 1997, Cutting Edge Press.

Renner P: *The art of teaching adults,* Vancouver, Canada, 1994, Training Associates.

Robertson A: *Empowering women—teaching active birth in the 90's,* Camperdown, Australia, 1994, ACE Graphics.

Romalis S: *Childbirth alternatives to medical control,* Austin, Tx, 1981, University of Texas Press.

Rooks J: *Midwifery and childbirth in America,* Philadelphia, 1997, Temple University Press.

Rorden J: *Nurses as health teachers: a practical guide,* Philadelphia, 1987, W.B. Saunders.

Rothman B: Awake and aware or false consciousness: the co-optation of childbirth reform in America. In Romalis S, editor: *Childbirth alternatives to medical control,* Austin, Tx, 1981, University of Texas Press.

Rothman B: *Recreating motherhood ideology and technology in a patriarchal society,* New York, 1989, Norton.

Rothman B: *In labor—women and power in the birthplace,* New York, 1991, Norton.

Rubin R: *Maternal identity and the maternal experience,* New York, 1984, Springer.

Sasmor J: *Childbirth education: a nursing perspective,* New York, 1979, Wiley and Sons.

Sequin L and others: The components of women's satisfaction with maternity care, *Birth J* 16(3):109-113, 1989.

Shaw N: *Forced labor: maternity care in the United States,* New York, 1974, Pergamon Press.

Sherwin S: *No longer patient: feminist ethics and health care,* Philadelphia, 1992, Temple University Press.

Simkin P, Whalley J, and Keppler A: *Pregnancy, childbirth, and the newborn: the complete guide,* Minnetonka, MN, 1991, Meadowbrook Press.

Sosa and others: The effect of a supportive companion on perinatal problems, length of labor, and mother-infant interaction, *N Engl J Med* 303(11):597-600, 1980.

Starck M: *Women's medicine ways: cross-cultural rites of passage,* Freedom, Calif, 1993, Crossing Press.

Strychar IM and others: How pregnant women learn about selected health issues: learning transaction types, *Adult Educat Q* 41(1): 17-28, 1990.

Tew M: *Safer childbirth?,* London, 1990, Chapman and Hall.

Timm M: Prenatal education evaluation. *Nursing Res* 28(6):338-342, 1979.

Wertz R and Wertz D: *Lying-in: a history of childbirth in America,* New Haven, Conn, 1989, Yale University Press.

Wheeler C and Chinn P: *Peace and power,* ed 3, New York, 1991, NLN.

# CHAPTER 14

# Providing Care and Support During Labor and Delivery

*"We bring to childbirth our histories, our relationships, our rituals, our needs and values that relate to intimacy, our sexuality, the quality and style of family life and community, and our deepest beliefs about life, birth, and death."*

— JUDITH DICKSON LUCE

*How do we demonstrate a "collaborative partnership" approach to care during the process of labor and delivery?*

*What options does a woman have to enhance her comfort during labor and delivery?*

*How might her choice affect the length, outcomes, and quality of the experience for her and her infant?*

*What must be considered when choosing a method of fetal surveillance during labor and delivery?*

*What nursing assessments and interventions take priority during labor?*

*What strategies can we use to enhance a family's well-being as a new member is added?*

Women conceive, grow, and produce the babies that become our next generation. During most of this process, they are the primary caretakers of themselves and their developing child. During the hours of the labor and delivery process, nurses join with women to assess their needs and provide supportive attention and care to both them and their families. This chapter describes the process of labor and delivery and how we may engage in a collaborative partnership with a woman and her family to provide a climate of confidence that allows the woman to feel affirmed and cared for as she shapes her birthing experience.

This period of time will be forever etched in the memories of the participants, with stories told and retold about the experience. Therefore we have the re-

sponsibility of providing the best experience possible for each family, each time. For us, it may be an 8-hour job with the normal rewards, frustrations, and coffee breaks, but it is a day of miracles for the family!

Working with clients through labor and delivery presents a unique challenge. First, we must realize that as caregiver, we are providing care for two clients—the mother and the unborn child. Our assessments, interventions, and evaluations must consider the well-being of both.

Secondly, labor and delivery is a "family affair" that takes place over a very short period of time. We must be able to develop a collaborative relationship with the woman rather quickly and provide care, taking into consideration her preferences, as well as her safety and that of the fetus. During this time, we must include and consider other family members (e.g., siblings, grandparents, and friends) of the woman. We also act as a patient advocate, communicating with other nurses, the nurse midwife, or the physician to ensure that the mother and fetus are receiving the best care possible.

 ## ESTABLISHING A COLLABORATIVE ENVIRONMENT

A woman approaches childbirth concerned about her ability to function within the normal limits established by others before her, to maintain control of her body and her behavior and situations within her control, and survive the experience intact (Mercer, 1995). Labor and delivery are a process through which the nurse, the woman, and the woman's support network move together with the end result being a healthy family. The labor environment, whether it is a hospital, birthing center, or home, should be one of collaboration. All participants bring information, expertise, skills, and expectations into the birthing process. Together, health care providers and family members can produce a positive birth experience for all.

To develop a collaborative partnership, we must be aware of how we interact with the woman and her labor support people and realize that we do not always "know best." Furthermore, what is "routinely" done for most women in labor is often based on tradition rather than research and may be in conflict with what a laboring woman needs or prefers. In other words, we must seek input, on an ongoing basis, from the woman and her significant others about their preferences while providing a research-based practice for a safe labor and delivery.

### Framework for Developing a Collaborative Partnership

There are four dimensions of collaboration that are easily applied in the labor setting: support, facilitate, inform, prescribe (Pugach and Johnson, 1995). While caring for laboring women and their families, we enter into a variety of interactions. The approach we take during these interactions determines if we are being collaborative or authoritarian. Using a collaborative approach assumes that both the nurse and the woman bring something unique and meaningful to the labor process and have something important to contribute. Each of these dimensions will be described and examples provided (Box 14-1).

#### Inform

Sharing information is a basic dimension of collaboration. We come to the labor experience with a broad knowledge base, a variety of patient experiences, and information about expected policy and procedures. Sharing this information, as well as keeping the woman and

family informed of progress and concerns, is essential in this relationship. The woman can use this information to make informed choices, but this information exchange remains a two-way process.

The woman also comes with information from childbirth classes, reading, etc., as well as the expectations of her culture and her personal experiences. Encouraging her to share this information promotes understanding between participants. An example of information giving is the nurse telling the patient the advantages and disadvantages of regional anesthesia, or the woman telling the nurse about her desire to remain in her own clothing during labor.

#### Support

This dimension can be defined as caring and being there for the woman whenever needed. Support is more than "just being caring and kind." Being supportive assumes that both the nurse and the woman are working towards some common goal and includes the following: sharing the woman's feelings and concerns; praising and recognizing her efforts during the labor process; talking her through difficult situations, giving her confidence to get through the labor; and mentoring her through the labor. We use our therapeutic communication skills to validate the woman's feelings and reflect her thoughts, and use touch to communicate a sense of caring and concern to her. Support is a necessary component of the collaborative process. Laboring women find comfort in knowing that they have a knowledgeable care provider who cares how they are feeling and demonstrates ongoing support for them. Examples of support during labor include talking the woman through a contraction and praising her breathing techniques; discussing a woman's feelings when she learns she must have a surgical delivery (cesarean delivery); or caring for the partner by praising his or her supportive actions with the woman and asking about his or her needs during the birthing process.

#### Facilitate

This dimension is very different than information-giving or supporting and allows the woman to use skills that

---

**BOX 14-1   *Four Dimensions of a Collaborative Relationship***

1. **Inform**—Share information
2. **Support**—Display kind and caring actions for the purpose of attaining a common goal
3. **Facilitate**—Assist the couple, using each other's strengths and expertise to attain a common goal
4. **Prescribe**—Direct the client because she is unable to make decisions or the situation is beyond her expertise

she has not used before. In this dimension, we help the woman with some tasks that she cannot do independently. For example, if a woman desires to have an unmedicated childbirth but finds that she is losing control of the pain, we facilitate her experience by suggesting other pain-relief methods (i.e., changing breathing patterns, changing position, using a focal point) and helping implement these methods. By "suggesting another way" to relieve pain, we are sharing our knowledge, providing her with additional skills, and facilitating the process so that the woman can achieve her goal.

### Prescribe

The final dimension of collaboration is prescription and is the most directive. Within such a collaborative relationship, we become prescriptive to meet the needs of the woman and her fetus—not the needs of the providers. This dimension is appropriate for emergency situations. An example of prescribing may be telling the woman she needs to wear the oxygen mask because "the baby needs more oxygen" (i.e., when the fetal heart rate is bradycardic). The interaction is still done in a caring fashion, giving a brief rationale for why the prescription is critical. If the woman understands that it is part of the process to meet her needs, she will be able to view the interaction as collaborative rather than authoritarian.

It should be noted that although each of these dimensions has a characteristic description, they are rarely used in their pure forms. We often move back and forth through the dimensions in any one interaction. For example, we might give the woman some information, so that she may make an informed decision, and then support and facilitate the woman in achieving her goal.

## Implementing the Collaborative Partnership

### Initiating the Partnership

We are often the first person to greet and assess the woman and the people who will be accompanying her through the birth process. A woman may wish to have her partner, mother, best friend, or a combination of people with her during the labor and delivery process.

Our initial encounter sets the tone for the labor and delivery experience. During this first encounter, we should make a conscious effort to be calm, confident, caring, and cooperative while engaging the woman and her support network. A first step is to review the birth plan. Many women have developed a written birth plan that outlines their cultural and personal preferences for labor and delivery. Examples of common preferences on birth plans include the following: the desire to maintain individuality by wearing her own clothing during labor; minimal invasive procedures (including vaginal examinations and internal monitoring); the number of individuals in the room during the birth; no routine episiotomy; do not cut the umbilical cord until it stops pulsating; do not refer to baby by name or describe its beauty (Box 14-2).

If the family does not have a written plan, encourage  them to express their preferences during the admitting procedures. We might make a statement such as, "I know that this is a very special time in your life, and I want to help make it how you want it to be. Please tell me how you picture this going. Do you have any special requests?" This type of interaction will allow the family to feel comfortable in expressing their desires. Many women may not be aware of the choices they have during the labor and delivery process. It is our responsibility to inform them of their options throughout the course of the labor and answer their questions about

---

### BOX 14-2   *Sample Birth Plan*

We are writing this birth plan to tell you our preferences during the birth of our baby. We understand that emergency situations may arise, and this plan may be altered— we rely on your expertise at this time. We would like to have an unmedicated delivery and minimal interventions. We also would prefer that no time limits be placed on the duration of this labor, as long as the baby and mom are doing alright. If possible, please discuss any deviations you may make from this plan with us. Below are our requests:

- Minimal vaginal examinations
- Freedom to eat and drink as desired
- Flexibility to change positions throughout labor
- Use of massage, showers, birthing ball, music, and dim lights
- No oxytocin
- Minimize interruptions and knock before entering room
- Spontaneous, open-mouth bearing down

- Use of gravity-enhancing pushing positions
- No episiotomy unless emergency arises for the baby
- Allow partner to "catch" the baby
- Baby to my chest immediately after delivery
- Postpone any newborn care (e.g., weighing, eye medication, etc.) until after we have had sufficient time to bond with our baby
- Delay clamping and cutting the cord until it has stopped pulsating
- Let partner cut the cord
- Deliver placenta without intervention (We view the time between the delivery of the baby and the delivery of the placenta as quiet time to bond—please be as unobtrusive as possible during this time.)
- We would like at least one parent to remain with the baby at all times

advantages and disadvantages. Once a woman has stated her preferences, it is our role to support and facilitate these preferences through the birth process, incorporating the woman's desires into the plan of care.

### Helping the Family Adapt to the Labor and Delivery Process

Family members are often very anxious about the birth process because it involves the health and well-being of the mother, who is already a part of their lives, as well as the health and well-being of a yet unknown new member of their family. Family members often want to be supportive but are unsure of how to provide support. We can provide information and demonstrate how they may be part of the process. Family members who remain in another room, away from the laboring woman also appreciate being kept informed about the labor progress. They often drop their normal activities and stay nearby for many hours, so anything we can do to acknowledge them in the process will be greatly appreciated by the woman and her family.

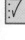

Ask the woman to ascertain the type and amount of involvement she wants other family members to have. Some women prefer to have the family gather in another room away from her, but others want them involved in the labor care as much as possible. Some women only want specific members of the family (e.g., her mother and/or sister) involved. If the woman wants family members involved in the care, include them in as many tasks as possible (e.g., getting ice chips, assisting with positioning or back massage, etc). Allow the family to help the woman as they see fit, as long as the woman approves and their actions do not pose a safety risk for the woman or fetus. At any time during labor, the woman may change her mind about this involvement and our role is to help her meet these needs by assisting in the additional inclusion or exclusion of family members. If the labor is occurring in a hospital or other facility, offering family members who are not directly involved coffee and informing them where the cafeteria or comfortable waiting areas are located will be appreciated.

### Facing Ethical and Legal Issues within the Collaborative Partnership

As client advocate and a member of the health care team, we often encounter ethical and legal dilemmas in our practice. One theme running through our collaborative partnership is that the nurse, the woman, and her family are working toward a common goal. Sometimes, the way the woman and her family have chosen to achieve that goal—or even the goal itself—may be different from what we would want for ourselves. It is also possible that provider decisions during the labor and delivery process conflict with patient rights and choices. Women have the right to refuse medical tests and procedures, providers, and interventions. We have the professional responsibility to navigate a course that sup-

ports a woman's legal rights while also meeting her care needs.

***Ethical Issues.*** Maternal/fetal issues arise because the rights and safety of two individuals must be considered, although only one has the ability to make the decisions. Sometimes what is in the best interest of the mother may not be most beneficial for the fetus, and vice-versa. Some of these issues include refusing a life-saving intervention such as a cesarean delivery or a therapeutic abortion. Ethical issues may also arise in the area of what services are provided and the ability of the patient to pay for services. In some states, Medicaid will not pay for epidural anesthesia for low-risk labor patients. Surgical delivery for other than medical indications is another occurrence that is often faced. We may also face issues where legal and ethical issues conflict.

***Legal Issues.*** Every woman expects to have a "normal" baby. When this expectation is not met or the family feels that the labor and delivery process has harmed the baby or mother, they often blame the nurses and physicians. Sometimes this leads to legal action. We need to be aware of our responsibility to practice in a legally defensively manner. We must accurately and in detail document all patient assessments and responses, interventions, physician contact, and outcomes while providing at least the minimum recommended standard of care.

***Cameras in the Labor Room.*** Many parents wish to videotape the labor and delivery of their child for a family memento. Although to date, it is very rare that these tapes are used in subsequent litigation, the possibility exists. Videotaping our care can be very intimidating, and these feelings increase when sound/voices are also taped. If videotaping is allowed by the facility, we should make an effort to balance the request of the woman with our task of providing care, as long as the taping does not interfere with the safety of the mother or fetus. There may be a compromise position that allows periodic taping during the long process, taping without the sound, taping from a certain position, still photography, etc.

By accommodating parents' wishes to record or photograph the birth, two things are accomplished. First, we demonstrate our confidence in our abilities if we are willing to be "captured on tape" providing care. Second, this willingness helps to establish rapport and a caring, congenial relationship with the clients—which is the single most important measure in preventing a malpractice claim (Cesario, 1998). Box 14-3 provides strategies for reducing liability in regard to videotaping and photographing births.

### Cultural Preferences and the Collaborative Partnership

Cultural attitudes toward the achievement of birth; methods of dealing with the pain of labor; recommended positions for delivery; the preferred location for birth; the role of the father, the maternal grandmother, and "the family or social support network; and the expectations of the health care provider all vary. The beliefs and rituals surrounding labor and delivery are based on customs, religious beliefs, and individual preferences" (Andrews and Boyle, 1995).

Do not ask a woman or her family to share their cultural beliefs with you. This question assumes that they know not only the expectations of their culture but also those of your culture or the culture they have entered for care. Most of us cannot easily separate our beliefs and expectations into cultural preferences and personal preferences. Cultural expectations are incorporated and internalized to such a degree that we are often only able to identify them when we compare our activities and expectations with those of other cultural groups.

Instead, ask the woman about her preferences concerning care providers and procedures upon admission. She will then share with you how you may provide care that is consistent with her personal and cultural beliefs. Identify how much personal control and involvement she and her family desire during this birth experience. The care plan you develop with them will reflect their needs. For example, Muslim women wear long-sleeved gowns and hair coverings (khimar) during labor, exemplifying that modesty is very important to them (Hutchinson and Baqi-Aziz, 1994). If we are not aware of this or do not initially ask about cultural preferences, an important concept the Muslim woman upholds will be violated when she is told to put on a short sleeved, open-backed hospital gown. Ignoring the possibility of cultural preferences inhibits the collaborative relationship and the comfort or ease that the woman and her support system feel.

Another example relates to the cultural practices of the Navaho Indians. Navaho women are very reluctant to deliver in the hospital. One reason for this is that hospital policy often states that no jewelry can be worn during birth or in the operating room. This conflicts with the desire of Navaho women to wear a "birthing necklace" to help them have a "safe birth." If a Navaho woman came to a hospital for a surgical delivery and was told to take off her necklace, she would feel violated in an environment where she might not be comfortable to begin with. A simple statement such as "Please tell me about your labor preferences," communicates to the family that you want to collaborate with them and provide care that is culturally appropriate.

 ## THE ESSENTIALS OF ASSESSMENT

During the labor process, we focus our assessments in three general areas: the progress of the labor, maternal well-being, and fetal well-being. All three areas must be considered simultaneously in order to provide safe care for all involved. The **progress of labor** includes assessments related to the cervix, the contractions, the position of the fetus in utero, and the maternal pelvis. The assessment of **maternal well-being** depends upon historic, physical, psychosocial, and spiritual data. **Fetal well-being** is primarily assessed by listening to the fetal heart rate and interpreting fetal well-being based on the patterns of the heartbeat. Each of these areas will be discussed in detail here.

### Assessing Labor Progress

There are several assessments that must be made to assess the progress of labor. As labor progresses, the cervix softens, thins, and dilates and the fetus descends lower into the birth canal. The cervical changes and fetal descent can only occur in the presence of regular contractions of moderate to strong intensity. We are responsible for assessing the progress of the labor and keeping the birth attendant notified of such. Our ongoing assessments related to labor progress include cervical effacement and dilation; fetal station; frequency, duration, and intensity of contractions; and the pattern of the contractions. Much of this assessment data is obtained while timing contractions, palpating the abdomen during contractions, listening to reports from the mother about what she is feeling and where she is feeling it, observing pressure on her anus and pelvic floor, and performing a sterile vaginal examination.

### Sterile Vaginal Examination

Cervical effacement, dilation, and fetal station are assessed by performing a **sterile vaginal examination.** Vagi-

## BOX 14-4    *Steps in Performing a Sterile Vaginal Examination*

1. Obtain the needed supplies: a single, packaged sterile glove; lubricant; nitrazine paper, if indicated; a drape for privacy.
2. Allow the woman to empty her bladder before the examination. Explain the procedure to the woman and assure her that you will do the examination gently. Ask her if she is allergic to latex.
3. Wash your hands.
4. Position the woman comfortably and ensure her privacy (e.g., use a drape, close the curtain and door). Vaginal examinations are most often performed with the woman's knees bent and relaxed out, with feet together but can also easily be performed with the woman lying on her side with her top leg raised and supported.
5. Open the package of water-soluble, sterile lubricant.
6. Open the single glove package, and don the glove on your dominant hand.
7. With your non-dominant hand, place the lubricant on the middle and index fingers, being careful not to touch the lubricant package to the glove. (If using nitrazine paper, do not use the lubricant until after the nitrazine test is complete.)
8. Speaking softly to the woman, encourage her to take some slow, deep breaths. Talk to her as you perform the examination: tell her what you are doing, and what you are finding.
9. Wait until the woman is in between contractions before inserting your fingers. Insert the two lubricated fingers along the posterior wall of the vaginal canal. When you reach the cervix, turn your fingers up and feel for its length and thickness.
10. Move your fingers slightly higher to locate the internal cervical os. Spread your fingers to estimate dilation.
11. Feel for the presenting part of the baby. Gently push on it to determine if it is ballotable. Feel for the ischial spines in the woman's pelvis.
12. Be aware of feeling membranes or a bulging bag of water.
13. Gently remove your fingers and remove and dispose of your glove.
14. Encourage the woman to move so that she is off of her back and comfortable.
15. Wash your hands.
16. Ask the woman if she has any questions or concerns.
17. Document your findings.

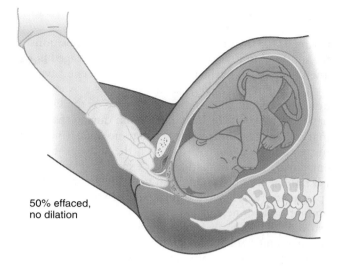

50% effaced, no dilation

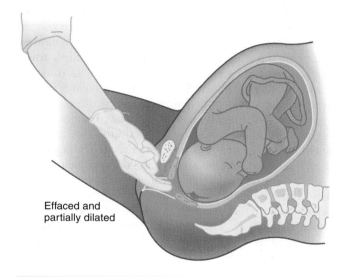

Effaced and partially dilated

*FIGURE 14-1* • Effacement.

nal examinations are performed by the nurse, midwife, or physician (Box 14-4). It is considered a "blind examination" because the assessments are made by feeling—not seeing—the cervix and fetal presenting part (Figure 14-1). Therefore if two people did an examination on the same patient, the assessment data may be slightly different. In order to obtain accurate assessments of pro-

gression, it is helpful if the same person performs the vaginal examinations. Also, vaginal examinations should only be performed when needed. Although they are considered "sterile" examinations, the gloves are the only things that are sterile. As the gloved finger is inserted in the vagina and moves up to the cervix, the organisms near the vaginal orifice are pushed up the vagina. Even using sterile gloves, it is always possible to introduce microorganisms into the uterine cavity, especially if the amniotic sac (sometimes referred to as membranes) has ruptured. A second reason that these examinations should only be performed when necessary is that they are uncomfortable for the woman. She is in labor and having contractions; having a finger or hand in her vagina is not only uncomfortable but also may make the contractions uncomfortable for a period of time afterwards. The woman also must often change the position or activity she has chosen for comfort (e.g., walking, rocking, squatting) and generally lies on her back for the examination. This is not only an uncomfortable position for the mother but also one that we have encouraged her to avoid to prevent occlusion of the inferior vena cava.

It is important to protect the patient's privacy when doing a vaginal examination. Be aware of the woman's desire to have visitors leave the room during the examination. Some cultures prefer that no men (including nurses and physicians)—not even the spouse—be present during the examination. For example, Hasidic Jewish fathers are not supposed to view the genitals of their spouse and will leave the room each time a vaginal examination is done. Chinese women are extremely modest and prefer that a female caregiver do examinations (Purnell and Paulanka, 1998).

A sterile vaginal examination is usually done when the woman first presents for care to help determine her stage of labor. A vaginal examination measures the cervical dilation and effacement and the fetal station and presentation of the fetus. These are important data to obtain to determine if it is necessary to request that the birth attendant come to the scene immediately, as well as to determine the presentation of the fetus (perhaps a surgical delivery is indicated for malpresentation). If a general assessment indicates that delivery is not imminent, this vaginal examination may be deferred until the mother is oriented to the area and other noninvasive assessments (e.g., vital signs and fetal heart rate) are completed.

When caring for laboring women who have been sexually abused, deliberate consideration is necessary before performing vaginal examinations (Roberts, Reardon, and Rosenfeld, 1999). Labor often brings back memories of abuse. The women may associate the touch of male health care providers with prior sexual assault or abuse from a man or men in the past. For this and other reasons, some women prefer female birth attendants. If a female attendant is not available, creative collaboration and a sensitive approach are required.

Establish trust with a woman before doing an invasive examination. Assure each woman that no one can do anything to her without her permission and that examinations will be done as gently as possible. Once the woman is given the power of granting permission, she may relax a little more about the procedures. After assuring the woman, you must then make sure that all health care providers (nurses, physicians, laboratory technicians, unlicensed personnel, anesthesia personnel, etc.) coming in contact with the woman treat her with sensitivity. Some women (even without a history of abuse) report feeling violated by their experiences during vaginal examinations. This is especially true in teaching facilities.

 Have a support person stand with the woman at the head of the bed to hold her wrist, stroke her arm, and/or breathe with her. Help the woman to do relaxation breathing. Prepare the woman for the sensations of the

examination. Tell her what you are doing it as you do it. Do examinations and procedures slowly, giving the woman time to adjust to what is being done and also allow her to request that the examination be stopped temporarily if she desires. Although this method of care is appropriate for all women, it is especially critical when caring for women with a history of sexual abuse.

This type of approach is also necessary when examining an adolescent. Vaginal examinations may be very uncomfortable for the adolescent due to the small size of her vaginal canal and her tendency to tense up and close her legs. As with adult women, having a support person with the teen during the time of examination and only doing examinations when necessary will make the labor process more tolerable.

### Effacement

The "taking up," shortening, or thinning of the cervix is known as **effacement**. During the first stage of labor, the cervix shortens in length from 2 cm to being almost paper-thin. This process starts before dilation in primigravidas and occurs after dilation begins in multiparas. The degree of effacement is assessed during a sterile vaginal examination and is documented in a percentage, with 0% being a long, thick cervix, and 100% being paper-thin (see Figure 14-1). Effacement is caused by uterine contractions and sometimes will result in expulsion of the mucous plug.

### Dilation

Cervical **dilatation** or **dilation** refers to the opening or widening of the cervix. It is measured in centimeters, ranging from closed to being 10 cm or "completely dilated" (Figures 14-2 and 14-3). Dilation can be felt during a vaginal examination by gently opening two fingers across the diameter of the cervix or by moving one finger around the circumference of the cervix. When the cervix is 10 cm or completely dilated, it can no longer be palpated by the examiner.

Cervical dilation is a result of uterine contractions and the pressure of the amniotic sac and presenting part on the cervix. Progress is occurring if the woman's cervix changes 1 cm every 1 to 2 hours (for a primigravida). The labor of a multigravida usually progresses much faster. Although these parameters may be used as guidelines to assess progress in dilation, we need to realize that the pattern and duration of each woman's labor is different and dilation times will vary from patient to patient.

### Station

**Station** refers to the relationship of the level of the presenting part with the ischial spines of the mother. If the lowest portion of the presenting part (e.g., the fetal head) is at the level of the ischial spines, the head is said to be at "zero station." The birth canal is divided into

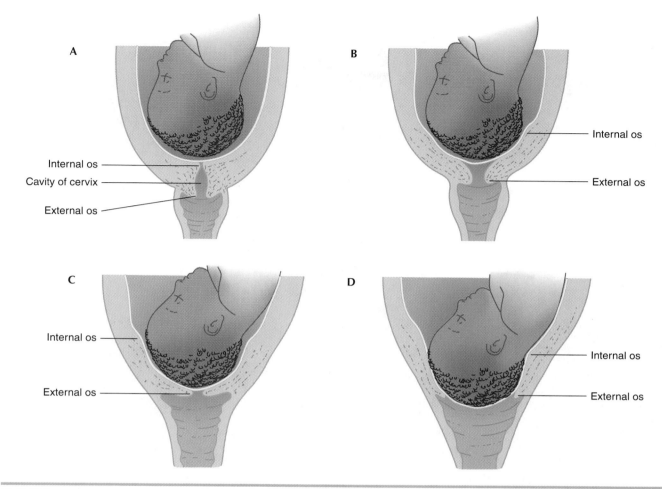

FIGURE 14-2 • Cervical effacement and dilation. **A,** No effacement, no dilation; **B,** Early effacement and dilation; **C,** Complete effacement, some dilation; **D,** Complete dilation.

fifths above and below the ischial spines. If the lowest portion of the presenting part is above the ischial spines, the station is a negative status; if the head is below the ischial spines, the station is a positive status. The station can range from −5 to +5 (Figure 14-4). If the head is 2 cm above the ischial spines, the station is −2; if the head is 1 cm below the ischial spines, the station is +1. It should be noted that if the fetal head is excessively molded or has a good amount of caput, the actual station might be higher than what is felt on the vaginal examination. When labor is progressing, the presenting part gradually descends through positive stations.

Friedman's curve is a graph of the average length of labors. Time is measured in hours on the horizontal axis. Dilation and station are plotted on two vertical axes in centimeters. When the labors of primigravidas and multiparas are plotted, the average differences in labor times can be easily seen (Figure 14-5). Keep in mind that Friedman's curve represents the average length of time of a woman's labors and not the expected length of

time of a specific woman's experience. Women will have shorter labors and women will have longer labors and still fall within the realm of normal.

Other assessments performed with a vaginal examination include the position of the cervix, determination of the presenting part of the fetus, the presence of ballottement, and detection of ruptured membranes. If the woman is in true labor, the cervix is usually but not always, anterior and can be easily found during a vaginal examination at the top of the vaginal canal. Often in preterm labor, false labor, and sometimes in early labor, the cervix is posterior, causing the examiner to reach farther in to find the cervix. Determining the dilation of a posterior cervix is very uncomfortable for the woman and should only be done when necessary.

### Presentation

The part of the fetus that appears at the cervical os is referred to as the **presenting part.** Upon entering a dilated cervix, the examiner should palpate the presenting part

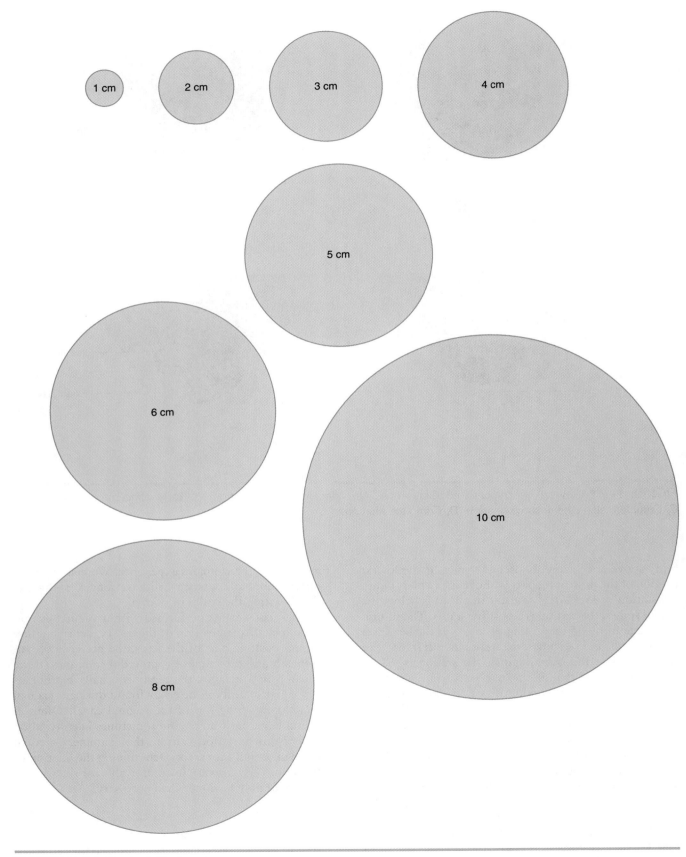

FIGURE 14-3 • Cervical dilation chart.

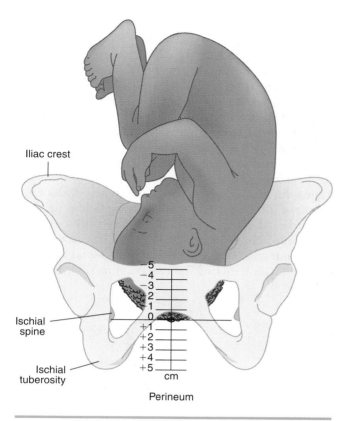

FIGURE 14-4 • Station. (Note how the station is determined by the relationship of the fetal head to the maternal ischial spines.)

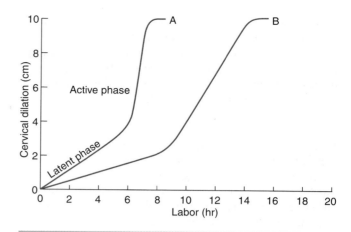

FIGURE 14-5 • Friedman's curve. (Note the difference in AVERAGE labor times for the primigravida **[B]** and multipara **[A]**.)

to determine if the position of the fetus is vertex, breech (buttocks, kneeling, footling), or some other presentation (e.g., face, brow, shoulder, or arm). See Figure 14-6 for several fetal positions. If the fetus is not vertex, the physician or midwife should be notified immediately. Chapter 18 discusses treatment of fetal malpresentations. Upon palpating the presenting part, the examiner should gently push to determine if the presenting part is well-applied to the cervix or if it is **ballotable** (i.e., floats away from the examiner's fingers upon palpation). This is an important assessment when the amniotic sac is ruptured; if the fetus is ballotable, and the amniotic sac is ruptured, the chances for a prolapsed cord increase with ambulation. The fetal attitude and lie are related to the presenting part.

### Attitude
**Attitude** is the relationship of the fetal parts to each other. Normal attitude for the fetus is flexion. The head is flexed on the chest, knees are flexed up to the abdomen, and arms are folded across the thorax (Figure 14-6, *A*). A deviation from the normal attitude of flexion can occur if the head is not flexed to the chest. Extension or hyperextension of the head can result in brow or face presentation (Figure 14-6, *B* and *C*). When this occurs, a larger diameter of the head must fit through the maternal pelvis.

### Lie
**Lie** is the relationship of the long axis or the spine of the fetus to the long axis or spine of the mother. The lie can be either longitudinal (vertical), in which the fetal spine is parallel to the maternal spine; or transverse (horizontal), in which the fetal spine is perpendicular to the maternal spine (Figure 14-6, *D*). An oblique lie, where the fetus is on a diagonal, is also possible; and such a lie will eventually move to a transverse or longitudinal lie. Fetal lie has implications for delivery. A transverse lie is almost always an indication for a surgical delivery. The lie can be assessed by Leopold's maneuvers, ultrasound, or a sterile vaginal examination.

### Position
After the presentation is identified, the examiner can then determine the fetal position. **Position** describes the relationship of the presenting part to the maternal pelvis. Three terms are used to describe the position. First is *left* or *right*, which refers to the maternal side that the "part" is facing (Figure 14-7). Second is the *part* of the fetus, which is sometimes referred to as the denominator or reference point. If the fetus is vertex, the *occiput* (i.e., the back part of the skull) is the denominator, or the term used to describe the position. *Sacrum* is used for breech presentations; *mentum* is used for face presentations; *frontum* is used for brow presentations; and *scapula* is used for shoulder and arm presentations. The third term describes which side of the maternal pelvis the part is facing: *anterior, posterior*, or *transverse* (Figure 14-8). A position of left occiput anterior (LOA) means that the fetal occiput is against the left anterior portion of the maternal pelvis. A position of right occiput transverse (ROT) means that the fetal occiput is against the right side of the maternal pelvis. When the occiput is against the mother's spine, it is in an occipitoposterior (OP) position.

The position is determined by doing a vaginal examination and palpating the triangular posterior fontanel, the diamond-shaped anterior fontanel, and the sagittal suture. Thus it is critical that we be able to feel landmarks of the fetal head (Figure 14-9). If the amniotic sac is still intact, this may be difficult.

### Status of Amniotic Membranes and Fluid

Intact membranes provide a barrier for infective organisms, preventing them from entering the uterus and reaching the fetus. During the 1970s, it became standard practice that once the amniotic sac ruptured—either spontaneously or artificially, the baby had to be born within 24 hours. More recent studies have demonstrated that infection rates do not relate to the length of time between membrane rupture and birth, provided that fingers and monitoring devices are kept out of the

vagina. During the 24 hours after the premature rupture of membranes (PROM), 60% to 95% of the women will start labor spontaneously. In some cases, women with ruptured membranes may be followed on an outpatient basis (Goer, 1995).

*Spontaneous Rupture of Membranes (SROM).* Ask the woman if she has noted any leakage of fluid. If she felt a gush of fluid, determine the time, the amount and color of the fluid, and if there was an odor noted. Sometimes it is obvious that the membranes have ruptured because the examiner can see amniotic fluid leaking from the vagina during an examination. Other times, it is not apparent or it is suspected that the leaking fluid is urine or leukorrhea and not amniotic fluid. There are two tests commonly done to determine if SROM has occurred.

The **nitrazine test** is based on the fact that amniotic fluid is alkaline (pH of 7.0 to 7.5, normally), whereas

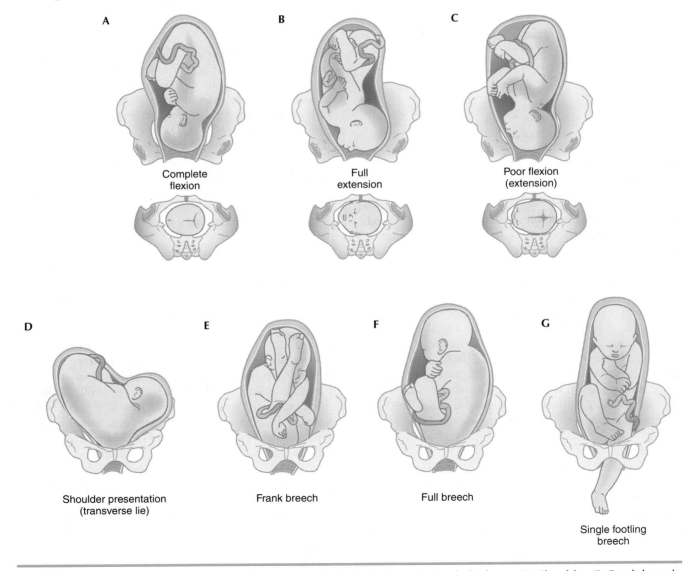

FIGURE 14-6 • Fetal presentation. **A,** Cephalic-vertex; **B,** Cephalic-face; **C,** Cephalic-brow; **D,** Shoulder; **E,** Frank breech; **F,** Complete breech; **G,** Footling breech (can be single or double).

vaginal secretions are acidic (pH of 4.5 to 5.5). Nitrazine paper is yellow and turns dark blue when touched to an alkaline substance such as amniotic fluid. To perform the test, a strip of the paper is placed in the fluid of the vagina. The color of the wet paper will designate if the fluid is alkaline or acidic. If there is a large amount of bloody show, the nitrazine test may show a false positive because blood is also alkaline.

The **fern test** is another commonly used test to determine if SROM has occurred. The midwife or physician performs this test, which involves inserting a sterile speculum into the vagina, swabbing the cervix with a sterile cotton-tipped swab, and then rubbing the swab on a slide. When the slide is viewed under a microscope, the appearance of "fern leaves" is seen if the membranes are ruptured.

## Maternal Pelvis

The maternal pelvis is the birth passage through which the fetus must pass. Maternal pelvises are discussed in Chapter 9 (see Figure 9-6). The gynecoid and anthropoid

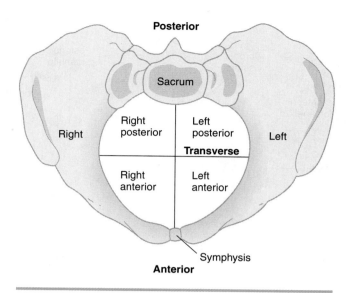

FIGURE 14-7 • Four quadrants of the maternal pelvis, used to describe fetal position.

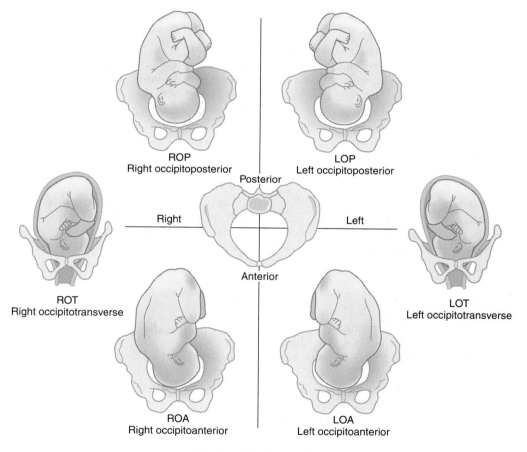

*Lie:* Longitudinal or vertical
*Presentation:* Vertex
*Reference point:* Occiput
*Attitude:* Complete flexion

FIGURE 14-8 • Fetal position.

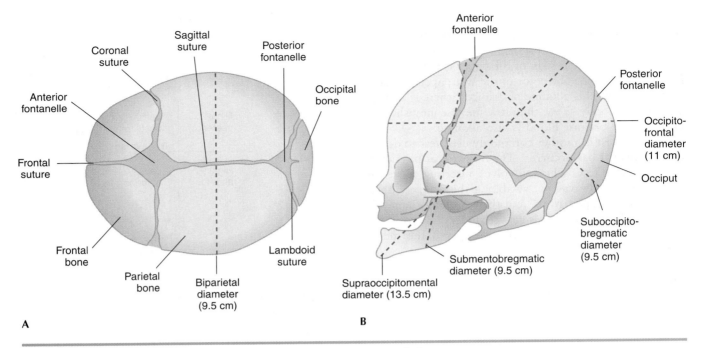

**FIGURE 14-9** ● Fetal head and landmarks. **A,** Superior view; **B,** Lateral view.

types are most common and are adequate to allow passage of the fetus. The android and platypelloid shaped internal pelvises provide less space and may not accommodate a full-term vaginal birth as easily. In some cases, the mother's coccyx has an increased curvature, which may also inhibit a vaginal delivery. If this is the case, the examiner can feel the head pushing against the coccyx during the second stage of labor.

### Contractions

Cervical changes and fetal descent cannot take place without uterine contractions. Contractions have a characteristic pattern; they gradually increase in intensity (increment) to a peak (acme) and then gradually decrease in intensity (decrement). We assess the frequency, duration, and intensity of contractions in order to assess the progress of labor (Figure 14-10).

The **frequency** of contractions is the time from the beginning of one contraction to the beginning of the next contraction, which is measured in minutes. The **duration** of a contraction is the time from the beginning of a contraction to the end of that contraction, which is measured in seconds. The **intensity** of contractions is a subjective assessment described as mild, moderate, or strong. To assess the intensity of contractions, firmly place your fingertips on the fundus and feel the tightening of the uterus. If the fundus feels like the tip of your nose, the contractions are labeled as mild. If the fundus feels like your chin, the contractions are labeled as moderate. If the fundus feels as firm as your forehead, the contractions are labeled as strong. If the woman has an internal uterine pressure catheter inserted (see the fetal

monitoring section of this chapter for more information), intensity becomes an objective measurement and is documented in units of millimeters of mercury (mm Hg).

Throughout labor, contractions gradually increase in intensity, come closer together, and last longer. For the labor to progress, the uterus must have moderate to strong contractions that last 60 to 90 seconds every 2 to 3 minutes.

Women feel these contractions differently. Some women experience almost no strong intensity and seem to have a labor of only two or three contractions. They are surprised when they are fully dilated and able to push. Other women experience intense contractions from the beginning of the labor process and require much more assistance in dealing with the labor process. All women, however, require sensitive nursing care to help them adjust to the reality of their own experience.

### Assessing Maternal Well-Being

Throughout the labor process, ongoing assessment of the mother is critical. Pregnancy and labor put additional stress on the body, which is well-tolerated by most healthy women. It is critical that we first obtain baseline assessment data and then monitor the mother's well-being as she moves through labor.

### Health History

A thorough health history—including information related to obstetrics, as well as other health issues—should be obtained. Ask the woman if she has any allergies. If so, protect her by following the protocol of

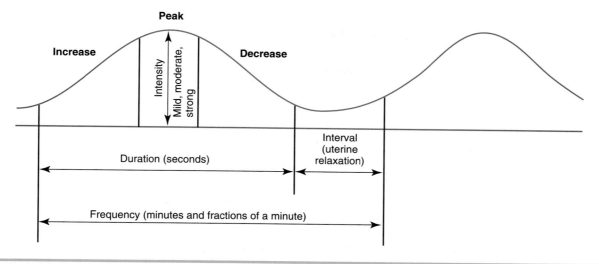

*FIGURE 14-10* • Characteristics of a contraction and uterine activity.

the facility (i.e., apply an institution allergy bracelet and document this information on the medication administration record, the admission form, the front of her chart, and the birth attendant's order sheets). Inquire about her previous medical history, including major illnesses, surgeries, etc. Ask about her family history of medical problems and conditions. Determine if she has any current medical problems that could affect the labor and delivery (e.g., asthma, epilepsy, cardiac problems). Determine if she is currently taking any medications and the last time she consumed herbal teas, drugs, or medications. This information is especially important for a woman who is an insulin-dependent diabetic or has a seizure disorder.

When obtaining her health history, be culturally sensitive and nonjudgmental. Ask about her dietary habits, food preferences, type of health care sought, and treatments used. Be alert to the possibility of any specific conditions (e.g., sickle cell anemia in women of African descent) or diseases.

### Obstetric History

Obstetric data should include the following: gravida and parity; date of the last menstrual period; estimated date of confinement (usually determined using Naegele's Rule and an ultrasound date or gestational wheel); and prenatal complications (e.g., bleeding, hypertension, gestational diabetes, preterm labor, etc). Inquire if any prenatal tests (e.g., a non-stress test) were done and learn the results. Also ask the woman about the occurrence and treatment of sexually transmitted infections before and during pregnancy. The questions about potentially sensitive issues (e.g., gravida and parity, as well as sexually transmitted infections) should be asked in private so that the woman may share accurate information.

The hospital or birthing center often has copies of prenatal records available. (We must protect the woman's privacy by keeping the contents of these records from her partner and family members.) Review these records to determine the frequency and duration of prenatal care. The later in the gestation the client entered prenatal care, the higher the risk for previously undetected complications manifesting during pregnancy, labor and delivery.

Ask the woman about any previous labors and deliveries. If she had a previous unpleasant or complicated labor and delivery, she may have increased anxiety during this labor. Also, some complications repeat themselves in subsequent labors. Obtaining this historic information can help us provide appropriate care. For example, if the woman has a history of a fetus in a posterior position and back labor, we should encourage her to avoid the supine position and to ambulate, assume different positions, and do the pelvic rock to increase the likelihood of the fetus turning to an anterior position. Knowing the length of prior labors may be helpful because subsequent labors are similar to or shorter than the first labor.

### Vital Signs

Follow protocol for how often vital signs need to be checked. **Temperature** is usually monitored every 4 hours, unless the amniotic sac is ruptured, in which case it is checked every 2 hours. Slightly elevated temperatures during labor usually indicate that the woman is dehydrated and needs to drink water or other liquids. Any temperature over 100.3° may indicate infection. An elevated maternal temperature accompanied by fetal tachycardia may be indicative of a uterine infection. The birth attendant should be notified because intravenous antibiotics and possibly a cesarean delivery are indicated. **Pulse rate** normally ranges from 60 to 100 bpm. An elevated maternal heart rate may result from stress, pain, dehydration, infection, or possible hemorrhagic shock. **Respiratory rate** ranges from 12 to 20 breaths/min and usually increases with painful contractions. Breaths are often rapid and shallow, causing hyperventilation. **Blood pressure** ranges from 100/60 to 140/90 mm Hg. When first taken, the woman's blood pressure may be high due to anxiety surrounding the labor. Determine what her blood pressure has been during the pregnancy. If she has a history of high blood pressure, it should be checked while she is lying on her left side. Hypotension may occur if the patient remains in the supine position, has epidural anesthesia, or with hypovolemia (Figure 14-11).

### Laboratory Tests

Examine all prenatal lab values. If the woman has had no prenatal care, the laboratory tests listed in Table 14-1 are usually done upon admission. Urine is dipped for glucose, ketones, and protein—substances that may indicate underlying diseases. A clean catch urinalysis is sometimes done, although some institutions only do a urinalysis if the patient presents with symptoms of a urinary tract infection or is in preterm labor.

Fewer blood tests are being routinely ordered for patients in labor if their prenatal course was unremarkable. However, a complete blood count (or hematocrit and hemoglobin) is still usually drawn as a baseline and is of-

ten a prerequisite to receive epidural anesthesia in many hospitals.

### Physical Assessment

A brief physical assessment is done. The assessment data upon admission are critical to establish a baseline against which to compare the woman's condition as labor progresses. Auscultate lungs bilaterally and the heart. Observe the woman's skin color, turgor, and nail blanching. Assess her deep tendon reflexes. Check her patellar and arm reflexes bilaterally. Reflexes are assessed on a scale of 1 to 4 with 2+ being normal, 0 absent, 1+ hyporeflexic, and 3+ and 4+ brisk.

Assess edema of the lower extremities, hands, face, and sacral area. Determine if pitting exists, and if so, determine the grade of pitting (Figure 14-12). Some edema is normal. Inquire if the edema has occurred suddenly, or if it was present throughout the pregnancy. Edema that occurs suddenly, especially in the face and sacral areas, can be a sign of pregnancy-induced hypertension (PIH), which is discussed in Chapter 18. Compare her prepregnancy weight with her current weight, and examine the prenatal records to determine the pattern of weight gain. Most weight is gained in the last 2 trimesters.

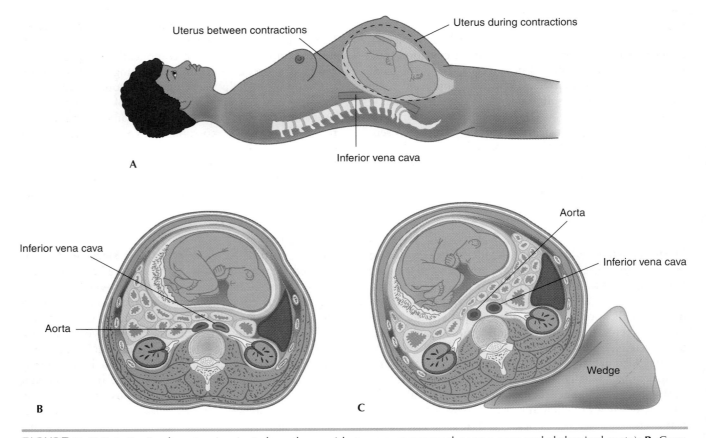

**FIGURE 14-11 • A,** Supine hypotension (note how the gravid uterus compresses the vena cava and abdominal aorta); **B,** Compression of aorta and inferior vena cava with the woman in a supine position; **C,** Compression of these vessels is relieved by placement of a wedge pillow under the woman's right side.

## Assessing Fetal Well-Being

The events of labor (i.e., contractions, maternal positioning, maternal anxiety, medications, etc.) place added demands on the fetus. Most healthy fetuses in uncomplicated pregnancies have no difficulties responding to these demands and can maintain adequate circulation of oxygenated blood throughout the labor process and quickly recover after being squeezed and forced against the cervix by each labor contraction. It is important that fetal well-being is monitored during labor. The type and frequency of monitoring depends on the acuity of the fetus and events of the labor process.

When women labor and deliver at home or in a birthing center, the fetus may be monitored using intermittent auscultation. When a woman labors in the hospital, the fetus is most often assessed using continuous electronic fetal monitoring (EFM). Each process offers advantages and disadvantages to the labor and delivery process of a healthy woman and her baby, and there is no documented difference in fetal outcomes (Vintzileos and others, 1993).

### Auscultation

The least invasive method of monitoring fetal well-being is by auscultation. This can be done with a fetoscope or, more commonly, with an ultrasound doppler device. The American College of Obstetrics and Gynecology (1995a) recommends that in labors void of risk factors, the fetal heart rate (FHR) should be auscultated every 60 minutes in early labor, every 30 minutes in active labor, and every 15 minutes while the woman is pushing. If there are risk factors present, more frequent monitoring is recommended. Fetal distress may be suspected if

### TABLE 14-1 *Prenatal Laboratory Tests and Their Significance in Labor*

| Laboratory test | Significance to labor |
| --- | --- |
| Blood type/rh factor | Needed if blood transfusion becomes necessary; evaluate if mother needs RhoGAM postpartum |
| Antibody screen | Screen for potential neonatal incompatibility disorders |
| Hematocrit/hemoglobin or complete blood count | Evaluate maternal oxygenation and fluid status; elevation of WBCs could indicate infection; low platelets could result in bleeding problems and may signal PIH |
| Rubella titer | If negative, mother is vaccinated postpartum |
| Venereal disease research laboratory (VDRL) (tests for syphylis) or rapid plasma reagin (RPR) | Fetal complications: inflammation and damage to spleen, kidneys, liver, adrenal glands, bone marrow, and presence of cutaneous lesions |
| Hepatitis B surface antigen (HBsAG) | Infant may develop acute hepatitis; preterm labor and intrauterine growth retardation (IUGR) is common; fetal immunization varies if mother is positive |
| Group beta streptococcus (culture) | Intrapartum antibiotic treatment required to prevent potential neonatal sepsis, meningitis, and respiratory distress |
| Gonnorrhea culture | Potential for neonatal orogastric infections, arthritis, septicemia, meningitis, vaginitis, and scalp abscess |
| Chlamydia culture | Neonatal conjunctivitis, pneumonia |
| Human immunodeficiency virus (HIV) screening | Infants are asymptomatic at birth, require retesting before 15 months |

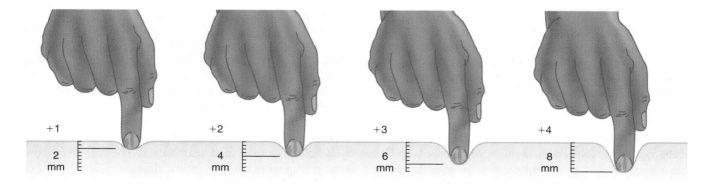

*FIGURE 14-12 •* Assessing for pitting edema.

the heart rate decelerates with and after the contraction is over or if there is bradycardia. When fetal distress is suspected, continuous electronic fetal monitoring should be used.

To determine the FHR using a fetoscope (similar to a stethoscope) or an ultrasound fetoscope or stethoscope, first perform Leopold's maneuvers to determine where the fetal back is located. Listen to the heart rate for 60 seconds, and record this number in "beats per minute" on the labor flow record. A normal fetal heart rate is 120 to 160 bpm, but some providers accept 110 as within the lower normal limit. Listen to the heart rate during and after the contraction ends. If the heart rate begins to decelerate with or after the peak of the contraction and does not return to the baseline rate until several seconds to minutes after the contraction is over, or if the heart rate is consistently below 110, the fetus may be in distress, and measures that may alter that status should immediately be implemented. Work with the mother to change her position, rehydrate her, empty her bladder, and reduce tension with conscious relaxation techniques. If available, an electronic fetal monitor may be applied to obtain a continuous visual recording of the fetal heart rate.

### Electronic Fetal Monitoring (EFM)

EFM produces a paper strip that shows the occurrence of contractions on the lower half of the strip and provides a continuous reading of the FHR on the upper half of the strip. EFM is based on the premise that different fetal heart rate response patterns occur with contractions if the fetus is hypoxic, stressed, stimulated, or receiving inadequate oxygenation. We are able to see how the fetal heart responds when the uterus contracts, when the fetus moves, when there is resting tone, when the mother changes positions or receives medications, etc. After interpreting these FHR patterns, we can implement interventions to maximize oxygenation of the fetus.

*Cautions.* When caring for labor patients on EFM, we need to be careful to not "care for the monitor" instead of the patient. Sometimes a nurse will enter a labor room and examine the monitor strip—rather than the patient. The EFM is a tool for us to use to assess fetal well-being. It tells us nothing about the status of the woman, even though what is happening with the woman may be affecting the fetal heart. The evaluation of the labor process must start with an evaluation of the woman.

Secondly, we need to use care when interpreting and documenting monitor strip information. We should seek out the opinions of other experienced nurses regarding strip interpretation and keep the birth attendant updated if there are any non-reassuring patterns on the strip. We must document interventions directly on the fetal monitor strip, at the time they are performed. Other notations that should be written on the strip are the patient's name, gravidity, parity, identification number, vital signs,

birth attendant visits and phone calls, spontaneous or artificial rupture of membranes (SROM or AROM), medications given, etc.

When EFM is being used, parents often ask, "Does everything look normal?" EFM does not give any information about the "normality" of the fetus. Be cautious about giving false reassurances to women and their families. EFM can only give us information about the apparent oxygenation status of the fetus. Note that there is also room for error due to machine malfunction.

Furthermore, the interpretation of the fetal monitor strip is only as accurate as the interpretive skills of the person reading it, and even experts may disagree on the same set of tracings. An incorrect interpretation will lead to inappropriate interventions being performed or necessary interventions being omitted. Thus, although EFM provides information, there is no guarantee of having a normal, healthy infant because of its use.

Because continuous EFM restricts a patient's ability to ambulate and move about, ask the birth attendant if the monitor can be removed intermittently to allow the patient to walk. Many facilities have fetal monitors with telemetry ability, which allows the mother to ambulate on the unit while obtaining a continuous tracing of fetal heart rate and uterine activity.

A final caution relates to teaching women and their families about how the monitor works. For example, inform them that if the heart rate disappears from the paper and the tone is no longer audible, the baby has probably moved and the transducer must be adjusted to pick up the heart rate again. It does not mean that the fetal heart stopped beating. As fascinating as the monitoring may be, remind the family members to focus on the woman doing the work of labor rather than the monitor tracing.

***Parts of the Fetal Monitor.*** Electronic fetal monitoring can be done externally or internally. External monitoring is easy and noninvasive. Internal monitoring provides more accurate information but is more difficult to apply than external monitoring devices. Parts of the external fetal monitor are discussed first here.

FHR is monitored using an **ultrasound transducer** that is placed on the maternal abdomen over the fetal back. Water-soluble conducting gel is placed on the transducer. The transducer is gently moved on the abdomen until a strong regular tone is heard (Figure 14-13). In addition to this audible tone, the monitor produces a digital reading and a flashing light on the face of the monitor. The transducer is held in place with an elastic belt or band. This transducer works on an ultrasound technique. High-frequency sound waves are transmitted through the abdomen and reflected back to the monitor by the opening and closing of the fetal heart valves. The FHR prints out on the upper portion of the monitor strip. The tracing of the FHR is dependent on the ultrasound waves aimed directly toward the fetal heart. Therefore minor variations in maternal positioning, fetal movement, and uterine

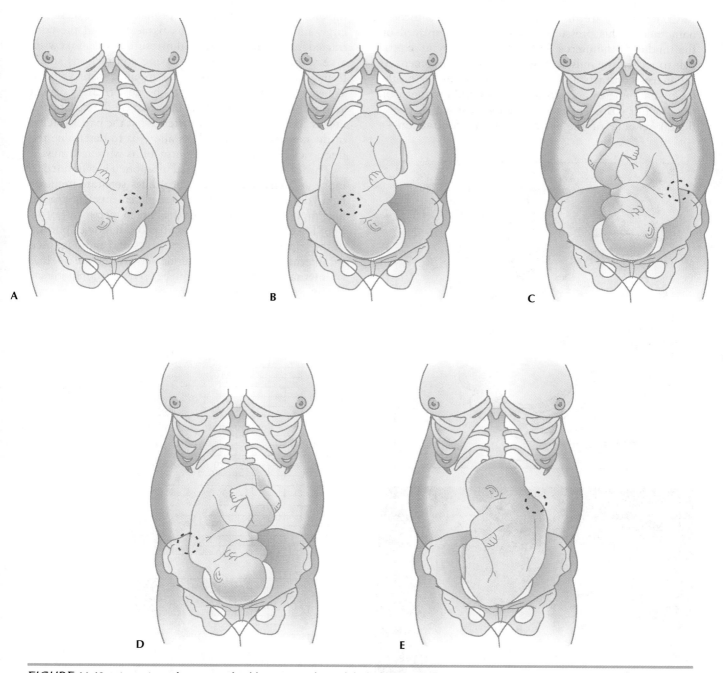

*FIGURE 14-13* • Location of strongest fetal heart sounds are labeled by fetal position. **A,** LOA; **B,** ROA; **C,** LOP; **D,** ROP; **E,** LSA.

contractions can affect the accuracy of the tracing. Before placing the transducer on the maternal abdomen, help the woman into a comfortable position. If the woman's position is changed after the monitor has been placed, the monitor may have to be readjusted (Figure 14-14).

Contractions are monitored externally by a **tocodynamometer.** This pressure-sensitive device is placed on the fundus of the uterus and held in place by an elastic belt to record the muscle movement of the abdomen. As the uterus contracts and becomes firm, it pushes on the tocodynamometer and produces a wavelike pattern on the monitor strip. The face of the monitor will display a digital reading of the intensity of the contraction—a number between 0 and 100. This number is not significant when an external monitor is used because a tocodynamometer does not have the ability to reflect the intensity of the contraction. If a woman is obese, she may be feeling the actual contractions as very strong, although the monitor depicts them as very mild because there is a large amount of subcutaneous tissue between the contracted uterus and the external pressure device. Likewise, a very thin person could be having contractions she is feeling as very mild, although the monitor displays them as being very strong. This occurs because there is a small amount of subcutaneous tissue between the contracted uterus and the tocodynamometer. What the paper tracing of the contractions does do is allow us to determine the frequency and duration of contractions with accuracy.

The fetal monitor paper used most often is calibrated to move at 3 cm/min. Dark vertical lines separate minutes; light vertical lines mark 10-second increments. Horizontal lines on the upper half of the paper are in increments of 10 bpm for the FHR. Horizontal lines on the lower portion of the paper are marked in increments of 5 mm Hg, used for internal monitoring of uterine activity (Figure 14-15).

**Internal monitoring** can only be used if the amniotic sac is ruptured. Because it is an invasive procedure, there is a

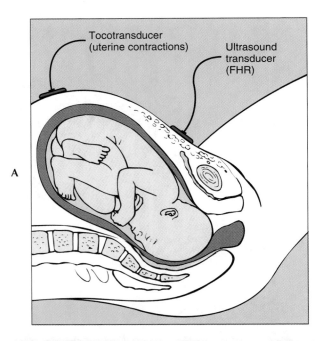

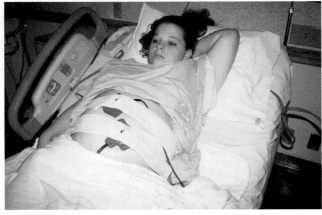

FIGURE 14-14 • **A,** External noninvasive fetal monitoring using tocotransducer and ultrasound transducer. **B,** Ultrasound transducer is placed below the umbilicus, over the area where fetal heart is best heard; and tocotransducer is placed on uterine fundus. *(B, Courtesy of Marjorie Pyle, RNC, Lifecircle, Costa Mesa, CA.)*

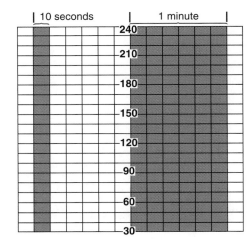

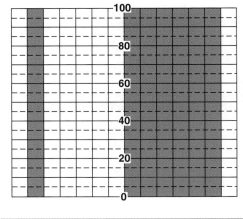

FIGURE 14-15 • Fetal monitor paper.

possibility of introducing microorganisms into the uterus and starting a process of infection. Strict sterile technique is required when inserting the electrode. The main advantage of internal monitoring is that it provides more accurate assessment data of the FHR and the contractions.

The FHR is monitored with a **fetal scalp electrode** or a spiral electrode. This electrode is attached in the fetal scalp (not over a fontanel or on the face) and then secured to a leg plate taped on the woman's thigh, and the wire is plugged into the monitor. The cervix must be dilated at least 2 to 3 cm before the electrode can safely be applied. Using a fetal scalp electrode is comparable to getting an ECG on the fetus. It provides long- and short-term variability, arrhythmias, and baseline heart rate. Indications for its use include suspected fetal distress and an inability to obtain an acceptable tracing with an external monitor, as well as any high-risk situation. Internal monitoring is often used with Pitocin inductions, especially if labor is prolonged. Families should be cautioned that if they suddenly cannot hear an FHR from the monitor, the electrode has probably become disconnected (Figure 14-16).

Contractions are monitored internally with an **intrauterine pressure catheter (IUPC).** This catheter is gently inserted inside of the uterus, along the side of the fetus. Great care must be taken during insertion to maintain aseptic technique and safely place the catheter in the uterus, while avoiding placing it on the placenta. This device has a pressure sensor at its tip and displays the intensity of the contractions (in millimeters of mercury) on the monitor strip. It also records the frequency and duration of the contractions, as well as the resting tone of the uterus. IUPCs have improved remarkably over the past 10 years and are very easy to use.

***Interpretation of Fetal Monitor Strips.*** It takes much practice and experience with fetal monitor strips to develop the skills of interpretation. Basic interpretation starts with an understanding of definitions. The definitions used in EFM terminology have recently been revised by a group of physician and nurse experts (National Institute of Child Health and Human Development Research Planning Workshop, 1997). To assure competency in strip interpretation, all nurses working with women on fetal monitors should annually take a 1-day refresher workshop on interpreting fetal monitor strips.

The FHR **baseline** is the approximate mean FHR rounded to increments of 5 bpm during a 10-minute segment; periods of marked variability or accelerations and decelerations are excluded from this assessment. Normal baseline is 110 to 160 bpm. The baseline is often recorded as a range (e.g., 130 to 140). Variations in the FHR baseline include variability, tachycardia, and bradycardia (Figure 14-17).

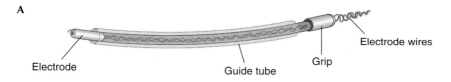

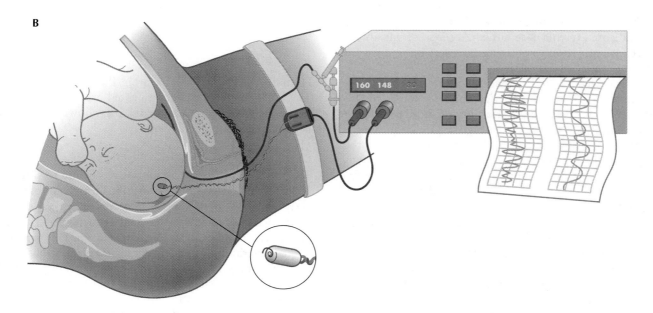

*FIGURE 14-16* • Internal spiral electrode and intrauterine pressure catheter. **A,** Parts of the fetal scalp electrode before it is applied. **B,** Fetal scalp electrode and intrauterine pressure catheter in place and connected to the bedside monitor unit.

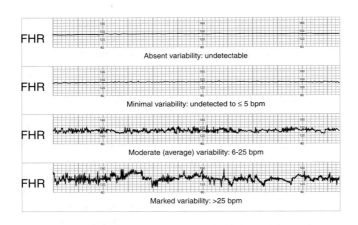

FIGURE 14-17 • Fetal heart rate baseline and variability.

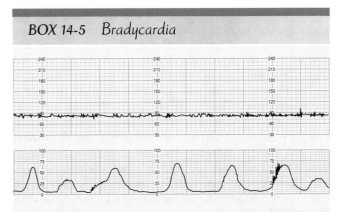

Bradycardia. *(From Tucker SM: Pocket guide to fetal monitoring, ed 4, St Louis, 2000, Mosby.)*

### BOX 14-5 *Bradycardia*

**DEFINITION**

Baseline heart rate below 120 bpm (or 110 bpm), or less than 30 bpm from the normal baseline for a duration of 10 minutes or more.

**CAUSES**

Causes include the following: late fetal hypoxia, beta-adrenergic blocking drugs, anesthetics, maternal hypotension, prolonged umbilical cord compression, fetal cardiac dysrhythmias, hypothermia, maternal systemic lupus erythematosus, cytomegalovirus, prolonged maternal hypoglycemia, congenital heart block.

**INTERVENTIONS**

* Place the mother on her left side.
* Increase maternal hydration. If the woman has an IV, the rate may be increased.
* Determine if the woman has hypotension.
* Administer oxygen by mask at 10 L/min.
* If oxytoxin (Pitocin) is infusing, stop it.
* Stimulate the fetus's scalp with an internal examination.

**Variability** is defined as fluctuations in the baseline FHR of at least 2 cycles per minute. The fluctuations are irregular in amplitude and rated as absent, minimal, moderate, and marked. Variability occurs as a result of an intact sympathetic and parasympathetic nervous system in the fetus. "Good" variability indicates normal neurologic control over the heart rate (i.e., the fetal brain is receiving adequate oxygenation) and is the primary indicator of fetal well-being and fetal reserve. Decreasing or "flat" variability is usually a sign of fetal hypoxia.

Causes of decreased variability include fetal sleep; drugs; hypoxia and acidosis; congenital anomalies; fetal cardiac arrhythmias; and extreme prematurity (i.e., <30 weeks). If variability is decreased due to fetal sleep, it should return to normal within 30 minutes and does not require any intervention. Narcotics, tranquilizers, barbiturates, anesthetics, and some anticholinergic drugs decrease variability; variability should resume as the medications metabolize. Treatment is generally not indicated in this case either. Absence of variability is seen on the monitor tracing as a flat line and is an ominous sign of fetal distress.

If decreased variability is suspected to indicate stress, an internal fetal scalp electrode should be applied. Interventions for decreased variability include turning the patient on her left side, increasing the IV rate, administering oxygen by mask at 10 L/min, and notifying the physician. If oxytocin (Pitocin) has been infusing, it is often decreased or discontinued. If the cause of the decreased variability is a narcotic and the delivery is pending, naloxone (Narcan) is administered intravenously to the mother before delivery and intramuscularly to the infant immediately at birth.

Other changes in baseline FHR that can occur include bradycardia; tachycardia; accelerations; and early, late, variable, and prolonged decelerations. Boxes 14-5 to 14-11 provide a definition of the change, the etiology, the nursing interventions, and a sample strip (Tucker, 1996; National Institute of Child Health and Human Development Research Planning Workshop, 1997). There are more complicated arrythmias and interpretations of fetal monitor tracings, however, that are beyond the scope of this book.

### Supporting Research-Based Practice

The purpose of using continuous electronic fetal monitoring is to identify non-reassuring heart rate patterns early in labor so that early intervention may produce better neonatal outcomes (i.e., fewer incidences of cerebral palsy, other fetal insults, or death). This purpose makes several assumptions. First, it assumes that there is such a thing as "non-reassuring heart rate pattern." That is, there exists some pattern that occurs, which is highly correlated with fetal hypoxia. Second, it assumes that health care providers readily identify these patterns. Third, this purpose assumes that interventions

## BOX 14-6  *Tachycardia*

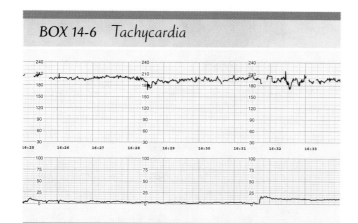

Tachycardia. *(From Tucker SM: Pocket guide to fetal monitoring, ed 4, St Louis, 2000, Mosby.)*

### DEFINITION
Fetal heart rate above 160 bpm or more that 30 bpm from the normal baseline for a duration of 10 minutes or more.

### ETIOLOGY
Fetal hypoxia, maternal fever, parasympatholytic drugs, betasympathomimetic drugs, illicit drugs, amnionitis, maternal hyperthyroidism, fetal anemia, fetal heart failure, fetal cardiac arrhythmias.

### INTERVENTIONS
- Determine the woman's temperature.
- Give the woman fluids to hydrate her; provide cool clothes, ice chips, and antipyretics.
- Give woman oxygen at 10 L/min via face mask.
- Tests may be ordered to determine if maternal or fetal infection is present.

## BOX 14-7  *Accelerations*

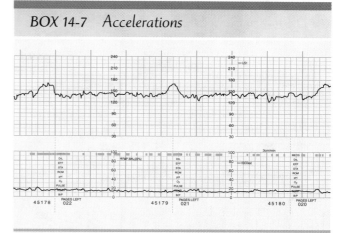

Accelerations. *(From Tucker SM: Pocket guide to fetal monitoring, ed 4, St Louis, 2000, Mosby.)*

### DEFINITION
Visually apparent abrupt increase of at least 15 bpm of the fetal heart rate from the baseline; the increase must last for at least 15 seconds or more (15 × 15 Rule), but less than 2 minutes from beginning of the acceleration.

### ETIOLOGY
Fetal movement, scalp stimulation (which can occur with vaginal examinations or electrode application), uterine contractions, abdominal palpation.

### INTERVENTIONS
- None required; considered a favorable change and evidence that the sympathetic nervous system is intact.
- Continue to monitor both the fetal heart and laboring woman.

will correct the insult, preventing cerebral palsy or another type of brain injury from occurring. Fourth, it is assumed that electronic fetal monitoring is superior to intermittent auscultation in producing better birth outcomes. Such was the thinking in the 1970s, when the use of EFM became common practice in this country.

Recently, the usefulness of continuous EFM compared with that of intermittent auscultation has been examined. Studies have shown that there is no difference in the perinatal outcomes of labors using EFM or intermittent auscultation (Vintzileos and others, 1993). Furthermore there is disagreement over EFM interpretive terminology, which causes concern about the identification of non-reassuring patterns. Bradycardia is the unquestionable non-reassuring FHR tracing that is easily seen on the monitor strip and requires immediate intervention, which is one benefit of EFM. If the fetal monitor tracing is being observed, a low heart rate is seen immediately and interventions can be implemented to help the fetus. The timing of intermittent auscultation could allow a fetus to have a below normal heart rate for a prolonged period of time, allowing hypoxia to occur.

Twenty-five years after electronic fetal monitoring became part of intrapartum care, however, it has not proved to be valuable in predicting or preventing fetal neurologic morbidity (Rosen and Dickinson, 1993). If EFM is not improving the health of neonates, why use it? It is expensive and usually forces the woman to stay in the bed and in a position that may not be comfortable or preferable to her but allows for the FHR to be picked up; the abdominal belts are uncomfortable; and it takes time and energy—that could be better used to support the woman and her family—to interpret the strips and document. Despite the wealth of data questioning the usefulness of EFM, its use in labor and delivery units in this country continues. We must be aware of the research data and advocate for research-based practice for our clients and discuss options for best practice in fetal surveillance techniques with our colleagues.

## BOX 14-8 *Early Decelerations*

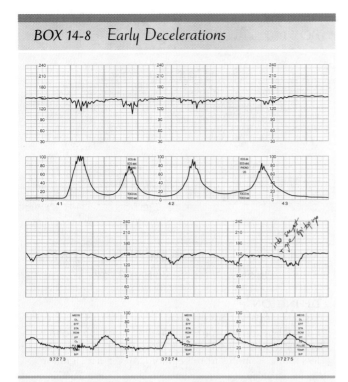

Early decelerations. *(From Tucker SM: Pocket guide to fetal monitoring, ed 4, St Louis, 2000, Mosby.)*

### DEFINITION
A visually apparent gradual decrease (defined as onset of deceleration to the nadir greater than or equal to 30 seconds) in the fetal heart rate that mirrors the contraction (i.e., the deceleration begins when the contraction begins; the lowest point of the deceleration occurs with the acme of the contractions; and when the contraction ends, the heart rate has returned to the baseline).

### ETIOLOGY
Direct vagal stimulation of the temporal baroreceptors as a result of head compression.

### INTERVENTIONS
• None required, is a benign pattern.
• Continue to monitor both fetal heart and laboring woman.

## BOX 14-9 *Late Decelerations*

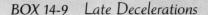
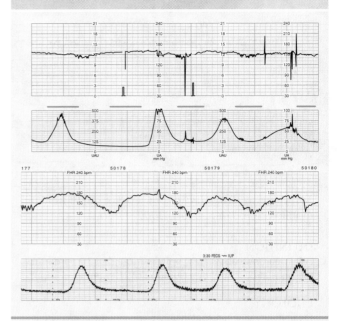

Late decelerations. *(From Tucker SM: Pocket guide to fetal monitoring, ed 4, St Louis, 2000, Mosby.)*

### DEFINITION
A visually apparent gradual decrease of the fetal heart rate that begins with or after the acme of the contraction and does not return to the baseline until after the contraction is over (late onset, late recovery, thus the name late deceleration). The deceleration does not necessarily mirror the intensity of the contraction; in fact, it is often a very subtle change.

### ETIOLOGY
Uteroplacental insufficiency, which can result from numerous factors including the following: placental deterioration, uterine hyperactivity, maternal hypotension, maternal anemia or cardiac disease, placenta previa or abruption, SGA, PIH, and many other conditions.

### INTERVENTIONS
• Position the woman on her left side.
• If she is receiving Pitocin, stop it.
• Administer oxygen at 10 L/min per mask.
• Determine if the woman is experiencing hypotension.
• Increase the IV rate.
• Notify the nurse midwife or physician.
• Prepare for a possible vaginal examination and scalp stimulation.

The ongoing research to determine accurate assessment of fetal well-being is critical. Research on nomenclature, methods, and determination of what constitutes best practice continues. Physicians agree upon what constitutes a tracing of a well-oxygenated fetus: baseline between 110 and 160 bpm, moderate variability, presence of accelerations, and absence of decelerations. Most physicians also agree that recurrent (i.e., occurring with at least 50% or more of the uterine contractions in any 20-minute segment) late or variable decelerations and substantial bradycardia, with absent variability, indicate current or impending fetal asphyxia. Many fetuses do not fit either of these two extremes; interpretation of the data and determining appropriate interventions for most cases that fall in the middle require more research.

## BOX 14-10   *Variable Decelerations*

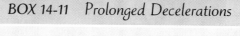

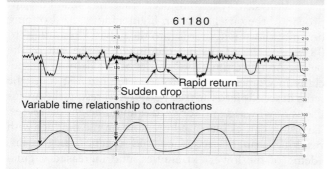

Variable decelerations. *(From Tucker SM: Pocket guide to fetal monitoring, ed 4, St Louis, 2000, Mosby.)*

### DEFINITION

A visually apparent abrupt decrease of the fetal heart rate below the baseline that varies in intensity, duration, and onset and can occur with or without a contraction. The decrease below the baseline is greater than or equal to 15 bpm, lasts 15 or more seconds but less than 2 minutes; and is often shaped like a U, V, or W; if it occurs with a contraction, the heart rate returns to the baseline when the contraction is over; often occurs with pushing.

### ETIOLOGY

Transient umbilical cord compression that may be due to maternal position, nuchal cord, a short cord, a knot in the cord, or a prolapsed cord.

### INTERVENTIONS

#### If Mild or Severe

* Change maternal position to relieve pressure on cord.

#### If Severe

* Put woman in knee-chest position with buttocks higher than hips to relieve pressure on the cord.
* Administer oxygen at 10 L/min via mask.
* Discontinue oxytocin.
* Administer a vaginal examination to check for a prolapsed cord.
* Notify physician.
* Amniofusion (i.e., normal saline infused into the uterus to provide fluid around the umbilical cord and keep it from being compressed) may be done.

## BOX 14-11   *Prolonged Decelerations*

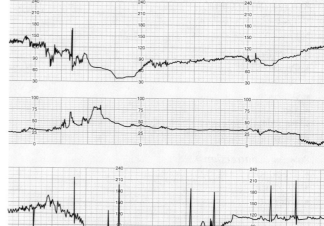

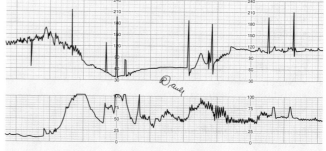

Prolonged decelerations. *(From Tucker SM: Pocket guide to fetal monitoring, ed 4, St Louis, 2000, Mosby.)*

### DEFINITION

Visually apparent decrease in the fetal heart rate below the baseline; the decrease must be 15 beats or more and last from 2 to 10 minutes; if the deceleration lasts longer than 10 minutes, it is termed bradycardia.

### ETIOLOGY

Occult or frank prolapse of umbilical cord; maternal hypotension; hypertonic uterine contractions; maternal hypoxia; rapid fetal descent.

### INTERVENTIONS

* Discontinue oxytocin to reduce the strength of contraction.
* Administer oxygen via mask.
* If caused by a prolapsed cord, reposition the woman and manually push the fetus off of the umbilical cord.
* If the woman is experiencing hypertonic contractions due to Pitocin, administer .2 mg of terbutaline SQ.

Research is currently being conducted on fetal oxygen saturation monitoring as a new and more accurate method of assessing fetal well-being during labor. A sensor placed on the fetal cheek or temple area is connected to a monitor. The EFM tracing displays the $FSaO_2$ with the contractions and the FHR. It is hoped that by using $FSaO_2$ and electronic fetal monitoring, health care providers will more accurately determine when an FHR pattern is non-reassuring and aggressive

interventions are needed to obtain positive outcomes. Furthermore, this means that unnecessary interventions will be avoided (Simpson, 1998).

## Summary of Labor Assessments

Many critical assessments related to the progress of the labor, maternal well-being, and fetal well-being are made

## BOX 14-12   *Summary of Labor Assessments*

***Passage (Birth Canal)***
- Type of maternal pelvis
- Placement of coccyx

***Passenger (Fetus)***
- Presentation
- Position
- Attitude
- Lie
- Estimated weight
- Fetal heart rate

***Powers (Contractions)***
- Frequency
- Duration
- Intensity
- Pattern

***Psyche (Emotional State)***
- Maternal well-being
- Ability to tolerate pain
- Support system

***Position (Maternal Position)***
- Mobility
- Pushing position

***Progress of Labor***
- Dilation
- Station
- Effacement
- Range of motion

 throughout the labor. These assessments are often categorized under the *P*s of factors that affect labor (Box 14-12). This organization presents a way of organizing the assessment data. It is important to discuss these assessments with the woman and her labor supporters and explain their significance so that they understand why so many things are being done. It is also important for us to put together these assessment pieces and not look at each one in isolation. Labor is a complicated—but a natural—process. We must combine our knowledge of assessment data and the art of practice to obtain this data and develop a collaborative plan of care.

##  THE FOUR STAGES OF LABOR

The labor process is divided into four stages: dilation of the cervix, delivery of the infant, expulsion of the placenta, and recovery with return to the nonpregnant state. In this section, each stage is described in detail using a nursing process approach. Assessment data that support nursing diagnoses, as well as appropriate interventions, are presented.

## Onset and Theories of Labor

Several physical symptoms occur that may signal the approach of the onset of labor. **Lightening** is the dropping down of the gravid uterus into the pelvis. Up until 36 to 38 weeks, the uterus has continued to rise out of the pelvis. At approximately 2 weeks before delivery—especially in women carrying to term for the first time, the fetus descends into the true pelvis. As a result, the uterus drops downward and forward. Fundal height decreases. This shift causes increased pressure on the bladder with resulting urinary frequency and urgency. Leg pains, edema of the lower extremities, and increased vaginal secretions (leukorrhea) also result from this shift. As the fetus descends, there is less pressure on the lungs and diaphragm, allowing the woman to breathe easier and experience less shortness of breath. Heartburn may also decrease.

Some women report feeling a burst of energy approximately 24 hours before going into labor. They may direct this energy toward cleaning the house and preparing for the baby. This phenomenon is referred to as the **"nesting instinct"** and may be a psychologic premonition of upcoming labor. When women do feel this burst of energy, they should rest rather than extend themselves, so that they conserve their energy for labor. Other signs that labor is nearing include a 1 to 3 pound weight loss and an increase in back discomfort. Sometimes diarrhea, nausea, and vomiting occur as labor is beginning, and the woman can mistake this for the "flu."

**Labor** is defined as "uterine contractions that bring about demonstrable effacement and dilation of the cervix" (Cunningham and others, 1997). It is often difficult to discern between true labor and false labor. Is the patient having strong Braxton-Hicks contractions or true labor contractions? Did her amniotic sac rupture or is she having excessive leukorrhea and urinary incontinence (Table 14-2)?

Labor usually begins between the thirty-eighth and forty-second week of gestation. Although the exact cause of labor onset is unknown, several theories are suggested:

- There is a decrease in the amount of progesterone available to the myometrial cells. Progesterone has a "relaxant" effect on the uterus throughout the pregnancy.
- The effects of estrogen increase. Estrogen increases the sensitivity of the uterus to oxytocin and simulates prostaglandin production. Oxytocin and prostaglandins both have the effect of stimulating smooth muscle contraction.
- The uterus is stretched and distended at term, which irritates the uterine muscles and causes subsequent production of prostaglandins.

**TABLE 14-2   Comparison of True and False Labor**

| False labor | True labor |
|---|---|
| No cervical change over several hours. | Cervical change in dilation and effacement noted. |
| Amniotic bag is intact. | Amniotic bag may be intact, ruptured, or bulging. |
| No bloody show is noted. | Blood show noted (in the absence of a recent vaginal exam). |
| Contractions are felt in the lower abdomen, similar to menstrual cramps. | Contractions begin in the lower back and radiate to the front of the abdomen. |
| Contractions are not regular in frequency, duration, or intensity. | Contractions become regular, last longer, and become stronger. |
| Contractions may stop with a change in activity, a warm shower, lying on left side, hydration, or sedatives. | Contractions will not stop with a change in activity, sedatives, or other relaxation measures. |

* The fetus produces more cortisol, which in turn decrease progesterone secretion and increases prostaglandins.

Because no specific process has been found, it is assumed that labor probably results from a combination of these factors.

## Stage One: Dilation of the Cervix

The first stage of labor is defined by cervical dilation and begins with the first sign of true labor and ends with complete dilation. It is the longest stage of labor, lasting 8 to 18 hours for a primigravida and 8 to 12 hours for a multipara. Because contractions may not be felt by women during the early part of labor, it is very hard to predict or measure an actual length.

The first stage of labor is divided into three phases: early (or latent) labor, active labor, and transition. Each stage is defined by the amount of dilation and has contractions of a characteristic frequency, duration, and intensity. Duration of each phase is influenced by a variety of factors, such as parity, maternal position, position of fetal presenting part, and the mother's activity level. Women who walk during labor, assume an upright position, and change position frequently during labor tend to experience a shorter first stage.

The guidelines describing the three phases of labor are presented in Box 14-13. We must remember that these are just guidelines. Every labor will not follow this "textbook" picture. Generally speaking, if the contractions become closer together, last longer, and increase in intensity, the labor is progressing. As this happens, the fetus descends lower in the birth canal, and the cervix dilates.

### Nursing Care in the First Stage

The nursing care provided during the first stage of labor focuses on the psychosocial, spiritual, and physical aspects of labor and its effect on the health and well-being of the mother and fetus. Common concerns are pain, anxiety, fluid volume deficit, risk for infection, and risk for fetal injury.

*Pain.* As nurses, we understand that a woman's pain is as mild or severe as she perceives it to be. We also understand that measures to deal with and control pain vary from woman to woman. In keeping with the collaborative nature of the labor process, we must be open to a woman's preferences for pain-relief methods and support her intent with our expertise. Informing women of additional methods along with their benefits and risks allows them to make informed choices. In keeping with the mandate that the labor nurse is caring for two patients—mom and fetus, we also need to keep the safety of both the mother and fetus in mind when implementing interventions for pain relief. The goal is to identify the method preferred by the woman that is safe for both mother and baby and provides the most effective pain relief for the mother (Simkin, 1995).

*Assessment.* Discomfort in labor has many causes. The obvious cause is muscle contractions of the uterus. This pain often begins in the back and radiates to the abdomen (Figure 14-18).

Many labor patients also have severe, nonradiating back pain, which is often created by the fetus being in a posterior position. The fetal back pushes up against the mother's back, and this pain worsens each time the uterus contracts and pushes on the fetus. Women in labor become more uncomfortable when their ability to change position is limited and they have to deal with fetal monitor belts and other events (e.g., IVs or placement of Foley catheters) while the contractions continue.

Women may express their pain in different ways. Some are very vocal, moaning or screaming in response to contractions. The level of vocalization is not directly related to the amount of pain a woman is feeling but is more often a factor of cultural expression.

Other women go through labor without making a sound. Still others indicate the ebb and flow of contractions by the rhythmic snapping of their fingers. Some may try to keep their discomfort to themselves (Purnell and Paulanka, 1998). Often women report feeling a loss of control as the labor intensifies and progresses towards transition. Some become very belligerent toward family members or care providers.

## BOX 14-13   *Overview of the Four Stages of Labor*

### STAGE 1: DILATION OF THE CERVIX

#### Stage 1, Phase 1: Early or Latent Labor
*Dilation*: 0 to 3 cm

*Effacement*: 100% for primiparas; 50% for multiparas

*Length*: 8 to 12 hours for primaparas; 4 to 6 hours for multiparas

*Contractions*:
- Frequency—5 to 10 minutes apart
- Duration—30 to 45 seconds
- Intensity—mild to moderate

*Possible Physical Symptoms*:
- Nausea, vomiting
- Small amounts of bloody show
- Possible rupture of membranes
- Back pain
- Mild to moderate discomfort
- Urinary frequency

*Possible Emotional State*:
- Excitement, relief that labor started, smiling
- Anxiety, talkative
- Wants information/able to follow instructions/eager to answer questions

*Nursing Activities*:
- Orient the woman and family to the care environment. If a home delivery, the nurse should orient himself or herself to the home.
- Review the birth plan.
- Obtain consents.
- Start documentation.
- Verify a reassuring fetal heart rate.
- Complete assessments/admission forms.
- Determine cervical dilation, effacement, and station.
- Notify midwife/physician of the woman's admission status.
- Review information about labor, breathing, etc.
- Encourage ambulation and position changes.
- Encourage fluids.

#### Stage 1, Phase 2: Active Labor
*Dilation*: 4 to 7 cm

*Effacement*: 100% for primiparas; 75% to 100% for multiparas

*Length*: 4 to 6 hours for primiparas; 3 to 5 hours for multiparas

*Contractions*:
- Frequency—3 to 5 minutes apart
- Duration—60 seconds
- Intensity—moderate to strong

*Possible Physical Symptoms*:
- Nausea, vomiting
- Increased amounts of bloody show
- Possible rupture of membranes
- Back pain
- Moderate to strong discomfort
- Urinary frequency

*Possible Emotional State*:
- Difficulty adjusting to stronger contractions
- Irritability
- Anxiety
- May lose temper
- Requests pain medication

*Nursing Activities*:
- Review birth plan as needed.
- Assist with comfort measures of the woman's choice.
- Make suggestions that support her birth plan.
- Monitor the fetal heart rate.
- Continue documentation.
- Do sterile vaginal examinations only as needed.
- Notify the midwife or physician of the woman's progress or difficulties.
- Review information about labor, breathing, etc. with the woman and her family.
- Assist the family and labor supporters as needed.

#### Stage 1, Phase 3: Transition
*Dilation*: 8 to 10 cm

*Effacement*: 100% for primiparas; 75% to 100% for multiparas

*Length*: 1 to 3 hours for primiparas; ½ to 1 hour for multiparas

*Contractions*:
- Frequency—1½ to 3 minutes apart
- Duration—45 to 60 seconds
- Intensity—strong

*Possible Physical Symptoms*:
- Nausea, vomiting
- Increased amounts of bloody show
- Spontaneous rupture of membranes
- Back pain
- Moderate to strong discomfort
- Urinary frequency
- Hyperventilation due to speed of breathing
- Rectal pressure and the urge to bear down

*Possible Emotional State*:
- Restless, wants to quit
- Irritability (i.e., asks for drugs or a cesarean section to "get it over with")
- Sense of helplessness and loss of control
- Does not want to be left alone but does not want to interact
- Difficulty concentrating on activities outside of herself, following instructions, and understanding information
- May forget this phase later when recalling her labor

*Nursing Activities*:
- Review birth plan as needed.
- Assist with relaxation and breathing techniques and other pain-relief methods of the woman's choice that are appropriate to this stage of labor.
- Monitor the fetal heart rate.

## BOX 14-13   *Overview of the Four Stages of Labor—cont'd*

- Document labor findings on appropriate forms.
- Perform a sterile vaginal examination only as needed.
- Notify the midwife or physician of the woman's progress or difficulties.
- Give instructions to the woman in short phrases.
- Praise and encourage her, do not leave her alone.
- Assist the labor supporter and family as needed.
- Encourage panting or spontaneous gentle pushing if appropriate.

### STAGE 2: DELIVERY OF THE INFANT

*Dilation*: 10 cm

*Effacement*: 100% for primiparas; 100% for multiparas

*Length*: 30 min to 3 to 4 hours for primiparas; 5 to 60 minutes for multiparas

*Contractions*:
- Frequency—2 to 3 minutes apart
- Duration—60 to 90 seconds
- Intensity—very strong

*Possible Physical Symptoms*:
- Renewed energy with pushing efforts, then may doze between contractions due to fatigue
- Rectal pressure and the spontaneous urge to bear down
- Increased amounts of bloody show
- Spontaneous rupture of membranes
- Back pain, especially if the fetus is posterior
- Extreme discomfort as baby descends birth canal that is somewhat relieved by pushing
- Reports perineal "burning" and "splitting" sensation

*Possible Emotional State*:
- Introspective
- Calmer
- Sense of control returns
- Willing to accept guidance on pushing

*Nursing Activities*:
- Review birth plan as needed.
- Offer the woman encouragement.
- Assist with pain-relief methods of the woman's choice.
- Assist woman in assuming pushing position of choice.
- Monitor fetal heart rate.
- Do perineal support and massage, if the woman desires.
- Notify physician or midwife of the woman's progress or difficulties.
- Assist labor supporters and other family as needed.
- Note the time of birth.
- Document delivery information.

### STAGE 3: PLACENTA EXPULSION

*Dilation*: closing

*Effacement*: not applicable

*Length*: 5 to 30 minutes

*Contractions*:
- Frequency—intermittent
- Duration—brief
- Intensity—mild, cramping

*Possible Physical Symptoms*:
- Renewed energy
- Gush of blood as the placenta becomes detached
- Rise of fundus in abdomen
- Perineal discomfort

*Possible Emotional State*:
- Talkative
- Anxious to interact with infant
- Relieved

*Nursing Activities*:
- Provide woman and family the care desired.
- Document the time the placenta was delivered.
- Administer oxytocin if ordered by birth attendant.

### STAGE 4: RECOVERY

*Length*: 1 hour after vaginal delivery; 2 to 3 hours after surgical birth

*Expected Physical Symptoms*:
- Uterine cramping
- Perineal soreness
- Exhaustion
- Hunger, thirst
- Fundus midline and firm at the umbilicus

*Possible Physical Symptoms*:
- Slightly elevated temperature due to dehydration
- Shaking, chills

*Expected Emotional State*:
- Relieved
- A "different person"
- Emotional with tears, gratitude, and happiness

*Possible Emotional State*:
- Excited to have infant (determined by cultural beliefs)

*Nursing Activities*:
- Monitor vital signs, fundus, bleeding, and episiotomy.
- Assess bladder and assist woman to void.
- Provide woman with clean clothing, bedding, face cloths, and towels.
- Answer the woman's questions and listen to her excited conversation.
- Encourage breastfeeding and parental-infant interaction.
- Monitor the infant's well-being.
- Provide perineal care.
- Offer food and drink.
- Provide family support.

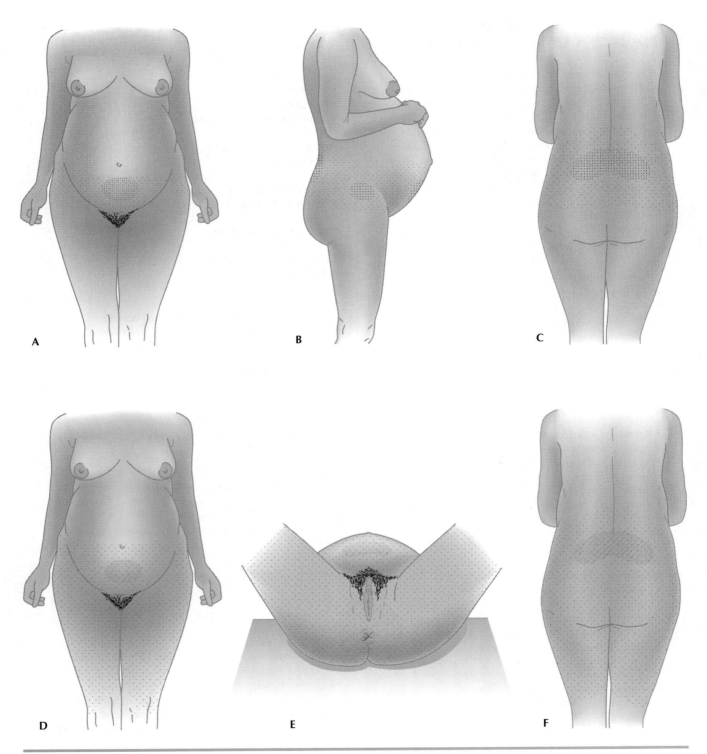

FIGURE 14-18 • **A-C,** Distribution of pain during the early phase of the first stage of labor. **D-F,** Distribution of labor pain during the latter phase of the first stage and the early phase of the second stage.

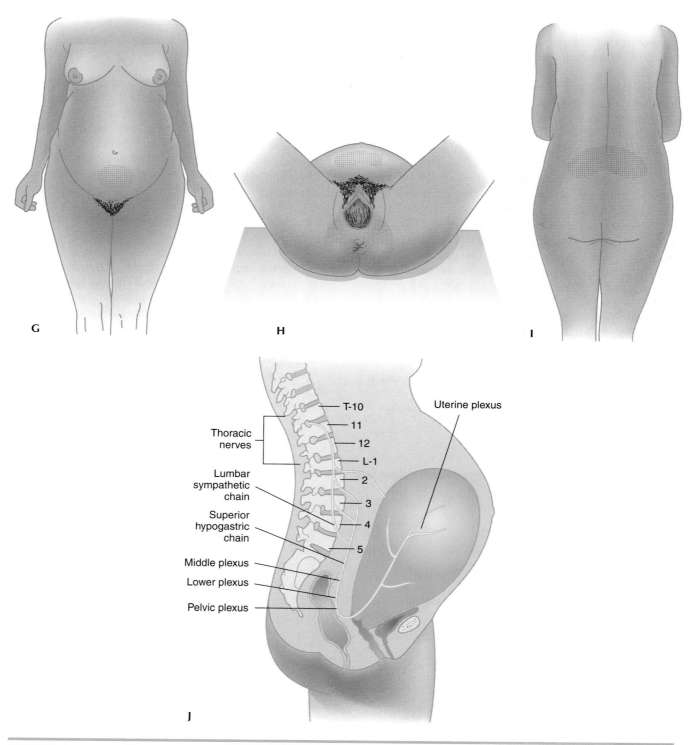

G

H

I

Thoracic
nerves

Lumbar
sympathetic
chain

Superior
hypogastric
chain

Middle plexus

Lower plexus

Pelvic plexus

T-10

11

12

L-1

2

3

4

5

Uterine plexus

J

*FIGURE 14-18—cont'd* • **G-I,** Distribution of labor pain during the latter phase of the second stage and actual delivery. **J,** Pain pathway from uterus to spinal cord. Nerve impulses travel through the uterine plexus, pelvic plexus, inferior hypogastric plexus, middle and superior hypogastric plexus, and lumbar sympathetic chain and enter the spinal cord through the 12th, 11th, and 10th thoracic nerves.

Adolescents often have a difficult time with the pain of labor. If they have not attended any childbirth classes, they do not understand and become frightened and overwhelmed as the labor process takes over their body. Developmentally, adolescents are self-centered and during labor are often most concerned with maintaining their own comfort and unable to think of the infant's well-being (Elkind, 1984). They may also feel alone due to family conflicts and lack of support from key individuals in their lives. Furthermore, labor may be difficult if they are still struggling with a decision to keep the infant or give the child to adoptive parents. Delivery will force the decision to be made. All of these factors have an effect on a teenage girl's ability to cope with the labor. Additional support, teaching, and patience are needed to successfully assist young pregnant clients through labor so that they do not blame the fetus for the pain.

Historically, a variety of pain-relief methods have been used (Box 14-14). Today, labor patients have a variety of choices of pain-relief methods, each with advantages and disadvantages. Many of these methods are noninvasive, easy to administer by the woman's labor supporters, low-cost, and pose little, if any, risk to the mother and fetus. Others that may provide a higher degree of pain relief are invasive and costly; require skill and ability to manage; and have the potential to adversely affect the mother, fetus, and progress of the labor. Several of these methods are discussed here, and information on the role of the nurse is incorporated with each.

***Positioning.*** The easiest method to ease discomfort is to be creative in maternal positioning. Lying in a hospital bed for 12 hours having contractions is not conducive to minimizing the discomfort of labor. Suggest a variety of positions to the woman and allow her to choose what works best for her. Most laboring women are more comfortable ambulating, especially in early labor, and many walk right up until second stage. Early ambulation has the benefit of increasing the frequency of contractions and using gravity to assist with fetal descent. When a woman is walking with her partner and a contraction comes, she may lean against the wall or have her partner support her as she handles the contraction.

If a woman is having back pain, assuming any position in which the fetus "drops" away from the maternal spine is recommended (e.g., on hands and knees or kneeling over a support). If she is walking, she may lean forward at the waist. Being upright often helps the baby turn during labor, and then the constant pain of back labor stops. The key is to encourage a woman to try a variety of positions until she becomes more comfortable.

Women can assume different positions with the use of a birth ball. A birth ball is a strong, plastic ball, approximately 30 inches in diameter, designed to hold the weight of an adult. Sitting on the ball and slowly rock-

---

### BOX 14-14 *Pain Relief in Labor: A Historic Perspective*

**1600s**
A physician in Salem, Mass. attempted to relieve labor pain with a remedy of ant eggs, red cow's milk, and a lock of virgin's hair.

**Early 1800s**
In France, alcohol intoxication was used during labor.

**1806**
Doctoral research by Peter Miller employed emetics (vomiting would distract the woman from her pain), vigorous exercise, starvation, and bloodletting (to relieve pelvic congestion).

**1831**
Hypnosis used in France.

**Mid 1800s**
Ether and chloroform are used in Scotland.

**1847**
First documented use of ether in childbirth (to the wife of Henry Wadsworth Longfellow).

**1900**
Cocaine used in spinals and epidurals in Switzerland.

**1902**
Morphine sulfate used.

**1906**
Morphine and scopalamine used together to produce "twilight sleep" in Germany.

**1933**
Grantly Dick-Read proposed natural childbirth in Great Britain.

**1938**
Meperidine used in Germany because it was thought to cause less respiratory depression in newborns.

**Early to mid-1900s**
Barbiturates used.

**1944**
Use of continuous epidurals began.

**1947**
Psychoprophylaxis (now called the Lamaze method) introduced in Russia.

From Stampone D: The history of obstetric anesthesia, *J Perinat Neonat Nurs* 4(1):1-13, 1990.

ing allows the women to assume a squatting position. Kneeling on the floor and laying her arms, chest, and head over the ball facilitates a hands-and-knees position. Gently rocking in this position can help to rotate the fetus into the posterior position. Care should be taken to avoid maternal injury. Having a support person nearby and keeping the ball free of fluid that might cause it to become slippery will help to avoid injury (McCartney, 1998).

Some positioning requires support from the birth partner, which also gives the woman the sense that she is not alone in this process (Figure 14-19). This support also helps to make the birth partner feel like an active participant in the labor process. These are easy measures to teach the labor partners and the mother. Having a choice of positions helps the woman have a sense of control over her labor.

*Heat/Cold.* Heat and cold application has long been used to promote comfort. A warm bath or shower, a warm blanket over her body, and/or a heating pad or heated rice pack to the lower back or abdomen relax the woman, allowing her to better deal with the contrac-

tions. Ice packs on the perineum, back, or abdomen create a numbing effect. We must use care when using heat/cold in order to avoid thermal injury to the woman. We should also be aware that some cultures (e.g., Chinese, Vietnamese, and Iranian) avoid cold or anything that might cause a chill during the labor process and should be sensitive to their wish not to use it.

*Hydrotherapy.* **Hydrotherapy** has become a popular method of easing pain during the labor process. Hot tubs and whirlpools, when thoroughly cleaned and maintained at a safe water temperature, are an effective way to relax laboring women, as well as ease the extreme discomfort of contractions. Many hospitals that are remodeling or adding labor rooms are installing some form of hydrotherapy facilities. If units do not have hot tubs available, a child's swimming pool can be used. Several studies have reported benefits of hydrotherapy, such as lowering elevated blood pressure, decreasing pain, increasing relaxation, necessitating less pharmacologic analgesia, decreasing stress, improving contraction efficiency, and improving patient satisfaction (Aird and others, 1997). Although all of these benefits have not been consistently replicated, hydrotherapy shows much promise in effectiveness and has become a popular means of pain relief during labor.

Hydrotherapy works on the hydrokinetic principle of buoyancy. When the body is immersed in water, it weighs less due to hydrodynamic lift. Therefore it is easier for the woman to support her body and relax her muscles. Hydrotherapy does not take away the perception of pain but relaxes the woman, allowing her to cope with the pain of contractions more effectively. Contraindications to using hydrotherapy include fetal malpresentation, Pitocin (oxytocin) induction/augmentation, large or small for gestational age, preterm labor, premature rupture of membranes, and presence of meconium (Figure 14-20).

The woman can get in the water at any time during the labor. Increased infection rates were not found in

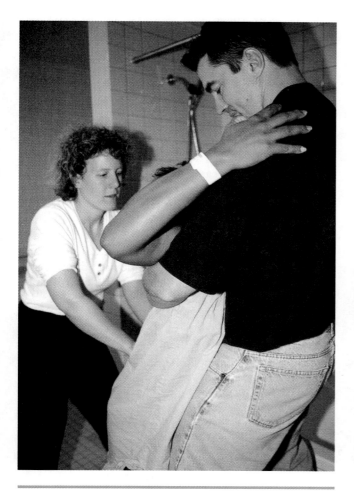

FIGURE 14-19 • Assisting with back labor. *(Courtesy of Caroline E. Brown.)*

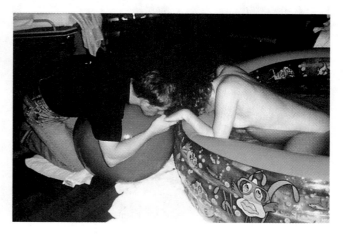

FIGURE 14-20 • Hydrotherapy. *(Courtesy of Caroline E. Brown.)*

women using hydrotherapy with ruptured membranes. The woman can stay in the water as long as no complications (e.g., bleeding, increased temperature, or fetal distress) exist. If the birth is not going to take place in the tub, the woman should move to the place of delivery upon complete dilation. Ultrasound stethoscopes and fetal monitors for underwater use are available. The woman can also lift her abdomen out of the water if a waterproof monitoring device is not available. The fetal heart rate should be checked every 30 minutes or per the facility's policy. The water temperature should be maintained at 35.6° to 36.6° C. If the water temperature is too hot, the woman will perspire, causing fluid loss that in extreme cases may cause poorer placental perfusion, hyperthermia, and fetal tachycardia. The room should be kept warm, quiet, and private to enhance relaxation. Ice chips and/or clear liquids should be offered to the woman. Assist the woman into a comfortable position of her choice and involve her support person if possible. Vaginal examinations can be done in the water if needed. Observe for dizziness, restlessness,

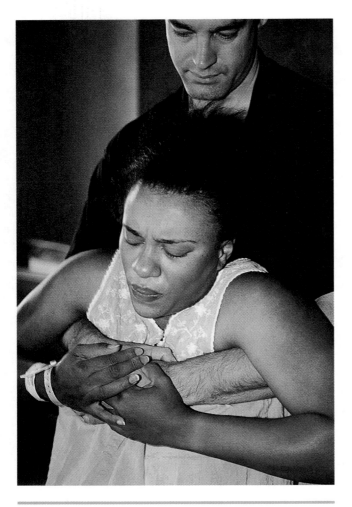

FIGURE 14-21 • Controlled breathing. (*Courtesy of Caroline E. Brown.*)

and pallor. Check vital signs hourly or per the institution's policy.

*Relaxation.* A woman can consciously relax her body. When the woman relaxes her body, it will produce endorphins that block pain reception. They will help her to feel exhilarated during labor and provide a sense of mellowness and peace between contractions. Endorphins do not make labor painless but do make it endurable (Boston Women's Health Book Collective, 1998).

Progressive relaxation involves releasing voluntary muscle groups, such as the muscles of the forehead, jaw, neck, chest, shoulders, upper arms, lower arms, wrists, fingers, abdomen, hips, thighs, calves, ankles, and toes. Some women will have learned this skill during childbirth preparation classes, but others we may teach during labor. Arms, legs, back, and hands must be supported and flexed slightly during contractions. We should provide extra pillows or rolled blankets to make the woman more comfortable as she stands and sits in the chair or bed. To facilitate the relaxation process, she should take a deep breath and then exhale slowly as she focuses on each muscle group in turn.

Focusing on a picture or mental image may also help the relaxation process. Some women think about their favorite peaceful place, while others visualize their cervix gradually opening. "In south India, birth attendants place a flowerbud next to the laboring woman; as its petals unfold, her cervix opens, and when the flower is in full bloom, they know it is time to push" (Boston Women's Health Book Collective, 1998). A flower may be a helpful visualization tool.

Provide the woman verbal assurance that she is relaxing well. Note areas that appear tense and massage (or have the labor support person massage) the area while the woman relaxes into the hands.

*Controlled Breathing.* As discussed in Chapter 13, there are different breathing patterns the woman can use to help in reducing anxiety, promoting relaxation, and relieving pain (Figure 14-21). The important thing for the woman is to follow a breathing pattern that is helpful

---

**BOX 14-15** *Doulas*

A doula provides the following:
- Physical, emotional, and informational support
- Help with breathing, relaxation, massage, and positioning
- Assistance to families in gathering information about labor
- Continuous emotional reassurance and comfort
- Assistance to partners who want to help the woman by using nonpharmacologic pain-relief measures

Doulas of North America

to her. Using these techniques does not necessarily change her perception of the pain but does help her to relax and focus, so that she can better cope with the contractions. Often laboring women want direction in what to do. Encouraging her in her efforts and breathing with her are very supportive. Also encourage and support her labor partner as they work together.

If the woman is breathing too fast, she may hyperventilate and have symptoms of tingling in her hands and face, as well as lightheadedness. If this occurs, have the woman breathe into a paper bag or her cupped hands. This allows her to breathe carbon dioxide, and the hyperventilation symptoms will disappear. Teach the labor support person to firmly but kindly guide the woman's breathing and to breathe with her.

*Doula Support.* Some pregnant women—whether delivering at home, a birthing center or in a hospital—hire a doula to assist them during labor. **Doula** is a Greek word meaning "woman's servant." Doulas are professionally trained birth companions who provide emotional support and physical comfort measures to the woman and her partner during labor. The essential qualities of a doula are compassion, cultural sensitivity, patience, stamina, and understanding of the birth process (Doulas of North America, 2000). The emphasis is on providing a variety of supports to help the woman have what she defines as a safe and satisfying birth. The doula and the woman's partner work together to make the labor as comfortable and positive as possible. We should incorporate the expertise and support of the doula when implementing care just as the woman has incorporated the doula as a partner in her care (Box 14-15).

Research comparing birth outcomes of doula-attended and non–doula-attended births has found a statistically significant reduction in the number of epidurals, oxytocin inductions, forceps/vacuum extractor deliveries, and days in the neonatal intensive care unit (NICU) and/or increased newborn hospital stays when a doula assists with labor (Kennel and others, 1991). Other studies support that doula involvement increases maternal-infant attachment (Landry and others, 1998) (Figure 14-22).

*Massage.* A simple technique such as massaging the lower back can provide comfort, especially if pressure is applied during a contraction. The labor support person can massage with his or her hands or with any other massage device (e.g., tennis balls in a cotton sock or wooden handheld ball devices). **Effleurage,** a gentle stroking down the middle of the abdomen and around the sides (see Figure 13-8, *A*), is useful to promote comfort and relaxation. Maximum benefits from effleurage can be obtained if the woman does not have fetal monitoring devices strapped across her abdomen.

*TENS.* **Transcutaneous electrical nerve stimulation (TENS)** is a method often used by physical therapists to treat back pain. This method involves a TENS unit, which is a small hand-held, battery-operated box connected to four electrode pads that are placed on the women's back. The woman can control the amount of electrical stimulation applied, increasing the voltage during a contraction. This device works best if the woman has had training in how to use the TENS unit prior to the labor. Although not widely used, TENS is of benefit for some women during labor (Figure 14-23).

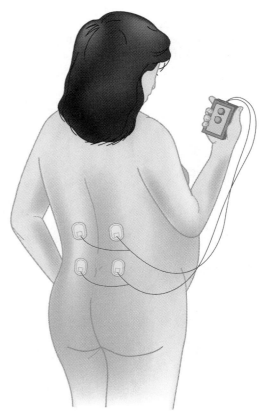

FIGURE 14-23 • Placement of a transcutaneous electric nerve stimulation unit (TENS) during labor.

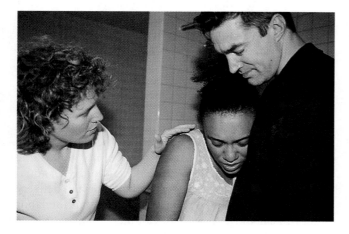

FIGURE 14-22 • Doula support. *(Courtesy of Caroline E. Brown.)*

*Other Methods.* Women may have music, chants, songs, or specific foods or teas to help them relax with the labor. They may also have the desire for aromatherapy with aromatic oils, incense or candles. Some traditions also have specific items, such as beads or clothing, that help a woman relax and do the work of her labor.

We should encourage the woman to use these methods even though they may seem unusual to us. This is part of respecting her individual and cultural beliefs and sharing our implementation expertise with her. Our role is to facilitate a conducive environment for the practice of helpful techniques that will not harm the woman or fetus. Dimming the lights in the room, discouraging an influx of visitors, disconnecting the phone, playing soft music, and speaking to the woman in calm soothing tones are also helpful. If EFM is being used, ask the woman if she prefers the volume for the FHR turned down or off to help her relax.

Acupuncture and acupressure may reduce the woman's experience of pain (Figure 14-24). Intravenous analgesics and epidurals or regional anesthesia may also be used for pain relief. Because these methods can have a negative effect on the process of labor and delivery, they are discussed in more detail later in this chapter.

In summary, pain is a very personal and individual perception. In recounting their labor experiences, some women speak in great deal about the pain they endured and how they survived, while others hardly mention the pain and focus more on the process they encountered. Women will have different preferences as to what interventions they want to use during labor to relieve pain. Whatever pain relief method the patient chooses, it is important that we support and facilitate the woman in her decision and involve any supportive family members or friends in the process.

*Anxiety.* Women going into labor—especially first-time mothers—are often anxious about the whole labor process. They wonder if they are going to be able to cope with contractions and maintain some sense of control. They probably have heard versions of their friends' labors that have not been positive experiences. They also may worry about the health of their newborn. Furthermore, labor and delivery are often the first time the mother has ever been admitted to a hospital.

Anxiety and fear will cause the woman to secrete adrenaline into her bloodstream, in a "flight or fight" response. This adrenaline will also cause her to tense up, making the labor more painful and slowing it down. In some cases, high levels of adrenaline will stop the labor process. Too often, we get caught up in "physical" care of the laboring woman and neglect her emotional side. When this occurs, we are doing the woman a tremendous injustice.

Postpartum women have reported that the following were the most supportive nursing behaviors: (1) made me feel cared about as an individual; (2) praised me; (3) appeared calm and confident giving me care; (4) assisted me in breathing and relaxing; and (5) treated me with respect (Bryanton, Fraser-Davey, and Sullivan 1994). Making the woman feel physically comfortable and giving pain medication were ranked fifteenth and eighteenth respectively. This study emphasizes the importance of interventions that support the emotional side of the patient. These findings are consistent with previous studies that have been done (Field, 1987; Kintz, 1987; Salmon, Miller, and Drew, 1990).

Lowe (1989) interviewed 134 laboring patients when they were an average of 5 cm dilated and were contracting every 3 minutes to examine factors that affect a woman's pain during labor. Maternal confidence in the ability to handle labor was the most significant predictor. Our encouragement and praise of the woman's efforts during labor can increase her ability to cope with pain.

*Assessment.* We must take time to discuss with the mother the concerns that are increasing her anxiety. We should ask open-ended questions or reflect back our observations of her anxious state. The support person should be as involved as possible in the dialogue and providing care because this is someone whom the woman trusts and has chosen to depend on. We should assess the woman's knowledge of the labor and delivery process and continue to teach her throughout the labor process. Fear of the unknown can increase anxiety.

*Nursing Intervention.* Knowing what is going to happen will help decrease these fears. Involve the woman and her support person in the decision-making process. Have the woman make her choices whenever possible.

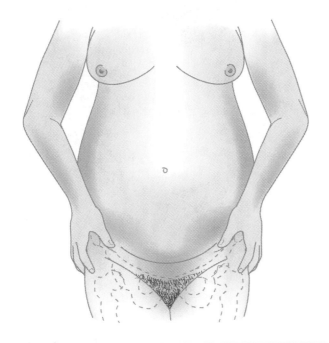

FIGURE 14-24 • Use of abdominal pressure points during transition.

When needed, explain the advantages and disadvantages of options. Making informed decisions allows her to feel like she has a sense of control over her body and the interventions available during labor. The woman's anxiety about the labor process often decreases as she develops trust and faith in her nurse. Knowing that she has a competent, caring individual to work with her during the labor is very comforting. We should present ourselves as caring and knowledgeable and be available to the woman as much as possible. We should encourage the woman and her support person to use whatever coping mechanisms and relaxation techniques they find work for her.

***Risk for Infection.*** Both the mother and fetus are at risk if **chorioamnionitis**, an infection of the amniotic membranes, develops. Risk factors include anemia; low socioeconomic status; poor nutritional status; presence of an IV or invasive monitoring devices; previous cervical cerclage; urinary catheterization; ruptured membranes; prolonged rupture of membranes; and frequent vaginal examinations.

*Assessment.* One of the first signs that might appear during care of a laboring woman is an elevated maternal temperature. Elevated maternal heart rate and fetal tachycardia may also occur. Sometimes malodorous amniotic fluid is noted, or the woman will complain of uterine tenderness. Blood work may reveal white blood cell counts elevated above 25,000.

*Nursing Inteventions.* Monitor the woman's temperature every 4 hours or hourly if the membranes are ruptured. Monitor the FHR; fetal heart rates over 160—especially when accompanied by decreased variability—may indicate maternal infection. Use good hand washing techniques when providing care. Always use sterile technique during vaginal examinations, and keep these examinations to a minimum after ROM has occurred.

***Fluid Volume Deficit.*** During the labor, several events can lead to fluid volume deficit. Women may have their intake restricted by standing protocols (i.e., "ice chips only"). Women lose moisture through the breathing techniques they use for pain management and heavy perspiration. Many women vomit during labor, and some may have diarrhea. Some may also have a complication that results in an increased blood loss. Along with fluid loss, electrolytes are also lost.

Women laboring in their homes or birthing centers are generally allowed to drink and eat as they desire. In hospitals, women are often restricted to ice chips during labor. Historically, fluids and foods were restricted during labor to prevent aspiration in the event that general anesthesia would become necessary. With modern anesthesia practices, however, aspiration is rarely a complication, although the tradition continues when each laboring woman is seen as a presurgical patient. In these situations, the women are expected to do the most physically difficult work of their life while receiving no nourishment or even water (Goer, 1995). If labor were considered an athletic event, good nutrition and good hydration, as well as periodic carbohydrate intake would be expected for optimum performance (Hazle, 1986). Based on the research, we should advocate for our patients by supporting policies that allow adequate nutrition and hydration and evidence-based practice.

*Assessment.* Assess the woman's skin and lips for signs of dehydration. Lips and mucous membranes often become dry when the woman is using mouth breathing patterns. Monitor vital signs as necessary. Dehydration usually causes an increase in temperature and an increased heart rate. If fluid volume deficit is related to blood loss, the patient will exhibit signs of shock (e.g., decreased blood pressure; increased heart rate; increased respiratory rate; pallor; cool, clammy skin; and a change in level of consciousness). Assess the fluid and electrolyte status by monitoring intake and output, skin turgor, and lab values. With severe dehydration, the hematocrit level will increase due to the concentration factor. Urine output and emesis must be measured and recorded.

*Nursing Interventions.* Prevention occurs through a conscious effort to maintain adequate fluid intake early in labor so that she is well hydrated before the heavier work of active labor. Although the simplest intervention is to encourage the woman to drink fluids during the labor, this may not always be possible.

Biting on a damp face cloth, having a cool cloth over the forehead, applying salve to the lips, and changing a woman's clothing as it becomes damp from diaphoresis, are comfort measures we and/or the support person can offer to the woman. Encouraging a woman who is lying in bed to lie on her left side will increase cardiac output and kidney perfusion, increasing urine output.

If fluids are needed, an IV—usually of lactated ringers solution—is started. Monitor the insertion and maintenance flow of the IV carefully. Pain and inflammation may develop at the insertion site. Too rapid infusion may cause fluid overload, resulting in pulmonary or cerebral edema. IV glucose solutions may cause diabetic levels of maternal hyperglycemia, leading to feelings of tiredness and illness and may slow labor. The fetus may become hypoglycemic (Newton, Newton, and Broach, 1988; Goer, 1995).

***Risk for Fetal Injury Due to Gas Exchange***

*Assessment.* The fetal heart tracing on the monitor strip is used to hypothesize on the oxygenation of the fetus. Assess the fetal heart monitor strip for rate, variability, decelerations, and accelerations. If problems are noted, several interventions are indicated.

*Nursing Interventions.* Turning the patient to her left side takes the uterus off of the inferior vena cava and aorta, allowing for increased cardiac output and greater placental perfusion. If the problem noted on the strip was variable decelerations, which are caused by cord compression, turning the patient on the opposite side may alleviate pressure on the cord. Increasing the rate of the IV increases maternal blood volume and also improves placental perfusion. Administering oxygen by mask at 8 to 10 L/min increases the oxygen concentration in the blood supply that is delivered to the fetus. There is usually a protocol stating that if fetal distress is noted the nurse can increase the IV rate and administer oxygen in place. If oxytocin is infusing, it should be decreased or discontinued. When the uterus contracts, there is a decrease in placental perfusion. Decreasing the number and intensity of contractions allows for greater placental perfusion.

Inform the birth attendant of the tracing on the fetal monitor strip that concerns you, as well as of any interventions provided. Document both what you told the birth attendant and any new orders you received. Contacting the birth attendant is critical. Even though you are there monitoring the progress of the woman, the birth attendant is the leader of the care team and must be part of the assessment, evaluation, and intervention process. If the problem with the tracing continues, a surgical delivery may be done. Furthermore, nurses must cover themselves legally by keeping the birth attendant apprised of progress and problems as necessary. If fetal distress is noted, a sterile vaginal examination to check dilation can be useful. If the woman is completely dilated, a vaginal delivery may be achieved more quickly than a surgical birth. On the other hand, if fetal distress is noted when the woman is in early labor, it is unlikely that the fetus will be able to resume homeostasis without constant care of the mother and her labor process.

When a monitor tracing indicates the possibility of fetal distress, you may need to intervene in a hurry. This is when it is appropriate for the nurse to "prescribe" in the collaborative relationship. Keep the woman and support person calm while performing the interventions. Your approach and attitude will determine how they respond. Explain that several things must be done to improve the fetal heart tracing. The support person will often help with repositioning the woman and offering her support and reassurance. Keep the woman informed of improvement and concerns. With a position change, oxygen administration, and adequate hydration of the mother, the tracing may return to the expected pattern. Evaluate the heart rate frequently, and observe for a recurrence of the problem.

## Stage Two: Delivery of the Infant

The second stage of labor is the "pushing" stage. This stage begins when the patient is 10 cm dilated or the cervix is pulled back around the head of the fetus and ends with the birth of the infant. The woman will often have a renewed energy at this time because of a burst of adrenaline, the knowledge that she may now work with her body to push the baby out, and that soon she will hold her child.

Contractions now come every 2 to 5 minutes and are very intense. The head pushing down in the rectal area may cause the woman to feel as if she wants to have a bowel movement. In fact, if during labor, a woman mentions that she feels as if she has to have a bowel movement look at the shape of the pelvic floor and determine if the anus is protruding. A vaginal examination may reveal that the baby has moved down the vagina. Bloody show usually increases during the second stage due to rupturing of capillaries in the cervix.

The length of this stage varies from minutes to hours due to several factors. Multiparity, the absence of epidural anesthesia, and pushing while in an upright or non-lithotomy position are factors that shorten this stage significantly. Primigravidas who have had epidural anesthesia may push for 2 or more hours.

Between contractions, we must review the birth plan with the woman to ensure that the management of this stage of labor and preparations for delivery continue to reflect her preferences.

### Collaborating with the Woman and Her Labor Partners

The woman has several choices during this stage: when and how to push; who will be in attendance during the birth and what role they will play; and in what position she will deliver. When pushing begins, often the perineum is exposed to check descent of the fetal head. Although a woman may have the urge to bear down, some may hold back because of fear, pain, or embarrassment at the thought of defecating (Roberts and Woolley, 1996). Asking the woman her position preferences, informing her of the normalcy of the process, and providing tactful hygienic care will help her relax and be a more effective pusher as she works with her body.

***Who Will Be in Attendance?*** Early in labor, ask the woman whom she would like in the room during this time. Now discuss privately with the woman who she wants in attendance. Some women may now only want one support person in attendance but may feel uncomfortable asking others to leave. If family members are asked to leave, assure them that you or the support person will keep them informed of the progress. Some facilities have waiting areas for family and friends.

Discuss the role of each support person who will be in the room. For example, in one delivery, the woman's spouse and three young sons were present. The spouse put on gloves and caught the newborn as it was born, the oldest son cut the umbilical cord, the middle son called the time of birth, and the youngest son called out the sex of the infant. The siblings had attended a special class prior to the delivery and were prepared and "debriefed."

***Which Pushing Position?*** The AWHONN Second Stage Research Utilization Project examined over 3,000 deliveries at 33 hospitals in the United States and Canada;

1,519 nurses completed questionnaires. The results showed that most patients are placed in the horizontal position for pushing and delivery (Shermer and Raines, 1997). The value of both the dorsal position, where the woman lies flat on her back, and the lithotomy position, where she lies on her back with her legs up in stirrups, have been challenged in the last 100 years. Since the decline of the use of scopolamine and morphine for "Twilight sleep," the trend in the United States has been to encourage women to use lateral and reclining positions to give birth, but such practices are not universal. Most cultures throughout the world, however, use—or have used—kneeling, squatting, sitting, and standing for labor and delivery (Dundes, 1987).

Discuss with the woman and her support person their desired pushing position. The position that the woman chooses to push in can shorten or lengthen this stage. Choosing a more upright position, which allows gravity to help with fetal descent, is preferable (Figure 14-25).

The lithotomy position neither uses gravity nor is comfortable for the woman. It is commonly used if the patient is on continuous EFM or has had an epidural. Continuous EFM often requires that the mother lie fairly still in one position, so that the monitor can detect the fetal heartbeat. Epidurals decrease the strength and mobility of the lower extremities and cause postural hypotension. These two symptoms make it very difficult to assume an upright position for pushing. When in the lithotomy position, you and the support person may bring the woman's legs back towards her body to give leverage and open up the pelvic area more.

Depending on where the birth is occurring, a squatting bar, birthing chair, or other device may be available to help a woman deliver in an upright position. Some women may choose to deliver on their hands and knees, especially if they are having back pain.

***When to Push?*** Ideas related to the best practice on when to push have evolved and will vary in different institutions and with different birth attendants. Historically, most practitioners believed that, to avoid trauma to the cervix, patients should not begin to push until they are 10 cm dilated. This is often difficult for women who begin to feel an urge to push at 8 or 9 cm but may have an hour or more of contractions until the cervix completely dilates. Women have also been told to begin pushing when they were completely dilated, regardless of the station. In

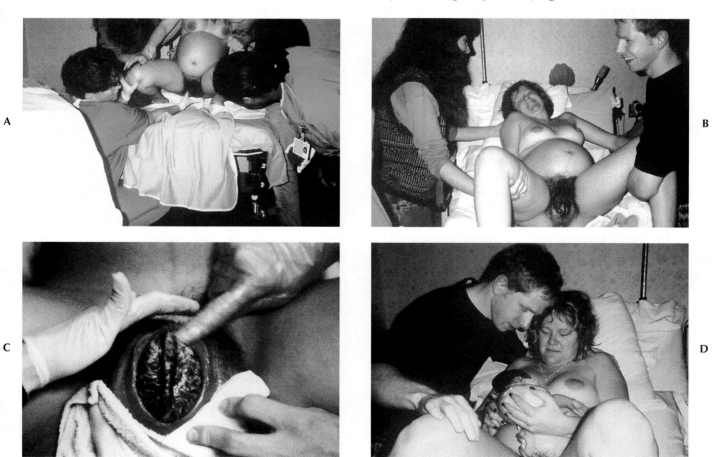

**A**  **B**  **C**  **D**

*FIGURE 14-25* • Second stage. **A,** Squatting on bed. **B,** Semi-reclining. **C,** Supporting vulvar. **D,** Getting acquainted. *(Courtesy of Caroline E. Brown.)*

other words, if dilation is complete—whether the presenting part is at −2 or at +2, the woman is told to push. In this situation, the mother becomes exhausted, discouraged, and frustrated at the slow progress of fetal descent. On the other hand, if the baby has come down the birth canal and the birth attendant is not in the room, some nurses will tell the mother not to push until the attendant arrives, but this does not stop the uterus from contracting.

 Each of these three scenarios ignores the fact that the woman has a natural urge to bear down. Current thought on commencement of pushing is that women should not push until they have the urge to do so (Ferguson's reflex) and are feeling rectal pressure. This reflex may occur when they are completely dilated or when they are 8 cm with a low station (Petersen and Besuner, 1997). Women who push by gently bearing down before complete dilation and have a soft pliable cervix and fetus at a plus station suffer no cervical trauma, are less fatigued and frustrated, and are more comfortable during stage two (Roberts and others, 1987). If the woman's cervix is completely dilated but she has no urge to push, waiting will conserve her energy; she will also push more effectively when she is doing it in harmony with her body.

*How to Push?* Methods of pushing also vary. Some women are told to use the **closed-glottis method** (also called Valsalva-type or "purple pushing"), which involves giving the following instructions: (1) when the contractions begins, take two deep cleansing breaths to allow the contraction to build; (2) take a third breath in and hold it while the support person slowly counts to 10; (3) during this count to 10, push out your bottom like you are trying to have a bowel movement; (4) at the count of 10, release all the air, take another deep breath in, hold it, and push again; (5) do this for three to four counts of 10; (6) take a final, deep, cleansing breath, and then relax. There is no scientific basis for this method of pushing. It is very tiring for the woman and takes her out of the control position.

The **open-glottis method** is a more effective method of pushing that allows the woman to push when she feels the urge to do so, rather than when someone is counting and telling her when to push. Women are encouraged to slowly blow air out of their mouths as they are bearing down. This helps to position the abdominal muscles so that they apply pressure to the uterus, while enabling the mother to relax her perineum and let the fetus come through. It is also acceptable for women to moan or yell. This open-glottis method makes women less tired and places less stress on the fetus.

We can encourage the woman by positioning a mirror so that she can see the fetal head as it is descending, placing her hand on the fetal head, and praising her efforts. We can increase her comfort by placing a cool cloth over her forehead and giving her ice chips or sips of water while she rests in between contractions. Some women actually nap between contractions.

Facilitating the progress of the second stage of labor has its advantages for mother and baby. The mother will conserve energy and feel better (i.e., more capable of breastfeeding and bonding with her infant) in the immediate postpartum period. Pushing for a shorter time may decrease the likelihood and size of hemorrhoids and may also cause less perineal trauma and decrease the likelihood of an episiotomy. Decreasing the time needed for pushing decreases the stress placed on the fetus. During this second stage, the process of pushing naturally decreases placental perfusion and decelerations of the FHR may become more pronounced.

The key to a better maternal and fetal response is to shorten the duration of the time the woman is engaging in active pushing (Roberts and Woolley, 1996). Rather than push immediately upon complete dilation, *the woman should begin to push after she is completely dilated and has the urge to bear down.* Rest periods between contractions must be respected.

### Nursing Care in the Second Stage
#### *Fluid Volume Deficit*
*Assessment.* Assess the fluid status of the woman and monitor her intake and output. She should be encouraged to sip liquids or take ice chips during this time, especially if she does not have an IV. Observe for increased vaginal bleeding. It is normal for bloody show to increase during pushing due to the rupturing of the cervical capillaries. Distinguish between a normal increase in bloody show and abnormal blood loss.

*Intervention.* If an abnormal blood loss is noted, notify the birth attendant immediately, monitor the patient for signs of shock, and start or maintain an IV line.

#### *Pain*
*Assessment.* Ongoing assessment of how the woman is tolerating the discomfort of labor is necessary. Some women express a decrease in discomfort and pressure because they are able to push. Others may have a hard time pushing because they are in pain.

*Interventions.* Nonpharmacologic pain-relief measures are called for at this time. Comfort measures consist of back massage, ice chips, a cool cloth on the forehead, perineal massage, and talking the patient through each contraction. She also may want to try different positions for pushing. The support person can be very active during this stage of labor, coaching the mother through contractions and encouraging her to rest in between contractions.

Pain medications are not indicated because they will depress the infant's respiratory system. Redosing of epidurals (discussed later in this chapter) is also not recommended because the patient loses the ability to push effectively and has a higher risk of needing forceps or a vacuum extractor for delivery. If the woman does not have an epidural and is having a lot of discomfort early in this stage, the physician or midwife might offer her a **pudendal block** to eliminate vaginal and perineal discomfort. Before cutting an episiotomy, a **local infiltration anesthetic** is more commonly used—not for the pain of the episiotomy but for the pain incurred when stitching the tissues (Figures 14-26 and 14-27).

### *Risk for Fetal Injury Due to Impaired Gas Exchange and/or Failure to Descend*

*Assessment.* If continuous fetal monitoring is being used, look at the monitor strip to assess the FHR baseline, variability, and presence of accelerations and decelerations every 5 minutes. Early and/or variable decelerations are often seen during pushing because the head and cord can be compressed with fetal descent. It is not uncommon to see the FHR drop to the 90s, but it is critical for heart rate to return back to the normal baseline when the contraction is over. The force of pushing coupled with strong contractions increases the likelihood that such decelerations will occur. Most healthy fetuses are able to tolerate this stress.

*Interventions.* Perform interventions as indicated in the labor section to correct any abnormal patterns (e.g., position changes, oxygen administration, increasing IV fluid rate) seen on the strip. Suggest that the woman pant through a few contractions or push very gently to give the fetus a brief rest. When deemed necessary, gently examine the woman to measure the progress of the fetal descent. If after a significant amount of pushing you note no progress in fetal descent, discuss a different pushing position and/or method of pushing with the woman. Continue to have the woman empty her bladder every hour to give the fetus more room to

descend. Evaluate if the heart rate maintains a normal baseline in between contractions, and if some variability is present. As fetal descent occurs, you should be able to gently separate the labia and see more of the fetal head with each push.

### Responsibility of the Nurse during Delivery

We must incorporate the woman's preferences into the delivery process and advocate for the woman's wishes by informing other members of the health care team of her desires and the possible modifications in the routine procedures of the facility. A woman may want either more or fewer interventions than the facility generally provides. Ongoing assessments of both mother and fetus are important because all interventions should be based on assessments.

It is also our responsibility to notify the birth attendant in enough time so that he or she may be present for the delivery. This occurs more often when a physician is to attend the delivery. Nurse-midwives generally spend more time with the woman when she is in labor and often remain with her through the second stage.

We should also be sure that the necessary supplies and equipment are prepared for the delivery. Just before the delivery, the woman's perineum should be cleansed, per the physician/midwife's preference. Some facilities use povidone iodine (Betadine) and then rinse gently with warm sterile water. The actual prep desired depends on whether the birth attendant anticipates the surgical procedure of an episiotomy (Figure 14-28).

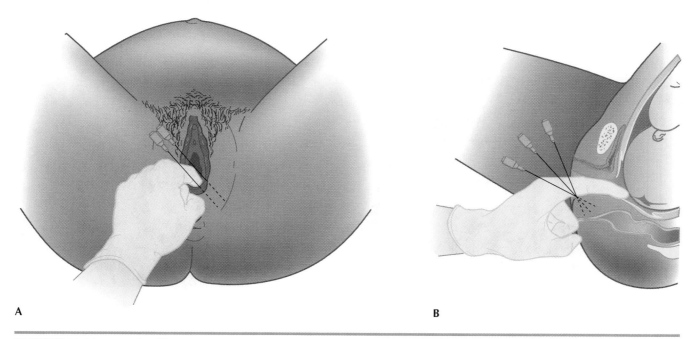

**A**                                                            **B**

*FIGURE 14-26* ● Local infiltration anesthesia. **A,** Technique of local infiltration for episiotomy and repair. **B,** Technique of local infiltration showing fan pattern for the facial planes. *(From Bonica JJ: Principles and practice of obstetric analgesia and anesthesia, Philadelphia, 1972, Davis.)*

### Episiotomy

An **episiotomy** is an incision of the perineum during the delivery of the infant. They are considered a surgical procedure and can only be performed by physicians and midwifes; nurses are not allowed to perform episiotomies. "Routine episiotomy has a ritual function but serves no medical purpose (Davis-Floyd, 1992; Goer, 1995). Not all women need (or want) an episiotomy.

Ask your patient her preference regarding episiotomies and communicate this to the physician or midwife. Although there is little scientific evidence to support the benefit of an episiotomy, some physicians continue to use them judiciously.

Physicians may prefer to do an episiotomy because they were trained that it is easier to repair an episiotomy than a jagged tear if one occurs. Research has found that this is not true; an episiotomy is not easier to repair than a second-degree tear (Hofmeyr and Sonnedecker, 1987). "In addition, episiotomies do not prevent tears into or through the anal sphincter or vaginal tears. In fact, deep tears almost never occur in the absence of an episiotomy" (Goer, 1995).

Another long-theorized benefit of episiotomies, although never documented, is that perineal muscles maintain better tone over the years if they are not stretched as much during delivery. This speculation appears to be untrue because many women today having repairs of cystoceles, rectoceles, or urinary incontinence had liberal episiotomies. Episiotomies should not be done because postoperative pain is decreased and healing is better. These advantages have not been documented in the literature.

Current thinking, although not implemented in general practice, is that episiotomies should not be performed routinely but rather preserved for deliveries involving shoulder dystocia, breech presentation, forceps or vacuum extraction, and occiput posterior position (Lede, Belizan, and Carroli, 1996). Ideally, the woman would have discussed this with her prenatal provider and chosen a provider who shares her philosophy. If that has not happened, we should learn her preference. If she prefers not to have an episiotomy, it is our responsibility to facilitate this. We can encourage pushing and birthing positions (e.g., lateral Sims, squatting, hands and knees) that reduce the need for an episiotomy. In addition, perineal massage with spontaneous, open glottis pushing techniques can decrease the need (Maier and Maloni, 1997). We must also remind the physician of the woman's desire not to have an episiotomy at the time of delivery.

There are two types of episiotomies—midline and mediolateral—based on where each is cut (Figure 14-29). **Midline episiotomies** involve an incision straight down from the vaginal os. Although this type of episiotomy is easy to repair, generally heals well, and is anatomically consistent, the major disadvantage is that the episiotomy can extend or tear into the rectum. **Mediolateral episiotomies** involve an incision at about 4:00, and go against the natural longitudinal pattern of the musculature of the perineum. They are more difficult to repair, and women have more postoperative pain. Extension to the rectum is rare. Most episiotomies are cut at the time the fetus is crowning. If the episiotomy is cut too soon, increased bleeding occurs (Cunningham and others, 1997).

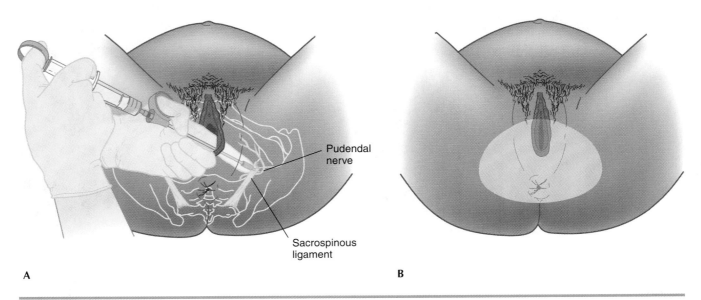

A

B

*FIGURE 14-27* • **A,** Technique of transvaginal pudendal block showing the needle extended beyond the needle guard and passing through the sacrospinous ligament to reach the pudendal nerve. **B,** Area of perineum affected by pudendal block.

## Understanding the Delivery Process

A nurse who works with laboring women must sometimes assist the woman in the delivery of her child. Keep in mind that this is a process that has gone smoothly for thousands of years. All that is required is to help the woman as she fulfills this natural process.

During the delivery process, the fetus goes through a series of movements, referred to as the **cardinal movements,** to fit through the pelvic outlet. We need to understand these movements in the event that we must support the child's head and body as the woman pushes and delivers the infant. All labor and delivery nurses should know how to support the woman's perineum and assist both her and her infant as it emerges (Figure 14-30).

First, the fetus flexes its chin to chest and descends into and engages the maternal pelvis. These three movements are **flexion, descent,** and **engagement,** which overlap. The fetal head then rotates internally from left occipitoanterior position (LOA)/right occipitoanterior position (ROA) to a midline occipitoanterior position (OA), **internal rotation.** The next movement is **extension** of the fetal head, and the head is outside the birth canal. After the head is out the fetus turns from OA to LOA/ROA (**restitution**), and then to ROT/LOT, which is referred to as **external rotation.** The final movement is **expulsion** where the anterior shoulder, posterior shoulder, and body is delivered. Some babies fulfill these movements rather rapidly and are completely expelled in one smooth motion. The progress of other babies is stopped momentarily

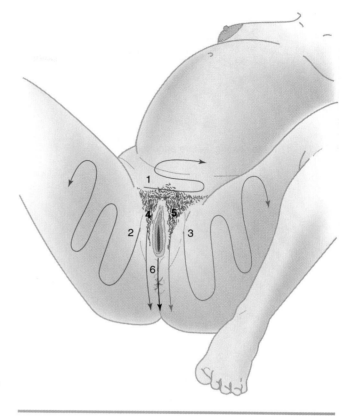

FIGURE 14-28 ● Delivery preparation. (Follow the numbered steps, use a clean sponge for each step.)

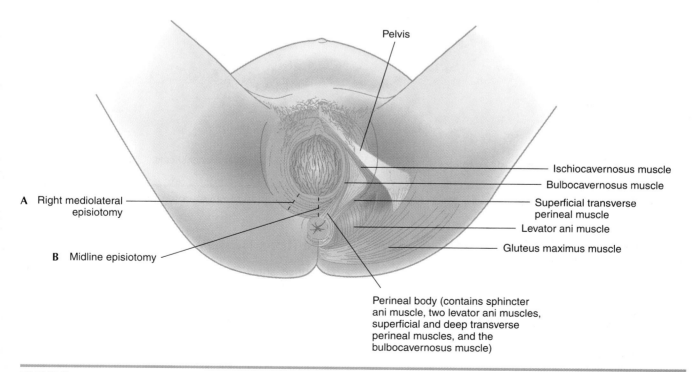

FIGURE 14-29 ● The two most common types of episiotomies are midline and mediolateral. **A,** Right mediolateral; **B,** Midline.

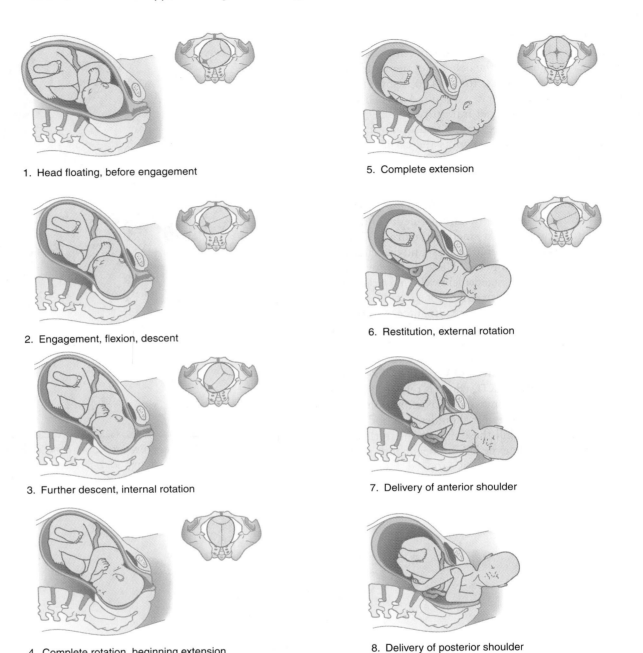

1. Head floating, before engagement

2. Engagement, flexion, descent

3. Further descent, internal rotation

4. Complete rotation, beginning extension

5. Complete extension

6. Restitution, external rotation

7. Delivery of anterior shoulder

8. Delivery of posterior shoulder

FIGURE 14-30 • Primary movements of a fetus in left anterior occiput position as it moves down the vagina and under the pubic bone.

after the head is out, and the birth process is finished with the next contraction (Box 14-16).

During the process of labor and delivery the mother and fetus are cared for as a unit, each of their responses to the process of labor is monitored individually, but generally by the same person. Once the infant is born the physical requirements of their symbiotic relationship are accomplished. Each receives care as an individual, simultaneously by two different individuals. The care of the woman is discussed in this chapter. The care of the newborn is discussed in Chapter 16.

### Stage Three: Delivery of the Placenta

The third stage of labor is the "delivery of the placenta." This stage begins after the baby is born and ends with the delivery of the placenta. The placenta is usually delivered within 5 minutes of the baby, but it can be up to 30 minutes later. The placenta can separate in two ways. If the placenta separates from the uterine wall in the center, with its edges releasing last, the shiny fetal side is seen first (Figure 14-31). If the placenta begins to separate on an edge and continues to separate across,

---

**BOX 14-16   *Steps to Deliver a Baby in a Normal Birth***

1. As the head crowns, support the perineum to minimize trauma to it.
2. After the head is out, instruct the mother to pant as you feel for a nuchal cord. If it is loose, slip it over the baby's head. If it is tight, double clamp and cut the cord.
3. Suction out the baby's nose and mouth with a bulb syringe.
4. Support the head as it rotates to the OT position. Gently assist if it does not do so on its own.
5. Support the baby as the anterior shoulder comes through.
6. Support the posterior shoulder.
7. Support the rest of the body.
8. Double clamp and cut the cord.
9. Dry and stimulate the infant to cry.
10. Place the infant on the mother, using skin-to-skin contact for warmth, and then cover both with a blanket.
11. Obtain cord blood.

---

the maternal surface of the placenta, which is dark, rough, and bumpy, presents first.

### Procedure

Usually, the placenta will separate from the uterus spontaneously and pass down through the introitus. Signs that placental separation have occurred are as follows: the uterus becomes globular and firmer; a sudden gush of blood may occur; the uterus rises in the abdomen because the placenta pushes it upward; and the umbilical cord protrudes farther out of the vagina (Cunningham and others, 1997). The birth attendant may ask the mother to push to help expel the placenta.

It is never appropriate to pull the umbilical cord to deliver the placenta because this can result in an inverted uterus (i.e., the uterus is pulled inside out), which is an obstetric emergency that can result in shock, hysterectomy, or maternal death. Occasionally, a placenta will not separate spontaneously and the birth attendant must remove it manually. Complications with placental delivery are discussed in Chapter 18. Once delivered, the placenta is inspected by the birth attendant to determine that it is all there and no part has been retained in the uterus. Retained placental fragments can prevent the involution of the uterus and cause a postpartum hemorrhage.

### Nursing Responsibilities

The nurse's responsibility during this stage is to note the time that the placenta was delivered and record it on the delivery record. Immediately after the placenta is delivered, you may be asked to gently massage the fundus to help it contract. If the mother is planning on breastfeeding, the baby may be put to her breast. The stimulation of the breast by the baby will release oxytocin within the woman's body and cause the woman's uterus to contract.

Some birth attendants may routinely order administration of an oxytocic medication intramuscularly (IM) or intravenously (IV). This medication is given to help the uterus to contract, creating vasoconstriction of the uterine spiral arteries. Pitocin, 10-20 units diluted in 1000 mL of IV fluid (e.g., lactated Ringer's solution or normal saline), may be used. If the woman does not have an IV, an oxytocic drug can be given intramuscularly if needed. Ergonovine or methylergonovine use calls for 0.2 mg IM every 2 to 4 hours for up to five doses. Then if the need continues, it may be given orally. If Pitocin is chosen, 10 units are given IM.

### Disposal of the Placenta

When caring for women of diverse cultures, we must be sensitive to requests about disposal of the placenta. In this country, the placenta is disposed of as human waste, sent to the lab for pathologic testing, or the amnion is removed and used in the care of burn patients. Several cultures (e.g., Mexican, Northern Indian, Nigerian, and Malaysian) bury the placenta for good luck in protecting the child's health (Kakar and others, 1989; Vincent, 1995; Specter, 1996). The Chinese make a soup with the placenta, which is supposed to improve the quality of the breast milk when eaten by nursing mothers. Other cultures have other rituals. Some families in the United States take the placenta home and bury it under a young tree in honor of the child. Honoring rituals of placental disposal is important, and failure to do so can have a negative affect on the parents' emotional well-being (Schneiderman, 1998).

## Stage Four: Recovery

The fourth stage of labor is referred to as "recovery" and begins after the placenta is expelled and ends when the woman is stable and has adjusted to a nonpregnant state. For the first hour or two after giving birth, a woman is generally alert and excited even if she hasn't slept well in days. After this initial excitement wears off, she will be ready for sleep.

In a home or birthing center, the return to maternal homeostasis is monitored while the woman relaxes with family members and friends and starts to get to know her baby. In a hospital environment, a woman is generally monitored for approximately 1 hour and then transferred to "postpartum" care. During this time the baby, family members, or friends may or may not be with her. If unexpected situations arise, this monitoring period is extended until the woman is stable.

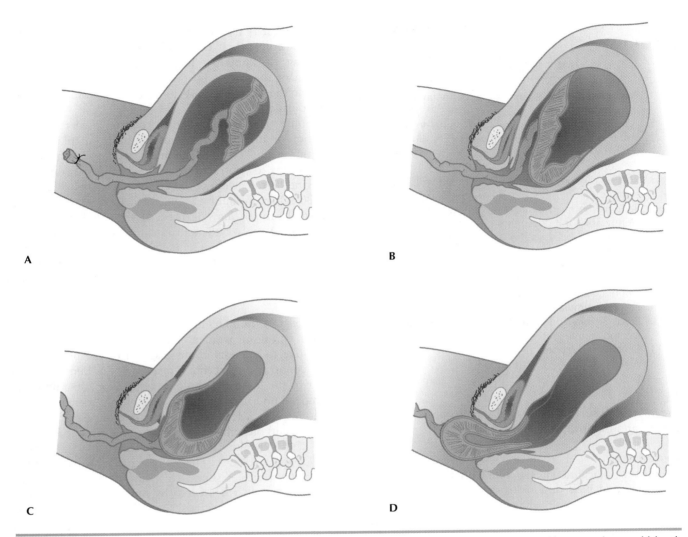

**A**

**B**

**C**

**D**

*FIGURE 14-31* • Third stage of labor. **A,** Placenta begins to separate in central portion accompanied by retroplacental bleeding. Uterus changes from discoid to globular shape. **B,** Placenta completes separation and enters lower uterine segment. Uterus is globular in shape. **C,** Placenta enters vagina, cord is seen to lengthen, and there may be an increase in bleeding. **D,** Expression (delivery) of placenta and completion of third stage.

We have two primary responsibilities during this stage. First, because the woman's body is rapidly adjusting to the nonpregnant state, we must monitor her physical well-being. Secondly, because infants are also usually alert and awake during the first hour of life, we should enable bonding and parental interaction with the infant to the degree the woman's personal and cultural expectations require. This section discusses maternal assessments and the interventions performed by the nurse during the fourth stage of labor. Chapter 15 presents a more detailed description of the ongoing changes that occur during the postpartum period and the postpartum care that is provided. Chapter 16 discusses care of the newborn.

### Assessments and Care

With the birth of her child, a woman takes on the task of maternal role identity. Any assistance or teaching

that she is offered should focus on empowering her in this role. "Physically and socially, she has become a mother; however, psychologically, she has much more work to accomplish before she has integrated the mother role into her self-concept" (Mercer, 1995). The taking-in process begins during the immediate postpartum as the woman starts to talk about her experience of childbirth and tries to integrate the thoughts, feelings, and physical experience that she just encountered. She will want to talk with someone who was there with her, whether it is a care provider or labor support person. She may have questions like, "Did I really scream at you?" or "Who was it that was rubbing my back there at the very end?" She may want to thank those who worked with her. Answer her questions. Give her positive reinforcement about her role and choices in labor and delivery. If her infant is not with her, she will have questions about the infant and its well-being (Mercer, 1995).

The priority physical assessment is the contracting of the uterus through the assessment of vaginal bleeding and fundal checks. After delivery, the uterus contracts to prevent excessive blood loss. We should palpate the fundus of the uterus to determine its placement, how high it is in the abdomen, and how firm it is (Figure 14-32). Normal assessment findings include the fundus at the level of the umbilicus, firm, and midline. If the fundus is "boggy" or relaxed, increased bleeding will occur. If you feel a boggy uterus, fundal massage will cause the uterus to become firm and bleeding will decrease. If the fundus does not become firm with massage, the birth attendant should be notified; the woman may need more oxitocin, either through nipple stimulation or medication. If the fundus is palpated above the umbilicus or displaced to the right or left side, it is likely that the patient has a full bladder.

Observe the amount, color, odor, and consistency of vaginal discharge. The amount is usually described as large or heavy (i.e., one peripad saturated within 2 hours), moderate (i.e., <15 cm of saturation on peripad), small or light (i.e., <10 cm of saturation on peripad), and scant (i.e., <2.5 cm of saturation on peripad). Some charting provides the space to diagram the amount of discharge as well as describe it. Normal discharge is usually dark red and can contain small to moderate size clots. We should report malodorous discharge, excessive amounts, and large clots to the birth attendant.

The woman's temperature should be checked at least one time during the first hour. A slightly elevated temperature, no higher than 100.3° F, is probably due to dehydration. Temperatures 100.4° F and above should be reported to the birth attendant because infection may be the cause. Intake of fluids should be encouraged. The woman may drink juices, water, sports drinks, etc.

Maternal heart rate, respiratory rate, and blood pressure may be checked every 15 minutes. Decreased blood pressure, increased pulse, and increased respiratory rate are signs of the hypovolemic shock that results from excessive blood loss.

Assess for the woman's bladder fullness by palpation and by noting the level of the fundus in relation to the umbilicus as noted above. A full bladder can prevent the uterus from contracting down, resulting in increased blood loss. Before getting the woman up to the bathroom, assess her ability to ambulate and tolerate a vertical position. Women may become lightheaded when they first ambulate due to hypovolemia from blood loss and dehydration. Have the woman sit on the side of the bed and dangle her legs for a few minutes, then help her to the bathroom. If she appears faint, have her sit again. Women who have had epidurals may not have control over their lower extremities and are unable to ambulate soon after giving birth.

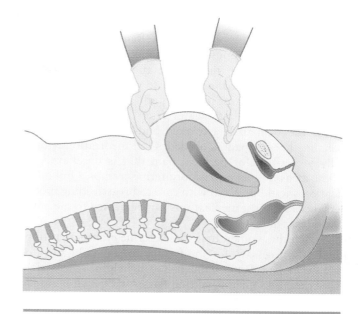

FIGURE 14-32 • Suggested method of palpating the fundus of the uterus during the fourth stage. The left hand is placed just above the symphysis pubis, and gentle downward pressure is exerted. The right hand is cupped around the uterine fundus.

Ideally, the woman will be able to void on her own, although some women cannot void immediately after delivery even when their bladder is full. The process may be facilitated if the woman sits on a toilet seat rather than uses a bedpan, is able to relax and given some privacy, smells oil of peppermint, listens to running water, has warm water flow over her perineum, or sits in a warm tub or bath. If none of these interventions work, an order for a straight catheterization may help.

Policies regarding food intake right after delivery vary. Most women are hungry at this time, especially if they have not eaten during labor. A woman usually starts with something light (e.g., soup, a sandwich, and some fruit). Some women have a special or ritual meal they eat after they deliver a baby, and this should be honored.

Assess the woman's comfort level. Women may complain of perineal discomfort, uterine cramps, muscle aches, and overall fatigue. Her perineum should be inspected for **R**edness, **E**dema, **E**chymosis, **D**rainage, and **A**pproximation (i.e., how well any separations or lacerations come together) (**REEDA** [acronym for assessment related to perineum]). If she has had an episiotomy, make sure that the stitches are intact. Also inspect the rectal area for hemorrhoids.

There are several interventions to enhance the woman's comfort level. First help the woman to sit in a firm chair or lie on her side in a lateral tilt. If the woman tightens her buttocks before sitting, she will be more comfortable. Apply an ice pack to the perineum; cold decreases edema by causing vasoconstriction and decreases pain by numbing the area. Remember that some cultures may be opposed to using cold to relieve pain. The birth attendant may order Tucks medicated pads and/or a hydrocortisone cream to soothe and decrease inflammation. Caring for the perineum by rinsing the perineal area off with water from a peri-bottle often helps the woman feel relaxed and more comfortable. Change her peripad as needed. Oral medication is usually prescribed for perineal pain that is unrelieved by these measures, as well as for uterine cramps. Oral medication should be given with care to breastfeeding mothers, because most medications can be passed to the baby via breast milk.

 Teach the woman that some uterine cramping is normal and necessary for the fundus to stay firm and decrease in size. Some women find it helpful to envision that their abdomen is getting flatter with each contraction. Cramping also occurs during breastfeeding because nipple stimulation causes the posterior pituitary to release oxytocin, which causes the uterus to contract. The amount and intensity of cramping increases with parity because the uterus must work harder to contract down due to its decreased tone from multiple pregnancies.

### Supporting the Family

As soon as the delivery is over, remove all soiled linens and unnecessary equipment. Give the parents time alone to interact with each other and their infant. Be around to answer their questions and ensure their comfort with the infant as it adjusts to extrauterine life but do not intrude on the new family. Keep nursing care as unobtrusive as possible. If you leave the room, make sure that they can easily reach you.

If family and friends are coming in to visit, the mother and baby must be clothed and appropriately covered. The woman may want a fresh nightgown or "johnny" on. The area also needs to be clean and safe. Be cognizant of anything that might be harmful to younger siblings who may be visiting their new brother or sister. Grandparents may ask questions or want to compare their birthing experiences to the present. Give them time to share this information, and help them get to know their grandchild.

Some parents prefer to be left alone with the infant for a time. If the mother is planning on breastfeeding, help her to put the baby to breast. Most infants are very interested in breastfeeding at birth; it will help the mother to make this contact with the infant. However, she may feel awkward breastfeeding if family and friends are in the room.

Talk the mother through the process of putting the baby to breast, supporting her efforts and her success. Gentle assistance will help the mother and the infant adjust to this new event. Even if the mother has breastfed before, this is a new infant who is learning its own way in the process. Some infants will lick the nipple and others will latch on as if they are famished. Time and patience with individual preferences are the key to long-term success.

Do not teach the woman the numerous principles of breastfeeding (e.g., positioning, latching on, feeding times, removing the baby from the breast, etc) at this time. She is not capable of taking in all of this information. Just help her with the basics and once the excitement has passed and she has seen family and friends, had fluids and food, and rested, she will be able to learn. Involve her partner as much as possible. He or she can help the mother with positioning the infant, supporting the mother with pillows, and ensuring that she is comfortable and has something to drink while feeding the baby.

The mother's physiologic status generally becomes stable within an hour. If she is in a hospital, she may move to a postpartum room, where her care is transferred to a different nurse. In other facilities, she will remain in the same room with the same staff until she is discharged. If the baby was born at home, the woman stays within her environment, receiving care from the same providers. All women should be encouraged to rest as much as possible when the baby sleeps, so that they are refreshed when the baby awakens and requires care.

## CIRCUMSTANCES AFFECTING A LABOR AND DELIVERY

Most women of term gestation will go into labor naturally and deliver vaginally. Most women also have single gestations. Sometimes, however, the birth attendant will determine that a woman's labor should be started artificially or that a woman needs to have a surgical birth rather than a vaginal delivery. It is our role to ensure safe passage of the infant and well-being of the woman, as well as to support her and her family as they adjust to these circumstances so that the birthing experience is a positive one for all.

### Artificial Rupture of Membranes (AROM)

An **amniotomy** or artificial rupture of membranes (AROM) is the procedure whereby the midwife or physician ruptures the amniotic sac (Figure 14-33). First a vaginal examination is done, and then a sterile amniohook is advanced (hook side down) along the examiner's fingers until the bag is reached. The hook is then rotated upward to "snag" the membranes. The examiner will immediately see an outpouring of amniotic fluid. AROM may be done as an attempt to induce or augment labor or if internal fetal monitoring is necessary. During this procedure, we must monitor the FHR because the umbilical cord can prolapse (i.e., fall in front of the presenting part) during this procedure. This is suspected if the FHR suddenly decreases.

In addition to monitoring the fetal heart rate, we should also record the Time the amniotic sac was

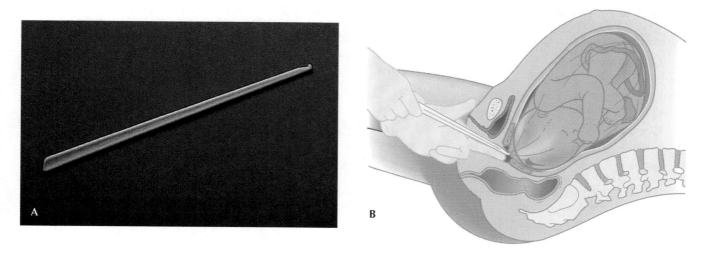

FIGURE 14-33 • Amniotomy. **A,** Disposable plastic membrane perforator; **B,** Technique for artficial rupture of membranes.

ruptured, the **A**mount of amniotic fluid, the **C**olor of the fluid, and presence of an **O**dor (**TACO** is an acronym for assessment related to rupture of membranes). **T**—the time is documented for future reference. **A**—excessive amounts of amniotic fluid (hydramnios) or very small amounts of amniotic fluid (oligohydramnios) are associated with congenital abnormalities and kidney problems, respectively. **C**—amniotic fluid is normally clear and may be mixed with bloody vaginal discharge or contains white flecks of vernix caseosa. If the fluid is "stained," it can range in color from a light tan to thick "split pea soup" green, and the birth attendant should be notified. Stained fluid indicates that at some time the infant had a bowel movement in utero. These situations are discussed in Chapter 18. From this point on throughout the labor, the woman will continue to leak amniotic fluid. She must be provided with a pad to catch the fluid and maintain her comfort.

Amniotomy early in labor appears to have little value and may actually have an adverse effect on the process of the labor and the tolerance of the fetus to labor. If done late in labor, amniotomy may provide treatment for slow progress by shortening labor by an hour or two (Goer, 1995).

## Induction/Augmentation

**Induction** of labor is defined as stimulation of contractions before spontaneous onset of labor, with or without ruptured membranes. **Augmentation** refers to the stimulation of contractions when spontaneous contractions are not causing progressive dilation or descent (Cunningham and others, 1997).

There are several ways that labor may be induced or augmented. Some traditional methods are taking a ride over a bumpy road, ingesting castor oil, eating a heavy meal, and sniffing pepper (Purnell and Paulanka, 1998). Herbs (e.g., black cohosh tea, cumin seed tea, or cinnamon tea) may be used to start or augment labor contractions (Spector, 1996).

Breast stimulation and intercourse are also helpful to induce or augment labor. Prostaglandins cause the uterus to contract, and semen has a high proportion of prostaglandin. The woman should position herself so that when the man ejaculates the semen is deposited as close to the cervix as possible. Breast stimulation may produce strong uterine contractions near the end of pregnancy and may initiate labor if the woman's body is ready. Nipple stimulation has also been found to be effective in augmenting labor (Kitzinger, 1980). To be successful, the woman and her partner may need to have you leave the room and provide them with time and privacy.

Induction or augmentation of contractions may occur through the stimulation of the release of natural oxytocin within a woman's body or the addition of oxytocin to a mother's system via the drug Pitocin (Box 14-17).

Since 1987, hospital admissions for induction of patients at 40 weeks of gestation have increased 100% (Ventura and others, 1997). According to the American College of Obstetricians and Gynecologists (1995b), induction of labor is indicated when the benefits to the mother and/or the fetus outweigh the risks of continuing the pregnancy. Providers do vary in the practice of oxytocin inductions when the pregnancy is thought to be of more than 40 weeks' duration, or past due.

### Indications

A non-stress test may be done to assess fetal well-being if the woman is past due. If accelerations are noted with fetal movement and all other maternal assessments are within normal limits, the woman is not induced at this visit. If the non-stress test is non-reactive, the woman is

---

## BOX 14-17   *About Oxytocin*

**Generic Name**
oxytocin

**Trade Name**
Pitocin, Syntocinon

**Classification**
oxytocic

**Action**
Acts directly on myofibrils to produce uterine contractions; stimulates mammary smooth muscle, enhancing milk ejection from breasts

**Usual Dosage and Routes**
*Labor and delivery*: 10 units in 500 to 1000 mL of D5W or 0.9% NaCl; administer 1 to 2 units/min; may increase q15 to 30 min until contraction pattern is similar to spontaneous labor, not to exceed 20 mU/min

*Postpartum*: 10 to 40 units/100mL of D5W or 0.9% NaCl given at rate of 20 to 40 milliunits (mU)/min, or 10 units IM after the placenta is delivered

*Breastfeeding*: 1 spray to one or both nostrils 2 to 3 minutes before nursing or pumping breasts

*Oxytocin should never be given IV push.*

**Onset**
IM, 3 to 7 min; IV, 1 min; Nasal, minutes

**Duration**
IM, 1 hr; IV, 30 min; Nasal, 20 min

**Half Life**
IM, 12 to 17 min; IV, 12 to 17 min

**Side Effects**
*Maternal*: hypotension; tetanic contractions; nausea, vomiting; constipation; dysrhythmias; increased pulse; abruptio placenta; decreased uterine flow; rash; hyperbilirubinemia; water intoxication, seizure, coma and death can occur with prolonged infusion and excessive fluid volume

*Fetal*: dysrhythmias, jaundice, hypoxia, intracranial hemorrhage

**Contraindications**
Hypersensitivity, serum toxemia, CPD, fetal distress, hypertonic uterus; anytime a vaginal delivery is contraindicated; nasal oxytocin is contraindicated during pregnancy

**Interactions/Incompatibilities**
After use of vasopressors, concurrent use with cyclopropane anesthesia

From Hodgson BB and Kizior RJ: *Saunders nursing drug handbook 1999*, Philadelphia, 1999, W.B. Saunders.

---

often induced. Physicians vary on their practice of induction based on postdates. Poor results on fetal tests during the prenatal period—especially those that suggest placental insufficiency—are an indication for induction. Diabetics often require inductions due to placental deterioration or macrosomia evident prior to 40 weeks. Other indications for inductions include the following: PIH, PROM, chorioamnionitis, any suspected fetal jeopardy (i.e., IUGR or Rh isoimmunization problems), maternal medical conditions in which continuation of pregnancy would jeopardize maternal long- or short-term health, fetal demise, and some individualized circumstances (e.g., the woman has history of rapid labors and lives a long distance from the hospital).

## Contraindications
Contraindications include any fetal malpresentation that would prohibit a vaginal delivery (e.g., a transverse lie). Oxytocin should not be administered to women of high parity or those who have had a classical (vertical) uterine incision from an earlier surgical delivery because it may place the woman at greater risk for a uterine rupture. Oxytocin is often avoided or used very cautiously in cases where the uterus is overdistended (e.g., multiple gestation, hydramnios, or an excessively large fetus) or the FHR is non-reassuring but does not require immediate delivery, or if maternal cardiac disease exists.

## Cervical Ripening
In some cases, an induction of labor is indicated, but the cervix is not "ripe" for labor (i.e., it is thick and hard). The woman's cervix may be softened chemically with semen (as described earlier) or a prostaglandin gel or suppository, or mechanically with laminaria tents made of seaweed or synthetic dilators. Local application of prostaglandin E2 gel or suppository softens the cervix and may start effacement and dilation. With the gel in place, a woman may be discharged home until the next day or the start of labor. The suppository is placed in the posterior fornix of the vagina and removed 12 hours after insertion or upon the onset of active labor. Thirty minutes after the vaginal suppository is removed, intravenous administration of oxytocin can begin (Figure 14-34).

The mechanical methods of dilation are inserted into the os of the cervix. As the laminaria tent absorbs fluids, it causes the cervix to dilate. After 6 to 12 hours, they are removed and the extent of cervical dilation is assessed. The process many be repeated until the necessary amount of dilation is achieved, at which point the intravenous administration of oxytocin is started.

Monitor and chart the woman's physiologic response as her system absorbs the prostaglandins. Maintain a record of the time of insertion and the type and amount of intervention used.

## Induction Procedure

Oxytocin infusion is the most common method of inducing labor. Before an infusion is begun, a birth attendant must be readily available and the nurse-patient ratio on the unit must allow for close supervision of the patient. The woman must have an open intravenous line and a fetal monitor attached.

Physicians usually have protocols or standard orders for their preferences on oxytocin inductions. Typically, 10 units of oxytocin is mixed into 1000 mL (or 500 mL if the preference is to have the patient receive less IV fluids) of lactated Ringer's solution. This mixture is piggy-backed into the mainline at the port closest to the patient. This medication should only be infused by an infusion device. It is not appropriate to administer this medication by gravity or IV push. The infusion is usually started at 0.5 to 2 mU/min, and the dose is increased 1 to 2 mU every 15 to 60 minutes until a regular contraction pattern is established. The rate is increased or decreased based on assessments of fetal and maternal status.

### Assessments and Care

We are responsible for several ongoing assessments. The contraction pattern caused by the infusion of Pitocin is of vital importance. If contractions last longer than 60 to 90 seconds and there is less than 1 minute of resting tone between contractions, the oxytocin infusion should be decreased and/or discontinued until contractions are occurring every 2 to 3 minutes. Hyperstimulation of the uterus can result in fetal distress or uterine rupture.

Assess the fetal heart rate for changes in baseline and variability and the occurrence of decelerations. Continuous electronic fetal monitoring is always used for women receiving oxytocin. If problems are noted, the following interventions are indicated: (1) discontinue the oxytocin; (2) turn the woman on her left side; (3) cautiously increase the rate of the primary IV line; (4) administer oxygen by mask at 10 L/min; and (5) notify the physician of the problem and that the oxytocin has been discontinued.

Assess the woman's blood pressure and heart rate; oxytocin can cause these two vital signs to increase. Because oxytocin has an antidiuretic effect, monitor intake and output. If large amounts of fluid are administered with high dosages of oxytocin, water intoxication can result, leading to convulsions, coma, and even death (Cunningham and others, 1997). Careful monitoring and timely interventions based on our assessments will decrease the likelihood of complications.

Assess the woman's comfort and emotional well-being. Assist with pain-relief interventions, as discussed earlier in this chapter. Involve the family in supporting the woman, who may be upset because induction of labor was not something she wanted to occur. Allow her to express her feelings and concerns about the process. Explain the procedures and what she can expect during

*Simple to administer.*

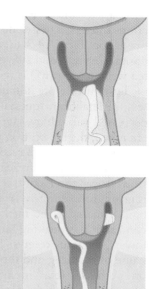

**1 Position Cervidil vaginal insert securely between the index and middle fingers.**

Does not require syringe, speculum, or stirrups.

**2 Place transversely in the posterior fornix of the vagina.**

Patient should be kept supine for 2 hours after insertion and then may ambulate.

*Simple to remove.*

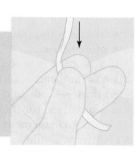

**3 To stop prostaglandin E₂ release, pull retrieval string to remove the insert.\***

Irrigation and wiping are not necessary. Oxytocin may be administered at least 30 minutes later.

FIGURE 14-34 ● Placement of a prostaglandin suppository in the posterion vagina. Simple to adminster: (1) Position CERVIDIL vaginal insert securely between the index and middle fingers. This does not require syringe, speculum, or stirrups. (2) Place transversely in the posterior fornix of the vagina. Patient should be kept supine for 2 hours after insertion and then may ambulate. Simple to remove. (3) To stop prostaglandin $E_2$ release, pull retrieval string to remove the insert.* Irrigation and wiping are not necessary. Oxytocin may be administered at least 30 minutes later. Uterine activity, fetal status, and the progression of cervical dilation and effacement should be carefully monitored. *CERVIDIL should be removed 12 hours after insertion, after onset of active labor, or should uterine hyperstimulation occur. (Courtesy Forest Pharmaceuticals, Inc., subsidiary of Forest—Laboratories, Inc., St. Louis, 63045.)

the induction. Allow her to make as many decisions as possible during this process.

## Pharmacologic Pain Relief

### Medications during Labor

Intramuscular or intravenous medications can also provide pain relief. These medications provide the best relief when a woman is in early labor, when the contractions are not as intense. A lesser degree of relief is obtained in active labor. Table 14-3 lists commonly used medications, dosages, effects, and side effects. A medication order (often written as "prn") is required for a nurse to give these medications. Before administering the drug, carefully assess the fetal heart tones; if any non-reassuring signs (e.g., decreased variablility, late decelerations, or bradycardia) are noted, the medication should not be given.

**Administration.** It is recommended that when administering intravenous medications, the dosage be pushed in slowly over three contractions. Because the medication is given intravenously, some of the drug enters the fetus' bloodstream. If the medication is pushed in when the contraction is peaking (and the perfusion to the baby is lower), the fetus receives less medication. Document the name of the drug and the dosage, route, and time given on both the fetal monitor strip and the medication record. Stay with the woman for at least 15 minutes after administration and monitor her respiratory status and fetal heart tones. If several doses of medication are needed to obtain small amounts of pain relief, you should assess the possibility that the woman has a history of drug use.

If a woman is an opiate, heroin, or methadone user, this has implications for the medication she can be offered during labor and delivery. Narcotic pain medication is indicated for these women. Stadol cannot be used for pain management because its partial antagonist properties will allow withdrawal to occur.

**Pain Relief.** After the medication is administered in early labor, the woman can expect fair pain relief for approximately 2 hours before the medication wears off. During this time, the mother may fall asleep between contractions and then wake up abruptly when a contraction is moving into its peak. To prevent this disruption, have the support person monitor the contractions and gently rouse the woman and help her breathe through the contraction before returning to sleep. This process is much more restful to the woman and helps her maintain her comfort. Talking to the woman in a soft voice, keeping the room dim and quiet, and encouraging her to relax with the medication will enhance the pain relief obtained from intravenous medications. If the woman relaxes well for 2 hours, the cervix may often relax and dilate, and the woman awakens rejuvenated and better able to handle labor.

**Side Effects for the Fetus.** Intravenous medications are not without side effects. It is recommended that continuous electronic fetal monitoring be used if medications are given. Decreased long- and short-term variability are often seen. This decrease is the result of the central nervous system (CNS) depression caused by the narcotics. If necessary, keeping the woman in the side-lying position and administering oxygen by mask can increase fetal oxygenation. Narcotics can cause respiratory depression in both the mother and the fetus; and infants born when the narcotic is peaking are more likely to have respiratory depression than those born before or after the peak effect. Infants affected by narcotics have lower Apgar scores at birth, decreased muscle tone, decreased respiratory rates, and poor crying efforts.

These effects can be improved by administering naloxone (Narcan) intramuscularly to the infant immediately at birth or intravenously to the woman immediately before birth (because the medication will go directly to the infant). The preferred method is to administer the medication to the infant after birth because the effects will last longer. No long-term fetal side effects have been noted to be caused by narcotic administration, so narcotics are considered a safe method of pain relief for women who prefer to use pharmacologic methods for pain relief during labor.

**Side Effects for the Woman.** Narcotics given intravenously can cause nausea and vomiting in the woman. These are more likely to occur if the medication is administered too quickly. Sometimes antiemetics (e.g., promethazine or hydroxyzine) are administered concurrently with the narcotic to prevent nausea and vomiting and promote rest.

---

### TABLE 14-3 Analgesics Commonly Used in Labor

| Medication | Dosage/route | Cautions |
|---|---|---|
| Meperidine (Demerol) | 25 mg IV q3 to 4 hr<br>50 to 100 mg IM q 3 to 4 hr | • Maternal respiratory depression, nausea, vomiting<br>• Can halt labor if given too early in labor<br>• Fetal respiratory depression, decreased long- and short-term variability<br>• Keep naloxone available to reverse respiratory depression in mother and infant |
| Butorphanol tartrate (Stadol) | 1 to 2 mg IM or IV q 3 to 4 hr | • Same as above<br>• Although rare, can cause urinary retention |
| Nalbuphine (Nubain) | 10 to 20 mg SQ or IV q 3 to 6 hr | • Same as above<br>• Fetal sinusoidal heart rate pattern |

## Epidurals

An epidural is a very effective method of obtaining pain relief during labor. Epidurals are included in this discussion because they can affect the length and type of the woman's delivery. An epidural consists of administering an anesthetic agent into the epidural space, producing pain relief across the abdomen and lower back. Pain relief varies in intensity, so some woman may feel a mild cramp when a contraction occurs (often described as what is felt during menstruation), while others are totally unaware that contractions are occurring. Most women who receive epidurals receive excellent pain relief. In some cases, the epidural is only effective on one side or is ineffective—often because of catheter placement. In addition to being the most effective pain relief available to labor patients, an epidural is also considered relatively safe for both the woman and infant. Having a skilled provider place the epidural and following this with conscientious nursing care will minimize any complications.

Although epidurals provide the most effective pain relief to laboring women, there are disadvantages. The woman with an epidural is confined to bed with an IV, fetal monitor, blood pressure cuff, and urinary catheter in place. Each of these may have a negative effect on the labor process or provide the woman with additional risk factors. The woman loses sensation in the lower half of her body and is able to move the lower extremities minimally, if at all. Thus she is unable to move around in the bed, ambulate, or assume any upright positions that facilitate delivery. She is unable to void on her own and must have intermittent straight catheterizations (or, if the labor is long, sometimes a Foley catheter is used) to keep her bladder empty. The woman may also lose her sensation to push, thereby increasing the length of the second stage of labor and the likelihood of delivery with forceps or vacuum extractor

or a surgical delivery. Rare complications may lead to maternal and/or fetus death.

***Insertion.*** Epidurals are inserted by a nurse anesthetist, an anesthesiologist, or sometimes by an obstetrician. Prior to insertion, 1000 mL of IV fluid is infused to fully hydrate the patient. Anytime an anesthetic is injected into the epidural space, hypotension is possible. Adequate hydration decreases the likelihood and severity of the hypotension. Additionally, some anesthesia departments require that a hematocrit and hemoglobin level are drawn prior to placement.

Getting the woman positioned properly and comfortably during epidural insertion is critical to successful placement of the epidural needle but difficult because the woman is still dealing with labor contractions. The woman is placed in one of two positions: sitting upright tailor style, or with legs hanging over the side of the bed, or lying on her side, curled up in the fetal position. In either position, it is critical that the woman "round" her back to separate the vertebrae. The anesthetist works behind the woman, and the woman's support person should sit down on a chair facing her. Encourage the support person to hold the woman's hand during the procedure and talk her through contractions (Figure 14-35).

The anesthetist begins by finding the insertion point on the patient's back, usually below L-2, which is the point where the spinal cord ends. Her back is then cleaned with cool povidone iodine (Betadine) on a sponge stick. A local anesthetic is administered. The epidural needle is inserted and advanced until a syringe of normal saline can be easily pushed in, indicating that the needle is in the epidural space. A fine catheter is then advanced into the epidural space through the needle. The needle is removed, and the catheter is taped up the woman's back and brought over her shoulder. A syringe of anesthetic is attached to the catheter, and a test dose

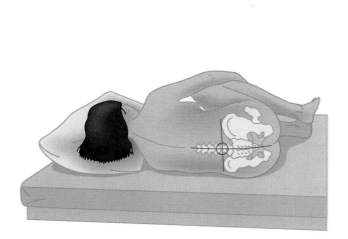
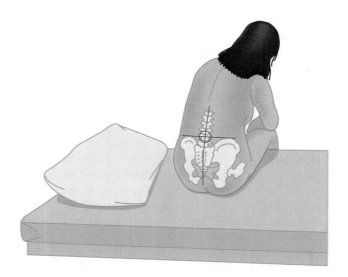

*FIGURE 14-35* ● Position for epidural insertion.

is given. If the catheter is in a vein, the woman will experience tinnitus and have a metal taste in her mouth. A drop in blood pressure and increase in heart rate will also occur. If the woman tolerates the test dose, a bolus dose is given. Finally, a 50 to 100 mL bag of anesthetic mixture is infused via pump through the catheter to provide ongoing pain relief. This is called a continuous epidural. Intermittent epidurals occur when the woman is given a dose every couple of hours as the anesthetic is wearing off, and there is no continuous infusion running. Continuous epidurals have the advantage of keeping the pain under control more effectively.

Opiates or opiate/anesthetic combinations have recently been given via epidural to decrease labor pain. These narcotic epidurals have the advantage of maintaining a woman's mobility, while decreasing the sensation of pain. In a study of 130 women receiving epidural fentanyl or an ultra low dose bupivacaine-epinephrine-fentanyl regimen, 70% of the women ambulated safely during the labor while experiencing satisfactory analgesia. One third of these women could also void on their own, which is rare with the typical epidural (Breen and others, 1993). Side effects of this procedure are pruritus (80%), urinary retention (55%), nausea and vomiting (45%), and headaches (10%) (Herpolsheimer and Schrententhaler, 1994). Respiratory depression is rare but is a potential complication. Naloxone can be given to reverse the side effects.

*Nursing Care.* AWHONN (1996) issued a position statement delineating what a registered nurse (RN) can and cannot do in regard to epidurals. Insertion, initial dosing, and re-bolusing are reserved for anesthesia personnel; RNs can replace empty infusion bags or pump syringes, stop the infusion, and remove the catheter when anesthesia is no longer needed.

During the procedure, monitor vital signs, support the patient, and watch the fetal monitor strip. After the test dose is given, follow the facility protocol in monitoring the woman. For example, her blood pressure is checked frequently, usually by automatic means. The pattern is usually every 2 minutes for 10 minutes, every 5 minutes for 10 minutes, and then every 15 to 30 minutes. Expect the woman to experience a drop in blood pressure. Maintaining the IV flow at 125 mL/hr helps keep blood pressure within normal limits. The most severe decreases occur in the first 10 to 20 minutes (Stem, 1997). If the systolic blood pressure drops more than 20% or below 100 mm Hg, put the woman on her left side, increase the flow of the IV, place the woman in a 10- to 20-degree Trendelenburg position, and notify anesthesia personnel. Ephedrine is often given; its vasoconstrictive effect raises the blood pressure.

Use pillows for support and to help maintain proper body alignment. Turn the woman (she will have difficulty moving herself) from side to side hourly because the epidural works by gravity. If she is left to lie on one side too long, she may begin to experience pain on the opposite side. Never leave her in the supine position.

Continue to assess the woman's level of comfort.  Even with a continuous epidural, additional medication is often needed. Explain to the woman that the epidural does not take away all feelings of pressure caused by fetal descent. It is desirable that the woman feel this pressure because it will help her when pushing. Check the level or degree of the anesthesia (dermatone level) by seeing if the woman can feel the touch of a cool alcohol swab on her abdomen. The level of pain blockage should start at around the umbilicus.

Palpate the woman's bladder and monitor her intake and output. She will lose her ability and urge to void, so she must be straight catheterized every 2 to 4 hours throughout labor. A full bladder can decrease the amount of room in the pelvis for fetal descent and prevent the cervix from dilating. If a forceps delivery is planned, catheterizing the woman before applying the forceps will give more room for delivery and decrease the likelihood of trauma to the bladder from the forceps.

Assess how the woman is doing emotionally. With the loss of sensations, she may feel unattached to the labor process and more like an observer of her body. She may not have planned to have an epidural and may now be afraid that the medication will harm her baby or lead to other procedures that may cause harm. Some women feel like a "failure" when they have not achieved an unmedicated childbirth. The woman may now also feel very dependent upon health care providers because she cannot move herself in bed, urinate on her own, or turn over. Involving her labor support person in positioning and caring for her may help her feel less dependent on health care providers.

*Complications.* The most common complication is hypotension. Sympathetic tracts are blocked, resulting in vasodilation, which leads to hypotension and decreased cardiac output. The occurrence of these effects is decreased when patients are bolused with 1000 mL of lactated Ringer's solution prior to epidural insertion. The systolic blood pressure is monitored and if necessary, ephedrine is given via IV push because of its vasoconstrictive effectiveness.

Another complication relates to insertion of the epidural. If the epidural needle is inserted through the dura, the woman will receive a spinal block, which can result in a postspinal headache due to the trauma caused by the dural puncture and possible leakage of cerebral spinal fluid. This headache is almost intolerable if the woman is in a vertical position and virtually unnoticeable when she is supine. If a spinal headache occurs, the woman must maintain strict bed rest in the horizontal position and be encouraged to force fluids. If the headache does not resolve in 34 to 48 hours, a blood patch is done. This procedure involves injecting the woman's own blood at the spinal puncture site in an effort to block it. Immediate relief may be obtained with a blood patch. If the woman is not in a supine position, hydration, medication, and repeat blood patches are done until the woman gains relief.

A high level block is also a complication of an epidural. If this occurs, the woman may experience difficulty breathing, weakness of the hands, and temporary paralysis until the epidural wears off. This is a life-threatening emergency, therefore oxygen, suction, and resuscitation equipment should be readily available for all women receiving an epidural.

When problems are assessed during the administration of an epidural, the infusion pump must be turned off immediately and anesthesia personnel notified. The woman must not be left alone. An epidural may also be used for pain management during a surgical delivery (Figure 14-36).

### Spinal

A spinal refers to a subarachnoid block, in which local anesthetic is injected through the third, fourth, or fifth lumbar interspace into the subarachoid space. Administered by a nurse anesthetist or an anesthesiologist, a spinal is used for delivery. Given as a single injection when delivery is imminent (i.e., 1 to 5 contractions away) it relieves the pain of the last part of the second stage of labor. The nursing care is as stated for a woman with an epidural. A spinal may also be given for a surgical delivery.

## Delivery by Surgical Birth (Cesarean Section)

A surgical birth or cesarean section (CS) is the delivery of an infant through an incision made in the woman's abdominal wall and uterus. This type of delivery occurs in cases where a vaginal delivery is questionable or a condition warrants immediate delivery for the well-being of the infant and mother. Cesarean section is the most common operation performed in the United States (VanTuinen and Wolfe, 1992). As a result, the United States has one of the highest CS rates in the world.

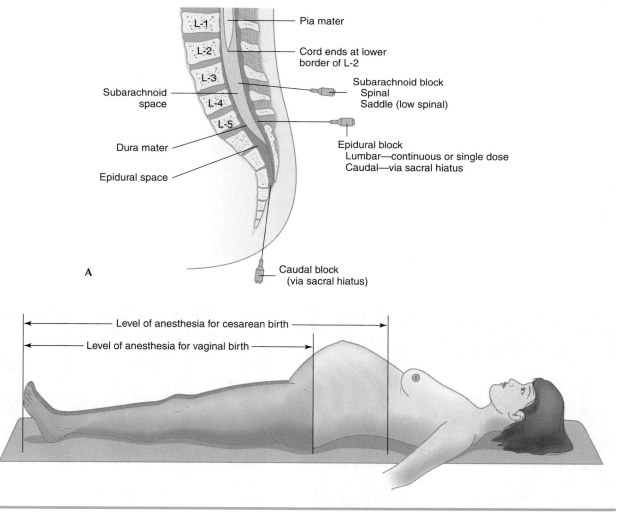

FIGURE 14-36 • Placement and nerve pathways for epidurals and spinal. **A,** Regional block analgesia and anesthesia in obstretrics; **B,** Anesthesia levels for vaginal and cesarean births.

Because there is no documented relationship between cesarean rates and perinatal mortality and morbidity rates and a cesarean delivery increases maternal risk, a deliberate effort is being made to reduce the number of surgical deliveries (Goer, 1995).

In 1965 the CS rate in this country was 4.5%. This rate increased to almost 25% by 1988 (Taffel and others, 1991) but had dropped to 20.8% in 1997 (Curtin and Park, 1999). "There remains a wide variation in cesarean rates among states ranging from 26.7 in Mississippi to 15.3 in Colorado" (Curtin and Park, 1999). Efforts to reduce the rate of surgical deliveries continue across the country.

Several reasons have been cited for the increase in the cesarean rate (Cunningham and others, 1997). The use of continuous electronic fetal monitoring, which began in the early 1970s in the United States, gives the provider a tracing that may indicate a problem with the fetus. The increase in the use of continuous fetal monitoring and the increase in cesarean rates have shown parallel growth. Physicians concerned about malpractice litigation may be choosing cesarean delivery when there is a disturbing monitor tracing, therefore contributing to this high rate. Further research has shown that cesarean rates depend on factors having nothing to do with medical indications. The factors are the following: "individual philosophy and training, convenience, the patient's socioeconomic status, peer pressure, fear of litigation, and possibly financial gain" (Goer, 1995).

### Indications

There are several medical conditions and emergency circumstances where a surgical delivery is indicated. Possible problems with the health of the fetus (e.g., fetal distress, as indicated on a fetal monitor strip, or a poor fetal capillary pH) may require removing the infant immediately.

A fetal scalp sample measures the pH of the blood in the capillaries as a measure of fetal compromise. A nurse-midwife or physician obtains the sample. Working up through the woman's vagina and cervix, the fetal scalp is swabbed with a disinfecting solution. Then a puncture is made in the scalp, and a blood sample collected. Because of the invasive procedure of taking a blood sample from the fetus and its failure to provide definitive information, this procedure is declining in use (Goodwin, Milner-Masterson, Paul, 1994). If a measure of fetal status is needed, fetal scalp stimulation may be used instead. Created with finger pressure or pinching, the stimulation may create a fetal heart rate increase. If the fetus has a 15 beat/minute acceleration that lasts at least 15 seconds, it is reassuring.

There are naturally many organisms in a woman's vagina. When a woman has a sexually transmitted active infection, it is sometimes dangerous for the fetus to descend. For example, because of the potential transmission of herpes from mother to infant during a vaginal delivery, active herpes is a contraindication to a vaginal delivery and a surgical delivery may be planned.

*Conditions of this Pregnancy.* Cephalopelvic disproportion (CPD) is when the fetus is judged to be too large to fit through the maternal pelvis. **Failure to progress (FTP)**, an arrest in the dilation process that places the fetus or mother in danger, is another indication. Events such as CPD and FTP are often classified as labor dystocia. Another indication is transverse or breech presentation that prevents the fetus from entering the birth canal (Figure 14-37). Some birth attendants with experience in the procedure will attempt to deliver a baby in a frank breech or complete breech presentation vaginally. The size and position of the baby's head are major considerations.

Placenta previa and abruptio placentae may lead to surgical delivery. **Placenta previa** is when the placenta or a portion of the placenta is covering the cervical os. As the cervix begins to dilate, bleeding and fetal distress can occur. **Abruptio placentae** occurs when the placenta becomes detached from the uterus prior to delivery of the infant. These conditions are covered in detail in Chapter 18 along with other problems of pregnancy and labor.

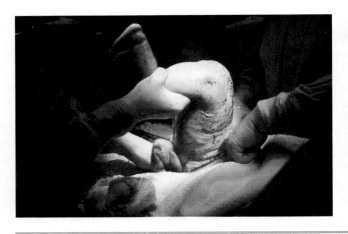 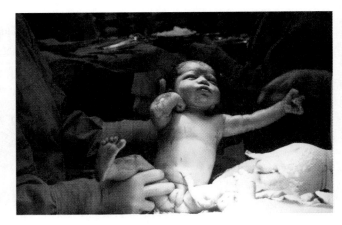

*FIGURE 14-37* • Baby in breech position born via surgical birth. *(Courtesy of Caroline E. Brown.)*

Depending on the number, presentation, and gestational age of the fetuses, a multiple gestation may warrant a surgical delivery. Other complications that occur during the labor process and contribute to the cesarean rate are a prolapsed cord when the amniotic membranes rupture and the occurrence of a uterine rupture.

### Repeat Surgical Deliveries

If the woman had a previous surgical delivery with a vertical uterine incision, she will generally not be allowed to attempt a vaginal delivery and risk rupturing the scarred area. Women who have had a previous surgical delivery with a horizontal uterine incision are encouraged to prepare for a **vaginal birth after cesarean (VBAC)**. Of the women who have had a previous surgical delivery, 27.4% are having vaginal deliveries (Curtin and Park, 1999). VBACs are often successful because the *P*s of labor (i.e., passage, passenger, powers, psyche, position, and power [uterine contractions]) are different each time. Each pregnancy produces a different combination of these factors so if the prior problem does not reoccur, the woman may complete a vaginal delivery.

### Contraindications

Unless a uterine infection is present, the risk of a surgical delivery is contraindicated in the case of a fetal demise. Other contraindications are based on the fetus's gestational age and condition. Maternal contraindications occur when the mother is experiencing medical problems (e.g., problems with blood clotting) that place her life at risk if she undergoes surgery.

### Preoperative Nursing Care

When a surgical delivery is scheduled, our role is to prepare the woman and her family physically, mentally, and emotionally for birth of the baby. Remember that if a woman is in labor, she continues to need our support in dealing with that, in addition to her new anxiety about surgery and the preparations she must now undergo. Therefore it generally takes two nurses to prepare a laboring woman for a surgical delivery.

Obtain informed consent from the woman for the surgical procedure. Be sure there is a comprehensive health and obstetric history, as described earlier under labor admission. If the woman has had any previous surgeries, inquire about surgical or anesthetic complications. Perform a physical assessment. Inquire about her most recent oral intake. Assess the status of the fetus. If a fetal monitor is not on, apply one and obtain a 30-minute strip. Obtain the necessary lab work, which usually includes blood type, antibody screen, Rh, and complete blood count.

***Physical Preparations.*** An IV must be in place and infusing. Perform an abdominal scrub and shave per institutional policy. A Foley catheter must be placed before the surgery begins, although this is often done after

the spinal anesthesia has been administered so that the woman does not feel the catheter being inserted. Administer any preoperative medications ordered. Medications are often ordered to dry up secretions (ranitidine), neutralize gastric acids (sodium citrate/citric acid), and prevent vomiting (metoclopramide). Discuss the operating room procedures with the woman's labor support person. Usually, when someone accompanies the woman into the operating room, he or she must wear scrubs, a hat, mask, and shoe covers. Instruct the support person on how and when to prepare, where to stand once in the room, and how he or she may help the woman. Also, tell them not to touch anything on the tables in order to maintain sterile technique. Answer any questions the patient and family may have.

If this is not a planned surgical delivery, assess how the woman and her partner are dealing with the idea of surgery. Often women are afraid that they will lose the baby. Partners may be afraid that they will lose both the woman and the baby. Women may express disappointment at not being able to have a vaginal delivery, but such feelings are generally not expressed until after the surgery.

Be sensitive to the fact that the time from when a birth attendant determines that there is a problem requiring a surgical delivery until the surgery actually starts will seem like forever to the woman and her labor supporters. They will be concerned about the status of their baby during that time and wonder why everyone is taking so long. Keep them aware of the preparations that are taking place and the condition of their baby, and try not to leave them alone.

Once preparations are complete, notify the physician and other operating room personnel. Transport the woman and her support person to the operating room. Arrange to be with them during the surgery or to return to see them after the birth. Speaking with them after the delivery will help the family bring closure to the process.

### Operative Nursing Care

The patient is placed on the operating room table, usually wedged in the left lateral position and covered with warm blankets. A fetal monitor continues to document the presence of fetal heart tones before the surgery begins. A grounding tape is applied to the leg, and suction machines are connected and turned on. Another abdominal prep is done; the type depends on the institution. Alcohol or Betadine are commonly used. A scrub technician or a scrub nurse is present. The role of scrub nurse is to remain sterile and pass instruments and supplies to the surgeon. Another nurse functions as a circulating nurse. The circulating nurse documents the surgery and places necessary supplies onto the sterile operating room table. A third nurse or a member of the neonatal team is present to care for the infant. Anesthesia personnel administer all medications to the woman.

### The Procedure

An incision large enough to deliver the infant is made through the abdominal wall. Most often a Pfannenstiel or low transverse incision is used. At one time a vertical incision, often called a "classical" incision, was used, but now this type of incision is reserved for emergency situations. A comparison of these two types of incisions can be found in Table 14-4. Once the uterus is seen, retractors are placed and a similar incision is made through the lower segment of the uterine wall. Then the infant is delivered. The mouth and nose are suctioned, the cord is double clamped and cut, and the infant is then handed off to a nurse or pediatrician for assessment and immediate care. Cord blood is obtained, and the placenta is delivered manually and inspected. At this time, the uterus is often placed on sterile drapes outside of the abdominal cavity to be repaired. After repair, the uterus is placed back in the abdominal cavity, and then the abdominal layers are repaired. The skin incision may be closed with staples or a running suture, as determined by physician preference. A dressing is firmly applied over the incision. The patient is then transferred to the recovery room.

### Postoperative Care

Care of a woman after a surgical delivery requires additional assessments when compared with a vaginal delivery. During the surgery, vessels are cauterized and much drainage is suctioned out of the uterine cavity. Just as after a vaginal delivery, vital signs and bleeding must be monitored and the fundus checked every 15 minutes. Sometimes the woman's temperature is below normal limits due to the low temperatures in the operating room. Placing warm blankets around her will help her relax and increase her body temperature. If the fundus is boggy, gently massage it until firm. Remember that the uterus now has stitches in it to hold the incision together.

Vaginal bleeding post-uterine surgery (hysterotomy) is usually less than that following a vaginal delivery. Blood vessels are cauterized during the surgery, and fluids in the uterus have been removed with suction. To remove the discharge that is occurring, rinse the perineum with warm water from a peribottle (a squeeze bottle) and then apply a clean, dry peripad to help the woman feel refreshed and more comfortable.

Wound care during the first hours involves inspecting the dressing every 15 minutes for new drainage. If drainage is noted, do not remove the dressing but outline the drainage on the dressing and record the date and time. If drainage is excessive, notify the surgeon. Reinforcing the dressing is often preferable to removing it.

Most women are placed on a cardiac monitor and pulse oximetry, especially if they received regional analgesia for the surgery. An oxygen saturation of over 90% is desirable. The nurse assessing the recovery of the woman after surgery must be skilled in interpreting ECG readings to determine if the patient has a normal cardiac rhythm.

If the woman had regional anesthesia, assess her ability to move her lower extremities as she regains feeling. She will need assistance in moving to a comfortable position because she probably does not have the ability to move her lower extremities. Keeping the side rails up provides her with the assistance of the rails as she moves and promotes her safety. Make sure the call light is in reach.

Due to the surgery, the woman's breath and bowel sounds must be assessed. If she had regional analgesia, closely observe her respiratory rate, which can be depressed. Also ask her if she is experiencing nausea or pruritis, which are two common side effects. Monitor her peripheral perfusion by noting her skin color and temperature.

---

**TABLE 14-4** *Comparison of Low Transverse and Vertical Incisions*

|  | Low transverse (pfannenstiel) | Vertical (classical) |
|---|---|---|
| Location | • Across the lower uterine segment | • Into the body of the uterus, above the lower uterine segment and reaching to the fundus |
| Advantages | • Requires only a modest dissection of the bladder from the myometrium<br>• Results in less blood loss<br>• Repair is easier and stronger<br>• Less likely to rupture in subsequent labors<br>• Less chance of adherence of bowel to incision<br>• Cosmetic advantage | • Quickest to make, allowing for rapid delivery in emergency situations<br>• Provides greater view of fetus and interior of uterus<br>• Can be extended upward if more room is needed |
| Disadvantages | • Takes longer to do, so it may not be the incision of choice in an emergency<br>• View is limited | • More blood loss<br>• More extensive dissection of the bladder is necessary<br>• If the incision extends downward, the tear can involve the cervix, vagina, and bladder<br>• More likely to rupture during subsequent labors than a transverse incision<br>• Skin incision cosmetically undesirable |

Ask the patient to rate her pain level on a scale of 1 to 10. Most women are very comfortable during this recovery period because the surgical anesthesia is still effective. Check the physician's postoperative orders. Medications are usually ordered for pain and nausea.

Assess urinary output; the patient will have an indwelling Foley catheter in place. Encourage ice chips or clear fluids if ordered and as tolerated by the patient. Maintain the IV line; the physician often orders oxytocin to be mixed with the first postoperative IV bag. Maintain accurate intake and output records.

Although concern for the woman's physical well-being is critical, we must also consider the woman's psychologic status. Some women may be disappointed and feel they have failed by having a cesarean section instead of a vaginal delivery, especially if the surgery was unplanned. Allow the woman and her support person to express their feelings. Listen to and validate their feelings. If the baby is stable, encourage parental interaction with the newborn. Sometimes the mother may have been given sedative drugs during the surgery and is sleeping. If so, support the significant other in bonding and becoming acquainted with the infant. If the mother is able, encourage holding and breastfeeding. Added pillows for comfort and support of the infant during breastfeeding may be needed. The football hold is recommended for breastfeeding after a cesarean delivery because the infant will not put pressure on the tender abdomen and incision.

### Legal and Ethical Considerations

There are several issues that emerge regarding the legalities and ethics of surgical deliveries. These issues are grounded in the fact that there are two patients—a mother and a fetus—involved. Cesarean deliveries may be against a woman's religious or cultural beliefs. When the cesarean section offers the possibility of saving a life and the woman refuses to consent, the rights of the fetus are violated (Johnson, 1992). Court action may be instituted to force the surgery. An alternative situation may occur when a woman is asked to consent to surgical delivery even though it is not medically indicated. Then the woman is needlessly placed at risk for complications. As nurses, we must be prepared to act and follow valid steps of ethical decision making.

### Cultural Considerations

Although surgical deliveries are considered a common procedure in the United States, this does not apply to all cultures. The surgical delivery rate in Iran, for example, is only 4%. Therefore if an Iranian patient is told she needs to have surgery, she may be very frightened, mistrustful, and skeptical of the diagnosis. In such cases, we should spend extra time with the woman to explain the circumstances and answer her questions and those of her family.

## Multiple Gestation

Multiple gestation refers to the conception of more than one ovum. In the United States, twins account for approximately 1 in 80 deliveries, and this number is increasing, probably due to the increased use of fertility drugs (Cunningham and others, 1997). The higher the gestation, the higher the risk for preterm delivery, and thus the higher the incidence of complications. Women with multiple gestations are at increased risk for pregnancy-induced hypertension, preterm labor, hyperemesis gravidarum, and iron and folate anemia; and the fetuses are at increased risk for intrauterine growth restriction and congenital anomalies. Care of the woman at high risk is covered in Chapter 18.

Many women with twin fetuses have uncomplicated labors and deliveries, however, the following precautions may need to be taken: (1) continuous electronic fetal monitoring (one twin can be monitored internally if ROM has occurred); (2) continuous intravenous fluids; (3) a blood type and crossmatch with blood or packed RBCs on hold if needed; (4) two skilled obstetricians (or an obstetrician and a nurse midwife), an anesthesiologist on call in case surgical delivery is needed, and two teams (including a neonatalogist if possible) skilled in neonatal resuscitation immediately available for delivery; (5) all equipment should be double-checked to ensure proper working condition; and (6) one-on-one nursing care.

### Admission Assessments

Upon admission in labor, the presentations of the fetuses are confirmed by ultrasound. Several combinations are possible (Figure 14-38). (The obstetrician will usually discuss method of delivery at this time with the woman.) If the position is cephalic-cephalic, a vaginal delivery is usually done. Surgical deliveries are often done for any other presentation. Sometimes the first twin is cephalic and can be delivered vaginally. If the second twin is transverse, it may rotate to a cephalic or breech presentation, allowing a vaginal delivery in some cases. Some obstetricians will attempt a version, in which the twin is manually rotated—internally or externally—to allow a vaginal delivery (Figure 14-39). Other obstetricians will deliver a breech presentation vaginally under ideal circumstances. The woman should be informed of options, advantages, and risks in each method. Three or more fetuses are almost always delivered by abdominal surgery.

### Nursing Assessments

The fetal heart rates should also be assessed immediately upon admission. Fetuses should be monitored simultaneously to ensure that two different heart rates are heard.

In addition to assessing fetal presentation, we must accurately determine the gestational age of the fetuses.

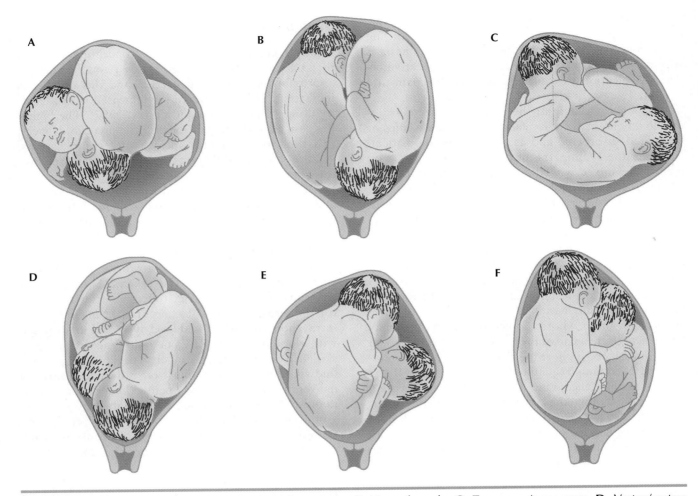

FIGURE 14-38 • Twin presentations. **A,** Vertex/transverse; **B,** Vertex/breech; **C,** Transverse/transverse; **D,** Vertex/vertex; **E,** Breech/transverse; **F,** Breech/breech.

Find in the chart the estimated date of delivery documented by dates, as well as prenatal ultrasound examination. Ultrasound data obtained when confirming the presentation can often also provide an estimate of fetal size and/or weight.

Other admission assessments and procedures discussed earlier in this chapter are also appropriate for the woman with multiple gestation: health and obstetric history, physical and emotional assessment, status of contractions, cervical examination, and status of membranes.

When admitting a woman with multiple fetuses, be aware that she might be very anxious. Take every opportunity to let her and her family voice their concerns and offer realistic assurances as needed. Let them know that the babies will be monitored closely and that they will be kept informed of all progress. The woman may also be worrying about how she will handle, care for, and provide for more than one infant. Discussing such concerns early in labor, before she is involved with the active work of labor, may help her relax and focus on the present, better able to deal with labor and delivery.

Discuss with the family the probable course of events following delivery based on the age and anticipated condition of the infants. For example, one or more of the infants may be taken to a nursery, NICU, or kept in the delivery room. Inform the family of possible procedures that will be done to the infant (e.g., suctioning, positive pressure ventilation, etc.) so that they are prepared. Because the delivery room will be too crowded with additional personnel and equipment, more than one family member often cannot be present at delivery. At that time, others will be directed to a comfortable place to wait and kept posted on the progress of the labor and delivery.

### Ongoing Nursing Care

Ongoing nursing assessments and care of the woman are similar to those of other laboring patients, although we must be alert to potential complications. Continue to monitor each fetus—simultaneously, if possible—to ensure that two different heart rates are being heard. Because the gravid uterus will be larger, a woman with multiple gestation will have more difficulty positioning herself and getting comfortable. The supine position is

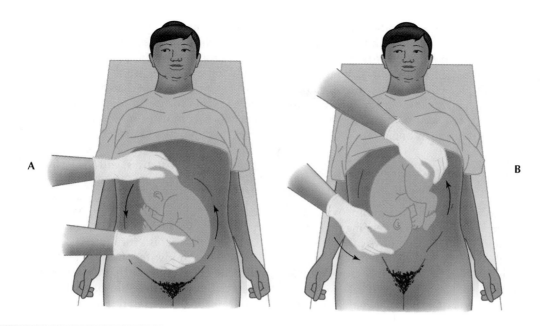

**FIGURE 14-39** • External version of fetus from breech to vertex presentation. This must be achieved without force. **A,** Breech is pushed up out of pelvic inlet while head is pulled toward inlet. **B,** Head is pushed toward inlet while breech is pulled upward.

generally uncomfortable and should be avoided. Encourage a variety of positions that promote comfort and relieve back discomfort.

Observe the contraction pattern closely. If the uterus is overdistended, the contractions may be less effective. Oxytocin for induction or augmentation will be used very cautiously because the woman is at an increased risk for uterine rupture. An amniotomy to augment labor will also be done cautiously because of the possibility of a prolapsed cord if the presenting fetus is in a breech presentation.

Monitor vital signs and urine output closely. Assess the woman's reflexes and note the presence of or an increase in edema. Ongoing comprehensive monitoring will allow you to identify any complications in a timely manner.

Special attention must be given to the supportive needs of the family. With the additional technology, equipment, personnel, and assessments necessary, the time spent supporting the woman and her labor support person can easily be overlooked. Develop a collaborative relationship with them and facilitate the process by incorporating as many of their preferences as possible into the labor and delivery experience.

### Delivery

Delivery may take place in an operating room, whether the expected method of delivery is vaginal or abdominal. Although the homelike atmosphere of the birthing rooms is missing, some birth attendants feel more comfortable there. The room should be strategically arranged to allow all health care providers space to work. All resuscitative equipment should be checked again before delivery. The average time between delivery of the twins is 30 minutes for a vaginal birth and 1 minute for a cesarean delivery. As the infants are born, place identifying bands on them immediately; the infants are identified with letters by birth order. After the placentas are delivered, they may be sent to the lab to verify chorionicity and zygosity (Ellings, Newman, and Bowers, 1998).

### Recovery

The woman's recovery following the delivery of multiples is similar to the care already discussed in the section on stage 4 and/or surgical delivery. Careful monitoring is critical due to hyperextension of the uterus during the pregnancy. Palpate the fundus at least every 15 minutes and massage it if boggy. An order is generally given to infuse an IV solution with oxytocin to aid the uterus in staying contracted. Monitor bleeding and vital signs closely.

Help the mother to breastfeed. (Nipple stimulation during breastfeeding helps the uterus to contract and control bleeding, reducing the mother's risk for a postpartum hemorrhage due to increased placental surface and an overdistended uterus.) She may choose to feed the infants one at time at the beginning so that she can get to know them as individuals. As she becomes rested and more adept to the process of breastfeeding and the babies each become better at it, she can choose to feed them both at the same time.

Refer her to a local chapter of Mothers of Twins, a national support organization. Having and raising more than one infant is a unique experience only truly understood by those who have been through it. Contact with other mothers of multiples will help her adapt to this new role. Also assure her that she can receive help from lactation consultants experienced with helping mothers who are breastfeeding more than one infant.

## SUMMARY

Entering into a collaborative partnership with the woman and her family in labor is challenging and critical. We must consider the mother's physical and emotional state, cultural preferences, age, family, and birthing plans while providing safe care. We must be both knowledgeable and caring.

Each woman and her family approach the birth of their baby with personal and cultural preferences. Birth attendants also have preferences regarding when, where,

and how they like to provide care. We must collaborate with both, while also fulfilling our responsibility to advocate for the best interest of our clients.

When caring for labor patients today, it is important for nurses to realize that many routine protocols (i.e., NPO except for ice chips, continuous EFM, begin pushing when complete) may not be based on research or even best practice. Furthermore, research studies published in reputable medical journals, as well as discussed in *William's Obstetrics*, call for a change in the practice of labor and delivery.

In a collaborative, collegial role, we can advocate for the women and their families to prevent harm to them. We must explore and discuss revisions in routine protocols for low-risk obstetric patients. Physicians, midwifes, nurses, and patients all want a healthy baby and mother. Empowered to work within a horizontal relationship of mutual trust, we can fulfill our professional nursing responsibility and improve the experience and the outcomes for women and their families.

## Care Plan · The Woman in Labor

NURSING DIAGNOSIS   **Pain** related to uterine contractions
GOALS/OUTCOMES   Will maintain optimal level of comfort *(see "Evaluation Parameters")*

### NOC Suggested Outcomes
- Comfort Level (2100)
- Pain Control (1605)
- Pain: Disruptive Effects (2101)
- Pain Level (2102)

### NIC Priority Interventions
- Analgesic Administration (2210)
- Conscious Sedation (2260)
- Pain Management (1400)

### Nursing Activities & Rationale
- Ask client which pain-relief measures she prefers; provide information as needed. *Allows her to have control over her labor and use measures she feels will benefit her.*
- Monitor for effectiveness of pain-relief measures (see parameters in "Evaluation"). *As contractions become more intense, different pain-relief measures may be needed.*
- Provide basic comfort measures (e.g., maintaining dry linens and providing a cool cloth on forehead, lip balm, and ice chips). *If otherwise comfortable, the couple can focus on self–pain-control measures, such as breathing techniques, effleurage, etc.*
- Involve the partner or coach as much as possible. *Emotional support decreases anxiety and therefore pain; because the couple may have practiced techniques together, the support person may be better able to meet the woman's needs.*
- Monitor for side effects of pharmacologic pain relief measures (e.g., respirations and level of consciousness for narcotics; blood pressure and level of numbness for epidural analgesia/anesthesia). *Close monitoring is needed in order to achieve a balance between pain relief and dosages that create unwanted or dangerous side effects.*

### Evaluation Parameters
- No change in pulse and respirations
- Focuses and breathes effectively during contractions
- Reports acceptable comfort level
- Demonstrates minimal restlessness and muscle tension

## Care Plan · *The Woman in Labor—cont'd*

**NURSING DIAGNOSIS   Risk for Fetal Injury** related to decreased fetal oxygenation

**GOALS/OUTCOMES**   Fetus will maintain good oxygenation and intact central nervous system function *(see "Evaluation Parameters" for indicators of goal achievement)*

### NOC Suggested Outcomes
- Neurological Status (fetus) (0909)
- Safety Status: Physical Injury (fetus) (1913)

### NIC Priority Interventions
- Electronic Fetal Monitoring: Intrapartum (6772)
- Intrapartal Care (6830)

### Nursing Activities & Rationale
- Obtain baseline maternal vital signs and monitor them regularly. *Must have baseline rate for comparison as labor progresses. Maternal blood pressure must be adequate to ensure good blood flow to the placenta.*
- Obtain baseline FHR. *Must have a baseline rate to use for comparison as labor progresses to assess fetal tolerance of labor.*
- Monitor FHR frequently. Note variability and periodic changes in response to uterine contractions, medications, and procedures. *Fetal status is reflected in the FHR and pattern, which can change instantly.*
- Monitor progress of labor. *Labor is stressful to the fetus. Complications such as prolonged labor, uterine rupture, maternal exhaustion, and maternal anxiety place the fetus at greater risk for hypoxia.*
- Avoid the supine position. *The gravid uterus compresses the vena cava and abdominal aorta in this position, decreasing venous return and, subsequently, maternal cardiac output and placental perfusion.*
- Maintain good hydration via IV fluids and/or offering clear liquids to drink. *Increasing circulating blood volume promotes adequate blood pressure for maintaining placental perfusion.*
- Note FHR and color of fluid when membranes rupture. *After membranes rupture, there is increased chance of cord compression by fetal parts, reducing circulation to the fetus. Meconium-stained fluid may be a sign of fetal distress.*
- On rupture of membranes, assess for visible cord in vagina. *When membranes rupture, the gush of fluid may carry the cord with it, resulting in cord prolapse (an obstetric emergency).*
- If cord prolapse occurs, elevate the woman's hips or have her assume a knee-chest position; wrap cord in sterile saline-soaked gauze; do not attempt to replace cord in vagina! Notify physician; prepare for emergency cesarean birth. *These are not preventive actions for the diagnosis of "Risk for Injury." If cord prolapse occurs, these nursing activities are intended to prevent injury until medical intervention can be obtained.*
- If FHR pattern is nonreassuring, position the woman in left lateral position, shut off oxytocin (if it is being administered), administer oxygen at 10 L/min per facemask, and provide fetal scalp stimulation. Notify physician. *Note that these are not preventive actions for the diagnosis of "Risk for Injury." They are meant to promote feto-placental circulation, increase the oxygen content of the circulating blood, and stimulate the fetus.*
- Explain interventions to parents. *Decreases anxiety. Maternal anxiety results in increase of catecholamines, which can cause vasoconstriction of uterine arteries and a decrease in uterine blood flow.*

### Evaluation Parameters
- FHR 120 to 160 bpm
- Good baseline variability
- FHR acceleration with fetal movement
- No late or variable decelerations

**NURSING DIAGNOSIS   Anxiety** related to unmet needs, situational crisis, knowledge deficit *(Note: A possible alternative diagnosis is Ineffective Individual Coping)*

**GOALS/OUTCOMES**   Reports anxiety is at a manageable level; no behavioral manifestations of anxiety *(see "Evaluation Parameters" for indicators of goal achievement)*

### NOC Suggested Outcomes
- Anxiety Control (1402)
- Coping (1302)
- Psychosocial Adjustment: Life Change (1305)

### NIC Priority Interventions
- Anxiety Reduction (5820)

*Continued*

## Care Plan · The Woman in Labor—cont'd

**Nursing Activities & Rationale**
- Orient the couple to the unit and staff; give information about what to expect during labor. *Information may reduce stress and anxiety.*
- Assess knowledge of and prior experience with childbirth. *This allows the nurse to individualize anxiety reduction interventions.*
- Inform the couple of labor progress, options, policies, procedures, etc. *Understanding events and options will decrease anxiety.*
- Encourage woman to express feelings, concerns, and fears. *Verbalization of anxiety can help to relieve it.*
- Ask the woman's permission to perform examinations and procedures. *This gives her a sense of control.*
- To the extent possible, support and involve the partner/coach in the woman's care. *Women in labor may feel dependent; the partner's involvement provides a feeling of safety. The partner may be anxious and in need of support, as well. Some partners need reassurance that their participation is helpful.*
- Dim the lights, decrease interruptions, play soft music, adjust room temperature as needed. *A calm, soothing environment will help the woman to concentrate on breathing and relaxation techniques and prevent sensory overload.*
- Keep the same nurse throughout labor, if at all possible. *Continuity of care decreases stress.*
- Provide privacy (e.g., drape the perineum during a vaginal examination). *Helps keep client from feeling depersonalized or objectified.*
- Help client to focus on the positive aspects of the experience: talk about choice of infant names, experiences during pregnancy, etc. *Serves as a diversion and demonstrates caring.*
- Assess and provide for diversional needs (e.g., cards, television, walking about the unit). *Provides diversion from anxious thoughts; helps time to pass more quickly; walking may promote cervical dilation and shorten labor.*
- Monitor physical and psychological manifestations of anxiety (see "Evaluation Parameters"). *To plan for and evaluate success of interventions.*

**Evaluation Parameters**
- Reports decreased anxiety, appropriate to labor situation
- Uses breathing and relaxation techniques effectively to stay in control with uterine contractions
- No change in vital signs (especially pulse and blood pressure)
- Able to focus and follow directions
- Communicates needs appropriately

---

NURSING DIAGNOSIS    **Risk for Fluid Volume Deficit** related to reduced intake and increased metabolic needs

GOALS/OUTCOMES    Maintains adequate fluid balance and hydration during labor *(see "Evaluation Parameters" for indicators of goal achievement)*

**NOC Suggested Outcomes**
- Fluid Balance (0601)
- Hydration (0602)

**NIC Priority Interventions**
- Fluid Management (4120)
- Fluid Monitoring (4130)
- Intravenous (IV) Therapy (4200)

**Nursing Activities & Rationale**
- Monitor color and amount of urine output. *Decreased, concentrated urine is a sign of fluid deficit.*
- Maintain accurate intake and output record. *Knowledge of intake amount allows the nurse to evaluate the adequacy of the output and detect fluid volume deficit.*
- Monitor hydration (see "Evaluation Parameters"). *To assess adequacy of fluid volume.*
- Monitor vital signs. *Mild temperature elevation is a sign of dehydration; decreased blood pressure and increased pulse are signs of fluid volume deficit.*
- Administer and monitor IV fluids as ordered. *Medical orders may require NPO during labor; IV fluids provide needed fluid volume.*
- Encourage clear oral fluids as appropriate. *If not contraindicated by medical order, supports fluid balance. Limit to clear fluids because vomiting is common in labor.*

**Evaluation Parameters**
- Exhibits good hydration: mucous membranes moist; skin turgor good; pulse volume full
- Urine output in proportion to fluid intake and not concentrated
- Does not experience abnormal thirst
- Pulse, temperature, and blood pressure in normal range for client

# CASE STUDY

Bonita, a 24-year-old woman, gravida 1, para 0, at 40 weeks of gestation, arrives at the birthing center having contractions every 10 minutes. She states that they have become more uncomfortable in the last hour. Each time her uterus contracts, she bends over and moans, complaining of back pain.

Bonita has received regular prenatal care from a nurse-midwife affiliated with the birthing center and states that she has had no complications. Her partner is with her and appears anxious but very supportive. Bonita states that she felt a trickle of fluid running down her leg in the past hour and noticed a watery bloody vaginal discharge the last time she urinated. The couple has collaborated with the nurse-midwife to develop a birth plan requesting an unobtrusive labor environment and an unmedicated delivery. Bonita prefers not to have an episiotomy and would like to have her partner as involved as possible in her care during the labor and delivery.

With the goal of setting the tone for a collaborative partnership during the labor, you begin the admitting procedures.

- What actions will you use to show the couple that you are being collaborative?

Bonita states that the well-being of her baby should be given top consideration during the labor. She wonders if continuous fetal monitoring would be better than intermittent auscultation in obtaining positive outcomes for the infant.

- What would you tell her?

  Bonita states that she feels a trickle of fluid.

- What could this mean, and how would you determine what it is?

- What has Bonita told you during the admission interview that leads you to believe that this is true labor?

You continue to interview the couple, update Bonita's history since the last visit, and begin part of the physical exam. Your findings are unremarkable. A vaginal exam determines that Bonita is 4 cm dilated, 100%, and at 0 station. The nitrazine paper turned blue, and there was a flow of vaginal fluid during the vaginal exam.

You listen to the FHR and determine the baseline to be between 130 and 140 bpm. You and the parents hear the heart rate increase with fetal movement.

- The couple asks what this means? What would you tell them?

Bonita is sitting up in bed, having an increasingly difficult time dealing with her contractions.

- Based on your assessment data and the couple's birth plan, what interventions would you offer?

Four hours later, Bonita has been ambulating, sitting in the rocking chair, and doing pelvic rocks while on her hands and knees. Her partner has been massaging her back. She says, "I don't know how much longer I can do this."

- What would you do?

A vaginal examination reveals that she is 100% effaced, 8 cm dilated, and at +1 station.

- What phase of labor is Bonita in and what behaviors may she exhibit now?

- Bonita tells you she feels like she wants to have a bowel movement. What will you do?

Bonita chooses to use a squatting bar to assist her while pushing. Once she is fully dilated, you and her partner help her to a squatting position and guide her with her pushing.

- Because Bonita does not want an episiotomy, what suggestions could you give her during pushing that would decrease the need for an episiotomy?

Bonita's baby begins to crown after 15 minutes of pushing. Unfortunately the midwife is next door attending to the birth of another baby, so you have to assist Bonita. You call in another nurse to collaborate with you, Bonita, and her partner in the birth of their baby. Bonita decides to lie on her side. Her partner is holding up her top leg. The infant's head extends and is born, as you support her perineum.

- What are the next steps in this birth process?

The midwife enters the room and takes over.

- What stage of labor is the woman in at this time? What are your responsibilities?

Examine the occurrences of Bonita's labor.

- What was atypical of the labor?

- How would receiving an epidural have affected Bonita's labor?

# Scenarios

**1.** Bethany calls the office to report that she thinks she is in early labor. You remember her from her visits for prenatal care but pull up her chart on the computer screen.

- What specific subjective and objective information do you need before you respond?
- What nursing diagnoses could apply? How will you validate these?
- What goals might be developed? How will these be prioritized?
- What interventions may you offer?
- How will you evaluate the effectiveness of your interventions?

**2.** Lindsay, who is 27 years old, G 1, P 0, and at 40 weeks of gestation, and her partner Brian are admitted to the labor, delivery, recovery room (LDR). They were sent over from their nurse-midwife's office, where they had gone to be checked for extent of effacement and dilation. They didn't want to rush to the hospital too early in the labor process. As you orient them to the room and start your admission assessment, Brian says, "We worked out a birth plan and are concerned that what we want won't happen."

- What specific subjective and objective information do you need before you respond?
- What nursing diagnoses could apply? How will you validate these?
- What goals might be developed? How will these be prioritized?
- What interventions may you offer?
- How will you evaluate the effectiveness of your interventions?

**3.** Lindsay hands you the report the midwife sent over with her. It reports that in the office a half hour ago she was 80% effaced, 4 cm dilated, and at −2 station. The amniotic sac appeared to be still intact. Her contractions were 5 minutes apart and lasting 60 seconds. As you take Lindsay's vitals, she becomes concerned because her contractions are now spaced at 10 minutes apart. She becomes concerned and says, "What is happening? I want this baby to come!"

- How will you respond?
- What nursing diagnoses could apply? How will you validate these?
- What goals might be developed? How will these be prioritized?
- What interventions may you offer?
- How will you evaluate the effectiveness of your interventions?

**4.** Fetal monitoring reveals that the FHR is 140 with good variability. With the onset of a contractions, simultaneous accelerations are noted. The FHR returns to baseline after the uterus relaxes. This pattern repeats itself over a half-hour period, during which Lindsay experienced 5 contractions.

- At this stage of labor, how often should the FHR be evaluated? Why?
- What nursing diagnoses could apply to the fetus?
- What nursing diagnoses may apply to Lindsay and Brian with regard to fetal monitoring? How will you validate these?
- What goals might be developed? How will these be prioritized?
- What interventions may you offer?
- How will you evaluate the effectiveness of your interventions?

**5.** As Lindsay's labor progresses and she reaches 6 cm of dilation, she decides to stop walking and rest before the labor becomes more difficult. The contractions are coming every 3 minutes and lasting about 60 seconds. She has been maintaining comfort by walking and doing conscious relaxation breathing. Brian has assisted her by supporting her during contractions, with her arms wrapped around his neck, and rubbing her back.

- How will you support her decision to rest?
- What subjective data do you need to obtain?
- What nursing diagnoses could apply? How will you validate these?
- What goals might be developed? How will these be prioritized?

- What interventions may you offer?
- How will you evaluate the effectiveness of your interventions?

---

6. Lindsay has now been in labor for approximately 14 hours, 4 hours of which have occurred in the LDR. Your shift is ending and you have to give a report to the nurse who will be assuming your role with Lindsay and Brian.

- What data are vital to give the nurse coming on?
- What are your responsibilities to the nurse replacing you?
- What are your responsibilities to Lindsay and Brian?
- What nursing diagnoses may occur because you are leaving? How will you validate these?
- What goal will you have during this transfer of care?
- What interventions may you offer?
- How will you evaluate the effectiveness of your interventions?

---

7. Lindsay and Brian have been working with the new nurse for the past hour, and things are going well. Contractions have been predictable in time and intensity, although the last three contractions lasted longer and longer. Lindsay starts to cry, "Okay, enough already! I'm changing the birth plan, I want pain medication." Brian places another wet face cloth on her head as he has for the last hour. She takes the cloth off and throws it in the sink, turns to him and says, "Leave me alone." Brian gives you a look of concern.

- What do you think is happening? How will you respond?
- What specific objective information do you need before you give a definitive answer?
- What nursing diagnoses could apply for Lindsay? How will you validate these?
- What nursing diagnoses could apply for Brian? How will you validate these?
- What would your goal be?
- What interventions may you offer?
- How will you evaluate the effectiveness of your interventions?

---

8. The nurse-midwife determines that Lindsay is fully dilated and is now in second stage. She has moved herself into a squatting position on the bed, supported by a bar. Brian says, "Good. Now we will have the baby real soon."

- How will you respond to Brian?
- How will you encourage Lindsay in her efforts of pushing?
- What assessments are you responsible for during stage 2 of labor?
- What nursing diagnoses could apply? How will you validate these?
- What goals might be developed? How will these be prioritized?
- What interventions may you offer to help Lindsay through stage 2?
- How can you measure the movement of the fetus down the birth canal without vaginal examinations?
- How will you evaluate the effectiveness of your interventions?

## REFERENCES

Aird and others: Effects of intrapartum hydrotherapy on labour related parameters, *Austrail New Zeal J Obstet Gynaecol* 37(2):137-142, 1997.

American College of Obstetrics and Gynecology: *Fetal heart rate patterns: monitoring, interpretation, and management,* ACOG Technical Bulletin No. 207, Washington D.C., 1995a, The College.

American College of Obstetricians and Gynecologists: *Induction of labor,* Technical bulletin No. 217, Washington D.C., 1995b, The College.

Andrews MM and Boyle JS: Transcultural concepts in nursing care, ed 2, Philadelphia, 1995, Lippincott.

Association of Women's Health, Obstetric and Neonatal Nurses (AWHONN): *Position statement: role of the registered nurse in the management of the patient receiving analgesia by catheter techniques (epidural, intrathecal, intrapleural, or peripheral nerve catheters),* Washington D.C., 1996, The Association.

Boston Women's Health Book Collective: *Our Bodies, ourselves for the new century,* New York, 1998, Simon and Schuster.

Breen T and others: Epidural anesthesia for labor in an ambulating patient, *Anesth Analg* 77:919-924, 1993.

Bryanton J, Fraser-Davey H, and Sullivan P: Women's perceptions of nursing support during labor, *J Obstet Gynecol Neonat Nurs* 23(8):638-644, 1994.

Cesario S: Should cameras be allowed in the delivery room?, *MCN* 23(2):87-91, 1998.

Cunningham FG and others: *Willliams obstetrics,* ed 20, Stamford, CT, 1997, Appleton & Lange.

Curtin SC and Park MM: Trends in the attendant, place and timing of births, and in the use of obstetric interventions: United States, 1989-97, *Nat Vital Statist Rep* 47(27), 1999, www.cdc.gov/nchs.

Davis-Floyd RE: *Birth as an American rite of passage,* Berkley, CA, 1992, University of California Press.

Doulas of North America: www.dona.com, January 26, 2000.

Dundes L: The evolution of maternal birthing position, *Am J Pub Health* 77(5):636-641, 1987.

Elkind D: *All grown up and no place to go: teenagers in crisis*, Reading, MA, 1984, Addison-Wesley.

Ellings JM, Newman RB, and Bowers N: Intrapartum care for women with multiple pregnancy, *J Obstet Gynecol Neonat Nurs* 27(4):466-472, 1998.

Field PA: Maternity nurses: how parents see us, *Internat J Nurs Studies* 24:191-199, 1987.

Goer H: *Obstetric myths versus research realities: a guide to the medical literature*, Westport, CT, 1995, Bergin and Garvey.

Goodwin T, Milner-Masterson L, and Paul R: Elimination of fetal scalp blood sampling on a large clinical service, *Obstet Gynecol* 83:97, 1994.

Hazle NR: Hydration in labor: is routine intravenous hydration necessary?, *J Nurse Midwife* 31(4):171-176, 1986.

Herpolsheimer A and Schretenthaler J: The use of intrapartum intrathecal narcotic analgesia in a community-based hospital, *Obstet Gynecol* 84:931, 1994.

Hodgson BB and Kizior RJ: *Saunders nursing drug handbook 1999*, Philadelphia, 1999, Saunders.

Hofmeyr G and Sonnedecker E: Elective episiotomy in perspective, *S Africa Med J* 71(6):357-359, 1987.

Hutchinson MK and Baqi-Aziz: Nursing care of the childbearing Muslim family, *J Obstet Gynecol Neonat Nurs* 23(9):767-771, 1994.

Johnson S: Ethical dilemma: a patient refused a life-saving cesarean, *MCN* 17(3):121-125, 1992.

Kakar DN and others: Beliefs and practices related to disposal of human placenta, *Nurs J India* 80:315-317, 1989.

Kennel JH and others: Continuous emotional support during labor in a US hospital: a randomized controlled trial, *JAMA* 265:2197-2201, 1991.

Kintz DL: Nursing support in labor, *J Obstet Gynecol Neonat Nurs* 16:126-130, 1987.

Kitzinger S: *The complete book of pregnancy and childbirth*, New York, 1980, Knoph.

Landry SH and others: The effects of doula support during labor on mother-infant interaction at 2 months, *Pediatr Res* 43(4):11-13, 1998.

Lede RL, Belizan JM, and Carroli G: Is the routine use of episiotomy justified?, *Am J Obstet Gynecol* 174:1399, 1996.

Lowe NK: Explaining the pain of active labor: the importance of maternal confidence, *Res Nurs Health* 12:237-245, 1989.

Luce JD: Birthing women and midwife. In Holmes HB, Hoskins B, and Gross M, editors: *Birth control and controlling birth: women centered perspectives*, Clifton, NJ, 1980, Humana Press.

Maier JS and Maloni JA: Nurse advocacy for selective versus routine episiotomy, *J Obstet Gynecol Neonat Nurs* 26(2):155-161, 1997.

McCartney PR: The birth ball—Are you using it in your practice setting?, *AWHONN Lifelines* 23(4):218, 1998.

Mercer RT: *Becoming a mother*, New York, 1995, Springer.

National Institute of Child Health and Human Development Research Planning Workshop: Electronic fetal heart rate monitoring: research guidelines for interpretation, *J Obstet Gynecol Neonat Nurs* 26(6):635-640, 1997.

Newton N, Newton M, and Broach J: Psychologic, physical, nutritional, and technological aspects of intravenous infusion during labor, *Birth* 15(2):67-72, 1988.

Petersen L and Besuner P: Pushing techniques during labor: issues and controversies, *J Obstet Gynecol Neonat Nurs* 26(6):719-726, 1997.

Pugach MC and Johnson LJ: *Collaborative practitioners: collaborative schools*, Denver, 1995, Love.

Purnell LD and Paulanka BJ: *Transcultural health care: A culturally competent approach*, Philadelphia, 1998, FA Davis.

Roberts JE and others: A descriptive analysis of involuntary bearing down efforts during the expulsive phase of labor, *J Obstet Gynecol Neonat Nurs* 25:48-55, 1987.

Roberts J and Woolley D: A second look at the second stage of labor, *J Obstet Gynecol Neonat Nurs* 25:415-423, 1996.

Roberts SJ, Reardon KM, and Rosenfeld S: Childhood sexual abuse: surveying its impact on primary care, *AWHONN Lifelines*, 3(1):39-45, 1999.

Rosen MG and Dickinson JC: The paradox of electronic fetal monitoring: more data may not enable us to predict or prevent infant neurologic morbidity, *Am J Obstet Gynecol* 168(3 Pt 1):745-751, 1993.

Salmon P, Miller R, and Drew N: Women's anticipation and experience of childbirth: the independence of fulfillment, unpleasantness and pain, *Brit J Med Psychol* 63:255-259, 1990.

Schneiderman JU: Rituals of placental disposal, *MCN* 23(3):142-143, 1998.

Shermer RH and Raines DA: Positioning during the second stage of labor: moving back to basics, *J Obstet Gynecol Neonat Nurs* 26(6):727-734, 1997.

Simkin P: Reducing pain and enhancing progress in labor: a guide to nonpharmacologic methods for maternity caregivers, *Birth* 22(3):161-171, 1995.

Simpson KR: Intrapartum fetal oxygenation saturation monitoring: ongoing clinical research explores partnering new method with electronic fetal monitoring, *AWHONN Lifelines* 2(6):20-24, 1998.

Spector RE: *Cultural diversity in health and illness*, Stamford, CT, 1996, Appleton & Lange.

Stampone D: The history of obstetric anesthesia, *J Perinat Neonat Nurs* 4(1):1-13, 1990.

Stem J: Flirting with disaster: do RNs go too far with epidurals?, *AWHONN Lifelines* 1(1):31-35, 1997.

Taffel SM and others: 1989 U.S. cesarean section rate steadies—VBAC rises to nearly one in five, *Birth* 18:73, 1991.

Tucker SM: *Mosby's pocket guide series: fetal monitoring and assessment*, St Louis, 1996, Mosby.

VanTuinen I and Wolfe M: *Unnecessary cesarean sections: halting a national epidemic*, Washington, D.C., 1992, Public Citizen Health Research Group.

Ventura SJ and others: *Births and deaths: United States, 1996*, Monthly Vital Statistics Report 46(suppl):1-40, 1997.

Vincent P: Traditional and modern thought about the placenta, *Midwives* 108:325-327, 1995.

Vintzileos AM and others: A randomized trial of intrapartum electronic fetal heart monitoring versus intermittent auscultation, *Obstet Gynecol* 81(6):899-907, 1993.

# Vaginal Delivery Clinical Pathway

## INTERDISCIPLINARY PATIENT/FAMILY EDUCATION RECORD

Patient Identification

**Learning Assessment:** Able to read: ☐ Yes ☐ No | **TEACHING GUIDELINE UTILIZED:**

**Barriers to Learning:** (Circle all that apply)

| None | Culture | Religion | Hearing | Language _____ |
| Vision | Cognitive | Emotional | Physical | Financial |
| | | Other: _____ | | |

**Learning needs identified by patient:** _____

| Date/ Time | Readiness to Learn | | Learning Needs/Content | Teaching Method | Evaluation | Status of Plan | Comment | Init. |
|---|---|---|---|---|---|---|---|---|
| | 1. Attentive<br>2. Denies need<br>3. Uncoop.<br>4. Clinical status interferes<br><br>Pt = Patient<br>F = Family/ Other | | **Examples**<br>• Medication<br>• Food/drug interaction<br>• Diet<br>• Equipment<br>• Community resources<br>• Psychosocial<br>• Personal care<br><br>**Expected Outcomes**<br>• Learner will state/ demonstrate knowledge of: | Circle preferred teaching method<br><br>A = Audio-visual<br>R = Role play<br>E = Explanation<br>D = Demon-stration<br>G = Group class<br>H = Handout | P = Partial understanding<br>R = Retains content<br>D = Demonstrates with cues<br>RD = Can return demonstration<br>N = No evidence of learning | 1. Reinforce content<br>2. Reteach<br>3. Needs practice<br>4. Outcome achieved | | |
| | PT | F | | | | | | |
| | | | Orient to LDR | E | | | | |
| | | | Visitor Policy | E | | | | |
| | | | Initial Plan of Care | E | | | | |
| | | | FHR/UA Monitoring | D | | | | |
| | | | Activity/Positioning | E | | | | |
| | | | Pain Management Options | E | | | | |
| | | | Pushing Techniques | E | | | | |
| | | | Induction/Augmentation | E | | | | |
| | | | Amniotomy/Infusions | D | | | | |
| | | | Catheterization | D | | | | |
| | | | Oxygen | D | | | | |
| | | | Orient to MBU* | E | | | | |
| | | | Lochia Patterns | E/A | | | | |
| | | | Peri Care/Sitz Bath | D/A | | | | |
| | | | Incision Care | D/A | | | | |
| | | | Intake/Output | E | | | | |
| | | | Activity/Rest | E | | | | |
| | | | Engorgement Care | E/A | | | | |
| | | | S/S to Report—Maternal | E/A | | | | |
| | | | Follow-up Care—Maternal | E | | | | |
| | | | Sexual Relations/Family Planning | E | | | | |
| | | | | | | | | |

*Mother-baby unit

Patient Identification

| | Discipline | | | | |
|---|---|---|---|---|---|
| RN | Registered Nurse | RT | Respiratory Therapy | CC | Care Coordination |
| OT | Occupational Therapy | SS | Social Service | PC | Pastoral Care |
| PT | Physical Therapy | NT | Nutrition Therapy | LC | Lactation Consultant |
| ST | Speech Therapy | MD | Physician | RPh | Pharmacy |

| Signature | Init. | Signature | Init. | Signature | Init. |
|---|---|---|---|---|---|
| | | | | | |
| | | | | | |
| | | | | | |
| | | | | | |
| | | | | | |

## Patient Education

| Date/Time | Readiness to Learn PT | Readiness to Learn F | Learning Needs/Content | Teaching Method | Evaluation | Status of Plan | Comment | Init. |
|---|---|---|---|---|---|---|---|---|
| | | | Safety ID (Security) | E | | | | |
| | | | Newborn Characteristics | E | | | | |
| | | | Bulb Syringe | D | | | | |
| | | | Hunger Cues | E | | | | |
| | | | Feeding Frequency | E | | | | |
| | | | Assessing Intake | E | | | | |
| | | | Positioning | D | | | | |
| | | | Burping | D | | | | |
| | | | Cord Care | D | | | | |
| | | | Circ care/diapering | D | | | | |
| | | | Elimination Patterns | E | | | | |
| | | | Bathing | A | | | | |
| | | | Temperature Taking | D | | | | |
| | | | Formula Preparation | E | | | | |
| | | | Breast Pump | D | | | | |
| | | | ODH Requirements | E | | | | |
| | | | S/S to Report Newborn | E/A | | | | |
| | | | Car Seat Safety | E | | | | |
| | | | Follow-Up Care—Newborn | E | | | | |
| | | | | | | | | |
| | | | | | | | | |
| | | | | | | | | |
| | | | | | | | | |
| | | | | | | | | |
| | | | | | | | | |
| | | | | | | | | |
| | | | | | | | | |
| | | | | | | | | |

Time of Delivery _____

| PATIENT FOCUS | DATE _____<br>Care Coordination<br>Pre-Hospital Phase | DATE _____<br>PT. OUTCOME Active Labor<br>(evaluate after birth) | DATE _____ TIME _____<br>PT. OUTCOME Birth-2 Hours |
|---|---|---|---|
| **Tissue Perfusion Management** | | ____ **RN** Pt. has no active bleeding<br>____ **RN** Pt. temp. is < 100.4°F<br>____ **RN** Pt. has no palpable bladder | ____ **RN** Pt. has ≤ moderate lochia<br>____ **RN** Pt. fundus is firm<br>____ **RN** Pt. has PACU PAR score of ≥ 8<br>____ **RN** Pt. has no palpable bladder |
| **Patient Education** | | | ____ **RN** Pt. verbalizes knowledge of safety limits |
| **Physical Comfort Promotion** | ____ **CC/RN** Pt. can discuss comfort measures and exercise appropriate for pregnancy | ____ **RN** Pt. utilized comfort options/alternative methods during progression of labor | ____ **RN** Pt. states she is comfortable |
| **Childbearing Care** | ____ **CC/RN** Pt. can discuss hospitalization process related to obstetrical management (i.e., birth options) | ____ **RN** Pt. stated individual preferences for birth experience were discussed<br>____ **RN** Pt's identified support systems/significant others available | ____ **RN** Breastfeeding initiated with 60-90 min of delivery<br>☐ N/A if bottle feeding<br>____ **RN** Pt. and significant other exhibit bonding behaviors (eye contact, touching, holding)<br>____ **RN** Identified support systems available |
| **CARE CATEGORIES** | | | |
| **Assessment:** | Breast assessment 20-24 weeks<br>Initiate anesthesia assessment form | FHR/uterine activity q 30 min., q 15 min. active labor second stage<br>VS q 1 hr, temp q 4 hrs; if ROM, temp q 2 hours<br>Review prenatal course<br>I&O q shift with 24 hrs totals<br>Bladder assessment q 2 hrs | Check lochia, fundus, VS q 15 min. × 4<br>Check voiding q 2 hrs |
| **Patient/Family Education:** | By 20-24 weeks:<br>• MRG given and reviewed<br>• Health/safety pamphlets given, reviewed<br>• Discuss benefits to breastfeeding | Support mother in birth plan<br>Review clinical pathway<br>Discuss comfort options<br>Instruct in use of pain scale 0-10 | Initiate parent and infant contact<br>Initiate breastfeeding<br>Self care starting, begin self care education<br>Instruct on safety measures |
| **Discharge Planning:** | PCC follow-up explained<br>Home visit info given<br>Identify pediatrician by 20-24 week visit | | |
| **Tests:** | DAU7 if indicated per policy | HBsAg if not done prenatally<br>CBC<br>Cervical exam prn<br>Notify MD if missing prenatal tests | |
| **Interventions:** | Pt. problem screen completed and sent to MD<br>Circumcision permit signed<br>Pt. preregistered<br>Register for appropriate classes<br>36 week follow phone call | Straight cath prn<br>Fetal monitoring<br>IV if applicable | Ice to perineum prn<br>Straight cath prn |
| **Consults:** | Referrals, if needed: lactation, social services, grief counseling, anesthesia | Anesthesia<br>Social Service if needed | |
| **Medications/IVs:** | | Analgesia<br>Epidural if applicable<br>Optional IV | Analgesia<br>IV DC |
| **Nutrition:** | Review "Healthy Beginnings"<br>Diabetes referrals | Optional po ice chips or fluids | Diet as tolerated |
| **Activity/Safety:** | | Activity as tolerated<br>Encourage ambulation in early labor<br>Instruct pt in activity level R/T anesthesia/analgesia | Up with assistance × 1, then activity as tolerated |

| DATE _____ TIME _____<br>PT. OUTCOME        PT. OUTCOME<br>**Postpartum 2-6 Hours** | DATE _____ TIME _____<br>PT. OUTCOME<br>**6-24 Hours** | DATE _____ TIME _____<br><br>**Time of Discharge** |
|---|---|---|
| ____ **RN** Pt. has ≤ moderate lochia<br>____ **RN** Pt. fundus is firm<br>____ **RN** Pt. has no orthostatic hypotension<br>____ **RN** Pt. voids spontaneously | ____ **RN** Pt. has ≤ moderate lochia<br>____ **RN** Pt. fundus is firm<br>____ **RN** Pt. temp. < 100.4°F<br>____ **RN** Pt. voiding spontaneously | ____ **RN** Pt. has temp ≤ 101°F<br>____ **RN** Pt. voiding spontaneously |
| ____ **RN** Pt. identified own learning needs regarding self & infant<br>____ **RN** Pt. demonstrates use of self medication | ____ **RN** Pt. initiates care for self and infant<br>____ **RN** Pt. demonstrates safe use of medications | ____ **RN** Pt. states understanding of discharge instructions and has questions answered<br>____ **RN/SS/CC** Pt. states understanding of information regarding follow-up care and concerns (MD, lactation consultants, community resources) |
| ____ **RN** Pt. verbalizes knowledge of 0-10 pain scale | ____ **RN** Pt. states comfort measures are effective | ____ **RN** Pt. states comfort measures are effective |
| ____ **RN** Pt. verbalized positive birth experience<br>____ **RN/LC** Milk production is stimulated | ____ **RN** Family/sign. others exhibiting supporting behaviors (positive comments, assisting in care)<br>____ **RN/LC** Pt. achieves a latch score ≥ 7<br>☐ N/A | ____ **RN/SS/CC** Pt. states readiness for discharge (emotionally, assistance at home, car seat)<br>____ **RN** Pt. aware of home visit if applicable<br>____ **RN** Pt./significant other exhibits bonding behaviors |
| Assess lochia, fundus, check voiding, vital signs on admission, at 2 hrs, then q 6 hrs × 4 | Assess VS, lochia, fundus q 6 hrs × 4 then q shift if stable | Assess VS, lochia, fundus q shift if stable and at time of discharge |
| Reinforce education on self-care, breastfeeding, nipple integrity, infant care<br>Instruct in self-med program | Infant feeding<br>Review discharge plan | Instruct pt. on increasing fiber intake and hydration<br>Complete discharge instructions |
| Discharge class/film | Consider D/C | Discharge: follow-up appointments<br>Care coordination for home care/phone call |
| Rhogam work up if mom Rh negative (need results ASAP) | | |
| Perineal hygiene<br>Straight cath prn<br>Circ permit signed<br>Breast pump prn<br>Ice to perineum | Discontinue ice to perineum<br>Sitz baths | Sitz baths<br>Encourage self-care |
| If needed: Home health<br>　　　　　Lactation consultants<br>　　　　　Social service | Social service if needed<br>Consider community resources if applicable | |
| Analgesia<br>Rhogam | Rhogam (if indicated) | Rubella if not immune |
| Regular diet | Regular diet | Regular diet |
| Activity as tolerated | Up as tolerated | Up as tolerated |

# Abdominal Delivery Clinical Pathway

**INTERDISCIPLINARY PATIENT/FAMILY EDUCATION RECORD**

Patient Identification

**Learning Assessment:** Able to read: ☐ Yes ☐ No  **TEACHING GUIDELINE UTILIZED:** _____

**Barriers to Learning:** (Circle all that apply)  None  Culture  Religion  Hearing  Language _____
Vision  Cognitive  Emotional  Physical  Financial
Other: _____

**Learning needs identified by patient:** _____

| Date/ Time | Readiness to Learn | | Learning Needs/Content | Teaching Method | Evaluation | Status of Plan | Comment | Init. |
|---|---|---|---|---|---|---|---|---|
| | 1. Attentive 2. Denies need 3. Uncoop. 4. Clinical status interferes<br><br>Pt = Patient F = Family/ other | | Examples: • Medication • Food/drug interaction • Diet • Equipment • Community resources • Psychosocial • Personal care<br><br>Expected Outcomes: • Learner will state/ demonstrate knowledge of: | Circle preferred teaching method<br><br>A = Audio- visual R = Role play E = Explanation D = Demon- stration G = Group Class H = Handout | P = Partial understanding R = Retains content D = Demonstrates with cues RD = Can return demonstration N = No evidence of learning | 1. Reinforce content 2. Reteach 3. Needs practice 4. Outcome achieved | | |
| | PT | F | | | | | | |
| | | | Admission/Pre-op routine | E | | | | |
| | | | Visitor policy | E | | | | |
| | | | FHR/UA monitoring | D | | | | |
| | | | Positioning—operative | E | | | | |
| | | | Pain management options | E | | | | |
| | | | Surgical procedure routine | E | | | | |
| | | | Recovery routine | E | | | | |
| | | | Orient to MBU* | E | | | | |
| | | | Lochia patterns | E/A | | | | |
| | | | Peri care/Sitz bath | D/A | | | | |
| | | | Incision care | D/A | | | | |
| | | | Intake/output | E | | | | |
| | | | Activity/rest | E | | | | |
| | | | Engorgement care | E/A | | | | |
| | | | S/S to Report—maternal | E/A | | | | |
| | | | Follow-up Care—maternal | E | | | | |
| | | | Sexual relations/family planning | E | | | | |
| | | | | | | | | |

*Mother-baby unit

## Discipline

| | | | | | |
|---|---|---|---|---|---|
| RN | Registered Nurse | RT | Respiratory Therapy | CC | Care Coordination |
| OT | Occupational Therapy | SS | Social Service | PC | Pastoral Care |
| PT | Physical Therapy | NT | Nutrition Therapy | LC | Lactation Consultant |
| ST | Speech Therapy | MD | Physician | RPh | Pharmacy |

| Signature | Init. | Signature | Init. | Signature | Init. |
|---|---|---|---|---|---|
| | | | | | |
| | | | | | |
| | | | | | |
| | | | | | |
| | | | | | |

## Patient Education

| Date/Time | Readiness to Learn PT | Readiness to Learn F | Learning Needs/Content | Teaching Method | Evaluation | Status of Plan | Comment | Init. |
|---|---|---|---|---|---|---|---|---|
| | | | Safety ID (Security) | E | | | | |
| | | | Newborn Characteristics | E | | | | |
| | | | Bulb Syringe | D | | | | |
| | | | Hunger Cues | E | | | | |
| | | | Feeding Frequency | E | | | | |
| | | | Assessing Intake | E | | | | |
| | | | Positioning | D | | | | |
| | | | Burping | D | | | | |
| | | | Cord Care | D | | | | |
| | | | Circ care/diapering | D | | | | |
| | | | Elimination Patterns | E | | | | |
| | | | Bathing | A | | | | |
| | | | Temperature Taking | D | | | | |
| | | | Formula Preparation | E | | | | |
| | | | Breast Pump | D | | | | |
| | | | ODH Requirements | E | | | | |
| | | | S/S to Report—Newborn | E/A | | | | |
| | | | Car Seat Safety | E | | | | |
| | | | Follow-Up Care—Newborn | E | | | | |
| | | | | | | | | |
| | | | | | | | | |
| | | | | | | | | |
| | | | | | | | | |
| | | | | | | | | |
| | | | | | | | | |
| | | | | | | | | |
| | | | | | | | | |
| | | | | | | | | |

| PATIENT FOCUS | DATE _____<br>CARE COORDINATION<br>Pre-Hospital Phase | DATE _____<br>PT. OUTCOME<br>Preoperative | DATE _____<br>PT. OUTCOME<br>Intraoperative | DATE _____<br>PT. OUTCOME<br>Recovery |
|---|---|---|---|---|
| Tissue Perfusion Management | | ____ RN Patient has received an IV fluid preload of at least 1000cc<br>____ RN CBC WNL | ____ RN Surgical blood loss < 1000cc<br>____ RN Urinary output ≥ 30cc hour<br>____ RN O$_2$ saturation ≥ 96% or unchanged from pre-op | ____ RN Uterus firm; not more than one finger-breadth above umbilicus<br>____ RN Small to moderate amount of vaginal bleeding<br>____ RN Incision drainage WNL<br>____ RN Skin warm, dry; capillary refill brisk<br>____ RN Urinary output ≥ 30cc/hour |
| Physical Comfort Promotion | ____ CC/RN Pt. can discuss comfort measures and exercise appropriate for pregnancy | ____ RN Patient verbalizes understanding of pain options and potential side effects<br>____ RN Patient verbalizes use of 0-10 pain scale | ____ RN Patient expressed no pain during surgical procedures | ____ RN Patient states pain/discomfort is controlled |
| Childbearing Care | ____ CC/RN Pt. can discuss hospitalization process related to obstetrical management (i.e., birth options) | ____ RN Family is aware of visitation opportunities<br><br>____ RN Body temperature WNL | ____ RN Family holds/touches infant | ____ RN Family holds/touches infant<br>____ RN Breastfeeding initiated within 60-90 min of delivery<br>☐ N/A if bottle feeding |
| Infection | | ____ RN Lungs clear per auscultation/exam | | |
| Elimination Management | | | | ____ RN No ↑ surgical risk (i.e., lysing adhesions manipulation) |

**CARE CATEGORIES**

| | | | | |
|---|---|---|---|---|
| Assessment: | Breast assessment 20-24 weeks<br>Initiate anesthesia assessment form | I&O (including ice chips)<br>Preanesthesia score<br>Admission interview, VS's, physical exam, review lab results<br>Electronic fetal monitoring (including central surveillance and recording)<br>Anesthesia interview | Cardio pulmonary monitoring per anesthesia<br>I&O | VS q 15 minutes<br>Assess dressing, bleeding, fundus q 15 min.<br>Post anesthesia recovery score<br>I&O<br>Breast and nipple, assessment and latch score |
| Patient/Family Education: | By 20-24 weeks:<br>• MRG given and reviewed<br>• Health/safety pamphlets given, reviewed<br>• Discuss benefits to breast-feeding | Instruct patient in sidelying position<br>Orient to room, procedures and visitation<br>Anesthesia information and instructions given<br>Instruct in C&DB for scheduled C-sections | Patient oriented to operating room<br>Father/S.O. instructed on garb and oriented to operating room | |
| Discharge Planning: | PCC follow-up explained<br>Home visit info given<br>Identify pediatrician by 20-24 wk visit | Identify newborn physician caregiver on admission record | | |
| Tests: | DAU 7 if indicated per policy | RPR<br>Blood type and screen<br>CBC (cell profile)<br>Ultrasound | | |
| Interventions: | Pt. problem screen completed and sent to MD<br>Circumcision permit signed<br>Pt. preregistered<br>Register for appropriate classes<br>36-wk follow-up phone call | Operative permit/OR checklist done<br>Informed consent for permit<br>Determine OR availability<br>Consider need for pedi resuscitation team<br>Support parental-infant contact | Begin regional anesthesia procedure<br>Insert foley catheter<br>Consider need for pedi resuscitation team<br>Support parental-infant contact | Foley catheter maintained<br>Perineal hygiene<br>Epidural catheter removed<br>Transport to postpartum unit, pending par score ≥ 8 |
| Consults: | Referrals if needed: lactation, social service, grief counseling, anesthesia | Consider: Neonatology/pediatrics resident/2nd opinion<br>Social service | | |
| Medications/IVs: | | Initiate IV for 1000cc IV LR preload<br>Pre-op medications<br>1000cc IV lactated ringers | IV fluids maintained<br>Prophylactic antibiotics after cord clamped<br>Epidural/duramorph | IM/IV analgesics<br>Epidural/duramorph<br>Antiemetics<br>IV fluids maintained |
| Nutrition: | Review "Healthy Beginnings"<br>Diabetes referrals | NPO | NPO | NPO |
| Activity/Safety: | | Call light in reach | Safety belt after insertion of foley<br>Bovie/grounding pad on<br>Set up suction for patient and newborn<br>Wedge-left lateral position | Side rails up |

| DATE ___<br>PT. OUTCOME<br>Day of Delivery | DATE ___<br>PT. OUTCOME<br>Post-op DAY 1 | DATE ___<br>PT. OUTCOME Day 2 | DATE ___<br>TIME OF DISCHARGE |
|---|---|---|---|
| ___ RN Uterus firm; not more than one finger-breadth above umbilicus<br>___ RN Small to moderate amount of vaginal bleeding<br>___ RN Incision drainage WNL<br>___ RN Skin warm, dry, capillary refill brisk<br>___ RN Urinary output ≥ 30cc/hour | ___ RN Uterus firm; at or below the umbilicus<br>___ RN Small to moderate amount of vaginal bleeding<br>___ RN CBC WNL<br>___ RN I&O WNL<br>___ RN No bladder distention; voiding qs within 8° | ___ RN Uterus firm and below the umbilicus<br>___ RN Small to moderate vaginal bleeding | ___ RN Small to moderate vaginal bleeding |
| ___ RN Patient has periods of sleep during immediate post-op period<br>___ RN Patient states pain/discomfort controlled<br>___ RN Patient verbalize how to manage pain with ↑ activity | ___ RN Progressed to oral pain management<br>___ RN Patient states pain/discomfort controlled with oral medications<br>___ RN Patient verbalizes how to manage pain with ↑ activity | ___ RN Patient states pain/discomfort is controlled<br>___ RN Patient verbalizes how to manage pain with ↑ activity | ___ RN Patient verbalizes how to manage pain with ↑ activity |
| ___ RN Family holds/touches infant<br>___ RN/LC Milk production is stimulated | ___ RN Achieves latch score > 7 □ N/A<br>___ RN Family holds infant<br>___ RN Mother/infant display eye contact<br>___ RN Family provides infant care | ___ RN Family providing infant care<br>___ RN Family responds to infant's care needs<br>___ RN Latch score > 7 □ N/A | ___ RN Family providing infant care<br>___ RN Family responds to infant's care needs<br>___ RN Latch score > 7 □ N/A |
| ___ RN Body temperature < 100.8° F | ___ RN Body temperature < 100.4° F<br>___ RN Incision without extreme redness/purulent drainage | ___ RN Patient able to describe signs of infection | ___ RN Patient able to describe signs of infection |
| ___ RN Tolerates small amounts of clear liquids | ___ RN Tolerates soft diet<br>___ RN Bowel sounds present<br>___ RN Abdomen soft and minimally distended | ___ RN Patient passing flatus<br>___ RN Bowel sounds present<br>___ RN Tolerating diet | ___ RN Tolerating diet |
| VS on admission, at 2 hr, then q 6° × 24°<br>Physical exam/assessment<br>I&O (including ice chips)<br>Breast, nipple assessment and latch score | I&O (including ice chips)<br>Physical exam/assessment<br>Inspect incision<br>VS q 6 hours first 24 hrs. then q shift<br>Breast, nipple assessment and latch score | VS every shift<br>Physical exam/assessment<br>Breast, nipple assessment, and latch score | VS every shift<br>Physical exam/assessment<br>Breast, nipple assessment, and latch score |
| Preparation for self-care<br>Instruct/review for DB, coughing<br>See newborn pathway for care of infant | Reinforce self-care<br>Promote self-care learning<br>Discharge packet reviewed<br>Breast/bottle feeding instructions<br>Health channel/video education | Review self-care<br>Birth control/family planning<br>Review discharge instructions including signs and symptoms of infection<br>Reinforce breast-, bottle-feeding education | Review discharge instructions including signs and symptoms of infection<br>Reinforce breast, bottle-feeding education |
| Discharge packet given | Support system identified<br>Plans for home needs made | Instruction for follow-up appointments and prescriptions | Instruction for follow-up appointments and prescriptions |
| | CBC (cell profile)<br>□ Rh positive □ negative<br>Rho(D) Immune Globin given<br>Rubella □ Immune □ Nonimmune<br>Rubella vaccination given | Rubella □ Immune □ Nonimmune<br>Rubella vaccination given | Rubella □ Immune □ Nonimmune<br>Rubella vaccination given |
| Perineal hygiene<br>Check sensation in legs/passive leg exercise<br>Foley cath maintained<br>C and DB<br>Breast feed/pump q 2-3° for breastfeeding moms | Breast feed/pump q 2-3° for breastfeeding moms<br>D/C Foley catheter<br>Assisted with AM/hygiene care<br>DB, coughing qid<br>Circumcision permit checked by MD<br>Ice packs/support bra<br>Breast pump at bedside | Shower<br>DB, coughing qid<br>D/C Heplock | |
| Consider social service consult | Consider SS consult<br>Consider lactation consult | | |
| Pain managed by duramorph<br>IV fluids maintained for fluid balance<br>Antiemetics | Oral pain management<br>IV converted to saline lock or DC'd<br>Gas control/antacid<br>Laxative/stool softener | Oral pain management<br>Laxative/stool softener | Oral pain management<br>Laxative/stool softener |
| Sips and ice chips<br>Cl. liquids as tolerated | Advance diet as tolerated | Regular diet | Regular diet |
| Out of bed with assist as tolerated | Up ad lib | Ambulate up ad lib | Ambulate up ad lib |

# CHAPTER 15

## Care of the Well Woman During the Postpartum

*When you are a mother, you are never*
*really alone in your thoughts.*
*A mother always has to think twice,*
*once for herself and once for her child.*
— Sophia Loren

*What events affect the health of the woman in the fourth trimester?*

*What initial assessments must be made on the postpartum mother?*

*What concerns do women and their families express in the postpartum period?*

*What are the health risks for women and their families in the postpartum period?*

*What kinds of teaching and anticipatory guidance are required to prevent or reduce risks?*

*What sociocultural determinants affect the health of the woman in the fourth trimester?*

*What is our role in community-based postpartum care?*

*How can we assist with the developmental tasks of a family in transition?*

 **COLLABORATING DURING THE POSTPARTUM**

With the birth of her baby, the mother enters the 3-month postpartum period, during which the mother's body returns to its nonpregnant state, the infant adapts to its surroundings and settles into extrauterine life, and the psychologic adaptation to parenthood takes place. The first 6 weeks of the postpartum may be referred to as the **puerperium**. This chapter provides information about the postpartum care the mother requires whether she is in the facility where she gave birth or at home.

Several hours after the birth, the woman and her baby generally become less alert and fall asleep. This is the first step of recovery from the hard work and energy both have expended during labor and delivery. As the natural adaptation to a nonpregnant state continues, the mother gradually becomes more able to focus on taking on responsibility, and gradually assumes the care of the baby. Before the completion of the postpartum period, she will have adapted to her new role and integrated her other personal and family responsibilities. Our role is to provide nursing assessments, anticipatory guidance and teaching of self-care, support and encouragement, physical interventions, and referrals that will enable our clients to successfully achieve their desired health status and roles.

If the woman had a vaginal delivery she may receive from 8 to 48 hours of continuous nursing care after the delivery before discharge. If the baby was delivered surgically she may remain hospitalized from 48 to 72 hours

**587**

for nursing care. Most care required in the postpartum period, by necessity, occurs within the woman's home, with the woman and family members being responsible for ongoing assessment of physical and psychologic well-being. Excellent assessment, anticipatory guidance, and skill teaching must occur so that the woman and her family can provide appropriate self-care.

## Changes in the Health Care System

The transition of the family from a facility to home presents a challenge to health care providers. Since the 1950s, the length of stay for mothers and babies following a vaginal delivery has decreased from an average of 10 to 14 days to an average of 1.5 days in 1995 (Clinical Classifications for Health Policy Research: Hospital Inpatient Statistics, 1995). Since the early 1980s the length of stay following a surgical birth likewise has been reduced from 6.1 days to 4.0 days in 1992. Reports have been made of a postcesarean 2-day length of stay provided there were no complications during pregnancy and childbirth (Commission on Professional and Hospital Activities, 1991; 1993; Strong and others, 1993). This trend toward a short length of stay and the fact that more women are choosing to deliver their babies in birth centers and at home has moved most postpartum care from the hospital to the home.

Several issues have emerged from these changes: safety concerns for mother and baby, if they receive insufficient postpartum nursing care; the cost-effectiveness of early discharge; the degree of satisfaction with services; the effect on breastfeeding; the amount of time for teaching and learning; and the varied structure and content of early postpartum discharge programs (Brown, Towne, and York, 1996; Williams and Cooper, 1996). Preliminary research concerning the safety of early discharge has shown that following appropriate assessments, it is safe for mothers and infants. This includes families considered high risk. The impact of early discharge on cost is more complicated because most research has not included the cost of home programs (including the cost and time of providers), the liability of programs, and their development cost. Women and their families express satisfaction with early discharge. The impact on breastfeeding is difficult to measure because many women breastfeed successfully without assistance. Since many prenatal programs include breastfeeding information along with anticipatory guidance regarding the postpartum period, the effect on successful feeding and other aspects of learning is confounded (Brown, Towne, and York, 1996). Finally, the shortened stay has focused attention on the need to develop programs in the community that will meet the health needs of the emerging family. These programs include telephone follow-up, 2-week clinic visits, and home visiting programs and postpartum support groups (Box 15-1).

### Minimum Criteria for Shortened Length of Stay

The timing of the discharge for the mother and baby is a decision made by the providers in collaboration with the family and motivated by the limitations of the woman's insurance coverage. Ideally, the decision to discharge the maternal-infant dyad to home should be based on the relative risks and benefits of discharge to the health of the emerging family members. The length of postpartum stay should be determined by recommended standards of care, specific client needs for care, and the availability of appropriate support systems and community health care services to meet these specific needs (Fiesta, 1994). Although each agency is charged with development of their own guidelines for discharge, professional organizations have established minimum criteria for shortened stay.

The success of early discharge programs is based on the careful screening of mothers and infants who are at low risk for problems in the early postpartum (Box 15-2). "How care is provided and whether care meets the needs of individual mothers and babies should be the focus for determining the appropriateness of care, not where care is rendered or how many hours are spent in the hospital; and hospital and community-based systems of care should be responsive to patient health and information needs, designed to enhance access, timeliness, and personalization of services to mothers and families" (American Hospital Association, 1995).

### Legal Issues

Although nurses are not responsible for discharging mothers and babies, we do bear the responsibility for knowing the criteria for early discharge and following the discharge guidelines established by our facility. Some states have mandated insurance coverage for a length of stay, and we should be aware of laws within our area of practice (Koniak-Griffin, 1999).

## Goals to Be Accomplished with the Postpartum Woman and Family

We have several goals to accomplish with the postpartum woman and her family during the postpartum period. It is important to recognize that our priorities about what constitutes necessary care may differ from the woman's and her family's priorities. These differences need to be recognized and responded to in a flexible manner. Meeting the priority needs of the woman and her family is important to the establishment of trust and rapport. At the same time, it is important that our care for the woman and her family ensures the safety and well-being of the postpartum dyad (Schultz and others, 1998) (Box 15-3).

Postpartum care, including postpartum home care, should be designed to provide the necessary therapeutic supports required by the woman and her newborn.

## BOX 15-1   *Considerations for Shortened Length of Stay*

### MATERNAL CONSIDERATIONS FOR SHORTENED LENGTH OF STAY

Vital signs within normal limits

Amount and color of lochia appropriate

Uterine fundus firm

Adequate urinary output

Surgical repairs or wound has minimal edema, no evidence of infection and appears to be healing without complications

Able to ambulate with ease

No abnormal physical or emotional findings

Able to eat and drink without difficulty

Arrangements made for postpartum follow-up care

Has been instructed in self- and baby care, aware of deviations from normal, able to recognize and respond to danger signs and symptoms

Demonstrates readiness to care for self and baby

Pertinent laboratory results available, including hematocrit and/or hemoglobin

ABO blood type and D type known, D immune globulin administered if appropriate

Has received instructions regarding activity, exercises, and common discomforts and relief measures

Family members or other support persons available for initial postpartum

### NEONATAL CONSIDERATIONS FOR SHORTENED LENGTH OF STAY

Antepartum, intrapartum, and postpartum course for both mother and baby are uncomplicated

Vaginal delivery

Singleton birth at 38 to 42 weeks of gestation, birth weight appropriate

Vital signs documented normal and stable for 12 hours before discharge

### NEONATAL CONSIDERATIONS FOR SHORTENED LENGTH OF STAY—cont'd

Has urinated and passed stool

Has completed at least two successful feedings, documented sucking, swallowing and breathing while feeding

Physical examination with no abnormal findings requiring hospitalization

No evidence of bleeding from circumcision site for at least 2 hours

No evidence of significant jaundice in first 24 hours

Mother's knowledge, ability, and confidence in baby care documented and she has received instruction in: feeding, cord, skin, and genital care; recognition of signs and symptoms of illness, particularly jaundice

Infant safety (e.g., car seat, position for sleeping)

Family members or support persons who are familiar with newborn care and safety are present for assistance for first few days

Laboratory data reviewed (mother's syphilis and hepatitis B status, cord or infant blood type and direct Coombs' test)

Screening tests done in accordance with state regulations

Initial hepatitis B injection done or appointment scheduled

Physician-directed source of follow-up care identified and appointment made for 48-hour assessment

### FAMILY, ENVIRONMENTAL, AND SOCIAL CONSIDERATIONS FOR SHORTENED LENGTH OF STAY

No evidence of parental substance abuse

No parental or family history of abuse or neglect

No parental mental illness

Adequate social support for a single parent or adolescent parent

Stable living situation

From the American Academy of Pediatrics and The American College of Obstetricians and Gynecologists: *Guidelines for perinatal care,* ed 4, Washington, DC, 1997, The Academy.

We are typically responsible for planning care that meets the individualized needs of the woman, her infant, and the family. Our role often requires supervising and coordinating inpatient and outpatient services, documenting and communicating responses to care, acting as a client advocate, and directly providing therapeutic services.

A recent study indicated that during the initial hospital stay, postpartum women valued nursing care that focused on their physical needs for comfort. The high priority they placed on meeting their physical care needs during this period requires interventions beyond learning self-care tasks and baby care (Schultz and others, 1998).

Nurturing and protective care are also required by the new mother.

Primiparas, as might be expected, ask for more information about infant care in the postpartum period. Other topics of interest to them are fatigue, their body shape, and infant feedings. Among multiparas, fatigue is also a topic of interest because they are reacting to the changes created by an expanding family. For these women, information is also needed about their other children's response to the birth and new baby, increased emotional tension, child development, and meeting the multiple needs of their family (Moran, Holt, and Martin, 1997) (Box 15-4).

## BOX 15-2   Risk Factors that May Place a Mother and Baby at Risk in the Postpartum Period

**ANTEPARTAL FACTORS**

Hypertensive disease, hypertension and kidney disease including preeclampsia, eclampsia, HELLP syndrome

Anemia, clotting disorders, sickle cell disease

Chronic illness such as diabetes, thyroid disease, heart disease

Infections including toxoplasmosis, rubella, cytomegalovirus, herpesvirus type 2 (TORCH), transplacental infections, and human immunodeficiency virus (HIV)

**INTRAPARTAL FACTORS**

Hemorrhage and resulting anemia

Operative birth, cesarean section, vacuum-assisted birth, forceps-assisted birth

Multiple gestation

**INFANT FACTORS**

Birth anomalies and/or genetic diseases

Baby large or small for gestational age

Prematurity

**INDIVIDUAL AND FAMILY FACTORS**

Age less than 16 or over 35

High parity (greater than 5)

Interval between pregnancies less than 3 months or more than 8 years

Single mother

Smoker, or exposed to second-hand smoke

Drug and/or alcohol abuse

Late registration for prenatal care, missing visits

Family violence

Lack of family support

Poor home situation, including housing, food, transportation needs

Psychiatric illness or developmentally challenged

Body image disturbance

Adapted from Williams LR and Cooper MK: A new paradigm for postpartum care, *J Obstet Gynecol Neonatal Nurs* 25(9):745-749, 1996 and the American Academy of Pediatrics and The American College of Obstetricians and Gynecologists: *Guidelines for perinatal care*, ed 4, Washington, DC, 1997, The Academy.

## BOX 15-3   Nursing Priorities in Caring for the Postpartum Family

1. Promote health and well-being of the family members through use of the nursing process
2. Provide/reinforce health teaching and anticipatory guidance
3. Foster a positive family transition
4. Detect problems that might put the woman, her infant(s), and/or family at risk
5. Provide appropriate referrals or treatment

Adapted from Association of Women's Health, Obstetric, and Neonatal Nurses (AWOHNN): Guideline for home care of women and newborns. In *Standards and guidelines*, ed 5, Washington, DC, 1998, The Association.

## Initiating a Supportive Partnership Process

The word "collaborate" comes from the Latin, *collaborare*, meaning "to labor together." This term is particularly apt for describing the relationship between the hospital nurse and the nurse in the community and the postpartum family. Further, the term is typically used in health care to mean a process of joint involvement with others on a team with mutual goals and commitments (Henneman, 1995). For the postpartum family, team members include anyone they identify as family, their support network of friends, the providers involved in the birth of the infant, the postpartum nurse, and other members of community agencies. The characteristics of a good team are excellent communication skills, mutual respect, sharing, and trust (Henneman, 1995).

Team members should begin to foster these characteristics during the pregnancy, so that by the time of discharge to the home, all participants of the team are aware of the goals for the emerging family (Box 15-5). Sometimes the antepartal and intrapartal process leads to changes in the goals of the postpartum. When this is the case, communication skills, respect, sharing, and trust become crucial as postpartum care transitions to the home.

### Collaboration with Other Care Providers

When women leave the facility in which they gave birth, whether 8 or 48 hours later, the transition of care from the hospital to the home needs to be bridged. Inpatient nurses take on the role of both teacher and caregiver in preparing women for their transition to home and are instrumental in connecting them to programs in the community. Various services have been developed to facilitate the transition including telephone warm lines/hot lines that the mother calls and telephone follow-up by a nurse, home visits, postpartum classes, and reunions for childbirth groups. We are also resource persons who are aware of services available in the community and will be the agents of referral and collaboration.

---

**BOX 15-4** *Topics of Concern to the New Mother during the Postpartum Period*

**PHYSIOLOGIC CONCERNS**
Fatigue
Pain and discomfort
Pelvic floor relaxation
Sore nipples and engorgement
Weight gain

**PSYCHOLOGIC CONCERNS**
Emotional lability
Depression
Inspiration to improve self
Self-esteem issues
Body image

**PSYCHOLOGIC CONCERNS—cont'd**
Social support
Regaining a sense of control

**CONCERNS ABOUT SOCIAL ROLE FUNCTION**
Ability to parent
Balancing competing roles and responsibilities

**CONCERNS ABOUT SEXUAL FUNCTION**
Dyspareunia
Changing libido
Partner reaction
Family planning

From Kline CR, Martin DP, and Deyo RA: Health consequences of pregnancy and childbirth as perceived by women and clinicians, *Obstet Gynecol* 92(5):842-848, 1998.

---

In consultation with the agency and the family, we collaborate with the home-visiting agency. Depending on need, the visit might take place within the first 24 hours home or be delayed for several days. Referral mechanisms vary with agencies, but some basic information shared with the visiting nurse is:

1. Client demographics such as name, phone numbers, address/travel directions, source of reimbursement
2. Requested services such as laboratory specimens, vaccinations, education
3. Information from the hospital stay such as diagnoses and procedures, laboratory information, and baseline physical and psychosocial assessment data
4. Special instructions, including use of equipment
5. Discharge medications
6. Follow-up appointments
7. Hospital liaison to call for help if problems arise with discharge care or follow-up plans

## Collaboration with the Family

Developing trust is a nursing competency that is difficult to describe but is essential to gain entry to a home. Zerwekh (1992) described several processes that are considered integral to building trust with families:

- *Getting through the door* includes locating where the family lives and physically being invited into the home. It is important to recognize that the home is the personal territory of the family and we must be invited in. Further, we need to understand that we are guests in the family's home and are not there to impose control or take over.

- *Backing off* refers to recognizing and responding to the family's cues that they need some physical and/or emotional space.
- *Listening* is central to the collaborative process. Listening means being open to discovering the concerns of the family, not fulfilling one's own expectations or agenda.
- *Making connections* between the families expressed needs and the care, services, or referrals that the nursing can provide. When a match is made, a relationship can usually begin.
- *Affirming strengths* is a crucial part of building a trusting relationship. No matter how difficult the family's circumstances are, existing strengths need to be affirmed.
- *Maintaining a nonjudgmental stance* or being accepting of whatever is shared is sometimes a difficult task, but it is an essential part of building and maintaining trust.
- *Persisting* means that the process of building trust takes time and may never occur; however, continuing to do the visible, concrete, practical tasks that the family needs done reminds them that we can be trusted.

When the time comes to terminate the collaborative nurse-family relationship the trust that has been built between us and family should provide the family with a sense of reassurance that nurses can be relied upon in the future should the need arise. Through positive collaborative relations, the family is given the opportunity to learn and build on their strengths. Further, as part of the collaborative process the family may be referred to other community resources to assist them in meeting their ongoing needs.

---

## BOX 15-5 *An Innovative Early Discharge Program*

**Right From the Start** is an innovative discharge program, conceived and developed by nurses at the Bassett Birthing Center in rural Cooperstown, New York to meet a community need. It was designed to follow the client from the entry into prenatal care through delivery and back to the community. Input into the design of the program came from clients and care providers, including obstetricians, pediatricians, nurse-midwives, registered nurses in the clinic and community, and community agencies. The philosophy of the program parallels the philosophy of the obstetric department ". . . we believe that care offered in a client-directed, educationally-oriented manner will empower women to make choices which will improve their overall health and that of their families."

### Goals of the program include the following:
1. To provide a discharge plan for all families, regardless of length of stay, that meets family needs and ensures the health and safety of both mother and newborn as they become a new family unit.
2. To streamline the delivery of obstetric care across the continuum.
3. To make the most of birthing center resources, with an emphasis on the delivery of safe, professional care to the families we serve.
4. To ensure that our practice is congruent with current New York state legislation regarding reimbursement for maternity care.
5. To meet the recommendations of the American Academy of Pediatrics and the American College of Obstetricians and Gynecologists regarding discharge criteria.
6. To respond to the desires and special needs of those patients requesting discharge before 48 hours after a vaginal delivery, and before 96 hours after delivery by cesarean section.
7. To promote effective working relationships with referral agencies.

To meet these goals, care providers discussed discharge criteria and using the professional guidelines, developed the criteria for the department. Each home care agency was involved in the project. They discussed the referral process, including the information received and how it would be received. Staff members from the agencies were oriented to postpartum issues and to the care and teaching being done at the birthing center. Clients were educated about the program during their prenatal care through discussion and educational materials. They were asked to identify the agency to which they would like referral. A quality assurance process was developed to evaluate the referral process.

From the Department of Obstetrics and Gynecology: *Right from the start*, Bassett Birthing Center, Department of Nursing, Bassett Healthcare, 1997, Cooperstown, New York.

---

## The Postpartum Home Visit: Nursing Process

Based on the information received with the referral, we develop expectations for the home visit. Several tasks are involved (Clark, 1999):

1. Preparatory assessment: Review available data from the woman's physical, psychologic, social, and environmental system.
2. Diagnosis: Identify actual or potential nursing diagnoses based on assessment.
3. Planning:
   - Review previous interventions to discover what has been done and the effectiveness of those interventions.
   - Prioritize expected client needs on the basis of the potential to threaten the health and welfare of the client.
   - Develop goals and objectives for each area of recognized need.
   - Consider acceptance and timing of the visit. If the family is preoccupied with other activities, they may be unable or unwilling to deal with health needs.
   - Specify nursing activities to be accomplished such as teaching, providing care, referral to other service agencies.
   - Obtain necessary supplies and equipment.
   - Plan evaluation of the client outcomes of the visit.
4. Implementing the planned visit:
   - Validate assessment and diagnoses. Unanticipated new problems or issues may be found, or some problems may have resolved.
   - Identify additional needs through the assessment of the physical, psychologic, and social situation of the client.
   - Modify the plan of care as the individuals or family situation dictates.
   - Perform nursing interventions.
   - Deal with distractions from the environment or the client's behavior. In addition, be aware that your presence may be responsible for creating this distraction through their fears, preoccupations, and personal reactions to different lifestyles.
5. Evaluating the home visit: This is done using criteria developed during the planning phase. Often evaluation may occur during subsequent visits, as the results of the teaching become apparent. Evaluate your effectiveness in use of the home visit process.
6. Documentation: Documentation is important. It is the record of the client assessment and

identified needs, the care given, and the response to the care. The record will be used for continuation of care. It is a legal record, and it is necessary for reimbursement.

### Legal Issue

We may be charged with abandonment if clients are not provided with adequate notice of the termination of care. Planning for discharge from services from the first visit prevents a feeling of abandonment. Clients should be aware of plans for discharge and be connected to community resources for continuing care.

## POSTPARTUM PHYSIOLOGIC ASSESSMENT

Whether in the hospital, birthing center, or home, the same assessments must occur. After 48 hours, follow-up screening may also be conducted over the phone (Table 15-1).

**Involution** is the process whereby the reproductive organs return anatomically to a normal nonpregnant state. The process of physical involution takes approximately 6 weeks (the puerperium), while the accompanying psychosocial changes may take months. Our assessment and care during this process focuses on promoting healing, assisting the mother to understand the changes that she is or will be experiencing, and detecting any signs that may indicate potential or actual complications. The most common physical complications during the puerperium include infection (breast, urinary bladder, wound, or endometrial), hemorrhage, and coagulopathies.

Before conducting a physical examination, encourage the woman to empty her bladder to promote her comfort and ensure an accurate assessment of the involution of her uterus. The examination should be performed in an orderly and consistent manner so as to promote her confidence, minimize her discomfort and provide a thorough examination. As you perform the examination, it is important that you communicate to the woman what you are doing and that you take measures to preserve her sense of modesty and privacy. Furthermore, it is important to discuss your findings with the woman and provide reassurance, encouragement, and related incidental teaching as you go (e.g., "Empty your bladder every few hours to allow your uterus to move back down and decrease your bleeding."). Following the assessment, when the woman is more comfortable and fully clothed, more in-depth teaching may occur. Additionally, elicit and respond to her concerns and questions during and following the examination.

Keep in mind that undressing for an examination and personal touch may have different meanings for women of different cultures and that some women may be extremely modest about being examined. These differ-

ences may require altering the manner in which you conduct the examination.

### Legal Issue

It is important to remember that before touching a patient, you must get her permission to do so. When a woman is sitting within her home, she may feel more empowered to set limits regarding what you may do and how you may do it. Without her consent to touch and/or examine her, you may be open to legal charges of assault (the threat of touching) and battery (actual touching) if you proceed (Brooke, 1995). Most home care agencies have a woman sign a "consent to treat" form that protects against legal liability for performing nursing actions related to care.

### Vital Signs

While the postpartum woman should be hemodynamically stable before discharge, the ongoing monitoring of her vital signs serves as an indicator of potential health problems that may have emerged since her discharge from the hospital or birth center. Also, the vital signs are a familiar part of a professional examination and may serve as an "ice breaker" in moving from the more informal aspects involved in gaining entry into the home to the formal aspects of the assessment.

#### Temperature

By 48 hours postpartum the woman should have had an opportunity to replace the large fluid losses that accompany the intrapartal experience and her temperature should be within normal range. A temperature of >100.4° F (38° C) may indicate the presence of an infection. Likewise, a persistent low-grade temperature may indicate the presence of an infection. Abnormal temperature readings warrant continued monitoring until the presence of an infection can be ruled out. Any elevated temperature should be monitored at least daily beyond the first 48 hours postpartum until it returns to normal. Be sure that the woman has a working thermometer. Teach her to take her temperature at the same time each day to prevent confusion of results from normal diurnal fluctuations. Provide her with written information regarding an acceptable temperature and when and who to notify if it goes higher.

#### Pulse

In the first several days postpartum, it is not unusual for the woman to experience a relative bradycardia, or slowing of the heart rate. Strictly speaking, bradycardia is a heart rate of less than 60 beats per minute, while a relative bradycardia is a slowing of the heart rate from the normal baseline. This slowing of the heart rate is related to the increased maternal blood volume that

TABLE 15-1  Guidelines for Telephone Follow-up

| Area of assessment | Suggested questions for screening |
|---|---|
| Perceptions of the labor and delivery experience | Tell me about your labor and delivery. How did it compare to what you expected? |
| Breastfeeding | How do you feel about the breastfeeding? Have you experienced any feelings of breast filling? Engorgement? Sore nipples? Let down? How do your breasts feel at the end of a feeding? Is the baby feeding well? How often are you feeding the baby? How long does the baby feed? When the infant is suckling have you noticed any tingling in your breasts or can you hear any swallowing sounds? How many wet/soiled diapers is the baby having in a day? Who would you call if you had a breastfeeding problem? |
| Breasts | Have you noticed any red, warm, tender areas on your breasts? When did you last do a breast self-examination? |
| Abdomen/gastrointestinal function | Have you been able to move your bowels since you delivered your baby? Have you had any abdominal discomfort or tenderness? If an incision is present, have you noticed any increased tenderness? Redness? Drainage? Do you have a return appointment to see your provider to follow-up on your healing? |
| Appetite | Who is preparing your meals? Can you tell me what you have had to eat in the last 24 hours? How many glasses of fluid have you had to drink in the last 24 hours? What kinds of fluids have you had to drink? |
| Lochia | How does the amount of vaginal flow you are currently experiencing compare to your periods? What kind of pads are you wearing? Are you saturating any pads? Are you passing any clots? What is the color of the flow? Do you notice a foul odor to the flow? |
| Perineum | How does your crotch area (bottom or some other familiar term) feel? Are you able to sit comfortably? Do you know how to perform Kegel exercises? Are you experiencing any rectal discomfort? |
| Voiding | Have you noticed any pain or burning with urination? Have you noticed any difficulty with passing a stream of urine? Do you feel as though your bladder is fully emptied after you urinate? Have you noticed any increased urgency or frequency of urination? Have you noticed any leakage of urine (e.g., when you cough, sneeze, or laugh)? |
| Extremities | Have you noticed any areas of swelling, redness, tenderness, or warmth? Does it hurt to walk? |
| Sleep-rest patterns | How many hours were you able to sleep last night? Did you take any naps yesterday or today? Are you sleeping when the baby sleeps? |
| Instrumental supports | Who is available to help you at home? What kinds of help are you getting? What other kinds of help, if any, would you find helpful? |
| Infant care | Before the birth of this infant, what kinds of experience did you have with newborn care? Feeding? Tell me how you are feeling about being able to care for the infant? Feed the infant? What kinds of things would you like me to explain to you about infant care? What worries you the most about taking care of the infant? |
| Family adjustments | What does your spouse/partner think about the baby? What do the other children think about the baby? How have you been able to involve them in the care of the infant? Since the birth of the infant, have you been able to get any time to yourself? What kinds of things are you doing for yourself? How are you and your partner getting along? Since the birth of the infant, have you and your partner been able to get any time alone? What do the infant's grandparents think about the infant? What kinds of advice are you getting from others? |
| Domestic violence | Having a new baby in the house can be overwhelming. We ask all new mothers, "Do you feel emotionally abused by your partner? Are you afraid of your partner? Do you feel your partner tries to control you? Has your partner ever hit, slapped, kicked, or otherwise physically hurt you? Has your partner ever forced you to participate in sex against your wishes?" (King and others, 1993) Do you have any questions for me? What phone numbers do you have to call if you have questions about yourself or the baby? |

Adapted from Varney H: *Varney's midwifery,* ed 3, Boston, 1997, Jones & Bartlett.

occurs once blood is no longer perfusing the placenta. With delivery of the placenta, the woman experiences as much as a 1000 ml autotransfusion.

The presence of tachycardia, or a heart rate greater than 100 beats per minute, may indicate hypovolemia, either as a result of dehydration or blood loss, or it may indicate the presence of an infection. In either case, the presence of tachycardia warrants further investigation. Discuss with the woman her need to be evaluated by her primary care provider. Problem solve with her how she might get to an appointment with her provider and who will care for the baby.

## Blood Pressure

By the fourth postpartum day, the blood pressure should be at approximately normal levels. Low or falling blood pressures may indicate either **orthostatic hypotension** or concealed or delayed hemorrhage. The woman experiencing orthostatic hypotension generally complains of accompanying dizziness or syncope with postural changes and a rapid heart rate (tachycardia). Orthostatic hypotension may also be related to inadequate fluid intake or excessive blood loss. Learn from the woman about her fluid intake and her lochia flow. Based on these reports, determine whether the woman should continue self-care and evaluation for a period of time or be seen by her primary care provider for a more thorough evaluation. If you determine that self-care and evaluation should continue, review with the woman what she should monitor and what events would indicate that she should be seen immediately. If you determine that the woman should be seen immediately, help her problem solve how she will do that.

## Breasts

During the course of pregnancy, under the influences of estrogen and progesterone, the breasts increase in size and functional ability to become ready for breastfeeding. Whether a woman decides to breastfeed or not, her body prepares for that possibility and manufactures colostrum and milk. Whether a woman chooses to breastfeed or bottle-feed, her breasts need to be assessed.

By the third postpartum day, secondary **lactogenesis** (milk production) is beginning to occur. This is heralded by a fullness of the breast tissues and venous distention. Size of the breasts is not an indication of a woman's ability to produce milk; however, the size and shape of the breasts generally make some feeding positions more favorable than others.

### Assessment of Breasts

Assessment of the breasts should include inspection for size, contour, asymmetry, engorgement, or areas of erythema, and palpation for any masses or areas of warmth or tenderness. Most women have mild asymmetry that is of no functional consequence; however, marked asym-

metry may indicate lack of functional breast tissue (Lawrence, 1998; Riordan and Auerbach, 1998).

### Assessment of Nipples

The nipples should be inspected for tissue integrity and protraction or ability to become erect. Flat nipples do not change with stimulation and may be difficult for the breastfeeding infant to grasp. Inverted nipples are rare; however, they retract when stimulated. If the inverted nipple is new, it may indicate an underlying problem and is reason for referral to the woman's primary care provider. Cracked, blistered, fissured, bruised, or bleeding nipples in a breastfeeding woman are generally indications of improper positioning of the infant at the breast. Nursing interventions can make the woman more comfortable and help remedy the situation (Lawrence, 1998; Riordan and Auerbach, 1998). Anticipatory guidance and interventions concerning breastfeeding are discussed later in this chapter.

### Affects of Prior Breast Surgery

Women who have had previous breast augmentation surgery may still be able to breastfeed as long as the milk ducts were not severed during the surgery. Breast reduction surgery may result in variable success in breastfeeding depending on the degree of functional tissue removed and the type of procedure performed and whether it interfered with the milk ducts and innervation to the nipple. In either case, it is important to consult the operative report and watch closely for signs of adequate milk transfer (Riordan and Auerbach, 1998).

Despite changes in the breasts during the postpartum period, postpartum women should be encouraged to continue to perform breast self-examination on a monthly basis. During our physical examination of the woman's breasts, we may elicit the woman's knowledge and comfort level about performing a breast self-examination and provide appropriate reinforcement and teaching.

## Respiratory System

Pulmonary function in the postpartum period is affected by changes in the thoracic rib cage and diaphragm. With expulsion of the fetus, the diaphragm descends and thoracic and abdominal organs gradually revert to their normal nonpregnant positions. Respirations are usually in the normal adult range of 16 to 24 breaths per minute. Changes in ventilation and acid-base balance return to prepregnant levels by 3 weeks postpartum (Bond, 1993).

Following delivery, changes in the respiratory rate or the presence of respiratory symptoms may be indicative of complications such as congestive heart failure, pulmonary edema, pneumonia, or atelectasis (a collapsed lung). Any woman who has a history of smoking, chronic disease (e.g., heart, renal, or respiratory disease), pregnancy-induced hypertension, or who has undergone an operative procedure is at greater risk for such pulmonary complications. During the postpartum, assess the quality and rate of respirations along with auscultation of the lung fields for the presence of any adventitious breath sounds.

## Genitourinary System

### The Uterus

Following childbirth, involution of the uterus involves changes in the body of the uterus, the endometrium, and the placental site, as the uterus returns to a healthy, nonpregnant state. Immediately after delivery of the placenta, strong **myometrial** (uterine muscle) contractions begin a rapid decrease in the size of the uterus.

*Height of Fundus.* Within 24 hours, the fundus of the uterus is located just below the umbilicus. After 2 days, the uterus begins to shrink approximately 1 to 2 cm per day, so that within 2 weeks, it is within the cavity of the pelvis (Figures 15-1 and 15-2).

*Contractions.* The "afterpains" (uterine contractions) present in the immediate postpartum period are often less noticeable at this time. Breastfeeding, multiparity, or conditions such as multiple gestations or polyhydramnios that create overdistention of the gravid uterus may increase the presence of afterpains. By 4 weeks postpartum, the uterus reaches its nonpregnant size. During involution, the total number of muscle cells does not decrease appreciably, rather the size of the cells decreases. The weight of the uterus decreases from 1000 g, just after delivery, to 100 g or less (Cunningham and others, 1997).

*Endometrium.* The separation of the placenta during the third stage of labor creates changes within the uterus. Two to 3 days after the birth of the baby, the **decidua** becomes differentiated into two layers. The outer layer becomes necrotic and is sloughed off in the lochia. The remaining basal layer contains the endometrial glands, the source of new endometrial tissue. By the end of the first postpartum week, the surface of the uterine cavity is covered by epithelium, and by 3 weeks postpartum, the entire endometrium is restored to its normal state (Cunningham and others, 1997).

The area where the placenta was located, the **placental site**, takes longer to regenerate. Immediately after the expulsion of the placenta, uterine contractions pinch off the blood vessels entering the area, preventing bleeding and sealing the site. The site is irregular in appearance and thick with blood vessels. This process of **subinvolution,** whereby the blood vessels become sealed off, or ligated, is critical. Failure to do so can result in a late postpartum hemorrhage. Through the process of vessel ligation, **thrombi** (clots) form, and the placental area is sealed. Healing takes place not by absorption of these clots, which would leave scar tissue, but by the process of **exfoliation.** The placental site is regenerated by extension and growth of the endometrial tissue from the margins of the site and upward growth from the endometrial glands left in the basal layer of the decidua. The newly formed endometrial tissue completely covers and heals the area, leaving no scar tissue. Healing occurs

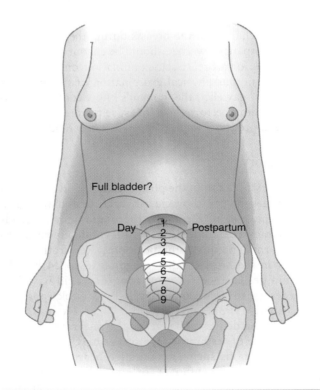

*FIGURE 15-1* ● Involution of the uterus.

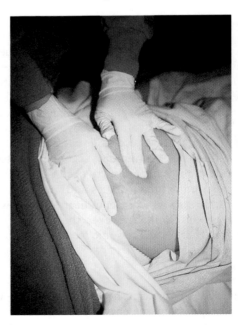

*FIGURE 15-2* ● Palpation of the uterus. *(Courtesy of Caroline E. Brown.)*

rapidly and by the end of the second postpartum week, the placental site is 3 to 4 cm in diameter. It is completely healed by the sixth postpartum week (Cunningham and others, 1997).

*Lochia.* The vaginal discharge of the puerperium is known as **lochia**. It is similar to a menstrual flow and is composed of decidua, erythrocytes, epithelial cells, and bacteria. By 48 hours postpartum, the woman should be experiencing a light to moderate flow. In the initial postpartum period, the lochia contains sufficient blood and occasional small clots so that the color is red—**lochia rubra**. After 3 to 4 days, it becomes paler pink in color, with a serosanguineous consistency—**lochia serosa**. Lochia rubra and serosa may have a characteristic fleshy odor. After about 10 days, the discharge becomes mucousy and the color becomes white or yellow-white—**lochia alba**. It is not unusual for lochia to cease by 3 weeks, but it may also persist until 6 weeks postpartum.

*Nursing Role.* Estimating the amount of lochia is subjective, but an attempt has been made to standardize the description of the volume as either scant, light, moderate, or heavy (Jacobson, 1985; Bond, 1993). Ask to see a pad and help the woman evaluate the amount of the flow. She will have more confidence in doing further evaluations after she has done one with you. (See Chapter 14, for an explanation of perineal pad measurements.)

A slight increase in lochial flow may occur during ambulation or with breastfeeding, and women should be counseled to expect these findings. Women who experience saturation of a perineal pad within 15 minutes are encouraged to lie down, put their feet up, and perform gentle fundal massage. The presence of bright red vaginal bleeding after lochia rubra has stopped, additional saturation of a perineal pad, or the presence of any steady bleeding may represent a delayed postpartal hemorrhage due to lacerations, uterine atony, or retained placental fragments. These symptoms require immediate medical attention.

Postpartum women should be instructed to report any foul-smelling lochia and any flow that is unusually heavy or steady or the continued presence or return of bright red bleeding and clots. Verbal instruction and written instructions listing signs and symptoms that should be reported, whom they are to be reported to, and how soon she is to report them should be left with the woman.

Signs and symptoms of endometritis are as follows:

* Tender, enlarged uterus
* Prolonged, severe cramping
* Foul-smelling lochia
* Fever

*Cervix.* Following delivery, the cervix contracts slowly, remaining slightly open for several days. By the end of the first postpartum week, the cervical opening has narrowed, the cervix has thickened, and a cervical canal is re-formed. At the end of the puerperium, if it was a vaginal delivery, the external os will not resume the primiparous circular opening, but will appear wider, with the os slightly open and slitlike. This change will not be observable without a vaginal examination, something that is not generally done until at least 6 weeks postpartum after recovery from birth has taken place.

*Vagina.* Following a vaginal delivery, the vagina is soft and distended beyond its normal size. The **rugae**, or skin folds that normally line the vaginal walls, are absent, leaving the walls thin and smooth. During involution the size of the **vagina** and **introitus** diminishes, but remains larger than their former nonpregnant dimensions. Rugae reappear by the third week (Cunningham and others, 1997). The speed of involution of the vagina depends on the stimulation of estrogen and will take relatively longer if the woman is breastfeeding. Breastfeeding women may find that their vaginal walls remain friable while nursing, and they may experience some bleeding during intercourse. Generally, normal mucous production returns with the onset of ovulation.

*Nursing Role.* Encourage the woman to continue to do  Kegel exercises to improve vaginal muscle tone. Also teach the woman about the use of a water-soluble lubricant during vaginal intercourse to reduce friction, improve comfort, and decrease the incidence of bleeding during intercourse. Some couples resume sexual intercourse as soon as 1 or 2 weeks after delivery, or when the woman feels comfortable.

*Perineum.* Depending on the circumstances of the delivery, the woman may have an **episiotomy** or laceration repair involving the perineum. In addition, the pressure on the perineum during the delivery process may have resulted in **ecchymosis** (bruising) or **edema** (tissue swelling). Women may experience pain because of a **hematoma** (distention of tissues caused by bleeding into the tissues) or tissue edema.

Ask the woman to lie on her side and flex her upper leg, bringing her knee up towards her chest. Observe the perineal area for redness, edema, ecchymosis, drainage, and **wound approximation** (how well the wound edges come together).

*Nursing Role.* Perineal healing and comfort may be enhanced by measures that improve circulation to the distended tissues such as sitz baths or use of warm soaks.  Encouraging the woman to avoid sitting on soft surfaces and using local comfort measures such as anesthetic ointments or soaks (witch hazel, Magnesium Sulfate or Epsom's Salts in water or a weakened tea solution) may also improve perineal comfort.

*Hemorrhoids.* Many women develop hemorrhoids during pregnancy, as the result of venous dilation, the pressure of the gravid uterus, and slowed peristalsis. Hemorrhoids appear as spherical bluish masses at the anal rim. The overlying skin may be edematous and tense. Pain and **pruritis** (itching) may accompany the presence of hemorrhoids. Hemorrhoids may be individual or may appear in clusters. During the expulsive phase of labor, the hemorrhoids may increase in size or become **thrombosed** (blood clots in the subcutaneous tissue of the hemorrhoid).

In the postpartum period, the hemorrhoids may cause considerable pain or may only be painful upon **defecation** (movement of the bowels). Thrombosed hemorrhoids are bluish-purple in color, hard, and painful. Women with thrombosed hemorrhoids report that they feel as though they are sitting on a hard object such as a stone or marbles. As the hemorrhoid heals, it becomes smaller, less tense, and assumes a normal skin tone. Measures should be taken to prevent further constipation, provide pain relief, and promote healing.

*Nursing Role.* Encourage the women with hemorrhoids to drink lots of water and eat a high-fiber diet with plenty of vegetables and grains. Applying witch hazel (cotton pads presoaked in witch hazel such as Tucks) or using hemorrhoidal cream, herbal sitz baths with comfrey leaves and calendula flowers, or herbal salves made of horse chestnut help soothe and shrink hemorrhoidal tissues. If dietary measures to ensure regular bowel movements are not successful, use of a mild laxative may be appropriate. Stool softeners; regularly scheduled times for bowel movements; and the complementary therapies of acupuncture, Qigong (a system of gentle exercise, meditation, and controlled breathing), reflexology, and yoga may also be advantageous (Dollemore, 1998; Nurse's Handbook of Alternative and Complementary Therapies, 1998). If the hemorrhoid is thrombosed, it may require incision and drainage to prevent tissue **necrosis** (death). Women should be encouraged to notify their primary care provider if they notice hemorrhoid pain increasing rather than improving.

*Urinary Tract.* In the immediate postpartum period trace proteinuria may persist related to the catabolic effects of the intrapartum. **Diuresis** begins within 12 hours after delivery and continues through the first postpartum week. It is not unusual for a woman to experience diuresis with urinary excretion reaching volumes of up to 3000 ml of urine per day. This diuresis is the result of decreasing aldosterone production and subsequent declines in sodium retention.

*Nursing Role.* Because her bladder may have experienced edema and hypotonia during labor, the postpartum woman is at risk for urinary retention and subsequent infections of the urinary tract. It is important during this period to encourage the woman to frequently and completely empty her bladder to prevent uterine atony. Counsel the postpartum woman to report any difficulties with urination, burning with urination, feelings of incomplete emptying, or difficulties with initiating a stream of urine.

To prevent urinary tract infections or stress incontinence, encourage the mother to:

- Ambulate. Gravity prevents urinary stasis. Improved circulation increases renal blood flow.
- Drink ample (6 to 8 glasses) fluids. Avoid excess use of caffeinated beverages or alcohol, which are bladder irritants and may cause excessive diuresis.
- Empty bladder frequently to prevent overdistention of the bladder and urinary stasis.
- Perform Kegel exercises.
- Practice hygienic measures to prevent skin irritation or fecal contamination of the healing perineum.
- Thoroughly clean the perineal area at least once per day with a mild soap and warm water.
- Wash hands before and after performing perineal care.
- Use a perineal bottle (i.e., plastic squeeze bottle) filled with warm water to squirt water over her perineum after voiding or defecating. Avoid touching the nozzle to the skin.
- Pat the perineal area from front to back to prevent fecal contamination.
- Change perineal pads frequently. Apply the pad from front to back, and avoid touching, and therefore contaminating, the inner surface of the pad. Wrap soiled pads and place in a covered waste container.
- Wear cotton underwear and avoid wearing tight or restrictive clothing.
- Monitor and report any signs (e.g., pain or burning) that might indicate a urinary tract infection.
- Discuss any ongoing stress incontinence with a health care provider.

## Cardiovascular System

### Hypervolemia

**Hypervolemia** occurs in late pregnancy and results in a 40% to 50% increase in blood volume at term. This increase allows women to tolerate the blood loss of delivery. By 1 week postpartum, the blood volume will return to normal levels. Between the third and seventh postpartum day, the hematocrit begins to rise and usually returns to normal levels by the fourth to eighth postpartum week. An additional protection against excessive blood loss during delivery is the pregnancy-related increase in plasma fibrinogen that is necessary for clotting. This elevation usually lasts through the first postpartum week (Cunningham and others, 1997).

### Leukocytosis

An additional protective mechanism is **leukocytosis** (increase in white blood cell [WBC] count), which occurs during and after labor. The WBC count sometimes reaches 30,000 per mm³ (Cunningham and others, 1997). This increase is in response to the stress of labor and is protective against invading organisms during labor, delivery, and the initial postpartum period. A sudden increase of more than 30% in a 6-hour period or the presence of **bands** (immature forms of WBCs) in the differential white count suggests the presence of an infection.

### Heart Sounds

It is not unusual to hear a split first heart sound ($S_1$), an $S_3$, or a systolic murmur at the left sternal border during pregnancy and in the immediate postpartum period. A split $S_1$ will disappear if you ask the woman to hold her breath. An $S_3$ heart sound is best heard with the stethoscope over the mitral area and the woman in a left lateral decubitus position. An $S_3$ heart sound may be the first clinical sign of a pathologic state such as congestive heart failure, but is a normal physiologic sound in a high output, high volume state such as the third trimester of pregnancy and the immediate postpartum; however, once diuresis has occurred the split $S_1$ and $S_3$ sounds should disappear. An innocent murmur should not radiate throughout the precordium and should not be accompanied by other cardiac symptoms such as palpitations, extreme diaphoresis, dizziness, dyspnea, edema, syncope, chest pain, or numbness or tingling in the extremities. The new onset of any of these findings requires consultation with the woman's nurse midwife or physician.

### Clot Formation

Thrombus or clot formation may occur in the postpartum period because of a disruption in the balance between blood-clotting activators and blood-clotting inhibitors. Three contributing factors are stasis of blood flow, an injured venous wall, and the hypercoaguability of blood. The presence of this triad (Virchow's triad) of conditions may lead to thrombophlebitis or thromboembolism.

**Thrombophlebitis** is an inflammation of the blood vessel due to the presence of clots in the vessel and/or unrelieved pressure on vessel walls. Typically this condition affects the veins of the legs, thighs, and pelvis. Symptom onset is usually rapid and includes pain or tenderness of the affected area, along with swelling, redness, and warmth. If the thrombophlebitis occurs in a woman's legs, she will generally exhibit a positive Homan's sign (pain upon dorsiflexion of the foot). Early detection of thrombophlebitis is essential to prevent life-threatening complication of a thromboembolism such as a pulmonary embolus.

**Thromboembolism** constitutes a health emergency that usually presents when the clot dislodges and travels to the lungs. Typically the woman has a dramatic and sudden onset of symptoms of chest pain, dyspnea, tachypnea, fever, tachycardia, and profound diaphoresis.

***Nursing Role.*** Tell the woman to call her primary care provider as soon as she feels a warm or painful area in her leg. Findings that indicate a possible thrombophlebitis require immediate referral and treatment to prevent a thromboembolism.

To prevent thrombus formation, encourage the woman to:

- Ambulate and change positions frequently.
- Avoid crossing the legs, flexing the legs at the groin, or standing or sitting in one position for a prolonged period.
- Perform leg exercises when the need for sitting or standing for a long period occurs.
- Rotate the ankle in a circular fashion.
- Perform alternating extension and flexion of the legs and feet.
- Wear antiembolism hose if she has varicose veins or a previous history of thrombophlebitis.
- Notify her care provider immediately if she notes any tenderness in the legs, groin, or pelvis with accompanying redness, warmth, and swelling of the overlying tissues.

### Varicose Veins

Pregnant women are more likely to develop varicose veins because of the vasodilating effects of progesterone on the blood vessel walls and the decreased venous return from the lower periphery that accompanies later pregnancy. Varicosities commonly occur in dependent areas such as the legs, groin, or perineal area. A family history of varicose veins, women whose occupations require long periods of standing or sitting, and weight gain and compression of vessels from the gravid uterus increase the woman's risk.

During the postpartum period, this condition should improve. Her varicosities should be assessed for retrograde filling or the presence of hard, palpable cordlike veins and the presence of any thrombosis (see thrombophlebitis). Normally, when a vein is occluded it will fill from below the occlusion; following release of the pressure, no additional filling should occur because competent valves in the vein prevent backflow. A varicose vein that fills from above upon release of pressure is an abnormal finding and should be discussed with the woman's care provider.

***Nursing Role.*** To prevent varicose veins, encourage the mother to:

- Avoid:
   unnecessary pressure on the leg or groin veins from prolonged sitting or standing.
   heavy lifting or straining.
   excessive weight gain.
   crossing her legs.
   wearing tight or restrictive clothing.
   using oral contraceptives or estrogens.

- Stop smoking or decrease as much as possible, if applicable.
- Wear support stockings.
- Elevate her feet when sitting.
- Exercise by walking.
- Report worsening, painful varicose veins.

### Pregnancy-Induced Hypertension

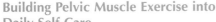

By 48 hours postpartum, if the woman had pregnancy-induced hypertension (PIH), the major risks have generally passed. If the woman experiences a headache, epigastric discomfort, or blurred vision, however, she should call her provider immediately.

## Musculoskeletal System

During the first days postpartum, many women experience muscle aches and strains as a result of their exertion during labor. The effects of relaxin, the hormone that relaxed ligament and cartilage during the end of pregnancy, gradually subside and her joints return to their prepregnant positions. The abdominal wall muscle fibers shorten but the abdominal musculature will remain soft and flabby as a result of the prolonged distention of pregnancy. During the postpartum period there may be marked separation or **diastasis recti** of the longitudinal muscles of the abdomen. Return to normal state is aided by exercises (Cunningham and others, 1997).

The muscles that comprise the pelvic floor provide support for internal reproductive, urinary, and bowel structures. These muscles stretch and thin during the second stage of labor as the fetus descends and rotates. During the postpartum period, these muscles may be bruised or torn and lack tone. Pelvic muscle relaxation refers to the lengthening and weakening of pelvic muscles. Because of the importance of good muscle tone for organ support and urinary continence, the restoration of pelvic floor muscle tone is of prime importance for postpartum women. Women with greater antepartal pelvic muscle strength retain greater pelvic muscle strength after vaginal delivery. In addition, women who do pelvic muscle strengthening exercises in the postpartum period have greater improvement in muscle tone than those who do not do pelvic exercises. Kegel muscle exercises have been recommended as a way to strengthen pelvic muscles (Sampselle and Brink, 1990). Many women learn these exercises as preparation for childbirth. Remind them of how helpful Kegel exercises are in the postpartum period and encourage them to do them every time they do perineal care. (See Chapter 13 for teaching of Kegel exercise.)

### Building Pelvic Muscle Exercise into Daily Self-Care

Exercise of pelvic floor muscles in the postpartum period aids in increasing comfort and recovery of the perineal area. Kegel exercises can be started in the first few days following delivery. If a woman incorporates this form of exercise into an ongoing self-care initiative, it may help prevent future urinary incontinence and enhance sexual enjoyment (Sampselle and Brink, 1990).

## Integumentary System

### Excessive Perspiration

Many postpartum women experience excessive perspiration or **diaphoresis**. This is a common occurrence, particularly at night, and it is one of the ways in which the body attempts to rid itself of excessive fluid volume that is no longer needed to support the placental and fetal circulation. This diaphoresis may cause some women distress because of hygienic concerns.

*Nursing Role.* Reassure women that this is a normal, transient state. When caring for women during this initial postpartum period, we should be sensitive to the bathing rituals that may be a part of her culture. There may be restrictions regarding when and how she bathes. Take your lead from the woman regarding how she wishes to clean and freshen herself.

### Changes in Pigmentation

Pregnancy is associated with several skin changes. These changes are so common, they are considered a part of normal pregnancy. During the postpartum period these changes will resolve to varying degrees. Hyperpigmentation of the skin such as the **linea nigra**, is believed to be the result of the effects of estrogen and progesterone on the epidermis during pregnancy. This generally fades in the postpartum period. **Chloasma,** or the mask of pregnancy, usually resolves after delivery, but for some women may persist in some degree for months or years, particularly if the woman chooses to use oral contraceptives. New **melanotic nevi,** or a change in existing nevi, may also occur during pregnancy (Rapini, 1999).

### Changes in Structure

Another normal change of pregnancy is the dilation  and proliferation of blood vessels. This is often seen in the skin as **telangiectasias** and **spider angiomas.** Both lesions may regress spontaneously postpartum. **Striae,** the stretch marks of pregnancy, are tears in the dermal connective tissue and during pregnancy appear as red or purple bands on the abdomen, breasts, thighs, buttocks, groin, and axillae. Despite many claims of effective therapy, none exists that will prevent or affect their course. Ordinarily these will fade during the postpartum period. **Skin tags** are another change in connective tissue and are common in pregnancy. They may often persist after pregnancy unless removed (Rapini, 1999).

Many postpartum women will also be alarmed by or notice hair loss on the comb or after washing. This also may be due to the effect of pregnancy hormones on the growth cycle of hair. The severity of the loss varies greatly, but regrowth normally occurs by 9 months after delivery (Rapini, 1999).

### Breaks in the Skin

Postpartum women may have wounds as a result of surgical interventions (episiotomy or surgical delivery) or birth-related trauma. REEDA (**r**edness, **e**dema, **e**cchymosis, **d**rainage, **a**pproximation) is a scoring system that may be used to assess perineal wounds or surgical wounds resulting from a cesarean section or postpartum tubal ligation. Each element is rated on a scale of 0 to 3, depending on the severity of findings. Normally, scores should range from 0 to 6 on the first postpartum day, 0 to 8 on the second postpartum day, 0 to 7 after 1 week, and by 2 weeks postpartum, 0 to 1 (Davidson, 1974).

***Nursing Role.*** Assess the integrity of the woman's skin. Use the REEDA scoring system as part of the documentation of your findings. Explain to the woman the healing process and the self-care that may facilitate the healing process. Review with her what findings should be reported immediately. The woman should report the following:

- Oral temperature >100.4° F (38° C)
- Increased redness, edema, wound tenderness, or drainage from the incision
- Breakdown or separation of the incision line

If the woman had a surgical delivery, her ability for self-care may be delayed. Box 15-6 provides additional areas of assessment.

## Neurologic System

Many postpartum women report the occurrence of headache, especially during the first week postpartum. These are generally mild, bifrontal, and are either self-limiting or respond to mild analgesics (Creasy and Resnik, 1999).

Women who have had spinal or epidural anesthesia during labor may experience a spinal headache resulting from leakage of cerebrospinal fluid from the site of puncture. Typically this headache is experienced when the woman lifts her head or is in the upright position. It generally improves by the third postpartum day and in most cases is absent by the fifth postpartum day (Scott and others, 1990; Cunningham and others, 1997). Treatment includes non-narcotic analgesics, bedrest, caffeine and increased fluid intake (Scott and others, 1990). However, some women experience the headache and auditory and visual problems for weeks (Scott and others, 1990; Cunningham and others, 1997). The woman who experiences severe symptoms requires further assessment by her primary care provider and specific interventions.

**Carpal tunnel syndrome** is common during pregnancy, probably as a result of fluid retention. Symptoms

generally clear within about 3 months postpartum. For symptoms that are intolerable, do not remit spontaneously, or resolve with physical therapy, surgery may be indicated (Aminoff, 1999).

## Gastrointestinal System

Various symptoms and complaints related to gastrointestinal functioning are common in pregnancy. These include heartburn, constipation, nausea and vomiting, alteration in appetite, and feelings of bloatedness after eating. Elevated levels of progesterone are thought to contribute to these problems, and with the return of progesterone to prepregnant levels in the postpartum, these symptoms may be expected to resolve.

Regardless of the method of delivery, many women experience a delay in return of their normal bowel function. It is determined that normal bowel function has occurred when the woman is able to tolerate a regular

---

### BOX 15-6   *Nursing Care Considerations Related to Surgical Delivery*

1. Assess ability to care for self. Mothers who are postpartum after a surgical delivery are experiencing the effects of anesthesia, decreased strength and endurance, and physical discomfort as well as the normal activities of maintaining a home and caring for a newborn and family. (To judge if she is doing too much, ask yourself, would we be expecting her to take on the same level of care of an infant and her family if she had just had a laparotomy for any other reasons? If not, help her to receive assistance.)
2. Ascertain the severity/duration of her discomfort. The discomfort of surgery may affect her emotional and behavioral responses making it impossible for her to focus on self-care activities until her need for comfort is met. Pain also saps a person's energy and makes it difficult to sleep.
3. If the woman received a spinal or epidural, also assess for the presence of spinal headache. The upright position may be associated with an intense headache. If so, her activities need to be modified and additional assistance provided.
4. Assess psychologic status. Physical and mental pain interfere with her desire, motivation, and ability to assume independent self-care.
5. Determine availability of support from family and friends. Having help at home lessens the burden on the mother, leaving her with more energy for self-care activities.
6. Refer to and collaborate with community agencies for ongoing assistance in the home.

From Doenges ME and Moorhouse MF: *Maternal/newborn plans of care: guidelines for individualizing care,* ed 3, Philadelphia, 1999, FA Davis.

diet and has experienced her first bowel movement. Factors contributing to a delay in normal bowel functioning might include the administration of a cleansing enema at admission, diminished abdominal muscle tone, alteration of intraabdominal pressure, and insufficient fluids or food. If a woman has a perineal wound or hemorrhoids, she may be afraid of the pain a bowel movement might create and hold back.

 ***Nursing Role.*** Learning a woman's fluid and food intake is the first step. Discussing the subject of bowel movements and any concerns the woman might have helps reveal her concerns. Several activities may help her be comfortable as she returns to a pattern of normal bowel movements. To prevent or treat constipation, encourage the mother to:

- Ambulate and/or exercise as tolerated.
- Avoid use of medications that have constipating side effects, if possible; consider nonpharmacologic relief measures when possible (e.g., acupressure, massage, progressive relaxation).
- Drink ample fluids (6 to 8 glasses per day of noncaffeinated, nonalcoholic beverages).
- Drink apple juice. It contains sorbitol, a natural sugar with laxative properties.
- Eat a diet high in fresh fruits and vegetables, whole grain cereals, or breads.
- Discuss any fears that she may have about pain.
- Use relief measures to prevent or relieve pain related to defecation (e.g., local anesthetics, sitz baths [soaking her perineum in a warm bath]).
- Use stool softeners as indicated (in the case of extensive repairs or hemorrhoids) to assist defecation.
- Take a glycerin suppository, bisacodyl suppository, or milk of magnesia if unable to have a bowel movement within 2 to 3 days of instituting measures.
- Avoid bearing down to move bowels or use of rectal suppositories or enemas because these might produce breakdown of the healing suture line in those women with extensive perineal repairs.

## Endocrine System

### Resumption of Ovulation and Menstruation

Following the delivery of the placenta, the levels of gonadotropins and progesterone rapidly decrease. As progesterone levels drop, prolactin levels increase. The initiation of lactation further increases these levels. Low levels of follicle-stimulating hormone and luteinizing hormone are experienced in the lactating woman. The resumption of ovulation and menstruation depends on the frequency and duration of breastfeeding. Generally, if a woman does not breastfeed, her menses will return in 6 to 8 weeks; however, a specific date is difficult to determine because many women will bleed small amounts intermittently beginning soon after delivery. For the breastfeeding mother, menses may occur as soon as 2 or as late as 18 months after delivery, depending on the frequency and duration of breastfeeding (Cunningham and others, 1997).

The return of ovulation may occur as early as 36 days after delivery. Research has shown that breastfeeding may delay the return of ovulation; however, lactation does not prevent the possibility of ovulation. Findings indicate the following: (1) resumption of ovulation is frequently marked by normal menstrual bleeding; (2) breastfeeding episodes lasting 15 minutes seven times a day will delay ovulation; (3) ovulation can occur without menstrual bleeding; and (4) menstrual bleeding can be anovulatory (Cunningham and others, 1997). The practice of supplementing breastfeeding with formula or food may lead to the earlier return of ovulation, and women who breastfeed for less than 28 days may have a return of ovulation similar to women who did not breastfeed at all (Resnik, 1999). For these reasons, women should be encouraged to use some form of contraception in the postpartum period regardless of whether their menses has returned.

##  POSTPARTUM PSYCHOSOCIAL ASSESSMENT

The first pregnancy, in particular, and beginning motherhood, in general, call for major psychosocial adjustments. Assessment of the postpartum woman should include exploration of the psychosocial adaptation of the new mother to her role. As the woman begins to mother her newborn infant she is challenged with integrating the new role of motherhood into her identity. After giving birth, postpartum women experience various feelings. A variation in moods is the normal result of the many adjustments that go hand-in-hand with the transition to parenthood and the physical and emotional stresses of childbirth and involution.

### Postpartum Blues

The postpartum woman may report feelings of **emotional lability** that are particularly confusing to them. Women may find themselves crying and yet not understand why. Adding to this normal variation in moods, many women report having difficulty concentrating; being irritable, tearful, and/or anxious; feeling inadequate; and being physically and emotionally fatigued. Additionally, some women report sleep disturbances and changes in appetite. These symptoms are generally transient lasting from 1 day up to 2 weeks and have been labeled as "postpartum blues," "baby blues," or "maternity blues." The condition affects 75% to 80% of American women and has an early postpartum onset, generally beginning within a few days after childbirth, although the onset may occur anytime from 1 to 10 days following childbirth (Ugarriza, 1992).

Initially these symptoms were thought to be a manifestation of the hormonal changes experienced in the initial postpartum period; however, research has not substantiated this claim (Affonso, 1992; Beck, Reynolds, and Rutowski, 1992). Lack of social support, ego adjustments, fatigue, and physical discomfort have been found to correlate with these symptoms, but have not been proven causative (Affonso, 1992; Beck and others, 1992; Beck, 1993). Outward expression of these feelings may be upsetting to the new mother and her significant others, because these feelings are not consistent with ideal expectations of the "happy new mother." However, crying or some other form of tension release, sleep and emotional support, and "mothering" of the new mother have been shown to be helpful interventions.

Many women experiencing these symptoms feel guilty for not feeling the way they believe the happy new mother should be feeling. Moreover, they may think they are going crazy and worry that by sharing these thoughts someone will view them as an unfit mother. New mothers and their families need anticipatory guidance and support to understand that the blues are a normal, temporary, self-limiting state that will generally pass within 1 to 10 days (O'Hara and Engeldinger, 1989; Association of Women's Health, Obstetric and Neonatal Nurses [AWHONN], 1998; Epperson, 1999).

*Nursing Role.* Postpartum women need opportunities to discuss these often troubling symptoms and often benefit from speaking with other women who have experienced similar symptoms. We can usually approach the subject of the "blues" by using principles of universality, for example, "Many women in the initial postpartum period experience symptoms of. . . . Is this something of concern to you now?" This approach often opens a door to communication that might be too difficult for the woman to openly acknowledge. Additional assessment questions based on symptoms are found in Table 15-2.

Women with symptoms should be given reassurances that they are not alone and that these symptoms will pass. Use of this approach may also serve as a means of providing anticipatory guidance to those not experiencing symptoms.

We play a key role in assisting the new mother and family to adjust to the many postpartum changes and challenges that will be encountered. The woman and her family should be encouraged to assist us in developing a plan of care that will fit with their particular situation. Families should be encouraged to monitor for symptoms that may require further intervention. In developing a plan of care, it is important to be sensitive to the history and culture of the woman and the needs, beliefs, support systems, and resources of the family. Per-

sonal expectations, cultural beliefs, and differences in lifestyle affect each woman's postpartum psychologic course differently (Box 15-7). Although the postpartum blues are generally mild and transient, approximately 12% of women experience more significant symptoms of postpartum depression (Albright, 1993). Postpartum depression and postpartum psychosis generally manifest later in the postpartal period (see Chapter 20).

## PSYCHOSOCIAL ADAPTATION IN THE POSTPARTUM PERIOD

The psychosocial adaptation process involves the mother, the infant, other family members, and their support network. It is interactive and developmental, evolving through some predictable and assessable stages. Supportive care helps the individuals to become a family.

### The Parent-Infant Acquaintance Process

Over the last several decades a good deal of research has been generated to describe the parent-infant acquaintance process. Whether maternal- and paternal-infant acquaintance behaviors should be considered as separate or similar phenomena remains controversial; however, it seems that differences and similarities do exist (Jones and Lenz, 1989; Jordan, 1990). Research continues in this area and is based on an understanding of the significance of this acquaintance process to the development of a loving and nurturing parent-infant relationship. Further, it is recognized that a positive parent-infant relationship fosters the emotional and physical growth and development of the child. The terms bond-

| TABLE 15-2 *Assessment of Postpartum Blues* | |
|---|---|
| **Symptom** | **Question** |
| Dysphoric mood | How would you best describe your mood recently? |
| Labile mood | How easily do your moods change? |
| Crying | How frequently have you had crying episodes? |
| Anxiety | How much anxiety or nervousness have you been experiencing? |
| Insomnia | How difficult is it for you to sleep? How many hours of sleep are you getting per night? |
| Loss of appetite | How is your appetite? What did you have to eat today? Yesterday? |
| Irritability | How often have you felt irritated or angered lately? |

Adapted from O'Hara MW and Engeldinger J: Postpartum mood disorders, detection and prevention, *The Female Patient* 14:136-141, 1989.

---

**BOX 15-7**    *Nursing Care Considerations Related to Transition to Parenthood, Unsatisfactory Social Support, and Fatigue*

- It is important for the woman to recognize that she is not alone. Many women experience these symptoms. The woman needs reassurance that the symptoms are normal and will generally pass in 1 to 10 days.
- Encourage the woman to talk to others about the way she is feeling and what she does and doesn't find helpful:

  Partner, family, friends

  Support group members
- Encourage the woman to get plenty of rest:

  Create visiting hours

  Nap when the infant does if possible

  Get to bed early

  Avoid caffeinated beverages

  Use relaxation techniques to decrease anxiety
- Encourage the woman to eat a well-balanced diet to assist in the physiologic healing process:

  Allow others to make meals (e.g., family, friends, church groups, and civic groups)

  Eat "take-out"

  Eat simple, frequent, nourishing snacks
- Encourage the woman to take friends and family members up on offers of help.
- Assist the woman to understand that availing herself of help is not a sign of weakness or incapability; conversely, recognizing the need for help is a strength.
- Encourage the woman to accept offers of help to plan some time for meeting her own needs for rest and relaxation:

  Naps, exercise, meals, bathing

  An outing with your partner or friends
- Seek out and use available community resources to meet needs. Provide referrals as appropriate.
- Reinforce the importance of keeping her appointments. This allows for serial assessment of involution change, including the presence and progression or regression of depressive symptoms.
- Teach the woman and her family to call if she expresses thoughts about harming herself or her infant. This may be a sign of significantly worsening symptoms that could result in harm to the woman or her infant.

Adapted from Carpenito LJ: *Nursing diagnosis: application to clinical practice,* ed 7, Philadelphia, 1997, Lippincott.

---

ing and attachment are commonly used to describe the evolution of this relational process (Mercer, 1982; Klaus and Kennel, 1982, 1995) (Figure 15-3).

### Bonding

The term **bonding** has traditionally been used to describe the unidirectional attraction felt by the parent towards the infant. Allowing the parents and infant uninterrupted time together, particularly during the initial hour following birth can facilitate bonding. This time period is a so-called sensitive time period because the infant is in a quiet, alert stage. When medically possible, delay of initial procedures such as the prophylactic administration of medications, will allow this relational process to unfold. Initially, it was felt that the period immediately following birth was a critical time period in which bonding must occur. This misinterpretation of the research findings resulted in unwarranted fears that bonding would not occur if initial parent-infant contact was limited. It is now recognized that bonding and attachment can occur at a later point in time when necessary (Klaus and Kennell, 1982; Mercer, 1982; Mercer and Ferketich, 1994).

### Attachment

**Attachment** is an interactive process between the parent and infant through which an enduring parent-infant relationship develops. Attachment begins during preg-

nancy and continues through the first postpartum year. As dependent beings, infants depend on this relationship to meet their needs for growth and development. Ideally, through the process of attachment, parents experience pleasure and satisfaction in the parental role and learn to subordinate their own needs, accept infant care responsibilities, and establish an identity as a mother or father. Unlike bonding, attachment is a reciprocal relationship that requires the mutual and reciprocal exchange of signals between the partners in the process (Klaus and Kennel, 1982).

### Infant Behaviors that Facilitate Attachment

Infants are said to have a repertoire of behaviors and abilities that assist them in developing relationships with others. These abilities include signaling behaviors (crying, cooing, and smiling); making and maintaining eye contact; tracking objects in their visual field; grasping, enfolding, or cuddling; moving synchronously in response to the rhythms and patterns of a familiar voice (entrainment); and rooting, suckling, and latching on to the breast. These behaviors are felt to be crucial in bringing the parents into close physical proximity with the infant, as well as initiating and maintaining contact (Brazleton, 1986).

Likewise, through the reciprocal use of touch, spatial relations, positioning, gaze, and vocalization, parents transmit cues to the infant that assist in the attachment process. In order for attachment to proceed in a smooth

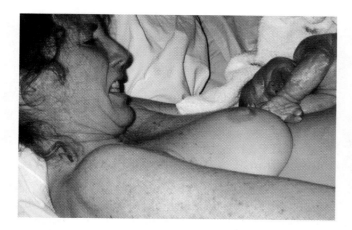

FIGURE 15-3 ● Mother begins bonding with newborn. *(Courtesy of Caroline E. Brown.)*

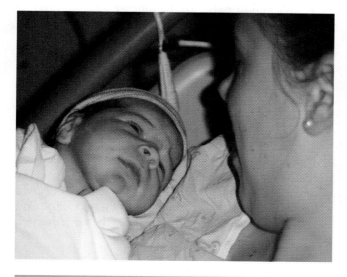

FIGURE 15-4 ● Mother and newborn gazing at each other, beginning the attachment process.

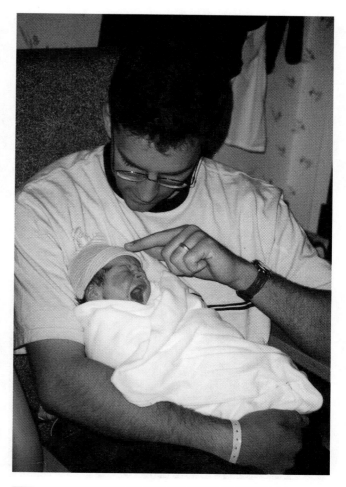

FIGURE 15-5 ● Father inspecting newborn.

fashion, the parent must possess the ability to trust, to communicate and provide care, and he or she must be within close physical proximity of the infant (Mercer, 1982; Brazleton, 1986).

Before the initiation of attachment, the parent "claims" the infant as a family member through identifying the features of the infant that are similar to those of other family members (Rubin, 1977). The progression of attachment will be aided by a congruence between the characteristics of the real infant and the ideal or imagined infant, including satisfaction of the parent with the sex of the infant, the infant's temperament, physical appearance, and state of health (Rubin, 1977; Mercer, 1982).

### Parent-Infant Communication

Studies of newborns indicate that they can purposefully react to stimuli, and therefore their behavior can provide significant cues regarding how they are feeling. In the initial postpartum period, social behaviors of the infant include crying, reflexive movements, and visual attentiveness to objects within the field of gaze. These social behaviors act as cues for the parents to respond to and serve as the basis of the emerging parent-infant relationship. In a pattern of reciprocal cues, infants respond to the care and attention that the parents give to them and, likewise, parents' attitudes and responses toward the infant are shaped by these responses. Further, through this interactional process, the parents form perceptions of their self-competence in performing parenting skills.

Signs of positive bonding behaviors include maintaining close physical contact, making eye-to-eye contact, speaking in soft, high-pitched tones, and touching and exploring the infant. Attachment behaviors include reciprocal responses from the infant to the parent's solicitations and vice-versa. For example, as the mother or father gazes into the eyes and face of the newborn, the alert newborn returns the gaze and studies the face of the parent (Figures 15-4 to 15-6).

Likewise, as the infant cries, the parents respond to the cries and offer comfort, care, or feeding. **Synchrony** or the "fit" between response and cue between the parent and infant is mutually rewarding and enhances the parent-infant attachment (Klaus and Kennel, 1995).

Parents and infants may likewise exhibit cues that inhibit attachment (Gerson, 1973; Klaus and Kennel, 1982, 1995). Caution must be applied, however, when interpreting the bonding and attachment behaviors of parent-infant dyads because the process proceeds in a very individualized manner, depending on several health and cultural variables. Infants that exhibit feeding difficulties, sleeping problems, congenital anomalies, or health problems may pose challenges in creating an attachment. Parents of these infants may need additional assistance

with interpretation of the infant's cues and making adjustments based on realistic expectations of the infant's characteristics and capabilities. Likewise, parents who are developmentally challenged or who have physical or psychologic problems of their own may need further assistance in developing a mutually satisfying and positive parent-infant relationship (Table 15-3, Box 15-8).

## Maternal Factors that Influence Attachment and the Transition to Maternal Role

A considerable amount of research has been done on factors that influence maternal-infant attachment and the transition to the maternal role. In general, the findings of this body of research indicate that the following factors serve as influences on this parent-infant relationship:

- Age and/or parity of the mother
- Maternal health
- Maternal self-concept
- Culture
- Social support
- Socioeconomic status
- Birth experience
- Desire to bear children

### Age-Related Issues

Advancing maternal age is associated with increased physical risks that might affect the health of the new mother and her ability to establish a relationship with the newborn infant (Berkowitz and others, 1990). Conversely, older mothers are generally better educated,

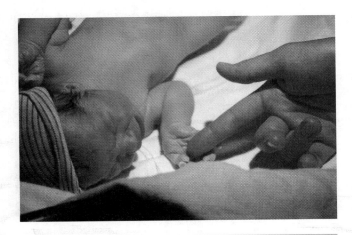

FIGURE 15-6 • Newborn grabbing father's finger.

---

**BOX 15-8** *Nursing Care Considerations for Parent-Infant Attachment*

1. Assess for risk factors, including a lack of support from family or significant others; multiple demands of home and family; excess fatigue; unrealistic expectations for self/infant/partner; presence of stressors such as financial, housing, or employment concerns; use of outside help or extended family.
2. Assess client/couple interaction with the infant. In American culture attachment is considered positive when parents make eye contact with the infant, call the infant by name, use an en face position, talk in a high-pitched voice, and hold the baby close.
3. Note the effect of culture on interaction. Different cultures have different values/beliefs about what constitutes positive attachment behaviors. Lack of culturally appropriate attachment behaviors places the infant at risk for abuse.
4. Assess client/couple strengths and weaknesses, maturity level, reaction to conception, and preparation for

parenting. These directly affect the ability to parent, the desire to gain comfort in the role, and the ability to be skillful in parenting.
5. Determine the client/couple perception of infant behaviors. When parents hold unrealistic perceptions of infant behaviors they are at higher risk for abusive or neglectful actions. Also parents who are unhappy about child care tasks such as diapering or feeding are at higher risk. These parents need more support and monitoring.
6. Refer to and collaborate with other community agencies to meet the needs of the client/couple for ongoing follow-up as needed.
7. Document your findings, the verbal and nonverbal responses as well as the positive or negative behaviors. Your record provides the assessment of the family situation, ongoing interventions, evaluation of progress and the path of collaboration with community resources.

From Doenges ME and Moorhouse MF: *Maternal/newborn plans of care: guidelines for individualizing care*, ed 3, Philadelphia, 1999, FA Davis.

have more material resources, and a greater repertoire of human resources to deal with the challenges presented by parenting (Queenan, 1987; O'Reilly-Green and Cohen, 1993; Stark, 1997). However, many older mothers have invested considerable time and energy into

careers that may present role conflicts in the transition to parenthood. Adolescent mothers may experience greater health risks, developmental conflicts, and role conflicts related to the demands of parenting. Mothers of any age may find that role conflicts arise because of the

**TABLE 15-3   *Assessment of Infant Characteristics that May Influence Attachment***

| Area of assessment | Critical thinking | Questions |
|---|---|---|
| Sex of the infant | Did the parents have a strong gender preference? How did the infant's gender meet with their expectations? If applicable, how do they seem to be handling this difference between expectations and reality? | Were you hoping for a boy or a girl? Did the parents have a strong gender preference? Does this infant meet those expectations? |
| Gestational age of the infant | Is the infant viewed as vulnerable? Did the early or late arrival of the infant have a negative effect on the parents'/families' attitudes toward the infant? Do members of the family seem pleased with the arrival of the infant? | When was the baby due? How did you feel about the baby being late/early? Were you prepared for this? How did your partner react? How did your family react? |
| Health of the infant<br>• Do the parents take an interest in health care decision-making for the infant?<br>• Do parents visit the nursery, call the nursery, inquire about the infant?<br>• Do the parents partake of opportunities to care for the infant? | Have the parents been able to spend time with the infant since the birth? Does the health of the infant preclude physical contact or the ability to care for or feed the infant? Do the parents seem hesitant to create an attachment with the infant because of its condition or prognosis? | How much contact have you been able to have with the infant since he/she was born? How long is this separation expected to last? What have you been told about the infant's condition? Have you been given a long-term prognosis? |
| Physical appearance of the infant<br>• What remarks are made about the infant's appearance? | Does the infant bear a resemblance to someone in the family? How do they feel about this person (positively or negatively)? Do the parents have any pet names for the infant? | Who does the infant resemble? What do you think about that? or How do you feel about that? |
| Presence of anomalies<br>• Observe reactions to the infant<br>• Observe parent-infant interactions as well as interactions between parents and extended family<br>• Observe for signs of bonding and attachment | Does the infant have any outward physical anomalies? How are the parents reacting to this? What are their fears or concerns? | Do you have any concerns about the appearance of your baby? How do you feel about . . . ? |
| Temperament of the infant<br>• Observe interactions for signs of bonding and attachment<br>• Observe for reciprocity of cues<br>• Observe for signs of frustration | How does the temperament of the infant fit with the temperament of the mother? How does the temperament of the infant fit with the mother's partner? Do you sense any frustration or feelings of lack of parental competence? What terms do they use to describe the infant's behaviors? | How are things going between you and the baby? |

Adapted from Gerson E: *Infant behavior in the first year of life,* New York, 1973, Raven Press; Klaus MH and Kennell JH: *Parent-infant bonding,* St Louis, 1982, Mosby; Klaus MH and Kennell JH: *Bonding: building the foundations of secure attachment and independence,* Reading, Mass, 1995, Addison-Wesley; Denehy JA: Interventions related to parent-infant attachment, *Nurs Clin North Am* 27:425, 1992.

challenges that parenting places on personal aspirations; however, this is more likely to occur in the career woman or the young, adolescent mother. Both older and younger mothers are more likely to have misperceptions with regard to parenting the infant. Often the older mother has very high expectations of herself as a mother and has difficulty with adjusting to the lifestyle changes that occur in her partnership as a result of childbearing (Cain, 1994). Conversely, the adolescent mother often has unrealistic expectations of the infant and likewise may have difficulty adjusting to the lifestyle changes that occur in peer relationships as a result of childbearing.

### Maternal Health

The physical or emotional health of the new mother can have an effect on attachment behaviors. Women who are physically ill may not have the physical strength to engage in developing a relationship with the newborn. Likewise women who are experiencing emotional problems or a psychiatric illness may not be able to engage fully in a relationship. In particular, they may not recognize or be able to respond well to the infant's cues. In most cases, these women are not fully incapacitated and with support they can be assisted in the attachment process by continually cueing them into the infant's signals and/or assisting them to respond to the infant's needs. As far as is reasonably and safely possible, attempts should be made to involve the mother in the care of her infant (Klaus and Kennell, 1982; 1995).

### Maternal Self-Concept

As a woman begins mothering her infant, she is faced with the task of integrating the new role of motherhood into her self-concept. In doing this she must work through her feelings about the new role, define her conception of motherhood, and redefine her self-concept, both as she is and ideally would like to be (Dimitrovsky, Lev, and Itskowitz, 1998). Maternal self-concept, or how the mother feels about herself, may affect her adaptation to motherhood and her self-evaluation of parenting behaviors. In general, a positive self-concept has been correlated with positive self-evaluations of one's parenting skills. Parental perceptions of competence have been found to be important predictors of parental attachment behaviors in low- and high-risk situations (Mercer and Ferketich, 1990).

### Culture

Parental expectations and parenting actions vary, depending on cultural beliefs and practices. In any society, childbirth is of social significance and signals a time of transition in which realignment of roles, responsibilities, and relationships occurs. These rites of passage have been referred to as **matresence** (mother becoming) and **patresence** (father becoming) (Raphael, 1976).

Although western culture places primary emphasis on the event of birth, many cultures place greater emphasis on the postpartum period. Postpartum may be viewed as a state of impurity or pollution that requires ritual seclusion of the mother and infant and elimination of activity to reduce inviting misfortune. Proscriptions may exist against contact with others, contact with food or objects, and avoidance of sexual relations. These practices may serve to reduce risks of infection; promoted healing, lactation, and attachment; and prevented closely spaced pregnancies (Lauderdale and Greener, 1995; Andrews and Boyle, 1999).

A woman's cultural background influences how the woman behaves and interacts with her newborn during the postpartum period (Andrews and Boyle, 1999). Specific cultural assessments in the postpartum period should include information about postpartum rituals, the parent's beliefs with regard to the role of the mother and/or the role of the father, infant feeding practices, and parental expectations for the infant's behavior. Only by understanding and respecting the values and beliefs of each woman and her family can we make accurate assessments of parenting behaviors.

### Social Support

Support from the father of the baby and extended family has been shown to be associated with less maternal stress and greater feelings of parental competence (Friedman, 1998). Social networks of family and friends are an important aspect of social support in the initial postpartum period. Positive emotional relationships are critical to the enhancement of mothering skills (Crawford, 1985). Conversely, social networks can be a source of conflict, particularly when beliefs and values surrounding childbearing are in conflict because of cultural or generational differences, or when roles, relationships, and boundaries are blurred (Wright and Leahey, 1984; 1994).

### Socioeconomic Conditions

Socioeconomic status is often closely related to the mother's educational level and affect the human, material, and emotional resources available to the mother to deal with the stressors of parenting. Life experiences and education may influence how knowledgeable the mother is about child care and health and subsequently make the adaptation to the parenting role smoother (Friedman, 1998). In families where resources are inadequate or stretched thin by the addition of a new family member, considerable stress may be experienced that interferes with establishment of a positive attachment with the infant.

### Birth Experience

It is common for the postpartum woman to engage in critical reflection on the birth process (Rubin, 1977; Konrad, 1987). When the idealized birth varies greatly from the actual birth process, mourning the loss of expectations

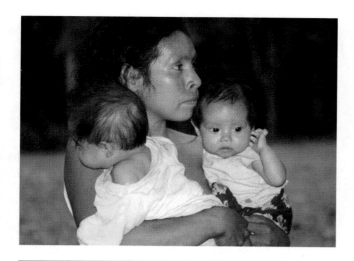

FIGURE 15-7 • When there are two infants, care and feeding become more complex. *(Courtesy of Caroline E. Brown.)*

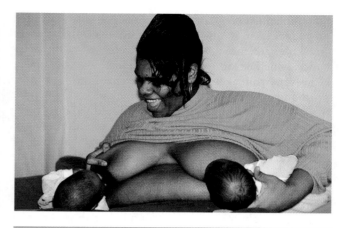

FIGURE 15-8 • Mothers of twins often breastfeed both babies at the same time. *(Courtesy of Caroline E. Brown.)*

must occur before adjustment to the actual birth experience can occur. Perceptions of the birth have been found to have a significant positive correlation with the woman's sense of gratification in the maternal role and with mothering behaviors (Deutscher, 1970). Relative factors found to have a positive influence on perceptions of birth include (1) earlier contact with the infant, (2) greater positive experiences in the year surrounding the birth, (3) greater social network, (4) greater physical and emotional support from a partner, (5) a higher positive self-concept, (6) fewer illnesses, (7) a healthier infant at birth, (8) a less complicated birth, and (9) positive feelings about the pregnancy (Mercer, 1981; Mercer, Hackley, and Bostrom, 1983).

### Birth of Multiple Infants

Even if expected, the birth of multiples may present challenges to the attachment process. The mother begins to attach to the infants as a unit, becoming comfortable with her celebrity status and role as a mother of multiples. She then attaches to each infant as an individual, spending a great deal of time learning their differences. Attachment is a highly individualized process; therefore, each infant develops a distinctive relationship with the mother. Obviously, it takes extra time and effort to get to know each infant as a separate and unique individual. The mother of multiples will benefit from use of extra formal and informal support systems during this transition (Gromada, 1992) (Figure 15-7).

If the mother is breastfeeding the infants, she may sometimes feed them together for expediency and sometime feed each of them separately for a little time alone with each of them. Some mothers of multiples find it helpful to feed the babies with a combination of breast and bottle feeding so that they can share the responsibilities of feeding with others (Figure 15-8).

With the development and increasing use of new technologies that improve fertility, we are more likely to encounter the family with twins, triplets, quadruplets, quintuplets, or even sextuplets. These pregnancies bring their own special health risks for both the mother and the fetuses (see Chapters 17 and 18 for discussion of higher risk pregnancy). In addition, the birth of multiples brings increased financial, emotional, psychologic, and logistic stresses to the postpartum family. These families may struggle with the financial needs incurred with loss of the woman's income during pregnancy and the additional expense of specialized care during the pregnancy and the obtaining of additional nursery supplies and equipment. Financial issues may also be faced in terms of an unexpected delay in returning to work.

The multiple gestation may have presented emotional issues such as the need to consider selective termination, concerns about maternal and fetal health, long periods of bed rest or curtailed activity, threats of preterm labor, and the process and timing of the birth itself. With the birth of the babies, the family now continues to invest emotionally as they adapt to the multiple personalities and needs of the babies. The family also needs to make decisions about how to relate to the babies in terms of their separateness or togetherness. The physical environment of the home may even be challenged with a loss of personal and family living space. To meet all of the needs of this postpartum family, support from others in their network may need to be mobilized. The organization of this support may involve identifying what tasks will be delegated, to whom, and for how long. Families may also benefit from referral to local groups such as Mothers of Twins or Mothers of Multiples, and LaLeche League; or to publications such as *Twins* (Walton, Collins, and Linney, 1994).

### Desire for Childbearing

Some pregnancies are planned, while others are unplanned or even, unwanted. It is important to understand that unplanned pregnancies are not necessarily unwanted pregnancies. It is also important to realize that most women experience ambivalence with regard to the pregnancy, whether or not it was planned or unplanned. However, women who have experienced prolonged or profound ambivalence about the pregnancy may exhibit **malattachment** or rejection of the infant in the early postpartum period (Lederman, 1996). This rejection may be demonstrated postpartally through limited handling of the infant; negative comments about the infant's appearance or behavior; failure to look at, touch, or name the infant; failure to demonstrate an interest in the infant's signals or care; or a failure to meet the infant's needs.

Interestingly, research has found that those couples who have experienced infertility may find the act of childbearing to have mixed psychologic consequences. On the one hand, while they are elated by the prospect of having a child, this may alienate them from other infertile couples who have been a source of social support to them through a difficult process. Likewise, they may have difficulty connecting to other childbearing couples who have not lived with the specter of infertility. Because of their long journey to childbearing, the couple may distrust their good fortune and have fears about their infant's health and well-being that can interfere with forming healthy attachments.

The state of altered parenting is one "in which one or more caregivers demonstrates a real or potential inability to provide a constructive environment that nurtures the growth and development of the child" (Carpenito, 1997). In any case, the role of nursing is to assist the family in forming healthy attachments, assist the childbearing woman or couple to acknowledge that a problem exists, provide a safe environment for the infant, and make the necessary referrals for assistance (Carpenito, 1997).

### Age-Related Issues: Adolescent Mothers

Adolescent parenting may present unique challenges to establishing healthy attachments. The egocentrism and concrete thinking exhibited in some adolescents may interfere with effective parenting (Tiller, 1991; Passino and others, 1993). The ability of the adolescent mother to parent effectively depends, to a great extent, on her ability to read her infant's cues and respond appropriately. Many factors may affect this ability such as the mother's emotional and cognitive development, educational level, past experiences, support systems, resources and stressors. While adolescent mothers have been shown to be capable of providing loving and attentive physical care, infants born to adolescent mothers are more likely to be neglected or to die as a result of accidents or domestic violence often because of ignorance, inexperience, and immaturity (McAnarney and Greydanus, 1989).

Studies reveal that pregnant adolescents often have poorer relationships with their families and peers (Passino and others, 1993); are often victims of abuse

or neglect themselves (Cappel and Heiner, 1990; Miller and Robertson, 1990; Aylward, 1992; Hall, Sachs, and Rayens, 1998; Williams and Vines, 1999); and exhibit more learning, social, or behavioral problems (East and Felice, 1990). Based on these findings, adolescent mothers are at greater risk for malattachment and its sequelae. In light of this, adolescent mothers and their families generally need special assistance as they transition to the parental role.

Although becoming an adolescent parent is not ideal and may have lasting negative consequences in terms of achieving developmental milestones, this need not be the case if timely and appropriate interventions are instituted (Roosa, 1983; Geronimus and Korenman, 1992; Or, Tari, and Fine, 1992; Arenson, 1994; Williams and Vines, 1999). Studies of adolescent mothers and their transition to motherhood have found that becoming a parent could, alternately, provide an opportunity for the adolescent to receive social support, build more positive family relationships, and develop greater ego strength (Arenson, 1994; Burke and Liston, 1994; Smith-Battle, 1995; Williams and Vines, 1999).

However, the adolescent mother may feel alienated from her peers and the activities they engage in. Therefore, added to the need to reconcile changes in their self-image and to subordinate their own needs for those of the infant, is the need for the adolescent mother to renegotiate other relationships.

In a small qualitative study of previously neglected or abused adolescent mothers, it was reported that these mothers viewed parenting as a "second chance for a successful and fulfilling life" and allowed them the opportunity to overcome difficult childhood experiences (Williams and Vines, 1999). Further, successful maternal-infant developmental outcomes were found when the adolescent lived with either her partner or the infant's grandmother. In these cases, the presence of a second caregiver appeared to be beneficial. These findings suggest that parenting presents an opportunity for us to work with adolescent mothers and their families to develop positive helping relationships that may have real and lasting consequences (Spieker and Bensley, 1994).

We must assess the adolescent mother's parenting abilities, including her ability to read and respond effectively to the infant's cues; her problem-solving abilities; her understanding of the infant's abilities; and her ability to meet the infant's physical, social, and emotional needs. An assessment of available social and instrumental supports needs to be made, including an assessment of anticipated needs. We need to develop an understanding of the meaning of the parenting experience to the young mother and her family, including how this is affecting their former roles and how they are dealing with issues related to the adolescent's needs for dependence versus independence. Additionally, identification of the individual and collective strengths and supports of the family needs to take place. After establishing a therapeutic relationship, the young mother and her family may be more receptive to teaching and connection with other support systems in the community.

## Maternal Adaptation Process

Following birth, the mother begins an exploration process that enables her to identify the features of the infant that make him or her similar to and different from other members of the family. This process leads to what has been termed **binding-in**. Binding-in, as described by Reva Rubin (1977), comes from the German *ein binding* and is used to describe the progressive and formative maternal-child relationship that occurs over a 12- to 15-month period, spanning from pregnancy to 6 months postpartum.

According to Rubin (1961), mothering is a set of skills that creates a social and physical environment that enables the optimal growth and development of the child. Development of the maternal identity and binding-in to the child are two processes that are said to occur concurrently through a dialectic process, "framed between the child and the mother's own significant world" (Rubin, 1977). Initial binding-in occurs during pregnancy through "awareness of" that is stimulated by fetal movements in utero and the changes in activities and lifestyle preferences that the pregnant woman makes in response to this growing awareness. Following delivery, binding-in accelerates significantly through identification of the infant as an objective human entity with its own characteristics and a claiming of the infant within the mother's social and familial context. That is, the mother comes to see the child as a member of her family. Identifying and claiming the infant allows the process of polarization to occur.

**Polarization** allows the mother to see herself physically, socially, and conceptually as a separate entity from the infant. The ability of the new mother to see herself as an intact, complete, and separate individual aids her in seeing the infant in a similar fashion. Likewise, this process allows the mother to reconstruct the family constellation to include the newborn as a member and accommodate to his or her own unique needs. Polarization proceeds slowly for the first several weeks postpartum and is said to be completed months later as the new mother recognizes her own needs for time and space and reasserts her needs as an individual person without losing sight of the infant's needs (Rubin, 1977).

### The Process of Adaptation to the Maternal Role

During the 1960s, Reva Rubin, a nursing theorist, identified phases that the postpartum woman goes through in the process of identifying herself as a mother. In the postpartum period these phases are defined as **taking in, taking hold,** and **letting go** (Rubin, 1961, 1977).

More recently, the length of these puerperal phases of adjustment have been called into question; however, it is still generally recognized that postpartum women do progress through phases of recovery, although this progression may occur more quickly than was previously thought (Ament, 1990). The three phases provide a useful guideline for assessing the postpartum woman and providing her with appropriate anticipatory guidance. In applying these guidelines, we need to consider individual circumstances such as current health and socioeconomic and cultural influences that may affect the woman's individual adaptation.

*Taking-in.* This phase typically occurs during the first day after delivery, although variation is normal (Ament, 1990). During this phase of adjustment, the woman is primarily concerned with her own physical and emotional needs. She may exhibit passive and dependent behavior and require assistance with self-care and decision making. The mother will often be very interested in the characteristics and behaviors of the infant, but may demonstrate little initiative in care taking and decision making with regard to the infant.

During this period the woman attempts to integrate the birth experience into a reality. The woman is often talkative and usually spends time recounting the details of the labor and delivery experience, particularly with those involved in the process, in an attempt to assimilate the details of the experience. Through this process the mother is able to accept that the pregnancy is over; and develops a sense of the infant as a separate and real individual. This recreation of events allows the mother to accept the reality of her current situation and begin her relationship with her infant. The mother's physical and emotional needs must be fulfilled for her to begin to recognize and meet the needs of her infant.

Because anxiety and preoccupation with her own physical and emotional needs may narrow a woman's perceptual abilities, information may need to be repeated. Additionally, physical discomforts common in the postpartum period can interfere with concentration, rest, and relaxation. In performing an assessment, we must elicit information about areas of discomfort because many women will hesitate to offer this information or ask for comfort measures, believing that pain is a normal part of the postpartum process and should, therefore, be accepted. Further, in planning the use of comfort measures, we need to consider the resources available and the woman's cultural beliefs.

The taking-in phase may be prolonged in those women who experience an unplanned surgical delivery or are dissatisfied with their birth experience. In these situations, women report having difficulty integrating the actual birth experience with the expected birth experience. These women often need assistance in understanding why certain interventions and decisions were necessary. Although the woman should have been given these explanations earlier, she may not have fully processed or understood what was happening because of anxiety, discomfort, or fatigue. This speaks to the need for postoperative or postpartum care that assists the woman to understand what she has experienced (AWHONN, 1998). It seems that the greater the perceived difference between the expected and the actual experience, the greater the dissatisfaction with the birth experience (Miovech and others, 1994). Helping the woman understand the circumstances that precipitated the need for a change in her expected birth plans may diminish this dissatisfaction. Additionally, it needs to be recognized that the woman that has experienced a surgical delivery will have increased dependency needs and require greater assistance with establishing a maternal-infant relationship (Reichert, Baron, and Fawcett, 1993).

***Taking Hold.*** This phase is said to peak on the second postpartum day and may last roughly 10 days. During this phase the woman will exhibit more independent behavior and begin to assume greater responsibility for her own self-care and the care of her infant. She moves from a state of relative self-absorption to one of interest in the events and people beyond herself. She begins to be more concerned with the health and well-being of her infant as manifested by making comparisons between her infant and other infants. Further, she is interested in learning about infant care and behavior. This period is often been referred to as the "teachable, reachable, and referable moment."

It is not uncommon during this period for the woman to verbalize anxiety about her abilities to resume some sense of control over her life and competence as a mother. During this period it is important for us to assist the woman to unveil her own capabilities as a mother. Mothers need opportunities to provide care for their infants and should receive praise and encouragement for their efforts. Resumption of responsibilities and unrealistic expectations of self may result in feelings of frustration, inadequacy, and exhaustion.

***Letting Go.*** "Letting go" is the period Rubin identified as one in which the woman lets go of idealized notions of the childbearing experience and past roles and relationships and begins to accept existing realities into her current life experience. Women may need to grieve the loss of idealized notions of their infant and their life. During this time they may also experience feelings of guilt and need sensitive, empathic care to help them understand that this is normal. This process requires readjustment of previously held roles and relationships. If childbearing is in conflict with other developmental needs or the pregnancy was unplanned, the feelings of loss and grief may be more acute and readjustment may be more difficult.

### Maternal Role Attainment

Ramona Mercer (1985, 1986, 1990), another nursing theorist, built on Rubin's work and described the process

of maternal role attainment. This process is said to begin before the birth of the infant and continue over a period of 3 to 10 months following the birth (Mercer, 1986). This process is a dialectic, requiring a continuous exchange between the mother and infant. The infant's continuous and evolving developmental behaviors and the mother's responses and adjustments to those changes punctuate this process. During this period, it is not unusual for the mother to doubt her maternal abilities.

According to Mercer (1986), the mother comes to the parenting experience with a relatively stable "core self," acquired through lifelong socialization processes. This sense of self determines how a mother defines, perceives, and responds to mothering. Additionally, the mother's developmental level and innate personality characteristics influence her behavioral responses toward the infant.

According to Mercer (1981, 1986) the immediate interpersonal environment is that in which maternal role attainment occurs and includes the family and factors such as family functioning, partner relationships, social support, and stress. These variables interact with one or more of the other variables in affecting maternal role. The infant is an individual embedded within the family system. The family system maintains semipermeable boundaries that allow control over the interchange between the family system and other social systems (Mercer, 1990). Ideally, through interchange between the mother, her infant, and their interpersonal environment, the required resources and supports are acquired to create a climate for maternal role attainment.

According to Mercer (1985, 1990), the transition to mothering or parenting occurs in four stages: **anticipatory, formal, informal,** and **personal.** Passage through these stages is said to result in attainment of the maternal role. The first stage, or **anticipatory stage,** begins during pregnancy when the pregnant woman chooses a provider for prenatal and intrapartal care. During this stage, the woman begins social and psychologic adjustment to the role. She begins to realize that she is thinking and acting for another. Many women start seeking out maternal role models and "study" the maternal behaviors of others in an attempt to learn the expectations of the role. Further, the mother fantasizes about herself in the role and begins to relate to the fetus in utero.

The **formal stage** begins with childbirth and continues for the next 6 to 8 weeks (Mercer, 1990). Maternal role behaviors during this stage are guided by consensual expectations and role modeling that are provided by significant others (e.g., health care professionals and significant others in the mother's social support system). Through interaction with the infant, the mother becomes acquainted with her infant's cues and responds. In this stage responses are formal (as if based on rules) laws or axioms that must be followed.

The **informal stage** begins once the mother has learned appropriate responses to the infant's unique cues. During this stage, the mother develops her own unique repertoire of parenting responses to the infant that are not taught by the social system.

Finally, the **personal stage** is attained when the mother feels a sense of harmony with the maternal role, enjoys the infant, sees the infant as a central priority in her life, feels confident and competent in the role, and has internalized the parental role. Most mothers achieve this sense of harmony by 4 months, although this may be variable (Mercer, 1986).

### Four Phases of the Adaptation Process

Additionally, Mercer identifies four phases to the mother's adaptation process that span the first year of the infant's life. These include the physical recovery phase, the achievement phase, the disruption phase and the re-organization phase. The **physical recovery phase** (birth to 1 month) is predominantly a time of biologic adaptation for the postpartum mother. This is often when the new mother is partially or fully reliant upon others for instrumental and/or emotional support (Mercer, 1986).

The second phase is the **achievement phase** (2 months to 4 or 5 months), and this is characterized by generalized feelings of physical well-being. During this phase psychosocial needs dominate. The infant may begin to settle into more predictable routines and mothers generally voice feelings of confidence and competence. These feelings are often reinforced by the blossoming social skills of the infant.

The **disruption phase** (6 to 8 months) may be a time of stress as the new mother tries to balance conflicting roles and relationships. The infant's developmental changes present new challenges to the mother's existing repertoire of parenting skills. Additionally, conflict may exist between the infant's and mother's developmental needs. This is a period when many new mothers are returning to roles that take them outside of the home.

The **reorganization phase** (beginning after 8 months and continuing to 12 months) is a time of increasing individuation between the mother and her infant. Biologic and developmental changes allow the infant to master his or her environment and develop greater autonomy. During this phase, mothers may experience restlessness with the burdens of motherhood manifested by a desire to be recognized as individuals and in roles other than that of mother; this may be particularly true for those mothers who formerly worked outside the home, but now have chosen to work in the home (Mercer, 1986).

## Adaptation of the Partner

The new mother's partner may be male or female. While the role of the mother as a nurturing parent has been recognized for some time, the role of the female partner or the father has been ignored. Tripp-Reimer (1991) lists several functions of fathers, which may form the basis of study of male partners:

1. Provision for the family
2. Protection: a sense of security and well-being for the family
3. Care-giving: child care, housework
4. Formative: a contribution to the formation of the child's character and personality; a father socializes his child in ways a mother cannot

### Historical Perspectives on Fatherhood and Families

Stearns (1991) reports that the study of fatherhood is a relatively new phenomenon generated by current interests in fatherhood as well as the changes in family life over time. Before the industrial revolution fathers had greater opportunities for interaction with children as they lived and worked together. Fathers were the heads of households and, as such, were held responsible for all aspects of a child's life, including the arrangement of training for a trade, moral teaching, and the control of economic resources. Families were geographically bound together by (vertical) patrilineal lines of property inheritance and horizontal kinship networks forged by women through the process of marriage.

Throughout the nineteenth century, economic and social changes resulted in the industrialization and urbanization of America. Changes in technology made farming a more efficient operation and the development of factories for the production of mass-produced goods required a labor force. These two changes resulted in a migration to urban areas. The ability to work for a wage outside of the home and/or community reduced the paternal control and authority over inheritance and property rights. This changed the balance of power between generations and allowed the younger generation to move away from home, particularly if family relations or economic resources were strained. The result was a change in the nature of relationships between the generations from one of economic dependence to one based increasingly on affectional ties (Osterud, 1991).

Movement from an agrarian to an industrial economy also changed the nature of daily interchange that occurred among family, friends, and neighbors in a community. No longer were work, family, and social life necessarily integrated. The net result was the separation of the extended family network, looser bonds of community, and the creation of separate spheres of home and workplace. With men leaving the home to work, mother's assumed increasing responsibility for the care and upbringing of children. This pattern continued into the middle of the twentieth century.

During the twentieth century, collective social movements such as the women's movement created a collective consciousness about the social inequities created by gender discrimination. This brought about changes in the family, including less rigidly proscribed rules for men and women. Social changes, changes in employment patterns, and a loosening of prohibitions against premarital sex and divorce have further affected the typology of families. Partners are now allowed a greater range of choice in terms of roles and the division of household labor; however, it should be noted that certain household arrangements have resulted in significant role strain. Women today are more likely to work what is known as a "double shift," taking on new roles while never shedding their traditional gender role. Comparatively, male gender role ascription has changed at a slower rate because of more rigid norms for masculine behavior.

A shift in gender roles requires that we rethink societal expectations in terms of power, resources, and prestige so that the costs of these changes do not continue to unduly burden women or shortchange men. Today's men's and women's movements have moved towards recognition of gender differences and the equal worth and value of the sexes while not permitting these differences to be the basis of unequal treatment. Practically speaking, this philosophic shift is pragmatic in recognizing innate biologic differences between the sexes that cannot be ignored, while allowing for greater choices in how gender roles are defined and the qualities that can and should be fostered.

Because of these changes, fathers are making more efforts to create nurturing relationships with their children and to share in their care. The "ideal" family continues to be an elusive and culturally relative term. Societal changes continue to exert an influence on the typology of families such that numerous definitions of family exist. Regardless of how one defines the term family, it continues to be the basic unit of society that occupies a position between the individual and society. Its basic purposes are twofold: (1) to meet societal needs for social reproduction of new members, and (2) to meet the needs (affective, socioeconomic, growth and development, and so on) of the individuals in it. As an agent of social reproduction, the family, in response to societal changes, continues to evolve in ways that will continue to influence gender roles. For nursing practice, the importance of this research lies in understanding the need to be sensitive to the various challenges that families of all types face today as they attempt to negotiate roles and responsibilities in response to childbearing.

### Theories of Paternal Bonding

Interest in the development of the maternal-infant bond preceded studies of the relationship between the father and newborn. Greenberg and Morris (1974) coined the term **engrossment** to describe the father's absorption, preoccupation, and interest in the infant. Engrossment is said to have several characteristics including sensory awareness of the infant, awareness of the distinct features of the infant, seeing the infant as perfect, developing strong feelings of attraction to the infant, and developing increased self-esteem.

Through **visual awareness** the father begins to see the infant as an individual who is attractive, pretty, or beautiful. **Tactile awareness** is experienced as a desire to pick up, hold, touch, and play with the infant as a means of knowing him or her (see Figure 15-5). **Awareness of the distinct characteristics of the newborn** is similar to the identification and claiming process described by Rubin and leads fathers to believe they could recognize their own baby. Fathers begin to see the unique features of the infant and the baby's resemblance to themselves. Through these actions, the father perceives the infant as perfect. A characteristic feature of engrossment is **the strong feeling of attraction to the newborn** that the father develops. This leads to his focusing attention on the infant. There is an experience of **extreme elation** often described as a **"high."** This is described regardless of their presence at the actual birth. Seeing the face of the infant seems to be the trigger for this elation. Finally, an **increased sense of self-esteem** results from these interactions. First-time fathers often describe themselves as being more mature, older, or proud after seeing their baby.

In a grounded study of expectant and new fatherhood, Jordan (1990) found that fatherhood begins as the pregnancy is diagnosed and the man "labors" to incorporate the paternal role into his self-identity. She describes three subprocesses in paternal role attainment: (1) **grappling with the reality of the pregnancy and infant**, (2) **struggling for recognition as a parent, and** (3) **plugging away at the role making of involved fatherhood.** Grappling with the reality of the pregnancy and newborn infant is a central process in the development of a paternal identity. Various "reality boosters" are said to assist in this process (Box 15-9).

The next step (**struggling for recognition**) in development of paternal identity is the recognition of the father as a parent by significant referent others. In this process, significant others are crucial in either allowing the father a role or keeping him in the wings. By their actions and information, the mother, others in her social network, and health care providers can reinforce the reality of the pregnancy and newborn infant as well as the role of the man as father. How we refer to him and include or ignore him during care affects the development of his paternal identity. The infant's ability to communicate with the father after birth is also a powerful stimulus in this stage of paternal role attainment.

Finally, in **plugging away at the role-making of involved fatherhood**, men search for role models and analyze their own experiences with their fathers. At this time, the reality of pregnancy or the infant is an impetus to action. Often lacking role models for involved fatherhood, the men cast about for assistance in this phase. Health care providers can help men gain knowledge and experience with child care and parenting skills. Actualization is said to occur when the father incorporates the paternal role into his self-concept. Many who reach this developmental stage cannot sustain the effort required to be an involved parent; however, those who do so find the experience rewarding.

### Experiences of New Fathers

The process of transition to fatherhood may be influenced by several factors, including participation in childbirth, relationships with significant others, competence in child care, and the method of infant feeding. During the preparations for the birth, fathers often participate in childbirth classes. The focus is on anticipatory guidance covering various labor and delivery scenarios. Some fathers believe that some of the information covered is unnecessary and will not pertain to them or their situations. Subsequently, fathers may enter labor and delivery with unrealistic expectations that clash with reality of their birth experience. This dissonance affects their postpartum bonding experience (Henderson, 1991).

Most research findings stress the importance of early contact for father and infant, as well as participation in child care activities (Greenberg and Morris, 1974). Research regarding the impact of a type of delivery has resulted in less consensus. It would appear that many factors besides the birth experience enter into creating the paternal bond. Prospective parents may not be ready to process information about the postpartum period until after the birth. Some advocate postpartum classes to help in the resolution of feelings generated by the birth (Tiller, 1995). Others try to help by providing information in childbirth classes that can help parents develop realistic expectations for childbirth. With the advance of liberal birthing and postpartum practices, the opportunities for fathers to interact with their newborns have increased. Information in both types of classes is best.

Fathers who reported good partner relationships also found these relationships provided a strong foundation for the transition to fatherhood (Hangsleben, 1983). The strength of the relationship rather than marital status or length of time together seems to be the determining factor for involvement with the pregnancy and the baby postpartum. For those couples who are not married or cohabiting, paternal role may be at risk if the mother does not want a high level of paternal involvement (Grant and others, 1997). A group most in need of intervention would be non-cohabiting couples in which the mother has high expectations for the involvement of the father in child care and decision making. These fathers need to be involved in prenatal visits, postpartum well-child visits, and father-focused community programs.

For fathers experiencing the stress and fatigue associated with childbearing, a decline in happiness has been found to resolve as the family becomes adjusted (Tiller,

---

## BOX 15-9   *Paternal Reality Boosters*

- Changes in the mother's behavior and body
- The "official" diagnosis of pregnancy
- Hearing the baby's heartbeat
- Seeing the baby on ultrasound
- Feeling the baby move
- Telling others about the pregnancy
- Giving the baby a nickname
- Nesting
- Seeing and holding the baby at birth
- Telling others about the baby
- Baby entering the home environment
- Assuming responsibility for the baby's care
- Getting to know the baby as a person

From Jordan PL: Laboring for relevance: expectant and new fatherhood, *Nurs Res* 39(1):11-16, 1990.

---

1995). As a part of childbirth classes, we might include postpartum stress-reduction techniques for women and their partners.

Prenatally, many fathers envision themselves being very involved in baby care activities. Fathers who report being competent and able to provide child care tend to be not only in good marital situations but also younger (Hangsleben, 1983). Encouraging fathers to stay with and hold their new baby after birth will help them feel more competent. Teaching child care skills in the postpartum will also help the new father feel comfortable in his role. Anticipatory guidance for new parents should include information about child growth and development.

Studies indicate that bottle-feeding tends to increase the involvement of the father while breastfeeding limits some child care activities by fathers. When fathers were unable to subordinate their own need for gratification for those of the mother-infant dyad, breastfeeding has actually generated negative paternal emotions (Hangsleben, 1983). Gamble and Morse (1993) studied fathers of breastfed infants and found that the happy ones were engaged in postponing their own feeding relationship with the infant in favor of the breastfeeding experience. Unhappy men measured their own relationship with the infant against the mother-child relationship and felt discouraged and frustrated when they could not compete. Fathers who were committed to breastfeeding for their infants reframed the situation so that it was more acceptable to them. Actions that reinforced postponing included examining the benefits of breastfeeding such as the health and emotional stability of the infant, the positive perspective of the mother, and the pleasure of seeing the infant nurse. In addition, they found other activities to increase their interaction such as bathing, putting the infant to bed, and changing diapers. After weaning, the fathers "caught up" to the point where they saw no difference in the infant's responses to the mother or father. Fathers who were unable to find positive activities related to breastfeeding were likely to express their dissatisfaction and put stress on the breastfeeding experience. Our prenatal and postpartum contacts with parents present the opportunity to discuss the couple's breastfeeding expectations. As the research suggests, fathers should be encouraged to accept their own different but equally important contributions to the infant.

## Cultural Variations in Fatherhood

The cultural background of the family influences the father's responses to childbearing and the paternal role. Paternal behaviors are culturally defined; therefore, it is important for us to refrain from making judgments about the father's involvement based on our personal or Western beliefs. Knowledge of individual cultural beliefs can assist us in making assessments about the father's postpartum adjustment. It is important to validate what practices are important to the father, since he may not adhere to the particular practices of his culture.

In the African-American family, the social and economic conditions of slavery were said to have destroyed family patterns, leaving a matriarchal organization with absent or only peripherally involved fathers. This stereotypical image of the African-American family is currently being challenged. African-American fathers have been found to be warm, loving, supportive, and sensitive to the needs of their children. In addition, other research has found African-American fathers to be actively involved in child care activities and to be equally involved in teaching, discipline, and decision making. African-American fathers have been found to be more authoritative than Anglo or Chicano fathers living in the same neighborhood (Mirande, 1991; Walters and Chapman, 1991).

Like the strong mother in the African-American family, the Latino father has been stereotyped as the "macho" head of the family, while the mother has been characterized as submissive. While the traditional view of the Latino family with respect for elders and male dominance is supported by some of the literature, an emerging family pattern is also described. In the new family pattern, the father is warm and provides significant positive experiences for the children and decision-making is shared between parents. In some Latino families, women are taking on more responsibility outside the home as breadwinners. Many of these current fathers may describe their own fathers as distant and aloof, but they intend to have a closer relationship with their children (Mirande, 1991; Walters and Chapman, 1991).

Like African-American's the economic history of Asians has impacted the family form; and like Latino's, the family is viewed along authority lines of "the older order the younger, and the men the women." Among Asian Americans there is great diversity but all have faced the need to adapt as they immigrated to America. In Chinese families, kinship traditionally has been organized along patrilineal lines but with the rise of Communism women were given legal equality. This change brought some alterations in traditional gender roles of men and women. Chinese immigrants to the United States may mix traditional and Western practices. In conducting postpartum assessments with Chinese-American families it is important to keep in mind that they may not be comfortable in displaying emotions in front of strangers, making eye contact or touching (Mirande, 1991; Walters and Chapman, 1991).

The Japanese have also experienced the need for adjustments related to their immigrant status. For some of these families, change has occurred over generations. Second-generation Japanese Americans tried to create a balance between the traditional family and their new homeland. This generation gave priority to conjugal over parent-child relationships. Male and female domains were maintained, but equal. Third-generation Japanese Americans are considered the most assimilated into American society. For Japanese, as well as other Asian-American families, the role of the father has been changed from the traditional head of the family to a more equal relationship with the mother (Mirande, 1991).

Very little research exists regarding paternal roles among Native Americans. To further complicate our understanding, there are 280 tribal groups and 161 different linguistic groups, thus resulting in vast cultural diversity. Native American family patterns have suffered extensively as a result of contact with the dominant Euro-American culture. Government policies toward Native Americans have consistently worked to destroy the traditional way of life among the native population. Policies toward Native American children have also served to fracture the family and deemphasize the parenting roles. Beginning in the 1800s and continuing until recently, children were removed from their families by the United States government and placed in boarding schools or Anglo families, often at a great distance from their own families. This policy was justified on the grounds that the children were socially deprived and could be better educated outside of the family in foster or adoptive families. Traditionally, most Native American families were matrilineal; however, changes in traditional roles have occurred with migration of members off the reservations, creating various cultural changes (Mirande, 1991; Still and Hodgins, 1998).

As a result of increased research on the role of the father, more has been learned about how ethnicity affects the perception of the father's role. A potential problem is to stereotype ethnic groups or to minimize the diversity within a group. However, a father's cultural identity does affect his perception and implementation of his role (Walters and Chapman, 1991) (Box 15-10).

Family roles and organization influence all other domains including head of household, gender roles, family goals and priorities, developmental tasks, and individual and family social status in the community. It is important to understand the family pattern of dominance when determining who to speak with in regard to health care decisions. An initial question about the roles of the men and women in the family will begin to provide insight into this matter.

## Adaptation of the Postpartum Family

### Developmental Tasks of the Childbearing Family

The birth of a child heralds a normative transition in the life cycle of any family. With the birth of the first child the family moves from a partnership to a threesome. This triad is said to endure, on some level, regardless of the outcome of the marriage (McGoldrick, Heiman, and Carter, 1993). Although this normative transition is one that some couples dream of, it requires changes in roles and relationships and is, therefore, often stressful (Martell and Imle, 1996). Relations within the partnership and extended family must be altered to incorporate the new family member and accompanying roles. In some cases, the changes that are called for in moving to this new developmental stage are so difficult that they lead to a family crisis (LeMasters, 1957; Clark, 1966; Hobbs and Cole, 1976). Because previous life experiences do not prepare most people for the parental role and idealized depictions of parenting create standards that most new parents cannot live up to, the potential for feelings of frustration and parental inadequacy exists even in normal transitions (Szafran, 1996). The most commonly identified stressors during this period include the personal loss of freedom associated with the demands of parenting, and the loss of time and companionship with the partner (Miller and Meyer-Wallis, 1983). Feelings of parental inadequacy, lack of social support, conflicting advice, ill health and fatigue may add to the stress experienced in emerging families.

According to family developmental theorists (Duvall and Miller, 1985; Carter and McGoldrick, 1989; Friedman and others, 1998), with the act of childbearing the family must work toward:

1. *Incorporating the newborn into the family system.* This requires identifying and claiming the infant as a family member.
2. *Reconciling the potentially conflicting growth and developmental needs of family members.* The dependency needs of the newborn create demands that need to be recognized and attended to. Partners must work at meeting the emotional and sexual needs of each other and sharing other parenting and household responsibilities. The unique needs of siblings

must be considered as well. Conflicting demands, pressures, and loyalties can create an emotional drain on the family.
3. *Maintaining a satisfying marital (partner) alliance.* New patterns of communication are established as partners learn to relate to each other as both partners and parents. The reestablishment of a strong and satisfying alliance is critical and communication is of key importance in this process. A strong marital alliance or partnership will bring stability to the family and allow the individual partners the energy to "give" to other roles.
4. *Establishing parental roles and a strong parental alliance.* This process of establishing parental roles should begin in the antepartal

---

### BOX 15-10   *Legal Issues for Fathers*

Like the social view of fathers, the legal issues of fatherhood have changed over time. Three issues—support, custody, and paternity—illustrate this change.

**Support**

Traditionally husbands acquired the property of their wives, but had the responsibility for the support of wives and children regardless of marital status. Despite state laws, which place responsibility for support on both parents, mothers were more likely to bear the burden for support because states did not actively pursue fathers who did not meet support responsibilities. However, noncustodial fathers were also more likely to be pursued for nonpayment than mothers. Although fathers may be required to pay support, mothers may deny access to children. Today the trend is shifting toward equal support as more women have access to well-paying jobs and men are arguing that they also have a nurturing role.

**Custody**

During the nineteenth century, social preference favored women as nurturers of the family. Fathers were unlikely to gain custody. Today maternal preference is giving way to the best interest of the child, which in the view of many courts is shared parenting.

**PATERNITY**

When a child is born of a married woman, it is assumed to be the child of her husband. This view spared the child any stigma of illegitimacy and relieved society of the responsibility of support. Today conclusive tests establish paternity. Although courts may favor "psychologic" parenthood by the mother's husband, biologic fathers have been successful in custody decisions when able to show involvement with the child.

From Walters LH and Chapman SF: Changes in legal views of parenthood: implications for fathers in minority cultures. In Bozett FW and Hanson SMH, editors: *Fatherhood and families in cultural context,* New York, 1991, Springer.

period as the individuals "try on" the parental role and imagine themselves as parents. How parental roles are fulfilled varies from family to family, from generation to generation, and from one culture to another. Fulfilling these roles fulfilled is often a negotiated process that occurs over time.

5. *Reestablishing boundaries with the extended family, including the establishment or maintenance of grandparenting and sibling roles.* Other family members need to develop relationships with the newborn and realign relationships with the new parents. This is an evolutionary process that requires good communication skills and an understanding and acceptance of differences in values and expectations. Tensions may result during this process.

### Factors Influencing Response of Family Members

How the family adapts to these changes is dependent on several factors, including family composition, cultural beliefs, quality and availability of social support, socioeconomic conditions, family resources, family roles, communication patterns, and environmental considerations. Several tools and approaches assess families.

Four commonly recognized approaches to family assessment include the structural-functional approach, the systems approach, the developmental approach, and the family-interactional approach. The **structural-functional approach** is concerned with how the structure of the family affects the function of the family. The **systems approach** encourages us to view the client as a member of a family constellation whose illness, injury, or normative transition affects and is affected by the family system (Wright and Leahey, 1994). The **developmental approach** encourages us to examine the evolution of the family over time as it confronts different stages of development (Duvall, 1977). The **family interactional approach** (Hill and Hanson, 1960; Rose, 1962; Turner, 1962) focuses on the interaction of personalities and family dynamics. Many nurses adapt an eclectic or integrated approach to family assessment that draws from multiple perspectives.

Three such integrated nursing assessment approaches exist: The Family Assessment Intervention Model and Family Systems Stressor Strength Inventory (Berkey and Hanson, 1991; Hanson and Mischke, 1996), the Friedman Family Assessment Model (Friedman, 1998), and The Calgary Family Assessment Model and Calgary Family Intervention Model (Wright and Leahy, 1994; Wright, Watson, and Bell, 1997). Genograms and ecomaps also serve as excellent assessment tools for determining the strengths and limitations of a family system (see Chapter 2 for further information).

### Family Composition

The composition of the family refers to those whom the family members identify as members of the family. Families today vary widely in their composition. These differences in composition may affect how the family is able to traverse the normative transitions related to childbearing and the postpartum period.

***Single-parent Families.*** Single-parent families may occur as a result of a conscious decision to bear a child alone or as the result of dissolution of a partnership or marital union. Single-parent families experience the same life cycle stages as two-parent families. The basic difference is the absence of a partner to carry a share of the burdens and responsibilities with respect to support, childrearing, and gender role modeling. Single parenting is particularly burdensome within the setting of a poor social support system (Carter and McGoldrick 1989). Increased rates of poverty and the single parent's need for employment add to the difficulties in child care and childrearing (Bowen, Desimone, and McKay, 1995). Single parents are often in need of increased social support during the normative transition of the postpartum period.

***Blended Families.*** The birth of a new family member in a blended family can result in renewed fears about emotional investment in a new family and hostile or upset reactions of children from previous unions, extended family, and the ex-spouse. Anticipatory guidance is helpful in working through these issues, if not before the birth of the infant then during the early postpartum period, to successfully negotiate realignment of relationships (Carter and McGoldrick, 1989).

***Lesbian/Gay Families.*** A growing number of children have at least one parent who is gay or lesbian. Estimates place the number of lesbian mothers at 3 to 5 million and 1 to 3 million gay fathers. Some of the children were conceived in heterosexual relationships, others are the result of adoption, foster parenting, or insemination with donor sperm. As with heterosexual families, new relationships are being formed, resulting in various parent roles (Perrin and Kulkin, 1996).

Although some research has been done, it is limited by the difficulties of small and potentially biased sampling. The outcomes however do demonstrate both similarities and differences from heterosexual families. In contrast to other families, homosexual couples face stigmatization upon disclosure of the nontraditional living arrangements. Efforts to prevent disclosure may be a contributing factor to family stress in dealing with the public and health care providers. In addition, the family may encounter legal barriers to equal parental rights in the case of separation or even in issues of consent for treatment of children (Perrin and Kulkin, 1996). Much of the research investigating gay/lesbian parenting has looked at child adjustment and found no differences in child rearing and adjustment (Patterson, 1995; Eliason, 1996; Perrin and Kulkin, 1996).

## Family Culture

The cultural orientation of a family may influence the family's behavior, values, and functions. Understanding the family's cultural beliefs and practices with regard to childbearing is critical to providing competent care. Differences between the beliefs and practices of the family and health care providers may result in a lack of rapport and differences in goals, communication styles, and the acceptance of ideas or recommendations (Coddy, 1975). For purposes of learning, it is important to understand the characteristics, beliefs, and practices of different cultural groups; however, when you are working with individuals or families, it is important to remember that these characteristics, beliefs, and practices refer to the aggregate only, and not to the specific family or individuals within that family. To understand a family, it is important to understand the cultural background of the family. Basic questions in any family cultural assessment should include the family's ethnic background, to what extent they have retained their cultural heritage (language, customs, affiliations, manner of dress, dietary customs, religion, health practices and beliefs, customs and beliefs about childbearing), and the family's religious practices and preferences.

By completing a general assessment, other cultural influences on family organization (roles, power, values and communication), child-rearing practices, affective responses, health care practices and beliefs, and coping strategies should be adequately determined (Friedman, 1998).

## Social Class

Social class and cultural background exert a strong influence on family values, priorities, behavior patterns, socialization practices, role expectations, and experiences. However, just as with culture, the assumptions are based on the aggregate and cannot be applied to a specific family or individual. Social class involves a complex interplay between the factors of a family's education level, occupational status, and income level. Each of these factors can only be raised through a process of raising the other two factors.

Questions relevant to understanding the social class of the emerging family include (Friedman, 1998):

1. Who is the primary wage earner in the family?
2. What kinds of supplementary assistance, if any, is the family receiving (food stamps, Women, Infants, and Children [WIC] Supplementary Food Program, Social Security, Disability, informal family support)?
3. Does the family consider its income adequate to meet its needs?
4. How does the family see itself managing with the birth of the infant?

Be careful not to assume that the social class of a family has an inverse relationship to need. Other than financial resources, the lower social class family might have greater resources on which to draw as they adjust to their infant and take on the role of parenting.

## Social Support

The quality and availability of social support can have a profound influence on the adaptation of the emerging family's ability to negotiate change and reestablish equilibrium following the birth of a child. Social supports can be internal or external, formal or informal. Three interactional dimensions of family social support are reciprocity (nature and frequency of reciprocal relations), advice/feedback (quality and quantity of communication), and emotional involvement (extent of intimacy and trust) in the social relationships. Social supports have been shown to buffer the negative effects of stress on health and have direct positive influences on health and well-being (Wills, 1985; Friedman, 1998).

A few well-directed questions and construction of an ecomap can assist in understanding the quality, strength, availability, and use of available social supports. Questions that might be relevant to understanding the social support network of the emerging family include the following (Friedman, 1998):

1. Who is available to help you with infant care? Household chores? Care of the other children? Running errands? Making meals? Decision-making? What kind of help do they give you?
2. If you had any problems with . . . whom would you talk to or get help from?

## Family Roles

The parental role is a set of behaviors that are normatively defined and expected of parents in a particular society. Role expectations of parents evolve and are defined within a particular societal context. The family is the agent for social reproduction of roles. It is in the context of one's family that parental roles are modeled, modified, and refined. Through the process of socialization, family members acquire a repertoire of roles through which they can act and interact with others.

During the pregnancy, expectant parents begin to try on the parental role and seek out role models (Rubin, 1977; Mercer, 1985). Roles are interdependent and patterned to interact with that of a role partner. Society specifies behaviors for each person in these reciprocal arrangements so that each person will know what is expected of the other. Role partners constantly influence each other's role behaviors. Whenever there is dissonance between role expectations and role performance, the potential for conflict and stress occurs.

Parental **role stress** occurs when very difficult, conflicting, or impossible demands exist for a parent within a family. Role stress results in subjective feelings of tension and frustration, referred to as **role strain** (Hardy and Hardy, 1988; Friedman and Heady, 1998). Parental role conflict occurs when the parent is confronted by incompatible expectations (Hardy and Hardy, 1988). **Role conflict** may involve interrole conflict, intersender role conflict, or person-role conflict (Friedman and Heady, 1998). **Interrole conflict** may be experienced by new parents as they adjust to the conflicting and consuming demands of being a parent, a partner, an employee, a housewife, a cook, a daughter, a sister, and so on, simultaneously (Hardy and Hardy, 1988).

**Intersender conflict** may occur as each partner tries on the new role of parent and their interpretation of the role does not meet with their partner's expectations (La Rocca, 1978). For example, the father may see his role as one of protector and financial provider, while his partner wants him to take on a more nurturing, care providing role.

**Person-role conflict** may occur as the partners evolve their parenting roles and a conflict occurs between the person's internalized values and the externalized values communicated to the person by referent others. Many breastfeeding women report that while lip service is given to the virtues of mothers who breastfeed, many friends and family members frown upon their breastfeeding in public.

Assessment of family roles in the postpartum should focus on role structure and the sociocultural, situational, and historical variables that affect role structure. The following four broad areas were identified as important to understanding the family role structure:

1. *Formal role structure* refers to the position and role of each family member.
   * What formal roles and positions do each of the family members fulfill (e.g. individual, partner and parent)? How are these roles carried out?
   * Are there any role conflicts or difficulties in carrying out these roles?
   * How do members perceive they perform their respective roles?
   * Is there flexibility in roles when needed?
2. *Informal role structure* includes the roles that one fulfills based on personality attributes (e.g., the clown, the scapegoat, the martyr, the organizer, parental child).
   * What informal roles exist in the family, who plays them, and how frequently or consistently are they enacted?
   * What purposes do the roles serve?
   * Are any of the roles detrimental to the family or family members in the long run?
3. *Role models* assist family members to see how past models influence current expectations and behaviors.

* Who are the role models that influenced the family members in their early life?
* Who acted as a role model for their partner in their roles as parents and as marital partners, and what were they like?
* If the informal roles are dysfunctional in the family, who enacted these roles in previous generations.
4. *Variables affecting role behavior:*
   * Social class: How does social class influence the formal and informal role structure in the family?
   * Ethnic influences: How do the family's ethnic and religious background influence the family's role structure?
   * Developmental or life cycle influences: Are the present role behaviors of family members developmentally appropriate?
   * Situational events, including changes in health or illness (this will hold true in the event of the illness of the mother or infant) How have health problems affected family roles? What reallocation of tasks has occurred?
     How have the family members who have had to assume new roles adjusted? Is there evidence of role stress and/or role conflict as a result of these shifts?
     How has the family member with the health issue reacted to her or his change or loss of a role(s)? (Friedman and Heady, 1998)

## Family Communication Patterns

The resultant change from the addition of a new family member necessitates positive communication patterns so that the needs of family members are fulfilled and frustrations or tension is minimized. Curran (1983) demonstrated that healthy families have the ability to communicate clearly and listen. Assessment questions to consider when analyzing a family's communication patterns during the postpartum include:

1. How firmly and clearly do family members state their needs and feelings?
2. To what extent do members use clarification and qualification in interactions?
3. Do members elicit and respond favorably to feedback?
4. To what degree do members use assumptions and judgmental statements in interactions?
5. Do members interact in an offensive manner to messages?
6. How frequently are emotional messages conveyed?
7. What types of emotions are transmitted?
8. Who talks to whom and in what manner?

9. What is the usual pattern of transmitting important messages? Does an intermediary exist?
10. Are verbal and nonverbal messages congruent?
11. What important family/personal issues are open or closed to discussion? (Friedman, 1998)

### Environmental Considerations

The nature and degree of interaction between the emerging family and its physical and psychosocial environment, in part, determine the health of the family. Exchanges that add to the human, material, or emotional resources of the family generally can be viewed positively, while those that serve as a drain on resources without adding value to the human, material, or emotional condition of the family generally can be viewed as negative (Wright and Leahey, 1994).

As the family experiences the normative transition of childbirth, it is important to assess for congruence between the family's needs and the environmental resources and supports available to meet those needs. An environmental assessment should include an ecomap and an assessment of the family's living conditions, neighborhood, and community (Friedman, 1998).

**Adaptation** is a process of managing the demands of stressors through the use of resources, coping mechanisms, and problem-solving strategies. To determine the degree of stress the family experiences during this normative transition, we should assess for the presence of other stressors, perceptions of the birth event, family resources, family coping, and how much the event has disrupted family functioning (Friedman, 1998). We can assist families through the requisite role changes demanded by the stress of childbearing by identifying the changes they can anticipate and the available coping mechanisms and resources they have to deal with the changes. We may assist the family in developing problem-solving strategies or acquiring the necessary resources to prevent or decrease stress (Wright and Leahy, 1994; Friedman, 1998).

## Sibling Responses to the Birth Experience

While the arrival of a new baby presents a transition for the parents, the presence of siblings in the family requires additional adjustments. During pregnancy, many women seek help in facilitating this transition for their other children. This represents a change that began taking place during the 1970s when "family centered childbearing" became popular. Today many families use services such as sibling classes, participation of the sibling at the birth, and visitation on the postpartum unit and at neonatal intensive care units to prepare the siblings for the new baby. Other families prepare their children themselves, often with the assistance of the care provider. Some of the methods these families use include reading books about infants, attending prenatal visits and/or childbirth classes, involving the child in preparations for the infant, sharing the child's own infant pictures with them, encouraging the child to feel fetal movement, and talking about what the newborn will be like and the changes the family will need to make with the arrival of the infant (Fortier, Carson, and Will, 1991) (Box 15-11).

Despite the interest, relatively little research exists to guide us in providing services to siblings in the postpartum family. According to Murphy (1993), sibling relationship has been viewed as one of rivalry and displacement of the older child. This theoretic perspective led to clinical practices, which emphasized means to reduce jealousy and negative behavior by the older child. More recently, the emphasis has been on the multiple developmental or ecologic processes within the family that influence sibling responses to a newborn. This perspective focuses on behaviors that are seen as teaching, imitating, protective, caretaking, and helpful (Figure 15-9).

While sibling relationships may begin early in the pregnancy, most interventions focus on the birth and the period following. Although some research has focused on the negative behaviors seen in children with a new sibling, other research has found that when considering positive and negative behaviors of a research

---

### BOX 15-11 *Suggested Readings for Expectant Parents and Siblings*

*The Berenstain Bears' New Baby*
Stan and Jan Berenstain
Random House, 1974

*Mommy's Lap*
Ruth Horowitz and H. Sorensen
William Morrow, 1993

*Sharing*
Nanette Newman
Doubleday, 1990

*My Baby Brother*
Harriet Hains and Doris Kindersley
Houghton Mifflin, 1992

*101 Things to Do With a New Baby*
Jan Ormerod
Mulberry, 1984

*Betsy's Baby Brother*
Gunilla Wolde
Random House, 1975

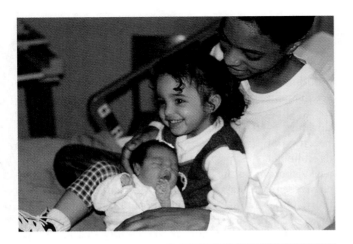

FIGURE 15-9 • Sibling meeting the newborn. *(Courtesy of Caroline E. Brown.)*

and a control group, few behavioral differences were seen in those children with a new sibling versus those without a new sibling. While younger children were more likely to have some toileting accidents when a new baby arrives, parents saw older children as becoming more independent. Researchers have also looked at what has previously been called "regression"; such as asking for a bottle or using baby talk and reconsidered it as imitation in which the child is "trying it out . . . seeing what it feels like to be the baby." Seen in this manner, these behaviors are more empathetic than regressive (Murphy, 1993).

Some individual factors that have been found to influence the sibling-newborn relationship include the age of the first child, their gender, and temperament.

### Age

Younger first-born children have been found to have more distress at the birth of a sibling than older children. Among toddlers, most mothers reported some regressive/empathetic behaviors, but less among children aged 3 to 4 (Sawicki, 1997).

### Gender

Research regarding gender is not conclusive. Some studies report that younger boys demonstrate more regressive and withdrawing behaviors than girls when a new baby arrives to gain a closer proximity to their parents. Other studies have suggested that rivalry between siblings is more prevalent among opposite-sex pairs of siblings (Sawicki, 1997).

### Personality and Temperament

Children who are more active and have a more impulsive temperament tend to have more behavior problems that can result in conflict with siblings (Sawicki, 1997). Seen in a family context, many variables may contribute to the interaction of a sibling with a new baby. Parental support is one. The distress reported after a

birth was higher for children who had less support from their mothers before the birth and from their fathers after the birth. Maternal fatigue surrounding childbirth and the accompanying need for fathers to provide more instrumental and emotional support for their partners may contribute to perceptions of less warmth in a mother-child interaction after the arrival of a newborn (Gottlieb and Mendelson, 1990).

Family communication is an important factor in sibling relationships. Siblings showed more positive interactions toward the newborn over a longer period of time when mothers talked to them about the baby as a person, with needs and feelings they could both meet. When these siblings were encouraged to participate in baby care, they were found to be more positive with the infant over time and to be more attuned to infant cues (Dunn and Kendrick, 1982). Longitudinal studies have shown that sibling interactions are not static, but change as the developmental tasks of the children change and the roles of the parents evolve. Initially relations may be positive as the sibling adjusts to the newborn and the parents adjust to their new roles. Relations will change as the newborn becomes mobile and disrupts the household stability. The third phase is characterized by the ability of the child to communicate, opening up new interactions with the sibling and parents (Kreppner, 1986).

Murphy (1992, 1993) describes a pattern of interaction between siblings that she called **sibling mutuality.** This is characterized by sensitivity and empathy in the interactions of the children with the newborn. In families in which this was observed, the children were allowed opportunities for uninterrupted interaction with the baby. Rather than critiquing the older child's behavior, the focus was on the feelings, behavior, and needs of the baby. Parents taught the sibling to interpret the cues and get feedback from the baby. The parents responded to the older children with respect for their feelings and needs. They were included in planning for the baby, sharing in the care of, and entertaining the baby.

Using this research as a base of knowledge, when involved in the postpartum care of families, we can be supportive in fostering positive relationships between siblings and the newborn. Parents may need to be reassured that the occurrence of occasional "babyish" behavior and squabbles is part of the process of sibling adjustment. Just as parents appreciate learning about infant states and cues, so can children learn to interpret feelings and respond appropriately. Children should not be coerced or forced to respond to the baby, but allowed to adjust at their own pace.

## Grandparent Adaptation

### Grandparenting Roles and Functions

Rather than being a family role with expected behaviors and functions, grandparenting is instigated and dictated by an interaction with other family members. Age, gender, ethnicity, and social class also influence the behavior and expectations of grandparents. Traditional grandparenting suggests an enjoyable extension of the parent role for older family members in which the grandparents enjoy visits with the family with little or no responsibility for child care. Grandparent roles have been studied in terms of symbolic and instrumental caregiving functions.

Several symbolic functions have been identified: (1) simply "being there," (2) acting as the national guard or family watchdog (protect and give care as needed), (3) being an arbitrator (between parents and children), and (4) being an active participant in the families' social construction of its history (Bengtson, 1985).

Grandparents also have an assistive role in the raising of children (Figure 15-10). Jendrek (1994) found grandparents assisting as daycare providers, live-in care providers (living in the home of the child and providing varying amounts of care), and as custodial in which the child lives with the grandparent.

Although precise figures are not available, it is estimated that in 1.1 million households, children live with grandparents with no biologic parent present. In some neighborhoods, as many as 8% of the children aged 12 and younger are being raised by grandparents (Kelley, Yorker, and Whitley, 1997). The most common reason for this alteration in family living relationships is child maltreatment, typically associated with substance abuse by one or both parents.

In the United States between 1985 and 1994, the reports of child abuse and neglect rose 24%. One result of this has been the increased number of children removed from their homes and placed in foster care, many being placed in kinship care with grandparents. In some cases, this is a formal arrangement, but for many more it is informal. Other reasons for this "parenting" arrangement are the death of a parent due to AIDS, homicide, incarceration, or mental illness (Kelley, Yorker, and Whitley, 1997).

### Issues Related to Grandparents as Parents

Kinship care raises some major issues that present challenges for grandparents. Because most children in this situation are there because of abuse and neglect, these children present a high risk for emotional and behavior problems. The grandparents, because of their age, are also at risk for multiple problems. Many report serious medical and health problems, often worsening after assuming the strenuous role of primary caregiver. Grandparents also suffer from psychologic distress. To protect their grandchildren, many have had to go to court and testify to the abusive and neglectful behavior of their own adult children. Many feel guilty that their own children have not become responsible parents (Box 15-12).

Parenting grandparents often suffer loss of social interactions with their own age group because of the child care responsibilities they have assumed. Most report

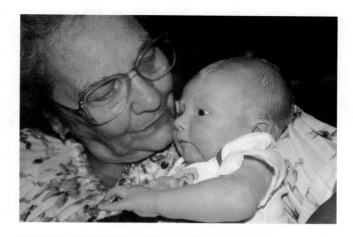

FIGURE 15-10 • Grandparent holding newborn. *(Courtesy of Caroline E. Brown.)*

feelings of depression. More than half report financial stress. At a time when their financial resources are limited, assuming responsibility for grandchildren stretches their money to the limit. Unfortunately, in many states they are not eligible for the financial support a nonkin foster parent would receive. Unless they are willing to relinquish custody to the state, they are not eligible for many of the programs available to state-approved foster parents (Kelley, Yorker, and Whitley, 1997). One intervention that has been found helpful is participation is support groups.

## POSTPARTUM PHENOMENON OF CONCERN: FATIGUE

Fatigue during the postpartum period has been well-documented (Affonso and others, 1990; Beck, 1993; Ruchala and Halstead, 1994; Milligan and others, 1996). The North American Nursing Diagnosis Association's (NANDA) (1999) definition of fatigue is "an overwhelming sustained sense of exhaustion and decreased capacity for physical and mental work at the usual level." Postpartum fatigue affects various aspects of the lives of postpartum women, including their relationships with significant others and the ability to fulfill household and familial responsibilities. In a study of postpartum fatigue by Ruchala and Halstead (1994), primiparas reported feeling uncertain, trapped, and overwhelmed by fatigue and a lack of experience in infant care. Although many of the multiparas in this study described their postpartum experience as being better than with previous births, this was primarily because of their comfort with caring for an infant. In this study, emotional concerns were a recurring theme, with mothers reporting feeling "down" and being tense, irritable, and depressed.

When a woman is discharged, she and her family may assume that she is back to normal. Therefore, it is important to help everyone understand that although the

---

## BOX 15-12 *Resources for Grandparents*

AARP Grandparent Information Center
Social Outreach and Support
601 East Street, NW
Washington, D.C. 20049
Phone: 202-434-2296
Fax: 202-434-6474

Grandparents as Parents (GAP)
PO Box 964
Lakewood, CA 90714
Phone: 310-924-3996
Fax: 714-828-1375
Contact person: Sylvie de Toledo

Grandparents Who Care
1 Rhode Island Street
San Francisco, CA 94103
Phone: 415-865-3000
Fax: 415-865-3099
Contact person: Evelyn Trowell

National Coalition of Grandparents
137 Larkin Street
Madison, WI 53705
Phone: 608-238-8751
Fax: 608-238-8751
Contact person: Ethel Dunn

Pacific Northwest Coalition of Grandparents
Raising Grandchildren
Pierce County Health Department
3629 South D Street
Tacoma, WA 98408
Phone: 206-565-4484
Fax: 206-627-3943
Contact person: Edith Owen

R.O.C.K.I.N.G./Raising Our Children's Kids
An International Network of Grandparents, Inc.
PO Box 96
Niles, MI 49120
Phone: 616-683-9038
Contact person: Mary Fron

Second Time Around Parents
Family and Community Service of Delaware County
100 W Front Street
Media, PA 19065
Phone: 610-566-7540,
Fax: 610-566-7677
Contact person: Michele Daly

---

new mother may be physiologically stable, she is not recovered and ready to resume her usual roles. It is important for the mother and the family to recognize her needs for rest and relaxation and to limit expectations. It is also important for us to assess the adequacy of the discharge plan and assist the mother and her family to determine if further interventions are necessary (Box 15-13). Use of the Fatigue Identification Form shown in Table 15-4 has been found helpful in assessing the degree of postpartum fatigue.

### ● POSTPARTUM PHENOMENON OF CONCERN: BODY IMAGE DISTURBANCES

According to Carpenito (1997), body image disturbance is a "state in which an individual experiences or is at risk to experience a disruption in the way he or she perceives his or her body image." Manifestations of a disturbed body image in the postpartum period may include negative verbal or nonverbal self-expressions about an actual or perceived change in body structure or function. Postpartum women with a disturbed body image may refuse to look at their bodies, hide or overexpose the body or body parts, avoid or change patterns of social or sexual involvement, become preoccupied with

their body image, and/or demonstrate self-destructive behaviors.

### Body Image

Changes in **body image** (the way the body appears to one's self) and **body boundaries** (the zone of perceived separation between one's self and objects or other people) can occur in anyone as a result of gradual (developmental) or abrupt (situational changes such as loss of a body part, ostomies, injuries, burns, surgical reconstruction and so on) changes in appearance or functioning. Developmental changes such as those that occur in pregnancy evolve over a period of time, can be anticipated, and may be shared with peers going through similar changes. Situational changes are more often sudden, unexpected, and set the individual apart from others as unique. Both types of changes involve alterations in body image, with the potential to influence a person's self-concept and self-esteem (Norris, Kunes-Connell, and Spelic, 1998).

People who have experienced changes in body image identify three phases of reimaging—**body image disruption, wishing for restoration,** and **reimaging the self.** In the phase of **body image disruption** the individual real-

---

### BOX 15-13   *Nursing Considerations for Fatigue*

1. Assess for risk factors such as physical and emotional demands of the infant and other family members, psychologic stressors, and continued discomfort.
2. Assess for signs of physical and emotional fatigue such as lack of energy, deep circles under the eyes, and statements indicating extreme fatigue.
3. Discuss risks for and signs of physical and emotional fatigue. Self-monitoring and awareness of a developing problem allows for timely intervention.
4. Allow opportunities for the mother to review intrapartal and early postpartal events. The need to work through the experience may help in overcoming emotions that are interfering with the ability to rest and relax. Cumulative sleep loss must be overcome as soon as possible to facilitate psychologic and physiologic recuperation.
5. Determine the infant's sleep-wake cycles. Encourage the mother to nap when the infant takes naps. As the infant gets older, suggest ongoing efforts to modify the infant's behaviors to promote more wakeful periods during the daytime. This helps the infant maintain progressively longer wakeful periods during the day and to sleep longer stretches at night. (Note: approximately 5 weeks are needed to regulate the infant's cycle.)
6. In the initial postpartum period, encourage restriction or lessening of outside activities and a limited number of visitors. Curtailing activities helps prevent overexhaustion.
7. Assess dietary intake and hematocrit. Provide information about daily iron and vitamin intake when applic-

able. Discuss the need for a balanced diet. Determine if the mother is able to meet her dietary needs. Provide appropriate referrals, if any, to formal support network (WIC, food stamps, community food pantries) or mobilize informal support network (e.g., family, friends, community groups, church members). A well-balanced diet, including the appropriate vitamins and iron, is needed to promote healing and overcome nutritional deficiencies that may contribute to feelings of excess fatigue and inadequate energy levels. Restoration of the hematocrit will increase the oxygen-carrying capacity of the blood and improve energy levels.
8. Determine the family structure and composition. Assess work capabilities, roles, and responsibilities of each member. Encourage the sharing of household tasks so that division of labor reduces the level of responsibility that the postpartum woman assumes and allows her to conserve energy.
9. Review the family's daily routine and assist the woman and her family in creative problem solving to identify times available for resting and napping throughout the day.
10. Assess the availability and use of formal and informal support systems. This assists in the identification of unmet needs and current means of physical and emotional assistance.
11. Encourage the woman to establish a quiet, relaxing routine before retiring (e.g., reading a book or having a glass of warm milk or wine) to aid in relaxation and promote sleep.

From Doenges ME and Moorhouse MF: *Maternal/newborn plans of care: guidelines for individualizing care,* ed 3, Philadelphia, 1999, FA Davis.

---

izes what has happened and begins the grieving process. Four responses characterize the body image disruption: surprise or shock, attempts to minimize awareness or deny the change, painful awareness of the change, and grieving the loss. As individuals are able to assimilate the change, awareness is established and participants begin grieving the loss.

Despite the severity of the physical or functional disruption that precipitated the change in body image, participants are found to experience a second phase defined by hope or a wish for idealized expectations. This **wishing for restoration** was so powerful that it prompted intense efforts on the part of individuals to mobilize their personal resources and maximize efforts to improve healing, appearance, or functioning. This idealization is disrupted by realism when the individual is confronted with the fact that they are not going to be the same as they had been or when restorative efforts are not yielding desired results. As these changes and their meanings are assimilated, the individual may experience intense emotional highs and lows.

In the third phase of **reimaging the self,** the subjects experienced events that prompted them to weigh the value of continued accommodation efforts against the costs in terms of time, energy, and effort. At this time, many began to replace idealized expectations with more realistic views of the self. In this phase the individual learns how to live a normal life that incorporates the physical changes.

Although the general characteristics of each phase are common to most participants, the intensity and duration of phases differed. Differences in response were said to be related to factors such as the value placed on appearance, the nature of the change, prior life experiences and self-esteem, social support and others' attitudes, and access to medical assistance (Norris, Kunes-Connell, and Spelic, 1998).

The ability to move through the reimaging process is facilitated by three actions: **assimilation, accommodation,** and **interpretation.** These three processes occur concurrently and are mutually reinforcing. **Assimilation** occurs predominantly in the first phase and

## TABLE 15-4    Fatigue Identification Form

Directions: I'm going to read a list of things you may have generally experienced since delivery. For each one, please answer "yes" if you have experienced it.

0 = No; 1 = Yes

|  | Yes | No |
|---|---|---|
| 1. My head feels heavy. | | |
| 2. My body feels tired. | | |
| 3. My legs feel tired. | | |
| 4. I yawn a lot. | | |
| 5. My brain feels hot and muddled. | | |
| 6. I am drowsy. | | |
| 7. My eyes feel strained. | | |
| 8. My movements are rigid or clumsy. | | |
| 9. I am unsteady when standing. | | |
| 10. I want to lie down. | | |
| 11. It's difficult to think. | | |
| 12. I get weary talking. | | |
| 13. I am nervous. | | |
| 14. I can't concentrate. | | |
| 15. I am unable to get interested in things. | | |
| 16. I am apt to forget things. | | |
| 17. I lack self-confidence. | | |
| 18. I am anxious about things. | | |
| 19. I can't straighten my posture. | | |
| 20. I lack patience. | | |
| 21. I have a headache. | | |
| 22. My shoulders feel stiff. | | |
| 23. My back hurts. | | |
| 24. It's hard to breathe. | | |
| 25. I'm thirsty. | | |
| 26. My voice is husky. | | |
| 27. I feel dizzy. | | |
| 28. My eyelids twitch. | | |
| 29. My legs or arms tremble. | | |
| 30. I feel ill. | | |

Scoring: low = ≤2.6; moderate = 2.7 to 11.7; high = ≥11.8

From Pugh LC and others: Clinical approaches in the assessment of childbearing fatigue, *J Obstet Gynecol Neonatal Nurs* 28(1):74-80, 1999.

involves an awareness of what has been lost and the initiation of the grief process. In the postpartum period this may parallel the need to assimilate the birth experience (loss of the pregnancy) and grieve the ideal versus actual birth.

This process continues through phase two as the woman attempts to assimilate the ideal body image with what she can reasonably expect her body to look like now that she has given birth. **Accommodation** is marked by efforts to live with the changes through development of coping strategies such as changing the manner of dress, using make-up, altering habits, and so on. Over time accommodation strategies change to fit the lifestyle of the individual and the restorative changes that have or have not occurred. Accommodation may also involve modifying goals or reprioritizing. These accommodations serve to redefine the individual's life.

**Interpretation** involves reflection on how one perceives the self, his or her situation, and others' responses to him or her. This interpretation influences the individuals' thoughts, feelings, actions, and overall adjustment. The final outcome of the reimaging process is reconciliation and normalization. Reconciliation is an outgrowth of the assimilation process and results in incorporation of the changes into the self-concept. Normalization is adapting goals and lifestyles to the limitations or losses of the changed body (Norris, Kunes-Connell, and Spelic, 1998). Further studies of the reimaging process are needed, particularly as it relates to the postpartum woman; however, it serves as a useful guide to understanding this process.

During pregnancy, women experience changes in **body image** and **body boundaries** (Fawcett, 1977). Values, cultural beliefs, and personality traits influence a woman's attitudes about her body and ideal body shape. How the woman feels about her body as the pregnancy progresses may influence the maternal-infant relationship, the decision to breastfeed, and feelings of self-esteem, self-satisfaction, and sexual desirability in the postpartum period.

Once the baby is born, concerns about excess weight gain and regaining a desired **body image** become common (Hiser, 1987). The woman may unrealistically expect her body to return to its prepregnant form. Although many women will feel better about their postpartum body than their pregnant body, they will have concerns about returning to their prepregnant form. Along with a generalized dissatisfaction with their postpartum body image, women will need to adjust to changes in body boundaries between themselves and their infants. Some women experience this separation as a loss of the intimate relationship that previously existed between themselves and the infant in utero and may report a sense of emptiness. Adolescent mothers are at particular risk for disturbances in body image because of the added biologic, psychologic, and maturational changes of adolescence.

### Postpartum Weight Gain

Following pregnancy, the average woman experiences a weight gain of 2.2 pounds (1 kg.) over their prepregnancy weight (Institute of Medicine, 1992); however, weight gain does vary and some women may become obese (Rossner, 1992; Williamson and others, 1994). In fact, one study reported that pregnancy carries a 40% to 60% risk of major weight gain. Such gains that are retained beyond 6 months postpartum are said to predict excessive weight gain years later. Based on studies of pregnant and postpartum women, a negative body image may occur due to dissatisfied feelings about weight during the postpartum period (Strang and Sullivan, 1985; Walker, 1998). Sustained weight gains have been found to be associated with increased health risks from chronic obesity, coronary heart disease, and breast cancer.

White women are less likely to experience weight gains at 6 months postpartum than women from other racial groups (Parham, Astrom, and King, 1990; Schauberger and others, 1992). These differences in postpartum weight gain may be related to cultural expectations, genetics, and lifestyle behaviors such as exercise, dieting, and smoking (Bouchard, 1991; Walker and Freeland-Graves, 1998). Maternal skill in regulating eating when under stress may be important during the postpartum period (Walker, Walker, and Walker, 1994). Some women may lose weight because of the level of stress they are experiencing as they take on this new role. Others may gain weight as they eat in response to stress.

Positive health behaviors including dietary and exercise patterns have been linked with higher feelings of self-esteem (Muhlenkamp and Sayles, 1986). Walker (1998) examined the extent of weight-related distress in postpartum women and discovered that more than 40% of the postpartum sample were mildly dissatisfied with their weight and an additional 8% experienced weight-related distress. Distress or dissatisfaction result from discrepancies between the ideal self and the actual self. Those women who had higher prepregnancy body mass index (BMI), larger gestational weight gain, higher postpartum BMI, less healthy lifestyles, and greater body image disturbance experienced more feelings of dissatisfaction and/or distress about their weight. In addition, as feelings about weight progressed along a continuum from satisfaction to distress, body image dissatisfaction increased and overall healthiness of lifestyle decreased (Walker, 1998) (Box 15-14).

## POSTPARTUM PHENOMENON OF CONCERN: DIET AND NUTRITION

Considerable controversy exists regarding the relationship of birth intervals, parity, prepregnancy weight or body mass index (BMI), height, and physical activity to maternal weight gain in pregnancy. The total amount of weight gained and the rate of metabolism differ among individual pregnant women (Suitor, 1997). Trends among U.S. women, and African-American women in particular, are towards increasing obesity and these gains correspond with increasing weight gain during pregnancy (Taffel, Keppel, and Jones, 1993; Kuczmarski and others, 1994;

---

> **BOX 15-14**  *Nursing Considerations for Body Image*
>
> 1. Assess for risk factors.
> 2. Establish a trusting nurse-client relationship.
> 3. Encourage expression of feelings about self-perceptions and expectations of self.
>    - Anticipatory guidance can be helpful for women experiencing loss and grief or feelings of distress over the physical changes of moving from a pregnant to a nonpregnant state.
>    - Help the woman to understand that a process of reimaging occurs, with variations unique to the individual; this can help the woman feel less isolated in the process.
>    - Acknowledge the person's feelings and assist with developing methods for dealing with cognitive distortions.
>    - Provide reliable, realistic information about postpartum involution, weight loss, nutrition, and exercise.
>    - Clarify any misconceptions that the person has about herself and her care.
> 4. Promote social interaction.
>    - Encourage the postpartum woman to accept visits from significant others.
>    - Encourage the postpartum woman to share feelings and concerns with other postpartum women.
>    - Encourage the postpartum woman to share her feelings and expectations of herself with others.
> 5. Assist the woman in developing alternative coping strategies.
> 6. Assist the woman in developing restorative goals.
>    - Nutrition
>    - Exercise
>    - Sleep-rest patterns
> 7. Evaluation of desired outcomes
>    The mother will:
>    - verbalize realistic perceptions of new body contours.
>    - report acceptance of self, speak of self in positive terms, and make no verbalizations of negative feelings about body.
>    - set realistic goals for change.
>    - initiate progressive, ongoing prescribed exercise and nutrition program.
>
> From Carpenitio LJ: *Nursing diagnosis: application to clinical practice,* ed 7, Philadelphia, 1997, Lippincott; Doenges ME and Moorhouse MF: *Maternal/Newborn plans of care: guidelines for individualizing care,* ed 3, Philadelphia, 1999, FA Davis.

---

Suitor, 1997). This is of concern because gestational weight gain is positively correlated with postpartum weight retention (Kucsmarski and others, 1994; Caulfield, Witter, and Stoltzfus, 1996; Suitor, 1997). Most postpartum women lose the majority of gestational weight during the first 3 months and continue to lose weight in smaller increments between 3 to 6 months (Brewer, Bates, and

Vannoy, 1989). However, women who retain excessive weight at 3 to 6 months postpartum are at risk for obesity (Rooney and Schauberger, 1995).

When the infant is born, most women experience an immediate weight loss of 10 to 12 pounds. In the initial 2 weeks of the postpartum period, additional weight loss occurs as the woman experiences postpartum diuresis and diaphoresis. In general, dieting for weight loss is not recommended until 6 weeks after childbirth. All women should be encouraged to eat a balanced and varied diet that includes 3 servings of dairy products, 3 servings of a lean protein source, 4 servings of fresh fruits, 4 servings of fresh or frozen vegetables, and 9 servings of unprocessed fibers. They should avoid or have minimal use of fat, oils, heavy sauces, and candy. Cooked foods should be baked, grilled, broiled, or steamed as opposed to fried or boiled (Institute of Medicine, 1992; Suitor, 1997).

All dietary instructions should be culturally sensitive. In working with women from diverse cultures, it is important to determine what foods form the basis for the particular group's diet. Additionally, we should determine the key sources of essential nutrients and the customary cooking methods the woman engages in. Useful sources of information are usually available from the state health department or WIC office.

Other concerns are the availability of foods and budgetary restrictions. Who will be doing the shopping and food preparation for the woman during the postpartum period? That person's knowledge and beliefs will have a strong influence on how and what the woman is eating. If the woman is cooking for herself, does she have the time and energy to care for herself and the baby and prepare appropriate foods? Perhaps she will need assistance in problem solving about how to be successful in this process.

In the immediate postpartum period, women should be discouraged from restricting calories (<1800 kcal of energy per day) and encouraged to increase their intake of calories or substitute foods rich in vitamins, minerals, and protein for empty calories. In some cases it may be necessary to recommend a balanced vitamin-mineral supplement. Women who are breastfeeding should be actively discouraged from use of liquid weight loss programs and appetite suppressants (Institute of Medicine, 1992).

Complete vegetarians should be advised to take a regular source of $B_{12}$, such as a $B_{12}$-fortified product or supplement. Postpartum women who are lactose intolerant should be advised of other dietary sources of calcium or should be encouraged to use low-lactose dairy products or take 600 mg of elemental calcium per day with meals. Those who live in areas where the exposure to sunlight (ultraviolet light) is limited or have low dietary intake of vitamin D should be counseled about vitamin-D fortified foods (milk, cereal) or to take a 10 $\mu$g supplement per day (Institute of Medicine, 1992).

All postpartum women should have their dietary patterns assessed. This may be accomplished with diet recall or a food frequency questionnaire. Diet recall requires that the mother recall everything she ate or drank in a specified period, usually the last 24 to 72 hours. In a food frequency checklist, the woman is asked how often she ate the foods on a list over a specified period of time, usually 1 week or longer. All women, regardless of appearances, should be asked if they need help in getting enough food to eat.

## Diet and the Lactating Woman

Data for U.S. women indicate that successful breastfeeding can occur regardless of the woman's body type. Most breastfeeding women eating self-selected diets typically lose weight at the rate of 0.5 to 1.0 kg (1 to 2 lbs) per month in the first 4 to 6 months of lactation; however, 20% may maintain or gain weight. This weight loss is felt to be a normal physiologic occurrence. Studies of healthy women in industrialized nations indicate that milk volume is not related to maternal weight, height, fluid intake, or fat indices. Rather, it is influenced by the infant's demands for milk, which in turn are primarily influenced by the size and health of the infant and the infant's intake of other supplemental foods. Studies of animals indicate that there may be caloric thresholds below which maternal intake is insufficient to allow milk production, but if this threshold exists in humans, it is unknown.

Generally speaking, maternal diets that are lacking in Recommended Daily Allowances (RDAs) of specific macronutrients will have little or no effect on the amount of that nutrient in the milk. This means, for the most part, that maternal diets lacking in specific nutrients will depend on maternal stores to provide the nutrient in the milk. Conversely, increasing maternal intake of nutrients to levels above the RDA does not result in higher levels of these nutrients in the woman's milk, with the exception of vitamin $B_6$, vitamin D, iodine, and selenium. The maternal dietary intake of fats is important. The fatty acids in human milk do vary with variation in maternal diet (Institute of Medicine, 1992).

If a breastfeeding woman is overweight and would like to lose weight, advise her that a weight loss of up to 2 kg (~ 4.5 lbs.) per month will not be likely to have an adverse affect on milk volume. However, rapid weight loss is not advisable. Women should be advised to pay special attention to eating a balanced, varied diet and to include foods rich in calcium, zinc, magnesium, vitamin $B_6$, and folate. Intakes below 1500 kcal/day are not recommended at any time during lactation (Institute of Medicine, 1992) (Box 15-15).

Contrary to popular belief, no scientific evidence supports that consumption of alcoholic beverages has a beneficial impact on any aspect of lactation performance. If a woman wishes to consume alcoholic beverages, she should do so immediately after feeding the infant or pumping her breasts, so that the maximum amount of time is allowed to metabolize the alcohol before the next feeding (Institute of Medicine, 1992).

## Referable Conditions: Weight-related Problems

Some weight-related problems may be indicative of pathophysiologic or psychologic conditions that fall outside of the purview of general nursing practice. If these problems are suspected or detected they should be referred to those with greater expertise and experience in handling these matter. Such problems may include the following:

* Slow infant growth in a breastfed infant despite frequent feeding and appropriate breastfeeding techniques
* Rapid postpartum weight loss
* Weight loss in the woman who is already below normal weight for her height
* A preoccupation with weight
* Obesity
* Postpartum weight gain

## Special Concerns for Low-Income or Homeless Women

Because of financial and social circumstances, some women may live in substandard housing or may even be homeless. These situations create unique barriers to proper nutrition, including:

1. *Lack of a safe or accessible water supply.* When the lack of a safe or accessible water supply is of concern, the woman should be encouraged to bring water jugs to the clinic to fill.
2. *Lack of refrigeration.* In these cases, one can explore the use of a cooler with ice or making an insulated cold box. Some communities also have a Salvation Army that might be able to assist with finding a serviceable refrigerator; however, that usually takes time. In these cases, it is important to suggest nutritious foods that don't require refrigeration, such as peanut butter, bread, fruit, vegetables, and canned or dry foods. Also, the family can be encouraged to obtain and prepare food in small quantities. However, when food is distributed through a food bank it is generally handed out in bulk amounts, making proper storage an ongoing problem for the family.
3. *No cooking facilities.* If the woman is on WIC, special food packages are available for these purposes. For those who are not homeless, explore potential use of a hot plate. Certainly,

---

> **BOX 15-15** *Dietary Recommendations for Lactating Women*
>
> 1. Obtain your nutrients from a well-balanced, varied diet rather than from vitamin or mineral supplements. Follow dietary guidelines that promote intake of nutrients from fruits; vegetables; whole-grain breads and cereals; calcium-rich dairy products; and protein-rich foods such as meats, fish and legumes.
> 2. Make an effort to eat vitamin-A-rich foods including carrots, spinach, or other cooked greens, sweet potatoes, and cantaloupe.
> 3. Drink plenty of fluids, particularly water, juice, and milk, to alleviate thirst. Forcing fluids is not necessary. If you drink caffeinated beverages, do so in moderation. Two servings per day are unlikely to harm the infant.
> 4. Elimination of a major nutrient source (e.g., all dairy products) to treat a presumed allergy or colic in the breastfed infant is not recommended without an elimination-challenge test (done under careful medical supervision) to determine sensitivity or intolerance to the food. Elimination-challenge tests generally involve elimination of the suspected food substance from the diet for a period of time (5 days) and reintroduction of the food substance on the morning of the sixth day to determine if the same reaction occurs. If it is necessary to eliminate a key nutrient source, you should be counseled on how to achieve adequate nutrient intake through food substitutions.
> 5. Avoid diets and medications that promise rapid weight gain. You need enough food (usually at least 1800 kcal/day) to maintain milk production.
> 6. It is best to avoid drinking alcoholic beverages, but certainly have no more than 2 to 2.5 oz. of liquor, 8 oz. of table wine, or 2 cans of beer on any 1 day.
> 7. Use foods or beverages containing sugar substitutes in moderation.
>
> From the Institute of Medicine, 1992.

---

in either case one could suggest community or church-based soup kitchens or shelters for a hot meal.

4. *Lack of money or food stamps to buy food.* Many families are not able to stretch their food or money resources enough to have food in the house from one check to another. In these cases, food pantries, soup kitchens, or shelters provide free meals. Further, the woman may need assistance with expediting her food stamp or WIC application or in applying to the program (Institute of Medicine, 1992).

Explore other options within your community. Local religious groups or community organizations may be helpful in supplying food to needy families. They may also be willing to store bulk amounts of food for a family.

### POSTPARTUM PHENOMENON OF CONCERN: ACTIVITY AND EXERCISE

Postpartum women and their families often have questions centering around when it is safe and reasonable to assume their activities of daily living and start to exercise and get back in shape. Some cultures (e.g., Mexican, Arab-American, Haitian, Russian) require new mothers to observe a specified period of bed rest or activity restriction during which female members of the family provide total care.

In general, it is important for the new mother to resume activities gradually and as she feels capable. Rest is advisable for the first week, if help is available, with the mother paying attention only to self-care and infant care. If no help is available, the woman should be advised to pace her activities and do only necessary light household chores and meal preparation. Lifting objects that weigh heavier than a grocery bag (15 lbs.) should be avoided until vaginal bleeding has stopped. Because of the weakness of the abdominal muscles, special attention to body mechanics is necessary to prevent back injuries. Climbing stairs should be limited for the first

week if there is an abdominal incision or if the woman experiences any dizziness. Overdoing with activities often leads to increased uterine bleeding; therefore, the woman should be advised that if she experiences an increase or resumption of bleeding once stopped, she should reevaluate what she is doing. She should rest for a while and monitor her bleeding (Cunningham and others, 1997; Varney, 1997).

Restrictions on driving a car should be discussed at the time of discharge. In general, following a vaginal delivery, if the woman is physiologically stable and feels safe and comfortable to drive, she may resume driving within a week. Women who have experienced a surgical delivery or postpartal tubal ligation should wait longer, certainly holding off until they are without pain. Insurance companies may also have specific restrictions that apply, particularly following an operative procedure; therefore, the woman should be encouraged to check with her auto insurance company before resumption of driving.

Returning to employment or educational pursuits should be discussed with the provider. The decision to return to these activities is often based on the health status of the woman and the type of activity in question. Most healthy postpartum women who have experienced a vaginal delivery can return to work or school

---

**BOX 15-16** *Recommended Exercises for the First Few Weeks Postpartum*

#### PATIENT TEACHING

1. *Abdominal Breathing*: Lie flat on your back with your knees bent. Take a deep breath in through your nose. As you breathe in keep your rib cage stationary and allow your abdomen to expand. Exhale slowly but forcefully and tighten your abdominal muscles, holding at the end of exhalation for a few seconds.
2. *Arm Raises*: Lie flat on your back with your arms at a 90° angle from your body (so you are in a T-shape). Raise your arms above your head moving in towards the center of your body until your hands touch. Lower slowly. Eventually these may be done with small hand weights.
3. *Cervical Range of Motion* (to relieve tension in the neck): While sitting tailor fashion, have the woman turn her head from side to side, looking over each shoulder.
4. *Poke and Tuck Exercises* (to relieve neck and subscapular tension): While sitting tailor fashion, have the woman jut her chin forward and then tuck it back, as if to create a double chin.
5. *Scapular Rotation* (to relieve tension in the neck and upper back): While sitting tailor fashion, have the shoulders rotated forward and up with inhalation, back and down during exhalation.
6. *Chin-to-Chest* (to strengthen the abdominal muscles): Lie flat on your back on a firm surface with no pillow

and raise your head onto the chest without using any other part of the body to assist you. Repeat 5 times, 3 to 4 times daily. Work up to 15 repetitions.

7. *Abdominal Crunches*: Lie flat on your back on a firm surface with no pillow, your knees bent and your arms folded across the chest or at the sides. Slowly raise yourself to a sitting position. Start by doing a few of these, 3 to 4 times daily. Work up to 10 repetitions.
8. *Knee to the Abdomen*: Lie flat on your back on a firm surface with no pillow, arms at your sides. Bend your foot at the knee until it touches your buttocks. Straighten your leg and slowly lower it. Repeat with your other leg.
9. *Buttocks Lifts*: Lie flat on your back on a firm surface with your arms down at your sides (palm down), knees bent and feet flat. Slowly raise your buttocks off the floor while arching your back. Slowly return to your original position.
10. *Double Knee Roll*: Lie flat on your back on a firm surface with your knees bent. Keep your shoulders flat and feet stationary. In a smooth rolling motion, bring your knees over to the left touching the floor or mat. Then turn to the left. Return to your starting position.
11. *Pelvic Tilt*: Lie on your back on a firm surface with your knees bent. Roll pelvis back by flattening the lower back on the floor or bed. Tighten the buttocks. Hold for a few seconds.

within 4 to 6 weeks, depending on the nature of the activity. Women who have had surgical deliveries need a longer recovery period, generally lasting at least 6 to 8 weeks (Tulman and Fawcett, 1990). Because of financial concerns, many women return sooner.

Exercises can be resumed gradually as well; however, vigorous exercise should be avoided for the first 3 weeks. In general, a program of postpartum exercise should concentrate on strengthening the pubococcygeal muscles and the abdomen as well as general toning of other muscle groups (Tulman and others, 1990). Kegel exercises should be incorporated into the daily routine of any woman, but the postpartum woman in particular should be encouraged to begin these exercises as soon as possible. Once the pelvic floor is able to withstand increased intra-abdominal pressure, abdominal strengthening exercises can begin. To test for this ability, the woman should be instructed to attempt to stop and restart urinary flow several times; once this ability is regained, abdominal toning can begin.

Postpartum women should be cautioned against leaning or bending forward when caring for the infant to prevent low back strain. Countertops or changing tables make a good working space for ease of bathing, diapering, and dressing an infant. Just as when pregnant, the mother should be instructed to bend her knees when picking up objects and to keep her spine in alignment. Heavy lifting should be avoided until the strength and tone of pelvic and abdominal musculature have returned.

Back strain from holding or carrying the infant may be minimized if the infant is held in one or both arms across the front of the body rather than in an upright position over the hip. Holding the infant over the hip may create an exaggeration of the natural lordosis of the spine. Additionally, breast engorgement and various nursing positions may create tension in the neck and upper back. In these cases, cervical range of motion exercises, neck exercises, scapular rotations, and the like have been found helpful (Box 15-16).

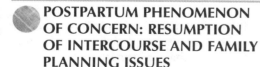

## POSTPARTUM PHENOMENON OF CONCERN: RESUMPTION OF INTERCOURSE AND FAMILY PLANNING ISSUES

Like all other areas of a couple's life, the birth of a child affects their sexual behavior. During the pregnancy, many couples report a decrease in sexual desire and frequency of intercourse. Many reasons are cited for this, including fear of miscarriage, discomfort, and the partner's fears that intercourse or orgasm will injure the fetus. After the birth of the baby, intercourse may be resumed when the lochia has stopped and sexual activity is comfortable. Resumption of intercourse in the postpartum varies with some studies reporting resumption as early as 3 weeks or as late as several months after the

birth with an average of 7 to 8 weeks. Reasons given for a delay include pain related to an episiotomy or laceration, vaginal bleeding or discharge, fatigue (Byrd and others, 1998), vaginal dryness, and involvement in infant care (Alteneder, 1997).

Breastfeeding has a significant impact on sexual desire and resumption of intercourse. In one study it was found that, at 1 month after birth, breastfeeding mothers were less likely to have resumed intercourse (14.9% vs. 28.7% of the bottle-feeding mothers) and their husbands less likely to report sexual satisfaction. By 4 months postpartum, breastfeeding mothers still reported less sexual desire; however, the number in the study still breastfeeding was much smaller, making comparison difficult (Byrd and others, 1998).

### Anticipatory Guidance

Many couples welcome, but are reluctant to initiate, a discussion regarding sexuality. By approaching the topic sensitively, we are in an excellent position to relieve anxiety, assist in adjustment, and prevent conflicts arising from misunderstandings or lack of information. Couples should be assisted to understand the changing nature of sexual satisfaction throughout the postpartum. They should be made aware of the decreased desire immediately postpartum and the variability in the timing of resumption of intercourse.

The PLISSIT model was developed to assist health care providers to identify and implement interventions for clients regarding sexuality issues. The letters in the acronym signify levels of intervention. We should be comfortable implementing the first three levels and in identifying when a referral to a specialist is needed for the fourth level (Annon, 1976). (Refer to Chapter 5 for a more in-depth discussion.)

Several nursing interventions may help dispel fears, encourage a positive relationship, and could be implemented in the PLISSIT model. Couples may need to be reminded that not all closeness and cuddling needs to lead to intercourse. Encouraging women and their partners to touch the perineum and to gently insert a clean finger may help reassure them of the integrity of the tissues. Other suggestions to decrease possible dyspareunia include use of water-soluble lubricants, warm baths, manual stimulation, and positions that allow for shallow penetration or positions that allow the woman to control the penetration such as side-lying or female superior. Instruct the woman to bear down and relax the pubococcygeal muscles to facilitate the ease of penetration (Bailey, 1989; Hampson, 1989; Fogel and Lauver, 1990; Alteneder, 1997).

Because child care becomes so consuming for a new family, finding the time to be alone and the energy for a sexual relationship becomes a challenge. In addition, sexual activity may be difficult until after the members of the extended family reduce their focus of care on the new family and resume their normal activities. The couple needs to be encouraged to find time when both are awake and interested and reassured that this time will become more frequent as time passes (Alteneder, 1997).

Because breastfeeding is considered advantageous for both mother and baby, these couples particularly need to understand that although resumption of sexual desire and activity may be delayed, there is no reason to believe it will not occur. Breastfeeding couples may also benefit from understanding that decreased sexual satisfaction and activity are normal and do not indicate a problem in their relationship. The responsible factors are:

1. Biologic: Estrogen, a hormone involved in maintaining a well-lubricated vaginal lining is suppressed during lactation, often making intercourse uncomfortable. Prolactin, which is associated with decreased sexual desire, is increased in lactation. Androgens, which are associated with increased sexual desire, are also lower during lactation.
2. Psychologic: Breastfeeding stimulates some women to orgasm. These women may then have less interest in sexual intimacy than their partners. Their partners report less sexual satisfaction because they are not engaging in satisfying sexual activity.
3. Fatigue: Breastfeeding mothers may be more fatigued (Byrd and others, 1998).

## Contraception Planning

As part of postpartum teaching, a plan for contraception should be discussed. All parents should understand the possibility of ovulation and subsequent pregnancy, even without a menstrual cycle, if no contraceptive method is employed. Most methods are initiated at the 4- to 6-week postpartum visit. However, for couples who may initiate sexual activity earlier, over-the-counter (OTC) methods such as foam and condoms provide a reliable and acceptable alternative.

The choice of product and time of initiation depend on whether the woman is breastfeeding or bottle-feeding, the presence of risk factors for a particular method, and personal preferences.

### Hormonal Preparations

Combined estrogen-progestin oral contraceptives (the pill) are an effective and popular method of contraception. For women who are breastfeeding, most providers agree that combination oral contraceptives should be discouraged until at least 6 months postpartum or when supplementary feedings are begun. This is based on the fact that the added estrogen may decrease the supply of milk. In the interim, progestin-only products may be used (the mini-pill).

A second hormonal preparation increasing in popularity is depomedroxyprogesterone acetate (DMPA, Depo-Provera, or "the shot"). Breastfeeding mothers can use this injection, which is given every 3 months. Women should be counseled regarding the most annoying side effect—unpredictable spotting and bleeding. A major advantage of this method is convenience.

Subdermal inserts of Levonorgestrel (Norplant) can be placed immediately postpartum or at the 4- to 6-week examination. Nursing mothers may also use them. The inserts may be left in place for 5 years. The long-term effects as well as convenience are advantages; the major disadvantage is irregular uterine bleeding.

### Intrauterine Devices

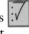

An intrauterine device (IUD) may be inserted at 6 weeks postpartum or with the first menses without any effect on breastfeeding. In some centers, IUDs are inserted immediately postpartum. Advantages of one type of IUD include safety for nursing mothers, a long period of effectiveness (10 years), and convenience. Disadvantages include a higher risk of pelvic infection, increased uterine bleeding and cramps, risk of ectopic pregnancy if a pregnancy does occur, and a low risk of uterine perforation at insertion.

### Barrier Methods

Condoms are a common method of choice in the immediate postpartum period until other methods are initiated. Women should consider using a spermicidal foam with the condom as extra protection if the condom slips or breaks. Diaphragms need to be sized for the mother and this can be done at the 6-week postpartum visit. Mothers should be aware that the diaphragm that fit before the pregnancy may not fit at this time and should not be relied upon as a contraceptive method. A different size diaphragm may need to be purchased. Instructions for use of barrier methods should be reviewed.

### Natural Family Planning

Natural family planning (NFP) refers to any method in which the woman is aware of the signs and symptoms of fertility and uses that information to avoid or achieve pregnancy. The two most common methods are the ovulation and symptothermal methods (Billings, 1987). Initiating this practice in the immediate postpartum is difficult even for the previously experienced couple. After the woman's body returns to its prepregnant state, it becomes more possible. When practiced by motivated couples, NFP can be highly effective. Advantages for couples include the absence of any chemicals, financial, and religious considerations, and interest in body awareness. Disadvantages include the investment of time and education in interpreting body changes (Trent, 1997).

**Surgical Contraception**

Surgery for a **bilateral tubal ligation (BTL or tubal)** may occur within 24 to 48 hours after the birth or at 6 weeks postpartum. The decision to proceed with a BTL should be made with care because it is considered a permanent procedure. Women need to understand that proceeding with a BTL can mean they will never become pregnant again. If a pregnancy is desired in the future, the possibility of reversal does exist, but this may fail. The efficiency of the method is an advantage; disadvantages include risks related to the surgery (bleeding, infection, anesthesia, injury to other organs) or failure of the procedure.

When the BTL has been done before postpartum discharge, we should incorporate an assessment of the incision into our visit. Characteristics of the healing BTL incision are similar to other wounds: presence of redness, discharge, or pain would necessitate notification of the provider. Mothers who have had a BTL may also delay beginning postpartum exercises until the incision area is healed and these exercises can be done comfortably. If the woman is planning to return to the hospital for tubal ligation at a later date, she should be questioned regarding the arrangements for returning for the surgery and her current method of contraception. If these have not been made, a call to the provider's office may smooth her way when she returns.

**Vasectomy,** or the surgical ligation of the male vas deferens, may be planned at any time during or after the pregnancy. Like the BTL, vasectomy is considered a permanent procedure that renders the male partner sterile. Once again, considerations for future pregnancies are important.

Because partners may change over the course of a lifetime, the decision for surgery must be a personal one. As a basic consideration, the person selecting the surgery should be the one who does not desire more children. When all else is equal, for a couple that has decided upon sterilization, the advantages of surgery in the male are the increased safety of this procedure and the lower cost. The success of the surgery may be determined by postoperative semen analysis.

*Legal Issues.* People who are considering either BTL or vasectomy and will be using Federal funds such as Medicaid for payment must be at least 21 years old. Providers also need to submit proof of client counseling, which includes knowledge of other methods that are reversible, awareness that the procedure means they will not become pregnant again, risks of the procedure, awareness that they may change their mind at any time before the surgery, and assurance that they are not being coerced in any way to submit to the procedure. The procedure may not be done within 30 days after the signing of this form, so that the person has time to change his or her mind.

**Emergency Contraception**

There may be situations in which we need to counsel the woman regarding emergency contraception after unprotected intercourse with no contraceptive method used or intercourse during which the method may possibly have failed (e.g., torn or slipped condom, torn diaphragm, errors in the practice of NFP, missed pills). When this occurs, the woman should notify her health provider because the method needs to be instituted within 72 hours of the unprotected intercourse. The most common method is a regimen of oral contraceptives, although the insertion of an IUD can also be done.

## POSTPARTUM PHENOMENON OF CONCERN: EXPECTED CHANGES WITH BREASTFEEDING

When the placenta is delivered following childbirth, estrogen and progesterone levels decrease and prolactin levels increase. Prolactin and oxytocin are necessary for the production and transfer of milk. Levels of prolactin and oxytocin are maintained through nipple stimulation. When the infant suckles at the nipple for several minutes, a complex interplay of hormonal and sensory messaging occurs between the mother and infant and the letdown (milk ejection) reflex is stimulated. During letdown the hormone oxytocin is released and this causes the alveoli to contract and milk to be ejected into the milk ducts and lactiferous sinuses and out through pores in the nipples. During the course of a feeding, several letdowns typically occur, but most women only notice the first. Maternal anxiety may inhibit the letdown reflex, so care should be taken to help the mother relax when she is breastfeeding the infant. Symptoms that may be indicative of a letdown include a sudden feeling of overwhelming thirst when the infant is at the breast, a tingling sensation in the breast tissue, ejection of milk from the opposite breast, and audible swallowing sounds from the infant.

Supporting the mother in the process of breastfeeding involves not only a positive attitude but also information about how to position the baby, how to present the nipple and bring the baby to the breast, the positioning of the nipple and the areola in the baby's mouth, and how to break the suction when the baby is to be removed from the breast. By helping the woman be comfortable and confident from the beginning, she will enjoy the process more and may prevent some of the possible problems that can occur (Figures 15-11 to 15-14).

At the time of delivery, the woman's breasts are generally soft and nontender, easy for a baby to latch on to for feeding. For the first few days postpartum, the breasts secrete **colostrum,** a rich concentrated form of breast milk that is high in calories and antibodies. Production of milk in the first few days postpartum occurs in all women, regardless of feeding method, as a result of changes in hormone levels that occur with the delivery of the placenta. On days 3 to 5 after the birth of an infant, **secondary lactogenesis** or production of transitional breast milk will occur. Transitional milk is thinner and less yellow than colostrum. During the second postpartum week, mature milk is produced. **Mature breast milk** contains a thinner, bluish white foremilk and a thicker hind milk, which is high in fat content (Lawrence, 1998; Riordan and Auerbach, 1998).

A fullness and firmness of the breast tissue, referred to as **engorgement**, generally precedes secondary lactogenesis. **Engorgement** is the result of swelling from venous distention and lymphatic congestion that accompanies this shift in milk production. With this shift in milk production, many women experience a transient flulike syndrome, reporting low-grade fevers and generalized chest aches and breast tenderness. Reassure her that this will soon pass. In addition the following information should be shared with the woman.

### Anticipatory Guidance: Prevention and Treatment of Breast Fullness

- Breast fullness is normal as the body moves from milk production that occurs solely as a result of hormonal changes to milk production that will occur because of nipple stimulation.

- When a mother has chosen to formula feed her infant, reassure her that milk production will not continue unless the nipples are stimulated either by the infant at the breast or breast pumping. Without stimulation, feelings of breast fullness and tenderness generally pass within a few days.
- When a mother has chosen to breastfeed, have her feed the baby or pump the breasts at frequent intervals to ensure continued milk production and avoid pathologic engorgement.
- During the first few days of this shift in milk production, some women may produce more milk than the infant requires and may experience discomfort associated with engorgement (Lawrence, 1998; Riordan and Auerbach, 1998).

### Breast Engorgement

Breast engorgement is a pathologic condition that may occur during the shift to secondary lactogenesis or anytime during the breastfeeding relationship when the breasts are infrequently or insufficiently drained. During engorgement, milk accumulates in the milk ducts and alveoli, producing tissue distention. The distention may be enough to result in hard and shiny breast tissue that is exquisitely painful. If the breast tissue becomes very distended, it may flatten the nipple tissue thus interfering with the ability of the infant to

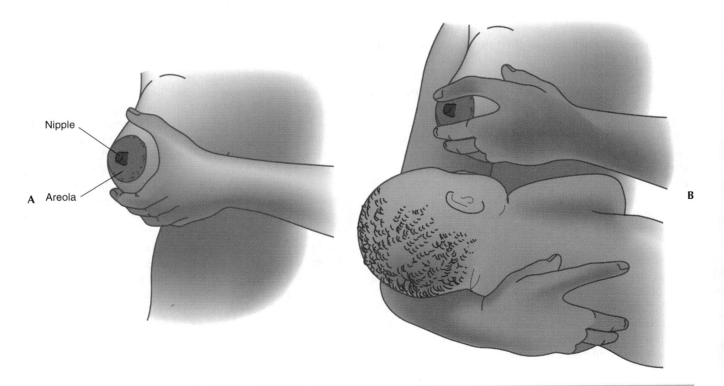

FIGURE 15-11 • To position breast and nipple. **A,** C-hold; **B,** Scissor.

latch on to the nipple and areolar tissue sufficiently to allow milk flow. Without taking the nipple and areolar into its mouth nipple trauma may occur (Figure 15-15). This places the woman at higher risk for mastitis. Pathologic engorgement requires symptomatic treatment in order to be reversed and prevent possible

further complications such as **mastitis**, or infection of the breast, or **breast abscesses.**

**Anticipatory Guidance: Breast Engorgement**

* Engorgement can be easily reversed through some simple measures such as frequent feeding at

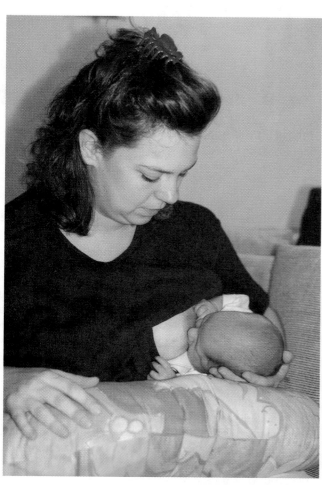

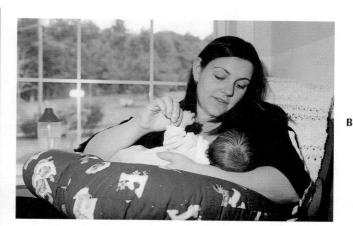

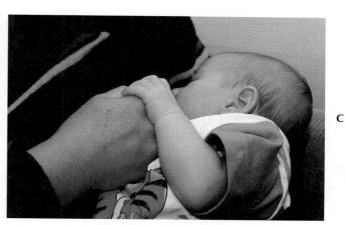

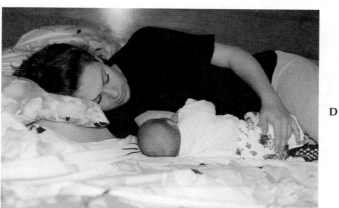

FIGURE 15-12 • Four common feeding positions. **A,** Football hold; **B,** Cradling; **C,** Across the lap; **D,** Lying down. *(Courtesy of Caroline E. Brown.)*

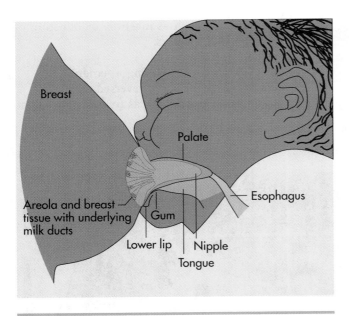

FIGURE 15-13 • Latching on.

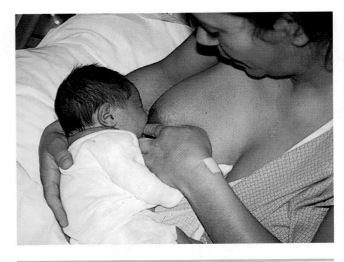

FIGURE 15-14 • Breaking the suction before removing infant from the breast.

the breast, beginning on the fuller breast until it is sufficiently drained and then having the infant switch to the opposite side to suckle enough to alleviate pressure.

- If the infant is too full or too sleepy to cooperate in this endeavor, apply warm packs to the full breast, or stand in a shower with warm water flowing over the breasts and manually express enough milk to alleviate feelings of back pressure or fullness.
- At the next feeding the infant should be offered the fuller breast first.
- Between feedings, ice packs wrapped in cloth may be applied to the breast tissue or axilla for periods of 10 minutes per hour.
- Use of a mild analgesic or antiinflammatory medication may be helpful in alleviating the aches that may accompany this period.

 Application of cool, raw cabbage leaves to alleviate breast engorgement has received some attention in the literature. Nikodem and others (1993) studied the use of cabbage leaves on maternal perceptions of breast engorgement. Mothers using the cabbage leaves tended to report less symptoms of engorgement than those mothers using routine measures, although the results were not statistically significant. Despite these limited findings, this intervention does not carry any known risks and could certainly be suggested in conjunction with other measures.

Women choosing to use this particular technique should be instructed to place washed, cool, raw cabbage leaves on the affected breast(s). Holes should be cut in the cabbage leaves to allow aeration of the nipple tissues. Cabbage leaves should be removed during feedings and every 2 hours or when they have wilted.

## Breastfeeding Support

Because breastfeeding has not always been popular in the United States, we often find that many women are breastfeeding without appropriate information on the subject and little family knowledge or support to draw upon. Most women who choose to breastfeed can be successful if they have adequate and informed support, and live in a sociocultural environment that is supportive of breastfeeding. We may be instrumental in providing breastfeeding women with the necessary support and encouragement. This requires that we recognize our role as advocates, be knowledgeable about breastfeeding, and work in ways that assist the breastfeeding relationship. We need to be aware of available lactation supports (i.e., hot lines, support groups) and provide the necessary information and referrals when necessary.

Many breastfeeding women need or desire to return to work and may need informational and instrumental support on how to combine breastfeeding and employment. This may require that she pump breast milk or supply formula for the baby to receive via a bottle when she is at work. In determining how best to combine these efforts, some important considerations include the woman's occupation, the number of hours that she plans to work, and the distance between the place of employment and the location of the infant's care provider. Some work settings are very accommodating to the needs of the breastfeeding employee while others are not. If these considerations have not been given thought during the antepartum

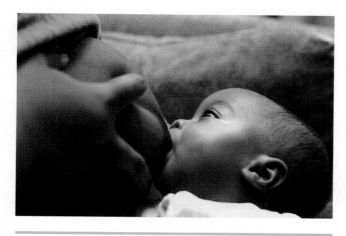

FIGURE 15-15 • Mother holding breast back so infant can breathe more easily while feeding. *(Courtesy of Caroline E. Brown.)*

period, they need to be explored now. If employment requires long periods of maternal-infant separation, the woman will need to learn about how to pump and store expressed milk. If possible, women should be encouraged to establish confidence with feeding their infants at their breasts and developing an internal milk supply before becoming focused on how to express and store milk.

### Anticipatory Guidance: Breast and Nipple Care

- Wear a firm, supportive bra to prevent undue tension on the breast tissue, particularly when they are feeling full and tender. Binding of the breasts is not considered helpful and may indeed be harmful.
- If you are breastfeeding, the breasts and nipples should be washed with plain water. Soap on the nipple area may be distasteful to the breastfeeding infant and will remove natural lubrication necessary to maintain the integrity of nipple tissues and prevent chapping and cracking.
- At the end of a breastfeeding, express a few drops of hind milk and massage it into the nipples to prevent or treat chapped nipples caused by the repeated exposure of nipple tissues to friction and moisture in the beginning breastfeeding period. Hind milk is high in fat content and has bacteriostatic properties that are helpful in protecting the integrity of nipple tissues.
- You may find the need to use a lubricant or emollient to the nipple tissue to treat chapped nipples. Several products are considered safe for these purposes.
- Use the least amount possible to achieve the desired outcome.

- A dot of the substance can be rubbed between the fingers and then gently massaged into the nipple tissue.
- Apply substances after feeding the infant and air drying a few drops of expressed hind milk on the nipples.
- There should be no need to remove the emollient or lubricant before the next feeding.

## Nipple Tenderness

Most women who breastfeed report some nipple tenderness. This tenderness is most likely to be apparent at the beginning of the feeding when the infant is suckling with the most vigor to initiate the **"letdown reflex"** and start the free flow of milk. Generally, once the letdown reflex occurs, the intensity of infant suckling efforts diminishes and the tenderness should subside. Normal nipple tenderness is transient, occurring at the beginning of each feeding for a week to 10 days. Initiating the letdown reflex before letting the infant latch on to the breast may alleviate tenderness. Stimulation of the letdown reflex may be accomplished through effleurage, use of relaxation techniques combined with visual or sensory imagery, or warm packing the breasts and doing some manual expression of the breasts before feeding.

**Effleurage** is a tactile technique of gentle stroking that uses the fingertips starting at the collarbone and working towards the nipple in a sweeping motion. Some women experience a "letdown" with this technique. Stimulation of the letdown reflex before the infant initiates latch on efforts, decreasing the amount of vigorous suckling required and thereby reducing discomfort.

### Anticipatory Guidance: Nipple Tenderness

- Stimulate a letdown reflex before initiating latch-on.
  - Practice effleurage of the breasts.
  - Use relaxation techniques.
  - Use visual and sensory imagery.
  - Provide warm packs to the breasts.
- Start the feeding on the unaffected side or the side that is less sore until the letdown reflex occurs.
- Alternate positions at each feeding to alleviate the pressure points on the sore nipple.
- Following a feeding, apply a wrapped ice pack to the nipple area for a few minutes.
- Wear ventilated breast cups (e.g., Woolrich cups) inside the bra to allow aeration of nipples and protect the nipples from chafing against clothing.
  - Remove cups and clean with warm soapy water, rinse, and dry before using them again.
- Empty the breast, but do not encourage sustained sucking as a pacifier.
- Normal tenderness resolves in 7 to 10 days and is present primarily at the start of the feeding.

## Nipple Soreness

Soreness of the nipple tissue is often due to incorrect positioning that has resulted in trauma to the nipple tissue, making the entire feeding session uncomfortable or even painful. Measures used to treat nipple tenderness may also be used to provide comfort when nipple soreness is present. Additionally, a thorough evaluation of maternal-infant positioning during the feeding is warranted.

Sudden onset of nipple soreness or prolonged, unrelieved soreness or pruritis that is apparent between feedings may be related to the presence of a yeast infection with *Candida albicans*. Women experiencing a yeast infection of the nipple typically report severe burning or stinging, which may radiate deep into the breast tissues with feeding. These feelings may persist between feedings. Typically the nipple has a hyperemic, shiny appearance with or without tiny papules. Yeast infections of the nipple often occur in the presence of a history of recent maternal and/or infant antibiotic exposure. Breastfed infants of women with these symptoms typically also manifest symptoms of thrush. The mother and infant should be referred for treatment and should be treated concurrently to eradicate the yeast infection.

## Blocked Milk Ducts

A blocked milk duct may occur because of inadequate drainage of an area of the breast in the presence of a plentiful milk supply or when an infant is persistently fed in the same position. A blocked duct will present as a smooth tender lump in the breast that does not change in consistency with feeding. Blocked ducts may lead to mastitis or a breast abscess if not adequately treated.

### Anticipatory Guidance: Blocked Milk Duct

- Before the feeding, apply moist heat to the affected area.
- Position the infant so that its nose is facing the affected area during the feeding.
- During the feeding, gently massage the area in a downward fashion, stroking towards the nipple.
- Report any flulike symptoms, increased breast tenderness, reddened areas, chills or fever.

### Mastitis

Mastitis is an inflammation of the breast that may occur at any time in the breastfeeding woman or in the initial postpartum period in the formula-feeding woman. In breastfeeding women, mastitis most often occurs sometime between the first two weeks and first two months postpartum. Mastitis is often the result of inadequate breast drainage due to missed feedings or engorgement and often occurs due to breaks in the nipple integrity. Symptoms are often sudden in onset and include a fever,

flu-like symptoms, and localized redness, warmth and tenderness of the affected breast. Mastitis is more often unilateral, but may occur bilaterally. Women with these symptoms should be referred immediately to a primary care provider and a lactation consultant.

## Breastfeeding Problems

To enable success in breastfeeding we should encourage the woman to seek out information whenever she is concerned. Written information and a telephone contact as well as a support group will be valuable as she seeks information or identifies misinformation. She should report the following breastfeeding problems:

- Unresolving breast engorgement or breast engorgement accompanied by difficulty initiating a latch-on.
- Cracked, traumatized nipples.
- Signs/symptoms of a yeast infection: sudden onset of nipple soreness that may be accompanied by fiery, red nipples, itching between feedings, and/or a burning sensation with feedings.
- Signs/symptoms of mastitis: temperature >101° F; flulike symptoms, accompanied by warm, tender, reddened areas on the breast.

## Nonlactating Engorgement

Women who formula feed their infant will experience shifts in hormones that will encourage milk production. Generally, secondary lactogenesis will cease with lack of nipple stimulation within 1 week; however, some women experience significant discomfort for a longer period of time. During this period of time, the woman should be encouraged to wear a firm, supportive bra, avoid any nipple stimulation, treat the condition symptomatically, and monitor for any signs of mastitis. Symptomatic treatment includes application of wrapped ice packs to the breasts and/or axilla to decrease venous congestion and the administration of analgesics. If the woman is amenable, cabbage leaves may also be used (see previous section on engorgement).

Many women will ask for a medication to assist in "drying up" the milk. Bromocriptine mesylate (Parlodel), Tace (an estrogen), and Deladumone (a combination of estrogen and testosterone) were routinely used in the past for this purpose. These drugs are no longer recommended (and may be prohibited in some states) because of the risks they pose to the health of the postpartum woman and the fact that engorgement may recur following discontinuation of the medication.

## Drug Use During Lactation

Few prescription drugs are contraindicated during lactation because of potential harm to the infant. Typically, drugs that are not compatible with breastfeeding can be avoided or replaced with safer ones. Breastfeeding women should consult with a care provider before taking any prescription or nonprescription medications to determine if the drug is compatible with safe breastfeeding.

Cigarette smoking and consumption of alcohol by breastfeeding women in excess of 0.5 g/kg of maternal weight may be harmful to the infant, partly because of the direct effects of nicotine and alcohol on the infant's central nervous system and partly because of potential reductions in milk volume. For a 60-kg (132-lb) woman, 0.5 g of alcohol per kg of body weight corresponds to approximately 2 to 2.5 oz. of liquor, 8 oz of wine or 2 cans of beer (Institute of Medicine, 1992). Heavy alcohol consumption in breastfeeding women has been associated with psychomotor retardation in the infant. The use of illicit drugs should be actively discouraged, and affected women, regardless of feeding method, should be assisted to enter a rehabilitative program that makes provisions for the infant. However, finding such a facility to assist the woman may be difficult, because available facilities are insufficient.

Caffeine intake should be moderated during breastfeeding to the equivalent of 1 to 2 cups of regular coffee daily. Some evidence suggests that caffeine may adversely affect the iron content of milk and the iron status of the infant (Institute of Medicine, 1992).

## POSTPARTUM PHENOMENON OF CONCERN: PERINATAL GRIEF

**Grief** is an alteration in mood and emotions related to an actual or perceived loss. Grief may accompany this period of attachment as the parents grieve the loss of an idealized child, give a child up for adoption, grieve the lost potential of a severely handicapped child, or experience the actual loss of an infant, whether anticipated or unanticipated. (Specific interventions to respond to the death of a fetus are presented in Chapter 19.) In the event of a critically ill infant, there may be anticipatory grief when the prognosis is poor. The parents may be reluctant to interact with or become more attached to the infant.

In doing postpartum home visits, we will encounter postpartum couples experiencing each of these types of grieving. The need for postpartum care of the woman continues no matter the outcome of the infant. The intensity and duration of the grief response are determined by perceptions of the loss, age, religious and cultural beliefs, ability to cope with the loss and the changes it brings about, and available support systems (Sanders, 1998). The grief response consists of many emotions including sadness, anger, guilt, fear, or relief. The goal in working with the individual or family experiencing grief is to encourage them to work through their grief while recognizing that grief is experienced in a highly individual manner.

### The Grief Process

The **grief process** has four dimensions that occur in varying and individualized patterns: **shock and numbness, searching and yearning, disorganization,** and **reorganization** (Davidson, 1984). Grievers may move back and forth between these phases or experience multiple dimensions of the grief process simultaneously. Time frames are general guidelines and should not be rigidly applied. **Shock and numbness** typically occurs in the first 2 weeks following awareness of the potential or actual loss and may be expressed as distress, disbelief, panic, or anger. The process of **searching and yearning** occurs at the time of loss, and activity generally peaks somewhere between 2 and 4 weeks later. This aspect of grief work is manifested by a search for answers, guilt, anger, and confusion over what was or was not done that might have caused this loss, and a yearning for what might have been. **Disorganization** peaks around 5 to 9 months as the bereaved moves to an awareness of reality. Physical and emotional symptoms occur that may result in a prevailing sense of a lack of well-being. As functional abilities return, self-confidence and self-esteem are restored and the bereaved person experiences **reorganization.** This period peaks at around 1 year following the loss and is manifested by an ability to experience the joys of life without guilt. The loss is still remembered, but it has been put into perspective and life has returned to "normal."

### Tasks of Perinatal Grief

Within the grief process, four tasks of perinatal grief work have been identified: **accepting the reality of the loss, working through the pain and grief, adjusting to the environment,** and **moving on with life** (Worden, 1991). As part of **accepting the reality of the loss** the family needs opportunities to see, hold, and touch their infant as a means of confirming the loss. Additionally, they need opportunities to tell their story about the events, experiences, and circumstances surrounding their loss. In **working through the grief** the bereaved need permission to express their emotions openly and will often benefit from referrals to bereavement support groups where they can share with others in a nonjudgmental environment. **Adjusting to the environment** includes learning how to live with the changes that the loss has caused. Issues about breaking the news to others, dealing with the empty nursery, returning to work, caring for other children, and getting pregnant again require some sensitive anticipatory guidance. Further, the bereaved often need an outlet for discussing how to deal with well-intended but insensitive friends, family, and coworkers. Worden's **"Moving on with Life"** (as cited previously) is consistent with Davidson's dimension of reorganization in the grief process.

### Factors that May Affect Perinatal Loss and Grief:

- *Ambivalence about the pregnancy.* Partners need assistance to understand that feelings of ambivalence during the pregnancy are normal and did not contribute to the pregnancy outcomes.
- *Motivations to become pregnant.* Some partners choose to get pregnant because they believe that the timing is right and they are ready to share and express their love through childbearing. Other partners may have chosen to become pregnant as a means of preserving a relationship, or they may have chosen to get married prematurely because of the pregnancy. Partners need assistance to understand that their motivations to become pregnant did not contribute to pregnancy outcomes.
- *Parent-fetal relationships.* Negative feelings toward the pregnancy or the fetus may contribute to feelings of guilt in the event of a loss. Conversely, positive parent-fetus relationships and enjoyment of the pregnancy may contribute to profound feelings of sadness in the event of an actual or perceived loss, regardless of the timing of gestation. In assisting these individuals or families, it is important to understand how they felt about and reacted to the pregnancy and developing fetus.
- *Social expectations related to childbearing.* Some individuals or partners may have experienced outside pressure from extended family members to become pregnant. This actual or perceived pressure may contribute to negative feelings toward those who pressured them during this grief process. These feelings need to be acknowledged and these family constellations may need assistance with working through these feelings together. Others may experience this loss as a threat to their procreative abilities and ability to fulfill their own developmental needs (Leaphart, 1985).

### Symptoms of Grief

Persons experiencing a grief response may exhibit various physical, emotional, and social effects. Physical effects include fatigue, sleep disturbances, anorexia, weight loss or weight gain, headaches, blurred vision, palpitations, vague aches, and a lack of physical strength. Emotional effects include mood disturbances, depression, difficulties in concentration, a sense of failure, and a preoccupation with the deceased. Social effects of grief include a withdrawal from normal activities and physical and/or emotional isolation from significant others (Box 15-17).

### Theoretical Framework of Caring in Perinatal Grief

Research has demonstrated that women and families experiencing perinatal grief benefit from nursing care that includes five components that were identified as knowing, being with, doing for, enabling, and maintaining belief (Swanson-Kauffman, 1986, 1988, 1990).

- *Knowing* requires asking questions and taking the time to understand the perceptions and meanings of loss in the lives of the bereaved.
- *Being with* involves using one's presence as a means of conveying acceptance of the feelings and perceptions of the bereaved. It is important to pay attention to what is said to avoid causing further distress. Responding to the feelings of the bereaved, genuine expressions of your sorrow over the loss or responding to the need of the bereaved to express feelings has been found to be helpful (e.g., "This must be difficult for you. How are you doing? I'm here if you would like to talk." "I'm sorry." "Tell me what I can do for you; I would like to help."). *Avoid statements* that negate the importance of the loss to the individuals (e.g., "You are young, you can have more children." or "This probably happened for the best.").
- *Doing for* refers to the performance of activities that provide for the physical and emotional needs of the bereaved (e.g., administration of medications, providing perineal care, making and fielding phone calls, and so on).
- *Enabling* involves offering informational support, anticipatory guidance, informed decision making, referrals, and support services that assist the bereaved to regain control over life. Local bereavement support services are often available through hospice (if the baby died) or mental health centers. Additionally, the parents may be referred to a local chapter of SHARE (Source of Help in Airing or Resolving Experiences), Resolve Through Sharing (RTS), or other perinatal bereavement groups.
- *Maintaining belief* involves assisting the bereaved to unveil or recognize their strengths and abilities as a means of beginning the healing process (Swanson-Kauffman, 1986, 1988, 1990).

## Counseling Techniques

Several techniques have been suggested to help the bereaved to express their grief, including:

- *Actualize the loss* through asking questions that allow expression of the experience of loss. It is important to refer to the infant by name, be familiar with the events surrounding the loss, and in the event of death, use the terms "death" and "dying" to make the loss real.
- *Help the bereaved identify and express feelings* by listening to the emotional tone of expressions and using communication techniques such as reflection to identify the feeling statements in verbal expressions (e.g. "You sound as if you feel guilty"). Offering answers regarding "why" the loss occurred does not assist the bereaved to work through their grief. It is important to assist the bereaved in this process and provide sensitive verbal and nonverbal support.
- *Provide time for grieving and the expression of feelings.* The bereaved need opportunities to ventilate their feelings with others.
- *Normalize feelings and symptoms consistent with the grieving process.* The grieving experience is foreign to many and the feelings and symptoms that are experienced may be disturbing if they are not normalized.
- *Allow for individual differences in the grieving process.* Because of these individual differences in grieving, it is not unusual for members of the bereaved family to have misperceptions about the feelings of others. Some family members may

hide their true feelings to protect others and, in the process, thwart their own grieving and create misperceptions of noncaring. In these cases, it is important to acknowledge how hard it must be for this person to meet everyone's needs at such a difficult time and invite them to share their hopes and personal feelings of loss. We can also assist family members to understand what one another is experiencing by acknowledging how difficult it has been for everyone (Worden, 1991).

### Complicated or Disabling Grief

There is no timetable for grieving; however, some individuals may experience incapacitating grief symptoms that do not allow them to resume usual activities of daily living. Symptoms of persistent anger, guilt, obsession with the loss, relationship difficulties, or suicidal ideation in the bereaved require referral to a qualified therapist. Because of the stigma associated with emotional difficulties, many persons are reluctant to seek therapy. We should make every effort to assist the individual with incapacitating grief to overcome perceived barriers to care.

## POSTPARTUM PHENOMENON OF CONCERN: DOMESTIC VIOLENCE

There are estimates that 1 of 4 to 1 of 10 women is in a violent relationship. This abuse may begin or worsen during the pregnancy or postpartum period, making screening for abuse an integral part of our care. All women should have the opportunity to be screened in a safe and private environment, and two or three questions will often elicit a positive response: "Is anyone physically hurting you?" "Has anyone ever hurt you physically?" and "Are you afraid of your partner?" (Furniss, 1993; King and others, 1993). If the woman answers positively to these queries, encourage her to talk about it (e.g., "Would you like to talk about what happened to you?" "How do you feel about it?" "What would you like to do about this?") and validate her experience (e.g., "You are not alone." "This is not uncommon even though it is against the law." "Would you like me to help you?") (New York State Office for the Prevention of Domestic Violence, 1992).

If the woman answers, "No" or will not discuss the topic, be aware of any clinical signs that may indicate abuse. Being sensitive to the potential of abuse may increase our awareness of behavioral cues such as excessive concerns about infant well-being, vague somatic complaints, acute anxiety during physical examinations, headaches, and weight loss (Furniss, 1993). If any of these clinical signs are present, make sure that the woman is alone and no one is listening, not even a child. Then ask more specific questions about how the injury happened (e.g., "Can you tell me how this happened?" or "I'd like to learn more about how this happened to you.").

If the woman denies abuse, document only your actual findings. Let her know that you are there to help. If she agrees, give her the names, locations, and numbers of area resources if should she need help. Do not leave this information with her unless she wants it. If she is being abused and the abuser finds the information, she will be at increased risk. Keep the lines of communication open and plan to see her again.

Many women, because of the stigma involved in domestic violence and/or their fear of the abuser, deny the existence of the problem. In these cases, it is often important to address issues of self-esteem and trust before the woman can openly admit to the problem (New York State Office for the Prevention of Domestic Violence, 1992).

Once the woman has confirmed the problem, learn from her what it is she would like to do. Remembering the steps of beginning intervention may be aided by using the simple mnemonic tool, ABCDES, developed by Holtz and Furniss (1993).

> **A**—Reassurance she is not **alone**. Abuse denigrates and isolates women; they need to know they have shared their story with a provider who can help. Knowledge that help is available may be the first step to a life without violence. Listen nonjudgmentally. This begins the healing process and gives you insight into what referrals are needed.
>
> **B**—Express the **belief** that violence is not acceptable, no matter what she has been told by the batterer. "No one has to live with violence." "You are not to blame." "You do not deserve to be treated this way." When she knows she should never be hurt, she may begin self-protection and setting boundaries.
>
> **C**—**Confidentiality** must be assured. She must be aware that the information will be confidential but will be documented in her chart in case it is needed for legal purposes.
>
> **D**—**Documentation** includes a statement by the woman about the abuse. Clear descriptions of the injuries and a history of the first, worst, and most recent incident are important. Saving evidence such as photographs should be done by agency protocol.
>
> **E**—**Education** about the cycle and possible escalation of violence is necessary. Women must be aware that protestations of remorse are mean-

ingless. Women need to have information about shelters, hot lines, and other community services.

> **S**—If a woman returns to the abuser, **safety** is an issue. Discussion of an escape plan, including a packed bag and identifying and locating important legal documents, is helpful. Women should also know the legal options they may take.

Understanding the process in which the woman is involved is not easy for health providers. The decision to leave is a dangerous and difficult process that the woman herself must make (Ulrich, 1993). Remember that the risk of being killed by her abuser is increased when the woman leaves.

## Legal and Ethical Issues in Postpartum Abuse

When confronted with the reality of domestic violence in the postpartum family, we face several legal and ethical dilemmas. The need for fidelity (confidentiality) must be balanced with the duty to care and protect from harm. From a legal standpoint, we must follow the mandated reporter laws in our state, which are usually limited to elder and child abuse cases. Some states also have mandated reporting of injuries from knives or gun shots. However, when violence occurs within a family, the children may be at a direct or indirect risk. We are put in the position of having to judge the dangerousness of the situation and to act as an advocate for the children. Yet this may compromise our relationship with the postpartum woman and place her in greater danger.

 **SUMMARY**

The postpartum period begins after the fourth stage of childbirth is complete (1 to 2 hours after the expulsion of the placenta). During the 3 months following the birth of her baby, the mother's body returns to its nonpregnant state, the infant adapts to its surroundings and settles into extrauterine life, and the psychologic adaptation to parenthood takes place.

Our care focuses on assessing the needs of the woman and her infant and responding with appropriate assistance as the woman, the baby, and the family adapt to new experiences. Collaborative care enables our clients to successfully attain their desired health status and adapt to new roles.

# Care Plan · The Well Postpartum Woman

For a well postpartum woman, nursing care focuses on assessing for and preventing potential problems and promoting adaptation. A comprehensive care plan would include assessments of all the physiologic and psychosocial parameters discussed in this chapter. This sample care plan merely lists those parameters to assess for all postpartum women. A more detailed plan is given for three nursing diagnoses that normal, healthy women commonly experience during the postpartum period.

## Assessments/Monitoring
- Vital signs (TPR, B/P)
- Breasts and nipples (for fullness and skin integrity)
- Breastfeeding (knowledge, adaptation)
- Uterus (height and firmness)
- Lochia (color, amount, odor)
- Perineum (incision approximation, bruising, hemorrhoids)
- Voiding (frequency, completeness, burning)
- Circulatory system (varicose veins, thrombophlebitis)
- Nutritional status and intake
- Mental-emotional status (e.g., "blues," depression)
- Parent-infant attachment
- Maternal and family adaptation

**NURSING DIAGNOSIS** **Risk for Ineffective Individual Coping ("blues" and depression)** related to transition to parenthood, unsatisfactory social support, and fatigue

**GOALS/OUTCOMES** Demonstrates ability to cope with and adapt to postpartum physiologic and psychosocial changes *(See "Evaluation Parameters")*

### NOC Suggested Outcomes
- Coping (1302)
- Decision Making (0906)
- Information Processing (0907)
- Role Performance (1501)

### NIC Priority Interventions
- Anticipatory Guidance (5210)
- Coping Enhancement (5230)
- Decision-Making Support (5250)
- Teaching: Individual (5606)F

### Nursing Activities and Rationale
- Assess for excessive mood changes, crying, anxiety, insomnia, loss of appetite, and irritability. *Depending on severity and duration, these may be symptoms of blues, depression, or postpartum psychosis.*
- Differentiate between transient postpartum blues, postpartum depression, and postpartum psychosis. *Most women experience some emotional lability immediately after childbirth, which usually passes without intervention. Depression occurs insidiously at about 2 weeks postpartum (or any time during the first year), is more severe, and lasts longer; it may include social isolation and thoughts of suicide. Postpartum psychosis is rare, has early onset, and includes functional impairment, confusion, hallucinations, and delusions.*
- Reassure woman and family that the symptoms of postpartum blues are normal and will usually subside within 1 to 10 days *to relieve anxiety and guilt over not being a "happy new mother" and to reassure her that she is not "crazy."*
- Promote rest (see care plan for "Fatigue"). *Fatigue has been found to be an etiology for depression.*
- Encourage the woman to eat a well-balanced diet *to enhance overall well-being.*
- Encourage the woman to talk to others about her feelings and what she does and doesn't find helpful *to allow for meaningful help and support.*
- Encourage the woman to accept offers of help from friends and family members; help her to understand that accepting help is not a sign of weakness or "poor mothering"; recognizing the need for help is a strength. *Postpartum physical and emotional changes together with the extra work of a new baby can be overwhelming.*
- Encourage the woman to plan time for meeting her own needs (e.g., exercise, an outing with partner or friends). *Promotes adaptation; allows for personal renewal so that she can resume caregiving activities.*
- Provide referrals to community resources as needed *to help meet the needs of the family and for social support if family and friends are not available or adequate.*
- Reinforce the importance of keeping her appointments, *which allows for serial assessment of depressive symptoms.*
- Teach the woman and family to call if she has or expresses thoughts about harming herself or the baby. *This may be a sign of significantly worsening symptoms that could result in harm to the woman of her infant.*

*Continued*

## Care Plan  ·  The Well Postpartum Woman—cont'd

**Evaluation Parameters**
- Verbalizes adequate support from family and friends
- Makes rational decisions about self-care and infant care
- Verbalizes plan for obtaining adequate rest
- Seeks and uses information about infant care, as needed
- Recognizes when stress is increasing and uses stress relief measures
- Talks to family and health professionals about her feelings
- Blues and depression are mild and limited in duration

NURSING DIAGNOSIS    **Risk for Fatigue** related to discomfort, physical emotional demands of infant and family, and emotional stressors

GOALS/OUTCOMES    Demonstrates energy level adequate for self-care and infant care and other activities of daily living *(See "Evaluation Parameters")*

**NOC Suggested Outcomes**
- Energy Conservation (0002)
- Psychomotor Energy (0006)
- Rest (0003)
- Sleep (0004)

**NIC Priority Interventions**
- Energy Management (0180)
- Sleep Enhancement (1850)

**Nursing Activities and Rationale**
- Assess risk factors (e.g., demands of infant and family, discomfort) *to individualize plan and address etiology of problem.*
- Assess for lack of energy, circles under the eyes, and statements of extreme fatigue, *which are signs of physical and emotional fatigue.*
- Discuss causes and symptoms of fatigue with the woman. *Awareness and self-monitoring allow for timely intervention if problem develops.*
- Allow opportunities for the mother to review intrapartal and early postpartal events. *The need to work through the experience may help overcome emotions that interfere with the ability to relax and rest. Cumulative sleep loss must be overcome as soon as possible to prevent additional problems such as Impaired Home Maintenance Management or Impaired Parent/Infant Attachment.*
- Explore with the mother what other responsibilities she must assume when the infant sleeps. Problem solve with her and encourage her to rest or nap when the infant sleeps. *Mothers sometimes must use the infant's sleep time to "catch up on" tasks they cannot attend to when the infant is awake.*
- Suggest efforts to modify the infant's sleep behaviors as the infant gets older, to promote longer waking periods during the daytime (Note: this may take several weeks). *This helps the infant maintain longer stretches of sleep at night and allows for more uninterrupted sleep for the mother.*
- During the first few days, encourage limits on outside activities and a limited number of visitors *to help prevent exhaustion.*
- Assess dietary intake and hematocrit; provide information about daily iron and vitamin supplements; teach content of a balanced diet; assess ability to meet dietary needs; provide referrals as needed (e.g., WIC, food stamps). *A well balanced diet is needed to promote healing and overcome nutritional deficiencies, which may contribute to fatigue and inadequate energy levels. An adequate hematocrit level is needed to maintain or increase the oxygen-carrying capacity of the blood and support energy levels.*
- Determine family structure; assess work capabilities, roles, and responsibilities of each member; encourage sharing of household tasks. *Division of labor reduces amount of responsibility that the woman assumes and helps conserve energy.*
- Encourage the woman to establish a quiet, relaxing routine before retiring (e.g., reading a book or having a glass of warm milk or wine), which *aids in relaxation and promotes sleep.*

**Evaluation Parameters**
- Balances activity and rest
- Recognizes energy limitations
- Maintains good nutritional intake
- Exhibits ability to concentrate
- Energy level adequate for ADLs and infant care
- Naps at least once a day
- Reports feeling rested after sleeping at night

## Care Plan · The Well Postpartum Woman—cont'd

**NURSING DIAGNOSIS**   **Pain** related to breast engorgement
**GOALS/OUTCOMES**   Will maintain optimal level of comfort *(See "Evaluation Parameters")*

### NOC Suggested Outcomes
- Comfort Level (2100)
- Pain Control (1605)

### NIC Priority Interventions
- Pain Management (1400)
- Teaching, Individual (5606)

### Nursing Activities and Rationale
- Teach signs and symptoms of breast engorgement and mastitis *to allow for early self-treatment of engorgement and prevention of a possible complication.*
- Assess for hard, shiny, painful breasts, *which are signs of engorgement.*
- Assess for unilateral (occasionally bilateral) localized redness, warmth, and tenderness of a breast with fever and flulike symptoms. *Signs and symptoms of mastitis should be referred immediately to a care provider.*
- If breastfeeding, offer the breast or pump the breasts at frequent intervals *to ensure milk production and alleviate pressure.*
- If infant is too full or sleepy to suck, apply warm packs to the full breast, or stand in a warm shower and manually express milk *to relieve pressure and fullness.*
- At the next feeding, offer the infant the fuller breast first *to relieve pressure where it is most urgently needed.*
- Between feedings, apply ice packs wrapped in cloth; apply to breast tissue or axilla for periods of 10 minutes per hour *to prevent further accumulation of milk in the ducts.*
- Apply washed, cool, raw cabbage leaves to the affected breast(s); cut holes in the leaves to allow air to the nipples. Remove leaves during feedings or when the leaves have wilted. *Some women have found this to relieve symptoms of engorgement; results are inconclusive, but the intervention carries no risks.*
- Suggest the use of a mild analgesic *to alleviate accompanying aches.*
- Assess for nipple redness or soreness. *If breast tissue is distended, it may flatten the nipple and interfere with the infant's ability to latch on to the nipple and areola properly, causing nipple trauma.*

### Evaluation Parameters
- Reports acceptable comfort level
- Reports resolution of breast tenderness and "aching" chest
- Reports reversal of engorgement

## CASE STUDY

Zoila is a 35 year old, G 2, P 2, who is now 7 days postpartum. Her husband, Tom, has brought her to the office today, Monday, because things had been going so well but this last weekend she has just been "crying." He says, "I don't remember her like this when our daughter was born 2 years ago. Then she cried in the hospital but not at home."

Zoila is college educated and worked as a research assistant before she left her job to work at home caring for their first child. She tells you that she is upset because she thinks she is "losing her mind." She can't remember where she puts things, she is irritable, and she just is not a good mother.

Zoila's recent pregnancy was uneventful. She had a vaginal birth for her first child, but this labor was protracted, complicated by a fetal distress, and their son

born with a surgical delivery. Her postpartum course in the hospital was routine, and during the last week she has had support and assistance from family members and friends. However, she feels very tired. She expresses dismay over her appearance, stating, "My body will never be the same again."

Zoila is breastfeeding the baby, and that is going well. Her pediatrician examined the baby before discharge from the hospital and said that he was healthy.

The last 2 days, Tom became concerned because Zoila just wanted to stay in bed. She cried and slept, feeding the baby when Tom brought him to her in bed. This morning he was concerned about leaving her and the children and going to work. His mother lives nearby but she is only able to help out three mornings a week. Zoila's mother died last year. Other family members

# CASE STUDY

and friends live nearby and have offered to help, but Zoila says she doesn't want to bother them or let them know that she "can't handle it."

- What subjective data do you have based on your interview?
- What other information would be helpful?
- What objective data would you want to obtain?
- Based on the information that you have, what do you think Zoila is experiencing?
- What factors support this diagnosis?

- What are other possible diagnoses that must also be considered?
- Develop short- and long-term goals.
- What interventions may be helpful to Zoila and Tom?
- How will you prioritize the interventions?
- How will you evaluate the effect of your care today?
- What will be the plans for care after Tom and Zoila leave the office today?

# Scenarios

**1.** Joy is 18 years old and delivered at your birthing center 3 days ago. She is now calling on the phone to tell you she just got up and is "passing clots."

- What subjective and objective information do you need before you respond?
- What nursing diagnoses could apply? How will you validate these?
- What goals might be developed? How will these be prioritized?
- What interventions may you offer?
- How will you evaluate the effectiveness of your interventions?

**2.** You are working in the clinic. Rose is there for her 6 week postpartum visit. As you weigh her, she expresses dismay over her weight—she has only lost 15 pounds since the birth of the baby. She is breast-feeding and very surprised she has not lost "a lot of weight."

- What subjective and objective information do you need before you respond?
- What nursing diagnoses could apply? How will you validate these?
- What goals might be developed? How will these be prioritized?

- What interventions may you offer?
- How will you evaluate the effectiveness of your interventions?

**3.** You are working in the WIC office. Maria comes in for a lactation consultation. Her baby is 2 weeks old. She is breastfeeding for the first time and having a problem with sore nipples.

- What subjective and objective information do you need before you respond?
- What nursing diagnoses could apply? How will you validate these?
- What goals might be developed? How will these be prioritized?
- What interventions may you offer?
- How will you evaluate the effectiveness of your interventions?

**4.** Your community health agency just received a phone call from a woman who wants information about emergency contraception because she thinks she may need it. She is 4 weeks postpartum, so she has not had her 6 week postpartum visit when her doctor talks about contraception. She and her husband went farther than they expected last night and had intercourse.

Now she is afraid she might be pregnant again. You are the nurse doing the telephone triage.

- What subjective and objective information do you need before you respond?
- What nursing diagnoses could apply? How will you validate these?
- What goals might be developed? How will these be prioritized?
- What interventions may you offer?
- How will you evaluate the effectiveness of your interventions?

5. Darcie gave birth to a healthy boy last night in the birthing suite. You are providing her care before she is discharged later today. She is filling out the birth certificate the clerk left on her bed and asks if she can ask you a question. She tells you that the man who went through labor and delivery with her is the father of her baby but not her husband. She is married, but she and her husband have been legally separated for some time. She wants to know if she can put the "real" father's name on the birth certificate.

- What other information do you need before you respond?
- What nursing diagnoses could apply? How will you validate these?
- What goals might be developed? How will these be prioritized?
- What interventions may you offer?
- How will you evaluate the effectiveness of your interventions?

6. Cynthia, a 21-year-old single woman living with her mother, gave birth to her first child in the birthing room yesterday and opted for discharge 8 hours later. You are doing a home visit this morning. It has been 48 hours since she gave birth to the baby.

- What assessments do you need to provide?
- What nursing diagnoses do you anticipate? How will you validate these?

- What subjective or objective data may indicate possible problems?
- What goals might be developed? How will these be prioritized?
- What interventions may you offer?
- How will you evaluate the effectiveness of your interventions?

7. You are making a home visit to Renee, age 34. Her referral states she is a G2 P2 002 who is now 4 days postpartum. She had a vaginal delivery and the repair of a second-degree perineal laceration. Renee is very concerned about having a bowel movement; she is afraid it will rip out her sutures.

- What subjective and objective information do you need before you respond?
- What nursing diagnoses could apply? How will you validate these?
- What goals might be developed? How will these be prioritized?
- What interventions may you offer?
- How will you evaluate the effectiveness of your interventions?

8. Yeona delivered her son yesterday and initiated breastfeeding during the first half-hour after birth. The baby has gone to the breast every 2 to 3 hours since then. He is now 24 hours old, and they will be going home today. Yeona tells you that she is a computer programmer and will be returning to work in 6 weeks. She asks what she should do when that time comes.

- What subjective and objective information do you need before you respond?
- What nursing diagnoses could apply? How will you validate these?
- What goals might be developed? How will these be prioritized?
- What interventions may you offer?
- What community referrals should be included?
- How will you evaluate the effectiveness of your interventions?

## REFERENCES

Affonso DD: Postpartum depression: a nursing perspective on women's health and behaviors, *IMAGE* 24(3):215-221, 1992.

Affonso DD and others: A standardized interview that differentiates pregnancy and postpartum symptoms from perinatal clinical depression, *Birth* 17(3):121-130, 1990.

Albright A: Postpartum depression: an overview, *J Counsel Dev* 71:316, 1993.

Alteneder R and Hartzell D: Addressing couples' sexuality concerns during the childbearing period: use of the PLISSIT model, *J Obstet Gynecol Neonatal Nurs* 26(6):651-658, 1997.

Ament LA: Maternal tasks of the puerperium reidentified, *J Obstet Gynecol Neonatal Nurs* 25(9):737-742, 1990.

American Academy of Pediatrics and The American College of Obstetricians and Gynecologists: *Guidelines for perinatal care,* ed 4, Washington, DC, 1997, The Academy.

American Hospital Association, Section for Maternal and Child Health: *Issue brief: maternal and newborn length of stay,* Washington, DC, 1995, Author.

Aminoff MJ: Neurologic disorders. In Creasy RK and Resnik R, editors: *Maternal-fetal medicine,* ed 4, Philadelphia, 1999, WB Saunders.

Andrews MM and Boyle JS: *Transcultural concepts in nursing care,* Philadelphia, 1999, JB Lippincott.

Annon J: *Behavioral treatment of sexual problems: brief therapy,* vol I, New York, 1976, Harper & Row.

Arenson JD: Strengths and self-perceptions of parenting in adolescent mothers, *J Pediatr Nurs* 9:251-257, 1994.

Association of Women's Health, Obstetric and Neonatal Nurses (AWHONN): *Guideline for home care of women and newborns. Standards and guidelines for professional nursing practice in the care of women and newborns,* ed 5, Washington, DC, 1998, AWHONN.

Aylward GP: The relationship between environmental risk and developmental outcome, *Dev Behavior Pediatr* 13:222-229, 1992.

Bailey VR: Sexuality before and after birth, *Midwives Chronicle and Nursing Notes* 102 (1212):24-26, 1989.

Beck CT, Reynolds MA, and Rutowski P: Maternity blues and postpartum depression, *J Obstet Gynecol Neonatal Nurs* 21(4):287-293, 1992.

Beck CT: Teetering on the edge: a substantive theory of postpartum depression, *Nurs Res* 42(1):42-48, 1993.

Beck CT: Screening methods for postpartum depression, *J Obstet Gynecol Neonatal Nurs* 24(4):308, 1995a.

Beck CT: The effects of postpartum depression on maternal-infant interaction: a meta-analysis, *Nurs Res* 44(5):296-304, 1995b.

Bengtson VN: Diversity in symbolism in grandparental roles. In Bengtson V and Robertson T, editors. *Grandparenthood,* Newbury Park, Calif, 1985, Sage.

Berkey KM and Hanson SMH: *Pocket guide to family assessment and intervention,* St Louis, 1991, Mosby.

Berkowitz GS and others: Delayed childbearing and the outcome of pregnancy, *N Engl J Med* 322, 659-664, 1990.

Billings JJ: *The ovulation method: natural family planning,* ed 5, Collegeville, Minn, 1987, The Liturgical Press.

Bond L: Physiology of pregnancy. In Mattson S and Smith JE, editors: *Core curriculum for maternal-newborn nursing,* Philadelphia, 1993, WB Saunders.

Bouchard C: Current understanding of the etiology of obesity: genetic and nongenetic factors, *Am J Clin Nutr* 53:1561S-1565S, 1991.

Bowen GL, Desimone LM, and McKay JK: Poverty and the single mother family: a macroeconomic perspective. In Hanson S and others, editors: *Single parent families: diversity, myths and realities,* New York, 1995, Howarth Press.

Brazleton TB: The behavioral competence of the newborn. In Avery GB, editor: *Neonatology: pathophysiology and management of the newborn,* ed 3, Philadelphia, 1986, JB Lippincott.

Brewer MM, Bates MR, and Vannoy LP: Postpartum changes in maternal weight and body fat depots in lactating vs nonlactating women, *Am J Clin Nutr* 49, 259-265, 1989.

Brooke PS: Legal context for community health nursing practice. In Smith CM and Maurer FA, editors: *Community health nursing,* Philadelphia, 1995, WB Saunders.

Brown LP, Towne SA, and York R: Controversial issues surrounding early postpartum discharge, *Nurs Clin North Am* 31(2):333-339, 1996.

Burke PJ and Liston WJ: Adolescent mothers' perceptions of social support and the impact of parenting on their lives, *Pediatr Nurs* 20:593-599, 1994.

Byrd JE and others: Sexuality during pregnancy and the year postpartum, *J Fam Pract* 47(4):305-308, 1998.

Cain M: *First time mothers, last chance babies: parenting at 35+,* Far Hills, NJ, 1994, New Horizon.

Campbell S and others: Course and correlates of postpartum depression during the transition to parenthood, *Develop Psychopathol* 4:29-47, 1992.

Cappel C and Heiner RB: The intergenerational transmission of family aggression, *J Fam Violence* 5:135-152, 1990.

Carpenito LJ: *Nursing diagnosis: application to clinical practice,* ed 7, Philadelphia, 1997, Lippincott.

Carter EA and McGoldrick M, editors: *The changing family life cycle: a framework for family therapists,* ed 2, New York, 1989, Gardner Press.

Carsoni D, David H, and Berthiaume M: Psycho-social correlates of postpartum depression. Paper presented at the 101st annual meeting of the American Psychological Association, August, 1993, Toronto, Canada.

Caulfield LE, Witter FR, and Stoltzfus RJ: Determinants of gestational weight gain outside the recommended ranges among black and white women, *Obstet Gynecol* 87:760-766, 1996.

Clark AL: Adaptation problems and the expanding family, *Nursing Forum* 5:98, 1966.

Clark MJ: The home visit process and home health nursing. In Clark MJ, editor. *Nursing in the community,* Stamford, Conn, 1999, Appleton & Lange.

Clinical Classifications for Health Policy Research: Hospital Inpatient Statistics, 1995. HCUP-3 Research Note. Agency for Health Care Policy and Research, Rockville, Md.. http://www.ahcpr.gov/data/his95/clinclas.htm

Coddy B: The therapist was a gringa. In Smoyak S, editor: *The psychiatric nurse as a family therapist,* New York, 1975, Wiley.

Collins NL and others: Social support in pregnancy: psychosocial correlates of birth outcomes and postpartum depression, *J Pers Soc Psychol* 65:1243-1258, 1993.

Commission on Professional and Hospital Activities: Hospital length of stay by diagnosis and operations in the U.S. (January-December 1990), Ann Arbor, 1991, Author.

Commission on Professional and Hospital Activities: Hospital length of stay by diagnosis and operations in the U.S. (January-December 1992), Ann Arbor, 1993, Author.

Crawford J: A theoretical model of support network conflict experienced by new mothers, *Nurs Res* 34:100, 1985.

Creasy R and Resnik R, editors: *Maternal-Fetal medicine,* ed 4, Philadelphia, 1999, WB Saunders.

Cunningham FG and others: *Williams obstetrics,* ed 20, Stamford, Conn, 1997, Appleton & Lange.

Curran D: *Traits of a healthy family,* Minneapolis, Minn, 1983, Winston Press.

Davidson GW: *Understanding mourning,* Minneapolis, Minn, 1984, Ausburg

Davidson N: REEDA: evaluating postpartum healing, *J Nurse-Midwifery* 19:6-8, 1974.

Denehy JA: Interventions related to parent-infant attachment, *Nurs Clin North Am* 27:425, 1992.

Department of Obstetrics and Gynecology: *Right from the start,* Bassett Healthcare, 1997, The Department.

Deutsher M: Brief family therapy in the course of first pregnancy: a clinical note, *Contemp Psychoanal* 7(1):21-35, 1970.

Dimitrovsky L, Lev S, and Itskowitz R: Relationship of maternal and general self-acceptance to pre-and postpartum affective experience, *J Psychol* 132(5):507-516, 1998.

Doenges ME and Moorhouse MF: *Maternal-Newborn plans of care: guidelines for planning and documenting client care,* ed 2, Philadelphia, 1994, FA Davis.

Dollemore D: *Natural healing remedies,* Emmaus, Penn, 1998, Rodale.

Dunn J and Kendrick C: Siblings and their mothers: developing relationships within the family. In Lamb ME and Sutton-Smith B, editors: *Sibling relationships: their nature and significance across the lifespan,* Hillsdale, NJ, 1982, Lawrence Erlbaum Associates.

Dunnewold A and Sanford D: *Postpartum survival guide,* Oakland, Calif, 1994, New Harbinger Publications.

Duvall EM: *Marriage and family development,* ed 6, Philadelphia, 1977, JB Lippincott.

Duvall EM and Miller BL: *Marriage and family development,* ed 6, New York, 1985, Harper & Row.

East PL and Felice ME: Outcomes and parent-child relationships of former adolescent mothers and their 12-year-old children, *Dev Behav Pediatr* 11(4):175-183, 1990.

Edwards DRL, Porter SM, and Stein GS: A pilot study of postnatal depression following cesarean section using two retrospective self-rating instruments, *J Psychosomatic Res* 38:111-117, 1994.

Eliason ML: Lesbian and gay family issues, *J Fam Nurs* 2(1):10-29, 1996.

Epperson CN: Postpartum major depression: detection and treatment, *Am Fam Phys* 59(8):247-254, 1999.

Fawcett J: The relationship between identification and patterns of change in spouse's body images during and after pregnancy, *Int J Nurs Studies* 14:199-213, 1977.

Field T: Early interactions between infants and their postpartum depressed mothers, *Infant Behav Develop* 7:517-522, 1984.

Field T and others: Infants of depressed mothers show "depressed" behavior even with nondepressed adults, *Child Develop* 59:1569-1579, 1988.

Fiesta J: Premature discharge, *Nurs Management* 25(4):17, 1994.

Fogel CI and Lauver D: *Sexual health promotion,* Philadelphia, 1990, WB Saunders.

Fortier JC, Carson VB, and Will S: Adjustment to a newborn, *J Obstet Gynecol Neonatal Nurs* 20(1):73-75, 1991.

Friedman MM: *Family nursing: research, theory and practice,* ed 4, Stamford, Conn, 1998, Appleton & Lange.

Friedman MM and others: Family developmental theory. In Friedman MM, editor: *Family nursing: research, theory and practice,* ed 4, Stamford, Conn, 1998, Appleton & Lange.

Friedman MM and Heady S: Family role structure. In Friedman MM, editor: *Family nursing: research, theory and practice,* ed 4, Stamford, Conn, 1998, Appleton & Lange.

Furniss KK: Screening for abuse in the clinical setting, *AWHONN's Clin Iss Perinatal Women's Health Nurs* 4(3):402-406, 1993.

Gamble D and Morse JM: Fathers of breastfed infants: postponing and types of involvement, *J Obstet Gynecol Neonatal Nurs* 22(4):358-365, 1993.

Gelfano D and Teti DM: The effects of maternal postpartum depression on children, *Clin Psychol Rev* 10:329-333, 1990.

Geronimus AT and Korenman S: The socioeconomic consequences of teen childbearing reconsidered, *Q J Econ* 4:1187-1214, 1992.

Gerson E: *Infant behavior in the first year of life,* New York, 1973, Raven Press.

Gottlieb LN and Mendelson MJ: Parental support and firstborn girls' adaptation the birth of a sibling, *J Applied Dev Psychol* 11:29-48, 1990.

Grant CC and others: The father's role during infancy, *Arch Pediatr Adolesc Med* 151:705-711, 1997.

Greenberg M and Morris N: Engrossment: the newborn's impact upon the father, *Am J Orthopsychiatry* 44(4):520-531, 1974.

Gromada KK: Maternal-infant attachment: the first step toward individualizing twins, *MCN Am J Matern Child Nurs* 6:129-134, 1992.

Hall LA, Sachs B, and Rayens MK: Mothers potential for child abuse: the role of childhood abuse and social resources, *Nurs Res* 47:87-95, 1998.

Hampson SJ: Nursing interventions for the first three postpartum months, *J Obstet Gynecol Neonatal Nurs* 18:116-122, 1989.

Hangsleben KL: Transition to fatherhood, *J Obstet Gynecol Neonatal Nurs* 15(4):265-270, 1983.

Hanson SMH and Mischke K: Family health assessment and intervention. In Bomar PJ, editor. *Nurses and family health promotion,* ed 2, Philadelphia, 1996, WB Saunders.

Harberger PN, Berchtold NG, and Honikman JL: Cries for help. In Hamilton JA and Harberger PN, editors: *Postpartum psychiatric illness: a picture puzzle,* Philadelphia, 1992, University of Pennsylvania Press.

Hardy ME and Hardy WL: Role stress and role strain. Managing role strain. In Hardy ME and Conway M, editors: *Role theory: perspectives for health professionals,* Norwalk, Conn, 1988, Appleton & Lange.

Harkness S: The cultural mediation of postpartum depression, *Med Anthropol Q* 1:194-209, 1987.

Henderson AD and Brouse AJ: The experience of new fathers during the first 3 weeks of life, *J Adv Nurs* 16:293-298, 1991.

Henneman EA, Lee JL, and Cohen JI: Collaboration: a concept analysis, *J Adv Nurs* 21:103-108, 1995.

Herz EK: Prediction, recognition, and prevention. In Hamilton JA and Harberger PN, editors: *Postpartum psychiatric illness: a picture puzzle,* Philadelphia, 1992, University of Pennsylvania Press.

Hill R and Hansen D: The identification of conceptual frameworks utilized in family study, *Marriage Fam Nurs* 22(4):299-311, 1960.

Hiser PL: Concerns of multiparas during the second postpartum week, *J Obstet Gynecol Neonatal Nurs* 16:195-203, 1987.

Hobbs DF and Cole SP: Transition to parenthood: a decade replication, *J Marriage Fam* 38(3):723-731, 1976.

Holtz H and Furniss K: The health care provider's role in domestic violence, *Trends in Health Care, Law, and Ethics* 8:47-53, 1993.

Institute of Medicine: *Nutrition during pregnancy and lactation. An implementation guide,* Washington, DC, 1992, National Academy Press.

Issokson D: Postpartum depression. Presented at Medical Grand Rounds, Bassett Healthcare, Cooperstown, NY, December 9, 1998.

Jacobson H: A standard for assessing lochia volume, *MCN Am J Matern Child Nurs* 10:174-175, 1985.

Jendrek MP: Grandparents who parent their grandchildren: circumstances and decisions, *Gerontologist* 34(2):206, 1994.

Jones CL and Lenz ER: Father-newborn interaction: effects of social competence and infant state, *Nurs Res* 35(2):149-153, 1989.

Jordan PL: Laboring for relevance: expectant and new fatherhood, *Nurs Res* 39(1):11-16, 1990.

Kelley SJ, Yorker BC, and Whitley D: To grandmother's house we go . . . and stay, *J Gerontol Nurs* Sept, 12-20, 1997.

Kennedy JC: The high-risk maternal-infant acquaintance process, *Nurs Clin North Am* 8(3):549-556, 1973.

Kitzinger S: *The year after childbirth,* New York, 1994, Scribner.

King MC and others: Violence and abuse of women: a perinatal health care issue, *AWOHNN's Clin Iss Perinatal and Women's Health* 4:163-172, 1993.

Klaus MH and Kennell JH: *Parent-infant bonding,* St Louis, 1982, Mosby.

Klaus MH and Kennell JH: *Bonding: building the foundations of secure attachment and independence,* Reading, Mass, 1995, Addison-Wesley.

Kline CR, Martin DP, and Deyo RA: Health consequences of pregnancy and childbirth as perceived by women and clinicians, *Obstet Gynecol* 92(5):843-848, 1998.

Koniak-Griffin K: Strategies for reducing the risk of malpractice litigation in perinatal nursing, *J Obstet Gynecol Neonatal Nurs* 28(3):291-299, 1999.

Konrad CJ: Helping mothers integrate the birth experience, *MCN Am J Matern Child Nurs* 12(4):268, 1987.

Kreppner K: Phases in family socialization after the birth of a second child. Paper presented at the Fifth International Conference on Infant Studies, Los Angeles, Calif, April, 1986.

Kruckman LD: Rituals and support: an anthropological view of postpartum depression. In Hamilton JA and Harberger PN, editors: *Postpartum psychiatric illness L A picture puzzle*, Philadelphia, 1992, University of Pennsylvania Press.

Kuczmarski RJ and others: Increasing prevalence of overweight among U.S. adults: the National Health and Nutrition Examination Surveys, 1960-1991, *JAMA* 274, 205-211, 1994.

LaRocca S: An introduction to role theory for nurses, *Supervising Nurse* 9(12):41-45, 1978.

Lauderdale J and Greener DL: Transcultural nursing care of the childbearing family. In Andrews MM and Boyle JS, editors: *Transcultural concepts in nursing care*, ed 2, Philadelphia, 1995, Lippincott.

Lawrence R: *Breastfeeding: a guide for the medical profession*, ed 5, St Louis, 1998, Mosby.

Leaphart E: Perinatal loss: strategies to facilitate bereavement, *NAACOG Update Series* 3(2), 1985, Princeton, Continuing Professional Education Center.

Lederman RP: *Psychosocial adaptation in pregnancy: assessment of seven dimensions*, ed 2, New York, 1996, Springer.

LeMasters EE: Parenthood as a crisis, *Marriage and Family Living* 19(2):352, 1957.

Locicero AK, Weiss DM, and Issokson D: Postpartum depression: proposal for prevention through an integrated care and support network, *Appl Prevent Psychol* 6:169-178, 1997.

Martell LL and Imle M: Family nursing with childbearing families. In Hanson SMH and Boyd ST, editors: *Family health care nursing: theory practice and research*, Philadelphia, 1996, Davis.

McAnarney E and Greydanus D: Adolescent pregnancy and abortion. In Hofman A and Greydanus D, editors: *Adolescent medicine*, Norwalk, Conn, 1989, Appleton & Lange.

McGoldrick M, Heiman M, and Carter B: The changing family life cycle, a perspective of normalcy. In Walsh F, editor: *Normal family processes*, New York, 1993, Guilford Press.

Mercer RT: A theoretical framework for studying factors that impact on the maternal role, *Nurs Res* 30(2):73-77, 1981.

Mercer RT: Parent-infant attachment. In Sonstegard LJ and others, editors: *Women's health*, vol 2, *Childbearing*, New York, 1982, Grune & Stratton.

Mercer RT: The process of maternal role attainment, *Nurs Res* 34(4): 198-204, 1985.

Mercer RT: Predictors of maternal role attainment at one year post birth, *West J Nurs Res* 8(1):932, 1986.

Mercer RT: *Parents at risk*, New York, 1990 Springer.

Mercer RT and Ferketich SL: Predictors of maternal attachment during early parenthood, *J Adv Nurs* 15:268-280, 1990.

Mercer RT and Ferketich SL: Predictors of maternal role competence by risk status, *Nurs Res* 43(1):38-43, 1994.

Mercer RT, Hackley KC, and Bostrom AG: Relationship of psychosocial and perinatal variables to perception of childbirth, *Nurs Res* 32(4):202-207, 1983.

Miller BG and Meyers-Wallis JA: Parenthood: stresses and coping strategies. In McCubbin HI and Figley CR, editors: *Stress and the family*, vol I, *Coping with normative transitions*, New York, 1983, Brunner/Mazel.

Miller JS and Robertson KR: Comparison of physical child abusers, intrafamilial sexual child abuser, and child neglect, *J Interpers Violence* 5:37-48, 1990.

Milligan R and others: Postpartum fatigue: clarifying a concept, *Sch Inq Nurs Pract* 10(3):279-291, 1996.

Miovech SM and others: Major concerns of women after cesarean delivery, *J Obstet Gynecol Neonatal Nurs* 23(1):53-59, 1994.

Mirande A: Ethnicity and fatherhood. In Bozett FW and Hanson SMH, editors: *Fatherhood and families in cultural context*, New York, 1991, Springer Publishing.

Monga M: Maternal cardiovascular and renal adaptation to pregnancy. In Creasy RK and Resnik R, editors: *Maternal-Fetal medicine*, ed 4, Philadelphia, 1999, WB Saunders.

Moran CF, Holt VL, and Martin DP: What do women want to know after childbirth? *Birth* 24(1):27-34, 1997.

Muhlenkamp AF and Sayles JA: Self-esteem, social support, and positive health practices, *Nurs Res* 35:334-338, 1986.

Murphy SO: Using multiple forms of family data: identifying pattern and meaning in sibling-infant relationships. In Gilgun J, Daly K, and Handel G, editors: *Qualitative methods in family research*, Newbury Park, Calif, 1992, Sage.

Murphy SO: Siblings and the new baby: changing perspectives, *J Pediatr Nurs* 8(5):277-286, 1993.

New York State Office for the Prevention of Domestic Violence. RADAR action steps developed by the Massachusetts Medical Society, 1992.

Nikodem VC and others: Do cabbage leaves prevent breast engorgement? A randomized controlled study, *Birth: Issues in Perinatal Care and Education* 20(2):61-64, 1993.

Norris J, Kunes-Connell M, and Spelic SS: A grounded theory of reimaging: body image, development and aging, *Adv Nurs Sci* 20(3):1-12, 1998.

North American Nursing Diagnosis Association (NANDA): *Nursing diagnoses: definitions and classifications 1999-2000*, Philadelphia, Penn, 1999, Author.

*Nurse's handbook of alternative and complementary therapies*, Springhouse, Penn, 1998, Springhouse.

O'Hara MW: *Postpartum depression: causes and consequences*, New York, 1995, Springer.

O'Hara MW and Engeldinger J: Postpartum mood disorders, detection and prevention, *The Female Patient* 14:136-141, 1989.

Or S, Tari A, and Fine M: A comparison of psychological profiles of teenage mothers and their nonmother peers: ego development, *Adolescence* 27(105):193-202, 1992.

O'Reilly-Green C and Cohen WR: Pregnancy in women aged 40 and older, *Obstet Gynecol Clin North Am* 20:313-331, 1993.

Osterud NG: *Bonds of community: the lives of farm women in 19th century New York*, Ithaca, NY, 1991, Cornell.

Parham ES, Astrom MF, and King SH: The association of pregnancy weight gain with the mother's postpartum weight, *J Am Diet Assoc* 90:550-554, 1990.

Passino AW and others: Personal adjustment during pregnancy and adolescent parenting, *Adolescence* 28(109):97-119, 1993.

Patterson CJ: Families of the lesbian baby boom: parents' division of labor and children's adjustment, *Dev Psychol* 31(1):115-123, 1995.

Perrin EC and Kulkin H: Pediatric care for children whose parents are gay or lesbian, *Pediatrics* 97(5):629-635, 1996.

Pugh LC and others: Clinical approaches in the assessment of childbearing fatigue, *J Obstet Gynecol Neonatal Nurs* 28(1):74-80, 1999.

Queenan JT: Managing pregnancy in patients over 35, *Contemp Obstet Gynecol* 29(5):180, 1987.

Raphael D: Matrescence, becoming a mother, and new/old rite of passage. In Grollig FX and Haley HB, editors: *Medical anthropology*, Paris, 1976, Mouton Publishers.

Rapini R: The skin and pregnancy. In Creasy RK and Resnik R, editors: *Maternal-Fetal medicine*, ed 4, Philadephia, 1999, WB Saunders.

Reichert JA, Baron M, and Fawcett J: Changes in attitude toward cesarean birth, *J Obstet Gynecol Neonatal Nurs* 22(2):159-167, 1993.

Resnik R: The puerperium. In Creasy RK and Resnik R, editors: *Maternal-Fetal medicine*, ed 4, Philadelphia, 1999, WB Saunders.

Riordan J and Auerbach K: *Breastfeeding and human lactation*, ed 2, Boston, 1998, Jones and Bartlett.

Rooney BL and Schauberger CW: *What happens to retained weight following pregnancy? A 4-5 year follow-up of a cohort of women*. Poster session presented at the annual meeting of the Society of Behavioral Medicine, San Diego, Calif, March, 1995.

Roosa MW: A comparative study of teenagers' parenting attitudes and knowledge of sexuality and child development, *J Youth Adolesc* 12:213-223, 1983.

Rose AM: *Human behavior and social processes,* Boston, 1962, Houghton Mifflin.

Rossner S: Pregnancy, weight cycling and weight gain in obesity, *Int J Obesity* 16:145-147, 1992.

Rubin R: Puerperal change, *Nurs Outlook* 9:753-755, 1961.

Rubin R: Binding-in in the postpartum period, *Matern Child Nurs J* 21(3):67, 1977.

Ruchala PL and Halstead L: The postpartum experience of low-risk women: a time of adjustment and change, *Matern Child Nurs J* 22(3):83, 1994.

Sameroff J, Siefer R, and Zax M: Early development of children at risk for emotional disorders, *Mono Soc Res Child Dev* 47:1-71, 1982.

Sampselle C and Brink CA: Pelvic muscle relaxation. Assessment and management, *J Nurse-Midwifery* 35(3):127-132, 1990.

Sanders CM: *Grief, the mourning after: dealing with adult bereavement,* New York, 1998, Wiley.

Sawicki JA: Sibling rivalry and the new baby: anticipatory guidance and management strategies, *Pediatr Nurs* 23(3):298-302, 1997.

Schauberger CW, Rooney BL, and Brimer LM: Factors that influence weight loss in the puerperium, *Obstet Gynecol* 79:424-429, 1992.

Schultz AA and others: Perceptions of caring: comparisons of antepartum and postpartum patients, *Clin Nurs Res* 7(4):363-378, 1998.

Scott JR and others: *Danforth's obstetrics and gynecology,* ed 6, Philadelphia, 1990, Lippincott.

Sheppard M: Postnatal depression, child care and social support: a review of findings and their implications for practice, *Soc Work Soc Sci Rev* 5(1):24-26, 1994.

Sherwen LN, Scoloveno MA, and Weingarten CT: *Maternity nursing. Care of the childbearing family,* ed 3, Stamford, Conn, 1999, Appleton & Lange.

Smith-Battle L: Teenage mothers' narratives of self: an examination of risk, *Adv Nurs Sci* 18(4):22-36, 1995.

Spieker SJ and Bensley L: Roles of living arrangements and grandmother social support in adolescent mothering and infant attachment, *Dev Psychol* 30(1):102, 1994.

Stark MA: Psychosocial adjustment during pregnancy: the experience of mature gravidas, *J Obstet Gynecol Neonatal Nurs* 26:206-211, 1997.

Stearns PN: Fatherhood in historical perspective: the role of social change. In Bozett FW and Hanson SMH, editors: *Fatherhood and families in cultural context,* New York, 1991, Springer Publishing.

Still O and Hodgins D: Navajo Indians. In Purnell LD and Paulanka BJ, editors: *Transcultural health care: a culturally competent approach,* Philadelphia, 1998, FA Davis.

Strang VR and Sullivan P: Body image attitudes during pregnancy and the postpartum period, *J Obstet Gynecol Neonatal Nurs* 14:332-337, 1985.

Strong T and others: Experience with early post cesarean hospital dismissal, *Am J Obstet Gynecol* 169:116-119, 1993.

Suitor CW: *Maternal weight gain: a report of an expert work group,* Arlington, Va, 1997, National Center for Education in Maternal and Child Health.

Swanson-Kauffman KM: Caring in the instance of unexpected early pregnancy loss, *Top Clin Nurs* 8(2):37, 1986.

Swanson-Kauffman KM: There should have been two: nursing care of parents experiencing perinatal death of a twin, *J Perinat Neonat Nurs* 2(2):78, 1988.

Swanson-Kauffman KM: Providing care in the NICU: sometimes an act of love, *Adv Nurs Science* 13(1):60, 1990.

Szafran KK: Family health protective behaviors. In Bomar PJ, editors: *Nurses and family health promotion,* ed 2, Philadelphia, 1996, WB Saunders.

Taffel SM, Keppel KG, and Jones GK: Medical advice on maternal weight gain and actual weight gain: results from the 1988 National Maternal and Infant Health Survey, *Ann New York Academy of Sciences* 678:293-305, 1993.

Tiller CM: Assessment of the potential for maladaptive parenting in expectant fathers with the adult-adolescent parenting inventory (AAPI), *J Child Adolescent-Psychiatric Mental Health Nurs* 4(2): 55-61, 1991.

Tiller CM: Fathers' parenting attitudes during a child's first year, *J Obstet Gynecol Neonatal Nurs* 24 (6):508-514, 1995.

Trent AJ and Clark K: What nurses should know about natural family planning, *J Obstet Gynecol Neonatal Nurs* 26:643-648, 1997.

Tripp-Reimer T and Wilson SE: Cross-cultural perspectives on fatherhood. In Bozett FW and Hanson SMH, editors: *Fatherhood and families in cultural context,* New York, 1991, Springer Publishing.

Tulman L and Fawcett J: Maternal employment following childbirth, *Res Nurs Health* 13:181-188, 1990.

Tulman L and others: Changes in functional status after childbirth, *Nurs Res* 39:70-75, 1990.

Turner RH: Role taking: process vs. confirmity. In Rose AM, editor: *Human behavior and social processes,* Boston, 1962, Houghton-Mifflin.

Ugarriza DN: Postpartum affective disorders: incidence and treatment, *J Psychosocial Nurs* 30(5):29-32, 1992.

Ulrich YC: What helped most in leaving spouse abuse: implications for interventions, *AWHONN's Clin Iss Perinatal Women's Health Nurs* 4 (3):385-390, 1993.

Varney H: *Varney's midwifery,* ed 3, Boston, Mass, 1997, Jones and Bartlett.

Walker LO: Weight-related distress in the early months after childbirth: weight research across the life span, *West J Nurs Res* 20(1): 30-44, 1998.

Walker LO, Walker ML, and Walker ME: Health and well-being of childbearing women in rural and urban contexts, *J Rural Health* 10:168-172, 1994.

Walker LO and Freeland-Graves J: Lifestyle factors related to weight and body image in bottle- and breast-feeding women, *J Obstet Gynecol Neonatal Nurs* 27(2):151-160, 1998.

Walters LH and Chapman SF: Cross-cultural perspectives on fatherhood. In Bozett FW and Hanson SMH, editors: *Fatherhood and families in cultural context,* New York, 1991, Springer Publishing.

Walton J, Collins J, and Linney J: Working together to meet the needs of multiple-birth families, *Health Visitor* 67(10):342-343, 1994.

Williams C and Vines SW: Broken past, fragile future: personal stories of high-risk adolescent mothers, *J Soc Pediatr Nurs* 4(1):15-27, 1999.

Williams LR and Cooper MK: A new paradigm for postpartum care, *J Obstet Gynecol Neonatal Nurs* 25(9):745-749, 1996.

Williamson DF and others: A prospective study of childbearing and 10-year weight gain in U.S. white women 25 to 45 years of age, *Int J Obesity* 18:561-569, 1994.

Wills TA: Supportive functions of interpersonal relationships. In Cohen S and Syme SL, editors. *Social support and health,* Orlando, Fla, 1985, Academic Press.

Worden WJ: *Grief counseling and grief therapy: a handbook for the mental health practitioner,* New York, 1991, Springer.

Wright LM and Leahy M: *Nurses and families: a guide to family assessment and intervention,* ed 1, Philadelphia, 1984, FA Davis.

Wright LM and Leahy M: *Nurses and families: a guide to family assessment and intervention,* ed 2, Philadelphia, 1994, FA Davis.

Wright LM, Watson WL, and Bell JM: *Beliefs: the heart of healing in families and illness,* New York, 1997, Basic Books.

Zerwekh JV: Laying the groundwork for family self-help: locating families, building trust, and building strength, *Public Health Nurs* 9(1):15-21, 1992.

Zuravin S: Severity of maternal depression and three types of mother-to-child aggression, *Am J Orthopsychiatry* 59:377-389, 1989.

# CHAPTER 16

# Care of the Newborn

*"A child is the root of the heart."*
— CAROLINA MARIA DE JESUS
BRAZILIAN WRITER

*What thoughts might fill new parents' minds as they look at their newborn?*

*What components of a newborn physical assessment are useful in teaching parents?*

*What clinical findings necessitate further evaluation by another professional?*

*What skills must a family have before assuming the total care of their newborn?*

*What anticipatory guidance will be included in the teaching?*

*How can we help a family unit integrate within the community?*

During the final moments before the baby's actual arrival, the excitement and exhilaration are immeasurable. For both the providers and the parents, nothing else matters for those few moments. We are concerned about the well-being of the baby, and the parents are concerned about the baby's gender and size. The parents are filled with questions: Will I make a good parent? Who will he or she look like? Will the baby be healthy? Will the baby be cute? First-time parents often have unclear expectations of what is to come.

Multiparous families often have other emotions to contend with. Questions about how they will fit this child into their current life and whether other family members will accept it may concern them. Having a prior experience to reflect on and compare it with, they wonder just how different or similar this child will be.

Women who have experienced a cesarean birth may worry they won't be able to adequately care for their new baby as they recover from this major surgery. Partners may wonder how they will care for both the newborn baby and the new mother as she recovers.

Chapter 15 presented information about the immediate postpartum, primarily from the mother and family's perspective. This chapter explores the postpartum experience for the infant and the care it requires during this time. It also provides anticipatory guidance to help the infant's caretakers assume the parenting role.

## MEETING THE NEEDS OF AN EXPANDING FAMILY

As a health care provider at the birth of a baby, our role is multifaceted. Awareness of the cultural needs and personal desires of the family is a requirement. When people have their cultural preferences met they feel valued and this increases their self-esteem (Leininger, 1997).

652

Addressing these needs can make the welcoming of a new member a fulfilling and memorable experience for the family. The actions and activities of these moments will be forever linked, positively or negatively, with this child in the minds of the family members.

If culturally acceptable, placing the baby on the mother's chest brings comfort to both the infant and the mother. The newborn can hear again its mother's heartbeat, something that has been part of its life up until now.

Cultural beliefs may dictate what may be said about the infant. Some Asian cultures believe that if the baby is described as beautiful, harm will come to it. They prefer that no positive comments be made about the child. To protect their child, some mothers will not look at their baby immediately after birth and express no desire to hold it. Other cultures do not name their child at birth. Some may have a name for the child, but do not share it. Because these behavior choices differ from the culturally accepted norms in the United States, some providers have erroneously labeled these parents as unfit. As providers we must set aside our own cultural biases, learn from our clients, and provide appropriate care that saves the family from unnecessary interventions and grief. Determine ahead of time the beliefs and desires of the new mother so that the experience is enjoyable for the family. Keep in mind that these moments are precious to the family and your comments and activities will long be remembered.

## NEW SENSATIONS TO A NEWBORN

This brighter, cooler environment that the baby enters at birth is a change from the wet warm, dark surroundings of a mother's womb. Once born, a baby is exposed to a whole new world of sounds, smells, and sensations. Those once muffled voices of family and friends heard while in utero are now much louder and clearer. The blanket placed across the baby to keep in body heat is relatively rough and slightly heavy. The sensations of being squeezed by the uterus down through the birth canal are gone. The baby is now free to move about in a whole new way. Adjusting to the different sensory stimuli may cause the newborn to cry or to close his or her eyes to block out the many external inputs.

## TRANSITION TO EXTRAUTERINE LIFE

The initial 24 hours of a newborn's life are the most critical, but the normal newborn negotiates this period satisfactorily. The changes in the infant's body follow a fairly predictable sequence of events as it recovers from the rigors of labor and adapts to extrauterine life. The sympathetic nervous system responds with changes in heart rate, skin color, respirations, motor activity, gastrointestinal (GI) function, and body temperature.

## Changes in the Newborn During the Transition

The transitional period for the newborn may be examined by looking at the three stages it involves. The **first stage** is when the infant is 0 to 30 minutes old—the first period of reactivity. When the infant is between 30 minutes and 2 hours old it enters the **second stage** of transitional process. At this time, the baby either sleeps or significantly decreases motor activity. The second period of reactivity, the **third stage**, begins at 2 hours old and lasts until the infant is about 8 hours old. This sequence of clinical behaviors is common to all well newborns regardless of gestational age or route of delivery (Thureen and others, 1999).

### First Stage (0 to 30 Minutes of Age)

During the first 30 minutes of extrauterine life the infant has what is termed the **"first period of reactivity."** If not experiencing the effects of maternal medication, the baby is alert and moving and may experience a startle reaction when it moves or is moved abruptly; it may have tremors and/or cry.

Moving its head from side to side, it will make eye contact and **gustatory movements** (pushing the tongue out, trying to taste). For these reasons, it is a particularly good time for the mother to put the baby to her breast if she is planning to breastfeed. The infant may not take in nourishment at this time, but it does connect the infant to the mother through smell and initiate the infant-mother connection (Thureen and others, 1999).

Most of the physiologic changes during this period are sympathetic. For 10 to 15 minutes the baby's heart rate increases from 160 to 180 beats per minute (beats/min). Then during the remainder of the 30 minutes, it gradually drops to a baseline rate of 100 to 120 beats/min.

After the baby takes its first breath, respirations are irregular for the first 15 minutes, but the highest respiratory rate is between 60 and 80 breaths per minute. Auscultation reveals rales as the lungs gradually make the transition from being fluid filled to air filled. Grunting, flaring, and retractions also may occur. The infant also may experience brief periods of apnea of less than 10 seconds duration.

As the baby becomes more accustomed to a world with gravity, muscle tone and generalized motor activity increase. At this time the production of saliva is minimal and bowel sounds are absent (Thureen and others, 1999).

### Second Stage (30 Minutes to 2 Hours of Age)

During the second stage, the infant begins to settle down and rests or goes to sleep; this is referred to as a **"period of decreased responsiveness."** The muscle becomes more relaxed, and the baby's responsiveness diminishes. The breathing pattern is fast, shallow, and synchronous at up to 60 breaths per minute without dyspnea. If well oxygenated, the baby's color should be good. With the breathing established, the shape of the chest gradually changes, increasing the anterior-posterior diameter. This is referred to as the "barreling of the chest" (Thureen and others, 1999).

With relaxation and rest, the heart rate falls into a range between 100 and 120 beats/min. It remains relatively stable and is less responsive to stimuli. The abdomen of the baby becomes rounded, and bowel sounds start to occur. Peristaltic waves may be visible (Thureen and others, 1999).

When loosely wrapped, the infant may experience spontaneous jerks and twitches, but it quickly returns to rest. It is difficult to rouse the baby and have it interact at this time.

### Third Stage (2 to 8 Hours of Age)

At about 2 hours of age, the baby generally becomes more responsive to exogenous and endogenous stimuli. This is labeled the **"second period of reactivity"** because the infant again interacts with its environment to the same degree, or even more than, as in Stage 1. It may be a brief period or last several hours (Thureen and others, 1999).

The infant's cardiac and respiratory systems are responsive with periods of tachycardia and rapid respirations. Changes in muscle tone and color may be abrupt. Oral mucus becomes more prominent and may be accompanied by gagging and vomiting. Bowel sounds are present and the baby may clear the bowel with the passing of meconium. At the end of this period of activity, the infant may settle down and become seriously interested in feeding (Thureen and others, 1999).

### Assessment and Care During the First Stage of Transition

As the baby emerges it is assessed for overall appearance, development, significant abnormalities, birth injuries, or cardiorespiratory disorders that may affect its adaptation to extrauterine life. Significant deviation from the normal sequence of events may result from various factors and may require specialized attention.

The results of this preliminary assessment determine whether the baby is placed on the mother's abdomen or removed to a warmer or prewarmed incubator. Assessment may continue in either place. A nurse, nurse practitioner, nurse midwife, or physician gently suctions the nose and mouth, decreasing the amount of fluid that the baby may draw in when it takes its first breath.

### Thermoregulation

Temperature regulation is imperative. Evaporative and conductive heat loss can cause a rapid decrease in an infant's body temperature. For this reason, the infant is dried with prewarmed blankets immediately after birth and a cap is placed on its head. The rubbing action of drying the infant can also serve to stimulate the infant to take the first breath and allow the assessment of both reflex irritability and muscle tone. Unnecessary procedures are avoided so that the infant does not become chilled. An understanding of the mechanisms of thermoregulation can be helpful during the initial stabilization of the infant and is important information to teach the parents as they assume the care of their infant (Table 16-1).

### Apgar Score

Respirations, heart rate, color, and overall appearance are evaluated and used to guide the need for further resuscitation efforts.

The **Apgar score** is an assessment process that results in a numerical score determined at 1 and 5 minutes immediately after birth. Dr. Virginia Apgar developed this scoring system in 1953 as a tool to evaluate the infant's transition to extrauterine life. Five parameters are assessed: (1) heart rate, (2) respiratory rate, (3) reflex irritability, (4) muscle tone, and (5) color.

**Heart rate** is the first and most important parameter assessed. In the first 15 minutes after birth, the average

---

**TABLE 16-1** *Mechanism of Thermoregulation*

| Name | Definition | Nursing interventions |
|------|-----------|----------------------|
| Evaporation | Heat is lost when fluids from the body turn to vapor. Fluids come from perspiration, pulmonary fluid, and insensible water loss. | Keep the baby dry. |
| Conduction | Heat is transferred from a warmer object to a cooler object by *direct contact*. | Keep baby from touching cold surfaces. |
| Radiation | Heat is transferred from a warm object to a cooler object by *indirect contact*. | Keep the baby covered. |
| Convection | Heat is lost from the warm body surface to cooler air currents. | Keep the baby away from a drafty window or fan. |

Adapted from MacLaren A: *Concepts and activities maternal-neonatal nursing,* Springhouse, PA, 1994, Springhouse.

heart rate is 160 beats/min, but this rate may vary from 120 to 190 beats/min. After 15 minutes, the average is between 120 and 140 beats/min, with a possible range between 90 and 175 beats/min. Consistently low or high heart rates may indicate a pathologic condition and require further evaluation (Thureen and others, 1999). The rate may be auscultated on the chest (Figure 16-1) or palpated at the base of the umbilicus (where the umbilical cord meets the abdominal wall).

**Respiratory rate** is the second system to be assessed by either watching the rise and fall of the chest or through auscultating breath sounds on the chest itself (Figure 16-2). The rate of respirations may range between 60 and 80, with the baby breathing room air. The baby may have mild retractions or experience brief episodes of apnea.

As the infant becomes stimulated through touch and temperature change, **reflex irritability** may be evaluated. A robust cry is a good example of a reflex response. Grasping the newborn's hand or foot and extending it out and then watching the degree to which the baby returns it from extension to flexion allows assessment of **muscle tone. Color,** is the last factor to be assessed. Optimally a newborn should be pink, but very few are completely pink even at 5 minutes.

As the newborn makes the transition to extrauterine life, the trunk may turn pink while the extremities remain more purple in color. A condition known as **acrocyanosis** is the result of a deficient amount of blood circulating to the infant's extremities. It is common to see the mottling of acrocyanosis for several hours after birth.

Using the Apgar score chart as a reference, each assessment measure is given a score based on the description in the chart. The higher the number, the better the condition of the infant. A score of 10 is the best and 0 is the worst (Table 16-2). An infant with a score of 7 or less may require resuscitative measures from a skilled team at the time of delivery. (Foster, Hunsberger, and Anderson, 1989). When the baby's condition warrants, interventions are initiated immediately and are not delayed until the completion of the Apgar at 1 minute of life. In the case of a depressed infant, although the Apgar score may not be helpful initially, it may offer objective information that reflects the effectiveness of the resuscitative methods (American Academy of Pediatrics, 1994).

Once it is determined that the infant's transition is going smoothly, the mother and others may wish to hold the infant. Bundling the baby within a warm blanket and a hat and then placing the infant into their arms is a moment they will long cherish.

If the mother desires, breastfeeding at this time is beneficial because the baby is probably alert and seeking the mother's breast. The oxytocin released when the

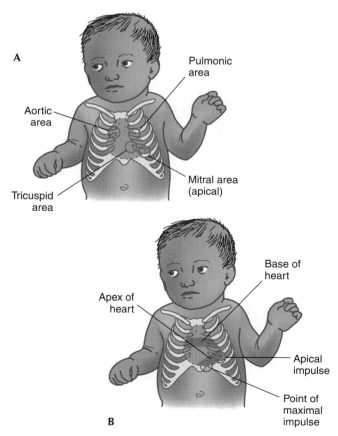

FIGURE 16-1 • Respiratory rate. **A,** Areas for cardiac auscultation. **B,** Location points of cardiac landmarks.

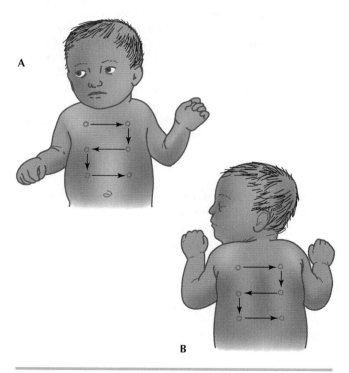

FIGURE 16-2 • Sequence for auscultation of the lungs. **A,** Anterior segments. **B,** Posterior segments.

**TABLE 16-2** *Apgar Score Chart*

| Observation | 1 | 2 | 3 |
|---|---|---|---|
| Heart rate | Absent | Slow (<100 beats/min) | >100 beats/min |
| Respiratory rate | Absent (apneic) | Slow, irregular, shallow | Good, sustained cry; regular respirations |
| Reflex irritability | No response | Grimace, frown | Sneeze, cough, cry |
| Muscle tone | Limp, completely flaccid | Some flexion of extremities; some resistance to extension of extremities | Active motion, good muscle tone, spontaneous flexion |
| Color | Cyanotic; pale | Body pink, extremities pale | Completely pink |

From Foster RL, Hunsberger MM, and Anderson JJ: *Family-centered nursing care of children*, Philadelphia, 1989, WB Saunders.

breasts are stimulated assists the mother because oxytocin also stimulates uterine contractions, promoting the delivery of the placenta and reducing the potential for postpartum hemorrhage (Mohrbacher and Stock, 1997).

At 15 minutes of age, the infant is again assessed. If it is experiencing difficulty adapting, it will be evident by assessing cardiac rate and rhythm, respiratory activity, color, muscle tone, and temperature. These parameters should be evaluated repeatedly and documented in the notes (Table 16-3).

## Assessment and Care During the Second and Third Stages of Transition

Because of the newborn's cycle of activity, in an apparently healthy baby the more complete examination is generally delayed until the baby is at least 30 minutes old and, depending on the parents' desire to hold the baby, until an hour of age. The examination involves the use of each technique of physical assessment: observation, auscultation, palpation, and percussion as every system receives a thorough evaluation. It is sometimes done with the mother and other family members present so that they may learn about the baby as the examination goes.

### Initial Observations
Observe color, approximate weight, and symmetry of development and extremities. This can be done by close observation without touching or awakening the baby. The initial observations will fine tune and focus the rest of the assessment.

### Respiratory Rate
The rate of respirations are between 30 to 60 breaths per minute with a prolonged expiratory phase. Coarse rales and moist tubular breath sounds may be heard until the lungs are completely cleared of fluid. During the first hours of breathing grunting and retracting (intercostal and/or substernal) may be present until the fluid clears the lungs (Thureen and others, 1999).

### Heart Rate
The normal heart rate ranges from 120 to 160 beats/min. However, this may drop to 80 beats/min when sleeping and rise to 180 beats/min when active and crying. Because of slight pulmonary hypertension during the first hours and days of extrauterine life, a loud second heart sound may be heard. There may also be a splitting of the second heart sound, but this is difficult to detect. Until the ductus arteriosus closes, a soft grade II/VI systolic murmur is present due to the left to right shunt of blood. Functional closure of the ductus arteriosus occurs within 15 hours of birth (Thureen and others, 1999).

### Temperature
After delivery, the infant's body temperature naturally drops. The mean low temperature is 35.6° C and occurs at the mean age of 75 minutes. After that time, it will rise again to the normal range of body temperature for a newborn: 36.5° to 37.0° C by axillary temperature or 36.0° to 36.5° C by skin temperature (Thureen and others 1999).

Because of this change, the infant's axillary temperature is checked every 30 to 60 minutes during transition. The first bath is delayed until the axillary body temperature has stabilized in the normal range. Once the bath is given, the baby's temperature is checked again 30 minutes later, and then an hour later. It is rechecked at least every 2 to 4 hours until stable, and then every 8 hours until discharged from care (Thureen and others, 1999).

### Blood Pressure
The newborn's blood pressure varies with birth weight; it tends to be lower in smaller babies. The range of normal for indirectly measured blood pressure is 65 to 95 mm Hg systolic and 30 to 60 mm Hg diastolic in term infants. Blood pressure may not be measured unless the newborn's heart rate is higher or lower than normal, or is irregular (Thureen and others, 1999).

### Umbilical Cord
The umbilicus should be positioned midway between the xiphoid process and the mons pubis. Assess that the

| TABLE 16-3 | *Normal Ranges of Vital Signs** |
|---|---|
| **Vital sign** | **Range of normal** |
| Heart rate | *After first 15 minutes* 120-140 bpm (range 90-175 bpm) |
| Respiratory rate | *After first 15 minutes* averages 60 breaths/min (range 60-80 breaths/min) |
| Temperature | *First bath is delayed until body temperature stabilizes at:* 36° C-37.2° C 96.8° F-99° F |
| Blood pressure | Range of normal for indirectly measured: 65-95 mm Hg/30-60 mm Hg in term infants |

*May vary with age in minutes and level of activity.

From MacLaren A: *Concepts and activities maternal-neonatal nursing,* Springhouse, PA, 1994, Springhouse; Bruno JP: Systematic neonatal assessment and intervention, *MCN Matern Child Nurs J* 20:21-24, 1995; Cusson RM, Madonia JA, and Taekman JB: The effect of environment on body site temperatures in full-term neonates, *Nur Res* 46(4): 202-207, 1997; Thureen PJ and others: *Assessment and care of the well newborn,* Philadelphia, 1999, WB Saunders.

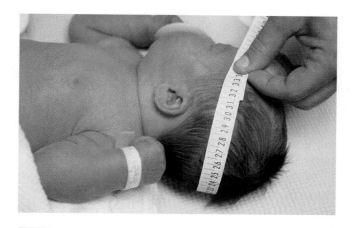

FIGURE 16-3 ● Measurement of head circumference. *(From Seidel HM, Benedict GW, and Ball JW:* Mosby's guide to physical examination, *ed 4, St Louis, 1999, Mosby.)*

cord is bluish/white in color and that it has two arteries and one vein. Within minutes after the cord is clamped, no discharge or blood should be oozing from it. It will start to dry and become shriveled and blackened within 48 hours.

### Anthropometric Measurements

After learning the gender, the height and weight of the infant are the next most requested information by parents.

*Weight.* The weight of the newborn is determined using an infant scale. Read the weight to the nearest 10 g or ½ oz when the infant is still. The weight is then plotted on the appropriate growth curve for age and sex. This allows the infant's weight to be tracked not only as it changes with regard to its own growth, but also in comparison to the population standard.

Healthy newborns weigh between 2500 g and 4000 g (5 lb 8 oz to 8 lb 13 oz). White infants are generally the heaviest, with black infants weighting 181 g to 240 g less. Babies of Asian, Filipino, Hawaiian, and Puerto Rican descent generally also weigh less than white babies. The greatest variety within a cultural group is with the babies of Native Americans. As much as 363 g separate the mean weights of babies of various tribes (Seidel and others, 1999).

*Recumbent Length.* The height measurement of an infant is actually the recumbent length. It is accomplished most easily when a newborn is laid on a measuring device. With the head at the top of the measuring tool, the in-

fant's legs are straightened at the knees, and the length is measured at the heel of the foot. The length is measured to the nearest 0.5 cm or 1/4 inch. The measurement is plotted on the appropriate growth curve for sex and age and can be compared to the population standard.

*Head Circumference.* The head is one fourth of the total length of the newborn, with the forehead being very prominent and the chin receding. To measure the actual size of the head accurately, a circumference is taken by placing a paper or cloth tape measure around the head. Accurate placement is imperative. Place the tape measure above the eyebrow and around the most prominent part of the occipital bone on the back of the head (Foster, Hunsberger, and Anderson, 1989). This measurement is called the **occipital frontal circumference (OFC)** and can range from 31 cm to 38 cm. Sometimes this measurement needs to be taken a few times with some adjustment to the tape measure so that a baseline is established. Plot this measurement on a growth chart for comparison to the weight and height (Tappero and Honeyfield, 1993). An increase or decrease in circumference outside the range of normal could signal a neurologic problem (Figure 16-3).

### GI Function

Bowel sounds usually are audible within a few hours after birth (MacLaren, 1994). During the second stage of the transition observe to see if peristaltic waves are visible. Listen to see if bowel sounds are audible. They may be heard as early as 15 minutes after birth.

The bowels may be cleared of meconium by the end of the third stage (MacLaren, 1994). Approximately 70% of normal newborns pass meconium during the first 12 hours, 25% between 12 and 24 hours, and the remaining 5% by approximately 48 hours. The time of the initial stool should be recorded.

## Urinary Function

Approximately 68% of normal newborns urinate within 12 hours of birth. Some even urinate within minutes of birth. By 24 hours of age, 93% will have urinated, and by 48 hours, all normal infants will have urinated. The time of the initial urination should be recorded.

If the baby does not urinate with 24 hours of birth, the possible reasons must be investigated. It may be caused by an obstruction or a prerenal condition.

## Appearance

### Discolorations

**Petechiae** (minute, pinpoint size, purplish red hemorrhages) may be apparent on the baby's face or presenting part. Facial bruising may be seen on an infant born in the vertex position after a rapid second stage of labor or if the umbilical cord was wrapped tightly around the baby's neck. If they appear on the torso they may be the result of thrombocytopenia or congenital infection (Thureen and others, 1999).

**Molding** (shaping) of the baby's head to the size and shape of the birth canal may occur as it passes through. This generally resolves within a few hours or after several days (Figure 16-4).

**Deformities** may be observed in the extremities. They may have been caused by the position of the baby within the uterus and resolve with birth, or they may be more permanent in nature. Others may have been created because of environmental conditions or genetic influence. A full evaluation is required to determine cause and a plan of possible interventions.

### Skin

Up until 35 weeks, the baby is coated with vernix. After that time, it gradually decreases. At full-term, some of this white, moist, cheeselike substance may still be found on the infant's skin and in the folds of the body. A post-term infant who has lived longer in the watery environment of the amnionic sac without this protection against the fluid may have dry, shriveled, peeling skin.

"Transient puffiness of the hands, feet, eyelids, legs, pubis, or sacrum occurs in some newborns. It has no discernable cause and should not cause concern if it disappears within 2 or 3 days" (Seidel and others, 1999) (Figure 16-5).

## Screening and Prophylactic Interventions

### Glucose Screening

If the infant is at risk for hypoglycemia or is exhibiting symptoms that could be secondary to hypoglycemia (i.e. jitteriness, hypothermia, apnea), a glucose screening is done between 30 and 60 minutes of age using capillary whole blood on a ChemstripbG or Dextrostix.

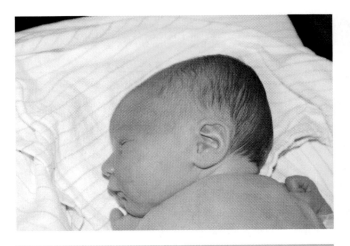

FIGURE 16-4 • Molding of baby's head. *(Courtesy of Caroline E. Brown.)*

An infant is considered at risk if it has experienced asphyxia, cold stress, respiratory difficulties or possible sepsis because these conditions increase metabolism and therefore increase glucose use. Other infants are screened if they are small for gestational age or premature because they have reduced stores of glucose. Infants who are large for gestational age or have diabetic mothers are screened because of the possibility of hyperinsulinemia when they are no longer receiving glucose from the mother.

Some facilities do one glucose screen on all newborns. Generally, a screening glucose result of less than 40 mg/dl is abnormal (Thureen and others, 1999).

### Eye Care

Prophylactic treatment for **ophthalmia neonatorum** caused by *Neisseria gonorrhoeae* is with 1% silver nitrate solution, 0.5% erythromycin ophthalmic ointment, or 1% tetracycline ophthalmic ointment. The erythromycin or tetracycline also works prophylactically for *Chlamydia trachomatis*.

Each infant has his or her own tube of ointment. The ointment is placed into the conjunctival sac within 1 hour of birth. When silver nitrate is used, many infants experience a reaction and develop chemical conjunctivitis. When treatment is mandated, the use of erythromycin or tetracycline is preferable (Figure 16-6).

### Vitamin K

Newborns are at risk for bleeding if they have a vitamin K deficiency due to the absence of intestinal flora, low liver stores of vitamin K, or immaturity. Because vitamin K is necessary to promote the synthesis of vitamin K–dependent clotting factors, vitamin K in the form of AquaMEPHYTON is given to infants as a prophylactic measure.

In England and Canada it is administered orally. However, the American Academy of Pediatrics (AAP) does not

DATE:

TIME:

| | | | | | | |
|---|---|---|---|---|---|---|
| **ACTIVITY** | ✓ | ACTIVE | | | | |
| | + | Activity decreased | | | | |
| | + | Tires easily | | | | |
| | + | Lethargic | | | | |
| | + | Floppy | | | | |
| | + | Irritable | | | | |
| | + | Pacifier required | | | | |
| | + | Frantic | | | | |
| | + | Swaddled | | | | |
| | + | Tremors | | | | |
| | + | Rigid | | | | |
| | + | Opisthotonos | | | | |
| | + | Moro poor or absent | | | | |
| **APPEARANCE** | ✓ | COLOR STABLE | | | | |
| | + | Pallor | | | | |
| | + | Plethora | | | | |
| | + | Mottled | | | | |
| | + | Harlequin syndrome | | | | |
| | + | Jaundice | | | | |
| | + | Dusky | | | | |
| | + | Cyanosis: Generalized | | | | |
| | + | Circumoral | | | | |
| | + | Circumocular | | | | |
| | + | Extremities | | | | |
| | + | Tearing | | | | |
| | + | Eye discharge | | | | |
| **FEEDINGS (GASTROINTESTINAL)** | ✓ | HUNGRY | | | | |
| | ✓ | DEMANDING | | | | |
| | ✓ | SUCKS WELL | | | | |
| | + | Sucks poorly | | | | |
| | ✓ | GAVAGED WELL | | | | |
| | ✓ | Gavaged well/slowly | | | | |
| | + | Gavaged poorly | | | | |
| | + | Gavage resisted | | | | |
| | + | Mucus on tube | | | | |
| | + | Mucus, other | | | | |
| | + | Drooled | | | | |
| | + | Gagged | | | | |
| | + | Regurgitated | | | | |
| | + | Vomited | | | | |
| | + | Abdomen distended | | | | |
| | cm | Abdomen, circumference | | | | |
| | + | Hiccoughs | | | | |
| | + | Sore buttocks | | | | |

DATE:

TIME:

| | | | | | | |
|---|---|---|---|---|---|---|
| **RESPIRATIONS** | ✓ | CRY GOOD | | | | |
| | + | Cry high-pitched | | | | |
| | + | Cry weak | | | | |
| | + | Sneezes | | | | |
| | + | Stuffy nose | | | | |
| | + | Yawning | | | | |
| | + | Hoarseness | | | | |
| | + | Stridor | | | | |
| | ✓ | RESPIRATIONS: Regular | | | | |
| | + | Shallow | | | | |
| | + | Labored | | | | |
| | + | Deep | | | | |
| | + | Irregular | | | | |
| | + | See saw | | | | |
| | + | Periodic breathing | | | | |
| | + | Rest periods        10 sec | | | | |
| | + |                  10–30 sec | | | | |
| | + | Apnea          30 sec | | | | |
| | + | Alae nasi dilated | | | | |
| | + | Cough | | | | |
| | + | Grunting | | | | |
| | + | Retraction | | | | |
| **SKIN** | ✓ | SKIN NORMAL | | | | |
| | + | Dry and peeling | | | | |
| | + | Irritated | | | | |
| | + | Petechiae (area) | | | | |
| | + | Ecchymosis (area) | | | | |
| | + | Bleeding (area) | | | | |
| | + | Dehydrated | | | | |
| | + | Edema | | | | |
| | + | Pustular rash | | | | |
| | + | Erythema toxicum | | | | |
| | + | Other rash (specify) | | | | |
| | + | Abscess (area) | | | | |
| | + | Sclerema | | | | |
| | + | Umbilical redness | | | | |
| | + | Umbilical oozing | | | | |

Completed by the nurse, this checklist indicates
the presence of findings (✓), severity (+, ++, +++),
timing (ac, pc) etc. Capitalized items indicate
normal findings. Each column signifies a period of
observations. Significant additional data are
recorded in the progress notes.

FIGURE 16-5 ● Checklist of significant observations in newborns. *(From Lubchenco LO: Checklist of significant observations in newborns,* Pediatr Clin North Am *8:471, 1961.)*

yet recommend oral administration, so we provide it as a single dose intramuscular injection within 1 hour of birth. If the infant weighs less than 1.5 kg, it receives 0.5 mg intramuscularly; if the weight is greater than or equal to 1.5 kg, 1.0 mg is given (Thureen and others, 1999).

### Hepatitis B Vaccine

The Centers for Disease Control and Prevention (CDC) and the AAP recommend that all newborns and infants be given hepatitis B vaccine (HBV) regardless of the mother's hepatitis B surface antigen (HBsAg) status. If the mother's HBsAg status is positive or unknown, hepatitis B immune globulin (HBIG) should be given within the first 12 hours of life. If delayed, the efficacy decreases, and it is of no value if given after the first 7 days of life (Thureen and others, 1999).

In some states and some institutions, parental consent is required before providing these interventions. No serious side effects have been documented with the use of the vaccine or the immune globulin.

Immunization with HBV is recommended for the newborn, after the infant's first bath, with an additional dose to follow 1 to 2 months later, and a third dose at 6 to 18 months of age. If HBIG is to be given, it should also be administered as soon as possible after the first bath. If the mother is breastfeeding her infant, the first feeding should be delayed until after the infant has had its first bath and received the necessary injections.

When the infant receives HBIG, it has passive protection from hepatitis B for 6 weeks. The HBV, with its protocol of three injections, provides active immunization for long-term protection. When a newborn is treated with HBV and HBIG, its risk of developing hepatitis B is reduced to about 5% to 15%.

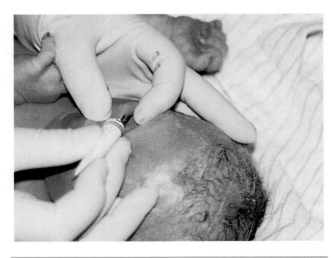

FIGURE 16-6 • Instillation of medication into eye of newborn. *(From Lowdermilk DL, Perry S, and Bobak IM: Maternity nursing, ed 5, St Louis, 1999, Mosby. Courtesy Marjorie Pyle, RNC, Lifecircle, Costa Mesa, CA.)*

## Feeding

An infant can be fed at anytime during the transition period if evaluations are within normal limits and the infant demonstrates a desire. If not interested before, most are ready to eat by the end of the transition period (8 hours old).

Before an infant may be fed, it must first be determined that it has the ability to suck and swallow. If it has been swallowing mucus, there will not be an excessive amount in the oropharynx. It should also not have vomited. If vomiting has occurred, a more complete evaluation must occur before the baby is fed.

The baby should have settled into a normal breathing pattern, with a rate of less than 70 breaths per minute. The nares should be unobstructed, so that the baby can breath while feeding and swallowing.

Normal color and perfusion indicate that cardiac functioning is adequate. Bowel sounds indicate that the GI tract is ready to receive food. In addition, the abdomen should not be distended and the anus must be patent.

| TABLE 16-4 | *Maternal, Obstetric, and Neonatal Conditions That Increase the Risk for Abnormal Transition* |
| --- | --- |
| Maternal factors | Chronic hypertension |
| | Pregnancy-induced hypertension |
| | Diabetes mellitus |
| | Renal disease |
| | Infection |
| | Abuse of tobacco, alcohol, or illicit drugs |
| | Collagen vascular diseases |
| | Homozygous hemoglobinopathies |
| | Certain maternal medications |
| Obstetric factors | Rh or other isoimmunization |
| | Fetal growth retardation |
| | Decreased fetal movements |
| | Multiple gestation |
| | Oligohydramnios or polyhydramnios |
| | Premature rupture of membranes |
| | Third-trimester bleeding |
| | Delivery by cesarean section |
| Neonatal factors | Prematurity (<37 weeks) |
| | Postmaturity (>42 weeks) |
| | Small for gestational age |
| | Large for gestational age |
| | Infection |
| | Metabolic abnormalities |
| | Birth trauma |
| | Major malformations |
| | Apgar 0–4 at 1 minute or need for resuscitation at delivery |
| | Anemia |

##  ABNORMAL TRANSITION

Significant deviation from the normal transition to extrauterine life may result from various influences. The challenge for the provider is to be able to distinguish between the early signs of a problem in an infant that will become high risk and the rapid changes that occur within the normal range of responses for a healthy infant. Understanding factors that may cause a difficult transition period helps the provider prepare for the unusual (Table 16-4).

##  THE NEWBORN EXAMINATION

Within 12 to 18 hours after birth, sometimes at 24 hours, a detailed and thorough examination of the infant is performed. A thorough examination combined with a history contributed by the family helps put the true status of the infant into context. Conducting the physical examination in the presence of the family allows the opportunity to gain history about the prenatal course and any family traits as questions arise. Knowledge of these may confirm or assist in potential diagnoses.

Early identification of abnormalities allows for early intervention and helps the family start to adjust to the situation (Bodurtha, 1998). A general rule of thumb is that if three or more minor anomalies with no known cause are discovered, chromosome testing is warranted. If at any time during the assessment unusual or abnormal characteristics are identified, an additional evaluation by a specialist may be required.

The examination starts with an overview of the infant. It is very common for the newborn baby to exhibit one of two distinct moods: irritability or quiet alertness, so timing of the examination is important. Choose a period of quiet or a sleep state because this is a perfect time to assess overall appearance, respirations, and normal skin color. Listening to the heart and lungs is also easier when the infant is peaceful (MacLaren, 1994).

### Behavioral State

While the physical assessment is being conducted, the infant's behavioral state should be observed simultaneously. **Behavioral state** refers to the baby's level of alertness at any given time. A baby may experience six states, ranging from a deep sleep to a very active, crying state (Table 16-5).

Information regarding the infant's various states is  helpful for the family. Explain to the family the baby's current state and then the different states the baby assumes during the examination.

### Assessment of Skin

Skin assessment can be incorporated into daily care when that care is provided by a professional nurse. The baby's skin should be soft, smooth, slightly opaque, and warm to the touch.

**Lanugo,** fine downy hair, may be found along the back of the neck or the back of the newborn. Preterm infants generally have more distribution of hair. In other infants, the extensive distribution of hair is a family trait. The hair will disappear on its own (Figure 16-7).

#### Color

Within the first few hours of life, the skin color should become less ruddy or red. This erythematous color is

| TABLE 16-5 *Behavioral States* | |
|---|---|
| **State** | **Observable behaviors** |
| Deep sleep | Few jerky type movements; no rapid eye movement (REM); arousable for only a few seconds; rhymic breathing patterns |
| Light sleep | REM may be observed, more spontaneous movement of extremities; varied breathing patterns |
| Drowsy state | Sluggish response to stimuli, more movement of arms and legs; may open eyes |
| Alert state | Awake but quiet; limited movement |
| Active alert | Responds to external stimulus by moving the entire body |
| Crying state | Cries without stopping; responds to all stimuli |

From MacLaren A: *Concepts and activities maternal-neonatal nursing,* Springhouse, PA, 1994, Springhouse.

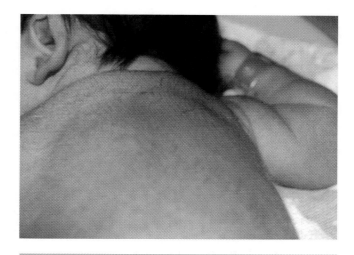

FIGURE 16-7 • Lanugo. *(Courtesy of Caroline E. Brown.)*

temporary and should fade. If the redness persists, the overfilled blood vessels, referred to as **plethora,** may indicate an overoxygenated or overheated infant or an elevated hemoglobin. If environmental factors are not the cause, it should be assessed thorough serum blood work. Some acrocyanoses may remain, but this color is due to a high level of hemoglobin, capillary stasis, and some vasomotor instability and also will fade over time.

Babies with **physiologic jaundice** have skin with a yellow coloring. In some babies it may be more easily detected in the oral mucosa or sclera of the eyes. Physiologic jaundice may be present in as many as 50% or more of newborn infants. It usually starts after the first 24 hours of life and disappears by the eighth to tenth day.

When examining a baby for hyperbilirubinemia, place the baby in natural daylight and look at the whole infant. "Jaundice begins on the face and descends. The bilirubin is not high if only the face is involved. However, the bilirubin may well be at a worrisome level if the jaundice descends below the nipples" (Seidel and others, 1999). In some babies, the jaundice may persist for 3 to 4 weeks.

If the jaundice occurs earlier than 24 hours, is intense in color, involves more than the face, or persists, it requires further investigation. It may be caused by the baby receiving too much water to drink, extensive bruising during delivery, liver disease, blood group incompatibility, or an infection (Seidel and others, 1999).

**Cyanosis** is a blue or dusky appearance of the skin that may occur because of various causes, ranging from trivial to life threatening. It is best detected when the infant is quiet or sleeping, by observing the color of the tongue, oral and buccal mucosa, and peripheral areas (Thureen and others, 1999). A systematic evaluation should be used to determine cause.

Another color change is **cutis marmorata,** a lacey red or bluish mottling of the skin. It may be seen in a

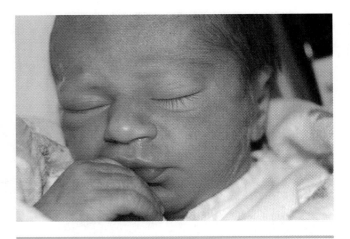

*FIGURE 16-8* • Face of normal newborn: milia on nose, lanugo in front of ears, slightly puffy eyelids. *(Courtesy of Caroline E. Brown.)*

normal infant or one with cold stress, hypovolemia, or sepsis. It is a result of dilated capillaries (Tappero and Honeyfield, 1993).

A phenomenon that may be seen in both sick and healthy infants, especially the low–birth-weight baby, is called the **Harlequin** color change. When the newborn is lying on its side, the dependent half of the body becomes red in color while the half of the body that is up is pale. Turning the baby to the other side alternates the color change to the other side. This is a temporary color change and is of no harm to the baby (Tappero and Honeyfield, 1993).

### Transient Cutaneous Lesions

Many skin variations are common in a newborn. They are not serious and resolve on their own. **Milia** are noted over the chin, bridge of the nose, forehead, and cheeks of 40% of full-term infants. These small (pinhead size), white papules (Thureen and others, 1999) are benign, sebum plugged sebaceous glans and disappear on their own within a few weeks (Seidel and others, 1999) (Figure 16-8).

**Sebaceous gland hyperplasia** is characterized by white or yellow macules and papules at the opening of pilosebaceous follicles (Thureen and others, 1999). It is most common on the forehead, cheeks, nose, and chin of the full-term newborn. It probably occurs as a result of androgen stimulation of the mother (Seidel and others, 1999).

These conditions are sometimes called "newborn acne." Parents will feel better if they understand that the conditions are normal and will disappear within 2 months or sooner, as the baby grows. Vigorous scrubbing of the skin is not recommended, and parents should be taught to just gently rinse the face.

**Erythema toxicum neonatorum** is a condition most often seen within the first 24 to 48 hours, but it may occur as late as 7 to 10 days after birth (Thureen and others, 1999). This skin variation is usually seen over the trunk and groin and is described as a rash of numerous areas of red skin that may be as large as 3 cm, each with a yellowish white papule in the center. They are most common on the thorax, back, buttocks, and abdomen. The rash resolves spontaneously 4 to 5 days after appearing (Figure 16-9).

**Telangiectatic nevi,** also called **stork bites,** salmon patch, vascular macule, nevus flammeus, and macular hemagioma, are most often seen around the neck, but may also occur on the eyelid, the bridge of the nose, or on the occipital bone. They are flat, deep pink or red areas caused by dilation of the capillaries. These birthmarks gradually go away within the first year of life. Sometimes the ones on the nape of the neck persist longer (Thureen and others, 1999) (Figure 16-10).

When an infant is in a warm environment, its sweat glands may become obstructed creating a condition called **miliaria** on its face and scalp. It may be one of two types: miliaria crystalline, which are tiny, superficial clear vesicles; or miliaria rubra (prickly heat), which are small, erythematous papules on a red base. These lesions disappear when the baby is placed in a cooler environment (Thureen and others, 1999).

### Vascular Lesions

Other vascular lesions are more troublesome to parents because they cover more area, last longer, and/or may indicate a more serious problem.

**Strawberry hemangiomas** are caused by dilated capillaries at the dermal or subdermal layer of skin. They may appear from birth to 2 weeks of age. They appear as red clusters raised above the skin and can grow for the first year. Although they may be visually upsetting, they eventually shrink but can take 7 to 10 years to do so. Large clusters may be indicative of further internal involvement and should be further evaluated.

**Mongolian spots** are often found on the buttocks or sacrum, predominantly among babies of Asian, southern European, Native American, Latin, or African descent. They are purple or bluish in color and disappear by school age without any treatment (Foster, Hunsberger, and Anderson, 1989; MacLaren, 1994). Inexperienced examiners often mistake the naturally occurring Mongolian spots for bruises.

**Nevus flammeus,** or port wine stain, may be a pale red to a deep purple area that blanches with minimal pressure. It is a permanent, sometime large birthmark caused by a capillary hemangioma. When they occur on the face, they may indicate the presence of Sturge-Weber syndrome and problems with vision and seizures. When they occur on the limbs or trunk, they may indicate the presence of Klippel-Trenaunay-Weber syndrome and visceral involvement, which may cause bleeding and/or limb hypertrophy, resulting in orthopedic problems (Seidel and others, 1999).

Various other skin lesions also may be present at or soon after birth. When they become apparent during a well-baby examination, each unusual or abnormal finding must be investigated further. The following are some examples. A tuft of hair (**Faun tail nevus**) overlying the spinal column in the lumbosacral area may be associated with spina bifida occulta. **Café au lait spots,** larger than 5 mm in diameter, may be associated with neurofibromatosis or miscellaneous other conditions. **Freckling in the axillary or inguinal areas,** may occur with Café au lait spots, and also are associated with neurofibromatosis. **Congenital lymphedema** may be associated with an absence of the X chromosome—Turner's syndrome. **Supernumerary nipples,** an extra nipple on the mammary ridge, may be associated with renal abnormalities. The occurrence of supernumerary nipples occurs much more often in blacks than in whites. **Persistent pruritus,** if not caused by skin disease, may indicate chronic renal failure, cholestatic liver disease, Hodgkin disease, or diabetes mellitus (Seidel and others, 1999).

### Skin Creases

The creases on the hands and feet of the newborn are examined because they provide several pieces of information. The number of creases on the fingers, palms, and soles reveals the maturity of the newborn—the more creases, the older the baby (Figures 16-11 and 16-12).

The pattern of the skin creases is also important. The most commonly known is the simian line, a single transverse crease across the palm. Although it occurs in individuals who are well, it may be an indication of Down syndrome (Seidel and others, 1999) (Figure 16-13).

### Temperature

Multiple sites can be used to assess the newborn's skin temperature. The skin should feel warm when touched and have a temperature range from 36.5° C to 37° C

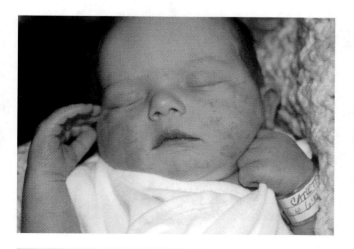

**FIGURE 16-9** • Erythema toxicum, or "newborn rash." *(Courtesy of Caroline E. Brown.)*

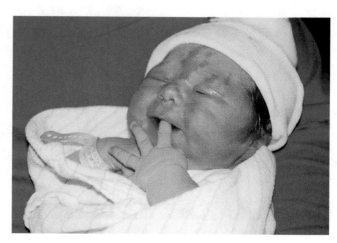

**FIGURE 16-10** • Telangiectatic nevi, or "stork bites." *(Courtesy of Caroline E. Brown.)*

(97.9° F to 98° F). Crying may increase the infant's body temperature slightly. The radiant warmer may give a false high axillary temperature (Wong and others, 1999).

Traditionally, the rectum and **axilla** (the armpit) have been the primary sites for assessing temperature in infants. Research now supports using the inguinal or tympanic area as alternatives to the rectum or axilla. Although the environmental temperature affects the tympanic temperature, it is considered a safe temperature screening method in the full-term infant in a bassinet. The inguinal temper-

ature offers a closer correlation to core temperature because of the vast blood supply and lack of brown fat in that area, and it may be a good indicator of temperature alterations (Cusson, Madonia, and Taekman, 1997). A temperature greater than 37.2° C (99° F) can be considered a fever or hyperthermia. A temperature of 35.5° C (96° F) can be a reflection of prematurity or poor perfusion (MacLaren, 1994).

## Examination of the Head

### Scalp

Starting at the head, assess for size, shape, symmetry, and general appearance. Inspect the hair for color, texture, distribution, and directional pattern. Hair color should be fairly uniform and in accord with the race of the baby. Reddish or blond hair on a dark skinned baby might indicate albinism. Other pigment defects or abnormalities may be familial in nature and normal or may indicate the condition of Waardenburg syndrome, with deafness and retardation (Thureen and others, 1999).

Observe for any molding, bruises, and demarcations. Unusual directional pattern or unruly hair may be an indication that further assessment of brain development is necessary.

Palpate the fontanels assessing whether they are flat or bulging. A sunken or flat fontanel may be due to dehydration. A bulging fontanel may occur when the baby cries or could be a sign of increased intracranial pressure or hydrocephalus (Figure 16-14).

Often times while inspecting the scalp, a small wound may be noted where the scalp clip used for fetal monitoring was placed. It is often toward the back or occipital region of the head. Instruct the family in how to keep it clean and dry and to watch for signs of infection (Figure 16-15).

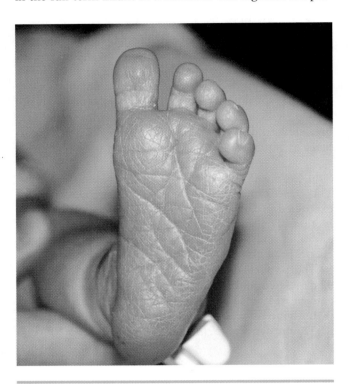

**FIGURE 16-11 •** Dry skin and creases on the sole of a very mature newborn. *(Courtesy of Caroline E. Brown.)*

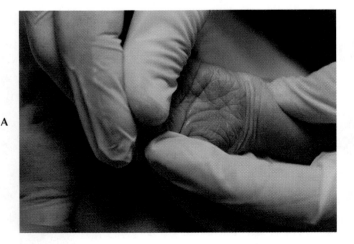

A

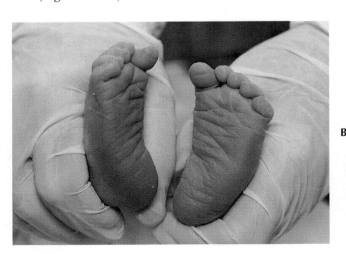

B

**FIGURE 16-12 •** Expected creases of a newborn's hand **A,** and feet **B.** *(From Seidel HM, Benedict GW, and Ball JW: Mosby's guide to physical examination, ed 4, St Louis, 1999, Mosby.)*

Some infants have swelling on the top of their heads. It may be one of the two common outcomes of labor and birth: caput succedaneum or cephalhematoma (Figures 16-16 and 16-17 and Table 16-6).

Parents may think that the swelling is unsightly and be sensitive to the way their child appears. A sympathetic response that normalizes the situation and an explanation that the condition is temporary and gradually will go away may help. The parents may also see that when the baby's head is covered with a hat, the condition is not as apparent.

### Face

Look at the face for symmetry, size, shape, and location of eyes, ears, nose, mouth, and chin. Also observe how the infant holds and uses them. An unusual appearance may be a familial trait or indicate that further investigation is necessary.

### Eyes

Although the eyes of the newborn are shut, they should be examined for symmetry and abnormalities. Parents should be taught that tears are not produced until 1 to 3 months of age. Any drainage that is other than clear is abnormal and requires further evaluation.

The eyes may be swollen for several days as a result of delivery and instillation of the prophylactic medica-

tion. Demonstrate to the family how to get the newborn to open his eyes. Gently position the baby upright and rock back and forth. Avoid bright lights and loud noises, which usually cause the baby to close its eyes tighter.

The sclera should be white. If a subjunctival hemorrhage is present because of delivery, it should clear in a few days. The iris of most babies is grayish or dark blue. This usually changes to a permanent color by 3 to

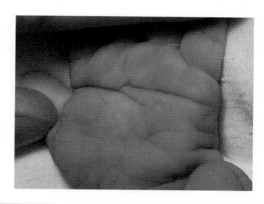

FIGURE 16-13 • Unexpected palmar crease. Simean crease in a child with Down Syndrome. *(From Seidel HM, Benedict GW, and Ball JW:* Mosby's guide to physical examination, *ed 4, St Louis, 1999, Mosby.)*

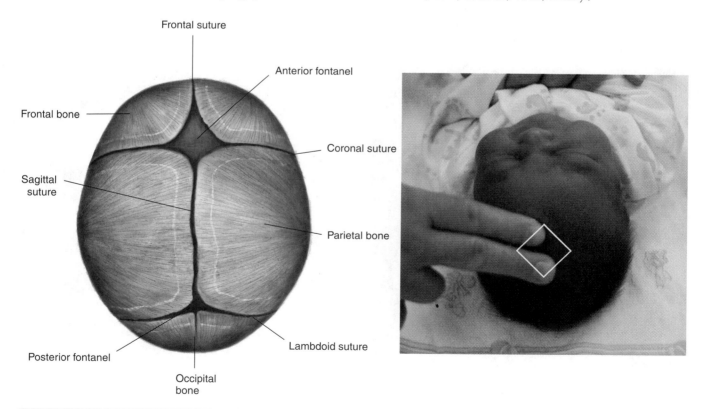

FIGURE 16-14 • Location and palpation of fontanels. *(From Wong DL and others:* Whaley and Wong's Nursing care of infants and children, *ed 6, St Louis, 1999, Mosby.)*

6 months. The presence of the red reflex indicates an intact lens. Its absence may indicate cataracts or other abnormalities (Thureen and others, 1999).

Observe the shape and position of the eyes as well as the tissue around them. Some variations are familial, but other times they may indicate a problem. An upward or downward slanting of the outer edge of the eyes may be indicative of several syndromes. Also observe for epicanthal folds—skin folds over the medial aspect of the eye—because it may be indicative of Down or other syndromes.

Observe for pupil response to light and symmetry of eye movements. At birth, the newborn is aware of light and dark and will close its eyes in the presence of bright light. Newborns are able to fixate on near objects from 3 to 30 inches away (Seidel and others, 1999).

### Ears

The position of the ears should be similar on both sides. The tip of the ear, or **helix**, should be at the level of the eye. Low-set ears may be a sign of a chromosomal abnormality or renal problem (Figure 16-18).

The ear structure is also a gestational age assessment tool. The cartilage of the term infant is not completely

formed and therefore the pinna, outside curve of the ear, can bend but will spring back. Skin tags and dimples are common.

If an infant responds to a soothing voice or turns toward a voice or a bell, it can probably hear. A more definitive evaluation will be done with a full screening physical.

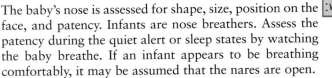

### Nose

The baby's nose is assessed for shape, size, position on the face, and patency. Infants are nose breathers. Assess the patency during the quiet alert or sleep states by watching the baby breathe. If an infant appears to be breathing comfortably, it may be assumed that the nares are open.

Flaring nostrils may be indicative of respiratory distress. Cyanosis, apnea, or noisy breathing also require further investigation. Demonstrate to the family how to use a bulb syringe to maintain clear and clean nares.

### Mouth and Chin

The shape of the mouth should be symmetric and open at equal angles bilaterally. Asymmetry may be the result of uterine position and neuromuscular activity. This will resolve spontaneously. Severe asymmetry may be related to nerve damage and must be investigated.

Optimize the alert active crying state to examine the tongue, buccal surfaces, palate, uvula, and back of the

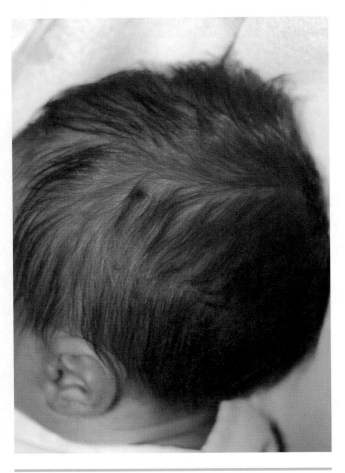

FIGURE 16-15 • Site of scalp clip for fetal monitor. *(Courtesy of Caroline E. Brown.)*

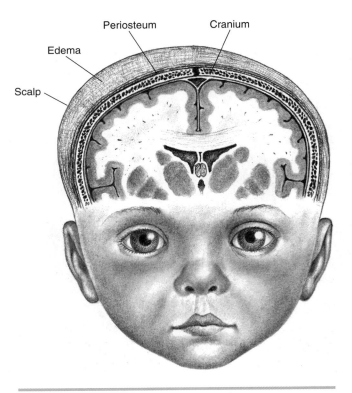

FIGURE 16-16 • Caput succedaneum. *(From Seidel HM, Benedict GW, and Ball JW: Mosby's guide to physical examination, ed 4, St Louis, 1999, Mosby.)*

mouth. While crying, the mucous membranes can be assessed for color and moistness. They should be pink and moist. A gloved finger can be used to palpate the gums and hard palate to assess for masses or defects and evaluate sucking and gag reflexes.

**Ankyloglossia**, or tongue-tie, is a relatively common condition in which the lingual frenulum limits movement of the tip of the tongue. In most infants with this disorder, the tongue can be extended beyond the lips and no therapy is necessary. Indications for surgical intervention include notching of the protruding tongue tip and the inability of the tongue tip to contact the maxillary alveolar ridge. Only rarely is surgical intervention required to correct difficulty in sucking and swallowing (Foster, Hunsberger, and Anderson, 1989).

**Epstein's pearls** are small white cysts that may cluster about the midline of the hard and soft palates. They are considered normal and resolve spontaneously with sucking.

## Neck

The infant should be able to open its mouth and move its head from side to side. This may be evaluated by brushing the infant's cheek, causing it to open its mouth and turn its mouth towards the finger (rooting reflex). Palpation of the neck should rule out hematomas, thyroid enlargement, thyroglossal duct cysts, webbing, and a redundant skin pouch at the base of the neck. The clavicles should be palpated for intactness because fractures sometimes occur during delivery.

## Respiratory and Heart Rates

Use a stethoscope to determine the cardiopulmonary status of the newborn. Auscultation of heart and breath sounds can be done at the same time.

The normal respiratory rate is 30 to 60 breaths per minute. Breath sounds should be done in sequence so that a comparison can be made from right to left, upper to lower, and anterior and posterior. Listen to breath sounds for 1 full minute because it is normal for infants to breathe irregularly and at varying depths. It is not unusual for an infant to go 10 seconds without breathing (Thureen and others, 1999).

Heart rate and rhythm may also fluctuate with the state of the infant. The heart rate of a normal newborn after the initial transition is 100 to 180 beats/min and usually is as high as 120 to 160 beats/min when awake and active (Thureen and others, 1999). Evaluate the heart rate for a full minute to compensate for the potential irregular heart rate (Bruno, 1995). Listen for possible defects in the heart, indicated by loud, harsh, or blowing murmurs.

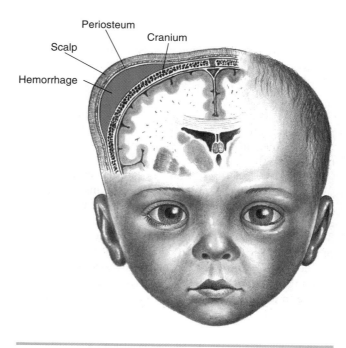

**FIGURE 16-17** • Cephalhematoma. Note that the swelling does not cross suture lines. *(From Seidel HM, Benedict GW, and Ball JW: Mosby's guide to physical examination, ed 4, St Louis, 1999, Mosby.)*

---

**TABLE 16-6   *Comparison of Caput Succedaneum and Cephalhematoma***

| Name | Cause | Location | Duration | Color | Demarcation |
|------|-------|----------|----------|-------|-------------|
| Cephalhematoma | Ruptured blood vessels between the skull bone and periosteum (layer just above skull bone) | Doesn't cross suture line because it only affects one bone | 2 to 3 weeks or longer | Ecchymotic | Clear edges |
| Caput succedaneum | Soft tissue edema due to continuous pressure during labor, which impedes venous return and lymph flow | May extend across suture lines; seen on presenting part | Fluid absorbs in a few days | Black/blue (ecchymotic) | Diffuse edges |

Developed by E. Lengetti from reference material.

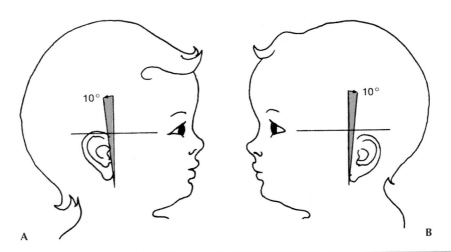

*FIGURE 16-18* • Ear alignment. **A,** Normal placement of ear. **B,** Low-set ear. *(From Barkauskas V and others:* Health and physical assessment, *ed 2, St Louis, 1998, Mosby.)*

Palpate the femoral, pedal, radial, and brachial pulses. Femoral pulses can be very difficult to detect. If not palpable, the blood pressure should be determined using the legs.

Capillary refill time in all extremities should be assessed. For 1 second, press one finger against the sole of the foot or the palm of the hand. Return of normal pink color should take 2 seconds. If it is delayed more than 3 seconds, it needs to be investigated. Measure in each of the extremities.

Tachycardia, abnormal pulses, wheezes and rales, or diaphoresis when feeding may indicate congestive heart failure in the infant.

### Abdomen

Abdomens of newborns rise and fall as they breathe. This occurs because most infants use their diaphragm more than the intercostal muscles.

Observe the area around the umbilicus. If intestinal muscles fail to close around the umbilicus, an umbilical hernia will occur. This is most common in babies of African descent. It may resolve naturally as the abdominal muscle becomes stronger, or it may require surgical repair (Figure 16-19).

Observe the umbilical cord. It should be starting to dry. Cord care includes the application of an antimicrobial ointment to the stump and on the skin surrounding the base of the cord. If edema is present around the base of the cord or a discharge, redness, or a foul odor is evident, it may indicate an inflammation of the umbilicus, **omphalitis,** or that there is a connection with the fetal bladder, **urachus.** Treatment is required.

Auscultation of the abdomen is completed similarly to the chest, in that you break the abdomen into four quadrants and compare right to left and upper to lower. Auscultation may reveal bruits over the liver or kidneys, both of which require further evaluation.

Palpation of a newborn's abdomen can be difficult because it is so small compared to an adult hand. To make it easier "place your right hand gently on the abdomen with the thumb at the right upper quadrant and the index finger at the left upper quadrant. Press very gently at first, only gradually increasing the pressure (never too vigorously) as you palpate over the entire abdomen" (Seidel and others, 1999).

Palpation starts in the right lower quadrant and progresses upward. The size of the liver is measured and uniformity of size is determined. Percussion at the midclavicular line will reveal a normal liver span of $5.9 \pm 0.8$ cm from the upper to the lower margins (Thureen and others, 1999). The spleen is rarely palpable.

### Genitourinary System

The kidneys are routinely palpable during the first 48 hours. During palpation, the infant normally demonstrates pain by grimacing, crying, or drawing up its legs. The bladder may be palpated 1 to 4 cm above the symphysis pubis. By 48 hours every infant should have urinated. The urinary stream should be strong. Dribbling or a reduced force may indicate a problem.

### Genitalia

The genitalia should be inspected for size and location. This is done most easily if the infant's legs are held in a frog position.

*Males.* The glans should be completely covered by the foreskin at birth. It is not fully retractable until at least age 3. Retract it just enough to determine the position of the urethral opening. The length of the nonerect penis in a full-term baby is 2 to 3 cm. Transitory erections commonly occur, during which the shaft of the penis is straight.

Using warm hands inspect the scrotum for color, size, and rugae. The scrotum of babies of black, Native American, and Hispanic descent appears darker than the

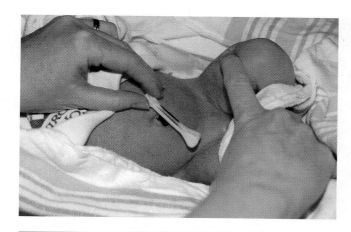

FIGURE 16-19 • Umbilical cord with clamp still on. *(Courtesy of Caroline E. Brown.)*

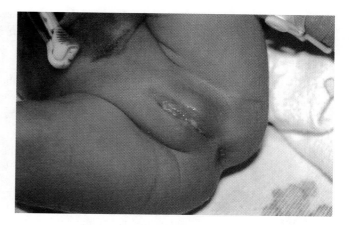

FIGURE 16-20 • Vaginal discharge. *(Courtesy of Caroline E. Brown.)*

rest of their skin. If the testes are discolored, it may indicate a hematoma or torsion. Unless it is superficial ecchymosis, it may require immediate surgical evaluation.

The proximal end of the scrotum should be the widest area. It will appear large compared to the rest of the genitalia. The presence of rugae indicates that the baby is at least 37 weeks of gestation.

Palpation determines if the testes have descended. If either of the testicles is not palpable, place your finger over the upper inguinal ring and push towards the scrotum. A soft mass, the testicle, may be felt in the inguinal canal. It may gently be pushed into the scrotum. Even if it then retracts, it is considered a descended testicle. A testicle that either is palpable but not movable or one that is not palpable is considered an undescended testicle (Seidel and others, 1999).

If the palpation of the scrotum indicates the presence of more than the testicle or spermatic cord, it must be determined if the scrotum is filled with fluid, gas, or solid material. Translumination may reveal a hydrocele, which may occur either unilaterally or bilaterally. If the mass does not transilluminate, it may be a hernia. Further evaluation must occur immediately because an incarcerated hernia is a surgical emergency.

***Females.*** The maternal hormones affect the female's genitalia causing them to swell. This is transient and should disappear within a few weeks. The labia, clitoris, meatus, and vaginal opening should be inspected for size and location. In a term infant, the labia majora will cover the labia minora, clitoris, urethral meatus, and external vaginal vault. The labia majora should be palpated for masses.

The vaginal orifice should be pink, moist, and intact. Many infant girls have a creamy white or slightly blood-tinged discharge (Figure 16-20). The central opening of the hymen is usually about 0.5 cm in diameter. Make no effort to stretch it. The perineum should be smooth.

***Ambiguous Genitalia.*** Sometimes the external genitalia do not clearly indicate whether the infant is a male or a female. Any ambiguous appearance or unusual orifice in

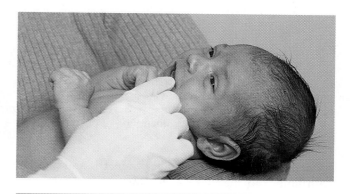

FIGURE 16-21 • Rooting reflex. *(From Seidel HM, Benedict GW, and Ball JW: Mosby's guide to physical examination, ed 4, St Louis, 1999, Mosby.)*

the vulvar vault or perineum must be explored before the infant is assigned a gender. This can be a very difficult time for parents because the first question everyone asks is, "Is it a boy or a girl?" An answer of "We don't know," is uncomfortable.

In a presumed male infant, the scrotum or inguinal canal is palpated for testes. In a presumed female infant, the labia may be palpated for testes.

### Anus and Spine

In all newborns, the anus should also be midline and free of any tufts of hair or dimpling.

When the newborn has passed its first stool, it should be recorded.

After checking the anus, turn the infant over to reveal the spine. The alignment and intactness of the spinal column is assessed and the area is observed for dimples, sinuses, or any abnormal growths (MacLaren, 1994).

## Neurologic Examination

Observations during the physical examination provide indirect evaluation of the cranial nerves. The infant's

---

**TABLE 16-7**    *Indirect Cranial Nerve Evaluation in Newborns and Infants*

| Cranial nerves | Procedures and observations |
|---|---|
| CN II, III, IV, and VI | Optical blink reflex; shine a light at the infant's open eyes. Observe the quick closure of the eyes and dorsal flexion of the infant's head. No response may indicate poor light perception.<br>Gazes intensely at close object or face.<br>Focuses on and tracks an object with both eyes.<br>Doll's eye maneuver: see CN VIII. |
| CN V | Rooting reflex: touch one corner of the infant's mouth. The infant should open its mouth and turn its head in the direction of stimulation. If the infant has been recently fed, minimal or no response is expected (Figure 16-21).<br>Sucking reflex: place your finger in the infant's mouth, feeling the sucking action. The tongue should push up against your finger with good strength. Note the pressure, strength, and pattern of sucking. |
| CN VII | Observe the infant's facial expression when crying. Note the infant's ability to wrinkle the forehead and the symmetry of the smile. |
| CN VIII | Acoustic blink reflex: loudly clap your hands about 30 cm from the infant's head; avoid producing an air current. Note the blink in response to the sound. No response after 2 to 3 days of age may indicate hearing problems. Infant will habituate to repeated testing.<br>Moves eyes in direction of sound. Freezes position with high-pitched sound.<br>Doll's eye maneuver: hold the infant under the axilla in an upright position, head held steady, facing you. Rotate the infant first in one direction and then in the other. The infant's eyes should turn in the direction of rotation and then the opposite direction when rotation stops. If the eyes do not move in the expected direction, suspect a vestibular problem or eye muscle paralysis. |
| CN IX and X | Swallowing and gag reflex. |
| CN XII | Coordinated sucking and swallowing ability.<br>Pinch infant's nose; mouth will open and tip of tongue will rise in a midline position. |

---

spontaneous activities should be symmetric and smooth, with limbs moving in an alternating fashion. The way the infant blinks, focuses on your face, turns its eyes toward sound, sucks, swallows, turns toward a touch on its cheek (rooting reflex, shown in Figure 16-21), and responds to its environment are indications of its neurologic abilities (Table 16-7).

The primitive reflexes provide information about the infant's nervous system and state of neurologic maturation. Some reflexes, such as rooting and sucking, must be present so that the infant is able to take in nutrition. Others, such as gagging, coughing, and sneezing, improve the infant's chance of survival. The assessment of the primitive reflexes must be done within the first 48 hours of birth. After that time, abnormal responses may be missed, and clues to possible future developments are lost (Table 16-8) (Figure 16-22). A summary of the assessment of the newborn is found in Table 16-9.

## Gestational Age

In addition to the previously stated components of assessment, determining the gestational age of the newborn is also necessary. The tool most often used is the Maturational Assessment of Gestational Age (New Ballard Score) (Ballard and others, 1991). This tool looks at six maneuvers that evaluate neuromuscular maturity and six factors to evaluate physical maturity. When data are collected from an infant of more than 20 weeks of gestation, the scoring can accurately determine gestational age within 2 weeks (Figure 16-23).

A newborn's growth pattern and size for gestational age can be determined once the gestational age is determined. Thereafter, standardized growth curves are used to plot the growth. Variations outside the normal, alert the provider to the possibility of problems.

## Behavioral Response

How the newborn reacts to the world around it is called a **behavioral response**. Expected behaviors are separated into six categories: habituation, orientation, motor maturity, variations, self-quieting ability, and social behaviors. **Habituation** refers to the newborn's ability to block out external stimuli once it has become used to the activity. This is why some babies can sleep anywhere. **Orientation** reflects the newborn's response to auditory and visual stimuli by moving the head and eyes. **Motor maturity** depends on gestational age and evaluates posture, tone coordination, and movements. This is best assessed during the alert state. The frequency of skin color changes, state, and activity level all reflect what is called **variation**. The newborn's ability to stop crying on its own whether through oral stimulation or in response to visual or auditory stimuli allows the observer to assess the **self-quieting ability** of the baby. **Social behaviors** are such things as snuggling into the arms of a parent or caregiver or crying to be fed. Any deviation in behavioral responses should be assessed

### TABLE 16-8   *Primitive Reflexes Routinely Evaluated in Infants*

| Reflex (appearance) | Procedures and findings |
|---|---|
| Palmar grasp (birth) | Making sure the infant's head is in midline, touch the palm of the infant's hand from the ulnar side (opposite the thumb). Note the strong grasp of your finger. Sucking facilitates the grasp. It should be strongest between 1 and 2 months of age and disappear by 3 months (Figure 16-22, *A*). |
| Plantar grasp (birth) | Touch the plantar surface of the infant's feet at the base of the toes. The toes should curl downward. The reflex should be strong up to 8 months of age (Figure 16-22, *B*). |
| Moro (birth) | With the infant supported in semi-sitting position, allow the head and trunk to drop back to a 30-degree angle. Observe symmetric abduction and extension of the arms. Fingers fan out and thumb and index finger form a C. The arms then adduct in an embracing motion followed by relaxed flexion. The legs may follow a similar pattern of response. The reflex diminishes in strength by 3 to 4 months and disappears by 6 months (Figure 16-22, *C*). |
| Placing (4 days of age) | Hold the infant upright under the arms next to a table or chair. Touch the dorsal side of the foot to the table or chair edge. Observe flexion of the hips and knees and lifting of the foot as if stepping up on the table. Age of disappearance varies (Figure 16-22, *D*). |
| Stepping (between birth and 8 weeks) | Hold the infant upright under the arms and allow the soles of the feet to touch the surface of the table. Observe for alternate flexion and extension of the legs, simulating walking. It disappears before voluntary walking (Figure 16-22, *E*). |
| Asymmetric tonic neck or "fencing" (by 2 to 3 months) | With the infant lying supine and relaxed or sleeping, turn its head to one side so the jaw is over the shoulder. Observe for extension of the arm and leg on the side to which the head is turned and for flexion of the opposite arm and leg. Turn the infant's head to the other side, observing the reversal of the extremities' posture. This reflex diminishes at 3 to 4 months of age and disappears by 6 months. Be concerned if the infant never exhibits the reflex or seems locked in the fencing position. This reflex must disappear before the infant can roll over or bring its hands to its face (Figure 16-22, *F*). |

further because it may be associated with more complex illnesses (MacLaren, 1994). All of the behavioral responses are excellent details to teach the family. The members can identify the individual cues of their baby and learn what stimuli are pleasurable.

## CARING FOR THE NORMAL NEWBORN

Caring for the newborn is both challenging and rewarding, and a task that the mother and her support system will completely assume within hours. Many opportunities are available for family participation in getting to know this baby and becoming comfortable in its care. A good mechanism to start with is *show and tell* while also gradually increasing the amount of care provided by the baby's care system.

### Washing

The baby's first bath is exciting for the family. A "sponge" bath may be given after the baby has maintained temperature stability for a few hours. Show how to start the bath at the face and head and work on down the body, saving the buttock and groin area for last. Explain how this technique allows for a total inspection of the baby's body and ensures thoroughness. A full bath in which the baby is submerged into a baby bath of tepid water in a draft free environment is not begun until after the umbilical cord falls off.

In addition, encourage the family to gently wash the baby's face after each feeding and to wash and dry the diaper area with each diaper change. Keeping the diaper area clean and dry is the best prevention for diaper rash.

### Cord Care

Cord care includes cleaning the umbilical cord, applying the antimicrobial ointment, and assessing with every diaper change. Review that the cord should be kept clean and dry until it falls off. Inform the family that the cord will remain intact for 5 to 10 days but will shrivel and dry as time progresses. It is common for a few drops of blood to be noted around the stump of the umbilical cord, especially after care, but redness, puss, or a foul smell should be reported to the health care provider immediately because they are signs of possible infection (Foster, Hunsberger, and Anderson, 1989).

Demonstrate how to roll down the top part of the diaper so that the umbilical cord can be kept dry from urine. The family also may be interested in knowing that, although they are not necessary, newborn diapers with an opening for the cord can be purchased.

### Handling the Baby

Each time you pick up the infant, you are demonstrating to the family the safest techniques. When picking

*Text continued on p. 678*

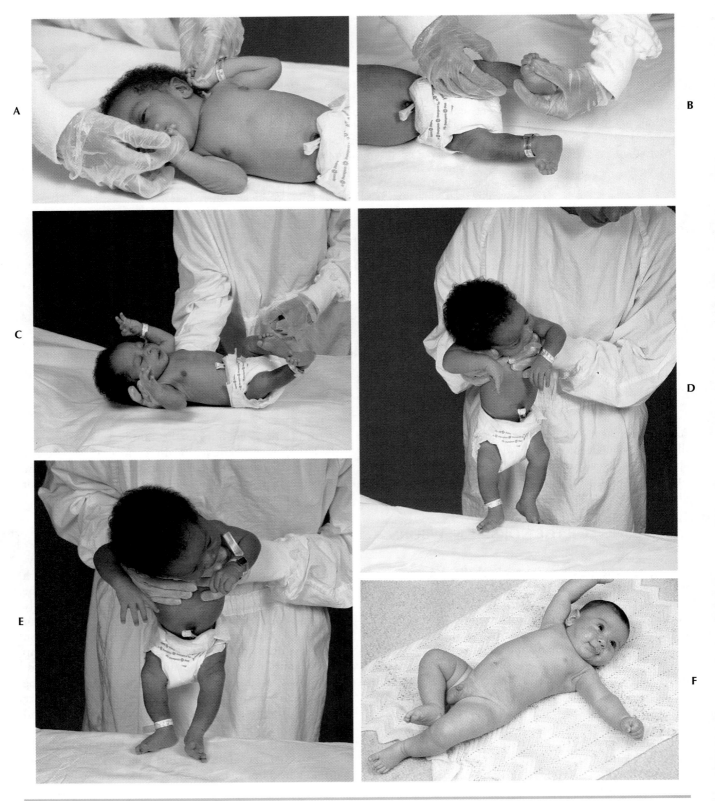

FIGURE 16-22 • Elicitation of the primitive reflexes. **A,** Palmar grasp. **B,** Plantar grasp. **C,** Moro. **D,** Placing. **E,** Stepping. **F,** Asymmetric tonic neck. *(From Seidel HM, Benedict GW, and Ball JW: Mosby's guide to physical examination, ed 4, St Louis, 1999, Mosby.)*

## MATURATIONAL ASSESSMENT OF GESTATIONAL AGE (New Ballard Score)

NAME _____   DATE/TIME OF BIRTH _____   SEX _____

HOSPITAL NO. _____   DATE/TIME OF EXAM _____   BIRTH WEIGHT _____

RACE _____   AGE WHEN EXAMINED _____   LENGTH _____

APGAR SCORE: 1 MINUTE _____ 5 MINUTES _____ 10 MINUTES _____   HEAD CFC _____

EXAMINER _____

### NEUROMUSCULAR MATURITY

| NEUROMUSCULAR MATURITY SIGN | SCORE | | | | | | | RECORD SCORE HERE |
|---|---|---|---|---|---|---|---|---|
| | −1 | 0 | 1 | 2 | 3 | 4 | 5 | |
| POSTURE | | | | | | | | |
| SQUARE WINDOW (Wrist) | >90° | 90° | 60° | 45° | 30° | 0° | | |
| ARM RECOIL | | 180° | 140°-180° | 110°-140° | 90°-110° | <90° | | |
| POPLITEAL ANGLE | 180° | 160° | 140° | 120° | 100° | 90° | <90° | |
| SCARF SIGN | | | | | | | | |
| HEEL TO EAR | | | | | | | | |

TOTAL NEUROMUSCULAR MATURITY SCORE

**SCORE**

Neuromuscular _____

Physical _____

Total _____

**MATURITY RATING**

| score | weeks |
|---|---|
| −10 | 20 |
| −5 | 22 |
| 0 | 24 |
| 5 | 26 |
| 10 | 28 |
| 15 | 30 |
| 20 | 32 |
| 25 | 34 |
| 30 | 36 |
| 35 | 38 |
| 40 | 40 |
| 45 | 42 |
| 50 | 44 |

**GESTATIONAL AGE (weeks)**

By dates _____

By ultrasound _____

By exam _____

### PHYSICAL MATURITY

| PHYSICAL MATURITY SIGN | SCORE | | | | | | | RECORD SCORE HERE |
|---|---|---|---|---|---|---|---|---|
| | −1 | 0 | 1 | 2 | 3 | 4 | 5 | |
| SKIN | sticky friable transparent | gelatinous red translucent | smooth pink visible veins | superficial peeling &/or rash, few veins | cracking pale areas rare veins | parchment deep cracking no vessels | leathery cracked wrinkled | |
| LANUGO | none | sparse | abundant | thinning | bald areas | mostly bald | | |
| PLANTAR SURFACE | heel-toe 40-50 mm: −1 <40 mm: −2 | >50 mm no crease | faint red marks | anterior transverse crease only | creases ant. 2/3 | creases over entire sole | | |
| BREAST | imperceptible | barely perceptible | flat areola no bud | stippled areola 1-2 mm bud | raised areola 3-4 mm bud | full areola 5-10 mm bud | | |
| EYE/EAR | lids fused loosely: −1 tightly: −2 | lids open pinna flat stays folded | sl. curved pinna; soft; slow recoil | well-curved pinna; soft but ready recoil | formed & firm instant recoil | thick cartilage ear stiff | | |
| GENITALS (Male) | scrotum flat, smooth | scrotum empty faint rugae | testes in upper canal rare rugae | testes descending few rugae | testes down good rugae | testes pendulous deep rugae | | |
| GENITALS (Female) | clitoris prominent & labia flat | prominent clitoris & small labia minora | prominent clitoris & enlarging minora | majora & minora equally prominent | majora large minora small | majora cover clitoris & minora | | |

TOTAL PHYSICAL MATURITY SCORE

FIGURE 16-23 ● Maturational assessment of gestational age (New Ballard Score). *(From Ballard JL and others: Maturational assessment of gestational age,* J Pediatr *119:417-423, 1991.)*

**TABLE 16-9** *Summary of Physical Assessment of the Newborn*

| Usual findings | Common variations/minor abnormalities | Potential signs of distress/major abnormalities |
|---|---|---|
| **GENERAL MEASUREMENTS** | | |
| *Head circumference*—33-35 cm (13-14 inches); about 2-3 cm (1 in) larger than chest circumference | Molding after birth may decrease head circumference | Head circumference <10th or >90th percentile |
| *Chest circumference*—30.5-33 cm (12-13 in) | Head and chest circumference may be equal for first 1-2 days after birth | |
| *Crown-to-rump length*—31-35 cm (12.5-14 in); approximately equal to head circumference | | |
| *Head-to-heel length*—48-53 cm (19-21 in) | | |
| *Birth weight*—2700-4000 g (6-9 lb) | Loss of 10% of birth weight in first week; regained in 10-14 days | Birth weight <10th or >90th percentile |
| **VITAL SIGNS** | | |
| TEMPERATURE | | |
| Axillary—36.5°-37° C (97.9°-98° F) | Crying may increase body temperature slightly | Hypothermia |
| | Radiant warmer will falsely increase axillary temperature | Hyperthermia |
| HEART RATE | | |
| Apical—120-140 beats/min | Crying will increase heart rate; sleep will decrease heart rate | Bradycardia—Resting rate below 80-100 bpm |
| | During first period of reactivity (6 to 8 hours), rate can reach 180 bpm | Tachycardia—Rate above 160-180 bpm Irregular rhythm |
| RESPIRATIONS | | |
| 30-60 breaths/min | Crying increases respiratory rate; sleep decreases respiratory rate | Tachypnea—Rate above 60 breaths/min Apnea >15 seconds |
| | During first period of reactivity (6 to 8 hours), rate can reach 80 breaths/min | |
| BLOOD PRESSURE (BP) | | |
| Oscillometric—65/41 mm Hg in arm and calf | Crying and activity increase BP Placing cuff on thigh may agitate infant; thigh BP may be higher than arm or calf BP by 4-8 mm Hg | Oscillometric systolic pressure in calf 6-9 mm Hg less than in upper extremity (sign of coarctation of aorta) |
| **GENERAL APPEARANCE** | | |
| *Posture*—Flexion of head and extremities, which rest on chest and abdomen | *Frank breech*—Extended legs, abducted and fully rotated thighs, flattened occiput, extended neck | Limp posture, extension of extremities |
| **SKIN** | | |
| At birth: bright red, puffy, smooth | Neonatal jaundice after first 24 hours | Progressive jaundice, especially in first 24 hours |
| Second to third day: pink, flaky, dry | Ecchymoses or petechiae caused by birth trauma | Cracked or peeling skin |
| Vernix caseosa | *Milia*—Distended sebaceous glands that appear as tiny white papules on cheeks, chin, and nose | Generalized cyanosis |
| Lanugo (see Figure 16-7) | | Pallor |
| Edema around eyes, face, legs, dorsa of hands, feet, and scrotum or labia | *Miliaria* or *sudamina*—Distended sweat (eccrine) glands that appear as minute vesicles, especially on face | Mottling |
| *Acrocyanosis*—Cyanosis of hands and feet (see Figure 16-8) | | Grayness |
| | | Plethora |
| *Cutis marmorata*—Transient mottling when infant is exposed to decreased temperature, stress, or overstimulation | *Erythema toxicum*—Pink papular rash with vesicles superimposed on thorax, back, buttocks, and abdomen; may appear in 24 to 48 hours and resolve after several days (see Figure 16-9) | Hemorrhage, ecchymoses, or petechiae persist |
| | | *Sclerema*—Hard and stiff skin |
| | | Poor skin turgor |
| | | Rashes, pustules, or blisters |
| | | *Café-au-lait spots*—Light brown spots |

TABLE 16-9 *Summary of Physical Assessment of the Newborn—cont'd*

| Usual findings | Common variations/minor abnormalities | Potential signs of distress/major abnormalities |
|---|---|---|
| **SKIN—cont'd** | *Harlequin color change*—Clearly outlined color change as infant lies on side; lower half of body becomes pink or red, and upper half is pale<br>*Mongolian spots*—Irregular areas of deep blue pigmentation, usually in sacral and gluteal regions; seen predominantly in newborns of African, Native American, Asian, or Hispanic descent (see figure at right)<br>*Telangiectatic nevi ("stork bites")*—Flat, deep pink, localized areas usually seen on back of neck (see Figure 16-10) | *Nevus flammeus*—Port-wine stain<br> |
| **HEAD**<br>*Anterior fontanel*—Diamond shaped, 2.5-4.0 cm (1-1.75 in) (see Figure 16-14)<br>*Posterior fontanel*—Triangular, 0.5-1 cm (0.2-0.4 in)<br>Fontanels should be flat, soft, and firm<br>Widest part of fontanel measured from bone to bone, not suture to suture | Molding following vaginal delivery<br>Third sagittal (parietal) fontanel<br>Bulging fontanel because of crying<br>*Caput succedaneum*—Edema of soft scalp tissue (see Figure 16-16)<br>*Cephalhematoma* (uncomplicated)—Hematoma between periosteum and skull bone (see Figure 16-17) | Fused sutures<br>Bulging or depressed fontanels when quiet<br>Widened sutures and fontanels<br>*Craniotabes*—Snapping sensation along lambdoid suture that resembles indentation of Ping-Pong ball |
| **EYES**<br>Lids usually edematous<br>Color—Slate gray, dark blue, brown<br>Absence of tears<br>Presence of red reflex<br>Corneal reflex in response to touch<br>Pupillary reflex in response to light<br>Blink reflex in response to light or touch<br>Rudimentary fixation on objects and ability to follow to midline | Epicanthal folds in Oriental infants<br>Searching nystagmus or strabismus<br>*Subconjunctival (scleral) hemorrhages*—Ruptured capillaries, usually at limbus | Pink color of iris<br>Purulent discharge<br>Upward slant in non-Asians<br>Hypertelorism (3 cm or greater)<br>Hypotelorism<br>Congenital cataracts<br>Constricted or dilated fixed pupil<br>Absence of red reflex<br>Absence of pupillary or corneal reflex<br>Inability to follow object or bright light to midline<br>Blue sclera<br>Yellow sclera |
| **EARS**<br>Position—Top of pinna on horizontal line with outer canthus of eye<br>Startle reflex elicited by a loud, sudden noise<br>Pinna flexible, cartilage present | Inability to visualize tympanic membrane because of filled aural canals<br>Pinna flat against head<br>Irregular shape or size<br>Pits or skin tags | Low placement of ears (see Figure 16-18)<br>Absence of startle reflex in response to loud noise<br>Minor abnormalities may be signs of various syndromes, especially renal |
| **NOSE**<br>Nasal patency<br>Nasal discharge—Thin white mucus<br>Sneezing | Flattened and bruised | Nonpatent canals<br>Thick, bloody nasal discharge<br>Flaring of nares (alae nasi)<br>Copious nasal secretions or stuffiness (may be minor) |
| **MOUTH AND THROAT**<br>Intact, high-arched palate<br>Uvula in midline<br>Frenulum of tongue | *Natal teeth*—Teeth present at birth; benign but may be associated with congenital defects | Cleft lip<br>Cleft palate |

*Continued*

**TABLE 16-9** *Summary of Physical Assessment of the Newborn—cont'd*

| Usual findings | Common variations/minor abnormalities | Potential signs of distress/major abnormalities |
|---|---|---|
| **MOUTH AND THROAT—cont'd**<br>Frenum of upper lip<br>Sucking reflex—Strong and coordinated<br>Rooting reflex (see Figure 16-21)<br>Gag reflex<br>Extrusion reflex<br>Absent or minimal salivation<br>Vigorous cry | *Epstein pearls*—Small, white epithelial cysts along midline of hard palate | Large, protruding tongue or posterior displacement of tongue<br>Profuse salivation or drooling<br>*Candidiasis (thrush)*—White, adherent patches on tongue, palate, and buccal surfaces<br>Inability to pass nasogastric tube<br>Hoarse, high-pitched, weak, absent, or other abnormal cry |
| **NECK**<br>Short, thick, usually surrounded by skinfolds<br>Tonic neck reflex | *Torticollis* (wry neck)—Head held to one side with chin pointing to opposite side | Excessive skinfolds<br>Resistance to flexion<br>Absence of tonic neck reflex<br>Fractured clavicle |
| **CHEST**<br>Anteroposterior and lateral diameters equal<br>Slight sternal retractions evident during inspiration<br>Xiphoid process evident<br>Breast enlargement | Funnel chest (pectus excavatum)<br>Pigeon chest (pectus carinatum)<br>Supernumerary nipples<br>Secretion of milky substance from breasts ("witch's milk") | Depressed sternum<br>Marked retractions of chest and intercostal spaces during respiration<br>Asymmetric chest expansion<br>Redness and firmness around nipples<br>Wide-spaced nipples |
| **LUNGS**<br>Respirations chiefly abdominal<br>Cough reflex absent at birth, present by 1-2 days<br>Bilateral equal bronchial breath sounds | Rate and depth of respirations may be irregular, periodic breathing<br>Crackles shortly after birth | Inspiratory stridor<br>Expiratory grunt<br>Retractions<br>Persistent irregular breathing<br>Periodic breathing with repeated apnea spells<br>Seesaw respirations (paradoxical)<br>Unequal breath sounds<br>Persistent fine crackles<br>Wheezing<br>Diminished breath sounds<br>Peristaltic sounds on one side, with diminished breath sounds on same side |
| **HEART**<br>Apex—Fourth to fifth intercostal space, lateral to left sternal border<br>$S_2$ slightly sharper and higher in pitch than $S_1$ | *Sinus arrhythmia*—Heart rate increases with inspiration and decreases with expiration<br>Transient cyanosis on crying or straining | *Dextrocardia*—Heart on right side<br>Displacement of apex, muffled<br>Cardiomegaly<br>Abdominal shunts<br>Murmurs<br>Thrills<br>Persistent cyanosis<br>Hyperactive precordium |
| **ABDOMEN**<br>Cylindric in shape<br>*Liver*—Palpable 2-3 cm below right costal margin<br>*Spleen*—Tip palpable at end of first week of age | Umbilical hernia<br>*Diastasis recti*—Midline gap between recti muscles<br>*Wharton's jelly*—Unusually thick umbilical cord | Abdominal distention<br>Localized bulging<br>Distended veins<br>Absent bowel sounds<br>Enlarged liver and spleen |

**TABLE 16-9   Summary of Physical Assessment of the Newborn—cont'd**

| Usual findings | Common variations/minor abnormalities | Potential signs of distress/major abnormalities |
|---|---|---|
| **ABDOMEN—cont'd**<br>**Kidneys**—Palpable 1-2 cm above umbilicus<br>**Umbilical cord**—Bluish white at birth with two arteries and one vein<br>**Femoral pulses**—Equal bilaterally | | Ascites<br>Visible peristaltic waves<br>Scaphoid or concave abdomen<br>Green umbilical cord<br>Presence of only one artery in cord<br>Urine or stool leaking from cord<br>Palpable bladder distention following voiding<br>Absent femoral pulses<br>Cord bleeding or hematoma |
| **FEMALE GENITALIA**<br>Labia and clitoris usually edematous<br>Urethral meatus behind clitoris<br>Vernix caseosa between labia<br>Urination within 24 hr | **Pseudomenstruation**—Blood-tinged or mucoid discharge (see Figure 16-20)<br>Hymenal tag | Enlarged clitoris with urethral meatus<br>Fused labia<br>Absence of vaginal opening<br>Meconium from vaginal opening<br>No urination within 24 hr<br>Masses in labia<br>Ambiguous genitalia |
| **MALE GENITALIA**<br>Urethral opening at tip of glans penis<br>Testes palpable in each scrotum<br>Scrotum usually large, edematous, pendulous, and covered with rugae; usually deeply pigmented in dark-skinned ethnic groups<br>Smegma<br>Urination within 24 hr | Urethral opening covered by prepuce<br>Inability to retract foreskin<br>**Epithelial pearls**—Small, firm, white lesions at tip of prepuce<br>Erection or priapism<br>Testes palpable in inguinal canal<br>Scrotum small | **Hypospadias**—Urethral opening on ventral surface of penis<br>**Epispadias**—Urethral opening on dorsal surface of penis<br>**Chordee**—Ventral curvature of penis<br>Testes not palpable in scrotum or inguinal canal<br>No urination within 24 hr<br>Inguinal hernia<br>Hypoplastic scrotum<br>**Hydrocele**—Fluid in scrotum<br>Masses in scrotum<br>Meconium from scrotum<br>Discoloration of testes<br>Ambiguous genitalia |
| **BACK AND RECTUM**<br>Spine intact, no openings, masses, or prominent curves<br>Trunk incurvation reflex<br>Anal reflex<br>Patent anal opening<br>Passage of meconium within 48 hr | Green liquid stools in infant under phototherapy<br>Delayed passages of meconium in very-low-birth-weight neonates | Anal fissures or fistulas<br>Imperforate anus<br>Absence of anal reflex<br>No meconium within 36 hr<br>Pilonidal cyst or sinus<br>Tuft of hair along spine<br>Spina bifida (any degree) |
| **EXTREMITIES**<br>Ten fingers and toes<br>Full range of motion<br>Nail beds pink, with transient cyanosis immediately after birth<br>Creases on anterior two thirds of sole<br>Sole usually flat<br>Symmetry of extremities | Partial syndactyly between second and third toes<br>Second toe overlapping into third toe<br>Wide gap between first (hallux) and second toes<br>Deep crease on plantar surface of foot between first and second toes<br>Asymmetric length of toes | **Polydactyly**—Extra digits<br>**Syndactyly**—Fused or webbed digits (see figure)<br>**Phocomelia**—Hands or feet attached close to trunk<br>**Hemimelia**—Absence of distal part of extremity<br>Hyperflexibility of joints |

*Continued*

**TABLE 16-9**    *Summary of Physical Assessment of the Newborn—cont'd*

| Usual findings | Common variations/minor abnormalities | Potential signs of distress/major abnormalities |
| --- | --- | --- |
| **EXTREMITIES—cont'd**<br>Equal muscle tone bilaterally, especially resistance to opposing flexion<br>Equal bilateral brachial pulses | Dorsiflexion and shortness of hallux<br>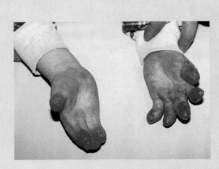 | Persistent cyanosis of nail beds<br>Yellowing of nail beds<br>Sole covered with creases<br>Transverse palmar (simian) crease<br>Fractures<br>Decreased or absent ROM<br>***Dislocated or subluxated hip***<br>  Limitation in hip abduction<br>  Unequal gluteal or leg folds<br>  Unequal knee height (Allis or Galeazzi sign)<br>  Audible clunk on abduction (Ortolani sign)<br>Asymmetry of extremities<br>Unequal muscle tone or range of motion |
| **NEUROMUSCULAR SYSTEM**<br>Extremities usually maintain some degree of flexion<br>Extension of an extremity followed by previous position of flexion<br>Head lag while sitting, but momentary ability to hold head erect<br>Able to turn head from side to side when prone<br>Able to hold head in horizontal line with back when held prone | Quivering or momentary tremors | ***Hypotonia***—Floppy, poor head control, extremities limp<br>***Hypertonia***—Jittery, arms and hands tightly flexed, legs stiffly extended, startles easily<br>Asymmetric posturing (except tonic neck reflex)<br>***Opisthotonic posturing***—Arched back<br>Signs of paralysis<br>Tremors, twitches, and myoclonic jerks<br>Marked head lag in all positions |

Adapted from Wong DL and others: *Whaley and Wong's nursing care of infants and children*, ed 6, St Louis, 1999, Mosby.

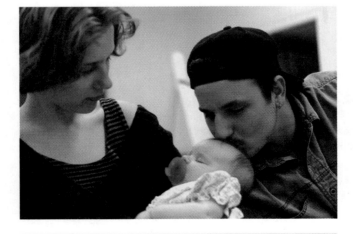

FIGURE 16-24 • Adolescent parents learning about their infant. *(Courtesy of Caroline E. Brown.)*

up the baby, support the back of the head and review that this is important because the head is such a large and heavy part of the newborn's body. Providing support prevents the possibility of injury to the infant's head or neck (Figure 16-24).

## Positioning

When laying the baby down in the bassinet to sleep or rest, tell them that all healthy newborns should be laid in a supine (on their back) position. Sleeping in the supine position has been shown to decrease the risk of sudden infant death syndrome (SIDS) as compared with sleeping in the prone position. This is reinforced by the "Back to Sleep" educational campaign begun by the AAP in 1996.

Side-lying is an alternative because it has been shown to have less risk then the prone position. However, unless supported, the infant has the potential of rolling over on the stomach. If side-lying is the position of choice, the arm on the infant's down side should be placed in the forward position to minimize the potential of rolling over.

Also emphasize that even though they are cute, soft bedding, stuffed animals, and pillows are not to be put in the area in which the baby sleeps (AAP, 1996). This recommendation may not be equally accepted by all families or comply with expectations or routines of all cultures. However, it is important to present the information in an unbiased and objective manner. Keep in mind that many of these infants' grandmothers were taught just as emphatically that they should place their infants face down to sleep because that was the protocol at that time. They did it and their infants grew up to now become parents themselves so how could it be wrong? Gently inform the family of the newly understood risks and set an example by positioning the infant in a supine position (Lockridge, 1997).

## Sleep Patterns

After the initial period of reactivity, the 30 minutes after birth, newborns generally sleep for 2 to 4 hours between feedings. They move from one state to the next, deep sleep to light sleep, to fussy and then alert or crying, to drowsy to light sleep to deep sleep. In the first week of life tell parents the baby may sleep as much as 20 to 22 hours per day. However, this varies according to the uniqueness of the individual child.

Explain to the mother and other infant caretakers that sleep patterns change during the first month. The baby will also gradually sleep less and less, so that it is more common to sleep 15 to 20 hours per day. The baby will gradually start to differentiate between day and night and sleep for longer periods at night and shorter periods during the day. As early as 2 weeks of age, some babies may sleep 5 hours at a stretch during the night. The process of sleeping more during the night and less during the day may be interrupted by illness, teething, and growth spurts.

## Dressing the Baby

One of the most common questions asked by mothers is "How should I dress my baby?" Tell her to use herself as the gauge. Whatever she is wearing plus adding one layer will do nicely for the baby. She will learn if the baby is too warm, it becomes sweaty or fussy. It is too cold if it develops a bluish color in its hands or feet (Foster, Hunsberger, and Anderson, 1989).

Some cultures have specific expectations of how a baby should be dressed. If the mother is concerned about blending her desires with familial or cultural expectations, help her explore how she may be empowered to do as she wishes with her baby.

When inside the home, the baby should be kept out of drafts. If the baby is going outside it should have a covering on its head. If it is windy, it should have protection for its face because the baby may have its breath blown away and be left gasping.

## Understanding the "Talk" of the Newborn

The cry of a newborn is the most common form of communication between the baby and caregiver. Knowing how to interpret each type of cry is an essential skill ac-

quired through trial and error as the caretaker responds to the baby. Over time, the caregivers learn to differentiate among cries of hunger, tiredness, being startled, boredom, and discomfort or pain.

The acoustic qualities of a cry may reflect the condition of the baby. Initially, during the first few weeks, the cry of a newborn is usually an attempt to balance both internal and external demands. Some hypotheses have been made on the positive and negative effects of crying. This information may be helpful in educating the family on how to interpret the cry of their baby.

Some of the positive effects of crying include the benefits of maintaining homeostasis and improvement in both the respiratory and cardiac systems. It may also help enhance the development of the vocal tract and serve to bring the baby nearer to the caregiver. Parents need to be reassured that they cannot "spoil" an infant by responding to its cries. Babies are not born manipulative. When they cry, it is for a reason, but not always for a reason we can understand or even fix. However, in responding to a newborn's cry, we can start to teach it to trust that they are not alone in this world.

Some of the negative effects of crying, especially that which is prolonged, may include the adverse effects on the cardiac system because of the increase in heart rate seen with continued crying. Persistent crying can also use up calories that could have been used for growth. Unfortunately, persistent crying can also cause negative feelings on the part of the caregiver. A feeling of inadequacy or being a poor provider can take over (Pinyerd, 1994).

Assure parents that all well-cared for, normal babies cry. Possible comfort measures that may be helpful, in no specific order are:

- Feed/burp (Figure 16-25)
- Change diaper
- Check clothing for comfort/warmth
- Swaddle or wrap securely if baby enjoys the restriction
- Hold close to chest so that baby can hear heartbeat until baby falls asleep
- Rock baby
- Walk with the baby
- Offer pacifier
- Decrease environmental stimulation by turning down the lights, decreasing noise, limiting activity in the room
- Place in baby swing
- Play soothing music
- Gently massage baby's body
- Carry in soft front baby carrier
- Take on stroller ride
- Put in car seat and take for a ride

These are suggestions that have worked for others. Empower parents by assuring them that they will learn what soothes their child the best. Encourage them to interact and learn additional techniques from other parents.

The newborn cries in response to many things, not just pain. Other indicators or changes in behavior help to identify and determine if the baby is uncomfortable or in pain. Such behaviors include facial grimacing, a higher pitched cry, arching of the back, or pulling an extremity away from the painful stimuli (i.e., a needle stick) (Bell, 1995).

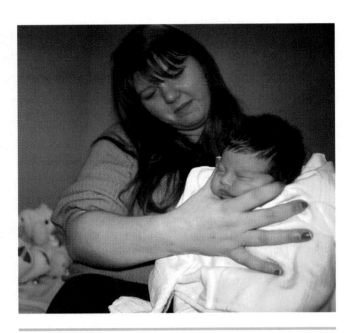

FIGURE 16-25 • Holding infant to burp. *(Courtesy of Caroline E. Brown.)*

## The Newborn's Senses

Parents have many questions about the their newborn's abilities. How much can they see? What can they smell? Can they taste? This again is an area for which different information has been given to different generations of mothers. Our understanding of newborns continues to increase. Currently we know that they come into our lives with a great many skills. Table 16-10 will assist in answering some of the questions that families will ask about how the newborn uses each of the senses. In addition, you might want to tell them of additional resources that will help educate those of other generations or increase their own spectrum of knowledge (see Table 16-10).

## Feeding the Newborn

Chapter 15 explored feeding the baby from the mother's perspective. Now the infant's needs are explored in a little greater detail. Breastfeeding is useful in developing the infants jaw development, but the process is harder work for the infant. Some infants prefer the bottle over the breast as a mechanism of delivery, because there is not as much work involved in obtaining the fluid. They may or may not care whether cow's formula, soy formula, or breast milk is coming out.

### Breast Milk

Human milk has been the food of choice that has evolved over thousands of years. It contains the elements needed for optimal growth in the proper proportions and is well tolerated and easily digested by the baby. In addition, it adjusts and changes to meet the needs of the

---

**TABLE 16-10**   *Developmental Level of Senses*

| Sense | Behavior | Observation |
|-------|----------|-------------|
| Vision | Fixate (looking at the same object with both eyes) | Can fixate for up to 10 seconds and refixates every 1-1.5 seconds |
| | Discriminate | Differentiates between shapes, sizes, colors and patterns |
| | Conjugation (use both eyes together) | Same as adult, but needs to refixate frequently |
| | Scanning (look over area to find the most pleasant object) | Prefers faces over objects<br>Prefers sharp light-dark contrasts |
| | Accommodate to distance | Unable to do this for the first month; focuses best at about 8 inches (about the distance from the elbow to the mother's face); at about 4 months, it is the same as the adult |
| Taste | | Can tell the difference between sweet and bitter; will push away with tongue when bitter is presented and will actively suck sweet tastes |
| Smell | | Present once the nares are clear of amniotic fluid; may differentiate and seek out mother's scent |
| Touch | | Present at birth; around the face is the most sensitive (i.e., rooting and sucking) |
| Hearing | Alerting (stopping to listen) | Within the first few hours after the amniotic fluid in the middle ear is absorbed, the baby may cry, startle or move its eyes to sounds |

Adapted from Foster RL, Hunsberger MM, and Anderson JJ: *Family-centered nursing care of children*, Philadelphia, 1989, WB Saunders.

infant both during the course of a day and as the infant grows. Evidence suggests that human milk also protects the infant against the development of food allergies and enhances its immune response. It is thought that human milk contains factors that influence brain growth and maturation (Wong and others, 1999) (Box 16-1).

## Cow's Milk

Whole (regular) cow's milk is unsuitable for infant nutrition because of the ratio among protein, fat, and calories. The choice for a parent who is selecting cow's milk is between the commercially prepared or evaporated milk formulas.

**Commercially prepared formulas** are used extensively in the United States. They are cow's milk that has been modified to more closely resemble the nutritional content of human milk. They are available in ready-to-use cans or bottles, a concentrated liquid that must be diluted with water, and a powered form that must be mixed with water. Cost varies from one brand to the next and by type of preparation. Encourage families to do comparative shopping.

The use of **evaporated milk formulas** is not extensive in the United States. However, it does have the advantages of being readily available in a can, needs no refrigeration until opened, is less expensive than commercial formulas, provides a softer, more digestible curd and contains more lactalbumin and a higher calcium/phosphorus ratio. However, it has low iron and vitamin C, excessive sodium and phosphorus, and poorly digested fat. To prepare for infant consumption, 13 oz of evaporated milk (not to be confused with condensed milk) are mixed with 17 oz of water and then 1 to 2 tablespoons of sugar or corn syrup are added (Wong and others, 1999).

## Goat's Milk

Some parents seek out **goat's milk** for their infants, hoping to reduce allergic milk reactions. However, infants that have had a reaction to the foreign proteins in cow's milk will also react to the foreign proteins in goat's milk. Goat's milk is unsuitable for infant nutrition because it is a poor source of iron and folic acid, and its protein content is too high for infants.

## Soy-Based Formulas

Some infants cannot drink formulas developed from a cow's milk base. They either have a milk protein sensitivity, a lactose intolerance, a lactase deficiency, or galactosemia. If not breastfed, they do well on soy protein–based formulas. Several soy formulas are now available commercially.

## Specialty Formulas

Other infants have malabsorption syndromes or other medical conditions for which special formulas or diet modifiers are given. Experts in infant nutrition must counsel mothers whose babies have very special needs. In addition, it must be determined that the recommended nutritional source is easily available and affordable.

Be aware of the mother's social and cultural situation and her medical history, and tailor feeding suggestions to fit her situation. Medical conditions in the mother that are contraindications to breastfeeding are hepatitis C virus, active tuberculosis, human immunodeficiency virus (protocol in the United States), and continuing maternal substance abuse. Also if the mother is experiencing a serious debilitating disease such as cancer or a cardiac problem, she will not have the reserves to provide for the infant. The infant cannot receive breast milk if it has **galactosemia** (lacks the enzyme to convert galactose to glucose) (Table 16-11).

---

### BOX 16-1 *Advantages of Human Milk vs. Cow's Milk Formulas*

**HUMAN MILK:**

Contains adequate (not excessive) protein; has greater quantities of certain amino acids, including cystine and taurine

Contains more lactalbumin (produces easily digested curds) than casein (produces large, hard curds)

Contains more lactose, which in the gut stimulates growth of microorganisms, which synthesize some B vitamins and produce organic acids that may retard growth of harmful bacteria

Contains more monounsaturated fatty acids, which enhance absorption of fat and calcium

Contains adequate (not excessive) minerals with exception of fluoride (low in both)

Amounts of iron and zinc are low but more readily absorbed

Contains less calcium and phosphorus but a more favorable ratio of the minerals, which prevents excessive calcium excretion

Contains adequate amounts of vitamins A, B complex, and E; vitamin C content depends on maternal intake; vitamin D is low but more readily absorbed (vitamins C, D, and E are low in cow's milk, but K is higher)

Contains growth modulators that modify growth or maturation

Offers several immunologic benefits: contains various immunoglobulins (Ig), especially IgA; macrophages, granulocytes, T- and B-cell lymphocytes, and other factors that inhibit bacterial growth

Has laxative effect

Is economic, readily available, and sanitary

Has psychologic benefits of a close bond between infant and mother during feeding

Adapted from Wong, DL: *Whaley and Wong's nursing care of infants and children*, ed 6, St Louis, 1999, Mosby.

### External Pressures

A woman may feel familial or cultural pressure to feed the baby in a specific manner. Her friends or the women in her family may voice strong opinions about what they liked or didn't like about their own choices. She may be aware of family members having a history of problems with the use of cow's milk. She may not feel comfortable with the choices she sees available to her and wish to explore alternatives. Information and empowerment to do what she feels is right will be very helpful (Children's Hospital of Philadelphia, 1998).

When a woman chooses to breastfeed, either for several weeks or for a longer term, nutritional counseling is important. This must be nutritionally sound and culturally acceptable. Often Hispanic women stay in bed for the first 3 days postpartum and may avoid eating such foods as pork, tomatoes, and chili. Their culture advocates avoiding extremes in temperature because of the belief that extreme heat can curdle the breast milk and extreme cold may decrease the flow (Mohrbacher and Stock, 1997).

### Bottle Feeding

 While in a facility, the bottle-fed infant will be given the product used there. During the preparation for discharge, help the parents determine where and how to obtain commercially prepared formula. Selecting the best nipple for the infant should also be discussed. A newborn nipple, with one or two small holes, will deliver the milk in a slow manner so that the infant will not choke as easily.

The daily intake for each baby increases with age and the amount offered to the baby changes over time. At first the baby will take about 30 to 60 cc (1 to 2 ounces) per feeding and may increase to 2 to 3 ounces by 2 weeks of age (Tsang and others, 1997). A bottle is offered every 3 to 4 hours. Assist the family in learning hunger cues. Crying or fussiness are the most common and are a good indicator that the infant is ready to eat.

 Help the person feeding the baby to get settled in a comfortable position, holding the infant before starting. Providing the newborn with nutrition is only one aspect of the feeding process. The other, equally important one, is that the baby is held closely and rocked so that it receives emotional nourishment also (Figure 16-26). Because infants need about 2 hours total time of sucking in a day, the feeding should not be rushed. If the baby has six feedings a day, that would mean that the baby should be allowed to suck for at least 20 minutes at each feeding to receive the necessary oral gratification.

An attempt to burp should be done about halfway through each feeding. This maneuver can be done by placing the infant on the shoulder or by sitting the newborn upright, supporting the jaw and head. If the baby tends to gulp or eat quickly, drawing additional air in while eating, more frequent burping may be necessary. Observe how the infant feeds and offer suggestions.

The temperature of the formula is the family's choice. Some may like to offer the formula warmed before feeding and some may offer it at room temperature. Either is acceptable. The important educational point to emphasize is that if they choose to warm it, they should do so with warm water. Microwave ovens can sometimes create hot pockets of formula in the center while the edges of the bottle still feel cool. Instruct the family that the safe way to heat formula is to warm it in a bowl of warm water a few minutes before feeding so that they may avoid scalding the baby's mouth.

### Breastfeeding

Chapter 15 provided information about the process of breastfeeding. If the mother chooses to breastfeed, the baby may have to be assisted in learning the process just as it has to learn how to bottle feed. If the baby is to receive both breast and bottle, it will learn two different sucking mechanisms in order to feed.

As the infant grows and requires additional human milk or a different proportion of nutrients, breast milk changes to meet the baby's needs. A baby will nurse as often as needed. The duration and interval varies with the age of the infant and the needs of the newborn.

The benefits of allowing the baby to nurse frequently in the early postpartum are many. Although the colostrum produced at this time is scant (a few teaspoons), it is rich in nutrients and immunities. Colostrum is a natural laxative, so allowing the baby to feed frequently helps prevent or diminish its chances of developing hyperbilirubinemia. Human breast milk is all that most infants need for the first 6 months of life (Mohrbacher and Stock, 1994).

### Determining the Adequacy of Nutrition

 The best indicator of adequate nutrition is the frequency and quality of the stool and urine in each diaper. Whether the infant is bottle fed or breastfed, the first stool passed before the final evaluation of the newborn is a thick, black or green, sticky substance called **meconium**. This stool is odorless and consists of a mixture of shed GI tract cells and amniotic fluid. The passage of the meconium stool occurs within the first 24 hours and confirms that the GI tract is patent (MacLaren, 1994; Tappero and Honeyfield, 1994).

Once fed, the GI tract begins to secrete enzymes to assist in the digestive process, and intestinal bacteria begin to colonize causing the stools to become transition stools that are green and less sticky (MacLaren, 1994). The infant will develop an elimination pattern that reflects the feeding method. Infants who are breastfed have two to five bowel movements per day, and the stool is either yellow, yellow-green, or tan. They are similar to pea soup in consistency and have little or no odor. Those infants who eat formula may have only one

*Text continued on p. 686*

## TABLE 16-11   Normal and Special Infant Formulas*

| Formula (manufacturer) | Protein source | Carbohydrate source | Fat sources | Indications for use | Comments (nutritional considerations) |
|---|---|---|---|---|---|
| **HUMAN AND COW'S MILK FORMULAS** | | | | | |
| **Human breast milk** | Mature human milk; whey/casein ratio—60:40 | Lactose | Mature human milk | For all full-term infants except those with galactosemia; may be used with low-birth-weight infants | Recommended sole form of feeding for first 5 to 6 months; nutritionally complete except for fluoride |
| **Evaporated cow's milk formulas** | Milk protein; whey/casein ratio—18:82 | Lactose, sucrose | Butterfat | For full-term infants with no special nutritional requirements; use of undiluted cow's milk after 12 months | Supplement with iron and vitamin C; A and D if not fortified; fluoride if fluoridated water is not used for formula preparation |
| **COMMERCIAL INFANT FORMULAS** | | | | | |
| **Enfamil** (Mead Johnson) | Nonfat cow's milk, demineralized whey; whey/casein ratio—60:40 | Lactose | Palm olein, soy, coconut, HOSun† oils | For full-term and premature infants with no special nutritional requirements | Available fortified with iron, 12 mg/L Also available in 24 cal/oz |
| **Improved Similac** (Ross) | Nonfat cow's milk; whey/casein ratio—48:52 | Lactose | Soy, coconut oils, and high-oleic safflower oil | For full-term and premature infants with no special nutritional requirements | Available fortified with iron, 1.8 mg/100 cal, nucleotides, 72 mg/L Also available in 24 cal/oz with iron |
| **Baby formula** (Gerber) | Nonfat cow's milk; whey/casein ratio—18:82 | Lactose | Palm olein, soy, coconut, HOSun† oils | For full-term and premature infants with no special nutritional requirements | Available fortified with iron, 12 mg/L |
| **Good Start H.A.** (Carnation) | Hydrolyzed whey | Lactose, maltodextrin | Palm olein, soy, safflower, coconut oils | For full-term infants | Manufacturer's claim regarding hypoallergenicity has been withdrawn |
| **Good Nature** (Carnation) | Nonfat cow's milk | Corn syrup solids | Palm, corn, oleic oils | For feeding older infants | Contains more protein and calcium than "starter" formulas |
| **Similac Natural Care Human Milk Fortifier** (Ross) | Nonfat cow's milk; whey protein concentrate | Hydrolyzed corn starch, lactose | MCT,‡ coconut, soy oils | For low–birth-weight infants; fed mixed with human milk or fed alternately with human milk; improves vitamin/mineral content of human milk | Protein, 2.7 g/100 cal osmolality—300 mOsm/kg water, 24 cal/oz |

*All formulas provide 20 kcal/oz except as noted in product information from the formula manufacturers. For the most current information, consult product labels or package enclosures.

†HOSun, high-oleic sunflower.

‡MCT, medium-chain triglycerides.

§L-Amino acids include L-cystine, L-tyrosine, and L-tryptophan, which are reduced in hydrolyzed, charcoal-treated casein.

||Ross Laboratories and Mead Johnson manufacture several specialty formulas for metabolic disorders for infants.

Adapted from Wong DL and others: *Whaley and Wong's nursing care of infants and children,* ed 6, St Louis, 1999, Mosby.

*Continued*

## TABLE 16-11 Normal and Special Infant Formulas* —cont'd

| Formula (manufacturer) | Protein source | Carbohydrate source | Fat sources | Indications for use | Comments (nutritional considerations) |
|---|---|---|---|---|---|
| **COMMERCIAL INFANT FORMULAS—cont'd** | | | | | |
| **Similac NeoCare with Iron** | Nonfat cow's milk, whey/ casein ratio— 50:50 | Corn syrup and lactose | MCT oils | Preterm infants, 22 cal/oz | Protein, 2.6 g/100 cal; Phosphorus, 62 mg/100 cal; Calcium, 105 mg/100 cal |
| **Enfamil Human Milk Fortifier** (Mead Johnson) | Whey protein concentrate, casein | Corn syrup solids | Trace | For low–birth-weight infants; fed mixed with human milk; increases protein, calories, calcium, phosphorus, and other nutrients | Used only as human milk fortifier, not as separate formula; one packet of powder supplies 3.5 kcal/ml and less than 0.1 g/dl fat |
| **FOR MILK PROTEIN—SENSITIVE INFANTS ("MILK ALLERGY"), LACTOSE INTOLERANCE** | | | | | |
| **Prosobee** (Mead Johnson) | Soy protein isolate | Corn syrup solids | Palm, soy, coconut, HOSun oils | With milk protein allergy, lactose intolerance, lactase deficiency, galactosemia | Hypoallergenic, zero band antigen; lactose- and sucrose-free |
| **Isomil** (Ross) | Soy protein isolate | Corn syrup, sucrose | Soy, coconut oils | With milk protein allergy, lactose intolerance, lactase deficiency, galactosemia | Hypoallergenic; lactose-free |
| **Isomil SF** (Ross) | Soy protein isolate | Hydrolyzed corn starch | Soy, coconut oils | For use during diarrhea | Lessens amount and duration of watery stools; contains fiber |
| **Lactofree** (Mead Johnson) | Milk protein isolate | Corn syrup solids | Palm olein, soy, HOSun oils | With lactose intolerance, lactase deficiency, galactosemia | Lactose-free |
| **Soyalac** (Loma Linda) | Soybean solids | Sucrose, corn syrup | Soy oil | With milk protein allergy, lactose intolerance, lactase deficiency, galactosemia | Lactose-free |
| **I-Soyalac** (Loma Linda) | Soy protein isolate | Sucrose tapioca dextrin | Soy oil | With milk protein allergy, lactose intolerance, lactase deficiency, galactosemia | Lactose- and corn-free |
| **FOR INFANTS WITH MALABSORPTION SYNDROMES, MILK ALLERGY (HYDROLYSATE FORMULAS)** | | | | | |
| **RCF** (Ross Carbohydrate Free) (Ross) | Soy protein isolate | | Soy, coconut oils | With carbohydrate intolerance | Carbohydrate is added according to amount infant will tolerate |

*All formulas provide 20 kcal/oz except as noted in product information from the formula manufacturers. For the most current information, consult product labels or package enclosures.

†HOSun, high-oleic sunflower.

‡MCT, medium-chain triglycerides.

§L-Amino acids include L-cystine, L-tyrosine, and L-tryptophan, which are reduced in hydrolyzed, charcoal-treated casein.

||Ross Laboratories and Mead Johnson manufacture several specialty formulas for metabolic disorders for infants.

## TABLE 16-11   Normal and Special Infant Formulas*—cont'd

| Formula (manufacturer) | Protein source | Carbohydrate source | Fat sources | Indications for use | Comments (nutritional considerations) |
|---|---|---|---|---|---|
| **FOR INFANTS WITH MALABSORPTION SYNDROMES, MILK ALLERGY (HYDROLYSATE FORMULAS)—cont'd** | | | | | |
| **Portagen** (Mead Johnson) | Sodium caseinate | Corn syrup solids, sucrose, lactose | MCT (coconut source), corn oil | For impaired fat absorption secondary to pancreatic insufficiency, bile acid deficiency, intestinal resection, lymphatic anomalies | Nutritionally complete |
| **Nutramigen** (Mead Johnson) | Casein hydrolysate, L-amino acids§ | Corn syrup solids, modified corn starch | Corn, soy oils | For infants and children sensitive to food proteins; use in galactosemic patients | Nutritionally complete; hypoallergenic formula; lactose- and sucrose-free |
| **Pregestimil** (Mead Johnson) | Casein hydrolysate, L-amino acids | Corn syrup solids, modified tapioca starch | MCT, soy, HOSun oils | Disaccharidase deficiencies, malabsorption syndromes, cystic fibrosis, intestinal resection | Nutritionally complete; easily digestible protein, carbohydrate, and fat; lactose- and sucrose-free |
| **Alimentum** (Ross) | Casein hydrolysate, L-amino acids | Sucrose, modified tapioca starch | MCT, oleic, soy oils | For infants and children sensitive to food proteins or with cystic fibrosis | Nutritionally complete; hypoallergenic formula; lactose-free |
| **SPECIALTY FORMULAS** | | | | | |
| **Lonalac** (Mead Johnson) | Casein | Lactose | Coconut | For children with congestive heart failure, who require reduced sodium intake | For long-term management, additional sodium must be given; supplement with vitamins C and D and iron; Na = 1 mEq/L |
| **Similac PM 60/40** (Ross) | Whey protein concentrate, sodium caseinate (60:40 ratio) | Lactose | Coconut, corn oils | For newborns predisposed to hypocalcemia and infants with impaired renal, digestive, and cardiovascular functions | Low calcium, potassium, and phosphorus; relatively low solute load; Na = 7 mEq/L; available in powder only |
| **DIET MODIFIERS** | | | | | |
| **Polycose** (Ross) | | Glucose polymers (corn syrup solids) | | Used to increase calorie intake, as in failure-to-thrive infants | Carbohydrate only; a powdered or liquid calorie supplement; powder, 23 kcal/tbsp |
| **Moducal** (Mead Johnson) | | Hydrolyzed corn starch | | Used to increase carbohydrate intake | Carbohydrate only; a powdered calorie supplement: 30 kcal/tbsp |
| **Casec** (Mead Johnson) | Calcium caseinate | | | Used to increase protein intake | Protein only; negligible fat and no carbohydrate |

*Continued*

TABLE 16-11 *Normal and Special Infant Formulas* —cont'd

| Formula (manufacturer) | Protein source | Carbohydrate source | Fat sources | Indications for use | Comments (nutritional considerations) |
|---|---|---|---|---|---|
| **DIET MODIFIERS—cont'd** | | | | | |
| **MCT Oil** (Mead Johnson) | | | 90% MCT (coconut source) | Supplement in fat malabsorption conditions | Fat only; 8.3 kcal/g; 115 kcal/tbsp |
| **FOR INFANTS WITH PHENYLKETONURIA ‖** | | | | | |
| **Lofenalac** (Mead Johnson) | Casein hydrolysate, L-amino acids | Corn syrup solids, modified tapioca starch | Corn oil | For infants and children | 111 mg phenylalanine per quart of formula (20 cal/oz); must be supplemented with other foods to provide minimal phenylalanine |
| **Phenyl-free** (Mead Johnson) | L-Amino acids | Sucrose, corn syrup solids, modified tapioca starch | Corn, coconut oils | For children over 1 year of age | Phenylalanine-free; permits increased supplementation with normal foods |
| **Phenex-1** (Ross) | L-Amino acids | Hydrolyzed corn starch | Soy, coconut, palm oils | For infants | Phenylalanine-free; fortified with L-tyrosine, L-glutamine, L-carnitine, and taurine; contains vitamins, minerals, and trace elements |
| **Phenex-2** (Ross) | L-Amino acids | Hydrolyzed corn starch | Soy, coconut, palm oils | For children and adults | Phenylalanine-free; fortified with L-tyrosine, L-glutamine, L-carnitine, and taurine; contains vitamins, minerals, and trace elements |
| **Pro-Phree** (Ross) | None | Hydrolyzed corn starch | Soy, coconut, palm oils | For infants and toddlers requiring reduced protein intake | Must be supplemented with protein; has vitamins, minerals, and trace elements |

*All formulas provide 20 kcal/oz except as noted in product information from the formula manufacturers. For the most current information, consult product labels or package enclosures.

†HOSun, high-oleic sunflower.

‡MCT, medium-chain triglycerides.

§L-Amino acids include L-cystine, L-tyrosine, and L-tryptophan, which are reduced in hydrolyzed, charcoal-treated casein.

‖Ross Laboratories and Mead Johnson manufacture several specialty formulas for metabolic disorders for infants.

stool per day, which may not be as loose or yellow in color. The baby should also have six to eight wet cloth diapers or five to six wet disposable diapers (MacLaren, 1994; Mohrbacher and Stock, 1997).

The instructions given to assess adequate nutrition should be clear and consistent. The parents should be instructed to notify their health care provider if the baby has changes from its normal bowel and voiding patterns, especially if accompanied by vomiting, abdominal distention, or irritability (MacLaren, 1994)

Weight loss of 5% to 7% from the birth weight is normal during the first few weeks of life. This is mostly

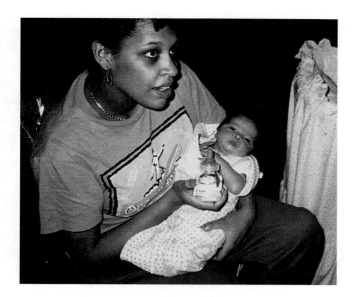

FIGURE 16-26 • Holding a bottle-fed baby. *(From Dickason EJ, Schultz MO, and Silverman BL:* Maternal-infant nursing care, *ed 3, St Louis, 1998, Mosby.)*

due to the passing of the meconium stool and loss of extra fluid from the tissues (Mohrbacher and Stock, 1994).

## The Choice of Circumcision

In addition to selecting a method of feeding, parents with male babies in the United States also must decide whether they will have their male infant circumcised. The AAP does not recommend circumcision as a routine procedure. Circumcision is not essential to a child's well-being. Parents should be given accurate information and are encouraged to discuss the benefits and risks of circumcision with their pediatrician and then make an informed decision about what is in the best interest of their child. It is legitimate for parents to consider cultural, religious, and ethnic traditions in addition to medical factors when making this decision.

Several reports about the advantages and disadvantages of circumcision have been in the popular press during the past 10 years. Parents may have some inaccurate notions about relative risk of having or not having a circumcision. The most current information that should be shared with parents includes the following:

- Although the relative risk of developing a urinary tract infection (UTI) in the first year of life is higher for baby boys who are uncircumcised, it is only a 1 percent risk. An uncircumcised male infant has at most about a 1 in 100 chance of developing a UTI, while a circumcised male has about a 1 in 1000 chance.
- Studies conclude that the risk of an uncircumcised man developing penile cancer is

more than three times greater than that of a circumcised man. However, in the United States only 9 to 10 cases of this rare disease are diagnosed per year per 1 million men. So although the risk is higher for uncircumcised men, their overall risk is extremely low.
- Circumcised men may be at a reduced risk for developing syphilis and human immunodeficiency virus (HIV) infections. However, behavioral factors are far more important in determining a man's risk of contracting sexually transmitted diseases than circumcision status.
- Circumcision is generally a safe procedure. Complications occur in 1 in 200 to 1 in 500 circumcised newborn males and are most often minor. The two most common are mild bleeding and local infection (AAP, 1999).

When parents are provided with the information about circumcision during pregnancy, they have time to think about their options and the procedure and to ask questions so that they are able to give informed consent. Information provided at prenatal classes allows the family ample time to learn about their options, explore their feelings, and make a decision.

Trying to make a decision about circumcision after delivery when the parents are in the midst of adjusting physically, mentally, and emotionally to so many changes makes careful consideration more difficult. Do not push them for a decision during the postpartum because it may make them be angry and regretful later.

Some parents are choosing not to have a son circumcised even though the father or older brother may be. Some may even express regret that they agreed to have an older child undergo the surgery. Reassure them that they made that decision based on the information they had at the time.

### Care of the Intact Penis

The intact penis should be cleaned with water during  every diaper change and bath. Teach the infant's caretakers that the foreskin is attached to the glans and not to force the foreskin back. Forceful retraction could damage the penis and cause pain, bleeding, and the possible development of scar tissue if the tissues are separated prematurely. By the time the child is 3 to 5 years old the foreskin will begin to retract. At that time they can teach the child to gently retract the foreskin during bathing.

### Male Circumcision

In the United States, 60% to 85% of parents continue to request circumcision of newborn male infants (Thureen and others, 1999). When asked an opinion by parents, providers should take a neutral position "that offers circumcision at the discretion of the parents (after informed consent) but not as part of routine medical care" (Thureen and others, 1999).

The decision for circumcision can be influenced by where someone lives, religious beliefs, or socioeconomic status. It is common for both the Islamic and Jewish faiths to perform a circumcision based on religious beliefs and cultural traditions. The Jewish custom is to perform the circumcision on the eighth day of life in a traditional ceremony called a *bris*. A trained person called a *mohel* is often brought into the home to perform the procedure (Harbinson, 1997).

Aside from religious or cultural beliefs, the decision to have a newborn circumcised is often based on personal bias. Whites in the United States tend to circumcise their males more than black or Hispanic families, supporting a preference among certain races and ethnic backgrounds (AAP, 1999) (Box 16-2).

If parents decide to circumcise their infant, it is essential that pain relief be provided. Analgesic methods include EMLA cream (a topical mixture of local anesthetics), the dorsal penile nerve block, and the subcutaneous ring block.

## BOX 16-2 Risks and Benefits of Neonatal Circumcision

**RISKS**
Complications:
Hemorrhage
Infection
Dehiscence (separation of approximated edges of skin)
Meatitis (from loss of protective foreskin)
Adhesions
Concealed penis
Urethral fistula
Meatal stenosis
Pain in unanesthetized infants (long-term consequences unknown, but short-term stresses include increased heart rate, behavior changes, prolonged crying, increased cortisol levels, and decreased blood oxygenation)

**BENEFITS**
Prevention of penile cancer and posthitis (inflammation of prepuce)
Decreased incidence of balanitis (inflammation of glans) and, possibly, urinary tract infection in infant males, as well as some sexually transmitted diseases later in life
Prevention of complications associated with later circumcision
Preservation of male's body image that is consistent with peers (in countries where procedure is common)

Adapted from Wong DL and others: *Whaley and Wong's nursing care of infants and children,* ed 6, St Louis, 1999, Mosby.

### Contraindications for Circumcision
The surgery should not be performed if one of the infant's parents has any hesitations. Delay always leaves the option open in the future, whereas, surgical removal of the foreskin cannot be undone later. Increasingly, some parents are deciding that because this surgery is unnecessary, the choice to have it performed actually belongs to the adult male the infant will become.

With regard to medical contraindications, circumcision should be delayed in preterm, sick, or unstable infants. **Anuria,** complete suppression of urine formation by the kidneys, hypospadias, epispadias, and chordee abnormalities all require further evaluation and possible correction. If the infant is at risk for herpes infection, the surgery is delayed until the cultures are negative. If the infant has a family history of bleeding disorders, the surgery also is contraindicated (Thureen and others, 1999).

### Methods of Circumcision
The principle of removal of the foreskin is the same regardless of the device used. Three types of devices currently are used in the circumcision process: the Mogen clamp, the Plastibell device, and the Gomco clamp. With the **Mogen** clamp, the **prepuce** (foreskin) is separated from the glans and then stretched out and pulled through a slit in the Mogen clamp before excision with a scapel. The penis is tightly wrapped to control bleeding. After separating the prepuce from the glans, the **Plastibell** (a small plastic ring) is inserted between the glans and the prepuce. "String is tied securing the prepuce to the Plastibell and creating stasis before excision with a scalpel. Skin remnants under the string necrose, allowing the string and Plastibell to fall off in 6 to 8 days" (Thureen and others, 1999). The use of the **Gomco** clamp also starts with the separation of the prepuce from the glans. The physician then pulls the prepuce over the metal cone-shaped device. A clamp is ap-

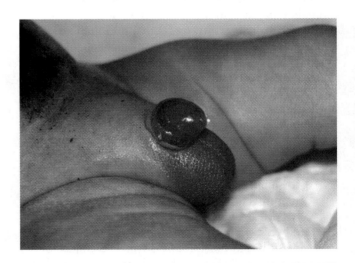

*FIGURE* 16-27 • Male penis after circumcision using Gomco clamp. (Yellow on abdomen is Betadine.) *(Courtesy of Caroline E. Brown.)*

plied around the metal cone and tightened to crush the blood vessels and provide for hemostasis. After 3 to 5 minutes, the foreskin is cut away with a scalpel (Figure 16-27).

### Pain Management

The most common time to be circumcised is in the neonatal period. The AAP recommends various types of analgesia to control pain and discomfort during the procedure and healing period. Often during the procedure, newborns exhibit pain by crying, an increased heart rate, and changes in both their blood pressure and oxygen saturation. Successful management of pain minimizes the adverse effects of this painful procedure.

A local **dorsal penile nerve block** may be administered at the base of the penis. For maximum anesthesia, there must be a wait of 5 minutes with lidocaine or 3 minutes with chloroprocaine. **Eutectic mixture of local anesthetics** (EMLA cream) provides a noninvasive form of local anesthesia. This cream consists of 2.5% lidocaine and 2.5% prilocaine. One to two g of cream is applied on the distal half of the penis and then wrapped in an occlusive dressing 60 to 80 minutes before the surgery. Once the procedure is completed, Tylenol or a glucose-dipped pacifier may be used as a method of calming (AAP, 1999).

### Complications

The most common complications are bleeding and local infection. Although both are fairly rare, early assessment for both is imperative.

Noting the first void after surgery and assessing the urine stream helps determine if meatal or meatitis stenosis occurred. Both are the results of inflammation narrowing the urinary orifice. Pain during urination and a thin stream of urine also may be indicative of these conditions.

The surgical procedure of circumcision is generally safe. However, inexperience or lack of attention may lead to serious complications such as the removal of too much or too little skin, which requires further surgery to correct the initial circumcision. The worst complication is that of penile amputation. (Harbinson, 1997).

### Nursing Responsibilities

General postoperative care includes assessment of the surgical site for bleeding during the first hour after surgery and evaluation of the first void for blood and forcefulness of stream. Unexpected amounts of bleeding and lack of urination must be reported. Bathing is not recommended for the first 24 hours.

### Care of the Circumcised Penis

Tell the parents that they may see small amounts of blood in the baby's diaper, especially during the first few diaper changes. Vaseline should be placed over the penis to prevent the head of the penis from sticking to the diaper. "If a plastic ring (Plastibell) was used for the circumcision Vaseline should not be used because it may cause the string to slip off. The Plastibell will come out as the site heals (approximately 7 to 10 days). It should not be pulled out" (Thureen and others 1999).

Have the newborn's caretaker wash the penis with clear water only as it is healing. Explain that during the healing process a light, sticky, yellow drainage will crust over the head of the penis. They should leave this alone because it is part of the healing process and will come off after the surgical site is healed. Ask the caretaker to call the child's healthcare provider if any other drainage, redness, swelling, or foul odor occurs.

## 🔷 COMMON COMPLICATIONS AND CONCERNS

An infant may encounter many common complications after delivery. These complications vary in severity and complexity. However, ongoing assessment of the newborn permits quick identification and early intervention.

### Difficulty with Feeding

Difficulty with feeding can cause a variety of complications in the newborn, most commonly dehydration and poor nutrition.

#### Breastfed Babies

Mothers who are breastfeeding for the first time may be unclear about what to expect. Home follow-up visits or telephone calls offer a perfect time to offer support, education, and early detection of potential or actual problems. Inquiring how the infant is latching on to the breast and how long each feeding is lasting provide helpful assessment information. Information about the number of voids and bowel movements are useful assessment data and reinforce to the mother how she may determine that the infant is receiving an adequate intake. Through supportive early intervention, complications such as dehydration and inadequate nutrition may be minimized or eliminated (Pascale and others, 1996).

#### Bottle-Fed Babies

Babies who are bottle fed may become dehydrated if not offered sufficient or frequent feedings. Poor nutrition may occur if formula is not used, or if the mixing of the formula is not done in the correct proportion. Bottle-fed babies are also at risk for illness and dehydration because of detrimental organisms that may be in the water used to wash bottles and nipples and prepare the formula for use.

### Orthopedic Disorders

Early identification of potential or actual orthopedic problems can help the family cope with the problem. Intrauterine ultrasounds are helpful for detection in utero. When the abnormality occurs during the first trimester, it is usually genetic in origin and is called a **malformation**. When abnormalities occur during the second or third trimester, they are classified as **deformations** (Fernbach, 1998).

### Developmental Dysplasia of the Hip

The diagnosis of **developmental dysplasia of the hip** (congenital dislocation of the hip) may be made during the initial physical examination of the newborn. The hip is manipulated with two maneuvers: the Barlow maneuver and the Ortolani maneuver. The **Barlow maneuver** assists in detecting the unstable dislocatable hip, that is in the acetabulum. The **Ortolani maneuver** assists in detecting the dislocated hip that can be repositioned into the acetabulum (Figures 16-28 and 16-29).

The diagnosis is described by the relationship between the head of the femur and the acetabulum. If the head of the femur is completely out of the acetabulum, it is considered dislocated. A partially positioned head is labeled a subluxation. An unstable hip is one the examiner may dislocate manually.

The goal of treatment is to maintain proper positioning of the head of the femur in the acetabulum as the child moves about normally. The most common treatment is to use a device called the **Pavlic harness,** which may be applied for 1 to 3 months. The device stabilizes the head of the femur in the acetabulum. This treatment modality is both inexpensive and easy for the family to learn (Fernbach, 1998).

### Brachial Plexus Injuries

Brachial plexus injuries are the most common intrapartum injuries. Such injuries manifest as an upper plexus palsy, ranging in severity from affecting the shoulder and elbow to including the function of the wrist and hand. This paralysis is the result of the force applied to the neck of the baby whose shoulder was manipulated during delivery.

The diagnosis is made through direct observation. When you visually assess a newborn, a baby with brachial plexus injuries exhibits limited movement on the affected side. The injury is often painless unless accompanied by a clavicle fracture or nerve damage. A thorough evaluation

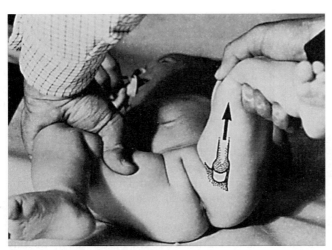
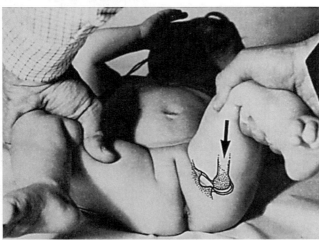

FIGURE 16-28 • Technique of Barlow maneuver. *(From Smith DW: Recognizable patterns of human deformations, Philadelphia, 1981, WB Saunders.)*

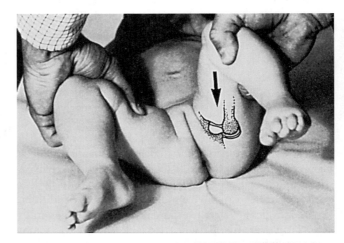
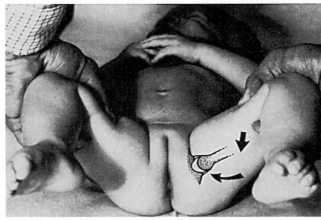

FIGURE 16-29 • Technique of the Ortolani maneuver. *(From Smith DW: Recognizable patterns of human deformations, Philadelphia, 1981, WB Saunders.)*

must be done to determine the extent of the injury and determine potential for and time frame of recovery.

Although the option of early physical therapy currently is being debated, standard treatment is that during the first 2 weeks the arm is immobilized to avoid further nerve damage. After this time, the family can be taught how to provide physical therapy to the affected area. Instructing them to do it with every diaper change is an easy way to remember to work it into a regular and frequent routine (Fernbach, 1998).

### Abnormalities of the Foot

The three most common abnormalities of the foot are metatarsus adductus, calcaneovalgus, and club foot. All three are identifiable by directly observing the foot's position, and each one varies in severity. The differential diagnosis among these three conditions is made by determining the curve of the foot when looking at it from the bottom and rear of the foot.

**Metatarsus adductus** is a forefoot abnormality. The forefoot angulates sharply inward while the heel and posterior half of the foot are normal, creating a c-shape. This is the most common congenital foot deformity and is usually a result of abnormal uterine position. It sometimes occurs with developmental dysplasia of the hip (DDH). More than 90% of these babies recover without intervention.

**Calcaneovalgus foot** is often associated with large-for-gestational-age infants (LGA). A side view of the foot reveals a check mark appearance and poor flexion, instead of the foot making an L shape. Family members exercising the foot will improve flexion. This may be done with every diaper change with good results.

**Club foot** is the most severe of these three foot abnormalities. The deformity affects the bone, muscles, and ligaments. Treatment is with manipulation and weekly casting of the affected foot for about a 2- to 3-month period. If this treatment modality is not successful, surgical intervention may be required (Fernbach, 1998).

## Hyperbilirubinemia

Hyperbilirubinemia is a common finding in the newborn and in most instances is relatively benign. **Hyperbilirubinemia** exists when an excessive level of bilirubin accumulates in the blood. **Bilirubin** is an orange bile pigment produced by the breakdown of heme and biliverdin. **Unconjugated** or indirect bilirubin is bound to albumin in blood and builds up in the body creating hyperbilirubinemia when uridyl diphosphoglucuronyl transferase (UDPGT) is insufficient to break down the bilirubin and allow it to be excreted via the bile to the intestines.

The level that is considered to be hyperbilirubinemia varies based on racial group, method of feeding, and gestational age. However, by the time a full-term infant is 14 days old it should have a normal value of less than 1 mg/dL. Levels that reach higher than 15 mg/dL place the infant at risk for serious injury. Hyperbilirubinemia can cause complications such as jaundice (yellowness of skin, sclerae, and excretions) or the more severe condition of bilirubin encephalopathy (kernicterus). Unconjugated bilirubin may be deposited in the brain cells and cause irreversible damage. Because multiple factors contribute to bilirubin neurotoxicity, knowing serum bilirubin levels alone does not predict the risk of brain injury.

### Types of Unconjugated Hyperbilirubinemia

Newborns may exhibit jaundice from one of four types of hyperbilirubinemia: hemolytic, nonhemolytic, physiologic, or breastfeeding-associated jaundice.

*Hemolytic.* **Hemolytic hyperbilirubinemia** may occur in both antibody-positive and antibody-negative situations. An antibody-positive reaction is when an ABO incompatibility occurs from the mother having type O blood and the baby being type A or B. As many as 33% of these babies will be antibody-positive, but only about 20% will develop serious jaundice. The antibody-positive reaction may also be caused when the mother is Rh-negative and the baby is Rh-positive (erythroblastosis fetalis). To prevent this difficulty, Rh-negative women are given RhoGAM immediately after a miscarriage, abortion, or delivery of an Rh-positive infant. The hemolytic condition may also be caused when other incompatibilities occur because of minor blood group antigens.

Hemolytic hyperbilirubinemia occurs in antibody-negative situations when the baby has red cell membrane defects, red cell enzyme defects, or alpha-thalassemia. These conditions have hereditary causes.

*Nonhemolytic.* The nonhemolytic hyperbilirubinemia category encompasses various causes. **Increased bilirubin production** may occur because of extensive bruising or an enclosed hemorrhage during the birth process. It also occurs when the process of bilirubin clearance is decreased. Bilirubin clearance may also decrease due to inborn errors of metabolism or hypothyroidism. Also, **unknown or multiple mechanisms** cause the condition. Where an infant lives makes a difference. Infants living at 10,000 feet or higher have more than twice the chance of developing a bilirubin level greater than or equal to 12 mg/dl than infants at 5200 feet and four times the likelihood than infants at sea level. The race of the child is a factor. A bilirubin level of greater than or equal to 12 mg/dl occurs in 4% of black newborns, 10% to 13% of white newborns, and 23% of Asian newborns. Gestational age at delivery also makes a difference. Infants born at 37 weeks of gestation are four times more likely to have a bilirubin level greater than or equal to 13 mg/dl than at 40 weeks. Bowel obstruction in an infant of any age can also lead to the development of hyperbilirubinemia.

***Physiologic.*** Many full-term newborns exhibit a bilirubin level that is less than 12 to 13 mg/dl. This **physiologic** hyperbilirubinemia may confer some biologic advantage that we currently are unaware of. We do know that bilirubin is a potent antioxidant compound even when bound to albumin. It may be important in protecting the newborn, who is deficient in most antioxidant substances such as vitamin E, catalase, and superoxide dismutase, from oxygen toxicity. Standards have been revised so that a bilirubin level of less than or equal to15 mg/dL for term, breastfed, or Asian infants who are otherwise healthy is now considered appropriate (Thureen and others, 1999).

***Breastfeeding-Associated Jaundice.*** Two syndromes exist within breastfeeding-associated jaundice: breast milk jaundice syndrome and breastfeeding or "lack of breast-milk" jaundice.

The **breast-milk jaundice syndrome** was first described in the 1960s. Full-term breastfed infants may exhibit persistent hyperbilirubinemia at a level between 10 and 30 mg/dl by 10 to 15 days after birth. If the breastfeeding continues, the hyperbilirubinemia may persist for 4 to 10 days and then gradually decline by the time the infant is 3 weeks to 3 months old. If breastfeeding is interrupted, the bilirubin level drops within 48 hours. It does not go back up when breastfeeding resumes.

**Breast-feeding jaundice** is thought to be due to low fluid intake. More breastfed infants have a high bilirubin than formula fed babies during the first days of life. If the baby is receiving inadequate time at the breast or inadequate amounts of fluid, he or she is physiologically less capable of reducing the levels of circulating bilirubin.

### Assessment of the Infant

When evaluating the infant, be aware of influencing factors. The color of the infant's skin, the time of day, and the amount of sunlight can all affect your observations. Other factors affecting the assessment include family history, the baby's age, and the possibilities of blood incompatibilities.

Traditional diagnosis of an elevated bilirubin is through a blood sample obtained from a heelstick. This test may be considered invasive and costly. An alternative is a jaundice meter that is noninvasive and less costly per unit of use. It is fairly simple to use because the meter is pressed into the infant's skin until it blanches. Using fiberoptic filaments, light is passed through the skin to the subcutaneous layer and then back to the instrument. The amount of yellow detected in the skin is evaluated. Research has found that it is as reliable as visual assessment of the infant (Ruchala, Seibold, and Stremsterfer, 1995).

### Human Immunodeficiency Virus

HIV may be vertically transmitted from an infected mother to her newborn. During the gestational period, a fetus passively acquires immunoglobulin and antibodies from the mother. Therefore the majority of the infants born to HIV-positive mothers will test positive for the HIV antibody at birth even though only 60% to 75% of the infants are not actually infected.

All infants should be handled with universal precautions, not just those born to identified HIV-positive mothers. Bathing the infant as soon as possible after birth and not giving the intramuscular injection of vitamin K until after the first bath can decrease an infant's risk of exposure. Mothers with HIV who have access to an uncontaminated water supply and formula are advised not to breastfeed their infant (Shannon, 1995).

## PREPARING FOR DISCHARGE FROM CONTINUING CARE

Whether receiving collaborative care from nurses in a hospital or home-visiting nurses, every baby and his or her caretakers are eventually discharged from care. The caretakers then become responsible for determining when and if a healthcare provider will see the infant for acute situations or periodic well-baby visits.

Parents should be given instructions about when and  how to contact a healthcare provider. A change in temperament; eating, elimination or sleeping habits; fever; or inconsolable crying means that the child should be seen immediately.

Understanding the value of well-baby visits is sometimes more difficult. When a parent has to take time out of work to take a seemingly well child to a healthcare provider and risk the child "picking up" an illness there, it is sometimes harder to be diligent about keeping the appointments. Be sure to share with the newborn's parents the long-term benefit of these ongoing evaluations and immunizations.

### Hearing Screening

The National Institutes of Health (NIH) have supported and advised universal hearing screening since 1993. Because hearing loss is the most common birth defect, early intervention holds the key to the infant's developmental success. Developmental delays may be minimized by detecting hearing loss and providing early intervention. It is suggested that all infants in a neonatal intensive care unit be screened before discharge and all other newborns be screened by 3 months of age (Sorenson, 1998).

Not all hearing loss is present or detected within the  first year. Often parents are not aware of defects or loss until about 2 years of age when developmental milestones are not achieved (i.e., speech). Education is the key. Teaching parents what to expect of their child developmentally can aid in the early detection of problems, including hearing loss or impairment (Sorenson, 1998).

## Genetic Screening

Newborn genetic screening is a requirement for all newborns before discharge. The actual inborn metabolic and inherited genetic diseases that are screened vary slightly from state to state. All states do include assessment for phenylketonuria (PKU) and congenital hypothyroidism. As with many other conditions, early assessment is the key to prevention of complications or actual disease manifestation. The best time to obtain this blood sample is within the first 48 to 72 hours of life. If the baby requires a blood transfusion or dialysis, the sample should be obtained before that procedure regardless of age. Any infant who is discharged at 24 hours of age should have a repeat assessment for PKU and congenital hypothyroidism as recommended by the AAP.

Awareness of state program requirements is the responsibility of the entire health care team. Educating the family about the tests provides an opportunity to obtain a more complete family history and assess the potential for familial transmission. Further evaluation and follow-up may be necessary as any actual or presumed positive test is repeated. Understanding the early signs and symptoms of the diseases are imperative so that prompt treatment may be obtained (Wallman, 1998).

 **SUMMARY**

The birth of a baby is exciting and challenging to the family it enters. We have the unique opportunity to influence the adaptation of the newborn within the care unit. Parenting preparation with the newborn fosters a relationship that may empower all members of the new family unit. Believe that each encounter presents the opportunity to advance understanding and support within caring networks of families and friends.

---

## Care Plan · The Infant Post-Circumcision

**NURSING DIAGNOSIS  Pain** related to trauma of surgical incision and irritation from diaper or urine
**GOALS/OUTCOMES**  Pain will be minimized *(See "Evaluation Parameters")*

**NOC Suggested Outcomes**
- Pain: Disruptive Effects (2101)
- Pain Level (2102)

**NIC Priority Interventions**
- Pain Management (1400)

**Nursing Activities and Rationale**
- Assess for signs of pain (e.g., crying, wakefulness, poor feeding). *The foreskin contains many nerve endings. Although there is controversy about the infant's pain experience, they do react to painful stimuli and, of course, cannot verbalize their pain. Acute pain should subside within an hour; however, some behavior changes may be seen for up to 24 hours.*
- Apply petroleum jelly and gauze dressing to the glans immediately after the procedure and at each diaper change for the first 24 hours. *Protects the area from irritation by urine and keeps diaper from sticking to the area.*
- Apply diapers loosely and change frequently *to keep the diaper from rubbing affected area and prevent burning and irritation from urine and stool.*
- Remove infant from restraints immediately after the procedure. *Being unable to move increases the infant's anxiety and therefore increases pain.*
- Wrap and cuddle infant after releasing restraints. Speak in a soft, calm voice. Give infant to parents to hold and comfort him. *Tactile stimuli provide distraction from pain. Cuddling promotes comfort.*
- Feed the infant. *Feeding provides opportunity for sucking, which may be comforting and promote relaxation.*
- Position infant on his side, not on abdomen. *Prevents pressure on and irritation to penis.*
- Cleanse area with clear water; avoid use of soap; protect from alcohol when cleansing umbilicus. *Soap and alcohol cause burning and irritation to the unhealed tissue.*

**Evaluation Parameters**
- Is consolable after crying
- Maintains normal feeding patterns
- Maintains normal sleeping pattern
- Demonstrates minimal restlessness and muscle tension

*Continued*

694   UNIT 3   Care and Support During Childbearing

## Care Plan · The Infant Post-Circumcision—cont'd

**NURSING DIAGNOSIS** **Parental Knowledge Deficit regarding care of circumcision** related to lack of previous experience or information

**GOALS/OUTCOMES** Parents demonstrate knowledge of care of the circumcised penis and knowledge of potential complications *(See "Evaluation Parameters")*

**NOC Suggested Outcomes**
- Knowledge: Infection Control (1807)
- Knowledge: Treatment Regimen (1813)

**NIC Priority Interventions**
- Teaching: Individual (5606)
- Teaching: Procedure/Treatment (5618)

**Nursing Activities and Rationale**
- Assess parents' level of knowledge related to circumcision care and complications *to establish database from which to individualize teaching.*
- Demonstrate procedure for dressing change, diaper change, cleansing the penis, and positioning the infant; have parents return demonstration. *Hands-on experience is the best way to learn psychomotor skills. Supervised practice increases the parents' comfort with the procedures and reassures them that they will not harm the baby.*
- Teach parents the signs of complications (i.e., bleeding, infection, and difficulty voiding) *to foster prompt reporting and immediate treatment.*
- If plastic bell procedure is used, teach parents to observe for displacement or failure of the plastic bell to fall off in 7 to 10 days *to foster prompt reporting and immediate treatment.*
- Teach parents that a yellowish exudate will form over the site, that it is normal and should not be removed *to help parents discriminate between normal healing and purulent drainage.*
- Teach parents comfort measures (see "Pain" diagnosis).
- Describe rationale for treatment regimen *to promote understanding and retention of information.*

**Evaluation Parameters**
- Parents demonstrate correct technique for dressing and diaper changes
- Parents position baby on back or side, not on abdomen
- Parents verbalize signs of infection
- Parents verbalize signs of excessive bleeding

**NURSING DIAGNOSIS** **Risk for Injury: Hemorrhage** related to deficient clotting factors at birth

**GOALS/OUTCOMES** Hemorrhage will not occur *(See "Evaluation Parameters")*

**NOC Suggested Outcomes**
- Coagulation Status (0409)

**NIC Priority Interventions**
- Bleeding Precautions (4010)
- Surveillance (6650)

**Nursing Activities and Rationale**
- Assess surgical site every 15 minutes during the first hour after surgery and then hourly for 12 hours.
- Report continued oozing or failure to form clot. *Slight bleeding and oozing is normal; saturated dressing or persistent bleeding requires treatment (e.g., Gelfoam or sutures) and may indicate a clotting disorder.*
- Cover site with petrolatum and gauze dressing (petroleum jelly should not be used with a Plastibell). *Keeps dried blood from adhering to the diaper and pulling the clot loose when diaper is removed.*
- If dressing or diaper stick to the site, soak with clear warm, water before attempting to remove it. *This prevents pulling the clot loose, causing subsequent bleeding.*
- If bleeding is more than oozing, use a sterile gauze pad to apply gentle pressure to the bleeding site *to physically prevent bleeding until clot can form.*
- If bleeding is persistent, Gelfoam or epinephrine may be applied (per medical order) to the bleeding area *to promote local platelet adhesion and clotting.*

**Evaluation Parameters**
- Clot will form at surgical site within 2 hours.
- Bleeding will be limited to a few drops on the dressing during the first 2 hours; none thereafter.
- Vital signs (i.e., pulse and respirations) are within normal limits.

## Care Plan · The Infant Post-Circumcision—cont'd

NURSING DIAGNOSIS   **Risk for Infection** related to break in primary defense (skin) secondary to invasive procedure
GOALS/OUTCOMES   Surgical site will heal in a timely manner without infection (*See "Evaluation Parameters"*)

### NOC Suggested Outcomes
- Infection Status (0703)
- Wound Healing: Primary Intention (1102)

### NIC Priority Interventions
- Infection Control (6540)
- Infection Protection (6550)
- Surveillance (6650)
- Wound Care (3660)

### Nursing Activities and Rationale
- Observe for whitish yellow exudate around the glans. Do not remove. *Exudate is usually seen 24 to 48 hours after the procedure. It is a sign of the granulation process and will disappear spontaneously.*
- Assess penis at each diaper change for redness, edema, or purulent drainage. *Timely detection of infection allows for treatment and prevention of sepsis.*
- Take axillary temperature every 4 hours. *Unstable temperature (either high or low) may indicate infection in a newborn.*
- Cleanse penis with warm, sterile water. *Removes contaminants (e.g., feces and urine) that may harbor microorganisms.*
- Teach parents to wash hands before changing infant's diaper *to prevent transmission of infectious organisms to infant.*
- If any signs of infection occur, review platelet and white blood cell count *to help confirm or rule out presence of infection. Normal WBC count for an infant is 15,000/mm³.*
- If signs of infection occur, obtain culture of the drainage, if present, *to identify the specific pathogen and guide medical treatment.*

### Evaluation Parameters
- No signs of infection such as fever or lower than normal temperature, redness, edema, and purulent drainage.
- Healing by first intention occurs within 7 to 10 days.
- If plastic bell method is used, prepuce and bell drop off within 7 to 10 days.

NURSING DIAGNOSIS   **Altered Urinary Elimination** related to tissue inflammation and edema of meatus
GOALS/OUTCOMES   Normal elimination pattern will be maintained (*See "Evaluation Parameters"*)

### NOC Suggested Outcomes
- Urinary Elimination (0503)

### NIC Priority Interventions
- Urinary Elimination Management (0590)
- Surveillance (6650)

### Nursing Activities and Rationale
- Note and record first voiding after circumcision. *Meatal edema could cause obstruction of urine flow.*
- Assess for inadequate urine stream and for hematuria. *Trauma from the procedure may result in edema of the meatus and urethra, blocking passage of urine.*
- Diaper loosely and do not place petroleum jelly directly over the meatus *because this may block the meatus and require more effort to void.*
- If no voiding occurs within 8 hours, place warm, damp cloth over lower abdomen, *which promotes voiding by causing muscle relaxation.*

### Evaluation Parameters
- Infant will void within 6 to 8 hours after the procedure.

## CASE STUDY

The Franklin family consists of Linda, age 36, and George, age 35. They are expecting their first baby. The estimated date of delivery is July 13. George works as an accountant and Linda is an elementary school teacher. They live in the suburbs and are anxiously awaiting the arrival of their first child.

On the morning of July 12 at 3:00 AM, Linda awoke with a bloody show and a slow leak of clear

## CASE STUDY

fluid vaginally. She telephoned her nurse midwife who instructed her and George to come to the birthing center next to the hospital.

Within 2 hours from the initial phone call, the Franklins arrived at the birthing center and were admitted. Linda was 100% effaced and 1 cm dilated. Linda was mildly uncomfortable with contractions about 8 minutes apart. She was instructed to walk to promote labor. After 8 hours, cervical dilation had progressed to about 3 cm.

After another 6 hours Linda's cervix was fully dilated. After 1 hour of pushing in second stage Linda gave birth to a full-term, 9 pound 11 ounce baby boy. His Apgar scores were 9 and 9.

You are providing care to the baby boy and his family during the transitional period. Based on your knowledge of the physiologic needs of the baby during this time, what might be appropriate nursing diagnosis(es)?

- What nursing diagnoses might be appropriate with regards to Linda? With regards to George?

The Franklins will be discharged home from the birthing center after 8 hours.

- How will you begin to prepare them for taking responsibility for the baby?
- What do they need to learn about their child?
- What would you include in your discharge teaching plan for this family?

Following birth center protocol, you also will provide the Franklins with three postpartum visits at home during the first week.

- What will you continue to assess when you visit this family in their home?

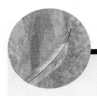

## Scenarios

1. A full-term baby girl has just been born in a labor/delivery/recovery room. This was an uncomplicated vaginal delivery. Because both parents were hot during labor, they had requested a fan for the room. With your initial assessment of the baby you note a decrease in the temperature.

- What subjective and objective data do you need before you answer?
- What nursing diagnoses could apply for the parents? For the baby?
- How will you validate these?
- What goals are necessary? How will these be prioritized?
- What nursing interventions can you do to warm the baby and prevent further heat loss?
- How will you evaluate the effectiveness of your interventions?

2. You are caring for a 2-hour-old baby boy. Tasha, the new mother, asks you to look at the hands and feet of her baby because they are a slight bluish color. She asks why that is happening.

- What subjective and objective data do you need before you answer?
- What nursing diagnoses could apply for the mother? For the baby? How will you validate these?
- What goals are necessary? How will these be prioritized?
- What nursing interventions can you offer?
- How will you evaluate the effectiveness of your interventions?

3. You are caring for a family who delivered a healthy baby boy 6 hours ago. The parents, Linda and Carol, ask you why the baby is sleeping so deeply in spite of their attempts to arouse and socialize with the newborn.

- What subjective and objective data do you need before you answer?
- What nursing diagnoses could apply for the parents? For the baby? How will you validate these?

- What goals are necessary? How will these be prioritized?
- What nursing interventions can you offer?
- How will you evaluate the effectiveness of your interventions?

---

4. During your morning assessment of an infant born the previous evening you notice that she has a very odd change in color. Half of the body is pink and the other is pale.

- What subjective and objective data do you need to further your assessment?
- What nursing diagnoses could apply for the baby? How will you validate these?
- What goals are necessary in explaining this to the mother of the baby?
- What nursing interventions are necessary?
- How will you evaluate the effectiveness of your interventions?

---

5. You are caring for a 1-day-old newborn and her family. Karen, the mother, has had a very long labor and was pushing for several hours. Both parents are now concerned with a black and blue mark on the side of the baby's head. They ask, "What's wrong with our baby? Will that go away?"

- What subjective and objective data do you need before you answer?
- What nursing diagnoses could apply for the parents? For the baby? How will you validate these?
- What goals are necessary? How will these be prioritized?
- What nursing interventions can you offer?
- How will you evaluate the effectiveness of your interventions?

---

6. You observe a new mother placing her newborn prone after completing the 12 noon feeding.

- How do you address this action and what will you teach the family?
- What subjective and objective data do you need before you act?
- What nursing diagnoses could apply for this mother? How will you validate these?
- What goals are necessary? How will these be prioritized?
- What nursing interventions can you offer?
- How will you evaluate the effectiveness of your interventions?

---

7. Preparing for discharge, the mother asks how to dress the baby to go home. The father is standing there with three blankets as instructed by his mother.

- How will you answer that question?
- What subjective and objective data do you need before you answer?
- What nursing diagnoses could apply for the parents? How will you validate these?
- What goals are necessary? How will these be prioritized?
- What nursing interventions can you offer?
- How will you evaluate the effectiveness of your interventions?

---

8. Claudia asks you how she will know if her baby is getting enough milk.

- How will you tell her to assess this?
- What subjective and objective data do you need before you answer?
- What nursing diagnoses could apply for the mother? How will you validate these?
- What goals are necessary? How will these be prioritized?
- What nursing interventions can you offer?
- How will you evaluate the effectiveness of your interventions?

## REFERENCES

American Academy of Pediatrics (AAP): *Textbook of resuscitation,* Elk Grove Village, Ill, 1994, The Academy.

American Academy of Pediatrics (AAP): Circumcision policy statement, *Pediatrics* 103(3):686-693, 1996.

American Academy of Pediatrics Task Force on Infant Positioning and SIDS (AAP): Positioning and sudden infant death syndrome (SIDS): update (RE9647). 98:1216-1218, 1996.

Ballard JL and others: New Ballard Score, expanded to include extremely premature infants, *J Pediatr* 119:417-423, 1991.

Bell G: Pain control: assessing pain in neonates, *Am J Nurs* 95(12): 15-16, 1995.

Bodurtha J: Assessment of the newborn with dysmorphic features, *Neonatal Network* 18(2):27-30, 1998.

Bruno JP: Systematic neonatal assessment and intervention, *MCN Matern Child Nurs J* 20:21-24, 1995.

The Children's Hospital of Philadelphia: Nursing standard—newborn care: breast and bottle feeding, Philadelphia, 1998, Author.

Cusson RM, Madonia JA, and Taekman JB: The effect of environment on body site temperatures in full-term neonates, *Nur Res* 46(4):202-207, 1997.

Fernbach SA: Common orthopedic problems of the neonate, *Orthoped Nurs* 33(4):583-593, 1998.

Foster RL, Hunsberger MM, and Anderson JJ: *Family-centered nursing care of children,* Philadelphia, 1989, WB Saunders.

Harbinson M: The arguments for and against circumcision, *Nurs Stand* 11(32):42-47, 1997.

Leininger M: Transcultural nursing research to transform nursing education and practice: 40 years, *Image J Nurs Schol* 29(4):341-347, 1997.

Lockridge T: Now I lay me down to sleep: SIDS and infant sleep positions, *Neonatal Network* 16(7):25-31, 1997.

MacLaren A: *Concepts and activities maternal-neonatal nursing,* Springhouse, PA, 1994, Springhouse.

Mohrbacher N and Stock J: *La Leche League International: the breastfeeding answer book,* Schaumberg, Illinois, 1997, La Leche League International.

Pascale JA and others: Breastfeeding. Dehydration, and shorter maternity stays, *Neonatal Network* 15(7):37-43, 1996.

Pinyerd B: Infant cries: Physiology and assessment, *Neonatal Network* 13(4):15-20, 1994.

Ruchala PL, Seibold L, and Stremsterfer K: Validating assessment of neonatal jaundice with transcutaneous bilirubin measurement, *Neonatal Network* 15(4):33-37, 1995.

Seidel H and others: *Mosby's guide to physical examination,* ed 4, St Louis, 1999, Mosby.

Shannon L: Clinical perspectives and current trends of HIV infection in the newborn and child, *Neonatal Network* 14(3):21-34, 1995.

Sorenson P: Universal hearing screening in the NICU: the Loma Linda University Children's Hospital Experience, *Neonatal Network* 17(7):43-47, 1998.

Tappero EP and Honeyfield ME: *Physical assessment of the newborn: a comprehensive approach to the art of physical examination,* Petaluma, Calif, 1993, NICU Ink Book Publishers.

Thureen PJ and others: *Assessment and care of the well newborn,* Philadelphia, 1999, WB Saunders.

Tsang RC and others: *Nutrition during infancy principles and practice,* ed 2, Cincinnati, 1997, Digital Educational Publishing, Inc.

Wallman C: Newborn genetic screening, *Neonatal Network* 17(3):55-60, 1998.

Wong DL and others: *Whaley and Wong's nursing care of infants and children,* ed 6, St Louis, 1999, Mosby.

# CHAPTER 17

# Care of the Woman at Risk During Pregnancy

*"I am never afraid of what I know."*

— ANNA SEWELL

*How can we help normalize a woman's pregnancy experience when she or her fetus is at risk?*

*What assistance can we offer women who enter pregnancy with preexisting conditions that place them at high risk?*

*What assistance can we offer women who develop conditions while they are pregnant that place them at high risk?*

*What interventions are necessary when a woman experiences trauma during pregnancy that places her at risk?*

*What care will a woman requiring surgery while pregnant require?*

*How may family members and friends provide assistance to a woman coping with a high-risk situation?*

When a woman has a pregnancy that places her health and well-being or that of her developing infant at risk for permanent injury or death, it is said that she is having a high-risk pregnancy. Pregnancy itself, under the best of circumstances, can be a stressful time. When medical conditions—whether preexisting or developing during pregnancy—occur, the stress and anxiety go even higher.

## COLLABORATIVE CARE STRATEGIES FOR A HIGH-RISK PREGNANCY

American society's view of birth as a joyful event, without recognizing the possibility of untoward events, leaves parents experiencing a high-risk pregnancy without a frame of reference from which to draw. Women experiencing a complicated pregnancy are faced with the physical, psychologic, social, and economic sequella imposed by the nature of treatment for their high-risk condition and the potential need for long-term home or hospital care. The literature exploring high-risk pregnancy primarily centers on the physiologic aspects of specific high-risk pregnancy conditions and the women's psychologic response to a high-risk pregnancy (Hales and Johnson, 1990; Maloni and Kasper, 1991; Mandeville and Troiano, 1992; Knupple and Drukker, 1993; Rich, 1996; Brown, 1997).

We are optimally positioned to play an important role in mediating some of the challenges facing high-risk antenatal women and their families. Intervention programs described in the literature are varied and involve some of the following components: discussion about the value of bed rest, components of childbirth education, communication tools, stress-reduction programs, and involvement of clients in their care (Hales and Johnson, 1990; Mandeville and Troiano, 1992; Rich, 1996; Brown, 1997; Gordin and Johnson, 1999).

## Education for the Woman at Risk, Her Family, and Her Support Network

### Information

Information is a critical resource for women experiencing a high-risk antenatal period (Brown, 1997). Information provides the catalyst for engaging women and their families to participate in their care and feel more satisfied with the overall experience. Families of women experiencing a high-risk antenatal period have the same informational needs as those of women with low-risk pregnancies but also need additional information about the woman's condition.

### Childbirth Preparation

Childbirth education, a vehicle for informational exchange, must be tailored to the individual needs of each woman with a high-risk condition. This type of childbirth education is best provided by a certified childbirth educator who specializes in helping women with high-risk pregnancies. Approaches for childbirth education may range from a group hospital or community-based formal class to an individual tutoring plan.

Education for the antenatal woman begins with an individual needs assessment. Learning activities are then planned considering learner readiness and implemented using the teachable moment, as well as structured timeframes. Evaluation of learning and adjustment of the teaching plan is an ongoing process. The educator must spontaneously adjust teaching plans to meet the individual needs of the woman at each teaching encounter. The teaching sessions should be documented in the woman's health care records, and any expressed concerns should be noted.

The goal of education for high-risk women is to improve their knowledge of the high-risk condition, enhance their knowledge of the birthing process and how the high-risk condition may affect their birth experience, facilitate their understanding of self-care recommendations, and increase their understanding of the ramifications of the condition for the newborn. Information on nonpharmacologic comfort strategies is appropriate for the woman and her partner because these comfort techniques can be used as the woman encounters painful antenatal procedures, as well as to reduce stress both at home and in the inpatient setting.

## EFFECT OF POTENTIAL RISKS ON THE WOMAN AND HER FAMILY

When experiencing a high-risk pregnancy, women are compelled to reorient their way of thinking about pregnancy and adjust their lifestyle. Being labeled as high-risk alters a woman's movement through the maternal psychosocial and developmental tasks of pregnancy (Rubin, 1984; Brown, 1997; Sather and Zwelling, 1998).

Women experience stress and anxiety during a low-risk or normal pregnancy. Researchers have demonstrated that perceptions of stress can be even higher in high-risk women when they believe their pregnancy is at risk for untoward outcomes (e.g., disability or death) (Kemp and Page, 1986).

A woman's self-esteem may also be negatively affected when she experiences a high-risk pregnancy (Kemp and Page, 1986). When a woman learns that there are possible problems or complications, she experiences myriad emotions and has to readjust to the notion of herself and her pregnancy (Gilbert and Harmon, 1998; Brown, 1997; Sather and Zwelling, 1998). Grief, denial, feelings of failure, self-blame, guilt, loss, increased dependence, helplessness, isolation, depression, stress, and anxiety are all possible emotional responses.

The family system is also affected when the mother is experiencing a high-risk pregnancy. Family members may become very concerned about the woman and the developing infant. If the mother is advised to reduce child care or household activities, stop employment, or must be hospitalized, the effect on the immediate and extended family system can be dramatic. The mother's responsibilities within the family system must be realigned, and when she is employed outside the home, her loss of income or health insurance could be devastating to the family. Any alteration in the mother's role in the family creates the potential for increased stress within the family and their network of friends as others take on additional responsibilities. Sometimes, the woman's concern about the family's response to these changes interferes with her desire or ability to follow the recommendations and advice offered by her health care provider.

### Effect on Prenatal Attachment

Attachment during the prenatal period is one of the maternal tasks to be accomplished. High-risk mothers exhibit patterns of prenatal attachment that are similar to those of mothers experiencing a low-risk pregnancy. And regardless of their risk status, all women develop a higher level of prenatal attachment to their unborn infants than their partners demonstrate (Kemp and Page, 1986).

### Effect on Psychosocial Adaptation to Pregnancy

A woman's ability to adapt to a high-risk pregnancy is strongly influenced by those around her—her friends, partner, family, and peers in the workplace (e.g., co-workers, colleagues, or other mothers at home). Problem-solving, coping skills, and social support networks also influence her adaptation. Individual and family coping potential involves the perception of the event, role expectations within the family system, situational support, and individual and family expectations.

A given family or individual's perception of an event influences the integration of the event into the current life context of the individual or family. For example, if the family does not believe an infant's status will be improved by alterations in maternal behavior, they will be less likely to assist in ways that would reduce the risk to the developing fetus.

Each family member's role within the family system is likely to be significantly affected by the high-risk pregnancy and affect the family's overall coping potential. For example, if the mother is the primary source of income and insurance for the family, a threat to her ability to carry out that role contributes negatively to the family's overall ability to cope. Situational support is a critical aspect of the overall coping potential, and if good situational support is present, it can strongly contribute to the overall coping potential of a family.

## Nursing Care

When working with a woman who is experiencing a high-risk situation, we assess her ongoing physical, mental, emotional, social support, and economic status. Appropriate nursing interventions promote her safety and well-being, as well of that of her baby, and empower her to participate to the degree that she desires in her care. In addition, we collaborate with her family and the other members of her health care team so that she receives the appropriate screening and medical interventions—whether she is in the hospital or at home.

### Home Care of the Woman with a High-Risk Pregnancy

The objective of perinatal home care is to monitor the effects of identified risk factors and prevent further problems from developing. Many women with at-risk conditions are now managing their own care at home with the assistance of their personal support system and periodic visits from community based nurses who specialize in both home visits and antepartal care of a woman and her family.

The change from automatic hospitalization to home care when a woman experiences difficulties during the perinatal period has occurred for a variety of reasons. First, consumer demand has forced health care organizations to develop treatment plans that are an alternative to hospitalization. Pregnant women facing prolonged hospitalizations have voiced concerns about the negative effect that separation has on family function. Second, technologies such as home uterine activity monitors and intravenous or subcutaneous infusion pumps have been developed to enable assessment and treatments to take place in the home. Collaborative self-care can be safely administered and activity restrictions may be maintained in the home setting with professional assistance and support. Finally, third party payers have demanded that the cost of maternity services be contained. Outpatient treatment and home care for many of the needs of a woman with a high-risk pregnancy are more cost-effective than hospitalization and just as effective, while also maintaining the integrity of the family unit.

The Association of Women's Health, Obstetric, and Neonatal Nurses (AWHONN) and the American Nurses Association (ANA) have developed the national standards of perinatal home care. The fifth edition of AWHONN's *Standards and Guidelines for Professional Nursing Practice in the Care of Women and Newborns* contains a section on home care of women and newborns (1998). These standards include the purpose of obstetric home care and the definition of terms used in this specialty practice. The standards also identify the woman and her family as partners in care planning and outline the nurse's responsibilities when providing this specialty care. The ANA, in conjunction with AWHONN, has also developed practice guidelines for perinatal home care. Other organizations that provide information concerning perinatal home care are the American College of Obstetricians and Gynecologists (ACOG) and the American Academy of Pediatrics (AAP).

To provide quality perinatal home care, communication and teaching skills, an understanding of individual and cultural needs of the woman, a high level of assessment skills, and the ability to work effectively with a multidisciplinary team are vital. The woman and her support system are responsible for providing the ongoing assessment and care that she requires. This assessment and care will only occur if women are partners in their care planning and understand how and when to perform certain activities. Individual and cultural beliefs must always be considered—no matter the location of care—because beliefs held across generations will not be forgotten just because the woman is instructed to do so. Periodic visits to the home enable us to assess the current status of the woman, her fetus, and her family. Assessment is holistic and includes physical, mental, emotional, and spiritual dimensions. Home visits also enable us to assess the need for additional anticipatory guidance. As the professional providing the assessments within the home, we are responsible for maintaining communication with the other members of the multidisciplinary team involved in the woman's care.

## Critical Care of the Woman with a High-Risk Pregnancy

Approximately 1% of the pregnant population requires critical care (Mabie, 1996). The notion of critical care obstetrics has triggered the development of very specialized nursing and medical care to respond to the unique needs of the critically ill perinatal woman. In some centers, a distinct critical care obstetrical care unit has emerged, while other centers continue to place critically ill pregnant women in a traditional critical or intensive care unit. A multidisciplinary approach to care is necessary regardless of where the woman is situated. The team consists of clinicians with critical care expertise and clinicians with perinatal expertise.

The challenge is to maintain a balance between pervasive use of technology and humanistic care for this population of high-risk and critically ill pregnant women. Because interfacing with technology is a reality for high-risk women, efforts must be taken to integrate technology within the conceptual framework of family-centered care. Women and families need information about the technology to allow them to make informed decisions and participate to the degree that they desire.

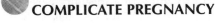

## PREVIOUS HEALTH DISORDERS THAT COMPLICATE PREGNANCY

### Cardiac Conditions

Women are reaching childbearing age with a history of cardiac disease yet are in relatively good health due to advances in surgical and medical management. Approximately 1% of pregnant women have cardiac disease.

The normal physiologic changes of pregnancy create demands on the cardiovascular system. This phenomenon places women with preexisting cardiac disease at greater risk during pregnancy. Maternal cardiac disease is associated with 25% of all cases of childbirth-associated mortality.

#### Congenital Heart Disease

*Etiology.* Women may be born with a heart condition due to a disease process in the mother, the ingestion of medication by the mother during pregnancy, or genetic factors. Multifactorial inheritance patterns contribute to 90% of congenital heart disease cases. Several maternal conditions are associated with the occurrence of congenital heart disease in offspring; diabetes mellitus has a 3% to 5% risk, systemic lupus erythematous carries a 30% risk, and maternal phenylketonuria has a 25% to 50% risk for offspring.

*Septal Defects.* **Septal defects** involve an opening in the heart between atria, ventricles, or as a congenital patency of the ductus arterosis. **Atrial septal defects (ASD)** are the most common congenital heart condition. Physi-

ologic increases in blood volume accompanying pregnancy can increase left to right shunting of blood through the ASD, increasing the overall demand on the right ventricle. Complications associated with artial septal defects include arrythmias (e.g., atrial fibrillation, atrial flutter, and superventricular tachycardia) and heart failure. Common treatment approaches include pharmacologic management, initially with digoxin and then moving to propranlol, and quinidine. Cardioversion is in less common use. Prophylactic antibiotics are often recommended to prevent bacterial endocarditis. Pregnancy and childbirth generally proceed without complications.

**Ventricular septal defects (VSD)** can yield more serious complications than ASDs. The size of the defect is a determinant of the associated complications. VSDs result in left-to-right shunting of blood in the heart. Complications include arrhythmias, congestive failure, pulmonary hypertension, and aortic regurgitation with larger defects.

**Stenosis** is the narrowing of a passage or orifice. **Pulmonic stenosis** can result in right heart failure. **Aortic stenosis** causes increased volume in the left ventricle during systole, and ventricular hypertrophy can occur.

**Ventricular hypertrophy** may be manifest clinically with a variety of symptoms including syncope, angina, congestive heart failure, and dysrhythmias. Treatment involves bed rest, digitalis, diuretics, and prophylactic heparinization. The therapeutic goal is to maintain preload (i.e., the end-diastolic stretch of the heart muscle fiber) and prevent tachycardia.

The condition called **Tetralogy of Fallot** is composed of a VSD, a displaced aorta that receives blood from both ventricles, stenosis of the pulmonic valve or artery, and right ventricular hypertrophy. This defect results in cyanotic heart disease because of right-to-left shunting. Systemic vascular resistance and venous return are decreased. This defect is most often corrected during early childhood, so women can proceed through pregnancy with good outcomes. If uncorrected, however, the risk of mortality is 15%.

**Patent ductus arteriosus (PDA)** occurs when the ductus arteriosus does not close at birth. This defect results in left to right shunting and may lead to pulmonary hypertension. PDA is most commonly identified in newborns and corrected by early childhood.

**Eisenmenger syndrome** involves a preexisting congenital septal defect with left-to-right shunting, with the development of pulmonary hypertension, resulting in bidirectional shunting. The syndrome can occur with an ASD but is more commonly seen with VSDs and PDAs, which create high pressure and flow in the heart. Mortality risk is 65% when the syndrome involves VSD, as compared with 33% with an ASD or PDA (Gabbe, Neibyl and Simpson, 1996). No surgical treatment is available; medical management centers on minimizing strain to the heart by decreasing preload and systemic vascular resistance. Termination of pregnancy is often recommended due to the high associated maternal mortality. Prophylactic heparinization may be indicated because of the increased risk of thromboembolsis.

**Ebstein anomaly** is a displacement of the tricuspid valve into the right ventricle, and an atrial septal defect may also be present. The result is an enlarged right atrium and a small left ventricle. Problems arise from the obstruction of the pulmonary value, resulting in right-to-left shunting through the defect and cyanosis. This congenital defect is associated with maternal ingestion of lithium during pregnancy.

**Marfan's syndrome** is an autosomal dominant genetic disease with a 50% recurrence rate in offspring. It is a disease of the connective tissue that is manifested in skeletal, cardiac, and ocular problems. The cardiovascular problems can include mitral valve prolapse, splenic artery aneurysms, aortic dissection, and aortic rupture. Pregnancy outcomes are related to the size of the aortic diameter, with a diameter of at least 40 mm being associated with increased maternal mortality.

### Acquired Heart Disease

*Rheumatic Fever.* **Rheumatic fever** most commonly results from inflammatory disease from a pharyngeal infection with group A streptococcus. The inflammation causes an infection in the heart. The damage is most often in the valves of the heart, with the mitral valve most commonly affected. Rheumatic fever can recur and cause more damage to the heart. Prophylaxis with antibiotics—penicillin or erythromycin—is indicated when a woman enters labor. Bacterial endocarditis is less common in pregnant woman but is associated with IV drug abuse and therefore is a potential source of acquired heart disease. This infection can lead to right-sided lesions in the heart, as well as pulmonic and tricuspid lesions.

*Mitral Valve Stenosis.* The most common sequella of rheumatic heart fever seen in pregnancy is **mitral valve stenosis**, which obstructs the blood flow from the atria to the ventricle. The obstruction decreases ventricular filling, causing a fixed cardiac output. Pulmonary edema and atrial fibrillation are two potentially life-threatening complications associated with mitral stenosis (Gabbe, Neibyl and Simpson, 1996).

*Aortic Stenosis.* Aortic stenosis occurs less frequently. The primary problem associated with **aortic stenosis,** narrowing of the aorta, is the difficulty in maintaining cardiac output. Pregnancy is generally well-tolerated, with the highest potential risk associated with the intrapartal period. Management strategies are aimed at avoiding fluctuations in the woman's cardiac output.

*Peripartum Cardiomyopathy.* **Peripartum cardiomyopathy** is the development of cardiomyopathy in the later part of pregnancy or in the early postpartum period. The cause is unclear, but several theoretic possibilities have been suggested. Autoimmune, viral, and genetic origins have been proposed (Cunningham and others,

1997). The woman may exhibit clinical signs of fatigue, dyspnea, and peripheral or pulmonary edema. Physical findings include signs of cardiac failure, jugular distention, rales, and an $S_3$ gallop. Management of peripartum cardiomyopathy involves a sodium-restricted diet, medications, and bed rest. Digitalis, diuretics, and potassium are the primary medications used.

*Myocardial Infarction.* Myocardial infarction (MI) in women of childbearing age is not common. The incidence is 1 in 10,000 pregnancies (Gabbe, Neibyl, and Simpson, 1996). MI results from ischemia within the coronary artery vessels. The common risk factors associated with the development of coronary artery disease in pregnancy are smoking, atherosclerosis, diabetes, and being over 35 years of age. Women with coronary artery disease experience prolonged chest pain accompanied by nausea, dyspnea, and diaphoresis that may or may not be associated with alterations in activity. These symptoms most commonly occur in the third trimester. Management for pregnant women is similar to that for non-gravid individuals, involving care in a coronary care unit (Box 17-1).

---

**BOX 17-1** *Maternal Cardiac Risk According to Defect*

**GROUP 1—ASSOCIATED WITH 0% TO 1% MORTALITY**
Atrial septal defect
Ventricular septal defect
Patent ductus arteriosus
Pulmonic or triscuspid disease
Fallot tetralogy, corrected
Bioprosthetic valve
Mitral stenosis, Class I and Class II

**GROUP 2—ASSOCIATED WITH 5% TO 15% MORTALITY**
Mitral stenosis, Class III and Class IV
Aortic stenosis
Aortic coarctation without valvular involvement
Fallot tetralogy, uncorrected
Previous myocardial infarction
Marfan's syndrome with a normal aorta
Mitral stenosis with atrial fibrillation

**GROUP 3—ASSOCIATED WITH 25% TO 50% MORTALITY**
Pulmonary hypertension
Aotric coarctation with valvular involvement
Marfan's syndrome with aortic involvement

Adapted from American College of Obstetricians and Gynecologists: *Cardiac disease in pregnancy,* ACOG Technical Bulletin No. 168, Washington, D.C., 1992, The College.

### Effect of Cardiac Disease on Pregnancy

Maternal cardiovascular disease affects the health of the growing fetus. The fetus's risk for morbidity and mortality is determined by the extent of disease in the mother. Specific risks can be attributed to altered oxygenation of the mother, alterations in blood flow to the uteroplacental circuit, and medications administered to the mother. Specific fetal risks include spontaneous abortion early in gestation, hypoxia, intrauterine growth restriction, prematurity, and death.

### Effect of Pregnancy on Cardiac Disease

The cardiovascular physiologic adaptations associated with pregnancy place a woman with preexisting cardiovascular disease at significantly higher risk for morbidity and mortality. The woman and her baby are at greatest risk during the twenty-eighth to thirty-second weeks of pregnancy, when blood volume is peaking and the demands on the cardiac system are the greatest.

### Clinical Presentation

Women may experience a number of subjective signs of cardiovascular disease that may be overlooked as they are very similar to the physiologic adaptations to pregnancy. The challenge is for the woman and provider to sort out and differentiate physiologic from pathologic alterations. Subjective signs of cardiovascular disease include fatigue, dyspnea, inability to breath, coughing, palpitations, chest pain, and peripheral edema (Box 17-2).

---

**BOX 17-2** *Functional Capacity Classification System*

**CLASS 1**
Normal activity causes no physical discomforts, no limitations of activity are indicated, and no symptoms of cardiac insufficiency or angina are experienced by the patient.

**CLASS 2**
Normal activity causes discomfort, dyspnea, fatigue, palpation, or angina; slight limitations of physical activity are required.

**CLASS 3**
Decreased activity is accompanied by discomfort, dyspnea, or angina; marked alterations in physical activity are required.

**CLASS 4**
Angina, dyspnea, and discomfort are experienced at rest; no physical activities can be accomplished without symptoms.

Adapted from Gilbert ES and Harmon JS: *Manual of high risk pregnancy and delivery,* ed 2, St Louis, 1998, Mosby.

---

Objective signs of cardiovascular disease include jugular vein distention, heart murmurs, tachypnea, tachycardia, abnormal lung sounds, cough, and cyanosis.

### Nursing Assessment

Assessments include particular attention to the woman's cardiovascular and pulmonary systems, as well as to the growth of the fetus.

The cardiovascular system assessment should include vital signs with particular attention to patterns over time and the maternal position (i.e., left or right lateral) while the vital signs are assessed; presence of chest pain with notation of precipitating factors, onset, duration, characteristics, and radiating qualities; auscultation of heart rate and rhythm for at least a minute and with the presence of murmurs; the inclusion of both apical and radial pulses; thromboembolic signs through general inspection and stimulation of Homan's sign; and the assessment of the presence and nature of edema. The pulmonary assessments should include auscultation for adventitious sounds; presence of a cough; presence of dyspnea; and cyanosis.

Obstetrical assessments occur more often for a woman with a cardiac condition and should include presence of premature onset of labor; presence of developing preeclampsia; and presence of hemorrhage complications. Fetal assessments should include fundal height as an indirect measure of fetal growth; fetal heart rate with attention to changes with advancing gestation and in response to fetal activity and spontaneously occurring uterine activity; and an assessment of fetal movements as an indirect measure of overall fetal oxygenation.

Psychosocial assessments are equally important in the consideration of a woman's adaptation to an at-risk pregnancy and her potential risks, as well as those of her baby. Specific assessments should determine anxiety; social support; adaptation to lifestyle changes for the pregnancy; and specific informational needs related to nutrition, exercise, and infection prevention.

### Possible Nursing Diagnoses

Nursing diagnoses for a woman dealing with pregnancy and a cardiac condition focus on her understanding of her condition and the implications it has for herself, her family, and the pregnancy. Her ability to implement the necessary self-care and follow the suggested regimen of activity will require guidance and appropriate referrals. Anxiety and disturbances within the woman's environment will also be an ongoing concern.

An example of a nursing diagnosis related to the woman is, Risk for altered health maintenance related to cardiac limitations and lack of role assistance. Because the woman's cardiac condition may decrease the flow of oxygen and nutrients to the placenta, the status of the fetus is also of concern. For the fetus, there is Risk for impaired fetal gas exchange related to the mother's cardiac condition, creating a diminished blood flow to the uterus.

## Expected Outcomes

Most women with cardiac disease are aware of their condition and have come to terms with the risks before becoming pregnant. Those who learn of the condition or develop the condition during pregnancy, however, must simultaneously go through the process of adapting to pregnancy and to a serious medical condition. The expected outcomes are that the woman will understand her condition, take medications as directed, modify her activities as necessary, and survive the pregnancy. During the pregnancy, the fetus will maintain a heart rate with a baseline between 110 and 160 bpm with normal variability and reactivity. Assessment will indicate a biophysical profile score higher than 6 and reactive nonstress tests. If it does not appear that the woman and/or baby will survive the pregnancy, the woman may be advised to terminate her pregnancy.

## Possible Interventions

Interventions offered to the woman will be both condition-specific and generalized. Care is accomplished through education of the woman and her support system, identification of fears of the woman and possible solutions to help her maintain control of care, periodic assessment of all involved systems, appropriate referrals, and anticipatory guidance in planning for potential problems and their solutions.

In general, interventions provided to a pregnant woman with cardiac disease include the following:

- Educational needs:
  Information about activity limitation.
  Information about nutritional needs and possible dietary changes (e.g., salt restricted to 1,000 to 2,000 g/day).
- Use of pharmacologic agents. "Common drugs used in cardiac disease and pregnancy are heparin, furosemide (Lasix), digitalis, beta-blockers such as propranolol (Inderal), antidysrhythmics such as quinidine, or disopyramide phosphate (Norpace). Drugs from newer classifications may be continued from the prepregnant state if stabilization of the mother has been difficult when she is taking the drugs just mentioned" (Gilbert and Harmon, 1998).
- Ongoing assessment for:
  Signs of cardiac decompensation, which may include increasing fatigue or dyspnea, tachycardia, progressive edema (particularly in lower extremities) associated with an increase in weight, rales and rhonchi, cyanosis, distention of the jugular vein, or hemoptysis.
  Understanding of condition and need for alteration in lifestyle.
  Adaptation of woman and her family to the reality of potential problems.

## Evaluation

Assess the woman's understanding of her condition and treatment plan. Have her explain how she will implement the necessary actions or restrictions. Measure the degree to which she is supported by her support network. Determine the level of anxiety being experienced by the woman and her support network.

## Summary

When a woman is experiencing a pregnancy complicated by cardiac disease, our primary goal is to work with her to reduce potential risks for complications. We are often in the best position to advocate for the woman and coordinate the multidisciplinary team that must be in place to provide her care.

# Respiratory Conditions

During pregnancy, a woman's pulmonary system is affected by hormonal changes, mechanical changes (with the progression of pregnancy), and prior respiratory conditions (e.g., asthma, cystic fibrosis, and infection). The incidence of onset of pulmonary disorders in pregnancy is low. Respiratory problems experienced during pregnancy are often the result of other systemic conditions (e.g., cardiac disease or thrombotic alterations) or from betamimetic drug therapy used in treating premature labor.

## Asthma

Asthma is a reversible hyperreactivity and bronchoconstriction of the airway to various stimuli. Asthma may complicate 0.4% to 1.3% of all pregnancies and accounts for most of the pulmonary disease seen in childbearing women (Gabbe, Neibyl, and Simpson, 1996).

The effect of pregnancy on asthma is unpredictable, with some women experiencing an improvement of respiratory symptoms and others experiencing a worsening of symptoms. Many women will continue through their pregnancies with their asthma symptoms unchanged from prepregnancy status. In women who have severe asthma predating pregnancy, their respiratory symptoms tend to worsen rather than improve. A woman's respiratory response during one pregnancy may or may not repeat in subsequent pregnancies.

The occurrence of upper respiratory infections will contribute to an exacerbation of symptoms. Lapse in medication use can also be related to the occurrence of exacerbations in the existing asthma (Gabbe, Neibyl, and Simpson, 1996).

Women experiencing asthma can present with respiratory symptoms including nonproductive cough, wheeze, chest tightness, and dyspnea. Women may complain of difficulty in catching their breath, shortness of breath, or not enough oxygen.

Respiratory assessment parameters for women with asthma should include the woman's history and subjective symptoms, followed by a comprehensive physical examination. The woman's lungs should be auscultated to assess the nature of respiration. The degree of accessory muscles used in breathing should be observed. The rate respirations and heart rate should be assessed. Significant laboratory data may be provided by a complete blood count (CBC) with differential (if an infection is suspected); blood gases (to assess maternal oxygenation); sputum culture; electrolytes; and chest radiography.

Treatment goals center around reducing the occurrence and severity of asthma attacks and optimizing maternal and fetal oxygenation. The initial focus is to identify the woman's triggers for the asthma attacks and prevent respiratory infection. If helpful, allergy desensitization is considered safe in pregnancy (Gabbe, Neybiel, and Simpson, 1996). In addition, the Centers for Disease Control (CDC) recommend that women with chronic asthma receive yearly influenza vaccinations. Because the influenza vaccine is not a live vaccine, it is considered appropriate for pregnant women (Gabbe, Neibyl, and Simpson, 1996).

Inhaled bronchodilators have become the primary pharmacologic approach for pregnant women with asthma. Albuterol and metaproterenol are the two most commonly used bronchodilators (Gabbe, Neibyl, and Simpson, 1996). Common side effects of these drugs include an increased heart rate and cardiac dysrhythmias. Glucocorticoids and antibiotics may be used if no response is seen with bronchodilators. Glucocorticoids are used to reduce the inflammatory response and mucous gland secretions.

### Cystic Fibrosis

Cystic fibrosis is an autosomal recessive condition. With this condition, the woman's respiratory system is compromised by chronic inflammation and excessive secretions that obstruct the airway. The disease is progressive, leading to multisystem involvement, respiratory failure, and death (commonly in the early 20s). The prevalence of cystic fibrosis is low in pregnant women. Progression of the disease can occur with pregnancy, although women entering pregnancy in stable health have had successful pregnancy outcomes (Gabbe, Neibyl, and Simpson, 1996). Management centers on careful assessment and support of the cardiopulmonary system, as well as nutritional counseling.

### Respiratory Infections

Respiratory infections occur more commonly in women who smoke. When a woman has a respiratory infection, it may be caused by viruses such as influenza; bacteria such as *Haemophilus, Streptococcus, Mycoplasma,* or *Chlamydia;* or tuberculosis. If a woman also has asthma or cystic fibrosis, she may experience more extensive respiratory complications (Gabbe, Neibyl, and Simpson, 1996; Gilbert and Harmon, 1998).

A woman with pneumonia will present with general malaise and respiratory symptoms. Other symptoms could include fever, chills, tachycardia, dyspnea, productive cough, hypoxemia, and chest pain, which is pleuritic in nature. Assessment may reveal bronchial breath sounds, chest dullness, decreased breath sounds, rales, or egophony. A chest radiograph may show infiltration and possible segmental or lobar consolidation. A complete blood count (CBC) may reveal leukocytosis.

With pregnant women, management usually involves hospitalization during the initial treatment period. Treatment includes IV antibiotics, adequate hydration, supplemental oxygen as needed, antipyretic medications, pain management, and respiratory therapy. Chest pain and reduced respiratory efforts can lead to **atelectasis** (a collapsed lung), a risk that is increased in the third trimester.

### Tuberculosis

Tuberculosis (TB) is an infection caused by *Mycobacterium tuberculosis* that is spread by droplets. TB is not common in the general childbearing population. Populations at risk for tuberculosis are immune compromised women and women originating from developing countries (or exposed to people from developing countries) where tuberculosis is endemic. Pregnancy does not alter the course of the disease, and the disease does not affect the outcome of the pregnancy (Gabbe, Neibyl, and Simpson, 1996; Gilbert and Harmon, 1998).

The tuberculin skin test, with purified protein derivative (PPD), is used for screening. TB is confirmed with clinical symptoms (i.e., lethergy and respiratory symptoms) and a chest radiograph. A positive PPD indicates previous exposure to TB or vaccination with Bacillus Calmette Guerin (BCG). A negative PPD indicates no exposure to TB.

The clinical presentation of a woman with tuberculosis includes general lethergy, systemic infection, and respiratory symptoms. Specific symptoms can include cough, night sweats, fever, anemia, weight loss, and changes in her chest radiograph.

Treatment during pregnancy involves supportive management and dual-agent therapy for a full 9 months. The standard regimen is isoniazid (300 mg/day) and rifampin (600 mg/day). If the woman demonstrates resistance to isoniazid, ethambutol (2.5 g/day) may be substituted. No other antituberculosis agents may be used. Women are also given Vitamin $B_6$ (pyridoxine) at 50 mg/day (Gilbert and Harmon, 1998). Significant complications of respiratory tuberculosis are renal and meningeal tuberculosis and the evolution of resistant strains.

Babies are placed at risk for infection when cared for after birth by an untreated mother.

Neonatal transmission can be as high as 50% if the pregnant woman is not treated. Management of an infected newborn involves daily medication similar to that for the mother. The uninfected infant may receive the BCG vaccine.

## Pulmonary Edema

Pulmonary edema occurs as a secondary condition in childbearing women. The cause may be attributed to cardiac disease, the use of beta-sympathomimetics (e.g., ritodrine [Yutopar]) to suppress premature labor, pregnancy hypertensive disorders, or an infection process (e.g., septic shock).

Clinical symptoms of pulmonary edema include tachycardia, dyspnea, orthopnea, hemoptypis, substernal chest pain, rales at lung bases, engorged jugular veins, $S_3$ gallops, cyanosis, and decreased or altered level of consciousness (LOC). Diagnostic tests for pulmonary edema include an EKG; chest radiograph; and laboratory assessment of electrolytes, oxygenation, and infection.

Management of pulmonary edema is an acute care process. An initial management step involves searching for the cause. Hemodynamic monitoring may be used to carefully assess a woman's hydration and fluid balance. Respiratory assistance with ventilation and oxygen therapy may be given. Pharmacologic therapy includes diuretics, digitalis, morphine, and vasodilators. The management goals are to stabilize the maternal cardiopulmonary system, thereby enhancing uteroplacental blood flow and fetal well-being.

## Effect of Respiratory Conditions on Pregnancy

By decreasing the flow of oxygen, maternal pulmonary disease can negatively influence the growing fetus. The fetus's risk for morbidity and mortality is determined by the extent of disease in the mother and the degree to which the disease alters the oxygenation of the mother. Specific fetal risks include intrauterine growth restriction, hypoxia with possible brain damage, and premature delivery.

## Effect of Pregnancy on Respiratory Conditions

Some women find that their respiratory conditions actually improve during pregnancy, while others find that the pregnancy has no effect of their condition or their condition becomes more complicated to manage.

## Clinical Presentation

Because women may experience a number of subjective signs of pulmonary disease that are very similar to physiologic adaptations to pregnancy, the challenge is for the woman and the provider to sort out and differentiate physiologic changes from pathologic alterations. Subjective signs of pulmonary disease include fatigue, dyspnea, inability to breathe, cough, and pleural chest pain. Objective signs of pulmonary disease include tachypnea, tachycardia, abnormal lung sounds, cough, clinical evidence of infection, respiratory secretions, cyanosis, and arterial blood gas valves (Tables 17-1 and 17-2).

## Nursing Assessment

Although condition-specific assessments are necessary, each should include attention to the woman's respiratory system and the growing fetus. Assessment should include vital signs with particular attention to patterns over time and maternal position; presence of chest pain with attention to precipitating factors, onset, duration, and characteristics; auscultation for adventitious sounds; presence of a cough; presence of dyspnea; nature of sputum; and presence of cyanosis.

Obstetrical assessments should focus on the condition of the fetus and the possibility of premature onset of labor. Fetal assessments include fundal height as an indirect measure of fetal growth, fetal heart rate, and the response of fetal heart rate to uterine activity and fetal movements as an indirect measure of overall fetal oxygenation.

Psychosocial assessments are important in considering a woman's adaptation to an at-risk pregnancy and the potential risks to both her health and well-being and that of her baby. Specific assessments should determine stress, fear, and anxiety levels; social support; adaptation to lifestyle changes for the pregnancy; and informational needs.

## Possible Nursing Diagnoses

Nursing diagnoses for the woman will generally focus on providing her knowledge and comfort, identifying a support system that allows her to receive the necessary treatment and rest to achieve sufficient levels of oxygenation and prevent complications. Possible diagnoses are as follows: Ineffective breathing pattern related to chronic disease (i.e., asthma, cystic fibrosis); Risk for infection related to presence of concurrent chronic disease; and Potential for fetal hypoxia related to degree and duration of maternal hypoxia.

## Expected Outcomes

Most women with respiratory disease are aware of their condition and have come to terms with the risks before becoming pregnant. Those who learn of or develop complications during pregnancy, however, must simultaneously go through the process of adapting to pregnancy and treating a serious medical condition. The

### TABLE 17-1  Arterial Blood Gas Values in Pregnant and Nonpregnant Women

|  | pH | PO$_2$ (mm Hg) | PCO$_2$ (mm Hg) |
|---|---|---|---|
| Pregnant woman | 7.4 | 100 to 105 | 30 |
| Nonpregnant woman | 7.4 | 93 | 35 to 40 |

Adapted from Gilbert ES and Harmon JS: *Manual of high risk pregnancy and delivery*, ed 2, St Louis, 1998, Mosby.

**TABLE 17-2    *Comparison of Pulmonary Values in Pregnant and Nonpregnant Women***

| Definition of terms | Nonpregnant | Pregnant | Clinical significance |
|---|---|---|---|
| Tidal volume (VT) = amount of air moved in one normal respiratory cycle | 450 ml | 600 ml | |
| Respiratory rate (RR) = number of respirations per min | 16/min | Slight increase | |
| Minute ventilation = volume of air moved per min; VT × RR | 7.2 L | 9.6 L | Increased $O_2$ available to fetus |
| Forced expiratory volume in 1 sec (FEV$_1$) | 80%-85% of vital capacity | Unchanged | Valuable to measure because there is no change |
| Peak expiratory flow rate (PEFR) | | Unchanged | Valuable to measure because there is no change |
| Forced vital capacity (FVC) = maximum amount of air that can be moved from maximum inspiration to maximum expiration | 3.5 L | Unchanged | If over 1 L, pregnancy usually tolerated well |
| Residual volume (RV) = amount of air that remains in lung at end of a maximal expiration | 1000 ml | Decreases to approx. 800 ml | Improves gas transfer from alveoli to blood |

Used with permission from Gilbert ES and Harmon JS: *Manual of high risk pregnancy and delivery,* ed 2, St Louis, 1998, Mosby.

expected outcomes are that the woman will understand her condition, be able to receive the necessary treatments, take all required medications as directed, modify her activities as necessary, and survive the pregnancy. During the pregnancy, the fetus will remain well-oxygenated, exhibiting normal growth and reactivity.

### Possible Interventions

Interventions involve the collaborative practice of nursing and medical care. Many of the specific medical interventions needed for each condition were presented when information about the condition was provided here.

In general, interventions provided to a pregnant woman with respiratory conditions include the following:

- Collaboration between pulmonary specialist and obstetrical specialist.
- Encouragement about health-promoting activities such as avoiding crowds or known sick people, using a cool mist humidifier at night to help the respiratory tract stay moist and intact, and maintaining proper hydration by drinking 8 ounces of fluid per hour.
- Information about the risks of exposure and encouragement to respond quickly to signs and symptoms of upper respiratory problems.
- Completion of ordered tests and incorporation of suggested treatment plan into the plans of the family.

- Information about monitoring for fetal movement and preterm contractions.
- Encouragement to have prenatal evaluation every 2 to 3 weeks to monitor fetal heart rate response and fetal growth.

### Evaluation

Assess the woman's understanding of her condition and treatment plan. Have her explain how she will implement the necessary actions or restrictions. Measure the degree to which she is supported by her support network. Determine the level of anxiety being experienced by the woman and her support network.

### Summary

When a pregnant woman has a respiratory condition, it can complicate the pregnancy, as well as the management of the disease. To reduce the possibility of negative outcomes due to respiratory complications, early incorporation of health-promoting activities, prompt response and assistance as necessary, and close collaboration with pulmonary specialists are required (Gilbert and Harmon, 1998).

## Conditions of the Urinary Tract

Asymptomatic bacteriuria effects 3% to 8% of pregnant women. Approximately 40% of women with bacteriuria go on to develop acute **cystitis** (inflammation of the bladder) or **pyelonephritis** (inflammation of kidney and renal pelvis). Infections of the renal system are associated with increased incidence of premature labor, premature birth, and low–birth-weight infants. The incidence of prematurity and pyelonephritis is decreased when asymptomatic bacteriuria is treated (Burrow and Ferris, 1995).

### Urinary Tract Infection and Acute Pyelonephritis

The occurrence of urinary tract infections (UTIs) in pregnant women is fairly common. Asymptotic bacteriuria occurs when there are bacteria in urine but no clinical symptoms of infection are perceived by the woman. *Escherichia coli* (*E. coli*) is the most common bacteria involved in UTIs.

Cystitis and pyelonephritis are the result of an ascending UTI. During pregnancy, pyelonephritis presents a serious threat to the mother and infant, requiring aggressive management.

**Effect of Urinary Conditions on Pregnancy.** Acute or chronic maternal renal disease can jeopardize the life of the woman and the pregnancy and influence the health of the growing fetus. The most common risk is premature labor and birth and the survival of the fetus.

**Effect of Pregnancy on Urinary Conditions.** The hormonally and mechanically mediated alterations in pregnancy predispose women to the development of renal infections in pregnancy.

**Clinical Presentation.** Women may experience a number of subjective signs of UTIs that mimic physiologic adaptations to pregnancy (e.g., as pregnancy advances, the mechanical pressure applied against the bladder reduces bladder capacity resulting in increased urination and incontinence). The challenge is for the woman and provider to sort out and differentiate physiologic from pathologic alterations.

Asymptomatic bacteriuria may be found in the urine of a woman who has no physical complaints but has a positive urine culture. When a woman experiences symptoms such as frequency of urination, burning, dysuria, and incontinence, she may have cytisis. Diagnosis is confirmed with a clean catch midstream urine specimen. A positive urinalysis culture reveals more than 100,000 colonies of bacteria per mL of urine.

Clinical symptoms associated with pyelonephritis include high fever; chills; costovertebral angle (CVA) flank tenderness; anorexia; nausea and vomiting; tachycardia; and hypotension. Physical examination will reveal suprapubic tenderness with cystitis and general malaise and flank pain with pyelonephritis. There is a high risk of premature labor associated with pyelonephritis.

**Nursing Assessment.** Condition-specific assessments include particular attention to the renal system and the prevention of premature labor. The assessment should include the presence of suprapubic or CVA pain with attention to precipitating factors, onset, duration, and characteristic of pain; amount and character of urine output; the frequency of urination; and general systemic symptoms.

Obstetrical assessments should focus on the signs and symptoms of premature labor. Fetal assessments should include fundal height as an indirect measure of fetal growth; fetal heart rate with attention to changes due to advancing gestation and in response to fetal activity and spontaneously occurring uterine activity; and fetal movements as an indirect measure of overall fetal well-being.

**Possible Nursing Diagnoses.** Nursing diagnoses for a woman dealing with pregnancy and conditions of the urinary tract will focus on her understanding of her condition and the implications it has on herself, her family, and her pregnancy. Her ability to implement the necessary self-care and follow the suggested regimen of activity will require guidance and appropriate referrals. Anxiety within the woman and her support network will also be an ongoing concern.

Examples of a nursing diagnoses related to the woman with alterations in her urinary tract are as follows: Altered urinary elimination related to urinary tract infection; Risk for urinary urge incontinence related to urethritis; Risk for fluid volume excess related to pyelonephritis; or Risk for ineffective coping related to life-threatening diagnosis. The woman's renal condition may have a negative effect on the health and growth of the fetus. There is a Risk for impaired fetal gas exchange related to the woman's UTI, renal cystitis, or pyelonephitus. There is also the Potential for inability to sustain spontaneous ventilation related to premature delivery if a term gestation is not achieved.

**Expected Outcomes.** The expected outcomes for a woman with urinary tract problems are that she will understand her condition, be able to take medications as directed, modify her activities as necessary, and survive the pregnancy. During the pregnancy, the fetus will maintain normal growth and activity with reactive nonstress tests and reach gestational maturity.

**Possible Interventions.** Treatment of urinary tract conditions are both condition-specific and generalized. Care  is accomplished through education of the woman and her support system, identification of the woman's fears and solutions to help her maintain control of her care, periodic assessment of all involved systems, appropriate referrals, and anticipatory guidance in planning for potential problems and their solutions.

Possible interventions include the following:

- Education of each woman about:
  The correct practice of perineal hygiene.
  Directions to report difficult or painful urination immediately.
  Drinking 3000 ml of fluid every 24 hours to reduce the chance of developing problems.

- Collaboration between urologist or renal specialist and obstetrical specialist.
- Antibiotic therapy:

Asymptomatic bacteriuria usually requires ampicillin for either 4 to 7 days or 7 to 10 days. Single-dose dosing schedules have been reported in the literature but have been shown to have a 20% to 30% of failure in therapy.

Cystitis usually requires ampicillin for 10 to 14 days. A test of cure reculture is done upon completion of the antibiotic therapy to document absence of bacteria. If there is continued bacterial growth, the course of antibiotics should be continued for 6 more weeks, at which time a reculture is done. If it still is positive, an antimicrobial (e.g., nitrofurantoin) may be given for the remainder of the pregnancy (Gilbert and Harmon, 1998).

Pyelonephritis requires acute care with intravenous antibiotic therapy, antipyritics, hydration, and obstetrical monitoring for premature labor. If the woman suffers acute renal failure, termination of the pregnancy may be recommended in order to save the life of the mother.

- Chronic renal disease requires the control of the frequently associated hypertension with antihypertensive drugs. The antihypertensive of choice is usually methyldopa (Aldomet) or hydralazine (Apresoline). The woman should be told to take the drug at the same time every day and warned that possible side effects are lightheadedness or extreme lethargy.
- Fluid overload is prevented through close monitoring of fluid intake and urinary output. Use of salt may be restricted. Diuretics may be given to aid in the excretion of fluids and prevent pulmonary edema, but then the woman's electrolyte balance must be closely monitored. The woman should be taught to eat bananas and citrus fruits because these are high in potassium.
- Anemia may develop due to the suppressed production of **erythropoietin** (a group of cytokines produced in the kidneys that stimulate the proliferation of red blood cells in the bone marrow). The woman may require increased intake of folic acid and iron supplementation.
- The woman and her family may have to consider terminating the pregnancy. "The effects of hypertension, loss of protein, and retention of sodium and water can create a life-threatening situation for the mother. If the fetus has little chance of surviving, the choice for terminating the pregnancy should be offered the mother" (Gilbert and Harmon, 1998).

- If the pregnancy continues, the woman will keep a daily fetal activity chart, ultrasound examinations will be done every 2 weeks from 24 weeks on to monitor the survival and growth of the baby, and stress tests will be done weekly after 26 weeks.
- Assistance in completion of ordered tests and incorporation of suggested treatment plan into the daily living activities of the woman and her family should be provided.

### Evaluation

Assess the woman's understanding of her condition and treatment plan. Have her explain how she will implement the necessary actions or restrictions. Measure the degree to which she is supported by her support network. Determine the level of anxiety that the woman and her support network are experiencing because of her condition.

### Summary

When a pregnant woman has bacteriuria, the goal of care is to prevent a symptomatic UTI and preterm labor. Prompt identification and treatment of a renal tract infection will reduce the possibility of negative outcomes for the woman or the baby (Gilbert and Harmon, 1998).

## Conditions of the Endocrine System

The two glands of the endocrine system may cause pre-existing disease in women of childbearing years and create major concern when a woman becomes pregnant. These glands are the thyroid, which may cause hyperthyroidism or hypothyroidism, and the pancreas, which may not produce enough insulin, leading to a **diabetogenic state** (causing diabetes).

### Conditions of the Thyroid

The thyroid is located in the anterior portion of the neck. The thyroid hormone controls the metabolic rate and indirectly influences growth and nutrition.

*Hyperthyroidism.* **Hyperthyroidism** is an increased production of thyroid hormone resulting in stimulation of the metabolic system. The most common cause of thyroid disease in pregnancy is Graves' disease. Toxic nodular goiter, acute thyroiditis, and hydatidiform mole can also result in thyroid disease but are less common causes.

Clinical symptoms of hyperthyroidism include fatigue, diaphoresis, heat intolerance, hyperactivity, weight loss, muscle tremors, palpitation, and tachycardia with a resting pulse rate of over 100. Laboratory values will demonstrate the stimulated state of the thyroid gland. The serum thyroxine $T_4$ is elevated, the free thyroxine index is elevated, and the level of free thyroxine is increased.

The clinical patterns associated with hyperthyroidism mimic physiologic changes occurring early in the gestational period. The woman and her health care providers are challenged with discerning the pathologic from the physiologic changes the woman is experiencing. Pregnancy is physiologically a hypermetabolic state with elevation in heart rate, basal metabolic rate, and heat intolerance as expected findings. However, women with elevated thyroid hormone levels and elevated HCG levels also experience an increased occurrence of hyperemesis (Gabbe, Neibyl, and Simpson, 1996).

Assessment parameters include vital signs, with attention to patterns and associated factors that may influence a woman's vital signs; neck examination for the size of the thyroid gland; eye examination for pathologic finding associated with hyperthyroidism including photosensitivity, tearing, and exophthalmos; deep tendon reflexes (with hyperthyroidism, hyperreactivity is present; with hypothyroidism, decreased reactivity is present).

Assessment for the development of thyroid storm is another important consideration for women with hyperthyroidism. **Thyroid storm,** caused by an excess of thyroid hormone, is an abrupt onset of fever, sweating, tachycardia, pulmonary edema or congestive heart failure, tremulousness, and restlessness. It is an uncommon but life-threatening complication that is associated with a 25% mortality rate. A thyroid storm may occur more frequently in women with undiagnosed thyroid problems or who are not using thyroid medications as directed. Clinical symptoms include a fever over 103° F, tachycardia, dehydration, and central nervous system agitation or stimulation. Treatment of thyroid storm includes giving propranolol to reduce the catecholamine effects triggered by the thyroid hormone excess; fluids; antipyretics; antithyroid medicine; intravenous sodium iodine; and possibly glucocorticoids.

***Hypothyroidism.*** Hypothyroidism is a lack of thyroid hormone and is less commonly seen in childbearing women because many women with hypothyroidism are infertile. Hypothyroidism is usually secondary to Hashimoto's disease but is also associated with thyroid neoplasm or surgery.

Clinical symptoms of hypothyroidism include weight gain; lethargy; weakness; irritability; cold intolerance; constipation; delayed deep tendon reflexes; and dry brittle skin, nails, and hair. Laboratory findings reveal reduced total thyroxine and free thyroxine and elevated thyroid stimulating hormone levels.

## Expected Outcomes

Therapeutic goals for management of hyperthyroidism and hypothyroidism are to establish and maintain stable thyroid hormone function and prevent premature labor.

## Possible Interventions

Stabilization of thyroid hormone function is generally accomplished with medical pharmacologic approaches.

***Hyperthyroidism.*** Stabilization of the thyroid hormone function is generally accomplished with medical or pharmacologic approaches.

- For hyperthyroidism, the medication of choice is an antithyroid drug, propylthiouracil (PTU), although this drug crosses the placenta and can result in fetal hypothyroidism. An alternative may be the surgical removal of the thyroid, but this is not an initial management approach.
- For hypothyroidism, management is aimed at replacing the thyroid hormone with a thyroid medication to achieve a euthyroid level. The drug commonly used is synthroid. The woman must be aware of signs of toxicity when she is given thyroid-replacement therapy. Signs and symptoms include palpitation, weight loss, tachycardia, and insomnia.

### Conditions of the Pancreas

The pancreas regulates carbohydrate metabolism by secreting the hormones insulin and glucagon. **Diabetes mellitus** is characterized by an alteration in carbohydrate metabolism due to reduced or absent insulin production by the beta cells of the islets of Langerhans of the pancreas. This altered pancreatic function can be due to genetic factors, acquired factors, or medications. Insulin regulates blood glucose levels by controlling the transport of glucose across cell membranes. Insulin facilitates fat formation and regulates glucose and protein storage. When insulin is lacking or a resistance to insulin is present, glucose cannot be stored in the tissues and hyperglycemia—increased glucose levels in the bloodstream—results. When the body cannot use glucose for energy, it begins to use fat and protein as an energy source. The metabolites of fat and protein are ketones and fatty acids, resulting in ketoacidosis and acetonuria.

### Effect of Pregnancy if a Woman Has Diabetes

Physiologic adaptations occurring within the woman's body facilitate nourishment of the growing fetus and the woman's own increased metabolic demands. These adaptations can create a diabetic state in a woman with no history of diabetes. Insulin production varies with the progression of pregnancy. During the first part of pregnancy, increases in estrogen and progesterone cause pancreatic beta cell hyperplasia, resulting in hyperinsulinemia. The increased insulin available allows for an increase in the uptake and storage of glucose. An end result of these changes is the increased incidence of hypoglycemia.

The later part of pregnancy is accompanied by increased cortisol secretion and production of prolactin and human placental lactogen (HPL). The change in these hormones is responsible for insulin resistance, which results in impaired glucose utilization. The alterations associated with pregnancy also create an accelerated starvation state when fasting.

## Effects of Diabetes on Pregnancy

The rate of maternal morbidity from preexisting diabetes is influenced by her ability to achieve **euglycemia** (a normal concentration of glucose in the blood) and the degree of preexisting vascular involvement. Women who have preexisting diabetes and become pregnant should meet with a team of high-risk perinatal care providers, including a perinatalogist and an internal medicine or endocrine specialist prior to conception. Glucose control, when achieved preconceptually and maintained during the first trimester, is associated with a reduced incidence of fetal anomalies (Moore, 1994).

A woman who incorporates management of the disease into her life and has the necessary support systems to facilitate her ability to comply with medical regimens can usually maintain good control throughout pregnancy. Because of the close monitoring, many women with diabetes are in better control when pregnant than when not pregnant. The diabetic condition of the woman does not deteriorate because of the pregnancy itself.

A pregnant woman with preexisting diabetes is at increased risk for complications such as hypoglycemia, UTIs, hypertension, polyhydraminos, ketoacidosis, and progression of retinopathy. A woman with gestational diabetes can be asymptomatic or may report recurrent candida vaginal infections, frequency of urination, excessive thirst, weight loss, hunger, or visual changes.

Morbidity and mortality of the fetus or newborn can be significantly influenced by maternal glucose control during the pregnancy. Specific risks to fetal and newborn health include **macrosomia** (i.e., an abnormally large body) and possible birth trauma, congenital anomalies,

## TABLE 17-3    *White Classification System of Diabetes in Pregnancy, Modified*

The White classification system uses the duration of diabetes and the presence of disease-associated complications to group women. This system places women in one of the following classes: B, C, D, E, F, R, RF, H, or T.

| | Age at onset | Duration of disease | Vasculopathy | Treatment |
|---|---|---|---|---|
| Class A₁ Gestational Diabetes (GDM) Abnormal glucose tolerance test (GTT) without other symptoms; fasting glucose normal | Any | Variable | None | Diet control |
| Class A₂ Gestational Diabetes Abnormal glucose tolerance test (GTT); fasting glucose elevated | Any | Variable | None | Diet and insulin |
| **PREEXISTING DIABETES (PRIOR TO PREGNANCY)** | | | | |
| Class B | At least 20 years | Under 10 years | None | Diet and insulin |
| Class C | From 10 to 19 years | From 10 to 19 years | None | Diet and insulin |
| Class D | Under 10 years | Over 20 years | Benign | Diet and insulin |
| Class E | Any | Variable | Pelvic vascular disease | Diet and insulin |
| Class F | Any | Variable | Nephropathy | Diet and insulin |
| Class R | Any | Variable | Proliferative retinopathy | Diet and insulin |
| Class RF | Any | Variable | Nephropathy and retinopathy | Diet and insulin |
| Class H | Any | Variable | Artherosclerotic heart disease | Diet and insulin |
| Class T | Any | Variable | After renal transplant | Diet and insulin |

Data from American College of Obstetricians and Gynecologists: *Management of diabetes mellitus in pregnancy,* ACOG Technical Bulletin No. 92, Washington, DC, 1986, ACOG Resource Center.

intrauterine fetal death (IUFD), respiratory distress syndrome (RDS) (in newborns), hypoglycemia, hypocalcemia, hyperbilirubinemia, polycythemia, intrauterine growth restriction (IUGR), prematurity, and asphyxia (Table 17-4).

## Classification of Diabetes Mellitus in Pregnancy

Classification of pregnant women with diabetes can be accomplished using either the White classification system or the National Diabetes Data Group system (NDDG) (Gabbe, Neibyl, and Simpson, 1996). The White Classification System is in Table 17-3. The NDDG of the National Institutes of Health classification system bases its definition on pathophysiology of the disease. The NDDG system gives the following three types: Type I is insulin dependent (IDDM); Type II is non-insulin dependent (NIDDM); and Type III is gestational diabetes (GDM).

## Screening for Altered Carbohydrate Metabolism

It may be learned that a woman has gestational diabetes through routine screening of urine or blood or through a more sensitive screening tool, the Glucola screen. Screening can be either universal—for all pregnant prenatal clients—or selective, based on risk factors (AAP and ACOG, 1997). Selective screening for diabetes may be based on the presence of the following risk factors: family history of diabetes, a previous infant with macrosomia (i.e., birth weight over 4000 g), congenital anomaly, an intrauterine fetal death, maternal hypertension, glycosuria, maternal age over 30 years, or a previous pregnancy with gestational diabetes.

***Initial Screening.*** Initial screening involves a Glucola screen between 24 to 28 weeks of gestation. To perform the test, 50 g of a cola-tasting beverage are given to the woman. Some researchers have found that giving the woman 18 jelly beans is an acceptable alternative to the Glucola (Boyd, Ross, and Sherman, 1995). One hour later the woman's blood sugar is tested. The 1-hour Glucola test is considered negative or within normal limits when the woman's blood sugar is less than 140 mg/dl. If the 1-hour glucose test reveals a glucose level of 140 mg/dl or greater, the screening is considered positive and a 3-hour glucose tolerance test (GTT) is indicated. It has been suggested that there is a normal variation in blood sugars between races and that the threshold indicating the need for further screening should be adjusted according to race (i.e., African-Americans, 130 mg/dl; Fillipinos, 145 mg/dl; and Asians, 150 mg/dl) (Nahum and Huffaker, 1993) (Boxes 17-3 and 17-4 and Table 17-5).

The diagnosis of gestational diabetes is made if two of the three glucose levels of a GTT are abnormal. If only one value is positive, the GTT will be repeated at 32 to 34 weeks of gestation. Women diagnosed with diabetes should be cared for by an interdisciplinary team including a perinatalogist, endocrinologist, nutritionist, and a diabetic nurse educator.

---

**TABLE 17-4   *Trimester Manifestations and Consequences of Diabetes***

|  | Insulin requirements | Blood glucose alterations | Complicating factors |
|---|---|---|---|
| First trimester | Reduced, related to inhibition of anterior pituitary hormones<br>Developing embryo is glucose drain<br>Decreased maternal caloric intake<br>Increased insulin production | Frequent low blood glucose levels leading to increased numbers of hypoglycemia episodes, increased incidence of starvation, ketosis, and ketonemia | Loss of appetite, nausea, or vomiting common in any early pregnancy<br>Recovery from an acidemic state is more difficult because of insulin antagonists |
| Second trimester | Increase related to placental hormones (cortisol, insulinase) and their antiinsulin properties | Hyperglycemia leading to ketonemia, aminoacidemia | Exaggerated ketone response to caloric restriction<br>Decreased renal threshold from increased blood flow makes urine sugar levels meaningless<br>Body produces lactose or milk sugar, which further increases urinary sugar |
| Third trimester | Marked increase related to increased placental hormones but level off after 36 weeks of gestation | Hyperglycemia leading to ketonemia, acidemia | Same |

Used with permission from Gilbert ES and Harmon JS: *Manual of high risk pregnancy and delivery,* ed 2, St Louis, 1998, Mosby.

## BOX 17-3  *3-hour Glucose Tolerance Test (GTT) — Instructions for the Woman*

Instructions to the woman before the test:
- For three days before the GTT, eat a diet of at least 150 mg of carbohydrates each day.
- After midnight the day before the test:
  —Do not eat.
  —Avoid all drugs that affect blood glucose levels. (This directive may require consultation between providers if the woman is on a regular regimen of medication for a chronic condition.)
  —Refrain from smoking and strenuous exercise.
- Explanation of the test procedures:
  —The test will take at least 3 hours (and up to 5 hours), so plan on being at the facility for 4 to 6 hours.
  —Before the test begins, a sample of blood will be taken to determine your fasting blood sugar.
  —You will be given a liquid to drink that is very sweet. (If you are unable to swallow the fluid, an IV will be inserted to administer the glucose and obtain the blood samples.)
  —After that, blood and urine samples will be collected at 30 minutes, 1 hour, 2 hours, and 3 hours. In some cases, the test will be extended and samples will be collected at 4 hours and 5 hours after the glucose was given.

Instructions during the test:
- Avoid strenuous exercise between the collection of urine or blood samples.
- Do not smoke during the test.
- If the second-voided specimen is used at the beginning of the test, you must void a half-hour before the required specimen is due to be collected.
- You will be given one glass of water to drink each time a urine sample is collected so that you have adequate urine output for the remaining specimens.

Instructions after the test is completed:
- Resume your usual diet, medications, and activities.

From Jaffe MS and McVan BF: *Davis's laboratory and diagnostic handbook,* Philadelphia, 1997, F.A. Davis.

## BOX 17-4  *3-hour Glucose Tolerance Test (GTT) — Implementation*

### GLUCOSE TOLERANCE TEST
- The glucose load may be provided either orally (OGTT) or intravenously (IVGTT).
- Results may be determined by collecting blood samples only or blood and urine samples. Urine samples should remain negative through out the test.

### ASSESSMENT
- Determine if the woman understands the reason for the test and how the procedure will be conducted.
- Determine if the woman has been able to comply with the instructions of eating at least 150 g of carbohydrates for the previous 3 days.
- Determine that the woman has had nothing to eat since midnight.
- Determine what medications she may have taken since midnight.
- Determine if she has smoked or participated in vigorous exercise since midnight.

### POSSIBLE NURSING DIAGNOSES
- Anxiety related to having blood drawn.
- Anxiety related to potential for learning of threat to heath status.
- Risk for impaired adjustment to threat to self-concept as being a healthy person.

### IMPLEMENTATION
- Using universal precautions, perform venipuncture and collect 7 ml of blood in a gray-top tube for determination of fasting blood sugar.
- If the woman is to receive IVGTT, insert the intravenous device that will be used to administer the glucose and to collect the blood samples.
- If a second void specimen is ordered, have the woman void and discard the sample. One half-hour later, have her void again and keep this sample.
- Administer the glucose load.
  —For an OGTT, the woman will receive 1.75 g/kg body weight or 75 to 100 g of carbohydrate in 15 to 20 minutes.
  —For an IVGTT, the woman will receive 50% glucose calculated according to body weight in 5 minutes.
- Be sure that the woman is comfortable and has something to occupy her time.
- Obtain blood and urine samples at 30 minutes, 1 hour, 2 hours, and 3 hours.
- Answer any questions as they arise.
- After the completion of the test, before leaving, be sure the woman knows:
  —How to care for the venipuncture site.
  —To resume her usual diet, medications, and activities.
  —How and when she will receive the results of her test.

Gilbert ES and Harmon JS: *Manual of high risk pregnancy and delivery,* ed 2, St Louis, 1998, Mosby; Jaffe MS and McVan BF: *Davis's laboratory and diagnostic handbook,* Philadelphia, 1997, F.A. Davis.

| TABLE 17-5 | *Normal Serum Values of 3-Hour Glucose Tolerance Test in Pregnancy* |
| --- | --- |
| **Time of measurement** | **Blood glucose (mg/dl)** |
| Fasting | <105 |
| 1 hour | <190 |
| 2 hours | <165 |
| 3 hours | <145 |

From The Expert Committee on the Diagnosis and Classification of Diabetes Mellitus: Report of the expert committee on the diagnosis and classification of diabetes mellitus, *Diabetes Care* 20(7):183-197, 1997.

### Nursing Assessment

The woman with diabetes requires ongoing assessment to evaluate her knowledge and ability to achieve glucose control and her obstetrical status. Determine her understanding of the signs and symptoms of hypoglycemia and hyperglycemia. Glucose control is assessed through self-glucose monitoring, urine testing for glucose and ketones, and laboratory testing.

Some endocrinologists screen for adequacy of control every 2 or 3 months using the blood test **glycosylated hemoglobin** (Hb $A_{1c}$) to determine the level of hemoglobin A that has become "sugar coated." The test reflects the adequacy of glucose control during the previous 4 to 6 weeks. If the Hb $A_{1c}$ levels are above 7, there is an increased risk of congenital anomalies in the fetus.

Obstetrical assessments include observations for signs of pregnancy-induced hypertensive disorders, renal infections, premature onset of labor, and fetal well-being. Assessments of fetal well-being typically begin at 28 weeks of gestation. Maternal assessment of fetal movement is used as a first line screening approach for women with at-risk pregnancies. Women become familiar with their infant's patterns of activity and, when they detect deviations or reductions in the fetal activity patterns, can inform their health care providers so that follow-up testing will be initiated.

The non-stress test is a preferred antenatal surveillance technique for women with diabetes. If the non-stress test is nonreactive (reflecting concern for fetal well-being), additional testing is indicated. A complete biophysical profile or the contraction stress test can provide additional information about fetal well-being. Serial ultrasound examinations may be used to monitor fetal growth, particularly when macrosomia is suspected.

### Possible Nursing Diagnoses

Whether a woman enters pregnancy with problems with her thyroid or her pancreas, the lack of the necessary hormones places the growth and development of her fetus at risk. Whether a woman with diabetes becomes pregnant or develops gestational diabetes while pregnant, both situations present a risk to the woman and her developing fetus. Nursing diagnoses focus on the understanding the woman has of her specific condition and the ways her health must be monitored, the treatment regimens that are required, and the potential long-term implications of the condition. Examples of possible nursing diagnoses are as follows: Anxiety related to threat to health status, Individual ineffective coping related to required changes in lifestyle, and Risk for impaired adjustment to altered self-concept related to a lack of necessary hormones.

### Expected Outcomes

The therapeutic goal promoting optimal maternal and fetal outcomes is to achieve and maintain hormonal patterns that are parallel to patterns considered normal with pregnancy. Desired glucose levels are between 60 to 120 mg/dl with variation within that range throughout the day. This goal is best achieved when the woman has the appropriate information, resources, and support to enact the therapeutic medical regime.

### Possible Interventions

Women are responsible for managing their thyroidism and diabetes because treatment generally requires integration of interventions into the context of daily living. Nursing interventions require that the woman understand her condition and the care she is expected to provide for herself, as well as the signs and symptoms that indicate that she should contact her provider immediately. It should be clear to the woman when she should contact her provider for obstetrical care and when she should contact her endocrinologist.

When a woman has diabetes, the following self-care considerations are especially important:

- *Record keeping*—A journal documenting self-blood glucose monitoring, insulin administration, exercise periods, diet, choices and patterns, and perceived stressors can help the woman and her health care providers determine possible challenges in her efforts to strive for glycemic control. Women may occasionally require hospitalization if acute circumstances arise so that their glucose levels may be stabilized (Box 17-5). These periods are generally brief but may be frightening to the woman and her family. The family may also need assistance in providing care to other family members while the woman is hospitalized.
- *Nutrition*—Maintaining proper nutrition is critical to management of diabetes in pregnancy. Consultation with a dietitian is critical for women with preexisting diabetes, as well for those with

BOX 17-5 *Indications for Antepartum Admission in Pregnant Diabetics*

Poorly controlled glucose levels
Inability to provide adequate self-care
Infection
Accelerating hypertension
Abnormal antepartum testing results
Diabetic ketoacidosis
Progressive cardiopathy

TABLE 17-6 *Desired Glucose Levels*

| Time | Glucose levels |
| --- | --- |
| Fasting | 60 to 90 mg/dl |
| Before meals and bedtime snack | 60 to 105 mg/dl |
| 1 to 2 hours after a meal (postprandial) | 100 to 120 mg/dl |
| 2 AM to 4 AM | 60 to 120 mg/dl |

Data from Gilbert ES and Harmon JS: *Manual of high risk pregnancy and delivery*, ed 2, St Louis, 1998, Mosby.

gestational diabetes. Dietary recommendations include three meals a day plus snacks; and calories derived from carbohydrates (50% to 60%), fats (20% to 30%), and protein (20%). Pregnant women require 300 additional calories per day beyond their nonpregnant nutritional needs in order to meet the maternal and fetal demands of the pregnancy. Recommended weight gain is based on prepregnancy weight, and weight loss is generally not recommended during pregnancy.

- *Exercise*—Exercise is an integral aspect of the therapeutic plan for women with well-controlled glucose levels. Controversy exists as to the risks associated with an exercise program in women with uncontrolled glucose levels because exercise in this case may increase her glucose levels (Gabbe, Neibyl, and Simpson, 1996). When glucose levels are controlled, exercise enhances the effectiveness of insulin (Mandeville and Troiano, 1992). Walking is considered to be an optimal form of exercise during pregnancy.
- *Monitoring of blood glucose*—Blood glucose monitoring significantly contributes to achieving and maintaining glycemic control as pregnancy progresses. Glucose levels are monitored before meals and at bedtime, and postprandial and nocturnal assessments can also be incorporated if problems are suspected (Table 17-6).
- *Monitoring of ketones*—The first voided urine specimen of the morning is checked for ketones with a dipstick at least 3 times per week. More frequent evaluation may be desired if the woman becomes ill or her blood glucose levels become elevated.
- *Insulin use to manage diabetes*—When required during pregnancy, a biosynthetic human insulin (Humulin) is used. Humalog (Lispro) works within 15 minutes, peaks in an hour and a half, and lasts 3 hours, matching the body's insulin needs at mealtime. Short-acting, regular Humulin takes 30 minutes to act, peaks within 3 to 4 hours, and has a duration of 5 to 8 hours. Intermediate-acting

Humulin (NPH, Lente) works within 2 to 6 hours, peaks between 4 and 15 hours, and lasts between 12 and 24 hours. During pregnancy both rapid- and intermediate-acting insulins are used (Gabbe, Neibyl, and Simpson, 1996).

The woman's 24-hour insulin dosage is usually calculated according to the trimester of the pregnancy. If the woman has gestational diabetes that requires insulin or Class B diabetes controlled with oral agents, the 24-hour insulin dosage is calculated according to the woman's weight and weeks of gestation (Table 17-7).

The type, amount, and scheduling of a woman's insulin will be modified based on a variety of factors, including weeks of gestation. Early in pregnancy, insulin requirements generally decrease slightly; as the pregnancy progresses, they increase gradually; by 36 weeks, they level off or decrease slightly.

When injections are the mode of delivery of the insulin, a woman's 24-hour insulin requirements are normally divided into two or four doses administered 30 minutes prior to meals if Humulin is used or just before the meal if Humalog is used.

If a two-dose regimen is followed, the breakfast dose reflects two thirds of the daily requirement (one-third is regular insulin and two-thirds is NPH), with the last third of her daily dose (one-half regular insulin and one-half NPH) being administered before dinner. This may be useful for the woman with gestational diabetes, but it is usually not effective for the woman with diabetes mellitus (Gilbert and Harmon, 1998).

If a three-dose regimen is followed, her morning dose will usually be NPH with or without regular insulin, regular insulin before dinner, and NPH at bedtime.

If a four-dose regimen is followed, regular insulin is given before each meal and NPH is given before the bedtime snack (Gilbert and Harmon, 1998).

| TABLE 17-7 | *Calculation Pattern for Insulin during Pregnancy* |
|---|---|
| **Trimester** | **Insulin dosage** |
| 1st trimester | 0.6 units/kg body weight |
| 2nd trimester | 0.7 units/kg body weight |
| 3rd trimester | 0.8 units/kg body weight |

Data from Heppard M and Garite T: *Acute obstetrics: a practical guide,* ed 2, St Louis, 1996, Mosby.

Subcutaneous infusion pump devices may also be used to administer insulin. Short-acting insulin is used with a basal infusion rate of approximately 1 unit of insulin an hour, with bolus dosing based on self-glucose monitoring results (Gabbe, Neibyl, and Simpson, 1996).

* *Identification of diabetic ketoacidosis (DKA)—* The occurrence of DKA in a pregnant woman is an emergency situation. DKA is a state of hyperglycemia and ketosis that can occur at lower blood glucose levels than found in the nonpregnant population. DKA occurs more commonly in newly diagnosed or women with difficult-to-control diabetes. DKA can be triggered by infection, inability to follow required regimen, or use of medicines such as corticosteriods and betamimetics.

A woman may describe or present with the following symptoms: exaggerated respiratory effort, fruity odor to breath, nausea and vomiting, altered mental state, and coma. Laboratory assessments will reflect hyperglycemia and acidemia. Treatment is aimed at correcting maternal glucose and electrolytes and seeking and managing the triggering event.

### Evaluation

Assess the woman's understanding of her condition and treatment plan. Have her explain how she will implement the necessary actions or restrictions and monitor the status of her condition. Measure the degree to which she is supported by her support network. Determine the level of anxiety she and her support network are experiencing because of her condition. Determine if she understands the signs and symptoms indicating that she needs medical assistance and if she can reach emergency care if needed.

### Summary

The ultimate goal of nursing care for a pregnant woman with endocrine problems is to minimize the risks and potential complications caused by the possible fluctuations. When the woman and her family understand her condition and have the support to provide the required self-care and implement the disease-management program, the outcome of the pregnancy can be positive for the mother, infant, and family.

## Conditions of the Digestive System

Conditions of the digestive system and its accessory organs can increase a woman's discomfort during pregnancy and interfere with her nutritional status if her intake is limited or the nutrients are not absorbed.

### Peptic Ulcer Disease

Peptic ulcers are ulcers that occur in the digestive tract, usually at the lower end of the esophagus or in the stomach. The woman may experience pain and bleeding from the damaged tissue.

When women with peptic ulcer disease become pregnant, most find that their symptoms decrease in severity during pregnancy, although they tend to relapse by the third postpartum month (Gabbe, Neibyl, and Simpson, 1996). It is thought that symptoms improve due to the influence of progesterone during pregnancy because it reduces gastric acid production and increases mucus production.

### Pancreatitis

**Pancreatitis** is an acute inflammation of the pancreas. There is a high association between pancreatitis and the development of **cholelithiasis** (gallstones) (Gabbe, Neibyl, and Simpson, 1996). Pancreatitis may be caused in pregnant women by preeclampsia or an infectious process, even though it is most commonly due to alcohol consumption in nonpregnant women. The occurrence of pancreatitis in pregnancy is attributed to the decreased emptying of the gallbladder.

The onset of this condition is more common in the third trimester, and the signs and symptoms are similar in pattern to those of nonpregnant women. Clinical presentation includes epigastric pain radiating to the flank or shoulders, nausea, vomiting, fever, and leukocytosis. Confirmation of the diagnosis during pregnancy can be challenging because the growing uterus can obstruct ultrasound views of the pancreas. As an alternative, a CT scan may be used. Laboratory testing will reveal an elevated serum amylase.

### Cholelithiasis

Physiologic adaptations of pregnancy set the stage for the development of cholelithiasis. The cause of gallstones during pregnancy is attributed to the increased levels of estrogen and progesterone and the net effects these hormones have on the gallbladder. These hormones cause a decrease in the emptying time of the gallbladder. The decreased emptying time results in increased biliary cholesterol saturation, predisposing the woman to gallstone formation.

The clinical pattern associated with cholelithiasis is an abrupt steady pain in right upper quadrant, radiating to the back. Women with gallstones may experience nausea, vomiting, anorexia, diaphoresis, fever, and leukocytosis. The onset of symptoms, which can last from seconds to hours, is 1 to 2 hours after meals.

### Inflammatory Diseases of the Bowel

Ulcerative colitis and Crohn's disease are inflammatory diseases of the bowel. The onset of these two conditions is typically seen during childbearing years. **Ulcerative colitis** is a disease involving the colon or rectum. Women present with clinical symptoms that are acute and include bloody stools, cramping, diarrhea, weight loss, and dehydration. **Crohn's disease** is an inflammation that can occur anywhere in the intestinal tract. Symptoms associated with Crohn's disease tend to be chronic in nature and include fever, diarrhea, and abdominal pain.

### Nursing Assessment

Assessment focuses on the description, onset, type, and duration of pain. Because the pain develops in the digestive track, the woman's fluid and nutritional intake must also be assessed. Evaluate for signs and symptoms of premature labor.

A variety of tests may be ordered to determine the cause of the woman's pain and other symptoms. Many of the same tests are done to identify any of these conditions. Assess the woman's knowledge of the reason for these tests and whether she is able to prepare for them appropriately. When a diagnosis is obtained, determine whether the woman understands the description of her disease, how she is to manage her condition, and its relationship to her pregnancy.

### Possible Nursing Diagnoses

Nursing diagnoses will focus on knowledge, pain management, and maintaining the necessary nutrition to adequately support the development of the fetus. Examples of possible nursing diagnoses are as follows: Pain related to caustic irritation of gastric tissues; Knowledge deficit related to potential complications of condition; Fluid volume deficit related to vomiting and nasogastric suctioning; and Altered nutrition, less than body requirements related to decreased oral intake.

### Expected Outcomes

With identification of the problem and appropriate intervention, it is expected that the woman's pain will be reduced. She will receive adequate nutrition for both her own needs, as well as those of the developing fetus. Premature labor will be prevented, and the fetus will go to full term.

### Possible Interventions

Treatment of the conditions of the digestive system is both condition-specific and generalized. Care is accomplished through education of the woman and her support system, identification of nutritional resources that will meet her requirements, periodic assessment of all systems involved, and assessment of the growth of the fetus.

*Peptic Ulcer.* During pregnancy, the treatment plan consists of oral antacids administered after meals and at bedtime and changes in diet so that the woman avoids alcohol, caffeine, and aspirin products.

*Pancreatitis.* The treatment plan for a woman with pancreatitis may include maintaining nothing by mouth (NPO); nasogastric suctioning when nausea is present; fluid and electrolyte replacement; and total parenteral nutrition (TPN) if dietary intake is inadequate. Pain management is with meperidine. A woman with pancreatitis is at risk for premature labor, which places the fetus at significant risk.

*Cholelithiasis.* Care for a woman with cholelithiasis involves fluid- and electrolyte-replacement, pain management, nasogastric suctioning, and antibiotics. Observation for pancreatitis is indicated because the two conditions are associated.

*Inflammatory Diseases of the Bowel.* Therapeutic management is similar for ulcerative colitis and Crohn's disease. With Crohn's disease, a low residue diet and a balanced nutritional intake are the foundations for management. With ulcerative colitis, a low roughage diet and general nutritional counseling are recommended. Stress reduction is an important aspect of care for both conditions because stress and emotional upset can trigger a flare-up of symptoms. A variety of medications, including narcotics, may be used to manage flare-ups of diarrhea. Steroids may be required for women who do not respond to the initial therapeutic plan. Fluid and electrolyte replacement may be indicated for longer episodes of diarrhea.

### Evaluation

Assess the woman's understanding of her condition and treatment plan. Have her explain how she will implement the necessary actions or restrictions and monitor the status of her condition. Measure the degree to which her support network provides for her. Determine the level of anxiety being experienced by the woman and her loved ones because of her condition. Determine if she understands the signs and symptoms that indicate that she needs medical assistance and if she can reach emergency care if needed.

### Summary

Conditions of the digestive system can be difficult to diagnose and resolve when a woman is not pregnant. When pregnant, the placement of the developing fetus can interfere with diagnostic tests. The condition must be resolved quickly so that the nutritional needs of two patients—the mother and the fetus—can be met.

## Neurologic Conditions

A woman who enters pregnancy with a history of migraine headaches or a seizure disorder may face a complicated course of care during her pregnancy. Some of the treatments normally available may not be options for pregnant women because of concern for the health of the fetus.

### Seizure Disorders

Seizure disorders are the most common neurologic disorder seen in pregnancy occurring in approximately .3% to .5% of the childbearing population. The objective of care is to keep the pregnant woman with a seizure disorder (e.g., epilepsy) seizure-free, while minimizing adverse effects on the woman and the developing fetus, including the possible teratogenic effects of medication (Burrow and Duffy, 1999).

Seizure disorders can be either acquired (15%) or idiopathic (85%). Seizures can be described as tonicoclonic, myoclonic, or focal. **Tonic-clonic** seizures are both tonic (i.e., persistent, involuntary, violent contractions) and clonic (i.e., alternately contracting and relaxing). **Myoclonic** seizures are the twitching of a muscle or group of muscles. A **focal** seizure can be seen when the woman's eyes become fixed as if she is staring at something. The best care is achieved through collaborate care with the woman, her partner, the perinatologist, and the neurologist.

Pregnancy has a distinct effect on the frequency of seizures; of women who have a history of seizure activity, 45% experience an increase during pregnancy. If a woman has experienced monthly convulsions in spite of following a anticonvulsant regimen, she should expect to experience more episodes when she becomes pregnant. If she has been seizure-free for the 9 months proceeding the pregnancy, she only faces a 25% chance of worsening. The longer her period of seizure control, the better her prognosis during pregnancy (Burrow and Duffy, 1999).

It is theorized that the exacerbations are due in part to hormonal changes and altered serum drug levels due to physiologic volume expansion seen in pregnancy. Also with increased plasma clearance during pregnancy, it is more difficult to maintain therapeutic drug levels. If the drug levels that were therapeutic before pregnancy are able to be maintained, only 10% of women will have their condition worsen during pregnancy. Insomnia, sleep deprivation, and stress increase a woman's risk for an increase in seizure activity (Gabbe, Neibyl, and Simpson, 1996; Burrows and Duffy, 1999).

The effect that seizure disorders have on pregnancy is related more to the use of antiseizure medications than to the seizure condition. Maternal age and parity, socioeconomic status, the degree of prenatal monitoring, and other maternal diseases have a greater effect on pregnancy than seizures. However, women with seizures should be prepared that they may experience more bleeding and have a higher chance of having a stillborn.

Metabolism is altered during pregnancy in a different manner for each drug. The risk of congenital malformation is determined by the time of exposure, the maternal dose, and the specific drug (Burrow and Duffy, 1999).

Some anticonvulsant medications are known teratogenic agents, with some increasing fetal congenital anomalies—especially cleft lip and palate and neural tube defects. The risk of malformation due to anticonvulsant medication becomes twice the population risk but is not 100%. Pregnant women with an active seizure disorder are therefore kept on their medication therapy. Prenatal diagnostic testing is then used to assess fetal anatomy and evaluate the fetus for evidence of malformations (Burrow and Duffy, 1999).

Maternal anticonvulsants can also affect the newborn by interfering with vitamin K production and increasing the risk of hemorrhagic complications. Additional risks associated with the occurrence of seizures include stillbirth, a small-for-gestational-age baby, and pregnancy-induced hypertension.

Folic acid supplementation (4 mg/day) is recommended for all pregnant woman to reduce the occurrence of neural tube defects. Folate, however, can alter the uptake of anticonvulsant medications so that if the woman takes the medication as prescribed she is at increased risk for seizures. Because most women on seizure medication do not take folic acid supplements, alphafetoprotein testing may be offered at 16 weeks of gestation to screen for neural tube defects.

### Migraine Headaches

Fifteen to twenty percent of women who become pregnant have a history of migraine headaches. Pregnancy is associated with an improvement in migraine headaches in approximately 80% of women. The clinical patterns associated with migraine headaches include photosensitivity, nausea, and headache.

Therapeutic strategies are aimed at providing supportive care. Episodic pain management can be achieved with narcotics or nonnarcotic analgesics. Nonsteroidal antiinflammatory agents (NSAIDs) should be avoided in the later part of pregnancy due their association with early closure of the ductus arteriosus and reduction of amniotic fluid volume with long-term use.

Attempts are made to determine the woman's headache triggers. Diet has been identified as a trigger for migraine headaches in some women. Dietary recall may help identify the precipitating events that may otherwise go unnoticed by the woman. Alcohol, hypoglycemia, cured meats, and monosodium glutamate (MSG) are commonly identified triggers.

### Nursing Assessment

Assessment focuses on the description of the incident, including onset, type, and duration of headache or seizure. Assess the woman's knowledge of her condition and the reason for tests or treatments. Determine if she has the capability of obtaining and storing her required medication. Learn what assistance she has to provide for her personal safety when either one of these conditions occur. Determine whether her family understands her condition and how to manage it, as well as its relationship to her pregnancy.

### Possible Nursing Diagnoses

Nursing diagnoses focus on the woman's knowledge, pain management, and safety. Examples of possible nursing diagnoses are as follows: Pain related to migraine headache, Visual disturbances related to migraine headache, Knowledge deficit related to potential complications of condition, and Risk for injury related to seizure activity.

### Expected Outcomes

With identification of the problem and the appropriate intervention, it is expected that the woman's pain will be reduced. The occurrence of seizures will be minimized, while the needed medication will provide the least amount of harm possible. Premature labor will be prevented, and the fetus will go to full term.

### Possible Interventions

Treatment of these neurologic problems is both condition-specific and generalized. Care is accomplished through the following:

- *Teaching*—Education of the woman and her support system about the condition and the care that is required.
- *Assessment*—Identification of triggers for the headaches or seizures and assistance in reducing their occurrence.
- *Nutrition counseling*—Assistance in determining what foods may be eaten to provide the necessary nutrients without including foods that may trigger the woman's condition.
- *Medication*—Use of appropriate medications to meet the needs of the woman and the developing fetus.
- *Assessment*—Ongoing assessment of the growth of the fetus.

### Evaluation

Assess the woman's understanding of her condition and treatment plan. Have her explain how she will implement the necessary actions or restrictions and monitor the status of her condition. Measure the degree to which her support network sustains her. Determine the level of anxiety she and her loved ones are experiencing because of her condition. Determine if she understands the signs and symptoms that indicate she needs medical assistance and if she can reach emergency care if needed.

### Summary

Conditions of the neurologic system can be difficult to treat when a woman is pregnant. Collaboration between the woman's specialists is necessary in order to have the best outcomes for both the mother and child.

## Hematologic Conditions

Nutrients and oxygen are supplied to the developing fetus via the blood flowing through the mother's circulatory system to the uterus. Alterations of the mother's platelets or erythrocytes not only place her health and life at risk but also that of her fetus.

### Thrombocytopenia

**Thrombocytopenia** (an abnormal decrease in the number of blood platelets) affects 4% of pregnant women, making it the most common hematologic condition seen in pregnancy (Gabbe, Neibyl, and Simpson, 1996). Thrombocytopenia has several forms and may be an inherited condition, a condition developed before or during pregnancy, or a result of an obstetric condition. The most common causes of thrombocytopenia found during pregnancy are immune or idiopathic thrombocytopenic purpura (ITP) and gestational thrombocytopenia.

Idiopathic thrombocytopenic purpura (ITP) is caused by drugs or a viral infection leading to immune sensitization of platelets. This results in peripheral destruction and sequestration of platelets. ITP carries substantial implications for the fetus because it may become sensitized. When a fetus develops thrombocytopenia, some clinicians believe that there is an increased potential for trauma and bleeding within the cranium. Some clinicians may recommend that the baby be delivered through abdominal surgery.

New-onset maternal thrombocytopenia of greater than 100,000/$\mu$l sometimes occurs during pregnancy. The underlying cause of gestational thrombocytopenia is not understood. Gestational thrombocytopenia generally requires no treatment, there is no threat of significant lowering of platelets in the fetus, and the outcome of pregnancy is good (Burrow and Duffy, 1999).

The cause of maternal thrombocytopenia should always be investigated because it may be a clue to other conditions developing in the woman's body. It may be an early indication of the development of eclampsia (Burrow and Duffy, 1999). Thrombocytopenia can also occur as a result of severe pre-eclampsia; the HELLP syndrome (i.e., hemolysis, elevated liver enzymes, and low platelet count); and disseminated intravascular coagulopathy (DIC) secondary to abruptio placenta, sepsis, hemorrhage, or a retained fetus after demise.

## Sickle Cell Anemia

Sickle cell anemia is an autosomal recessive disease of Mediterranean and African origin. The sickle cell trait is carried by 1 in 12 Americans of African or Mediterranean descent (Cunningham and others, 1997). Screening for sickle cell trait is recommended for all women at high risk for the condition.

Sickle cell anemia is the result of a defect in the hemoglobin molecule, causing the erythrocytes to be elongated and crescent-shaped. These sickled cells have a life span of 20 days, as compared with 120 days for normal erythrocytes.

Pregnant women with sickle cell disease are at higher risk for developing infections, particularly in the urinary tract. Sickle cell disease is associated with increased spontaneous abortions (up to 25% has been documented by some sources), prematurity, intrauterine growth restriction, pregnancy-induced hypertension (PIH), and stillbirth.

Sickle cell anemia is not a static condition. When a woman with sickle cell disease is exposed to a trigger event, sickling increases, leading to stasis of cells and a **vasoocclusive crisis** (sickle cell crisis). Events that may precipitate a sickle cell crisis include viral or bacterial infection, fever, acid-base imbalance, trauma, dehydration, exposure to cold, strenuous exercise, ingestion of drugs or alcohol, trauma with associated blood loss, severe emotional disturbance, air travel, or extreme fatigue. Vasoocclusive crises tend to occur more frequently during pregnancy.

### Clinical Presentation

***Thrombocytopenia.*** A woman may experience an increase in bruising or a prolonged bleeding time. Petechial lesions are the characteristic lesions in thrombocytopenic states. The presence of a low platelet count is determined with blood work. Immune thrombocytopenia is documented through the presence of antibodies. The indirect assay, a Western blot test, is a specific test for ITP that identifies specific antibodies. The direct assay, using platelet immunofluorescence, demonstrates the presence of immunoglobulins on the woman's own platelets. Although sensitive to identifying ITP, it is nonspecific (Burrow and Duffy, 1999).

***Sickle Cell Crises.*** Pain is the primary clinical presentation of women experiencing a vasoocclusive crisis. Pain can be acute and occur in joints and bones—particularly extremities, chest, abdomen, and spine. Additional symp-

toms range from general malaise, dyspnea, headache, visual changes, and nausea and vomiting (Cunningham and others, 1997). Physical examination may reveal jaundice, pale skin, altered visual acuity, and respiratory difficulty. Diagnosis is confirmed with hemoglobin electrophoresis.

### Nursing Assessment

Assessment focuses on the woman's knowledge of her condition and understanding of the reason for her tests or treatments. Learn what assistance the woman has to care for her family while she is hospitalized, as well as to care for herself when she returns home. Determine if she understands her condition and how to manage it and the connection between her disease and the type of care she requires because she is pregnant.

### Nursing Diagnoses

Nursing diagnoses will focus on knowledge; management of bruising, bleeding, and pain; prevention of exacerbation of the condition; and rapid interventions to limit the damage caused by the hematologic condition to the woman or the developing fetus. Examples of possible nursing diagnoses are as follows: Anxiety related to unknown cause of bruising and bleeding, Pain related to vasoocclusive crisis, Altered tissue perfusion related to interruption of venous flow, Knowledge deficit related to potential complications of condition, and Risk for fetal demise due to decreased profusion of the placenta.

### Expected Outcomes

With early identification of the problem and appropriate intervention, it is expected that the woman's bleeding and pain will be reduced and the fetus will grow. An appropriate level of platelets will be maintained. The occurrence of vasoocclusive crises will be minimized. Premature labor will be prevented, and the fetus will go to full term.

### Possible Interventions

Answer the woman's questions and address concerns about the possible effect this condition will have on the developing baby. Treatment of these hematologic problems are both condition-specific and generalized. Care is accomplished through education of the woman and her support system, identification of the cause of her condition, and the use of appropriate medications to meet the needs of the woman and the developing fetus. Periodic assessment of all systems involved and assessment of the growth of the fetus continue throughout the pregnancy.

***Thrombocytopenia.*** Treatment approaches for ITP during pregnancy are aimed at increasing the maternal platelet count and maintaining careful surveillance of the fetus. Administration of glucocorticoid drugs decreases the antibodies from binding with platelets, thereby halting platelet destruction. Treatment of ITP during pregnancy is not implemented until the mother's platelet count drops below 50,000/µl. Administration of steroids with a beginning dosage of 1 mk/kg of oral prednisone decreases the binding of antibodies with platelets, thereby halting platelet destruction. As soon as possible, the amounts of medication are gradually decreased to a dose that maintains the platelet count in the 50,000 µl range.

Some clinicians use IV immunoglobulins in place of steroids. An initial course of 1g/kg/day for 2 days usually elevates the platelet count for approximately 2 to 3 weeks. Although more expensive than the use of steroids, this allows the woman to escape the hypertensive, diabetogenic threat caused by steroid use (Burrow and Duffy, 1999).

Platelet transfusion may be used for acute emergencies. It is generally reserved for women with a platelet count of less than 50,000 cells/mm³ while waiting for the steroids or immunoglobulins to work or in preparing for surgery.

Splenectomy is an option during the second trimester of pregnancy. It is avoided during the first or third trimester to reduce the risk of a spontaneous abortion.

*Sickle Cell Anemia.* Counseling women with sickle cell anemia during pregnancy is a critical aspect of their care. Women can be assisted in determining how to avoid their personal triggers, as well as infections, dehydration, stress, high altitude, and hypoxia.

Encouragement of early entry into prenatal care and frequent visits—every 2 weeks until 20 weeks—has been recommended to enhance outcome and reduce the occurrence of vasoocclusive crisis (Cunningham and others, 1997). Folate and iron supplements are recommended (Gabbe, Neibyl, and Simpson, 1996). Prophylactic transfusions and exchange transfusions have been used to promote optimal oxygenation and improve perinatal outcomes.

If the woman experiences a sickle cell crisis, care is most frequently accomplished on an inpatient basis with the woman discharged home as soon as possible. During a sickle cell crisis transfusion, hydration, oxygen supplementation to maintain an arterial $PO_2$ over 70 mm Hg, and narcotics are commonly used. A systematic evaluation of possible precipitating factors is a critical aspect of future management and planning for ongoing care. Laboratory testing may include blood gases, hemoglobin electrophoresis, electrolytes, a complete blood count, and type and cross match of blood.

### Evaluation

Assess the woman's understanding of her condition and treatment plan. Have her explain how she will implement the necessary actions or restrictions and monitor the status of her condition. Measure the degree to which she is supported by those around her. Determine the level of anxiety she and her support network are experiencing because of her condition. Determine if she understands the signs and symptoms that indicate that she needs medical assistance and if she can reach emergency care if needed.

### Summary

Hematologic conditions can create a crisis situation when a woman is pregnant. Collaboration between the woman's specialists is necessary in order to have the best outcome for both the mother and child.

## Autoimmune Conditions

One of the most common autoimmune conditions to occur in women of childbearing age is systemic lupus erythematosus (SLE). When a woman with lupus becomes pregnant, careful management is necessary to address concerns for both the health and life of the mother, as well as that of the fetus.

### Systemic Lupus Erythematosus (SLE)

SLE is a chronic autoimmune inflammatory disease involving multiple organ systems. The disease has a period of exacerbation and remission. The name is derived from the commonly seen butterfly or malar rash that appears over the woman's nose and cheeks. The cause of SLE is unknown, but it is found in 1 in 750 women of childbearing age, with a higher occurrence—1 in 245—in black women (Gabbe, Neibyl, and Simpson, 1996).

### Effect of the Pregnancy on the Disease

The pregnancy does not affect the prognosis of the disease, although flare-ups may increase. If the woman has renal disease, the potential for irreversible damage exists.

### Effect of the Disease on the Pregnancy

SLE has the potential to negatively affect each trimester of the pregnancy. In the first trimester, the risk of miscarriage is increased. In the second and third trimesters, the risk of hypertension, premature labor, intrauterine growth restriction, and thrombolitic conditions is increased.

### Clinical Presentation

Clinical presentation is individualized, but early signs may include malaise, joint pain, and fever of unknown origin. Other symptoms are skin changes (present in approximately 80%); inflammation in joints, skin, kidneys, CNS, and serous membranes; butterfly rash; discoid rash; photosensitivity (skin eruptions triggered by light); oral or nasal ulcers; arthritis; pleuritis; pericarditis; nephritis with proteinuria; seizures; psychosis and organic brain disease; hematologic disorders; and immunologic disorders.

Common laboratory findings are a positive lupus erythematosus (LE) cell factor, positive immunoglobin antibody IgG, and false positive serology for syphilis.

Various increases in antinuclear antibodies may occur, depending on which body systems are affected.

### Nursing Assessment

Assessment focuses on the woman's knowledge of her condition and the reason for tests or treatments. Learn what assistance the woman has to provide care for her family while she is hospitalized, as well as care for herself when she returns home. Determine if she understands her condition, how to manage it, and its relationship to her pregnancy.

### Nursing Diagnoses

Nursing diagnoses will focus on knowledge, pain management, prevention of exacerbations of the condition, and rapid interventions to limit the damage caused to the woman's organs or systems and the developing fetus. Examples of possible nursing diagnoses are as follows: Pain related to inflammatory process affecting connective tissues, Impaired skin integrity related to chronic inflammation, Fatigue related to increased energy requirements caused by chronic inflammation, and Disturbed body image related to altered body function.

### Expected Outcomes

With early identification of the problem and appropriate interventions, it is expected that the woman's inflammatory process will be controlled and the fetus will grow to full term.

### Possible Interventions

Treatment of the SLE is dependent upon the symptoms that the woman is manifesting. Management approaches are individualized based on the systemic involvement of each woman. Possible interventions include the following:

- *Teaching*—We should educate the woman and her support system about her condition and the care that is necessary and ensure that she understands the role of medication in relieving her symptoms.
- *Medication*—Antiinflammatory agents are commonly used with prednisone as the drug of choice during pregnancy. Anticoagulant therapy may be initiated with heparin. Some researchers use salicylate, in the form of low-dose aspirin, because it is thought that the salicylate may counteract increased platelet adhesiveness.
- *Assessment*—All involved maternal systems should be periodically assessed, and the growth of the fetus should be assessed on an ongoing basis.

### Evaluation

Assess the woman's understanding of her condition and treatment plan. Have her explain how she will implement the necessary actions or restrictions and monitor the status of her condition. Measure the degree to which she is supported by her family and friends. Determine the level of anxiety she and her support network are experiencing because of her condition. Determine if she understands the signs and symptoms that indicate she needs medical assistance and if she can reach emergency care if needed.

### Summary

Autoimmune conditions can create a crisis situation when a woman is pregnant. Collaboration between the woman's specialists is necessary in order to have the best outcomes for both the mother and child.

## Malignant Neoplasms

The incidence of cancer in pregnant women is similar to that in nonpregnant women of the same age group. Because the risk for cancer increases with age, as more women delay the age of childbearing, the coincidental occurrence of pregnancy and cancer may increase (Burrow and Duffy, 1999). Currently malignant neoplasms are diagnosed in 1 in 1000 pregnancies. Breast cancer is the most common cancer encountered, with cervical cancer, melanoma, ovarian cancer, leukemia and lymphoma occurring in decreasing frequencies. Cancer during pregnancy represents a significant moral dilemma for women, families, and health care providers. The treatment of the cancer may be lethal to the developing fetus. The pregnancy may present an obstacle to the woman choosing chemotherapy and radiation treatment.

### Breast Cancer

The occurrence of breast cancer in women under the age of 40 is between 2% to 3%, with an incidence of 1 in 1300 to 3330 pregnancies (Copeland and Landon, 1996; Gabbe, Neibyl, and Simpson, 1996). Women who develop breast cancer in pregnancy are more likely to be nulliparous or have not previously breastfed. Breastfeeding has a protective effect on breast cancer.

Breast cancer screening should be encouraged in all childbearing women as an important aspect of early prenatal care. Identification of a breast lump will initiate prompt evaluation. However, assessing breast lumps in pregnancy can be difficult due to the physiologic breast changes associated with pregnancy. Mammography has a limited value in pregnancy because of the increased density of the breast tissue. Fine needle aspiration of a mass is the diagnostic approach of choice in pregnancy (Copeland and Landon, 1996).

The recommendation for a subsequent pregnancy in a woman treated for breast cancer with negative lymph nodes to wait for is 2 to 3 years. If the lymph nodes tested positively, it is recommended that future pregnancies be postponed for 5 years.

## Cervical Cancer

Cervical cancer complicates approximately 1 in 2200 pregnancies. Many women with cervical cancer are asymptomatic, while others describe some vaginal bleeding or vaginal discharge. Many have considered these events part of the changes that come with pregnancy.

Screening for cervical cancer with a Papanicolaou (Pap) smear is recommended during the initial prenatal examination. Follow up for an abnormal Pap smear involves a colposcopic examination of the cervix. Treatment for invasive cervical cancer is based on the stage of the disease. The survival rates for women with cervical cancer are unchanged due to pregnancy.

## Hodgkin's Disease

Lymphomas occur in 1 in 6000 pregnancies. Fertility is not affected early in the disease process. Pregnancy does not adversely affect the course of the disease. The clinical symptoms associated with Hodgkin's disease are enlarged cervical or axillary nodes, fever, night sweats, and weight loss. Staging of the disease process is important in deciding whether to delay treatment and proceed with the pregnancy. Treatment approaches are determined by the stage of the disease. Initial treatment approaches for early stage Hodgkin's involves radiation therapy; chemotherapy is added for treatment of later stages of the disease.

## Leukemia

Acute leukemia is diagnosed during pregnancy with estimates of 1 in 75,000 pregnancies. The frequency of acute lymphocytic leukemia is 60%, with myleoctic leukemia accounting for 30% of the cases. Chronic leukemia occurs infrequently, being present in only 10% of the cases.

Clinical symptoms include fatigue, fever, increased bleeding, recurrent infections, and petechiae. Laboratory findings reveal an increase in white blood cells (i.e., leukopenia). Diagnosis is confirmed with bone marrow biopsy. Treatment is aimed at correcting bone marrow failure. Pregnancy does not alter the course of the disease, but the prognosis for the woman's long-term survival with leukemia is guarded. Due to the medications used in treatment, leukemia places the fetus at risk for intrauterine growth restriction, prematurity, and still birth.

### Clinical Presentation

The clinical presentation of malignant neoplasms during pregnancy is dependent upon the type and location of the cancer. Among the most common symptoms are fatigue, appetite disturbance, and pain.

### Nursing Assessment

Assessment focuses on the woman's knowledge of her condition, the types of treatments available to treat her cancer, and the effect of these treatments on her fetus.

Learn the woman's beliefs about termination of pregnancy and if she considers it an option for herself. Determine if she has assistance to provide care for her family while she is hospitalized, as well as care for herself when she returns home.

### Nursing Diagnoses

Nursing diagnoses will focus on knowledge of her cancer and treatment options, as well as her beliefs about termination of pregnancy. Examples of possible nursing diagnoses are as follows: Anxiety related to threat of death, Anticipatory grieving for loss of developing fetus, Fatigue related to overwhelming psychologic and emotional demands, and Ineffective family coping related to threat of loss of mother and loss of fetus.

### Expected Outcomes

With early identification of the problem and appropriate intervention, it is expected that the woman's cancer will be treated and her chance of long-term survival will be increased. With some treatments, the fetus will also survive and grow to full-term.

### Possible Interventions

***Staging of the Cancer.*** The staging of a cancer is determined by studying the cancer itself and its location. In determining the stages of most cancers, imaging studies are used to establish both the local extent of the tumor and to search for secondary sites. "Imaging with plain x-rays, mammograms, computed tomography (CT) scans, and nuclear medicine studies expose the fetus and mother to variable amounts of radiation" (Burrows and Duffy, 1999). To avoid radiation exposure, ultrasound and magnetic resonance (MR) studies are preferred in most situations. Some staging may be done by visually examining sites via laparoscopy (i.e., abdominal exploration using a type of endoscope called a laparoscope) or **laparotomy** (i.e., surgical opening of the abdomen) and a series of node sampling.

The use of blood work to determine the level of organ functioning (e.g., liver function tests) or presence of specific antigens in the serum is not often helpful. Oncofetal proteins are expressed normally when there is a developing fetus and abnormally in the presence of a cancer. Therefore detecting otherwise useful tumor markers in a pregnant woman's serum is not helpful unless a distinction can be made between the fetal and the malignant expression of the antigen (Burrow and Duffy, 1999).

***Treatment Decisions.*** Treatment of the cancer is dependent upon the type of cancer and the degree to which it has progressed. "Anticancer therapies may be teratogenic and mutagenic, and in managing cancer in the pregnant woman the effects of therapy on the developing fetus are an important consideration. The prognosis, the risks of the cancer and the therapy to the mother, and the risks of pregnancy must also be taken into account in helping the patient make a decision about continuing the pregnancy and in managing both the pregnancy and the malignancy should she choose to continue the pregnancy" (Burrow and Duffy, 1999).

Care is accomplished by educating the woman and her support system and providing appropriate treatment to meet the needs of the woman. If termination of the pregnancy is necessary, the woman and her family will be offered assistance with the grief process.

***Surgery.*** Surgical removal of a cancer during pregnancy necessitates consideration of the possible effect of anesthesia. Although the anesthestic drugs are relatively safe to the fetus, the incidence of a surgical procedure does cause a risk for the pregnancy (i.e., it slightly increases the fetus's risk for premature delivery, intrauterine growth retardation, and neonatal death). The risk is higher when the procedure involves abdominal or pelvic surgery. Extraabdominal surgery is less likely to cause complications.

***Radiotherapy.*** Radiation places the fetus at risk for death, abnormalities, low birth weight, cancer in later life, and—theoretically—transmission of genetic abnormalities to future generations. The woman herself may be at increased risk for increased chromosomal damage when pregnant. This increased sensitivity reverts back to normal immediately after delivery (Burrow and Duffy, 1999).

***Chemotherapy.*** The long-term consequences of the use of chemotherapy during pregnancy are not known. Some predictions may be made based on known physiology and case reports. Most cytotoxic agents cross the placenta, and almost all of these are teratogenic during the first trimester. This increases the rate of fetal loss during the first trimester. Among the fetuses that survive, the incidence of fetal malformations is increased by as much as 20%. During the second and third trimesters, after organogenesis is complete, certain chemotherapy agents do not significantly increase the rate of fetal malformations. The use of chemotherapy at any time during a pregnancy, however, results in a baby of lower birth weight. The long-term effects of in utero exposure to chemotherapy are not know (Burrow and Duffy, 1999).

Chemotherapy for cancer commonly causes nausea and vomiting. Premedication with an antiemetic before chemotherapy, as well as supplying it to the woman to self-treat delayed emesis after she returns home, is important. Consistent data about the use of any antiemetic in pregnancy is not available.

***Nutritional Needs.*** A woman with cancer also often needs total parenteral nutrition. The need may be produced by the cancer itself or the treatment regimen put in place. For a pregnant woman, the need is especially important to prevent malnutrition.

### Evaluation

Assess the woman's understanding of her condition, treatment choices, and treatment plan. Have her explain how she will be able to free herself from her other responsibilities and implement the necessary actions or restrictions that her disease requires. Measure the degree to which she is supported by her support network. Determine the level of anxiety she and her support network are experiencing because of her cancer. Determine if she understands the signs and symptoms indicating that she needs medical assistance, as well as if she can reach emergency care if needed.

### Summary

Cancer and its diagnostic tests and required treatments cause a crisis situation when a woman is pregnant. Collaboration between the woman's various specialists is necessary in order to have the best outcomes.

 ## HEALTH CONDITIONS CREATED BY PREGNANCY

### Hypertensive States of Pregnancy

Hypertension is one of the most common medical complications of pregnancy. It affects the health of both the mother and the fetus and can have life-threatening consequences. If treated early and effectively, maternal mortality is low, although the pregnant woman may still suffer the morbidity of a stroke, acute cardiac decompensation, convulsions, coma, and renal failure. When a mother has either chronic or gestational hypertension, the fetus may experience a placental insufficiency with intrauterine growth restriction (IUGR), abruptio placenta, premature delivery, intrauterine growth retardation, or intrauterine death (Gilbert and Harmon, 1998; Burrow and Duffy, 1999).

When a woman has hypertension disorder during a pregnancy, it may have been a preexisting condition or it may have developed during the pregnancy (Table 17-8). **Gestational hypertension** includes hypertension or proteinuria that develops during pregnancy, generally after 20 weeks of gestation in the absence of a molar pregnancy and subsides after delivery. Another manifestation may develop within 7 days postpartum.

### Gestational Hypertensive Disorders

This section will focus on gestational hypertensive disorders, which are also referred to as pregnancy-induced hypertension (PIH). PIH includes four types of disorders: transient hypertension, gestational proteinuria, preeclampsia, and eclampsia. **Transient hypertension** is high blood pressure in late pregnancy without other signs of preeclampsia. Women who experience transient hypertension usually develop chronic hypertension later in life. **Gestational proteinuria** is the finding of protein in a woman's urine after 20 weeks of gestation when she has no history of it prior to the pregnancy and she does not have hypertension.

**TABLE 17-8** *Classification of Hypertensive States of Pregnancy*

| Type | Description |
|---|---|
| **GESTATIONAL HYPERTENSIVE DISORDERS: PREGNANCY-INDUCED HYPERTENSION (PIH)** | |
| Transient hypertension | Development of mild hypertension during pregnancy in previously normotensive patient without proteinuria or pathologic edema |
| Gestational proteinuria | Development of proteinuria after 20 weeks of gestation in previously nonproteinuric patient without hypertension |
| Preeclampsia | Development of hypertension and proteinuria in previously normotensive patient after 20 weeks of gestation or in early postpartum period; in presence of trophoblastic disease it can develop before 20 weeks of gestation |
| Eclampsia | Development of convulsions or coma in preeclamptic patient |
| **CHRONIC HYPERTENSIVE DISORDERS** | |
| Chronic hypertension | Hypertension and/or proteinuria in pregnant patient with chronic hypertension |
| Superimposed preeclampsia/eclampsia | Development of preeclampsia or eclampsia in patient with chronic hypertension |

Gilbert E and Harmon J: *Manual of high risk pregnancy and delivery*, ed 2, St Louis, 1998, Mosby.

**Preclampsia** is a systemic disorder that only occurs in pregnancy. It is the development of hypertension and proteinuria after 20 weeks of gestation (or in the early postpartum) in a woman who has previously been normotensive. It can occur before 20 weeks of gestation in the presence of trophoblastic disease (a molar pregnancy). **Eclampsia** describes the situation when a woman with preeclampsia develops convulsions or goes into a coma. Approximately 5% of women with preeclampsia develop eclampsia, but the mechanisms for the convulsions are not known. Preeclampsia and eclampsia cause the most complications for the mother and pose the greatest risk to the fetus so they will be covered in more detail (Gilbert and Harmon, 1998; Burrow and Duffy, 1999).

*Etiology.* The cause of preeclampsia remains unknown, although there are several common theories: nutritional deficiency, an immune response, or a genetic predisposition.

Dietary deficiencies have long been explored as causative factor for PIH because of the physiologic effect of specific nutritional elements. It is known that protein promotes cellular growth and maintains normal serum osmotic pressure, so it could be significant in preventing edema and elevated blood pressure. Calcium can decrease the contraction of the smooth muscles of the arteries and arterioles, therefore a deficiency might trigger preeclampsia. Magnesium causes vasodilation, so it might decrease the occurrence of preeclampsia. For these reasons, dietary deficiencies of protein, calcium, or magnesium have been explored. No adequate data, however, have supported a strong connection between the deficiency of these or other nutrients and the development of preeclampsia.

Some researchers suggest that preeclampsia develops when the woman's body develops an immune response to the placenta and fetus. This theory may partially explain why primigravidas, multigravidas who have changed partners, couples whose use only barrier contraceptive methods, and women who become pregnant through donor insemination programs are at higher risk for preeclampsia. The prevalence of preeclampsia is decreased in women who receive heterologous blood transfusions, practice oral sex, or have a long period of cohabitation with the father of the baby before the pregnancy occurred (Gilbert and Harmon, 1998; Burrow and Duffy, 1999).

Genetic patterns have also been explored in the etiology of PIH. Because a high percentage of daughters of mothers who had experienced preeclampsia also develop preeclampsia, the possibility that it is related to a single recessive gene is being explored.

What we do know is that a woman has a higher-than-normal chance of experiencing pre-eclampsia if any of following are true:

- It is her first pregnancy;
- She is younger than 19 or older than 40 years;
- She experienced preeclampsia in a prior pregnancy;
- Other women in her family have experienced preeclampsia;
- She is exposed to a superabundance of chorionic villi due to carrying more than one fetus or trophoblastic disease;
- She entered pregnancy with chronic hypertension, renal disease, or diabetes; or
- She has an Rh incompatibility with the fetus (Gilbert and Harmon, 1998; Burrow and Duffy, 1999).

### HELLP Syndrome

The **HELLP syndrome** is a condition of liver dysfunction during pregnancy marked by **hypertension, elevated liver** enzymes, and low platelets. It occurs in 2% to 12% of women with preeclampsia, most commonly in the third trimester of pregnancy. The woman has elevated transaminase levels and may experience subcapsular bleeding or hepatic rupture. HELLP syndrome can be a devastating illness, as the rate of mortality for the mother increases to 15% and perinatal mortality can be as high as 60% (Gilbert and Harmon, 1998).

Some of the women (10% to 20%) with HELLP syndrome maintain a normal blood pressure. Liver function may become impaired, resulting in hemorrhagic necrosis with right upper quadrant tenderness or epigastric pain, nausea, and vomiting. The elevated liver enzymes occur as the liver tissue becomes necrotic. Hyperbilirubinemia (jaundice) may develop as a result of the hemolysis of red blood cells.

## Clinical Presentation

***Preeclampsia/Eclampsia.*** Clinical manifestations of PIH are the classic triad of the following:

* Hypertension,
* Proteinuria, and/or
* Edema.

Systemic changes are manifested through clinical signs as the disease progresses. Pulmonary edema and respiratory distress are indications of pulmonary involvement. Central nervous system involvement is indicated by hyperreflexia (i.e., reflexes +4 with clonus) or severe, unrelenting headaches. Ophthalmic involvement creates visual disturbances (e.g., photophobia, blurring, or double vision). Alterations in hemostatsis may cause blood in the urine, bruising, and oozing from open wounds. Occasionally the coagulation system is inappropriately activated, and DIC develops. Hepatic involvement is indicated by right upper quadrant pain or epigastric pain and indicates that eclampsia is impending (Gilbert and Harmon, 1998).

***HELLP Syndrome.*** Women with the HELLP syndrome may experience the following:

* Epigastric pain or right upper quadrant tenderness,
* Nausea and vomiting,
* Headache,
* Nonspecific malaise jaundice, or
* Hematuria.

Women experiencing HELLP may have frank hypertension but many women demonstrate only a slight diastolic elevation. Perinatal morbidity and mortality are high with HELLP syndrome with mortality cited between 7.7% to 60% (Sabi 1990; Gabbe, Neibyl, and Simpson, 1996). Complications resulting from HELLP include maternal death, liver hematoma and rupture,

cerebral edema, renal failure, abruptio placenta, DIC, and pulmonary complications. Management for women experiencing HELLP follows similar patterns to the management of severe preeclampsia.

### Nursing Assessment

There is no specific diagnostic test available to detect preeclampsia. The signs and symptoms of hypertension, proteinuria, and edema are what lead to its detection. The most reliable diagnostic symptom is the rise in blood pressure.

***Hypertension.*** Measurement of maternal blood pressure should begin with positional considerations. Supine positioning results in supine hypotension and is not an appropriate position for assessing maternal blood pressure. Postural considerations are also important; with standing, both systolic and diastolic pressures are elevated (i.e., over sitting values). In lateral positions, hydrostatic pressure changes can affect maternal blood pressure readings.

Recommendations for measuring maternal blood pressure include having the woman sit with her right arm supported at approximately heart level or in a semi-reclining position (with adequate uterine displacement) (Gabbe, Neibyl, and Simpson, 1996). Consistency in maternal positioning is critical to ensuring accurate blood pressure measurements. The Korotkoff phases IV and V should be recorded because phase IV is 5 to 10 mm Hg higher than phase V (Gabbe, Neybiel, and Simpson, 1996).

If a woman has documented normotension in early pregnancy, the diagnosis of hypertension is easier to discern. The criteria for hypertension is one of the following:

* Systolic blood pressure $\geq$30 mm Hg or diastolic blood pressure $\geq$15 mm Hg from the normotensive readings.
* A reading of $\geq$ to 140/90 mm Hg after 20 weeks of gestation.

If the woman's prior blood pressure readings are unknown and she presents with a reading of 120/75 mm Hg at 25 weeks of gestation, this may appear to be normal. However, many young women have mid-pregnancy blood pressures as low as 90/60 mm Hg. Failure to appreciate that this woman may be experiencing hypertension with the 122/76 mm Hg reading is one reason that early diagnosis of preeclampsia is missed (Burrow and Duffy, 1998).

Also be aware that the hypertension associated with preeclampsia can vary widely from moment to moment, so two successive readings may be very different. The elevation in blood pressure must be sustained for two documented incidents with at least 6 hours between measurements.

*Mean Arterial Pressures (MAP).* The MAP should be calculated.

$$MAP = Systolic + (Diastolic \times 2) \div 3$$

A MAP value of 90 to 100 is considered normal. A MAP of 105 or higher or an increase of 20 or more is indicative of hypertension.

*Proteinuria.* The amount of protein excreted by a woman with preeclampsia may vary greatly, from barely abnormal to frankly nephrotic amounts. Proteinuria is diagnosed if one of the following occurs:

- If there is >0.3 g (300 mg) of protein per liter of urine in a 24-hour urine specimen.
- If random urine specimens are used, there should be > 0.1g (100 mg) of protein per liter in two or more random urine specimens collected at least 6 hours apart. The specific gravity must be 1.030 or less and the pH less than 8.
- If a dipstick is used, the reading is +2 or greater (Gilbert and Harmon, 1998).

The evaluation of urine for protein can be a false positive reading if the following are true:

- Vaginal discharge, blood, amniotic fluid, or bacteria get into the sample.
- The urine is alkaline or very concentrated (specific gravity > 1.030).

The evaluation of urine for protein can be a false negative reading if the following is true:

- The urine is dilute (specific gravity < 1.010) (Gilbert and Harmon, 1998).

Other assessments for renal function include monitoring the woman's weight, intake and output, specific gravity of her urine, and her blood urea nitrogen and creatinine levels.

*Edema.* Because edema is present in normal pregnancies, its presence is not definitive in diagnosing preeclampsia. Also, its absence does not mean that the woman is not preeclamptic. Some women experience what is called a dry preeclampsia, in which there is an absence of edema (Burrow and Duffy, 1999).

Monitor the presence of edema by evaluating whether it is dependent or generalized and the degree of pitting present. Monitor the woman's respiratory status, listening for breath sounds, the presence of rales, or shortness of breath. Observe her neck veins for distention.

Pathologic edema is indicated by the following:

- Nondependent edema of the face, hands, or abdomen that is nonresponsive to 12 hours of bed rest, or
- A rapid weight gain of more than 2 pounds in 1 week (Gilbert and Harmon, 1998).

*Fetal Assessment.* Fetal assessment is initiated when the diagnosis of PIH is confirmed or at between 24 to 28 weeks of gestation for women with preexisting hypertension. Alterations in uteroplacental blood flow create a threat to the growth and proper oxygenation of the fetus. Specific fetal surveillance techniques may include serial ultrasound to assess fetal growth patterns; biophysical profile; doppler flow studies; amniocentesis for lung maturity; contraction stress test; non-stress testing; and fetal movement counts.

*Diagnostic Tests.* There are diagnostic tests for specific body systems affected by PIH that are used to evaluate the severity and progression of the condition and the mother's response to the treatment. These tests may be ordered individually in response to specific symptoms or as a group (Table 17-9).

---

**TABLE 17-9** *Summary of Diagnostic Tests Affected by Pregnancy-Induced Hypertension*

| Condition evaluated | Diagnostic test | Significant finding |
|---|---|---|
| Kidney involvement | BUN (blood urea nitrogen) | >10 mg/dl |
| | Creatinine | >2 mg/dl |
| Reduced blood volume | Hematocrit | >40% |
| Disseminated intravascular coagulopathy (DIC) | Fibrin split products (FSP) | >40 μg/ml |
| | Platelet count | <100,000/mm³ |
| | Bleeding time | Prolonged |
| | Fibrinogen | <300 mg/dl |
| Uteroplacental involvement | Biophysical profile (BPP) | <8 |
| | Amniotic fluid index | <8 cm |
| Fetal lung immaturity | Lecithin/sphingomyelin (L/S) ratio | <2 |
| | Phosphatidyl glycerol (PG) | Not present |
| Hepatic involvement | Albumin | <2.5 |

Gilbert E and Harmon J: *Manual of high risk pregnancy and delivery,* ed 2, St Louis, 1998, Mosby.

## Possible Nursing Diagnoses

Nursing diagnoses will generally focus on the woman's knowledge and comfort, identifying a support system that allows her to receive the necessary treatment and rest while preventing complications as a result of her condition. Possible diagnoses are as follows: Fear related to lack of predictable outcome for self or fetus, Altered role performance due to hospitalization for treatment, Fluid volume excess related to pulmonary edema, Altered maternal tissue perfusion related to disease progression, and Risk for injury related to disease progression causing injury or aspiration if a seizure develops. With regard to the fetus, there is a Risk for impaired fetal gas exchange related to the effect of the disease on uterine blood flow.

## Expected Outcomes

It is expected that with the proper treatment, the woman's hypertension, edema, and/or proteinuria will be controlled. The fetus will have an adequate supply of oxygen and nutrients, and the placenta will stay intact. The ultimate goal is delivery of a mature, healthy infant, without compromising the woman's health.

## Possible Interventions

Birth is the definitive therapy for preeclampsia. When the disease occurs after the pregnancy has progressed to at least 36 weeks of gestation and fetal lung maturity is confirmed by a lecithin/spingomyelin (L/S) ratio of 2:1 in the amniotic fluid, birth is the treatment of choice. The hypertension of preeclampsia usually resolves with the first few days after delivery.

The disease often develops when the fetus is less than 36 weeks of age and the fetal lungs are immature, so the severity of the disease and the maturity of the fetus must be considered in determining when delivery should take place. If the HELLP syndrome develops or there are signs that the woman may develop eclampsia or her physical condition is worsening, immediate delivery of the fetus is virtually mandatory—no matter the gestational age— because the life of the mother is now of concern (Gilbert and Harmon, 1998).

Preeclampsia is usually categorized as mild or severe before the course of treatment is determined (Table 17-10). This may give a false sense of predictability, however, as women with mildly elevated blood pressure and even minimal proteinuria can rapidly progress to eclampsia (Burrow and Duffy, 1999).

*Mild Preeclampsia.* Conservative strategies are recommended for management of mild preeclampsia with no signs of deteriorating renal or hepatic function or coagulopathy. Aggressive monitoring of the woman and her fetus for progression of the disease must be maintained, either through home health care or frequent office visits. Research indicates that when a woman becomes normotensive with no significant proteinuria, similar outcomes occur with home management as with in-patient hospital care (Gilbert and Harmon, 1998) (Box 17-6).

*Severe Preeclampsia.* When it is necessary to administer antihypertensive therapy to maintain maternal blood pressure in a safe range, hospitalization is required. Inpatient care allows easier monitoring of the progression of the disease and rapid intercession if complications arise. Hospitalization also enables the status of the fetus to be frequently evaluated with nonstress testing, ultrasonography, and the development of a biophysical profile.

*HELLP.* Because the laboratory abnormalities of the HELLP syndrome can quickly reach life-threatening levels with profound thrombocytopenia and extremely elevated levels of hepatic enzymes, most obstetricians choose immediate delivery.

*Activity Restriction.* One of the first recommendations often given to a pregnant woman with hypertension is bed rest. The lateral recumbent position facilitates venous return by taking the gravid uterus off of the inferior vena cava. By increasing the circulating volume, the renal blood flow increases and the process of diuresis is enhanced. This may drop the woman's blood pressure and increase blood flow to the fetus. Women may also benefit from taking a rest period in the middle of the day and sleeping 8 to 9 hours each night.

Even though there may be benefits to reclining, determining how much of the day the woman should be lying down is controversial. There is no scientific research that supports the effectiveness of continuous bed rest when compared with the negative physical and psychologic effects of bed rest. In addition, if a woman is employed outside her home or has other children to care for, she may not be able to comply with this directive and feel guilty.

Documented physical effects of bed rest include the following:

* Skeletal muscle atrophy starts within 6 hours with the greatest progression in 3 to 7 days

| TABLE 17-10 | Comparison of Mild and Severe Preeclampsia | |
| --- | --- | --- |
| | **Mild** | **Severe** |
| Blood pressure | | |
|   Systolic | 140-160 mm Hg | >160 mm Hg |
|   Diastolic | 90-110 mm Hg | ≥110 mm Hg |
| Proteinuria (24 hr) | 0.3-4 g | ≥5 g |
|   Dipstick | +2/+3 | +4 |
| Urinary output | >30 ml/hr | <20 ml/hr |
| | >650 ml/24 hr | <500 ml/24 hr |
| Pulmonary edema | Not present | Can be present |
| Subjective signs | Not present | Can be present |
| HELLP syndrome signs | Not present | Can be present |

Adapted from Gilbert ES and Harmon JS: *Manual of high risk pregnancy and delivery,* ed 2, St Louis, 1998, Mosby.

## BOX 17-6    Home Health Care for Mild Preeclampsia

**CRITERIA SELECTION**

Blood pressure less than 150/100 mm Hg sitting and less than 140/90 mm Hg in the left lateral position

Proteinuria less than 500 mg/day

Platelet count more than 125,000/$\mu$l

Normal liver enzymes: AST less than 50 U/L; ALT less than 50 U/L; LDH less than 200 U/L

Serum creatinine less than 1.32 mg/dl

Reassuring fetal status with no intrauterine fetal growth restriction

No worsening signs present

A compliant patient

A reliable patient

**HOME CARE PROTOCOLS**

Limited home activity with 12 hours of sleep each night and rest periods during the day to facilitate renal and placental perfusion by mobilizing the movement of extracellular fluid back into the intravascular space

Balanced diet containing at least 60 to 70 g of protein; 1200 mg of calcium; adequate zinc and sodium (2 to 6 g); and 6 to 8 glasses of water per day

Blood pressure checked every 4 to 6 hours daily while awake

Daily weight at the same time each day

Urine for protein using first-voided specimen of the day

Instructed as to worsening signs and symptoms that should be reported immediately:

  Headaches

  Changes in vision

  Epigastric pain or RUQ pain

  Increased edema

  Vaginal bleeding or changes in vaginal discharge

  Severe abdominal pain

  Sudden gush of fluid

Home health nurse visits two times per week with daily telephone contact

Weekly prenatal visits

Initial and frequent diagnostic laboratory assessments

  Creatinine clearance

  Serum creatinine

  Serum uric acid levels

  Platelet count

  Hematocrit

  Serum albumin

  Liver enzymes

Fetal surveillance

  Daily fetal movement charts

  Frequent evaluations with BPP, CST, NST, and/or AFI

  Fetal growth by ultrasound every 3 weeks

Hospital admission for worsening status

*AST,* Aspartate transaminase; *ALT,* alanine transaminase; *LDH,* lactate dehydrogenase; *RUQ,* right upper quadrant; *BPP,* biophysical profile; *CST,* contraction stress test; *NST,* nonstress test; *AFI,* amniotic fluid index.

Developed from information in Grohar J: *J Obstet Neonatal Nurs* 23(8):687-694, 1994.

From Gilbert ES and Harmon JS: *Manual of high risk pregnancy and delivery,* ed 2, St Louis, 1998, Mosby.

- Weight loss despite reduced activities and increased caloric intake
- Plasma and volume decrease by approximately 7% of body weight
- Increased blood coagulation
- Increased heartburn and reflux
- Decreased cardiac output and stroke volume
- Increased glucose intolerance and insulin resistance
- Bone demineralization
- Muscle volume loss of more than 25% during 5 weeks of bedrest
- A lengthened postpartum recovery period due to loss of cardiovascular and muscle strength (Maloni and Kasper, 1991; Maloni, 1993; Goldenberg and others, 1994; Knupple and Drukker, 1993; Schroeder, 1996, 1998; Gilbert and Harmon, 1998).

Negative psychologic changes that may develop when a woman is placed on bed rest are as follows:

- Anxiety
- Depression

- Sensory disturbances
- Feelings of loss of control
- Reduced self-esteem
- Feelings of helplessness (Kemp and Page, 1986; Hales and Johnson, 1990; Maloni and Kasper, 1991; Mandeville and Troiano, 1992; Knupple and Drukker, 1993; Rich, 1996; Gilbert and Harmon, 1998).

Activity restriction, bed rest, and hospitalization also bring socioeconomic challenges to a woman and her family. These challenges center around the following:

- Social isolation due to displacement from family and community of origin
- Financial burden resulting from treatment costs and loss of income
- Alterations in preexisting patterns of personal and family functioning (Loos and Julius, 1988; Brown, 1997; Sather and Zwelling, 1998).

Because studies of outcomes for the newborn do not show improvement and some studies suggest deleterious physical and psychologic effects, the recommendation for expensive, prolonged antenatal home or hospital bed rest must be implemented cautiously (Gilbert and Harmon, 1998).

**Diet.** All pregnant women should eat a nutritious and balanced diet and drink 6 to 8 (8-oz) glasses of water or nutritious fluids per day. Restricting fluid intake to less than 64 ounces per day, unless the woman has a specific medical condition, can actually decrease the blood supply to the placenta. A diet high in protein, at least 60 g per day, will be therapeutic in replacing the protein lost in the urine and will also help pull the fluid from the intracellular spaces back into the circulatory system. Adequate calcium (1200 mg), magnesium, and vitamins are also important. Calcium supplementation has demonstrated initial benefit in research literature (Enkin, and others, 1995).

No evidence exists to recommend salt restriction for pregnant women with PIH. In general, instruct women to salt food to taste. An excessive intake (>6 g daily) will cause increased vasoconstriction and an inappropriate level of dietary sodium (<2 g daily) can reduce the blood volume and decrease placental perfusion. Only women with preexisting hypertension or other systemic conditions requiring a sodium-restricted diet before pregnancy should be advised to maintain their limited salt intake during pregnancy (Enkin and others, 1995; Gilbert and Harmon, 1998).

**Water Therapy.** In the presence of severe edema, research has demonstrated that shoulder-deep immersion in water can mobilize extravascular fluid; initiate diuresis; and decrease blood pressure. Therefore water therapy may be helpful in slowing the progression of preeclampsia (Gilbert and Harmon, 1998).

**Pharmacologic Therapy.** The goals of pharmacologic therapy center on the reduction or prevention of seizure activity and the stabilization of maternal blood pressure to achieve a diastolic reading of 90 to 100 mm Hg. Specific pharmacologic treatment may include the following: antihypertensive agents, anticonvulsants, sedatives, and diuretics. If delivery of the fetus is required, stimulants for development of fetal surfactant will be given.

**Anticonvulsive Therapy.** Magnesium sulfate is the drug of choice, in the United States, for prevention and management of seizures with preeclamptic and eclamptic women. Even though it is not an established anticonvulsant, clinical trials have demonstrated its superiority when compared to either phenytoin (Dilantin) or diazepam (Burrow and Duffy, 1999).

**Magnesium sulfate** ($MgSO_4$) is a neuromuscular blocker that blocks the release of acetylcholine at neuromuscular junctions and diminishes irritability of muscle fibers. In addition, magnesium sulfate reduces prostacycline production, causing smooth muscle relaxation and vasodilation, which increases blood flow to the

**TABLE 17-11   Serum Magnesium Levels**

| Magnesium levels (mEq/L) | Magnesium levels (mg/dl) | Interpretation |
|---|---|---|
| 1.5-2.5 | 1.7-2.1 | Normal |
| 4-7 | 5-8 | Therapeutic |
| 8-10 | 10-12 | Loss of deep tendon reflexes |
| 13-15 | 16-18 | Respiratory paralysis |
| 15-20 | 18-25 | Heart block |
| 20-25 | 25-30 | Cardiac arrest |

Data from Heppard M and Garite T: *Acute obstetrics: a practical guide,* St Louis, 1996, Mosby.

From Gilbert ES and Harmon JS: *Manual of high risk pregnancy and delivery,* ed 2, St Louis, 1998, Mosby.

uterus and can cause a transient drop in blood pressure for 30 to 45 minutes.

The dosage is an initial bolus of 4 to 6 grams by IV push over 15 to 20 minutes. A maintenance dose of 2 to 3 g/hr diluted in 5% dextrose and lactated Ringer's solution is administered via a continuous infusion pump. The medication dose is titrated based on the woman's response.

Although seldom done because the rate of absorption cannot be controlled and tissue necrosis may occur, the maintenance doses may also be given intramuscularly. The normal dosage is 5 g per buttock or a total of 10 g every 4 hours using Z-track technique with a 3-inch, 20-gauge needle. Because the injections are painful, a local anesthetic may be added to the magnesium sulfate solution. The site should be gently massaged to facilitate absorption.

Prepare the woman for the normal side effects of lethargy, sensations of heat or burning, headache, nausea and vomiting, blurred vision, and constipation. Excretion of magnesium sulfate is through the renal system; therefore if the woman is experiencing reduced output, her serum levels will become elevated. As serum magnesium levels rise, the neuromuscular and cardiac transmission of nerve impulses is increasingly blocked, causing a loss of deep tendon reflexes (DTR), the first sign of toxicity. Other early signs are nausea, a feeling of warmth, flushing, somnolence, double vision, slurred speech, and weakness. A continuing rise can lead to respiratory paralysis, heart block, and cardiac arrest (Table 17-11).

Assess any woman receiving magnesium sulfate for early signs of toxicity. If the woman is receiving the drug through an IV, her respirations, pulse, and blood pressure should initially be checked every 5 minutes and then every 15 to 30 minutes and her DTR should be checked every hour. If she is receiving intermittent therapy, her respirations, pulse, blood pressure, and DTR should be checked before each dose.

Monitor output closely because the magnesium is primarily excreted in the urine. If the woman is receiving continuous IV therapy, her output should be at least 30 ml/hr. When she is receiving intermittent therapy, her urinary output is measured over a 4-hour period and should be at least 120 ml over 4 hours.

To decrease the woman's risk of developing pulmonary edema, also monitor her input. Her total intake of fluids should not exceed 2000 ml within a 24-hour period.

Discontinue or withhold the magnesium sulfate and contact the physician if any of the following signs occur:

* A sudden change or loss of deep tendon reflexes
* Respirations <12 breaths/min
* Urinary output <30 ml/hr or 120 ml over 4 hours
* A significant drop in pulse or blood pressure
* Signs of fetal distress (Gilbert and Harmon, 1998).

Calcium gluconate is an antagonist for magnesium toxicity and should be readily available at the bedside of a woman receiving magnesium sulfate. Ten milliliters of a 10% solution (1 gram) is administered—generally by the physician—by IV push slowly over 3 minutes. If administered too rapidly, calcium gluconate can cause vasodilation, bradycardia, dysrhythmias, and ventricular fibrillation. It may also be administered intravenously at a rate of 1 g/hr if needed. The side effects of calcium gluconate include tingling, loss of flushing, transient decrease in blood pressure, and hypercalcemia.

The fetus experiences parallel side effects to the mother receiving magnesium sulfate. The maternal serum levels are indicative of the potential effect experienced by the fetus.

*Antihypertensive Therapy.* Hydralazine (Apresoline) is the most common agent used to reduce a diastolic blood pressure of more than 110 mm Hg or a systolic blood pressure greater than 180 mm Hg and decrease the risk of a CVA. Hydralazine is favored because it is most effective in reducing mean arterial pressure but does not affect uteroplacental blood flow in an adverse manner. When hydralazine is ineffective, labetalol hydrochloride (Normidyne), nifedipine (Adalat), or verapamil (Apo-Verap) may be used (Cunningham and others, 1997).

The dosage for hydralazine (Apresoline) is 5 to 10 mg by IV push over 10 minutes. The dose may be repeated every 15 to 20 minutes until the diastolic blood pressure is between 90 and 100 mm Hg. The diastolic pressure should not be allowed to fall below 90 mm Hg, or the blood flow to the placenta will be compromised. Hydralazine may be readministered whenever the diastolic blood pressure reaches 110 mm Hg. Side effects include headache, faintness, dizziness, tachycardia, palpitations, numbness, or tingling of the extremities (Gilbert and Harmon, 1998).

Assess the woman's blood pressure every minute for the first 5 minutes after administration and then every 5 minutes for the next 30 minutes. If an automatic blood pressure cuff is available, use it.

No adverse fetal or neonatal effects have been documented, but the drug is excreted in breast milk so if the baby is born the woman should not start breast-feeding until 48 hours after she received the last dose of medication.

Chronic hypertension is present in approximately 4% to 5% of all pregnant women, and 21% of these women develop preeclampsia (Gilbert and Harmon, 1998). All pregnant women with chronic hypertension must be taught the signs and symptoms of placenta abruption and be continuously monitored for superimposed preeclampsia. Antepartal fetal assessment in a woman with a history of chronic hypertension begins at 28 to 30 weeks of gestation as the risk of IUGR increases.

The first response to treat chronic hypertension is periodic bed rest of 45 minutes in the middle of the day and 1 hour before the evening meal (prepared by someone else) to promote uterine blood flow. A regimen of tapering and stopping hypertensive medication is usually tried simultaneously (Zuspan, 1996). When the diastolic pressure exceeds 90 to 100 mm Hg or there is left ventricular hypertrophy, however, drug therapy is initiated. The woman is usually given **methyldopa** (Aldomet), a centrally acting adrenergic inhibitor (Gabbe, Neibyl, and Simpson, 1996). For oral administration 250 to 500 mg are given 2 to 3 times a day and may be increased every 2 days as needed. The usual maintenance dose is 500 to 2000 mg/day administered in divided dose usually twice a day. If it is given intravenously, the dosage is 250 to 500 mg diluted in 100 ml of solution and infused over 30 to 60 minutes every 6 hours for a maximum dose of 1000 mg every 6 to 12 hours. Maternal side effects include sedation, decreased mental alertness, nasal stuffiness, orthostatic hypotension, bradycardia, diarrhea, and dry mouth. No fetal or newborn effects have been documented (Knupple and Drukker, 1993).

Monitor the woman's pulse and blood pressure frequently during the initial dose adjustment and periodically throughout the course of therapy. Monitor intake and output. Monitor weight and assess for edema daily. Assess the woman for depression or other alterations in her mental status. Monitor her temperature, especially at the beginning of therapy because a drug fever may occur shortly after the initiation of therapy. Notify the physician of any significant changes.

Alternative hypertensive drugs used to treat chronic hypertension during a woman's pregnancy are either beta-blockers or calcium channel blockers. Beta-blockers are labetalol (Trandate), atenolol (Tenormin), or pindolol (Visken). Nifedipine is a calcium-channel blocker.

*Stimulation of Fetal Surfactant.* If the fetus is of less than 34 weeks of age and the L/S ratio is less than 2, corticosteroids and thyrotropin-releasing hormones may be given to decrease the risk of neonatal respiratory distress. If the mother has diabetes or hypertension, the use of the steroids can aggravate the disorder. Betamethasone (Celestone) or dexamethasone is usually given as they cross the placenta unchanged, with betamethasone the favored drug. The dosage is two doses of 12 mg 24 hours apart. Forty-eight hours after the first dose, the full effect on maturing the surfactant is reached. Be sure that the woman gives informed consent for the medication and understands that this is preparing her baby for imminent delivery. Monitor the mother for infection. If she has diabetes be sure that she receives her insulin and has her blood sugar levels evaluated frequently for hyperglycemia. Closely monitor the fetus for signs of compromise.

***Sedatives.*** Sedatives are no longer used in the treatment of preeclampsia because they may mask the woman's ability to report symptoms. In addition, the fetus may experience CNS depression (Gilbert and Harmon, 1998).

***Diuretics.*** Unless the woman is experiencing heart failure, diuretics are no longer used. Research has shown that diuretics further decrease blood flow to the placenta by decreasing blood volume, disrupt the normal electrolyte balance, and create further stress on already compromised kidneys (Gilbert and Harmon, 1998).

***Information for Future Pregnancies.*** Because the cause of PIH is unknown, it has been difficult to determine ways to prevent it. There are several possibilities, however, that may be shared with the woman. Water therapy is being explored as a possible intervention to prevent the development of preeclampsia. Shoulder-deep immersion has been found to decrease levels of renin, angiotensin, aldosterone, and vasopressin.

Low-dose aspirin therapy (i.e., with acetylsalicylic acid [ASA]) is being used in research to reduce the development of PIH (Enkin and others, 1995; Gabbe, Neibyl, and Simpson, 1996). ASA inhibits thromboxane production, making the maternal vascular system less sensitive to vasopressors. Therefore it decreases blood pressure, mean arterial pressure, and the occurrence of proteinuria. The dosage used in the research was 60 to 81 mg/day (baby aspirin). One risk associated with ASA therapy now being investigated is an increased occurrence of placental abruption in women receiving aspirin (Gabbe, Neibyl and Simpson, 1996). When higher ASA dosing schedules are used, there is an increased occurrence of premature closure of the ductus arteriosus and the potential for maternal hemorrhage and newborn complications. These complications were not reported with the low dose schedule.

Calcium supplementation has been associated with a reduction in the development of PIH in low-risk women and women at risk for PIH (Lopez-Jaramillo 1990; Sanchez-Ramos, 1994). Calcium supplementation may be a preventative strategy. The doses of elemental calcium ranged from 1500 to 2000 mg/d (Gabbe, Neibyl, and Simpson, 1996 ).

### Evaluation

When PIH is detected, the woman may be overcome by the precautions she is given and the series of tests she must undergo. Assess the woman's understanding of her condition and treatment plan. Have her explain how she will implement the necessary actions or restrictions and monitor the status of her condition. Measure the degree to which she is supported by her support network. Determine the level of anxiety being experienced by the woman and her support network because of her condition. Does she understand the implications of her condition for her baby? Does she understand the signs and symptoms that indicate that she needs immediate medical assistance and can she reach emergency care if needed? Does she understand the implications for future pregnancies?

### Summary

The ultimate goal of nursing care for a pregnant woman with hypertension is to minimize the risks and potential complications. When the woman and her family understand her condition and have the support to provide the required self-care and follow the appropriate disease management program, the outcome of the pregnancy may be positive for the mother, the infant, and the family.

## Alterations in Amniotic Fluid Volume

Amniotic fluid volume gradually fluctuates over the course of pregnancy. The volume peaks at approximately 34 weeks of gestation, plateauing at approximately 750 ml until 38 weeks. Then it gradually declines at a rate of 8% per week, averaging only 400 ml at 40 weeks. Knowledge of these alterations in volume assists in the interpretation of fundal height and fetal growth patterns, as the gestation advances. Alterations in normal amniotic fluid volume can be associated with potential problems related to the fetus.

### Amniotic Fluid Volume

Evaluating amniotic fluid volume is an essential yet difficult task. Because of the complex shape of the fetus within the uterus, direct calculation of the volume of amniotic fluid surrounding the fetus is impossible. Available techniques only allow an estimate to be made.

**Hydramnios,** which is also known as polyhydramnios, is a situation where more than the expected amount of amniotic fluid is present. There are two types of hydramnios: acute and chronic. With chronic hydramnios, the amount of fluid gradually increases during the pregnancy but does not become a problem until the third trimester. Acute hydramnios is usually diagnosed between 20 and 24 weeks of gestation, at which time the amount of fluid increases over the period of a few days.

Hydramnios can be associated with maternal disease and fetal complications but can also be idiopathic in nature. The increased amniotic fluid volume may be created by an alteration in the fluid exchange within the fetus and uteroplacental unit. Some of the maternal or fetal conditions that may cause this to occur are as follows:

- Diabetes may cause hydramnios by altering the osmotic pressure with higher glucose in the amniotic fluid or possibly from fetal hyperglycemia (Blackburn and Loper, 1992).
- Multiple gestation is also associated with hydramnios particularly when there are monochorionic twins sharing the same amniotic sac.
- Gastrointestinal anomalies of the fetus may interfere with fetal swallowing or obstruct amniotic fluid in the fetal gastrointestinal tract. Gastrointestinal anomalies associated with hydraminos are atresia of the esophagus or duodenum, diaphragmatic hernia, abdominal wall defects (omphalocele and gastroschisis), and bronchial or pleural masses and effusions.
- Neural tube defects, chromosomal deviations, and hydrocephalus may influence amniotic fluid production and the ability of the fetus to swallow, thereby altering amniotic fluid volume.

**Oligohydramnios** is less than expected amniotic fluid and predisposes the fetus to increased risk of perinatal morbidity and mortality. Reductions in the amount of amniotic fluid decreases the ability of the fetus to move freely without risk of cord compression or entrapment and to engage in fetal breathing, which is critical for respiratory development. When the fetus experiences restricted breathing movement, pulmonary hypoplasia (underdevelopment) may result. With oligohydramnios, the fetus is also placed at increased risk for fetal death and intrapartal hypoxia due to increased risk of cord compression/entrapment.

Factors associated with the occurrence of oligohydramnios include utero placental insufficiency, fetal anomalies—particularly renal, and premature rupture of the membranes.

### Clinical Presentation

*Hydramnios.* Hydramnios commonly presents as a discrepancy between fundal height and weeks of gestation or as accelerated uterine growth. The woman may be short of breath due to pressure on her diaphragm and have edema in her lower extremities due to pressure on the vena cava. On physical examination, the fetal parts may be more difficult to palpate and the fetal activity may be perceived by the mother as increased. Diagnosis is accomplished with ultrasound examination and evaluation of amniotic fluid index and fluid pockets. Amniotic fluid amounts over 1700 to 2000 ml in the third trimester or a fluid pocket of greater than 8 cm is considered to be hydramnios (Burrow and Duffy, 1999).

*Oligohydramnios.* Oligohydramnios presents as a less-than-expected fundal height. Diagnosis includes obstetrical history, with information for dating of pregnancy, information about membrane integrity, and an ultrasound to estimate amniotic fluid volume and measure fluid pockets. When there is less than 500 ml of amniotic fluid, it is considered oligohydramnios. Oligohydramnios is diagnosed during the third trimester when there is less than 300 ml of fluid or the largest vertical pocket of amniotic fluid visible on ultrasound is 5 cm or less (Burrow and Duffy, 1999).

### Nursing Assessment

Hydramnios should be suspected when the fundal height appears to be out of proportion with the gestational age. If there is excess fluid, it may be more difficult to auscultate the fetal heart rate. If there is a large amount of fluid (e.g., 2500 to 3000 ml), the abdomen may appear to be severely stretched and tight. If an ultrasound is performed, large spaces of fluid will be identified.

*Oligohydramnios.* Oligohydramnios may be suspected when the uterus is small for expected time of gestation, the fetus is easily palpable and outlined, and the fetus is not ballottable. The fetus may be assessed with a nonstress test, biophysical profiles, and serial ultrasounds.

### Possible Nursing Diagnoses

Because of the increased size of the uterus with hydramnios, the woman will experience more discomfort than usual. She will also have concerns about her body and the health of her developing baby. Possible nursing diagnoses are as follows: Pain related to size of uterus, Sleep deprivation related to physical discomfort, and Risk for impaired gas exchange related to pressure on diaphragm. Because of the smaller-than-expected size of the uterus with oligohydramnios and the ongoing assessment of the fetus, the woman may be concerned about the health of her baby. Possible nursing diagnoses are as follows: Fear related to uncertainty about outcome of the pregnancy and Anxiety related to health of baby.

### Expected Outcomes

During the pregnancy, the woman and her family will understand the condition she is experiencing. They will receive the supportive treatment necessary to relieve the woman's symptoms. They will be aware of the results of all diagnostic testing and the implications it has for their baby. If the fetus is diagnosed with a congenital defect while in utero, the family will receive the psychologic assistance it desires.

### Possible Interventions

*Hydramnios.* Care of the woman experiencing hydramnios centers around ongoing assessment and an expectant approach. If the amount of amniotic fluid causes the woman pain and difficulty breathing, hospitalization and removal of excess fluid may be required. This may be done with amniocentesis or artificial rupture of the membranes (AROM). If AROM is used, there is a risk for prolapsed cord.

Another method is to decrease fetal urine output. A prostaglandin synthetase inhibitor (indomethacin) crosses the placenta and decreases amniotic fluid by decreasing fetal urine output.

The distention of the uterus places the woman at risk for premature labor and delivery. Serial ultrasound evaluations of the amount of amniotic fluid assist in evaluation. Careful ultrasound evaluations for fetal anomalies—particularly gastrointestinal—and general patterns of fetal growth should be done. Anticipatory counseling for premature labor and fetal defects is a critical aspect of the plan of care.

*Oligohydramnios.* Management of oligohydramnios involves serial ultrasound assessment of amniotic fluid volume and careful assessment of fetal anomalies—particularly of the renal system. Another aspect of management is to elicit a careful history and physical assessment to rule out membrane rupture. Antenatal testing should be initiated to follow utero-placental exchange and cord entanglement. Intrapartal management may include amnioinfusion, which is the transvaginal infusion of saline to compensate for the lost amniotic fluid.

## Evaluation

When there is a variation from the normal amounts of amniotic fluid, the fetus is at increased risk. Assess the woman's understanding of her condition and treatment plan. Have her explain how she will implement the necessary actions or restrictions and monitor the status of her baby. Measure the degree to which she is supported by her support network. Determine the level of anxiety being experienced by the woman and her support network because of her condition. Does she understand the implications of the condition for her baby? Does she understand the signs and symptoms that she needs medical assistance and can she reach emergency care if needed? If the fetus has been diagnosed with a congenital defect while in utero, has the family received the assistance it desires?

## Summary

The ultimate goal of nursing care for a pregnant woman with an alteration in amniotic fluid is supportive treatment. The woman and her family must understand her condition, the test and procedures she must undergo, the implications of the diagnostic findings, and the possible outcomes of the pregnancy.

# Hemorrhagic Disorders of Pregnancy

The more common hemorrhagic complications of pregnancy are placenta previa, abruptio placenta, and DIC.

**Hemorrhage** in pregnancy is defined as a rapid loss of blood of more than 1% of body weight or 10% of blood volume. (1 ml of blood = 1 gram of body weight, so if a woman weighed 110 lbs, 500 ml of blood loss would represent hemorrhage.)

Blood flows through the uteroplacental circuit at a rate of 500 ml per minute. During the second and third trimesters, the total maternal blood volume flows through the placenta every 8 to 11 minutes. Any uterine hemorrhage provides the possibility of a potentially catastrophic event for the mother and fetus. In addition, breaks in the fetal-maternal placental circulation at any time during the gestational period can lead to the process of isoimmunization.

Maternal-fetal **isoimmunization** is the immunization of an individual against the blood of an individual of the same species. It is of particular concern during prenatal care when the blood type or Rh of the woman and fetus differ.

## Placenta Previa

**Placental previa** is an abnormal implantation of the placenta in which the placenta attaches to in the lower segment of the uterus. The incidence of placenta previa is 1 in 200 pregnancies (0.5%) (Gilbert and Harmon, 1998). The primary risk to the mother and infant is related to the potential threat for significant hemorrhage.

A woman has an increased chance of developing placental previa if she has experienced endometrial scarring, has impeded endometrial vascularization, or has an increased placental mass. Endometrial scarring may result from a previous low implantation; previous surgical deliveries, uterine curettage, or endometriosis; multiple pregnancies; or closely spaced pregnancies. Endometrial vascularization may be impeded by medical conditions such as diabetes or hypertension, smoking or drug use, or if the woman is over 35 years of age. If there is a large placenta or multiple placentas because of the presence of more than one fetus, there will be an increased placental mass, increasing the chance that part or all of the internal os of the cervix will be covered (Gabbe, Neibyl, and Simpson, 1996; Gilbert and Harmon, 1998).

The classification of the placenta previa is determined by the position of the placenta in relation to the internal os of the cervix. The categories are as follows:

* *Type I—Low Lying*: Placental implantation is the lower uterine segment lying next to but not reaching the cervical os. As the gestation advances and the lower uterine segment stretches, the part of the uterus to which the placenta is attached moves away from the os.
* *Type II—Marginal*: Lower placental edge reaches but does not cover the cervical os.
* *Type III—Partial*: Placenta partially covers the cervical os.

- *Type IV—Complete*: Placenta is centrally located over the cervix (see Figure 12-6).

### Clinical Presentation of Placenta Previa

A woman with placenta previa typically presents after 24 weeks of gestation with *painless* bright red vaginal bleeding and a relaxed uterus (Gabbe, Neybiel, and Simpson, 1996). The woman's vital signs may remain normal even in the presence of severe blood loss. She may not even exhibit signs of shock until after she has lost 30% of her blood volume. Hypovolemia and shock are two major concerns. Anemia and infection are two ongoing concerns even after the bleeding is stopped (Gilbert and Harmon, 1998).

Auscultating for the fetal heart or gentle palpation may find the fetus malpositioned, commonly in a breech or a high cephalic position. No digital vaginal examinations should be done if placenta previa is suspected. Diagnosis is with ultrasound. The fetal heart rate will remain normal unless there has been significant blood loss or major placental detachment. The greatest cause of fetal mortality is prematurity due to the need to deliver the fetus in order to stop the bleeding. If the bleeding is stopped and the pregnancy continues, the fetus is at risk for being small for gestational age and having congenital abnormalities and anemia.

Medical interventions are dependent on the type of previa the woman is experiencing, the gestational age of the fetus, and the extent of the bleeding. No vaginal examinations are performed due to the associated risk of disturbing the placental bed and precipitating a hemorrhage. Once a diagnosis of placenta previa has been confirmed by ultrasound, the initial management involves preventing or controlling hemorrhage. Laboratory testing may include a blood type and cross match in preparation for a transfusion.

Women who have a low-lying placenta and are stabilized are managed at home by visiting nurses and scheduled for a repeat ultrasound between 30 and 32 weeks to determine the status of the placenta. If the pregnancy is less than 36 weeks, the bleeding is mild (i.e., less than 250 ml) and the woman is not in labor, the women may be kept in an inpatient setting. The purpose is to allow the fetus to grow while providing immediate intervention if necessary. The woman will generally be put on complete bed rest for 72 hours and then bed rest with limited activity—usually bathroom privileges. If bleeding continues, pad checks are done every hour. IV infusions with a 16- or 18-gauge needle will provide fluids and/or blood products. If bleeding is minimal, a heparin lock may be left in place for emergency access. The uterus will be monitored for signs of preterm uterine contractions. If delivery within 48 hours is anticipated, betamethasone may be ordered to enhance fetal pulmonary maturity.

Fetal well-being will be monitored through continuous fetal monitoring or assessment every 4 hours with Doppler ultrasound or fetoscope. Weekly nonstress tests and biophysical profiles may be ordered.

Whether an abdominal birth or vaginal birth is recommended depends upon the extent of the placenta previa. A surgical, abdominal birth is indicated for a complete previa. A trial vaginal birth with a double set up for a surgical birth may be recommended for a marginal or partial placenta previa. Fetal surveillance is an ongoing process to assess fetal oxygenation and viability. Once the placental situation is stabilized, fetal surveillance will monitor growth.

### Placental Abruption

**Placental abruption,** or abruptio placentae, involves premature separation of an otherwise normally implanted placenta. The incidence of placental abruption is approximately 2% of all pregnancies. Placental separation occurs in varying degrees from a small segment to the complete sheering of the placenta.

The nature of bleeding also varies from concealed to overt hemorrhage (Cunningham and others, 1997). The condition is normally classified as mild, moderate, or severe or as Grade 1, 2, or 3 (Table 17-12).

The primary cause of abruptio placenta is hypertension, either PIH or chronic hypertension. Hypertension is more likely to produce a more severe abruption than other causes. Other related factors are trauma (motor vehicle accident or maternal battering), cigarette smoking (a factor in approximately 40%), use of cocaine/crack, an aggressive oxytocin (Pitocin) induction, uterine fibroids, chorioamnionitis, maternal malnutrition, maternal vascular disease, and vena caval compression. If a woman has experienced a previous abruption, she has a 5% to 17% of it occurring again. If she has had two abruptions, she has a 25% chance of it happening again (Gabbe, Neibyl, and Simpson, 1996; Gilbert and Hanson, 1998).

Maternal effects depend upon the cause and degree of hemorrhage. With blood loss, the woman may develop shock and DIC. An Rh negative mother may become sensitized. The woman is at risk for anemia, development of infection at the placental site, and a possible hysterectomy if the uterus does not contract.

The fetus is at risk for hypoxia due to uteroplacental insufficiency, prematurity if it must be delivered early, being small for gestational age due to inadequate nutrition from decreased placental profusion, and neurologic defects due to lack of adequate profusion.

### Clinical Presentation of Placental Abruption

Women present with placental abruption in a variety of ways. Vaginal bleeding is the first sign with most women. The major difference between an abruption and a placenta previa is the fact that the woman experiences some degree of pain.

TABLE 17-12   *Comparison of the Classification of Abruptio Placenta*

| | Mild: grade 1 | Moderate: grade 2 | Severe: grade 3 |
|---|---|---|---|
| Definition | Less than one sixth of placenta separates prematurely | From one sixth to one half of placenta separates prematurely | More than one half of placenta separates prematurely |
| Incidence | 48% | 27% | 24% |
| Signs and symptoms | Total blood loss less than 500 ml<br>15% of total blood volume<br>Dark vaginal bleeding (mild to moderate)<br>Vague lower abdominal or back discomfort<br>No uterine tenderness<br>No uterine irritability | Total blood loss 1000-1500 ml<br>15% to 30% of total blood volume<br>Dark vaginal bleeding (mild to severe)<br>Gradual or abrupt onset of abdominal pain<br>Uterine tenderness present<br>Uterine tone increased | Total blood loss more than 1500 ml<br>Greater than 30% total blood volume<br>Dark vaginal bleeding moderate to excessive<br>Usually abrupt onset of uterine pain described as tearing, knifelike, and continuous<br>Uterus boardlike and highly reactive to stimuli |
| Hypovolemia | Vital signs normal | Mild shock<br>　Normal maternal blood pressure<br>　Maternal tachycardia<br>　Narrowed pulse pressure<br>　Orthostatic hypotension<br>　Tachypnea | Moderate to profound shock common<br>　Decreased maternal blood pressure<br>　Maternal tachycardia significant<br>　Narrowed pulse pressure<br>　Orthostatic hypotension severe<br>　Significant tachypnea |
| Disseminated intravascular coagulopathy (DIC) | Normal fibrinogen of 450 mg/dl | Early signs of DIC common<br>Fibrinogen 150 to 300 mg/dl | DIC usually develops unless condition is treated immediately<br>Fibrinogen less than 150 mg/dl |
| Fetal effects | Normal fetal heart rate pattern | Fetal heart rate shows nonreassuring signs of possible fetal distress | Fetal heart rate shows signs of fetal distress and death can occur |

From Gilbert ES and Harmon JS: *Manual of high risk pregnancy and delivery,* ed 2, St Louis, 1998, Mosby.

The clinical manifestations are as follows:

- Dark vaginal bleeding (80%)
- Uterine tone varying from uterine irritability (frequent low amplitude contractions) to uterine hypertonicity and rigidity.
- Pain—from restlessness to acute sharp stabbing sensations.
- Fetal heart pattern may remain normal or show signs of fetal distress (e.g., a rising heart rate baseline, absence of accelerations, reduced variability rate, and late deceleration pattern) (Gabbe, Neibyl, and Simpson, 1996).

A woman with mild abruptio placentae (Grade 1) will have the symptoms develop gradually and have mild to moderate dark vaginal bleeding without uterine tenderness. Her vital signs will be stable, and the fetus will not have signs of distress. This type of abruption may be self-limiting or may progress to a higher grade.

A moderate abruptio placentae (Grade 2) can develop either gradually or abruptly. The woman will experience persistent abdominal pain (or backache if the placenta is implanted on the posterior side of the uterus) and visible dark vaginal bleeding. The uterus may be tender or firm. The woman may exhibit signs of shock. Fetal distress depends upon the degree of separation of the placenta.

Severe abruptio placentae (Grade 3) usually comes on suddenly, causing the woman excrutiating, unremitting abdominal pain. The woman may describe it as knifelike. The uterus may be boardlike and tender. There may or may not be visible bleeding. If the woman is experiencing what is known as a "silent abruption", the blood may be trapped behind the placenta. In this case, the uterus will be enlarging. The woman may go into shock, although the signs of shock may seem to be disproportionate to the amount of visible blood. The fetus will exhibit signs of distress or death.

Actual diagnosis is made through patient history, clinical examination and ultrasound, which may detect a retrograde clot formation at the placental site. However ultrasound is not always conclusive, as 50% of the occurrences of placental abruption are not evident on ultrasound (Gabbe, Neibyl, and Simpson, 1996). A laboratory test that may assist in the diagnosis is the Kleinhauer-Betke test to assess for fetal cells in maternal circulation.

Medical management is contingent upon the extent of the separation. Women experiencing mild abruption may stabilize and continue the pregnancy. If the woman is experiencing a moderate or severe abruption, aggressive intervention works to stabilize the mother and prepare for a possible delivery.

Initial management involves controlling the hemorrhage, maternal surveillance to assess placental integrity and maternal response to bleeding, and fetal surveillance to assess oxygenation. Laboratory testing may include a blood type and cross match in preparation for a transfusion.

Evaluation of coagulation status is an important aspect of care for the woman with a severe abruption. To conduct an inexpensive bedside test of coagulation, place maternal blood in an unheparinized blood tube and observe the length of time it takes to coagulate. If the woman has normal coagulation function, a clot should form within 6 minutes.

The extent of the placenta abruption will determine whether a surgical or vaginal birth is recommended. A surgical, abdominal birth is indicated for a total abruption. A trial vaginal birth with double set up for a surgical delivery may be recommended in other situations depending on individual circumstances. Concern is for blood loss and fetal distress. Initial management of the newborn involves resuscitation needs and managing infant hypovolemia.

## Disseminated Intravascular Coagulation (DIC)

DIC is an abnormal activation of the coagulation system resulting in widespread microcoagulation throughout the vascular system which leads to depletion of fibrin in the blood and generalized hemorrhage. There are two categories if DIC—slow and fast. Slow DIC occurs after there has been a fetal death in utero. The clotting cascade appears to be released in response to the decomposing fetus. Fast DIC may be caused by an amniotic embolism, abruptio placenta, or clostridial sepsis (*Clostridium welchii* organisms). DIC may also occur as a result of PIH and HELLP Syndrome, hydatiform mole, or trauma.

## Clinical Presentation of DIC

A woman with DIC presents with evidence of frank bleeding. Generalized bleeding may be evident in the form of oozing, bruising, and petechiae on any mucous membrane, from incisions, IV sites, or the gastrointestinal or genitourinary systems. Laboratory tests will demonstrate coagulation defects.

Medical management for DIC begins with identification of the trigger event. The trigger is removed or treated, blood volume is maintained, and the woman is protected from further injury.

## Isoimmunization

The two most common blood components that are incompatible are blood type and Rh factor. **ABO incompatibility** results when a mother's blood type is O and the fetus's blood type is either A, B, or AB. The problem occurs when the mother develops anti-A or anti-B antibodies that interact with antigen sites on the fetal blood cells. Treatment is not typically indicated during the antenatal period, but the newborn is assessed closely for the development of hyperbilirubinemia.

**Rh isoimmunization** occurs when an antigen-antibody reaction occurs due to the mixing of Rh-positive fetal blood with the negative maternal blood. The Rh positive cells trigger the Rh negative maternal cells to develop antibodies against the fetal Rh positive cells. The triggering event is most commonly birth, but Rh sensitization can also occur as a result of trauma, amniocentesis, abortion, any pregnancy-associated bleeding event, ectopic pregnancy, or random breaks in the fetal-maternal placental circulation at any time during any gestational period.

The initial exposure is what causes the sensitization process to occur. When exposure occurs, it becomes a problem—not so much for the fetus in this pregnancy, but fetuses in subsequent pregnancies. Then the maternal antibody response is rapid and the potential for hemolysis of fetal cells is great. There is no effect on the mother, but the fetus is at high risk for hemolytic conditions, fetal anemia, and erythroblastosis fetalis. The maternal antibody response becomes more powerful with successive exposures to the positive fetal cells, and the effects of isoimmunization worsen in each subsequent pregnancy.

The incidence of isoimmunization has decreased dramatically as a result of antenatal and postnatal $Rh_o$-D immunoglobulin administration after any event in which blood transfer may have occurred. This prevents maternal sensitization by developing a process of passive immunity. Antibody-mediated immune suppression is achieved when an antibody is passively administered and consequently blocks active immunization from occurring. The fetal cells are coated by the administered anti-D and blocked from the maternal antibody response. If the woman has already developed an antibody response, the $Rh_o$-D will be of no benefit.

When men are Rh positive, an Rh negative woman has a distinct possibility of carrying an Rh positive infant. Antenatal sensitization occurs infrequently with an incidence of 1% to 2%.

As a precaution, when the father of the baby is Rh-positive, antenatal administration of Rh immunoglobulin is indicated for an Rh-negative woman at 28 weeks of gestation in the event of any identified risk trigger and after delivery when an Rh-positive infant. Timing of administration should be within 72 hours of birth.

Once a woman has been sensitized, management during future pregnancies centers around careful and ongoing fetal surveillance for developing hemolytic disease. Interventions are based on accurate gestational dating and guided in part by maternal anti-D antibody titers. A maternal anti-D titre of less than 1:8 is followed with monthly titers and serial ultrasound. A maternal anti-D titre of greater than 1:8 should be managed with serial amniocenteses. The amniocentesis allows for serial determinations of bilirubin in the amniotic fluid. Bilirubin levels correlate with the severity of fetal hemolytic disease. Serial determinations are critical to evaluating the effect on the fetus during the pregnancy.

Estimation of fetal hemolysis is calculated using spectrophotometric analysis. These serial calculations are plotted against Liley's curve, which identifies the disease as being in one of three categories: Zone I, mild disease; Zone II, moderate disease; and Zone III, severe disease.

Fetal blood analysis, using fetal blood obtained through percutaneous umbilical cord sampling (PUBS), which is also known as **cordocentesis,** can be tested for blood type, fetal Rh, and hematocrit level. This technique can also be used to give blood to a fetus by intrauterine transfusion. The use of cordocentesis is done cautiously because it presents the risks of maternal-fetal hemorrhage, fetal distress, persistent bleeding at the puncture site, and infection.

Ultrasound is used to observe fetal growth and guide invasive testing, such as intrauterine transfusion. The timing of birth is determined by the estimated gestational age and the extent of hemolysis. Intrauterine transfusion may be attempted to extend the fetal gestational age.

## Nursing Assessment

When a woman presents with bleeding, we must immediately respond. The signs and symptoms of placenta previa, placenta abruption, and DIC have both similar and differing characteristics, as follows:

- Determine if the woman is in pain. If she is experiencing vaginal bleeding with no pain, it is probably placenta previa and a vaginal examination should not be done.
- After the twentieth week of gestation, if the woman is experiencing abdominal pain (constant or rhythmic) with or without bleeding, she is probably experiencing abruptio placenta.
- If the woman is bleeding from her gums and has petechiae, eccymoses, and hematomas with or without vaginal bleeding, she is probably experiencing DIC.

## Nursing Diagnoses

A woman experiencing a hemorrhagic disorder has multiple needs for nursing interventions. Nursing diagnoses will focus on her physical and emotional needs. Examples of applicable nursing diagnoses are the following: Fluid volume deficit related to excessive blood loss, Fear related to the threat of death, Pain related to collection of blood between the uterine wall and placenta (abruptio placenta), and Pain related to bleeding into joints and muscles (DIC). If the woman is put on bed rest or hospitalized, there may be the concern of Risk for diversional activity deficit related to imposed activity restrictions or Altered role performance related to prolonged hospitalization. With regard to the fetus, there is the concern of Impaired fetal gas exchange related to decreased uteroplacental oxygen transfer.

## Expected Outcomes

The goal is to recognize and control the hemorrhage, prevent sepsis and if possible, maintain fetal gas exchange, and avoid premature delivery.

## Possible Interventions

In cases where there is no bleeding or minimal bleeding, bed rest may be advised. If the woman is allowed to return home after evaluation and stabilization, she should be instructed to limit her activity and avoid douching and coitus because they increase her risk of uterine infection. She should also avoid enemas and sexual orgasm because these may stimulate labor contractions. Ideally, the woman should live within 15 minutes of emergency care and have a telephone and transportation and the constant companionship of another adult. Because this is not always possible, explore with her other options that will facilitate her safety. Teach her how to monitor the status of her baby with daily fetal activity or kick count records. If there is ongoing vaginal bleeding, be sure that she knows how to monitor the flow and when to seek assistance. If intrauterine growth restriction is suspected, a weekly NST or biophysical profile may be ordered. Ensure that she understands the importance of these tests and facilitate her ability to comply.

When the woman remains hospitalized, monitor her vital signs, fundal height, and uterine contractions or tetany. Monitor the fetal heart rate and rhythm and determine fetal position and degree of engagement. Measure the amount of vaginal blood loss by weighing perineal pads. Record the amount of blood loss (i.e., the weight of a saturated pad minus the weight of a clean pad) and the time the pad was in place, as well as the character of the blood. Administer the prescribed IV fluids and medications through a large-bore catheter—either 16- or 18-gauge. Monitor urinary output through the indwelling catheter and monitor fluid balance. Encourage appropriate and adequate hydration and nutrition by ensuring that culturally appropriate foods and beverages are available for her selection.

As soon as the fetus is mature, excessive bleeding occurs, active labor begins, or other complications (e.g., an amniotic infection, fetal anemia, or hemolytic condition) develop, the pregnancy will be terminated. Prepare the woman and her family for the surgical delivery. If the fetus is already dead or has anomalies incompatable with life, or if labor has progressed rapidly and the fetal head is engaged, a vaginal delivery will be performed.

On the rare occasions that the uterus fails to contract after the delivery, an immediate hysterectomy may be required. This will necessitate teaching and support for the woman post-surgery, as she adjusts to her sterilization. If the baby was lost, this will be even more difficult.

### Evaluation

When a hemorrhagic emergency is detected, the woman may be overcome by the bleeding and intensity of the emergency care that she is given and the series of tests she must undergo. Assess the woman's understanding of her condition and treatment plan. While she is hospitalized, assess her ability to maintain connections with her family members and friends. If she is stabilized and discharged home, have her explain how she will implement the necessary actions or restrictions and monitor the status of her condition. Measure the degree to which she is sustained by her support network. Determine the level of anxiety or fear that she and her support network are experiencing because of her condition. Does she understand the relationship between her condition and the survival of her baby? If the baby was lost, is she grieving effectively? Does she understand the implications of this emergency on future pregnancies?

### Summary

The ultimate goals in the treatment of hemorrhagic disorders are early recognition and appropriate intervention to prevent hemorrhage and its resulting complications. With appropriate diagnoses and care, the best outcomes for the mother can be provided during these potentially life-threatening situations.

## Pregnancies with Multiple Fetuses

Twin gestations are the most common form of multiple gestations. Monozygotic (identical) twins occur in 4 in 1000 pregnancies. Dizygotic (fraternal) twinning occurs in 3 in 1000 pregnancies in women under 20 years of age, increases to 14 in 1000 in women 35 to 40 years of age, and declines in incidence in women over 40 years of age (Chitkara and Berkowitz, 1996).

Monozygotic twins develop from one fertilized ovum and carry the same genetic material. They occur randomly across race and age. Dizygotic twins, which are no more similar genetically than siblings, develop from two different ova. They may appear more often following a woman's family line as the tendency to ovulate more than one ovum at a time can be passed from mother to daughter. The highest frequency for dizygotic twins is in women of African descent and the lowest is in Asian women.

This variation may be based in part on the historic treatment of women giving birth to more than one baby at a time. In many African cultures, these women were thought to have special powers and were honored. In Asian cultures, women who gave birth to multiples were thought to have been unfaithful to their partners and were killed. Sometimes the children were also killed. These historic practices increased the genetic pool for African woman who ovulated more than one ovum at a time and decreased the genetic pool for Asian women. Generations later, the effect may still be seen. A recent increase in multifetal pregnancies in the United States is attributed to advances in infertility treatment.

Monozygotic twins result when one egg is fertilized and divides into two distinct embryos. If the cell division occurs early, before 2 to 3 days, amniotic membranes develop as a two chorions and two amnions (Moore and Persaud, 1998). If cell division occurs after 3 but before 8 days, amniotic membranes develop as a single chorion and two amnions. If the split occurs between the 8th and the 13th day, the result is a single chorion and single amnion. Splitting that occurs between the 13th and 15th days results in conjoined twinning. Twinning will not occur beyond 15 days.

Diazygotic twins occur with the multiple ovulation and fertilization of separate ova. The result is distinct placental development with individual amnions and chorions. One variation that may occur with dizygotic twins results from the proximity of the placental implantations. If the implantations occur in close proximity, the placental units may fuse together but continue to maintain distinct circulation systems.

Perinatal morbidity and mortality are approximately three times higher in twin gestations than in single gestations (Chitkara and Berkowitz, 1996). The primary cause is low birth weight due to prematurity and/or intrauterine growth restriction. Pregnancy-induced hypertension, obstetric bleeding, anemia, and umbilical cord entanglement or twin-to-twin transfusions in monozygotic twins are also contributing factors.

Higher numbers of fetuses may be any combination of monozygotic and dyzygotic twins. For example, triplets may have originated from two ova. After fertilization, one of the embryos may have divided, making two of the triplets identical twins and the third a fraternal twin. Perinatal morbidity and mortality increase as the number of fetus increases.

### Clinical Presentation

Twins are suspected with clinical assessment of rapid uterine growth patterns and alterations in expected laboratory findings and diagnosed with ultrasound examination. Once identified, the woman is followed closely with an emphasis on prevention of intervening complications, such as premature labor and pregnancy induced hypertension. The infants are closely followed for growth and development patterns.

### Nursing Assessment

Nursing assessment for a woman carrying multiple fetuses is the same as for carrying one. The difference is that there are parallel assessments and charts for each of the developing fetuses. Due to the increased possibilities of maternal or fetal difficulties, prenatal appointments may be scheduled more frequently. The woman will be offered additional testing, such as serial ultrasounds, biophysical profiles, and non stress testing to follow fetal growth patterns and fetal well-being.

### Possible Nursing Diagnoses

A woman who expected to be adjusting to a pregnancy with one fetus can be overwhelmed when she learns that she has more than one. She will immediately be concerned about the effect this will have on her body and if she will be able to provide for them both in utero and after delivery. If she experiences complications, she will have the same concerns as other women with a high-risk pregnancy. Possible nursing diagnoses are the following: Anxiety related to providing sufficiently for two or more fetuses, Altered nutrition less than body requirements due to multiple fetuses, Body image disturbance related to early enlargement of uterus, Risk for sleep deprivation due to the enlarged size of the uterus, and Risk for altered role performance related to need for activity restriction due to size of uterus.

### Expected Outcomes

The woman will be guided and supported in her efforts to adequately sustain the growing fetuses. The fetuses will be monitored for growth and development and early identification of problems.

### Possible Interventions

Continuity of care is recommended for women with twin gestations. Due to the additional concerns and increased physical discomforts associated with the physiologic changes of a multiple pregnancy, women need consistent anticipatory advice and social support to promote their adjustment to a twin gestation. In addition, they must learn the signs and symptoms of a problem (i.e., PIH, placenta previa, fetal inactivity) with the pregnancy and know how and when to seek care.

***Selective Reduction.*** When a woman has multiple fetuses developing in her uterus, she may be faced with a decision about selective reduction. This is a process whereby the development of selected fetuses is stopped so that the remaining fetuses have a better chance of reaching an age of viability. The choice is most often presented to women who have three or more fetuses, often as a result of infertility treatments. The irony is that after spending time and money to become pregnant, the woman must now decide if she will terminate some of the fetuses. The choice is not an easy one. If she does have the reduction, the procedure may induce labor and she will lose all of the fetuses. If she does not have the reduction in fetuses, she has an increased risk of premature labor and not having any fetuses reach viability. This is a personal decision that must be reached over time and after careful consideration by the woman and her partner. Her personal view about abortion may influence her decision about whether to proceed with the procedure. Either way, the woman will require ongoing support that whichever decision she made was the right one for her.

***Nutrition.*** Women who are carrying multiple fetuses  must increase their nutritional intake to meet their developing needs. A balanced, nutritious diet, with more protein than a regular prenatal diet should be suggested. As the pregnancy progresses and the uterus presses on her stomach, the woman will resort to eating smaller, more frequent meals. During the third trimester, she may have to plan how to meet her nutritional needs for the day and then eat in a pattern of "grazing", such as is done at parties (i.e., taking a few bites of food at a time all day long).

***Exercise.*** Because the changes of pregnancy are felt earlier in a woman carrying multiple fetuses, movement and exercise can become a problem as early as the second trimester. Explore ways that the woman can maintain her strength and some degree of activity while still incorporating adequate rest periods.

***Assistance.*** Explore with the woman what her daily responsibilities are and how they might be adjusted as her pregnancy progresses. Determine who will be able to assist her as her uterus increases in size. Many women with twins go to full term with a very large uterus and healthy babies. This is facilitated when the woman is able to have someone take care of her as she focuses on "growing the babies."

***Preparation for Labor.*** Because a woman with multiples is more apt to experience an early onset of labor, she should be aware of the signs and symptoms that must be reported immediately. Her care will then be determined based on the length of her pregnancy.

Women may deliver their twins vaginally or by abdominal surgery or one each way. Women with more than two babies generally experience a surgical delivery. To prepare for the delivery, the woman should experience childbirth preparation during the second trimester, if possible with other couples who have multiples. This allows the parents to interact with others who are having a similar experience. Childbirth preparation during the second trimester also ensures that the woman is more comfortable and better able to move about and that the couple will be prepared if they experience an early onset of labor.

### Evaluation

Assess the woman's understanding of her condition, treatment choices, and treatment plan. Have her explain what is occurring and her options for care. Determine her success in freeing herself from her other responsibilities and implement the necessary actions or restrictions that her stage of pregnancies requires. Measure the degree to which she is supported by her support network. Determine if she understands the signs and symptoms indicating that she needs further medical assistance and that she can reach emergency care if needed. If one or more of the fetuses has died, has she started the grieving process and is she aware of community services that might help her and her family members?

### Summary

A pregnancy involving multiple fetuses is a pregnancy that requires us to provide a normal, supportive response while also being alert to the increased possibility that problems may arise. When a woman is pregnant with multiple fetuses, prenatal care becomes more complicated due to the size and position of the uterus and because multiple patients are involved. When the fetuses are developing, the safest environment is generally in the uterus. When the mother's uterus can no longer meet the needs of the fetuses, delivery may be necessary. If the infants are premature, one or more of them may be in a life-threatening situation. Families benefit from assistance in dealing with these life and death concerns.

## EXPECTANT CARE FROM THE HOME TO THE HOSPITAL

A woman with a high-risk pregnancy may manage her entire pregnancy in her home with periodic visits to her health care provider or assessments and interventions provided by home health care nurses. Hospitalization may only occur for short-term crisis management, or it may be for a prolonged period. Home care has the advantage of reducing the effect of separation on the family, as well as reducing costs.

Expectant care of a woman experiencing a high-risk pregnancy requires careful assessment, therapeutic interventions, and anticipatory guidance and support. Assessment skills incorporate physical, nutritional, and psychosocial dimensions. Therapeutic interventions center around the particular underlying medical or obstetrical complication. Interventions may include urine testing, blood pressure assessment, fetal heart rate monitoring, contraction monitoring, physical assessment, obtaining

blood specimens, medication monitoring or administration, and weight assessment (Dineen and others, 1992).

Anticipatory guidance, education, and referral are also significant aspects of providing care in the home setting. Referrals to home health care aides, child care assistance, childbirth educators, doulas, and social service agencies are all of possible relevance for high-risk women.

### Bed Rest

The research evidence supporting the efficacy of bed rest as a therapeutic intervention in most high-risk pregnancies is unsubstantiated; in fact, more evidence exists suggesting that it is harmful rather than beneficial (Maloni and Kasper, 1991; Maloni and others, 1993; Goldenberg and others, 1994; Knupple and Drukker, 1994; Schroeder, 1996, 1998). The reality remains, however, that many obstetric texts recommend bed rest and it continues to be a pervasive clinical practice in management of high-risk pregnancies.

When ordered, compliance with bed rest is another facet of the bed rest controversy. Research has demonstrated that the rate of noncompliance to prescribed bed rest is 30% to 50% (Monahan and DeJoseph, 1991; Josten and others, 1995). Women's reasons for not engaging in prescribed bed rest included not perceiving the need for bed rest, no family support to aid compliance, needing to care for children or families, and employment demands. When women are counseled to include bed rest into a therapeutic plan, they should have the opportunity to understand the evidence substantiating that recommendation. With the lack of evidence supporting beneficial outcomes from bed rest with many high-risk pregnancy conditions, women should be offered a choice as to whether or not they would choose to incorporate such a recommendation and, if so, how and to what degree they will be able to participate.

### Prolonged Bed Rest and Hospitalization

Management of high-risk pregnancy often incurs long-term hospitalization and confinement to bed. Displacement from familiar surroundings coupled with disruption of prolonged hospitalization leaves these women experiencing anxiety and sadness at a time that is normally accompanied by joy and fulfillment of dreams (Brown, 1997). Prolonged hospitalization and confinement to bed places these childbearing women at high risk for developing serious physical health threats including thrombophlebitis, pulmonary emboli, and bone and muscle degeneration (Maloni and Kasper, 1991; Knupple and Drukker, 1994). The potential for side effects of bed rest developing is directly related to the degree of activity restriction (Maloni, 1993; Crowther, 1995; Schroeder, 1996, 1998).

## Assessment of Activity Levels

Maternal and fetal surveillance is the most fundamental reason for caring for a woman in the hospital for a prolonged period of time. Assessment centers on the underlying medical or obstetric condition, intervening complications, side effects of bed rest, and fetal response to the intrauterine environment. Interventions are then directed by the specific assessment findings.

Care of the woman on extended periods of bed rest should also assess and incorporate a plan of activity levels that are appropriate for her (Figure 17-1). This will reduce her potential for physical complications due to prolonged bed rest. A collaborative activity plan should be developed and incorporated into daily aspects of care for each antenatal woman based on the underlying medical or obstetrical complication requiring hospitalization.

The addition of appropriate range of motion exercises with the consultation of physical therapy is one way to help reduce the physical effects of bed rest. The research literature does not address activity interventions for pregnant women and offers no specific guidelines to date.

## Assessment of Psychologic/Social/Economic Needs

There are substantial psychologic, social, and economic ramifications of high-risk pregnancy and prolonged bed rest for families. Therapeutic approaches within the psychosocial and economic domain include engaging a doula, stress-reduction activities, assistance with child care referrals and household management, and referral to social services to assist with financial and employment concerns.

Assessment of the family's adaptation to the high-risk pregnancy and need for alteration in lifestyle is a critical aspect of high-risk antenatal care. An assessment will gauge the degree of disruption and reorganization that will be needed to accommodate the high-risk pregnancy. Internal coping mechanisms and family coping should be explored. The plan of care can then incorporate appropriate referral and mobilize external resources.

A "High-risk assessment form" can facilitate care planning. This assessment tool should be completed early in the woman's admission to the inpatient setting and provide the basis for the individual plan of care and educational plan. The assessment tool can also provide a mechanism for considering the multidimensional needs of this client group, thereby facilitating the development of a holistic intervention strategy.

### Diversional Activities

Include diversional and recreational activities in an attempt to mediate the boredom that occurs during prolonged hospitalizations. Materials for crafts, games, and

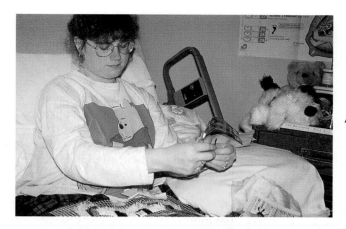

**A**

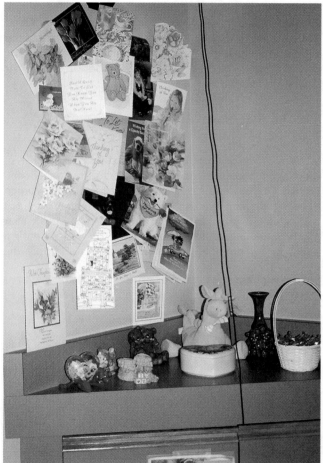

**B**

FIGURE 17-1 • **A,** Bed rest with restful activities during a high-risk pregnancy. **B,** If the woman must be hospitalized during the prenatal period, encourage her to personalize the environment. *(Courtesy of Caroline E. Brown.)*

puzzles can provide creative activities for the woman and help to pass time during a hospital stay. Reading and video materials can also provide diversional opportunities. The creation of a journal or diary, memory books, or a calendar can be incorporated to not only facilitate the woman's time orientation but also express her emotions, concerns, and anxieties during the stressful events of hospitalization.

An antepartum fun or resource cart with educational and diversional materials can centralize materials and provide the woman with choices as to what she would like to do. The materials and money to establish and maintain an "antepartum fun cart" can be solicited from hospital vendors with an interest in maternal and newborn health, as well as from hospital, church, and community groups.

Establish social networks to mediate the social isolation experienced by women displaced from their families. Volunteers from university, church, and community groups can provide a schedule of visiting and facilitate diversional activities. Depending upon the interest and skills of the individual volunteers, they can maintain actual contact with women on a weekly basis, provide phone contact, and/or participate in opportunities for diversional activities (Box 17-7).

## Maintaining Normalcy and a Woman-Centered Approach

Women's time orientation during bed rest in a high-risk pregnancy becomes focused on the future (Schroeder, 1996). This emphasis on passage of time allows women to set goals for getting through the pregnancy. Each week that the pregnancy continues reflects a hurdle that has been achieved. The goal of care for women with a high-risk pregnancy centers around maintaining the pregnancy until fetal maturity is achieved, which is often 36 to 37 weeks of gestation (Brown, 1997). Fetal development timelines provide a mechanism for women to see how their baby is developing and record events that are significant to them.

While she is hospitalized, a woman's patterns of daily life are surrendered and replaced with schedules imposed by the inpatient hospital environment. The inpatient environment is structured to meet the needs of the health care providers. Women experiencing prolonged hospitalization should be encouraged to request alterations in the schedule to help them establish more personal patterns. Simple alterations may begin with the routine, early morning waking; perhaps the woman can sleep to a time that is more normal for her or return to sleep after the early assessment before the 7AM shift change. Breakfast can be kept for her in the unit kitchen. Unless absolutely necessary, there will be no interruptions in sleep during the night. Small changes such as these will contribute to the woman's needed rest and can make a significant difference in her ability to cope with the hospital experience (Brown, 1997).

Creating an environment that is more homelike is another easy to implement strategy (Brown, 1997). Provide for the woman's privacy. She may want to be alone for part of the day or be assured that she and her partner will not be interrupted when visiting. If respected by all members of the health care team, a simple habit of knocking before entering and posting signs on doors requesting a period of privacy will help. Orientation of the bed to be able to see out a window is important for some women. The ability to see the natural progression of the day can be reassuring. Family and pet photos can be placed on walls. Music is important to some women, and a portable stereo is easily accommodated into the inpatient setting. The use of personal clothing and the changing of clothes for the days' activities and nights' sleep have been identified by women as additional ways to normalize the hospital experience (Box 17-8).

## ● ACUTE OR CRISIS CARE IN THE HOSPITAL SETTING

When the woman must be moved to acute care during a crisis period, it creates high levels of tension for

---

**BOX 17-7** *Suggestions for Diversional Activities for Women and Their Families*

Beautician visits
Wheelchair trip to an outside location or cafeteria
Crafts or Art work
Needle work
Crocheting
Journaling
Photo Journal of experience
Games
Crossword puzzles
Reading
Audiotaped music and books
TV with a VCR
Videotapes
TV-based games
Volunteer visitation programs
Scheduled group interaction time (e.g., a mother's tea)

---

**BOX 17-8** *Creating a Personal Space*

Personal clothing from home
Personal mementos and pictures from home
Private time in room
Changing the position of the bed in the room
Obtaining a private room
Playing of personally selected music

the woman, her family, and health care providers (Mandeville and Troiano, 1992). Women quickly experience a loss of their anticipated pregnancy and birth experience. Some women feel as if they have failed in performing a very basic feminine process. Women and their families are suddenly faced with technology and terminology, as well as providers, that are unfamiliar to them. Health care providers, operating in a crisis mode, quickly organize and manage the environment without realizing how unfamiliar and scary this is to the woman and her family. The environment in high-risk care may appear chaotic to parents who see many strangers suddenly converging on them, asking questions, and performing assessments. This type of environment is anticipated and seems normal to the team of providers but is frightening to the expectant parents. The continuous presence of one person with the woman can provide security, answers to questions, and anticipatory guidance will help alleviate or reduce parental fears.

---

## BOX 17-9   CPR in Pregnancy: ABCs

**AIRWAY**

Determine unresponsiveness.

Call for help.

Position on firm, flat surface.

Displace uterus manually or with wedge under one hip.

Perform open airway head tilt (i.e., chin lift).

**BREATHING**

Look, listen, and feel.

If absence of breathing is noted, give two slow breaths (1 to 1.5 seconds long).

If unsuccessful, reposition and attempt ventilation again.

***If foreign body obstruction***

Chest thrusts—not subdiaphragmatic thrusts—are used when doing the Heimlich.

**CIRCULATION**

Feel for carotid pulse.

If pulses are absent, begin external chest compressions. Rate 80 to 100/min.

- Reassess after every fourth cycle.
- If it is one-person CPR, the ratio of ventilation to compressions should be 2:15.
- If it is two-person CPR, the ratio of ventilation to compressions should be 1:5.
- If CPR is with an intubated client, compressions and ventilations are asynchronous and respirations are at a rate of 12 to 15 per minute.

Adapted from the American Heart Association: *Basic Life Support: heart saver guide*, Dallas, 1993, The Association.

---

## Maternal Resuscitation

### Cardiopulmonary Resuscitation (CPR) during Pregnancy

The functional mechanism of CPR is that blood flow and perfusion are produced by phasic fluctuations in intrathoracic pressure. CPR is achieved by direct compression of the heart between the sternum and spine, creating a pumping motion (AHA, 1993) (Box 17-9).

The process of CRP is affected by pregnancy due to the fact the gravid uterus mechanically compresses the vena cava and the aorta, causing diminished venous return and increased intrathoracic pressure. This has the most pronounced effect when the woman is in the supine position. In pregnancy, apnea results from rapid increases in $PaCO_2$ and decreases in PH and $PaO_2$, predisposing the mother to acidosis (Box 17-10).

The mechanism of arrest will determine the drug therapy to be initiated (AHA, 1993). The mechanisms of arrest are as follows: respiratory arrest, ventricular fibrillation, ventricular tachycardia, bradyarrhythmia, electromechanical dissociation (EMD), or asystole. Advanced life support treatment strategies include the following: defibrillation, endotracheal intubation, IV access, and medications. Common drugs used in a resuscitation effort may include epinephrine hydrochloride, lidocaine hydrochloride, bretylium tosylate, atropine sulfate, and sodium bicarbonate.

The route of medication administration is typically via a central vein because medications administered via a peripheral vein may take up to 300 seconds to reach a central artery. The intratracheal route also provides rapid uptake to central circulation. The medication is diluted in normal saline mix and administered via the endotracheal tube. The lungs are hyperinflated for 5 to 10 breaths for dispersal following medication administration.

---

## BOX 17-10   Complications of CPR in Pregnancy

**MATERNAL COMPLICATIONS**

Laceration of the liver

Uterine rupture

Hemothorax

Hemopericardium

Preterm labor

**FETAL COMPLICATIONS**

Dysrhythmia (due to maternal drugs and defibrillation)

Asystole

CNS depression (due to antidysrhythmic drugs)

Fetal distress (due to maternal oxygenation deficit)

Preterm delivery

The immediate focus of resuscitation is on maternal survival efforts. If it is evident that the mother is not responding well to resuscitative efforts, the infant's survival becomes the focus of the resuscitation and a **postmorteum or agonal cesarean delivery** is done. On occasion, the maternal response to resuscitation improves after the infant's birth.

The personnel to provide aggressive neonatal resuscitation should be present. The infant is at high risk for metabolic acidosis. Treatments including intubation, medications, umbilical line placement, and infant CPR are highly likely. A critical factor determining fetal survival is the length of time after maternal death (since onset of cardiopulmonary arrest). If it is less than 5 minutes, the chance of fetal survival is excellent; if it is between 5 and 10 minutes, the chance of fetal survival is good; if it is between 10 and 15 minutes, the chance of fetal survival is fair; if it is between 15 and 20 minutes, the chance of fetal survival is poor; and if it is between 25 and 25 minutes, the chance of fetal survival is unlikely.

Maternal and fetal care after successful resuscitation continues to require critical care expertise. The focus of maternal care is assessment, monitoring, and management of underlying cause of cardiopulmonary arrest. The focus of fetal care centers around determining the fetus's viability and gestational age (Box 17-11).

---

### BOX 17-11   *Maternal-Fetal Care after Successful Resuscitation*

**MATERNAL CARE**

**Cardiovascular System**
Cardiac output
Pulses
Hemodynamic monitoring
Vital signs
EKG
Skin color and temperature
Capillary refill

**Pulmonary System**
Oxygenation
Breath sounds
Character of respirations
Blood gases

**Neurologic System**
Level of consciousness
Glascow coma scale

**Obstetric System**
Uterine status
Vaginal bleeding
Membrane integrity

**FETAL CARE**

**Continuous Fetal Monitoring**
Baseline fetal heart rate, presence of accelerations, and presence and characteristics of decelerations

**Biophysical Profile**
NST, fetal tone, fetal activity, fetal breathing, and amniotic fluid volume

**Ultrasound Evaluation**
Amniocentesis
   Fetal pulmonary maturation
   Fluid character

---

## SURGICAL EMERGENCIES IN PREGNANCY

Surgical emergencies may be the result of an inflammatory process such as appendicitis, an obstruction in the intestines, or a traumatic injury such as a knife or gunshot wound.

### Medical Conditions Requiring Surgery

#### Appendicitis

Appendicitis is an inflammation of the vermiform appendix. The disease may be acute, subacute, or chronic. Surgery is usually required for acute appendicitis.

Appendicitis is the most common surgical emergency to occur during pregnancy, accounting for two thirds of all laparotomies in pregnant women. With a reported incidence of 1 in 1500 pregnancies, appendicitis can occur during any trimester. Because of the potential of fetal death if perforation occurs, it is important to have a high level of suspicion and an early diagnosis. The perforation rate is highest in the third trimester, when it is double that of the second trimester.

#### Intestinal Obstruction

Intestinal obstruction is the second most common nonobstetrical surgical intervention seen in pregnancy. The etiology of an intestinal obstruction is generally previous abdominal surgical incision. The incidence ranges from .0014% to .00054%.

#### Clinical Presentation

*Appendicitis.* A woman with a developing appendicitis may begin with vague, systemic complaints, such as nausea, vomiting, anorexia, and fever. Abdominal pain may be generalized or can be localized. Rebound tenderness is not a specific finding in pregnant women. Her temperature will be within normal limits, unless perforation has occurred.

After the third month of pregnancy, the appendix moves up the right side of the abdomen and reaches the level of the iliac crest by the sixth month. Given these changes, the woman may not feel the pain in the lower right quadrant but in some other location on the right side.

**McBurney's point** is a point in the lower right abdomen where pressure generally produces tenderness in acute appendicitis. As the gestational age of the pregnancy increases, this point shifts upward from the lower right quadrant.

To help determine the proper the diagnosis, Alder's sign can be used to differentiate uterine pathology from abdominal pathology. **Alder's sign** is elicited by localizing pain at the point of maximum intensity in the supine position and then repositioning the woman to the left lateral position. If pain decreases, it probably has a uterine cause; if it persists, it most likely has an abdominal cause.

In a nonpregnant woman with appendicitis, laboratory data will reveal an elevated white blood cell count (WBC), often over 18,000 cells/mm³. Since a pregnant woman may normally have a WBC count ranging from 6 to 16,000 cells/mm³ during pregnancy, an elevated WBC is not helpful in determining the diagnosis. Some women undergo ultrasound imaging to assist with the diagnosis.

***Intestinal Obstruction.*** If a woman is experiencing an obstruction of her intestines, clinical symptoms include nausea, vomiting, anorexia, constipation, and hyperactive bowel sounds.

### Nursing Assessment

Nursing assessment will focus on responding appropriately to a woman who reports signs and symptoms that may be the result of appendicitis or an obstruction. She needs an immediate consult with a physician to determine the cause of her nausea, vomiting, and pain. Focus on her ability to understand the tests that are necessary for determining her diagnosis; her level of anxiety with regard to the cause of her pain; who will provide her care before, during, and after her surgery; and possible concerns about how her baby will be affected by this medical emergency.

### Nursing Diagnoses

With a medical emergency such as appendicitis or intestinal obstruction, nursing diagnoses will focus on providing the woman with emotional and physical comfort while preparing her for medical interventions. Examples of possible nursing diagnoses are as follows: Pain related to inflammation in abdomen, Anxiety related to unidentified cause of pain, Fear related to effect of surgery on the development of the baby, and Impaired physical mobility related to abdominal surgery.

### Possible Interventions

Treatment for both acute conditions is surgical intervention. Because of the difficulty in determining that appendicitis is present in a pregnant woman, most large studies report a false laparotomy rate of approximately 20% to 35% for appendicitis. To prevent peritonitis, however, it is often determined to err on the side of caution and operate.

Premature labor may result from the surgery within the abdomen. However, the course of the pregnancy is generally not affected, and a vaginal birth is possible.

### Evaluation

Determine if a woman who reports signs and symptoms indicating the possibility of appendicitis or an obstruction understands the importance of further evaluation and her referral for care. Does she understand the tests that are necessary for determining her diagnosis? To what degree was her level of anxiety reduced? What arrangements were facilitated to provide her care before, during, and after her surgery? To what degree were her concerns about how her baby would be affected addressed?

### Summary

Appendicitis and intestinal obstruction place a pregnant woman in an emergency situation. Medical diagnosis of her problem and the necessary resolution are complicated by her pregnancy. Interventions require that she be prepared and supported as she faces uncertain diagnostic testing, surgery and a recovery period while maintaining her pregnancy and her role within her daily activities. The understanding and support of family members and friends is vital to her health and well-being.

## Traumatic Injuries that May Require Surgery

Trauma is the leading cause of maternal death during the childbearing years. The challenge is to determine the nature and extent of damage to the mother and fetus and provide appropriate care while dealing with the normal physiologic changes and risks caused by pregnancy.

The overall incidence of trauma during pregnancy is 7% (Huzel and Remsberg-Bell, 1996). The incidence of minor trauma increases as the pregnancy progresses, whereas the incidence of major trauma remains constant throughout the gestational period. The etiology of traumatic injury includes domestic violence, motor vehicle accidents (MVA), falls, burns, and shootings or stabbings. Maternal fatalities occur most frequently due to motor vehicle accidents or shootings.

The most common cause of fetal death is maternal death or sustained hypotension. Other causes are direct uterine trauma, abruptio placenta, hypoxia, pelvic fracture, and severe head injury.

### Blunt Non-Penetrating Trauma

Motor vehicle accidents are the most frequent cause of blunt, non-penetrating injury, followed by battering and falls. Ejection of the mother during a motor vehicle accident is associated with the highest rates of maternal and fetal morbidity and mortality. Head injury and internal hemorrhage are more frequent contributors to maternal mortality.

Blunt injury can also result from compression of the lap belt against the abdomen and from impact with the dashboard or steering wheel. Internal injury may also occur from organs hitting against the bony pelvis.

Potential damage includes a ruptured spleen or liver, anterior abdominal wall bruising, ruptured bladder, fractures in mother or fetus, and obstetrical complications. Rib fractures can increase the potential for respiratory compromise in a pregnant woman. When a woman sustains a fracture, there is a potential risk for infection and thrombosis due to coagulation changes in pregnancy.

There is a relatively high occurrence of placental abruption following both minor and major trauma, with the highest occurrence during the initial 48 hours following the accident. Abruptio placentae occurs when the placenta, a relatively fixed organ, shears away from the uterine musculature, an elastic structure.

Uterine rupture is a less commonly occurring obstetrical complication that results from blunt trauma. Women who experience a trauma that creates a uterine rupture typically also experience multisystem injury. Uterine rupture is caused by an abrupt increase in uterine pressure resulting from deceleration force during impact. With traumatic rupture, the fetal mortality rate is high especially if multisystem injuries are present.

Trauma may more easily lead to pelvic fractures in pregnant women. Hormonally influenced relaxation of the pelvic ligaments predisposes pregnant women to pelvic fracture, with the symphysis pubis a common fracture site.

Direct fetal injury is a less common occurrence, but intraventricular hemorrhage, skull fracture, and clavicular fracture have been reported. These occurrences are typically seen late in pregnancy when the fetal head is positioned within the confines of the bony pelvis.

A traumatic injury may cause maternal-fetal hemorrhage with the possibility of fetal anemia, distress, and potential for fetal maternal transfusion and Rh isoimmunization (Huzel and Remsberg-Bell, 1996). Fetal distress may occur as maternal blood pressure drops and uteroplacental blood flow decreases, resulting in oxygenation deficits to the fetus.

### Penetrating Trauma

Gunshot and stab wounds are the most common cause of penetrating injury seen in pregnancy. Stab wounds can cause maternal bowel and liver injury if the woman's upper abdomen is penetrated. If the abdomen is penetrated below the uterine fundus, the uterus and fetus are more prone to injury. When that happens, the outcomes for the mother are generally good because, the uterus and fetus act as a shield for the maternal internal organs.

Gunshot wounds are more common than stab wounds. Maternal outcomes are better than fetal outcomes when a woman is shot in the abdomen. Perinatal mortality rates range from 47% to 71%. The uterus and fetus again may shield the mother from sustaining a life-threatening injury.

### Clinical Presentation

Clinical presentation for any traumatic injury is directly related to the cause of the trauma. When a pregnant woman presents with a traumatic injury, it must be remembered that pregnancy alters the signs, symptoms, and clinical presentation. For example, shock may be present without expected clinical indicators due to the increased blood volume that occurs as a result of the physiologic changes associated with normal pregnancy. Hypovolemia is a common result of blunt or penetrating injury, however, the woman's vital signs may remain normal until up to 30% to 35% of her circulating blood volume is lost.

Pregnancy increases the complexity of the clinical presentation because fetal distress, premature rupture of membranes, premature labor, abruptio placenta, uterine rupture, DIC, and fetal distress are all potential complications.

### Nursing Assessment

Primary assessment of the mechanism of injury is vital, while simultaneously ensuring that a patent airway is maintained; breathing is assessed and controlled so that oxygenation and acid-base balance are maintained; and bleeding is controlled to maintain adequate circulation. If the woman is more than 24 weeks pregnant, evaluation of the fetus is also done immediately. Uterine contractions develop in 5% of women, but these usually stop spontaneously. If they do not, it can be a sign of abruptio placenta.

Once the woman is stable, provide a general review of systems and vital signs, assess skin color and temperature, auscultate heart and lung sounds, and observe chest wall motion and movement of extremities. Other assessments include medical and obstetric histories (Huzel and Remsberg-Bell, 1996).

Obstetric assessment include history; last menstrual period (LMP); estimated date of delivery (EDD), past labor and birth history; uterine size; membrane status; cervical status; and fetal activity. Obstetrical diagnostic approaches may include fetal monitoring and ultrasound.

### Possible Nursing Diagnoses

Nursing diagnoses for a woman who has received a physical trauma focus on immediate assessment and understanding of her condition and the implications it has on herself, her family, and the pregnancy. Once she is stable and out of danger, the woman's ability to implement the necessary self-care and follow the suggested regimen of activity will require guidance and appropriate referrals. In addition, anxiety and disturbances within her environment will be an ongoing concern. If the baby has been damaged or lost, grief work will be necessary for the woman and her family.

Examples of a nursing diagnoses are as follows: Decreased cardiac output related to hemorrhage, Risk for infection related to impaired skin integrity, Ineffective breathing pattern related to pain, and Impaired physical mobility related to broken leg. Other diagnoses may be developed that address the woman's fear of death, knowledge deficits related to her condition, concerns for her baby, concerns for her future fertility, concerns of family members about the survival of the woman and her baby, and the possible need for grief work.

Because the woman's injury may decrease the flow of oxygen and nutrients to the placenta, the status of the fetus is also of concern. An example of a diagnosis is Risk for altered tissue perfusion related to maternal hypovolemia from hemorrhage.

### Expected Outcomes

The expected outcomes are that the damage to the mother and/or her infant will be discerned in an emergent manner. Interventions will minimize the damage and, if possible, the pregnancy will continue. If the fetus is lost, the woman and her family will grieve the loss. If the woman losses her uterus and the prospect of future pregnancies, this loss will also be addressed.

### Possible Interventions

Aggressive maternal resuscitation improves the chances for the survival of both the woman and her fetus. Interventions for pregnant women with a traumatic injury, however, must be modified to accommodate the pregnancy. For example, careful attention to maternal positioning and the administration of medication must consider the possible effect on the fetus.

Initial stabilization of a pregnant woman follows the plan of "A," "B," "C," with the addition of a possible "D." It is ensuring an open *airway*, assessment of *breathing* and support, and *circulatory* support with control of known bleeding sites and prevention or management of shock. Assessment of the fetal heart may provide an indication of fetal distress due to abruptio placenta or death. Depending on the type of trauma, the fetus may have sustained a fracture or head injury. Evaluation of the fetus through auscultation, cardiotocographic monitoring or sonography may determine that surgical *delivery* is necessary. Two indications for emergent surgical delivery are as follows: (1) a distressed but live fetus if abruptio placenta or uterine rupture is suspected, or (2) a dying mother who is not responding to resuscitation efforts. Delivery may allow not only fetal rescue but also restoration of maternal venous return (Burrow and Duffy, 1999).

If the pregnancy is at more than 20 weeks of gestation, resuscitation is impaired because of the decreased venous return when the woman is placed in a supine position. The choice of supine positioning becomes a clear danger in pregnant women who require immobilization for a possible spinal injury after a motor vehicle accident. The danger becomes accentuated if the woman is experiencing a decreased blood volume because of hemorrhage.

***Blunt Trauma.*** Fetal maternal transfusion (FMT) is a risk after blunt abdominal trauma. "The Kleihauer-Betke test has been used to detect fetal hemorrhage into the maternal circulation, but its sensitivity is much less than the volume of fetal cells necessary to sensitize an Rh-negative mother with an Rh-positive fetus. As few as 0.01 ml of fetal red blood cells can trigger a maternal immune response; therefore it has been recommended that $Rh_o$ D immune globulin (RhoGAM) 300 $\mu$g, be given to all Rh-negative mothers without antibodies and without a known Rh-negative father who sustain abdominal trauma" (Burrow and Duffy, 1999). If the Kleihauer-Betke assay indicates that the fetus has transfused a large amount of its blood into an Rh-negative mother, the dose of $Rh_o$ D immune globulin may need to be increased in the proportion of 300$\mu$g/30 ml of fetal whole blood (Burrow and Duffy, 1999).

***Penetrating Trauma.*** If the woman has been knifed or shot, the entrance and exit sites will be located to determine the path of the knife or bullet. Further exploration will be immediately instituted if the woman's status is unstable, the gunshot wound penetrated the peritoneal cavity, the woman is eviscerating, or there are signs of peritoneal irritation.

If the woman is stable, it is assumed that the damage is localized and the wound is explored locally. This is also true of gunshot wounds that do not appear to penetrate the peritoneum. **Culdocentesis** (i.e., aspiration from the posterior vaginal cul-de-sac) and peritoneal **lavage** (i.e., washing of the cavity) are performed on all wounds of unknown extent or that penetrate the peritoneum to determine the presence and degree of internal bleeding.

When a woman is pregnant, the enlarged uterus is most often involved with a penetrating injury. Because of the low incidence of injury to other maternal organs, it is recommended that when the penetrating injury is below the uterine fundus, observation is the first course of action if the fetus does not appear compromised or is dead. If assessment of the fetus indicates that it may be injured, survival of the premature fetus is more likely in utero, unless it is in distress.

An exploratory laparotomy is recommended if the mother is unstable, the injury is above the fundus of the uterus, or there is evidence of maternal organ damage. A **hysterotomy** (i.e., surgical opening of the uterus) is only performed if fetal compromise is documented. Premature labor is a risk when uterine manipulation occurs.

## Evaluation

Assess the woman's understanding of her condition, treatment choices, and treatment plan. Have her explain what has occurred and the options for care. Determine her success in freeing herself from her other responsibilities and implementing the necessary actions or restrictions that her injuries require. Does she have the necessary options to increase her level of safety? Measure the degree to which she is supported by her support network. Determine if she understands the signs and symptoms that she needs further medical assistance and if she can reach emergency care if needed. If the fetus has been injured or died, has she started the grieving process and is she aware of community services that might help her and her family members?

## Summary

Traumatic injury is a situation that requires a rapid and supportive response. When a woman is pregnant, that response becomes more complicated due to the size and position of the uterus and because two patients are involved. When the fetus is premature, the safest environment for it is in the uterus. When the mother's uterus can no longer meet those needs, fetal death may be the outcome. Families benefit from assistance in dealing with these life and death concerns.

## Conclusions

Providing care to a woman experiencing a threat to her own health or her expected infant is a complicated task, yet one that can be very rewarding. The care the woman and her family receive will affect them for the rest of their lives as they remember those minutes or months that you collaborated with them to meet their physical, educational, and psychosocial needs.

## Care Plan · The Woman Experiencing Gestational Hypertension (PIH)

**NURSING DIAGNOSIS**   Risk for (or potential) complications of gestational hypertension: cerebral edema, coma, HELLP syndrome, pulmonary edema, renal insufficiency, fetal morbidity/mortality

**GOALS/OUTCOMES**   Will remain free of complications of gestational hypertension

**NOC Suggested Outcomes**
- Circulation Status (0401)
- Tissue Perfusion: Cardiac (0405)
- Tissue Perfusion: Cerebral (0406)
- Vital Sign Status (0802)
- Fluid Balance (0601)
- Urinary Elimination (0503)

**NIC Priority Interventions**
- Circulatory Care (4062)
- Cerebral Perfusion Promotion (2550)
- Respiratory Monitoring (3350)
- Fluid Management (4120)
- Risk Identification (6610)
- Fluid Monitoring (4130)

**Nursing Activities & Rationale**
- Identify women at risk for PIH. *The most effective therapy for PIH is prevention.*
- Obtain baseline maternal vital signs. *Must have baseline data for later comparisons to determine progression of disease and effectiveness of treatments. Hypertension is defined as a blood pressure greater than or equal to 140/90 mm Hg.*
- Monitor for weight gain. *Weight gain of more than 0.5 kg/week or sudden weight gain of 2 kg/week during the second or third trimesters is associated with PIH.*
- Monitor urine for protein. *Urine protein dipstick readings of 2+ or more are associated with preeclampsia. Severe preeclampsia is associated with dipstick readings of 3+ and 4+.*
- Monitor for distribution, degree, and pitting edema. *The presence of generalized fluid accumulation in the face, hands, or abdomen, that does not respond to 12 hours of bed rest is associated with preeclampsia. Dependent edema occurs in the lowest or dependent parts of the body. Pitting edema leaves a small depression following pressure applied to a swollen area.*
- Monitor lung sounds. *The presence of crackles may indicate pulmonary edema.*
- Monitor deep tendon reflexes. *Absence of DTRs is an early indication of impending magnesium toxicity (treatment for preeclampsia).*
- Monitor for signs of HELLP syndrome (platelet count less than 100,000/mm$^3$, elevated AST and ALT, intravascular hemolysis). *Early recognition of HELLP syndrome is essential in order to implement aggressive therapy and prevent maternal and neonatal mortality.*
- Monitor serum creatinine and blood urea nitrogen levels. *To determine the presence of renal compromise. As renal function becomes impaired, renal excretion of creatinine and other waste products, including magnesium sulfate, declines. When renal excretion declines, serum levels of creatinine, urea nitrogen and uric acid increase.*

# Care Plan · The Woman Experiencing Gestational Hypertension (PIH)—cont'd

- Monitor CBC, platelet count, clotting studies. *To determine the woman's potential for developing DIC, which is associated with a platelet count below 100,000/mm³.*
- Monitor liver enzymes (LDH, AST, ALT). *To determine the presence of HELLP syndrome.*
- Obtain baseline FHR. *Must have a baseline rate to use for comparison to determine effect of PIH and its complications on fetus. Uteroplacental perfusion is decreased in women with PIH, placing the fetus in jeopardy.*
- Monitor FHR frequently, noting variability in response to medications. *Fetal status is reflected in the FHR and pattern, which can change instantly.*

**Evaluation Parameters**
- Blood pressure within normal limits.
- CBC, liver enzymes, renal studies and coagulation studies within normal limits.
- Absence of peripheral, facial, and abdominal edema.
- Weight gain within normal limits for stage of pregnancy.
- FHR within 120 B 160 bpm with good baseline variability.

NURSING DIAGNOSIS  **Fear** related to lack of predictable outcome for self or fetus

GOALS/OUTCOMES    Will exhibit fear control (see "Evaluation Parameters")

**NOC Suggested Outcomes**
- Fear Control (1404)

**NIC Priority Interventions**
- Anxiety Reduction (5820)
- Coping Enhancement (5230)
- Security Enhancement (5380)

**Nursing Activities & Rationale**
- Assess woman's reaction to PIH and correct misconceptions. *To establish a baseline for care planning and determine the degree of intervention needed. Correcting misconceptions and supplying factual information may reduce fear and anxiety.*
- Assess the woman's understanding of the disease process. *To determine if teaching is needed. To allow for corrections of misconceptions.*
- Encourage verbalization of feelings, concerns and fears. *Verbalization of fears can help relieve them. Provides insight into the woman's individual needs.*
- Stay with the woman without requiring verbal interactions. *To promote feelings of security while fostering physical and emotional rest.*
- Explain all tests and procedures. *Knowledge can reduce fear and anxiety.*
- Provide reinforcement for use of positive coping strategies and relaxation techniques. *Such techniques allow the woman to gain control over her fears. Reinforcement increases the possibility that positive coping strategies, and relaxation will be used again.*
- Use a calm, reassuring approach. *To prevent transference of anxiety to the woman during stressful situations and to help the woman maintain control when feeling stressed.*
- Convey acceptance of the woman's perception of fear. *To encourage open communication with the woman regarding the source of her fear.*
- Encourage an attitude of realistic hope. *To help the woman deal with her feelings of helplessness by focusing on a positive but realistic outcome.*
- Reduce external stimuli in the environment. *To prevent external stimuli from increasing the woman's feelings of anxiety and to encourage rest.*

**Evaluation Parameters**
- Seeks information in order to reduce her fear.
- Uses relaxation techniques and positive coping strategies.
- Verbalizes fears and concerns freely.

NURSING DIAGNOSIS  **Altered role performance** related to need for tertiary management

GOALS/OUTCOMES    Demonstrates return to normal role performance

**NOC Suggested Outcomes**
- Coping (1302)
- Role Performance (1501)

**NIC Priority Interventions**
- Role Enhancement (5370)

*Continued*

## Care Plan  ·  The Woman Experiencing Gestational Hypertension (PIH)—cont'd

**Nursing Activities & Rationale**

- Assess current family situation and support systems. *To determine the ability of other family members to provide support and assume the woman's responsibilities during her illness.*
- Assist the woman in identifying her personal strengths. *Encourages the woman to focus on her abilities rather than her limitations.*
- Actively listen to the woman's concerns about her change in role. *Demonstrates concern and helps to establish trust between the woman and nurse.*
- Encourage the woman/family to verbalize their feelings about the woman's limitations. *Provides insight into the woman's/family's needs and allows the nurse to correct misconceptions.*
- Encourage the woman to accept dependence on others if necessary. *A woman needs to feel that it is okay to accept help from others in order to protect herself and her fetus.*
- Provide information about community resources as appropriate. *Ensures that the woman has the information necessary to access available community resources during her illness.*
- Explore with the woman how and when community resources will be approached. *The next step toward implementation is facilitated when the woman has assistance, time, and telephone access while still hospitalized.*

**Evaluation Parameters**

- Describes actual changes in function.
- Expresses willingness to use resources.
- Verbalizes feelings of usefulness and self-worth.

| | |
|---|---|
| NURSING DIAGNOSIS | **Knowledge deficit** regarding hypertension (PIH) management (e.g., Diet, medications, activity restrictions) |
| GOALS/OUTCOMES | Will adhere to dietary, medication, and activity restriction regimens |

**NOC Suggested Outcomes**

- Knowledge: Disease Process (1803)
- Knowledge: Diet (1802)
- Knowledge: Medications (1808)
- Knowledge: Prescribed Activity (1811)
- Knowledge: Treatment Regimen (1813)

**NIC Priority Interventions**

- Teaching: Disease Process (5602)
- Teaching: Prescribed Activity/Exercise (5612)
- Teaching: Prescribed Medications (5616)
- Teaching: Individual (5606)
- Teaching: Prescribed Diet (5614)

**Nursing Activities & Rationale**

- Teach the woman about her disease process and its potential effects on her and her developing fetus. *To enhance the woman's understanding, correct misconceptions, and gain compliance with prescribed therapies.*
- Teach the benefits of taking a rest period during the middle of the day and sleeping 8 to 9 hours each night, lying in the lateral recumbent position. *Facilitates venous return by removing the gravid uterus off the inferior vena cava. Increasing circulating volume increases renal blood flow and enhances diuresis, thereby lowering blood pressure. There is, however, controversy regarding the benefits of bed rest vs. the negative physical and psychologic effects of bed rest. Although bed rest is often one of the first recommendations given to a woman with PIH, there is no scientific research that supports the effectiveness of continued bed rest.*
- Teach the woman to drink 6 to 8 glasses (64 ounces) of water daily. *Inadequate fluid intake actually decreases the blood supply to the placenta.*
- Encourage a nutritious diet that is high in protein from a variety of available, affordable, and culturally acceptable sources. *To provide adequate vitamins and minerals and replace protein lost in the urine.*
- Teach the woman to avoid excessive intake of salt. *No evidence exists to recommend salt restriction in women with PIH. Excessive salt intake will, however, cause increased vasoconstriction, reduce blood volume, and decrease placental perfusion.*
- Prepare the woman regarding the side effects of magnesium sulfate therapy as appropriate (headache, sensations of heat or burning, nausea/vomiting, visual blurring, and constipation). *To reduce fear and anxiety should medication side effects occur.*

## Care Plan · The Woman Experiencing Gestational Hypertension (PIH)—cont'd

- Teach the woman about medication dosages and schedules and the need for adhering to prescribed medication regimens. *To ensure continued control of PIH and safety of mother and fetus.*
- Teach the woman about side effects of medications that need to be reported to the health care provider if they occur. *To detect side effects or toxicity in a timely manner so that the therapeutic regimen can be altered.*

### Evaluation Parameters
- Describes recommended diet.
- Selects foods recommended in diet.
- Describes need for increased fluid intake.
- Accurately describes medication dosage and schedule and side effects to be reported.
- Accurately describes benefit of lateral lying rest periods.

NURSING DIAGNOSIS   **Anticipatory grieving** related to possible effect of hypertension (PIH) on developing fetus
GOALS/OUTCOMES   Will express feelings of self-worth, productivity, and usefulness

### NOC Suggested Outcomes
- Coping (1302)
- Grief resolution (1304)

### NIC Priority Interventions
- Active listening (4920)
- Emotional support (5270)
- Grief work facilitation (5300)
- Hope instillation (5310)
- Support system enhancement (5440)

### Nursing Activities & Rationale
- Establish a trusting relationship. *Women must trust us in order to share personal concerns and feelings. Our demeanor and actions can facilitate or establish barriers to communication.*
- Provide positive affirmation of worth. *Focuses on strengths since the woman may feel that she is useless or of little worth if her illness compromises the life of her baby.*
- Encourage the woman to focus on what is known rather than what may occur. *To provide hope for a positive outcome. Focusing on what may happen rather than what is known increases anxiety.*
- Encourage the woman to identify her own strengths. *Focusing on those areas in which the woman feels in control will increase her sense of power over the current situation.*
- Assess the woman's knowledge of community resources. *Knowledge of available resources and how to obtain those resources increases the woman's feeling of power and/or control over her situation.*
- Assess the woman's comfort level with approaching community resources. *Knowledge of resources does not mean the woman feels comfortable approaching the service providers or participating in programs.*
- Assess the amount of emotional support provided by the woman's partner. *An adequate support system facilitates developmental tasks and adaptation; if partner support is not adequate, the nurse can make other recommendations for support.*
- Involve the partner and other family members (as woman desires) in care planning. *To strengthen family ties and provide emotional support for client.*
- Explain to her partner and family members how they can help. *Many times the partner and family members want to be helpful but need concrete suggestions for ways in which to do so.*

### Evaluation Parameters
- Relates fears and concerns about possible loss of baby.
- Client and partner express feelings freely with one another.
- Expresses optimism about outcome of current situation.
- Verbalizes self-acceptance and self-worth.
- Maintains eye contact.
- Communicates openly.
- The couple verbalizes realistic appraisal of their situation.
- The couple is involved in making decisions about treatment options.

# CASE STUDY

Tina is a 29-year-old G 2, P 1 who is 28 weeks pregnant. She works as a teller at a large bank to obtain health insurance for her husband and her 2-year-old daughter. She has come to the office because she has been experiencing periodic spotting of bright, red vaginal bleeding.

As you provide the initial assessment in the prenatal office, you determine that Tina is 5'4" and weighs 100 pounds. Her vital signs are within normal limits. She is experiencing no pain, and her uterus is relaxed. The position of the fetal heart is higher than expected. The fetal heart rate is regular.

- What do you anticipate may be causing Tina's symptoms?
- Until the cause of the bleeding is determined, what obstetric assessment technique must not be used?
- How will you respond to Tina's anxiety when she is told that she needs to be admitted to the hospital for further diagnosis and treatment?
- What will you say about the possible diagnostic techniques that may be used? How will you explain the laboratory testing that may be necessary?

The hospital nursing staff will then provide care.

- Once a diagnosis has been confirmed, what ongoing assessments will be necessary?
- What interventions will be used to prevent or control hemorrhage?
- What is the greatest risk to Tina? What is the greatest risk to Tina's baby?
- After the bleeding has stopped, what risks does the developing fetus still face?

- How may this medical emergency affect Tina's family?
- What may happen if Tina must miss work for an extended period of time?

Tina's condition is stabilized, and she is discharged home. A repeat ultrasound is scheduled for 32 weeks of gestation to monitor the status of the placenta. Weekly nonstress tests and biophysical profiles are ordered.

Sent out from the prenatal office, you will be doing daily home visits to Tina to monitor her status, as well as that of the fetus, and assess and intervene appropriately to the educational needs and emotional support required of the family. Anemia and increased risk of infection are two ongoing concerns even after the bleeding is stopped.

- Is early assessment of uterine contractions also necessary?
- What anticipatory guidance will assist Tina in her self-care?

Tina is told to stay off her feet and rest for the good of the fetus.

- What is difficult about the directive of this plan? What collaborative plan may be developed that Tina will be more able to achieve?
- What information do you need from Tina?
- What nursing diagnoses could apply? How will you validate these?
- What short-term goals might the two of you develop?
- What interventions may be possible?
- How will you evaluate the effectiveness of your interventions?

# Scenarios

1. Amie is a 28-year-old G 1 P 0 who is being seen in the office for a new prenatal visit. She has just moved from another part of the state and reports that she is 22 weeks pregnant. She has asked that her records be sent by her prior provider, but they have not yet arrived. While her past medical history is being taken, she reports that had scarlet fever at 9 years of age. This alerts you to possible complications that may occur in this pregnancy.

- What additional subjective data do you want to gather?
- What additional objective data may be required?
- What nursing diagnoses could apply? How will you validate these?
- What goals might be developed? How will these be prioritized?
- What interventions may you offer?

- How will you evaluate the effectiveness of your interventions?

2. Veronica, age 27, G 1 P 0, has just come to urgent care exhibiting difficulty breathing. She was diagnosed with asthma at the age of 10 and has successfully managed with self-care strategies and medication since that time. These are the first respiratory difficulties she has experienced since her pregnancy began 20 weeks ago. When you ask about her last use of her inhaler, she says, "I stopped using it when I got pregnant because I didn't want to hurt the baby."

- What additional subjective data do you want to gather?
- What additional objective data may be required?
- What nursing diagnoses could apply? How will you validate these?
- What goals might be developed? How will these be prioritized?
- What interventions may you offer?
- How will you evaluate the effectiveness of your interventions?

3. Sioban, a 31-year-old G 2 P 1, called 2 hours ago for an immediate appointment at the clinic because she is experiencing a 103° F fever, chills, nausea, and vomiting. When you do her admitting assessment, you determine that she has not felt like eating and is positive for costovertebral angle (CVA) tenderness.

- What do you suspect Sioban is experiencing?
- What additional subjective data do you want to gather?
- What additional objective data may be required?
- What nursing diagnoses could apply? How will you validate these?
- What goals might be developed? How will these be prioritized?
- What interventions may you offer?
- How will you evaluate the effectiveness of your interventions?

4. Bobbi is a 37-year-old woman, who is G 2 P 1, in the twelfth week of her pregnancy. Even though she was seen 2 weeks ago for her first prenatal visit, she came in today because she is concerned that she is tired all the time, has been perspiring, and cannot

stand the heat even though it has been a rather cool summer. She says that sometimes she feels like she is having palpitations. As you talk with her, you also take her vitals and find that her pulse is over 100.

- What may be causing Bobbi's symptoms?
- What will be necessary to differentiate between the physiologic changes that occur during the gestational period and a pathologic change?
- What additional subjective data do you want to gather?
- What additional objective data may be required?
- What nursing diagnoses could apply? How will you validate these?
- What goals might be developed? How will these be prioritized?
- What interventions may you offer?
- How will you evaluate the effectiveness of your interventions?

5. Tanya has been admitted to the high-risk prenatal unit this evening. She is 28 years old and in the third trimester of her first pregnancy. She has insulin dependent diabetes mellitus (IDDM) and has been able to carefully monitor and control her glucose levels with diet, exercise, and insulin therapy. She called her physician today and was admitted to the hospital because during the last 3 days she has not been able to maintain an optimal level of control. Tanya reports that the last blood glucose level that she obtained at home was 210 mg/dl. It is hoped that during the admission, her level of glucose can again be controlled with alteration in her therapeutic regimen.

- What additional subjective data do you want to gather?
- What additional objective data may be required?
- What nursing diagnoses could apply? How will you validate these?
- What goals might be developed? How will these be prioritized?
- What interventions may you offer?
- How will you evaluate the effectiveness of your interventions?

6. Amita, a 29-year-old woman of Egyptian descent, is at 16 weeks of gestation, G 3 P 0, SAB 2. She went to her primary care physician today because she has not felt well for the last 2 weeks. At first she thought

it was just the flu, but now it feels like a urinary tract infection except that she is experiencing acute pain in her fingers and doesn't have the energy to do anything. She was admitted to the hospital to determine the cause of her physical difficulty.

- Based on the information that you have been given in her report, what so you anticipate may be going on?
- What additional subjective data do you want to gather?
- What additional objective data may be required?
- What nursing diagnoses could apply? How will you validate these?
- What goals might be developed? How will these be prioritized?
- What interventions may you offer?
- How will you evaluate the effectiveness of your interventions?

---

7. Susan, a 37-year-old G 1 P 1 in the third trimester of her pregnancy, has been followed at home with twice weekly assessment visits since an elevated blood pressure of 135/92 mm Hg was discovered during a prenatal visit 2 weeks ago. She called her visiting nurse today, as directed, because she is experiencing severe epigastric pain, nausea, and vomiting. She was then admitted to the hospital.

- Based on this information, what might you suspect Susan is experiencing?

- What additional subjective data do you want to gather?
- What additional objective data may be required?
- What nursing diagnoses could apply? How will you validate these?
- What goals might be developed? How will these be prioritized?
- What interventions may you offer?
- How will you evaluate the effectiveness of your interventions?

---

8. Lesley, a 31-year-old G 3 P 2 at 30 weeks of gestation, comes to the emergency room because during the last 2 days she has been experiencing nausea, vomiting, anorexia, and fever. Today she experienced pain in the upper right quadrant. Her temperature is within normal limits.

- Based on this information, what may Lesley be experiencing?
- What additional subjective data do you want to gather?
- What additional objective data may be required?
- What nursing diagnoses could apply? How will you validate these?
- What goals might be developed? How will these be prioritized?
- What interventions may you offer?
- How will you evaluate the effectiveness of your interventions?

## REFERENCES

ACOG: *Cardiac disease in pregnancy*, ACOG Technical Bulletin No. 168, Washington, DC., 1992, ACOG Resource Center.

ACOG: *Management of diabetes mellitus in pregnancy*, ACOG Technical Bulletin No. 92, Washington, DC., 1986, ACOG Resource Center.

American Academy of Pediatricians (AAP) and American College of Obstetricians and Gynegologists (ACOG): *Guidelines for perinatal care*. Elk Grove, IL, 1997, The Association.

American Heart Association (AHA): *Basic life support: heart saver guide*, Dallas, 1993, The Association.

Association of Women's Health, Obstetric, and Neonatal Nurses (AWHONN): *Standards and guidelines for professional nursing practice in the care of women and newborns*, ed 5, Washington D.C., 1998, The Association.

Blackburn S and Loper D: *Maternal, fetal, and neonatal physiology*, Philadelphia, 1992, Saunders.

Boyd K, Ross E, and Sherman S: Jelly beans as an alternative to a cola beverage containing fifty grams of glucose, *Am J Obstetr Gynecol* 173:1889-1892, 1995.

Brown C: At the bedside: childbirth education tutoring for high-risk hospitalized antenatal women, *Int J Childbirth Educat* 12(3):20-21, 1997.

Brown C: Two women's experiences of prolonged hospitalization with a high-risk pregnancy, *Int J Childbirth Educat* 12(4):26-30, 1997.

Burrow G and Duffy T: *Medical complications during pregnancy*, ed 5, Philadelphia, 1999, Saunders.

Burrow G and Ferris T: *Medical complications of pregnancy*, ed 4, Philadelphia, 1995, Saunders.

Chitkara U and Berkowitz R: Multiple gestations. In Gabbe S, Neibyl L, and Simpson J, editors: *Obstetrics: normal and problem pregnancies*, ed 3, New York, 1996, Churchill Livingstone.

Copeland L and Landon M: Malignant diseases and pregnancy. In Gabbe S, Neibyl J, and Simpson J, editors: *Obstetrics: normal and problem pregnancies*, ed 3, New York, 1996, Churchill Livingstone.

Crowther C: Commentary on bedrest for women with pregnancy problems: evidence for efficacy is lacking, *Birth* 15(4):242-246, 1995.

Cunningham F and others: *Williams obstetrics*, ed 20, Norwalk, CT, 1997, Appleton and Lange.

Dineen K and others: Antepartum home care services for high-risk women, *JOGN* 21(1):121-125, 1992.

Enkin M and others: *A guide for effective care in pregnancy and childbirth*, ed 2, Oxford, England, 1995, Oxford University Press.

Expert Committee on the Diagnosis and Classification of Diabetes Mellitus: Report of the expert committee on the diagnosis and classification of diabetes mellitus, *Diabetes Care* 20(7):1183-197, 1997.

Gabbe S, Neibyl J, and Simpson J: *Obstetrics: normal and problem pregnancies*, ed 3, New York, 1996, Churchill Livingstone.

Gilbert ES and Harmon JS: Manual of high risk pregnancy and delivery, ed 2, St Louis, 1998, Mosby.

Goldenberg R and others: Bed rest in pregnancy, *Obstetr Gynecol* 84:131-136, 1994.

Gordin P and Johnson B: Technology and family centered perinatal care: conflict or synergy?, *JOGNN* 28(4):401-408, 1999.

Hales D and Johnson T: *Intensive caring: new hope for high-risk pregnancies*, New York, 1990, Crown.

Heppard M and Garite T: *Acute obstetrics: a practical guide*, ed 2, St Louis, 1996, Mosby.

Jaffe MS and McVan BF: *Davis's laboratory and diagnostic handbook*, Philadelphia, 1997, F.A. Davis.

Josten L and others: Bed rest compliance for women with pregnancy problems, *Birth* 22(1):1-12, 1995.

Kemp V and Page C: The psychological limits of a high risk pregnancy on the family, *JOGN* May/June:232-236, 1986.

Knupple R and Drukker J: *High-risk pregnancy: a team approach*, Philadelphia, 1993, Saunders.

Loos C and Julius L: The client's view of hospitalization during pregnancy, *J Obstetr Gynecol Neonat Nurs* 18:52-55, 1989.

Lopez-Jaramillo P and others: Dietary calcium supplementation and prevention of pregnancy hypertension, *Lancet* 335:293, 1990.

Mabie W: Critical care obstetrics. In Gabbe S, Neibyl J, and Simpson J, editors: Obstetrics: normal and problem pregnancies, ed 3, New York, 1996, Churchill Livingstone.

Maloni J: Bed rest during pregnancy: implications for nursing, *JOGN* 22(5):422-426, 1993.

Maloni J and others: Physical and psychological effects of antepartum hospital bed rest, *Nurs Res* 42(4):197-203, 1993.

Maloni J and Kasper C: Physical and psychological effects of bedrest: a review of the literature, *Image* 29(2):187-192, 1991.

Mandeville L and Troiano N: *High-risk intrapartum nursing*, Philadelphia, 1992, Lippincott.

Monahan P and DeJoseph J: The woman with preterm labor at home: a descriptive analysis, *J Perinat Neonat Nurs* 4(4):12-20, 1991.

Moore K and Persand T: *Before we are born: essentials of embryology and birth defects*, Philadelphia, 1998, Saunders.

Moore T: Diabetes in pregnancy. In Creasy R and Resnik R, editors: *Maternal-fetal medicine: principles and practice*, ed 3, Philadelphia, 1994, Saunders.

Nahum G and Huffaker B: Racial differences in oral glucose screening test results: establishing race-specific criteria for abnormality in pregnancy, *Obstetr Gynecol* 81:517-522, 1993.

Rich L: *When pregnancy isn't perfect: a layperson's guide to complications in pregnancy*, Rhinebeck, NY, 1996, Larata Press.

Rubin R: Maternal identity and the maternal experience, New York, 1984, Springer.

Sabi B: The HELLP syndrome: much ado about nothing, *Am J Obstetr Gynecol* 182:311, 1990.

Sanchez-Ramos L, Briones D, and Kaunitz A: Prevention of pregnancy induced hypertension by calcium supplementation in angiotension II sensitive patients, *Obstetr Gynecol* 84:349, 1994.

Sather S and Zwelling E: A view from the other side of the bed, *JOGNN* 27(3):322-328, 1998.

Schroeder C: Women's experience of bed rest in high-risk pregnancy, *Image* 28(3):253-258, 1996.

Schroeder C: Bed rest in complicated pregnancy: a critical analysis, *Maternal Child Nursing* 23(Jan/Feb):45-49, 1998.

Zuspan F: Chronic hypertension. In Queenan J and Hobbins J, editors: *Protocols for high-risk pregnancies*, ed 3, Cambridge, England, 1996, Blackwell Science.

# CHAPTER 18

# Care of the Woman at Risk During Labor and Delivery

*"You can't invent events. They just happen.*
*You have to be prepared to deal with them when they happen."*
— CONSTANCE BAKER MOTLEY

---

*When preparing for a high risk labor and delivery, what are the woman's needs?*

*What interventions will her partner and family require?*

*When a woman develops complications during what was expected to be a normal labor, what interventions are required?*

*What interventions are necessary when an emergency delivery is required?*

*What interventions assist parents after a stillborn baby is delivered?*

---

American society views birth as a joyful event, without recognizing the possibility of maternal or fetal morbidity or mortality. Parents are often surprised and unprepared when faced with a birth experience that is complicated by a condition that places the mother and the infant in danger and confronts the family with the possibility of adverse physical, psychologic, social, and economic sequelae. The rapidly changing events of labor and birth increase the parents' fears and anxiety. They are faced with a language and unfamiliar technology that makes them totally reliant on the health care providers for information and support. The environment during a high-risk labor or birth may appear chaotic to the parents who see many people converging when the crisis escalates or birth is imminent.

All families going through a birth experience require the care described in Chapters 13 and 14. This chapter provides the additional, specialized information needed to provide care to women and families experiencing a birth that places the mother and/or fetus at risk for morbidity or death.

##  PREEXISTING HEALTH CONDITIONS

### Cardiac Conditions

Labor can be a critical period in the care of a pregnant woman with a cardiac condition. The goal of care is to maintain an adequate cardiac output so that she may safely give birth.

#### Intrapartum Strategies

Vaginal birth is the optimal choice for birth unless an obstetric complication arises, necessitating a hysterotomy (cesarean/surgical) birth. Maintaining the woman

758

in a lateral position; sufficient pain management, especially with caudal or epidural anesthesia; comprehensive assessment; and medication administration, including antibiotic prophylaxis and anticoagulation are considerations when caring for the woman through the laboring process. For delivery, the woman may be offered an episiotomy and outlet forceps may be used to decrease the strain on the heart caused by prolonged pushing.

Uterine contractions increase cardiac output and stroke volume because of increased intravascular volume. This leads to an increased workload for the heart (Gilbert and Harmon, 1998). During the first stage of labor, cardiac output gradually increases from 15% to 30%, with an additional 15% increase during each uterine contraction. Second-stage labor has a 45% increase in cardiac output with the additional 15% increase continuing during each uterine contraction. Cardiac output peaks at a 65% increase at 5 minutes after the birth and continues at a 40% increase at 1 hour after birth (Gilbert and Harmon, 1998). Because of these changes, women who are susceptible to fluctuations in cardiac output are at greatest risk during second-stage labor and the immediate postpartum period.

### Assessment

Assessment, support, and reassurance during the intrapartal period are of critical importance. Assessment incorporates both cardiovascular and obstetric parameters.

***Cardiovascular Assessment.*** Assessment of the cardiovascular system includes vital signs, with particular attention paid to changes in patterns over time; the maternal position (left or right lateral) when vital signs are assessed; the presence of chest pain, with attention paid to precipitating factors, onset, duration, characteristics, and radiating qualities; auscultation of heart rate and rhythm for a minimum of a minute; the presence of murmurs; and assessment of apical impulse and radial pulses. Also assess for signs of a thromboembolism through general inspection and Homan's sign. Inspect for the presence and nature of edema. Pulmonary assessments include auscultation for adventitious sounds and presence of a cough, dyspnea, and cyanosis.

***Obstetric Assessment.*** Obstetric assessments include fetal heart rate (FHR), paying attention to changes in response to fetal activity and uterine activity, and fetal movements as an indirect measure of overall fetal oxygenation. Psychosocial assessments include stress adaptation, fear and anxiety levels, presence of helpful labor support, and informational needs. Fear and anxiety must be addressed because they directly affect the progress of labor and a woman's response throughout the intrapartal period.

## Respiratory Conditions

Women may enter labor with a chronic respiratory condition such as asthma or cystic fibrosis, or they may have a respiratory infection or develop the acute condition of pulmonary edema. The goals of care are to maintain a stable maternal cardiopulmonary system so that both the mother and the fetus are adequately oxygenated.

Pulmonary edema requires acute care and a search for the etiologic trigger. The development of pulmonary edema may be attributed to cardiac disease, $\beta$-sympathomimetic drug treatment for preterm labor, pregnancy hypertensive disorders, and infection such as septic shock. Clinical symptoms include tachycardia, dyspnea, orthopnea, hemoptysis, substernal chest pain, rales at lung bases, engorged jugular veins, $S_3$ ventricular gallops, cyanosis, and a decreased or altered level of consciousness (LOC). Diagnostic tests include an electrocardiogram (ECG); chest radiograph; and laboratory assessment of electrolytes, oxygenation, and infection. Hemodynamic monitoring assesses hydration and fluid balance. Respiratory assistance may be provided with ventilation and oxygen therapy. Pharmacologic therapy includes diuretics, digitalis, morphine, and vasodilators.

### Intrapartum Strategies

Helping the woman minimize inefficient levels of activity, remain calm, and continue appropriate breathing patterns during labor assists in maintaining required levels of oxygenation. For delivery, regional anesthesia is the anesthetic method of choice for asthmatic women. Severe bronchospasm can occur with intubation, and general anesthesia can be associated with fetal atelectasis and pneumonia.

### Assessment

Assessment should include vital signs, with particular attention paid to patterns over time; the mother's position (left or right side/head elevated versus flat) when vital signs are assessed; the presence of chest pain, with attention paid to precipitating factors, onset, duration, characteristics, and radiating qualities. Auscultate the woman's lungs to assess the nature of her respirations and for adventitious sounds. Observe the degree of accessory muscles used in breathing. Observe for the presence of a cough, dyspnea, or cyanosis. Determine the presence and nature of her sputum. Significant laboratory data to review may include a complete blood count (CBC) with differential if an infection is suspected; blood gases to assess maternal oxygenation; sputum culture; and electrolytes.

Fetal assessments should include FHR, with attention paid to changes in response to fetal activity and uterine activity, and fetal movements as an indirect measure of overall fetal oxygenation. Psychosocial assessments include stress adaptation, fear and anxiety levels, presence of helpful support during labor, and informational needs.

## Diabetes Mellitus

The goal of intrapartal care for a woman with diabetes mellitus (DM) is to maintain adequate glucose control during the process of labor, birth, and the immediate postpartum. The desired maternal glucose level for labor is between 70 mg/dl and 100 mg/dl. Maintaining the target maternal glucose enhances the infant's glycemic transition in the immediate period following birth, reducing neonatal rebound hypoglycemia.

### Intrapartum Strategies

A woman with well-controlled diabetes and no other complications does not have to deliver before term if the fetus is not macrosomic and the biophysical profile is reassuring. Delivery before term may become necessary if the woman has not had good glucose control, she has a previous history of stillbirths, she has developed pregnancy-induced hypertension (PIH) or vasculopathy, the fetus is becoming large for gestational age, or there is an indication that the fetus's health is being compromised (Gilbert and Harmon, 1998).

"Because of the danger of fetal compromise, it is not recommended to wait for spontaneous labor after 40 weeks of gestation" (Gilbert and Harmon, 1998). Elective induction or hysterotomy is commonly scheduled by 40 weeks of gestation (Gabbe, Neibyl, and Simpson, 1996).

An abdominal delivery is generally advised when the cervix is not favorable for the induction of labor or fetal **macrosomia** (birth weight above the 90th percentile on intrauterine growth curve) is suspected.

If the gestational age of the fetus is a concern, tests for fetal lung maturation help guide the decision to initiate the birth process and tests for fetal well-being provide a measure of fetal oxygenation. An amniocentesis can provide information about fetal lung maturation, specifically lecithin-sphingomyelin (L/S) ratio and phosphatidylglycerol (PG). For a woman with DM, the fetal lung is considered mature when PG is present (Gabbe, Neibyl, and Simpson, 1996). The L/S ratio is not a reliable indicator for women with diabetes.

Other tests for maturity are a Lamellar body count (LBC), foam stability index (FSI) and florescence polarization test (microviscosimetry). Lamellar bodies carry

surfactant, and the amount present gives an indication of the amount of surfactant available. Using the same laboratory equipment used to count platelets, 1 ml of amniotic fluid is examined to determine the number of Lamellar bodies. A **lamellar body count** of $30,000/\mu l$ to $55,000/\mu l$ is highly predictive of pulmonary maturity (Mattson and Smith, 2000).

**Foam stability index (FSI)** also uses amniotic fluid. Equal amounts of 95% ethanol, isotonic saline, and amniotic fluid are placed in a test tube and shaken. The formation of a complete ring of bubbles on the surface of the liquid after 15 minutes indicates a result signifying mature lungs (Mattson and Smith, 2000).

The **fluorescence polarization test** (microviscosimetry) uses the microviscosity of lipid aggregates in the amniotic fluid to indicate lung maturity. The amniotic fluid is mixed with a specific fluorescent dye. The intensity of the fluorescence created by polarized light is measured. A polarization value of 0.320 is an indication of fetal lung maturity (Mattson and Smith, 2000).

The evening before anticipated labor or planned birth the dinner and bedtime routine remain unchanged. The morning glucose monitoring is conducted. During labor, continuous insulin infusion or intermittent subcutaneous insulin is provided. Documentation of insulin administration and glucose levels should occur every hour. Glucose levels are maintained between 70 mg/dl and 90 mg/dl throughout labor

***Insulin Infusion.*** Obtain a baseline blood glucose level. An infusion of 10 U of regular insulin and 1000 ml of dextrose solution is administered at a rate of 100 to 125 ml/hr to infuse 1 unit of insulin per hour (Gabbe, Neibyl, and Simpson, 1996). To use a piggyback setup, 25 units of regular insulin is added to 250 mg of normal saline (NS) and then infused to the mainline IV of NS and lactated Ringer's solution (LR) of $D_5$ LR at a rate of 125 ml/hr (ACOG, 1994). The continuing rates of infusion are based on evaluation of blood glucose levels every 1 to 2 hours. Assess for urine ketones every 4 hours.

If urine ketones are present or blood glucose drops below 70 mg/dl, 5% dextrose is infused at a rate of 2.5 mg/kg/min (ADA, 1995). An infusion pump may be set up with the rate of infusion based on blood glucose levels (Table 18-1).

***Intermittent Subcutaneous Insulin.*** When intermittent subcutaneous injections are used, one third to one half of the woman's pre-pregnancy dosage of insulin may be given that morning. Generally, a rapid-acting or short-acting insulin is used rather than a long-acting insulin because of the immediate drop in insulin requirement after delivery. A continuous IV of 5% glucose is started, running at approximately 100 ml/hr. Supplemental insulin is given periodically, based on the glucose values measured every 1 to 2 hours. Urinary ketones are tested every 4 hours. If glucose levels warrant it, a continuous infusion may be started. If the woman becomes hypogly-

| TABLE 18-1 | *Insulin Dosage with Infusion Pump* |
|---|---|
| **Blood glucose (mg/dl)** | **Insulin dose (U/hr)** |
| <100 | 0 |
| 100-140 | 1.0 |
| 141-180 | 1.5 |
| 181-220 | 2.0 |
| >220 | 2.5 |

From Gilbert E and Harmon J: *Manual of high risk pregnancy and delivery,* St Louis, 1998, Mosby.

cemic, regular insulin may be administered in 2 to 5 U per dose to maintain the blood glucose levels between 70 and 90 mg/dl (Gilbert and Harmon, 1998).

***Hysterotomy (Cesarean) Birth.*** If a surgical delivery is required, it will be scheduled for early morning. As with all surgical preparation, the woman may have nothing to eat or drink after midnight. Because of this, her evening and morning dosages of insulin are also held. Her capillary glucose levels are checked before and immediately after the surgery. Glucose is administered through an IV.

***Changes at Birth.*** Insulin demands drop dramatically with the birth of the placenta and removal of human placental lactogen (HPL), which causes resistance to insulin during the pregnancy. For this reason insulin administration is discontinued at birth. Blood glucose levels and ketones continue to be monitored

### Assessment

***Assessment of Glucose Levels.*** The glucose levels of the woman with DM are periodically assessed during her labor and delivery—generally every 1 to 2 hours. Test for urinary ketones every 4 hours or as appropriate. If the woman is kept in a fasting state during labor, she may quickly move into a starvation state. Maintain continuous monitoring for the signs and symptoms of hypoglycemia.

***Obstetric Assessment.*** Obstetric assessments focus on evaluating electronic fetal monitor readings for the baseline FHR, variability, and response to contractions throughout the intrapartal period. Monitor and evaluate the progress of labor. Be alert to the possibility of dystocia or the arrest of descent of the fetus down the birth canal. If the progression of the labor process is inhibited, the woman may have a hysterotomy.

## Systemic Lupus Erythematosus

The multisystem inflammation that occurs with systemic lupus erythematosus (SLE) requires that a woman with this condition receive closer attention during her labor and delivery. The goal of intrapartal care for a woman with SLE is to provide focused care on the system or systems that have been attacked by the autoantibodies and minimize the chance of maternal system failure, especially cardiac, renal, and/or central nervous system (CNS) failure, and to achieve the birth of the fetus.

### Intrapartum Strategies

Care of a woman with SLE is focused on minimizing and managing complications so that her blood pressure, pulse, platelet count, and serum creatinine remain within normal limits. The woman's urine should remain free of protein, blood, and white blood cells. The specific gravity of her urine should remain between 1.010 and 1.030. Chest sounds should remain clear. The fetus should adapt to the labor process without exhibiting decelerations with contractions (Gilbert and Harmon, 1998).

### Assessment

***Assessment of Involved Systems.*** If the woman is experiencing hypertension, evaluate her renal function by assessing the amount of urinary output, specific gravity, and presence of proteinuria every 4 hours. Evaluate her pulmonary function every 4 hours by assessing breath sounds and asking about chest pain. If the woman is being given tocolytics to relax the uterus for a fetal version or to suppress preterm labor or if she has a history of pulmonary, cardiac, or renal involvement, do the pulmonary assessment more frequently. Be alert for signs and symptoms of disseminated intravascular coagulation (DIC) or late-onset preeclampsia (Gilbert and Harmon, 1998).

If the woman has a history of CNS involvement, assess for unexpected mood swings, seizure activity, or transient changes in her level of consciousness. If the woman has severe cardiac or renal complications or preeclampsia, noninvasive monitoring using an electrocardiogram (ECG) and conventional blood pressure may be ordered to monitor her hemodynamic status. If the situation is more severe, invasive hemodynamic monitoring may be ordered to assist in the assessment process (Gilbert and Harmon, 1998).

If the woman starts to exhibit pulmonary difficulties, be prepared to administer antibiotics, bronchodilators, intravenous heparin, or diuretics as directed and assess the effect of the medication.

 **HEALTH RISKS CREATED BY PREGNANCY**

## Pregnancy-Induced Hypertensive Disorders

For women who develop PIH, delivery is the definitive therapy. Occasionally previously normotensive, nonproteinuric women develop PIH during the labor process. Clinical manifestations of PIH consist of the classic triad of hypertension, proteinuria, and edema (Cunningham and Lindheimer, 1992). These three primary manifestations do not have to be present together to reflect the severity of the disease process.

Women may enter labor after having received medication to control the disease. Most commonly it is anticonvulsant therapy with magnesuium sulfate and/or antihypertensive therapy with hydralazine.

### Intrapartum Strategies

Termination of the pregnancy is indicated for a woman with PIH when any of the following conditions are met:

- Fetal well-being deteriorates.
- Treatment has not improved the mother's symptoms or laboratory results indicate continuing damage to her organs.
- The mother experiences eclampsia or warning signs of eclampsia.

Vaginal delivery is generally the preferred method. If labor is not already under way and the fetus's gestational age is at least 33 weeks, induction of labor contractions with an amniotomy and/or administration of oxytocin is attempted. In some cases, if the fetus is less than 33 weeks gestational age but the cervix is ripe (soft), labor induction is still attempted. Because the uterus may be more sensitive to oxytocin than normal, the contractions must be monitored for hypertonus.

A hysterotomy becomes the choice for delivery if (1) labor does not begin promptly and progress efficiently; (2) the fetus weighs less than 1500 g; or (3) vaginal delivery is contraindicated for other reasons such as fetal malpresentation or distress, a fetal gestational age of less than 33 weeks, and a firm cervix.

During labor, the care that the woman has received throughout the antepartum period is continued. The assessment parameters for the woman with PIH focus on a systemic evaluation for evidence of progression of the disease process and to determine the fetal response.

Pain management during labor is complicated for a woman with PIH. Analgesia during labor is limited to small doses and is withheld when the woman is within 2 hours of expected delivery. If the fetus is preterm, analgesics may be avoided to prevent further depression of the fetus.

Anesthesia also adds risks to the mother. When given an intrathecal or epidural block, there is a risk of hypotension that would decrease the profusion of blood to the placenta and oxygenation of the fetus. To treat the hypotension, large volumes of fluids are given to the woman intravenously—a clear danger to the woman experiencing PIH. A general anesthesia may elevate her blood pressure, especially during induction and awakening.

If the woman has experienced the HELLP syndrome (*h*emolysis, *e*levated *l*iver enzymes, and *l*ow *p*latelet count) during the pregnancy, her resulting low platelet count places her at risk of hemorrhage associated with an epidural or pudendal block. The administration of any anesthesia is done judiciously and requires ongoing and careful monitoring for its effect on both the woman and her baby (Gilbert and Harmon, 1998).

### Assessment

***Assessment for PIH.*** Blood pressure monitoring remains the fundamental assessment for altered cardiovascular status. Monitor renal function by measuring intake and output, urine specific gravity, protein in urine, and BUN and creatinine levels. Assess for edema and degree of pitting present. Listen to breath sounds and assess for pulmonary edema, presence of rales, tachycardia, shortness of breath, and distended neck veins. Assess CNS status by checking for hyperreflexia; clonus; and transient neurologic deficits, including visual alterations, altered level of consciousness, or vomiting. Be alert to the woman reporting nausea or an un-

relenting frontal headache. Assess for alterations in hemostasis with evidence of bleeding, bruising and other indications of DIC.

***Obstetric Assessment.*** The progress of labor must be monitored closely because the woman is being stimulated by an exogenous hormone. Assess her contractions for hypertonus.

Assess her anxiety and levels of pain because these may contribute to raising her blood pressure. Assess the woman's comfort level and support her labor partner in meeting her needs. If she is receiving analgesia or anesthesia, her response needs to be assessed more frequently.

Assess the FHR—baseline and in response to contractions. The uteroplacental blood flow was already compromised and the stress of labor may further compromise the infant. "Magnesium sulfate crosses the placenta readily. It can cause decreased beat-to-beat variability as seen on the fetal monitor strip. However, there is no indication that it adversely affects the fetus as long as the mother's serum magnesium level does not reach toxic levels" (Gilbert and Harmon, 1998). If the mother is receiving analgesia or anesthesia, assess the effect on the FHR.

## Hemorrhagic Disorders

The placental complications of placenta previa, abruptio placentae, and abnormal placental or umbilical cord development often lead to an emergency delivery of the fetus or are discovered during the delivery process. Each of them can lead to hemorrhage and a potentially catastrophic event for the mother and fetus.

### Intrapartum Strategies

***Placenta Previa.*** Placenta previa is an abnormal implantation of the placenta in which the placenta implant is in the lower uterine segment. Treatment depends on the gestational age of the fetus and the extent of the bleeding from the placenta. Delivery is delayed if the fetus is less than 36 weeks gestational age, the bleeding is mild (less than 250 ml), and the woman is not in labor.

If the fetus is mature, 36 weeks of gestation or more; the L/S ratio is 2:1; PG is present; excessive bleeding occurs, active labor begins, or other obstetric problems develop, the pregnancy is terminated.

Whether hysterotomy or vaginal birth is recommended depends on the extent of the placenta previa. A trial vaginal birth with the ability to do an immediate hysterotomy (known as a *double set up*) may also be selected for a marginal placenta previa. A hysterotomy is required for a total previa.

If the fetus is dead, has anomalies incompatable with life, or the delivery process has already advanced to the point where the fetal head is engaged, a vaginal birth is attempted.

***Abruptio Placentae.*** Placental abruption involves a partial or complete premature separation of an otherwise normally implanted placenta. If the woman has a moderate or severe abruption, the management is aggressive stabilization of the mother and delivery of the fetus if it is more than 36 weeks gestational age or at any age if it is in distress.

Whether an abdominal or vaginal birth is recommended depends on the infant and the extent of the placental abruption. If the fetus is mature and in cephalic presentation, induction of contractions with an amniotomy or a labor stimulant such as oxytocin may be attempted with a mild or moderate abruption. A trial for vaginal delivery can only be attempted when a double set up is also available for an immediate hysterotomy if further abruption or fetal distress occurs. Continuous fetal monitoring provides the status of the fetus during labor. An immediate hysterotomy is indicated in the following situations:

- There is a total abruption and the fetus is alive.
- The fetus is in distress.
- The fetus is not in cephalic position.
- Bleeding increases during labor.
- The uterus fails to relax during contractions.
- The labor process does not progress.

If the fetus is dead, the preferred method of delivery is a vaginal birth because it is less traumatic for the mother, with potentially less blood loss than surgery. If the bleeding from the placental site cannot be controlled, a hysterotomy may be performed.

***Abnormal Implantation of the Placenta.*** Alterations in the implantation of the placenta occur infrequently, with the incidence being approximately 1 in 12,000 births (Gabbe, Neibyl, and Simpson, 1996). Alterations in placental implantation are highly associated with placenta previa and are thought to occur as a result of implanta-

tion of the zygote in a nonreceptive or damaged part of the endometrial lining.

The four types of abnormal placental implantation are (1) placenta accreta, (2) placenta increta, (3) placenta percreta, and (4) placenta succenturiata. **Placenta accreta** occurs when the trophoblastic cells implant into the myometrium in the absence of the decidua basalis. Placenta increta and placenta percreta are more advanced forms of placenta accreta. **Placenta increta** is the invasion of chorionic villi into the uterine myometrium. **Placenta percreta** occurs when chorionic villi (trophoblastic cells) extend through the myometrium and into the uterine wall and other organs in close proximity. This can occur with the entire placental unit or with individual cotyledons of the placenta. **Placenta succenturiate** is implantation into the decidua with the separation of a cotyledon connected with a vascular supply to the larger placental unit (Figure 18-1).

Abnormal implantation of the placenta becomes evident in the third stage of labor when the placenta does not separate in an expected manner. Alterations in placental implantation lead to a high rate of maternal morbidity, with a high risk of postnatal hemorrhage and hysterectomy. The risk of maternal hemorrhage is high because the uterus cannot contract effectively as a result of the placental tissues remaining in the uterus. Treatment is often hysterectomy, although alternate surgical procedures may be attempted to preserve the uterus.

***Abnormal Attachment of the Umbilical Cord.*** Altered cord development and insertion occurs in 1 in 3,000 births. The etiology is not understood. This cord disorder presents a threat for hemorrhagic shock for the fetus.

Alterations in the insertion of the umbilical cord are velamentous insertion and battledore placenta. **Battledore placenta** occurs when the umbilical cord attaches at one edge of the placenta so that the placenta then resembles a paddle or battledore. This creates a potential problem because all fetal vessels transverse the placental

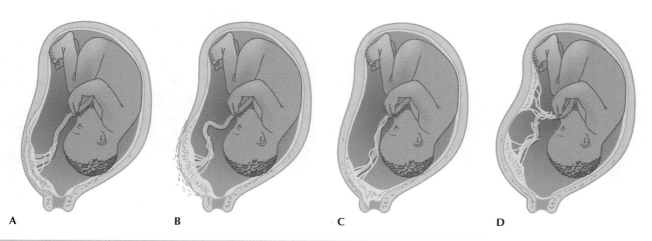

**A**   **B**   **C**   **D**

*FIGURE 18-1* • Abnormal implantation of the placenta. **A,** Placenta accreta. **B,** Placenta percreta. **C,** Placenta increta. **D,** Placenta succenturiate.

surface in the same direction. If pressure is applied to the placental surface near where insertion occurs by a fetal body part, most or all of the fetal blood supply will be diminished. If this occurs with a placenta in which the cord is attached in the middle only one half of the blood supply would be diminished. Because of the risk of interference with fetal circulation and nutrition, the chances of preterm labor are higher than normal. Hemorrhage during labor is also more likely because of vessel rupture. **Velamentous insertion** is the connection of the blood vessels of the umbilical cord to the placenta unprotected by Wharton's jelly as they travel between the amnion and chorion. A condition called **vasa previa** occurs when the velamentous vessels become positioned in front of the internal os ahead of the presenting part of the fetus. They can become easily compressed and rupture (Figure 18-2).

Both of these alterations place the fetus at risk for hemorrhage. They typically become evident when membranes rupture, triggering the release of amniotic fluid and compression of the umbilical cord. Treatment is the recognition of fetal compromise and an expedited birth.

*Uterine Rupture.* Uterine rupture is a rare occurrence. When it occurs during labor, it is most commonly associated with previous uterine surgery, especially a classic (vertical) uterine incision. Labor stimulated by prostaglandin and oxytocin is the second most common precipitating factor associated with uterine rupture (Cunningham and others, 1997). Uterine rupture is an obstetric emergency for the infant and mother.

A woman experiencing uterine rupture is likely to have sharp stabbing abdominal pain, often with vigorous uterine contractions followed by continued pain and cessation of uterine activity. Physical assessment reveals easily palpable fetal parts and signs of shock in the fetus and mother. Vaginal bleeding may or may not be present, and intraabdominal bleeding is suspected when the abdomen becomes distended and tense with referred pain to the shoulder. An emergency delivery and possible hysterectomy with neonatal resuscitation of a hypovolemic infant follows.

### Assessment

*Assessment of Hemorrhagic Emergency.* Monitor blood pressure, pulse, and respirations at frequent intervals. Assess peripheral pulses. Observe for restlessness or confusion because either may indicate decreased cerebral perfusion. Observe for signs of shock. Remember that because of the increased blood volume of pregnancy, the early warning is less pronounced. Monitor urinary output hourly because renal blood flow may be decreased as the body attempts to maintain cerebral and cardiac perfusion.

If signs of shock develop, place the woman in a modified Trendelenburg position with only her legs elevated. This increases blood return without contributing to respiratory impairment. Administer oxygen at 8 to 10 L/min by mask. Report changes to the physician immediately.

*Obstetric Assessment.* Check uterine contractions for duration, frequency, and uterine resting tone. Monitor for flow of blood from vagina. Observe amniotic fluid for meconium staining. Evaluate the FHR for tachycardia, bradycardia, late or variable decelerations, and loss of long- or short-term variability. Assess if the FHR is different if the mother is lying positioned on her left or right side, or on her back and tilted to the left with a blanket under her hip (Figure 18-3).

## Multiple Gestations

The management of the birth of more than one fetus depends on several factors, the primary ones being the positions and gestational ages of the infants. When the infants enter labor in a head down, vertex presentation

**A**                          **B**

FIGURE 18-2 • Abnormal insertion of the umbilical cord. **A,** Velamentous insertion. **B,** Vasa previa.

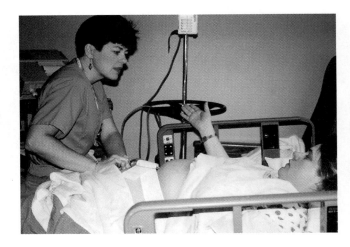

FIGURE 18-3 • Assessing fetal heart rate. *(Courtesy of Caroline E. Brown.)*

the possibility for vaginal birth of both infants is good. A hysterotomy (surgical birth) is often suggested when the first twin is not in a vertex position.

When the first infant is vertex and the second is breech or transverse, the recommendations for birth become less definitive. The vaginal birth of the first infant is followed by an attempt to turn the remaining infant with external version techniques. If the version is successful, a vaginal birth is recommended; if not, a hysterotomy is recommended. The second twin is considered to be at higher risk for associated birth-related morbidity and mortality (Knupple, 1993). Typical birth interval between the first and second twin is 15 to 30 minutes, yet there are case reports indicating much longer intervals (e.g., days or even weeks), particularly in preterm gestations.

### Intrapartum Strategies

Care during the intrapartal period continues to center around surveillance but at a heightened level. Continuous electronic fetal monitoring for each fetus is initiated when labor starts and continues through the birth. External and internal fetal monitoring techniques may be used simultaneously so that the assessment of the two or more fetuses can be conducted with less confusion. As soon as membrane rupture occurs, the fetal scalp electrode is placed on the presenting twin. The external ultrasound is used to monitor the second infant until the birth of the first twin. Then when membrane rupture occurs, the fetal scalp electrode is attached to monitor the second twin until its birth.

Preparation for an emergent birth and neonatal resuscitation is always necessary with a woman experiencing a multiple gestation. Excellent and open communication continues to be essential, and anticipatory guidance is helpful as the labor and birth process unfold. Often a multiple birth is associated with several people converging on the delivery area when birth is anticipated. The apparent chaotic nature of the birthing environment can be frightening for the woman and her support systems if they do not know the rationale behind what is occurring.

### Assessment

Assess the understanding of the woman and her partner about the status of their infants. Determine if they have developed any fears or misunderstandings due to "helpful" comments from family members and friends.

The assessment process for a woman in labor with more than one fetus is the same as during a regular labor and delivery. However, assessment is complicated because of the need to differentiate between the FHR and response of more than one fetus at a time.

Assess the anxiety and concern of the woman and her partner. Generally, concern is greater because the health and well-being of more than one fetus is involved.

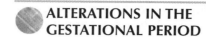

# ALTERATIONS IN THE GESTATIONAL PERIOD

## Preterm Labor and Birth

The rate of preterm birth is higher in the United States than in 18 other industrialized nations. Despite the availability of our technologic and pharmacologic resources to stop preterm labor, preterm births account for 75% to 85% of all neonatal morbidity and mortality. The cost of treating preterm babies is more than $5 billion annually.

**Preterm or premature labor** is when regular uterine contractions start between the twentieth and completion of the thirty-seventh week of gestation and the woman experiences cervical dilation. The extent of cervical dilation may be estimated with a digital vaginal examination. A more accurate determination is obtained by transvaginal cervical sonography that can measure the length of the cervix more accurately, determining the extent of effacement. An immunoassay test for fibronectin may be helpful to detect fetal fibronectins and predict the woman's labor status. **Fetal fibronectin** is a substance that is present in cervical and vaginal secretions early in the pregnancy at the time of implantation and again later when labor is to begin. When fetal fibronectin is found after the twentieth week of pregnancy, it may be a marker associated with preterm labor (Iams, 1996) (Box 18-1).

For 50% of the women who experience preterm labor, there is no discoverable cause. Factors that may alert a woman or provider to the possibility that it may occur are a past history, risky lifestyle practices, stress, altered uterine factors, and infection. Causes that have been identified as placing a woman at higher risk are multiple gestation; infection, especially urinary tract infections (UTIs); an illness with a raised body temperature; and abdominal surgery (Gilbert and Harmon, 1998).

When infants are born before reaching 37 weeks of gestation, their lack of physical maturity places them at an increased risk of trauma during the birth process.

---

### BOX 18-1   *Diagnosis of Premature Labor*

Cervical Changes
   cervical dilation >2 cm
    effacement or a cervical change of 1 cm
Transvaginal cervical sonography
   cervix <30 mm
Contractions
   4 in 20 minutes or 8 in 60 minutes
Fetal fibronectin present

Once born, they face difficulty because they are not fully prepared to handle extrauterine life. A preterm infant is at greatest risk for developing respiratory distress syndrome. Other risks are intraventricular or pulmonary hemorrhage, hyperbilirubinemia, anemia, infection, neurologic disorders, metabolic disturbances, and/or ineffective temperature regulation. The severity of problems depends on the developmental status of the fetus.

When a woman experiences early contractions, a major concern is for the well-being of her infant. Additional concerns will develop with regard to the side effects she and the fetus will experience after a treatment regimen is selected.

### Intrapartum Strategies

Once it has been determined that the woman is in active labor, the medical team must determine the cause of labor and the risks and benefits for the mother and the fetus to try to stop labor and continue the pregnancy or allow the process to go on to delivery. Various tests assist in the process of gathering data before the decision concerning intervention is made.

Diagnostic tests to determine the presence of an infection include a CBC with a differential and platelets; a urinalysis for culture and sensitivity to rule out a UTI; and cervical cultures for gonorrhea, group B streptococci, *Chlamydia*, *Bacteroides vivius*, and *Bacteroides fragilis*. A wet mount may rule out bacterial vaginosis.

An ultrasound examination assesses the approximate gestational age, presenting part, placental location, amniotic fluid volume, number of fetuses, and evidence of fetal or uterine abnormalities. In addition fetal monitoring is conducted to assess the fetal heart. If the fetus is between 32 and 36 weeks of gestation, tests for fetal lung maturity are done. A fibronectin evaluation is helpful. If the amniotic sac has broken, the amniotic fluid is evaluated for infection, using a Gram's stain and culture and sensitivity.

**Continuation of Labor.** In 20% of the cases, the decision is made not to intervene because of a medical or obstetric reason and labor is allowed to progress to delivery. Maternal reasons for allowing labor to continue are severe preeclampsia, heart disease, the occurrence of a hemorrhage, or the risk of hemorrhage from placenta previa or a placental abruption. Reasons related to the fetus that contraindicate stopping labor are fetal lung maturity, fetal compromise, intrauterine growth restriction (IUGR), intraamniotic infection, a fetal anomaly incompatible with life, or fetal death.

For the most part, the process of preterm labor parallels a woman's labor experience with a term infant. Evacuation of the lower intestines due to hormonal changes; membrane rupture; uterine activity; menstrual-like cramping; abdominal, thigh, or pelvic pain; dull backache, pelvic pressure, and increased vaginal discharge are signs of labor that a woman may experience

even though she is not yet at term. Options for pain relief during labor are determined by the mother's health and the status of the fetus. When a preterm birth is imminent, the focus becomes the resuscitation and stabilization of the compromised infant

**Labor Suppression.**

*Restriction of Activities.* Until recently, the first response when a woman became "crampy" was to put her on bed rest in the hospital or at home. As explained in Chapter 17, the cost/benefit ratio of this directive is questionable because it has negative physical and psychosocial consequences. Research has demonstrated that a plan of modified restful activities spaced between periods of activity is as effective without the negative complications and is more likely to be acceptable to the woman and her family (Box 18-2).

*Hydration.* Hydration is another common recommendation for women experiencing increased uterine activity. Hydration is thought to reduce uterine activity by inhibiting the secretion of antidiuretic hormone (ADH) and oxytocin. Hydration can be achieved with the oral intake of 8 to 10, 8-ounce glasses of water a day or the oral intake of fluids with nutritive calories, such as fruit juices, milk, and gelatin. The administration of intravenous fluids is sometimes done but is not an evidence-based practice. The risk is that if the woman does require therapy with tocolytic drugs, the complication of pulmonary edema is increased if large amounts of fluids have been given intravenously. Currently, research is not available to either support or refute this pervasive practice (Enkin and others, 1995).

*Stress Reduction.* Stress has a demonstrated association with the onset of preterm labor (Pagel and others, 1990; Janke, 1999). A nursing research study has determined that women who practice progressive relaxation on a daily basis experience longer gestational periods and larger birth weight infants. The use of progressive relaxation for women experiencing preterm onset of labor may also prolong their gestational period, resulting in increased infant birth weight and maturity (Janke, 1999) (Figure 18-4).

*Pharmacologic Agents.* Analgesics, narcotics, and sedatives have been used in the past with women experiencing preterm onset of labor. The underlying intent was reduction of uterine activity; however, no evidence supports this practice. Of concern are the implications of adding CNS depressants to an already compromised infant. This practice has the potential for serious ramifications including hypotonia and respiratory depression.

Drugs more commonly used to inhibit uterine activity are **tocolytic** pharmacologic agents. They may stop preterm labor and delivery when the woman is experiencing persistent uterine contractions and cervical changes have occurred or a vaginal examination finds that the woman's cervix has started to efface and is dilated 2 cm. The selection of a drug regimen to slow the

---

## BOX 18-2   *Suggestions for Women Attempting Modified Activity*

**Self-care**

Wear clothes during the day.

Be neat and clean and keep up your personal hygiene routine.

Set goals and keep them in mind.

Keep a journal.

Have a small cooler next to you so that you may satisfy needs for drinks and snacks.

Give yourself little treats such as a manicure, a facial, watching your favorite movie, or indulging in your favorite food.

Borrow books on tape from the library.

Do crossword puzzles, word searches, or jigsaw puzzles.

Keep a calendar and focus on how far you have come, not how far you have to go.

Focus on why you are doing this, not what you are doing.

**Care for your family**

Shop by phone using catalogs, the yellow pages, or the Internet.

Plan your menus and organize the grocery list so that someone else may shop.

Reorganize files, pay the bills, compile tax data, or update your address book.

Catch up on projects such as putting pictures in photo albums, doing the mending, or preparing holiday cards or birth announcements.

Make something for the baby or maybe someone else.

Arrange a "date" with your partner, having him bring home your favorite take-out food.

Have as much contact with your children as possible.

Do things that your children enjoy such as reading, talking, playing games, watching television, and doing puzzles.

If you do not have childcare, safety proof the room that you rest in so that it is like a giant playpen. This way you can bring the children in, shut the door, and not worry.

**Interactions with others**

When people ask what they can do, provide them with some suggestions. If they didn't want to help, they wouldn't ask.

Arrange for a childbirth preparation class in your home.

Call a friend, relative, or supportive person each day.

Invite visitors over to break up the day.

Utilize your support group for empathy and understanding.

Modified from Gilbert E and Harmon J: *Manual of high risk pregnancy and delivery,* ed 2, St Louis, 1998, Mosby.

---

labor is complicated because none are without serious, undesirable side effects and all have the potential for being ineffective.

Tocolytic agents are currently divided into four classes (1) the β-sympathomimetics, ritodrine (Yutopar) and terbutaline sulfate (Brethine); (2) magnesium sulfate; (3) the prostaglandin synthetase inhibitors, indomethacin or ibuprofen; and (4) the calcium channel blocker, nifedipine. The U.S. Food and Drug Administration has only approved ritodrine for suppressing labor. However, terbutaline and magnesium sulfate are used more frequently, are equally safe, and are less expensive. Prostaglandin inhibitors and calcium channel blockers are frequently reserved for treatment when the other drugs have failed to be effective in suppressing labor (Gilbert and Harmon, 1998). This may change in future practice because calcium channel blockers have fewer side effects and appear to work as well as the β-sympathomimetics and magnesium sulfate.

The **β-sympathomimetic** drugs may be administered either intravenously or orally. They supplement or mimic the effects of norepinephrine and epinephrine on the body's organs. Use of the drug can cause severe side effects and pose the risk of potentially life-threatening complications for the woman. If the woman has diabetes, PIH, cardiac disease, or hyperthyroidism or the fetus is experiencing IUGR, this is not the agent of first choice.

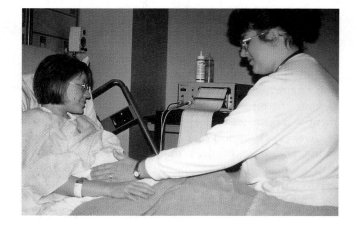

FIGURE 18-4 • Assessing preterm contractions. *(Courtesy of Caroline E. Brown.)*

Common side effects of the β-sympathomimetics are elevated heart rate, nervousness, widening pulse pressure, tremors, nausea and vomiting, hyperglycemia, decreased serum potassium, cardiac arrhythmias, and pulmonary edema. The experience of the woman is related directly to the dosage and route of administration. Oral doses have the potential for the same side effects as intravenous doses, although the effects are usually milder. The fetal side effects are thought to be the same as those the mother experiences because the drug crosses the placenta. Treatment is stopped when the maternal heart rate is greater than 140 beats/min, blood pressure drops to less than 90/60, the woman experiences chest pain or tightness, or she develops cardiac dysrhythmias or pulmonary edema.

The **subcutaneous terbutaline pump** provides a continuous subcutaneous infusion of small amounts of terbutaline. Delivering a small, continuous basal rate, usually 0.05 to 0.075 mg/hr, it also can provide a scheduled bolus of 0.25 mg. The maximum pump dose delivered in 24 hours is 3 mg, much less than the oral 24-hour dose of 15 to 30 mg. While allowing the woman to be at home, the pump offers the advantages of not relying on self-administration of medication, a reduction in unpleasant side effects, and an extension of the time before contraction breakthrough to as much as 6 weeks. The disadvantages are that the woman must learn how to operate the pump, the needle site is at risk for infection, and infusion therapy is more expensive than oral tocolytics (Gilbert and Harmon, 1998).

**Magnesium sulfate (MgSO₄)**, a smooth muscle relaxant, is used in the treatment of preeclampsia and preterm labor. Administered through an intravenous piggyback, the magnesium relaxes the smooth muscles of the uterus by substituting itself in place of the calcium. A secondary benefit is that the magnesium decreases arteriole pressure and increases uterine flow. A woman can tolerate a much higher dose of magnesium to stop preterm labor than the woman with preeclampsia because compromised kidney function is not a concern.

The side effects are sweating, flushing, nausea and vomiting, depressed deep tendon reflexes, flaccid paralysis, hypocalcemia, decreased cardiac function, and respiratory depression. Concurrent administration of a narcotic or sedative is inappropriate because it will potentiate the effect of respiratory depression. The treatment is terminated if the woman demonstrates signs of toxicity: a respiration rate of fewer than 12 breaths per minute, absence of deep tendon reflexes, severe hypotension, and extreme muscle relaxation. To reduce uterine contractions, therapeutic serum levels must be in the range of 4 to 7.5 mEq/L. Toxicity can develop with levels of 10 mEq/L or greater. Because of the risk of sudden onset of toxicity, CPR equipment and calcium gluconate (1 to 2 g), the antidote, must be readily available.

**Calcium channel blockers** block the movement of calcium into the smooth muscles. Administered either orally or subcutaneously, nifedipine (Procardia) and nicardipine (Cardene) have been demonstrated to be effective in stopping uterine contractions. The side effects are an insignificant decrease in blood pressure, fatigue, facial flushing, headache, nausea, dizziness, palpitations, and peripheral edema. Clinical trials have indicated that nifedipine is as effective as ritodrine or terbutaline in stopping uterine contractions, with significantly fewer adverse side effects (Mattson and Smith, 2000).

Prostaglandin is a natural agent in the body that is thought to cause uterine contractions and cervical ripening in term pregnancies. **Prostaglandin synthetase inhibitors,** such as indomethacin or ibuprofen (Motrin) inhibit prostaglandin synthesis. Because of the potentially serious side effects, prostaglandin inhibitors are currently used only with very immature gestations after other tocolysis has failed. Generally, the period of treatment is for 24 to 48 hours because of the risk of oligohydramnios due to impaired fetal renal function, premature closure of the ductus arteriosus, and increased risk of fetal pulmonary hypertension increase when the course of treatment is longer. The risk of premature closing of the ductus arteriosus increases with gestational age, so it is not used after the thirty-fourth week of gestation.

Prostaglandin synthetase inhibitors are contraindicated for women who have a peptic ulcer, a drug sensitivity to salicylates, poorly controlled hypertension, renal disease, vaginal bleeding, a coagulation disorder, or liver disease. The treatment plan is contraindicated when a fetus has chorioamnionitis, IUGR, oligohydramnios, a ductal-dependent cardiac defect, or twin-to-twin transfusion syndrome. The short-term use of indomethacin may delay the time of onset of preterm labor contractions to delivery, allowing for a course of antenatal steroids to be given to enhance fetal lung maturity (Simpson and Creehan, 1996) (Box 18-3 and Table 18-2).

*Home Uterine Monitoring.* **Home monitoring** of uterine contractions may be done with self-palpation or the use

---

**BOX 18-3** *Patient Selection for Tocolytic Drug Therapy*

A woman is considered for tocolytic drug therapy if any of the following occur:
- Gestational age is between 20 and 36 weeks.
- Uterine contractions occur (2 in 15 minutes).
- Cervical changes occur.
- Cervix is dilated <5 cm.

Tocolytic drug therapy is contraindicated if any of the following conditions are present:
- Infection
- Maternal bleeding
- Maternal cardiac disease
- Intrauterine fetal demise (IUFD)
- Pregnancy-induced hypertension (PIH)
- Severe intrauterine growth restriction (IUGR)
- Maternal hyperthyroidism
- Maternal history of migraine headaches
- Family history of diabetes

From Knupple R: *High-risk pregnancy: a team approach,* Philadelphia, 1993, WB Saunders.

## TABLE 18-2 *Common Medications for Tocolytic Drug Therapy*

### β-ANDRENERGIC AGONISTS
Mechanism of action: Stimulation of the β-adrenergic receptors in the uterus results in uterine relaxation. A secondary effect is increased uteroplacental blood flow.

| | ROUTE | DOSE/RESPONSE TITRATION | SIDE EFFECTS | |
| | | | Maternal | Infant |
|---|---|---|---|---|
| Ritodrine | IV with infusion pump | 0.05-0.30 mg/min<br>Increase by 0.05 mg/min every 10 minutes until<br>  1. Uterine contractions stop<br>  2. Intolerable side effect develop<br>  3. Maximum dose of 0.35 mg/min is reached<br>Maintained at effective dose for 12-24 hr, then tapered off and transferred to oral | Elevated heart rate<br>Widening pulse pressure<br>Nausea and vomiting<br>Nervousness<br>Tremors<br>Transient hyperglycemia<br>Cardiac arrhythmias<br>Pulmonary edema | Tachycardia |
| | PO | Initial dose 10-20 mg started 30 minutes before IV discontinued<br>Continued at 10-20 mg every 4 to 6 hours<br>Maximum dose is 120 mg/24 hr | | |
| Terbutaline | IV | 2.5-25 μg/min<br>Increase by 5 μg/min every 10-20 min until<br>  1. Uterine contractions stop<br>  2. Intolerable side effects develop<br>  3. Maximum dose of 80 mg/min is reached<br>Maintained at effective dose for 12-24 hr then tapered off and started on SC or PO | Elevated heart rate<br>Nervousness<br>Tremors<br>Nausea and vomiting<br>Transient hyperglycema<br>Decreased serum potassium<br>Cardiac arrhythmias<br>Pulmonary edema | Tachycardia |
| | SC or<br>PO | 0.25-0.50 mg q4hr<br>5.0 mg q6-8h *or* 2.5 q4hr | | |

Intolerable side effects for the mother: Tachycardia >140 beats/min
Drop in blood pressure to <90/60
Chest pain or tightness
Cardiac dysrhythmias
Potential complications for IV administration: Pulmonary edema
Subendocardial myocardial ischemia
Cardiac dysrhythmias
Cerebral vasospasm in women with a history of migraine headaches

### MAGNESIUM SULFATE
Mechanism of action: relaxes the smooth muscle of the uterus by substituting itself in place of calcium. A secondary effect is decreasing arteriole pressure and increasing uterine blood flow, which also may be helpful.

| | ROUTE | DOSE | SIDE EFFECTS | |
| | | | Maternal | Infant |
|---|---|---|---|---|
| Magnesium sulfate | IV piggyback (IVPB) with infusion pump | Loading dose 4-8 g/hr over 20 to 30 min<br>Maintenance dose 2-4 g/hr IVPB until contractions stop or signs of toxicity develop | Sweating<br>Flushing, hot flashes<br>Nausea and vomiting<br>Drowsiness<br>Blurred vision | CNS depression |

*IUGR,* intrauterine growth restriction; *PO,* by mouth; *SC,* subcutaneous.

*continued*

## TABLE 18-2 *Common Medications for Tocolytic Drug Therapy—cont'd*

| | | | |
|---|---|---|---|
| Magnesium sulfate—cont'd | | Signs of toxicity:<br>1. Respirations <12/min<br>2. Absence of deep tendon reflexes<br>3. Severe hypotension<br>4. Extreme muscle relaxation<br>Toxic serum magnesium level:<br>≤10 mEq/L | Flaccid paralysis<br>Hypocalcemia<br>Respiratory depression<br>Depressed cardiac function<br>Maternal side effects usually subside when the loading dose is completed |
| Magnesium gluconate | PO | 1 g q 2-4 hr to maintain tocolysis | Nausea and vomiting<br>Diarrhea |

### CALCIUM CHANNEL BLOCKERS

Mechanism of action: Calcium channel blockers work primarily by blocking the movement of calcium ions into cell membrane of the smooth muscle of the uterus. The lack of calcium decreases the activity of smooth muscle from contraction.

| | ROUTE | DOSE | SIDE EFFECTS | |
|---|---|---|---|---|
| | | | **Maternal** | **Infant** |
| Nifedipine | PO | Loading dose 30 mg *or* 30 mg then 20 mg after 90 min | Headache<br>Fatigue<br>Hypotension | Being investigated |
| | SC | 10 mg q20min × followed by 20 mg PO q4-8 hr | Dizziness<br>Facial flushing<br>Nausea<br>Palpitations<br>Peripheral edema | |

### PROSTAGLANDIN SYNTHETIC INHIBITORS

Mechanism of action: Prostaglandin synthetic inhibitors stop prostaglandin synthesis. Because of the seriousness of potential side effects, these are used only with very immature gestations in which other tocolysis has failed.

Contraindicated in (1) women who have a peptic ulcer or drug sensitivity to salicylates, poorly controlled hypotension, renal disease, active peptic ulcer disease, vaginal bleeding, coagulation disorder, and liver disease and (2) fetuses of more than 35 weeks gestation because the drugs will cause premature closing of ductus arteriosus, IUGR, oligohydramnios, chorioamnionitis, ductal dependent cardiac defect, and twin-to-twin transfusion syndrome

| | ROUTE | DOSE | SIDE EFFECTS | |
|---|---|---|---|---|
| | | | **Maternal** | **Infant** |
| Indomethacin | PO | Loading dose: 50-100 mg | Increased bleeding time<br>Potential exacerbation of hypertension | Oligohydramnios |
| | Suppository | Loading dose: 100-200 mg | | Premature closing of ductus arteriosis |
| | PO only | Maintenance dose<br>25-50 mg q4-6 hr for 24 to 48 hr<br>Treatment stopped after 48 hr | | Renal dysfunction<br>Increased risk of necrotizing enterocolitis<br>Increased risk of intraventricular hemorrhage |
| Ibuprofen | PO | 600 mg q6hr | | |

*IUGR,* intrauterine growth restriction; *PO,* by mouth; *SC,* subcutaneous.

From Knupple R: *High-risk pregnancy: a team approach,* Philadelphia, 1993, WB Saunders; Gilbert ES and Harmon JS: *Manual of high risk pregnancy and delivery,* ed 2, St Louis, 1998, Mosby; Mattson S and Smith J: *Core curriculum for maternal-newborn nursing,* ed 2, Philadelphia, 2000, WB Saunders.

of a home monitor unit that prints out the contractions a woman may be experiencing. Some units are designed so that the woman may download the monitor information to her provider over the telephone lines. There are two presumed advantages to the use of the monitors: (1) The units are more sensitive to some contractions than the mother may be and may detect contractions as much as 3 days earlier than the woman, and (2) physicians tend to respond to the objective data faster than to a woman's subjective report of contractions (Gilbert and Harmon, 1998). The earlier the response, the better the chances of initiating successful treatment before the woman experiences advanced cervical dilation.

Controversy exists regarding the efficacy and cost effectiveness of the home uterine monitor. Many studies have found that it is the frequency of comprehensive nursing visits that improves the outcomes and not just the use of the machine. The use of the machine is more beneficial than self-palpation by the woman and telephone reports to a nurse (Gilbert and Harmon, 1998) (Boxes 18-4 and 18-5).

***Stimulation of Fetal Lung Maturity.*** If labor continues and a fetus is to be born between the age of 28 and 34 weeks of gestation, respiratory distress syndrome is a high risk. Steroids may be given to the mother to stimulate the production of lecithin, a surface-active phospholipid that enhances normal alveolar function. The therapy reduces respiratory distress in the newborn by 40% to 60%. Betamethasone (Celestone) and dexamethasone are the steroids of choice

---

### BOX 18-4   *Home Visit Physical Assessment*

Vital signs, including blood pressure, respiratory rate, and temperature
Breath sounds
Fetal heart rate
Fetal activity
Cervical status
Fasting blood glucose because of possible drug-induced alteration in glucose metabolism
Weight
Fundal height
Urine for ketones, protein, and leukocyte esterase
Signs of pathologic edema

From Gilbert E and Harmon J: *Manual of high risk pregnancy and delivery,* ed 2, St Louis, 1998, Mosby.

---

### BOX 18-5   *Functional Health Pattern Assessment for Home Visit*

**HEALTH PERCEPTION/HEALTH MANAGEMENT ASSESSMENT**
Which prenatal health care resources (e.g., childbirth education classes, support groups, social service, and community agencies) have you used or do you plan to use?

**NUTRITIONAL ASSESSMENT**
What is a typical daily food and fluid intake?
Appetite?

**ELIMINATION ASSESSMENT**
Urinary elimination pattern: changes or problems (e.g., odor or burning pain on urination) perceived?
Bowel elimination pattern: changes or problems (e.g., flatulence or constipation) perceived?

**ACTIVITY/EXERCISE ASSESSMENT**
What activity level are you maintaining? What kinds of limited activity exercise are you doing?

**SLEEP/REST ASSESSMENT**
How do you feel after a night's sleep?

**COGNITIVE/PERCEPTUAL ASSESSMENT**
Describe your uterine activity pattern. How many contractions do you palpate during the assessment hour? What activities seem to stimulate contractions?
What kind of management problems have you experienced with the pump, home bed rest, or other recommendations?

**SELF-PERCEPTION/SELF-CONCEPT ASSESSMENT**
Describe how you and your family feel everything is going.

**ROLE-RELATIONSHIP ASSESSMENT**
How are all of your role responsibilities being managed while you are maintaining limited activity?
How are you dealing with boredom?

**SEXUAL/REPRODUCTIVE ASSESSMENT**
Have you experienced any warning signs of preterm labor? How are you and your partner dealing with the restricted sexual activity?

**COPING/STRESS TOLERANCE ASSESSMENT**
What are you most concerned or worried about at this time?
How are other family members dealing with their concerns, anxiety, or fear?

From Gilbert E and Harmon J: *Manual of high risk pregnancy and delivery,* ed 2, St Louis, 1998, Mosby.

because they cross the placenta unchanged. Because it has both short- and long-term activity, betamethasone is generally the preferred drug.

The usual dose of betamethasone is two intramuscular doses of 12 mg of the steroid, 24 hours apart. The dosing of dexamethasone may be 4 intramuscular doses of 6 mg at 12-hour intervals. Forty-eight hours after the first dose is given, the maximum response is achieved. If delivery does not occur within the week and the pregnancy is still less than 34 weeks of gestation, the treatment is repeated.

Medicating the fetus through the mother has potential side effects for the woman. They include increased risk of infection and delayed wound healing and, if the woman has diabetes or hypertension, aggravation of these conditions. If the amniotic sac has ruptured the risk of endometritis is increased. The benefit to the fetus is that in addition to decreasing the risk of fetal respiratory distress, steroid therapy also has been associated with reduced neonatal intraventricular hemorrhage and necrotizing enterocolitis (Enkin and others, 1995; Gilbert and Harmon, 1998).

 ### Assessment

Approximately 10% of pregnant women experience preterm labor. When a woman starts to experience regular rhythmic contractions, she is the first person who must decide whether action must be taken. If she is concerned, she should notify her provider or seek care in an emergency unit. Her health care providers then assume the tasks of further evaluation and determination of whether labor is progressing.

Place the woman in a left lateral position to maximize uterine blood flow. Evaluate the woman's vital signs and blood pressure. An elevated temperature or tachycardia may indicate dehydration or infection. Determine the amount and frequency of her fluid intake.

Assess the contractions using palpation and external fetal monitoring. The woman may experience the contractions as painful or painless, and she may feel them as lower back pain (a backache that comes and goes) or pelvic pressure. Determine if the amniotic sac is still intact using nitrazine paper and the fern test.

A digital examination of her cervix may reveal softening, effacement, dilation, or shortening of her cervix. Examinations should be done infrequently to minimize the risk of infection and by one examiner to allow a more accurate comparison to be made from one examination to the next.

Other possible physical findings are related to the possible cause of the contractions, such as an infection. Nitrites, leukocytes and/or white blood cells or red blood cells may be found in her urine. Costovertebral tenderness (CVAT), indicating kidney involvement, may be present. Vaginal secretions may contain fetal fibronectin. The FHR may demonstrate tachycardia.

The woman may demonstrate that she is feeling stressed through expression of anxiety or fear of the unknown or pregnancy loss. If she is overwhelmed by what is happening to her, she may be confused or restless, have difficulty communicating, and not be able to comprehend instructions. Assess whether she can verbalize her feelings. Determine the level of involvement she currently desires. Expect her desire for involvement to change as she becomes more comfortable with the situation.

If it is determined that the woman requires medication, administer the drugs as ordered and monitor the response of the woman and her fetus. Be aware of the expected side effects and prepare her for their occurrence.

If labor is continuing, assess the preparation of the woman and her support person. Determine what appropriate comfort measures and support they require during the process. Determine their need for information about the preterm labor and delivery process. Assess whether they understand the developmental level of their baby and the special needs it may have at delivery. If the fetus has been compromised or has died in utero, assess if they have been adequately prepared with realistic information.

If labor is stopped and the woman returns home, assess her understanding and ability to follow the prescribed self-medication process. Determine if she will be able to implement the recommendations for self-care, such as reduced stress and activity. Assess whether she will be able to recognize the return of preterm labor. Determine if she knows how to palpate for uterine contractions and to time them. Assess if she understands the procedure to follow if she thinks her labor has returned.

## Premature Rupture of Membranes

**Premature rupture of the membranes (PROM)** occurs when the amniotic membranes spontaneously rupture before the onset of labor. This can occur in either preterm or term gestations. The incidence of identified PROM in pregnancy is 5% to 10% (Knappy, McTigue, and Guzman, 1993).

The time interval between rupture of membranes and the onset of labor may be referred to as the latent period. At term the majority of women begin labor within 24 to 48 hours, 70% giving birth within 24 hours and 90% within 28 hours (Enkin and others, 1995). At 34 weeks of gestation 20% of women will experience a latent period of more than 1 week. At 24 weeks, 40% will have a latency period of more than a week.

The etiology of PROM is not known, but it is stongly linked to intrauterine infection. Other predisposing factors are early effacement and dilation of the cervix, genetic abnormalities, fetal malpresentation, multiple gestation, polyhydramnios, trauma, a history of PROM, and smoking.

The goal of treatment is to maintain the pregnancy until fetal maturity occurs, as long as the uterine environment stays healthy. If the uterine environment becomes infected or is detrimental to the developing fetus, the outcome for the fetus may be improved even with a premature delivery. For assistance with breathing, a neonate may be placed on a ventilator (Figure 18-5).

### Intrapartum Strategies

Diagnosis of PROM can be challenging. Gestational age of the fetus generally determines the plan of care. If the woman is at or near term or if there is fetal pulmonary maturity, delivery will generally be induced or augmented. Women with gestational periods farther away from term are at greater risk of developing an infection and neonatal morbidity.

The woman will report either a gush or small trickle of leaking fluid. Increased vaginal discharge and urinary incontinence should be ruled out. Physical examination may reveal frank fluid pooled in the vagina, but this can be difficult to assess at times because of cessation of an active leak and the simultaneous increase in vaginal secretions. A speculum examination may be helpful in assessing fluid pooling in the vagina and facilitate obtaining a nitrazine test. Amniotic fluid is alkaline and therefore turns nitrazine paper bright blue. A small amount of fluid can be placed on a slide and the fern test done. When amniotic fluid dries, microscopic examination reveals a characteristic fern pattern.

Management approaches for the woman experiencing PROM either can be expedited, in which the process of labor is facilitated, or expectant, in which observation for infection is the central focus of care while "buying time" for fetal maturity in premature gestations. Prophylactic antibiotics have been found to reduce the incidence of both maternal and fetal infection and to extend the birth interval by at least 1 week (Enkin and others, 1995).

The occurrence of PROM places the fetus and neonate at risk for infection, cord prolapse and compression, and deformities resulting from fetal exposure to an environment with reduced amniotic fluid. Fetal structural development may be interfered with by the development of **amniotic bands** (constrictions by multiple fibrous stands of amnion), a diminished fluid environment in which to move, and decreased respiratory "breathing" movement. Amnioinfusion may be ordered to increase the amount of fluid in the uterus.

### Assessment

Have the woman lie in a left lateral position. Assess the fetal heart and determine if it is within normal limits and responds to fetal or uterine activity. Monitor uterine activity for irritability or contractions. Palpate the abdomen for uterine tenderness. Assess the woman's vital signs because elevated temperature or tachycardia may indicate infection.

Do not do a vaginal examination! Even with the use of sterile gloves, organisms near the mouth of the woman's vagina can be pushed up toward the cervix, increasing the risk of infection from vaginal and enteric flora.

Ask the woman about the length of her gestation. Ask about the date and time of the rupture of the membranes (ROM). Does she feel any labor symptoms, including backache, pelvic pressure, or cramping. When the membranes ruptured did she experience a gush or a trickle? Did she notice an odor, flakes of vernix, blood, or meconium?

Why does she think the membranes ruptured? Did any event immediately precede the ROM? Has she had a UTI (urinary frequency, urgency, dysuria, or flank pain)? Has she had a vaginal or pelvic infection (change in vaginal discharge, pelvic pain)?

Assess whether she has an understanding of the possible risks for her baby. Assess her level of stress, preparedness for delivery, sense of guilt, and ability to cope with this unexpected event.

Determine if she understands the reason for the blood work (to indicate presence of an infection), nitrazine paper test (to detect amniotic fluid), and possibly amniocentesis (to determine presence of infection and fetal lung maturity).

Observe if amniotic fluid is still discharging and assess for purulence or odor. Observe vaginal discharge for purulence and odor.

If ordered, administer antibiotics and determine the woman's response to the drug. The woman may be placed on bed rest with a uterine and fetal heart monitor. If the head of the fetus has not engaged in the pelvis, the woman may be placed in a slight Trendelenburg position to decrease the risk of a prolapsed cord. Observe for evidence of cord compression as indicated by variable decelerations on the fetal monitor.

Emergency interventions begin when an individual discovers a prolapsed cord. A sterile vaginal examination

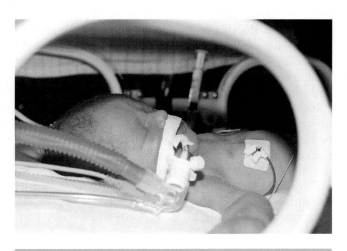

FIGURE 18-5 • Premie on ventilator. *(Courtesy of Caroline E. Brown.)*

and manual support of the presenting part to reduce pressure applied against the umbilical is critical. The mother is then placed in a position that facilitates gravity's ability to slide the fetus away from the prolapsed cord; elevating the hips is the therapeutic goal and this can be accomplished with a modified lateral position or knee-chest position. A Foley catheter may be inserted and the bladder filled to act as a block elevating the presenting part. If in use, all oxytocin drugs should be discontinued. A tocolytic agent may be ordered to reduce the contraction force against the prolapsed cord. Saline soaked gauze at body temperature may be applied to the cord if it has prolapsed beyond the vagina. A surgical delivery is expedited and a neonatal resuscitation team should be present at the birth.

If there was a leakage of amniotic fluid but no emergent danger for the fetus, the woman may be sent home. Assess whether she understands the signs and symptoms of infection (e.g., elevated temperature, foul-smelling amniotic fluid, a significant increase in vaginal discharge, or abdominal pain or tenderness), the signs and symptoms of labor, and when she should return to the hospital.

## Postterm Pregnancy

A **postterm** or prolonged pregnancy is one that has extended beyond 42 weeks since the first day of the last menstrual cycle, when the woman's cycles have been 28 days. A postterm pregnancy is associated with increased perinatal morbidity and mortality (Grub, Rabello, and Paul, 1992).

A **postmature** infant is one that has developed an abnormal condition resulting from a postterm pregnancy. The infant often has little or no vernix; an "old look" with a gaunt appearance, long nails and hair; reduced subcutaneous fat; meconium-stained, wrinkled, and peeling skin; and heightened alertness. Vernix caseosa, the oily substance that protects the skin of the fetus from the effects of being immersed in water in utero begins to disappear after the thirty-sixth week, allowing the skin to become shriveled and peel.

The effects of a postdate pregnancy on the fetus are related to changes in amniotic fluid and in the placenta and umbilical cord. Reduced amniotic fluid volume results in oligohydramnios that in turn predisposes the fetus to cord entrapment and compression. The passage of meconium into the amniotic fluid causes the fluid to thicken, inhibits the abnormal antibiotic properties of the amniotic fluid, and stiffens the umbilical cord by pulling fluids from the Wharton jelly. As the result of the stiffening of the cord, it becomes more susceptible to pressure and possible kinking (Gilbert and Harmon, 1998).

Degenerative changes in the placenta affect the diffusion of oxygen. It is not known if this affects fetal outcomes because most postterm babies continue to grow.

If the fetus continues to grow it can become macrosomic and at higher risk for birth injuries. Macrosomia occurs in 20% to 25% of postdates pregnancies.

### Intrapartum Strategies

Management of postdate pregnancies begins with accurate gestational dating.

Evaluation focuses on determining uteroplacental exchange and amniotic fluid volume. Fetal well-being is evaluated. Maternal fetal movement counts have been used as a general screening tool. A routine nonstress test is usually initiated at 41 to 42 weeks of gestation. The contraction stress test may be used to assess fetal oxygenation. Ultrasound provides information about amniotic fluid volume and the biophysical profile creates a general picture of the behavioral status of the fetus.

To initiate labor some women are encouraged to have sexual intercourse or engage in breast stimulation  with their partners. Women who are discouraged from these activities have a higher occurrence of postdate pregnancies (Crowley, 1995). The use of prostaglandin gel has been shown to increase the success of initiating labor. The prostaglandin gel causes effacement and softening of the cervix, thereby increasing cervical readiness to efface and dilate when labor contractions start.

Initiation of more active interventions such as the induction of labor with Pitocin is controversial. Some benefit for pregnancy outcome has been demonstrated with induction of labor at 41 weeks or greater gestation as compared to induction between 40 and 41 weeks of gestation when limited benefit has been demonstrated (Crowley, 1995).

### Assessment

Warning signs that a pregnancy is becoming postterm are maternal weight loss in excess of 3 pounds per week. This is a reflection of possible decreased amniotic fluid. With the decreased fluid will come a decreased uterine size. Measure the fundal height.

Assess the pregnancy dating using Naegele's rule, the timing of the positive pregnancy test, the timing of quickening, and the date when fetal heart tones were heard. Assess the woman's understanding about the use of an ultrasound examination to date the pregnancy.

Assess the woman's stress and anxiety concerning not having gone into labor yet. Determine how well she is coping with the normal discomforts of pregnancy.

Assess her understanding of the process and purpose of the diagnostic procedures such as fetal movement counts, amniotic fluid volume index, a nonstress test, a contraction stress test, and a biophysical profile.

Assess the knowledge and concerns of the woman and her partner concerning a postterm pregnancy. Determine their comfort in following a directive to stimulate labor through breast stimulation and sexual intercourse. Assess whether they understand and are comfortable with an intravenous induction procedure with Pitocin.

## Labor of Unusual Duration

A woman's labor may be labeled as precipitous or prolonged as compared to Friedman's curve, which diagrams the average labor experience. Women and providers alike often forget that this curve represents an average, with as many women having longer labor experiences as those having shorter labor experiences. The effect of the labor on the fetus and mother is the basis of intrapartum assessment and intervention.

### Intrapartum Strategies

**Precipitous labor** is a labor that is 3 hours or less in duration. It often is accompanied by rapid expulsion of the fetus through the birth canal. Risks of a precipitous labor for the mother involve soft tissue damage, lacerations of the birth canal, and increased risk of postpartum hemorrhage. Risks to the neonate involve birth trauma resulting from rapid descent through the birth canal.

**Prolonged labor** is one that is longer than expected. The fatigue that develops as the result of coping with unrelenting uterine contractions presents a challenge to the woman and her labor support. The lengthening can occur in the latent or the active phases of labor. Prolonged labors in low-risk pregnancies do not increase fetal distress (Enkin and others, 1995).

**Prolonged latent phase** is a latent phase that extends beyond 14 hours in the multiparous woman and 20 hours in the primiparous woman. Alterations in latent phase have demonstrated little relationship with perinatal outcome. The most significant concern is for the level of fatigue of the woman and her support system. Rest is the most commonly offered therapeutic intervention, most often with the administration of morphine. Amniotomy is not recommended, and rest induced with sedative agents is discouraged. These drugs are more slowly metabolized in the fetus, and the effects may extend into the newborn period. Optimal management centers around prevention with the provision of anticipatory guidance for women to avoid early admission to the hospital or birth center and ambulate freely.

A **protracted active phase** of labor is defined as cervical dilation in a nullipara of less than 1.2 cm per hour and of less than 1.5 cm per hour in the multipara. Secondary arrest of cervical dilation is defined as no cervical changes for 2 hours during active labor. Common contributing factors include malposition of the fetus (occiput posterior presentation), maternal fear or anxiety, maternal fatigue, regional anesthesia, and cephalopelvic disproportion. Initial management involves assessment of the underlying contributing factors. With a reassuring FHR tracing, rest, positional changes, movement, hydrotherapy, and acupressure can be used before

medical interventions are initiated. Pain management, oxytocin, and amniotomy may be initiated if the previous interventions do not create cervical change. A hysterotomy may be recommended if no cervical change occurs with the medical interventions.

**Uterine contractility** is another factor in the alterations of the length of labor. Uterine contractility patterns have been grouped as hypertonic and hypotonic. The assessment of uterine contractility becomes a determinant of oxytocin use. Iatrogenic factors, maternal fatigue, medications, distention of the uterus, and malpresentation of the fetus can alter uterine contractility. Hypertonic uterine contractions are most commonly seen with oxytocin administration but they also may be caused by iatrogenic factors. Pain management is often suggested to allow the woman to rest and to attempt to break the pattern of hypertonic contractions. If oxytocin is the causative agent, it should be decreased to obtain a more physiologic contraction pattern.

The hypotonic uterine contraction patterns are managed by attending to the causative factor and considering stimulation of uterine activity. This can be achieved with nonintervention techniques as a first-line approach. Maternal movement and nipple stimulation are two common approaches.

Second stage may be facilitated in several ways. Maternal position has a dramatic effect on second stage, with squatting positions expanding the pelvic diameter by 20% to 30%. A trend toward more liberal thinking on second-stage management is beginning to occur, with less tendency to time progress and more of a tendency to allow maternal efforts to continue when the FHR continues to be reassuring. Medical interventions including vacuum extraction and outlet forceps may be employed if the fetus develops a nonreassuring pattern or the mother cannot continue her expulsive efforts. A hysterotomy also may be chosen as the method of delivery.

### Assessment

Assessment of the physiologic response of the woman and the fetus to labor remains the same and is not dependent on the length of labor. Assessment of the emotional response of the woman and her labor support person to the events of labor is vital. Assess their concerns regarding the process being different than what they expected. Determine if they have fears for the health and well-being of the woman, the baby, or both.

## Amniotic Fluid Embolism

A rare respiratory emergency is created when a small amount of amniotic fluid enters the maternal circulation through a tear in the placental membranes. The amniotic fluid contains particles of debris that create blockages in the maternal pulmonary capillary and systemic circulatory system and may lead to acute respiratory distress and circulatory collapse. A vigorous labor, oxytocin, multiple gestations, and a hysterotomy are risk factors associated with amniotic fluid embolism. Although the exact incidence is unknown, this rare complication has a mortality rate as high as 80%. If a woman survives an amniotic fluid embolism, hemorrhage and DIC are two additional complications.

### Intrapartum Strategies

An amniotic fluid embolism is such a rare obstetric complication that there is no need to prepare the couple for the potential emergency. Be alert to the possibility of an amniotic embolism occurring if the woman experiences a rapid or vigorous labor or abruptio placentae. It also may occur as a side effect to an amnioinfusion. Therapeutic management involves an expedited birth and resuscitation of the mother with further care in a critical care setting if the mother survives. If an embolism occurs, after the woman has survived the event an explanation should be forthcoming (Mattson and Smith, 2000).

### Assessment

Acute onset of respiratory distress, often during the delivery process, is a sign of an amniotic fluid embolism. Observe for restlessness, dyspnea, cyanosis, frothy sputum, and chest pain. Cardiovascular collapse occurs with severe hypoxia, severe hypotension, and possibly hemorrhage and DIC.

## Shoulder Dystocia

Shoulder dystocia occurs when the infant's head is born spontaneously but the infant's shoulders do not slide under the pubic bone. Shoulder dystocia occurs in approximately 1% of births, increasing perinatal morbidity and mortality (Seeds and Walsh, 1996). A brachial plexus injury, a fractured clavicle, and/or asphyxia can occur as the birth of the infant is facilitated. Macrosomic infants are at highest risk for the occurrence of shoulder dystocia at birth.

### Intrapartum Strategies

Management centers around altering the pelvic diameter to allow more room for the infant to be born. The nurse midwife or physician may try to compress the infant's shoulders under the pubic bone by applying direct suprapubic pressure. Fundal pressure is contraindicated because it forces the shoulders against the pubic bone worsening the impaction.

### Assessment

The infant's head may appear to draw back towards the vagina because of the tension from the impacted shoulders. The second stage of labor appears to stop. Maintain assessment of maternal and fetal vital signs. Assess the woman's level of anxiety and respond appropriately.

## CARE OF THE FAMILY AFTER A LABOR AND DELIVERY WITH RISK

It is almost certain that every woman and her partner will need assistance in sorting out and dealing with the events that occurred during their labor and delivery experience. Things may have happened very rapidly at some points, without the parents having a full explanation or understanding.

They are also dealing with loss, often of an unexplainable and unexpected intensity. Women experience a loss of their anticipated birth experience and partners have lost their anticipated role during the process. Some women feel that their need for high-tech intervention means that they have failed at a very basic feminine process—giving birth. Family members are often not helpful or supportive in their responses, since they are just grateful that the woman is alive.

A woman may be grateful that she survived, yet grieve the loss of her fertility and ability to bear future children if her uterus had to be removed to stop bleeding. She may have a live, but disabled infant, and must grieve the loss of the perfect child she had envisioned welcoming into her family. If she was pregnant with multiples, she may now have to grieve the loss of one infant while welcoming the arrival of its sibling. The woman or her partner may feel responsible for creating the crises and be trying to handle this unnecessary guilt.

The experience for each woman and her partner is different. Respond in an individualized manner. Help them each "debrief" as they talk about the events and try to fill in their gaps in understanding. They may not know why a certain procedure was done or a certain specialist was called in to the care team. Respond to misconceptions or misinformation with accurate information. Identify and provide information that alleviates feelings of guilt. Enable the couple to collaborate in the development of the plan of care they require and help them make the appropriate connections for continuing care after discharge from the hospital.

## CARE OF THE FAMILY WHEN THE INFANT REQUIRES SPECIAL CARE

The birth of a live infant is a cause for rejoicing; however, depending on the baby's health, the parents may not get to meet the infant until after he or she has been stabilized and placed in a special care nursery for further observation and treatment. Approaching the nursery with its machinery, apparatus, and alarms can be frightening to parents. Seeing their baby so small and vulnerable in the incubator with intravenous tubing, leads attached to its body, or on a ventilator can be very disturbing. Briefly orient them and give them culturally appropriate encouraging words about their baby. Explain the apparatus, what each piece is, and how it is helping in the care of their baby. Encourage the parents to interact with their baby, reaching in and stroking the infant and/or talking to it. If culturally acceptable, ask the parents what the child's name is and role model talking to the baby, "Hey Peter, your Mommy is here. Remember her voice?" If the parents seem comfortable give them some privacy by moving away a little distance so they can talk to the baby more freely. If the infant dies, this may be the only time they can communicate with him or her. If there are siblings they may also be brought in to greet their baby (Figure 18-6).

If the baby requires minimal special care, such as oxygen, the mother may be able to interact and bond with him or her in the privacy of her hospital room. Gradually the father of the baby, if initially hesitant, also may become involved. Gentle encouragement and role modeling how to handle and hold the infant can help a hesitant father move from looking at the infant while the mother holds it to holding the infant himself. The amount of time for this process to occur varies and should not be rushed because it must be individualized to the father's needs and abilities. Some fathers feel more comfortable taking it in steps or waiting until the infant is larger or older (Figure 18-7).

## CARE OF THE FAMILY WHEN THE INFANT DIES

When an infant is born dead or not expected to survive, families are placed in a crisis situation for which they are often unprepared. For some, it is the family's first experience with a significant loss. When an infant dies at any point in the reproductive cycle parents may respond in various ways.

The attachment between the mother and her unborn infant occurs early in the pregnancy. The extent of the attachment mothers and fathers have with the developing fetus influence the way they experience the grief (Limbo and Wheeler, 1998). A mother and father can have very different reactions to loss in the perinatal period, or the same reactions although they occur in a different pattern. Siblings, grandparents, and other relatives also experience sadness and grief with the loss of the expected child. Information, referral, and compassion are necessary to help families as they begin the process of grieving their loss.

Some hospitals have instituted intervention strategies for parents experiencing loss in the perinatal period (Brown, 1992; Brown and Kozick, 1994). A guiding principle for these programs is to establish the reality of the infant's life and death (Harr and Thistlethwaite, 1990). Bereavement research has demonstrated that preserving memories of an infant's existence facilitates maternal expression of grief (Harr and Thistlethwaite, 1990; Brown, 1992). Perceptual confirmation of the infant's existence enables the mother to begin to accept the reality of her infant's life and death, a process central to grief work (Brown, 1992). Interventions such

as contact with the infant and obtaining photographs and mementos are most often seen in hospital-based perinatal loss programs.

### Caring for Families Following an Infant's Death

A first step in assisting parents through the grieving process is evaluating our own emotional response to

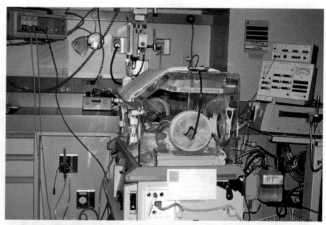
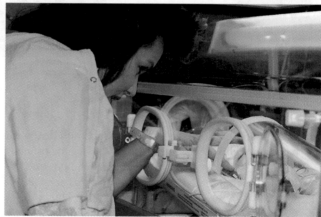
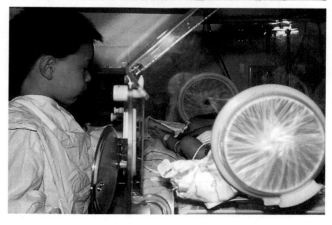

*FIGURE 18-6* • Seeing a baby on a ventilator can be a frightening experience for the parents and siblings. *(Courtesy of Caroline E. Brown.)*

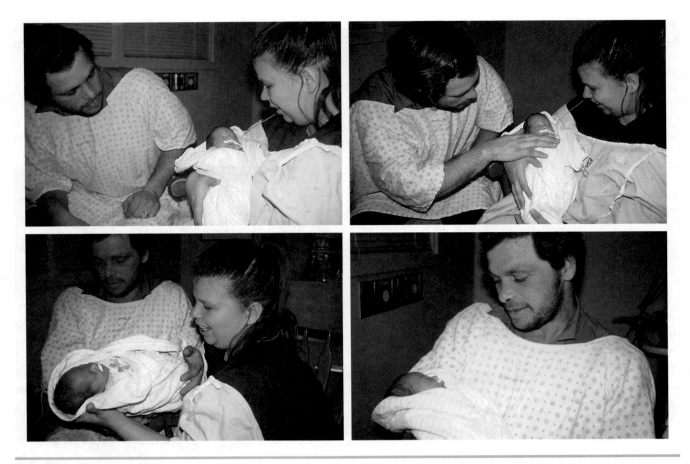

FIGURE 18-7 • Father's interaction increases. *(Courtesy of Caroline E. Brown.)*

perinatal loss. We must be able to recognize and deal with our personal feelings before effectively caring for others.

When an infant dies, the maternal attachment and future planning that had begun early in pregnancy is replaced with shattered hopes and dreams. The mother needs the opportunity to complete the attachment process before she can proceed to grieving. Attachment behaviors provide the mother with the opportunity to define the infant's reality in her own terms. To do this a woman may hold her infant, touch and caress the baby, and bathe and dress it.

New mothers confirm the acquaintance process with their newborn infant by achieving congruence between the images of the infant they created during pregnancy and the reality. At birth, maternal attention centers around confirmation of gender, health, and identifying characteristics such as hair and eye color. Identification of the infant then proceeds to visual inspection and touch, as the mother engages in exploration of the newborn infant. Touch begins with the finger tips and then progresses to the use of the palms to uncover, explore, and enfold the infant (Rubin, 1984). Exploration progresses from the outer aspects of the infant, moving in-ward to encompass the infant's body . The mother refines and develops confidence in her skills of touch through repeated contacts with the infant (Rubin, 1984).

It is clearly evident that seeing, touching, and holding are central to the attachment process for mothers with infants born alive or for stillborn infants. In actuality, these hours after the birth of a stillborn become a critical time because it is the only time they will have to develop a sense of knowing and parenting their infant.

Mothers with stillborn infants and those that die after birth should be offered the opportunity to spend time with their infant. Although this may be difficult for parents because it is unexpected, it is not morbid or an unusual behavior. When initially asked, parents may hesitate because they are unsure of the appropriate procedures or if they can deal with the interaction. Mothers and their partners are often immersed in shock, anger, and denial. The mother may still be feeling the effects from medications used during the birth process.

We play a critical role in guiding parents with gentle suggestions, reassurance, and support for taking their time to make decisions. Describe the infant to them so that anticipatory fears are restructured by reality. Par-

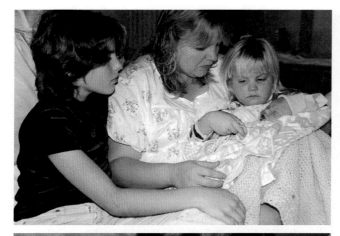

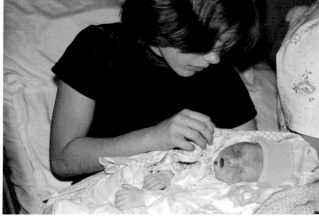

FIGURE 18-8 • Mother and siblings taking time to say goodbye. *(Courtesy of Caroline E. Brown.)*

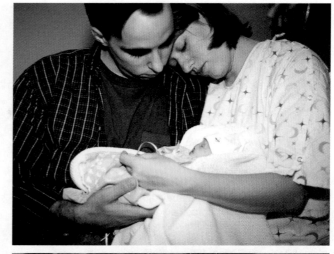

A

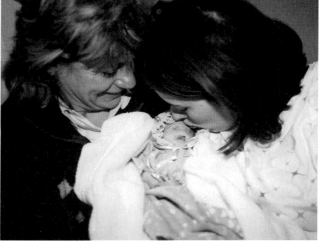

B

FIGURE 18-9 • **A,** Parents grieving together. **B,** Grandparents and other relatives also experience sadness and grief with loss. *(Courtesy of Caroline E. Brown.)*

ents may worry that their child looks terrible and not be sure they want that vision in their mind. Offer to spend time with the parents and infant more than one time. Gently share that being with the infant has been found helpful by other mothers later on in their grief process.

### The Initial Contact

The initial contact begins with a concrete description of the infant, including physical appearance and feeling of coldness that the infant may have. Bring the infant to the parents swaddled in a blanket and dressed. New mothers touch their newborns tentatively, fearful of hurting the infant and of not performing the mothering tasks correctly. This is also true of women who are interacting with their dead infant. We can model nurturing behaviors while teaching the new mother about her infant, thus easing her into this role.

New mothers often need permission to open the blankets and to explore their live infant; when an infant

has died, the need for permission can be intensified. Facilitate the process of acquaintance by highlighting features of the infant, recognizing size and development of hands and feet or simply recognizing the beauty of the infant. If family members are with the mother, include them in the process (Figures 18-8 and 18-9).

Some mothers and their support systems will want privacy and time alone to explore their infant while others will not want to be alone and prefer that we stay. Be sensitive to their needs as they spend time with the infant and adjust your plan accordingly.

Offer parents the opportunity to engage in any of the infant caretaking activities they would have done if the infant had been born alive. Some parents find it helpful to participate in bathing, dressing and diapering, cuddling, and simply being with the infant. It is important to allow the mother and her support person the

## BOX 18-6 *Considerations When Providing Care to a Family Facing Grief and Loss*

1. Family members and health care providers should support the woman throughout the labor process.
2. Ensure physical comfort during labor. Pain medication should be offered as needed. Sedatives are generally not offered because they tend to interfere with the establishment of the grief process. Provide basic nursing comfort measures.
3. Maintain privacy and confidentiality.
4. Do not separate mother and partner/prime support person and supportive family members.
5. Talk to parents together rather than individually.
6. Be sure that all providers provide consistent information.
7. Recognize the family's need for active participation in decision making.
8. Location after delivery. Offer parents the choice of being on the postpartum unit or transferred to another floor. Some mothers choose to stay on the postpartum floor as a way to begin facing the reality of their infant's death and facilitating the grief process; others may find it too painful.
9. A checklist can be a useful tool to communicate the plan of care within the health care team.
10. Remember, partners and support persons also need to be supported. If the partner's response is one of calm strength, it may be misunderstood and his needs not recognized or supported. Most men feel the need to maintain their strength and are socialized not to cry or show emotions.
11. Seeing and touching the baby can facilitate the grieving process by dispelling fantasies that may be more frightening. A verbal description of the infant's appearance will help prepare the parents.
12. Encourage parents to name the baby, using the name decided upon during pregnancy. It is best not to save it for another child.
13. Parents should be encouraged to have an autopsy done so that their questions of why this happened may be answered. This will facilitate future counseling and decision making for the parents.
14. Photographs of the dead were a common occurrence in previous generations. For parents of a dead infant at the initial time of loss it may be difficult to consider, but a picture can provide tangible evidence of the existence of a baby. Many commercial baby photo companies offer free photographs to parents when an infant dies.
15. Offer the option of baptism or other religious services for the family.
16. Have a religious leader of the parents' preference available to them.
17. Allay guilt feelings in each of the parents that they somehow caused this death.
18. Explain the grief process to them and ask them to be patient with themselves.
19. Describe the normal variation in the grief reaction between mothers and fathers.
20. Collect keepsakes the parents may desire: a lock of hair (taken with their permission); complimentary birth certificate with foot prints (if possible); identification wrist bracelet; and the record of weight, length, and head and chest measurements, with the time of birth.

opportunity to fulfill the early attachment behaviors they desire. Care should be directed at facilitating the same early experiences for this family that the family of a live-born infant would be offered, allowing each family to choose activities that meet their individual needs. Some families may desire a long period of time or repeat contacts with the infant. There is no right or wrong way for them to structure this "hello and goodbye" experience.

Assist the parents in planning how to include their family members and friends in the process. Some may wish to plan a funeral while others may desire a memorial service or graveside service. Because parents are not aware of their options and alternatives, they will require anticipatory guidance in developing a plan (Boxes 18-6 and 18-7).

We critically influence the parent's journey through grief with our actions and words. Supporting the perceptual reality of the infant's existence is very supportive. Maternal expression of grief is an intense and individual experience unique to each person within her own life context. Therefore each intervention must be individualized for the particular situation.

The process of grieving extends over a period of time. Before a woman is discharged from the hospital appropriate referrals and connections to community-based support services are vital. Few parents will have friends or family members with whom they can continue their grief work.

 **SUMMARY**

A woman who experiences an intrapartum period that presents risks to her or her child's health and well-being requires extensive physical and emotional care. The needs of the family also must be addressed as they experience the potential loss of the woman or the baby. Each intrapartum period ends with the delivery of a baby, either dead or alive. Helping the parents move through the final steps of the pregnancy process to its natural conclusion can be challenging yet satisfying.

## BOX 18-7   *Making Memories*

Confirmation of an infant's existence through concrete means has been shown to help a parent's process of grief. Reconstruction of a parent's vision of his or her infant establishes memories that serve to confirm the infant's life and death. Some ideas for helping mothers and fathers make memories of their infant follow.

### CREATE A MEMORY BOX
Place the following items in the box:
- Hand/foot prints: You can use the back ink printing system, inkless ink pads, or a bright colored paint.
- Baby cap
- Blanket
- Crib card
- ID bracelet
- Lock of hair
- Impressions of the hands and/or feet
- Baby clothing worn
- Tape measure that measured head circumference and length
- Diapers and any other items that came in contact with the infant

Be creative—the parents' desires and your imagination will guide you.

### IMPRESSIONING TECHNIQUE
Impressioning is another means of preserving memories (Brown and Kozick, 1994). The impressioning technique has been created for infants of varying gestational ages. The technique is effective in creating a memento of any stillborn infant, especially those who may be macerated. The impressions provide a tangible memento and help parents create an image of their infant they can easily share with family.

### HOW TO CREATE LASTING IMPRESSIONS OF BABY HANDS AND BABY FEET
**Materials Needed:**
Disposable gloves

Cups for mixing

Tongue blades or mixing spoon

Shallow containers for pouring molds

Impression powder-alginate regular set

Plaster/porcelain mix

Sea shells or other final containers

**Procedure:**
1. The impression material is mixed, using the coldest water possible to prevent the material from "setting up" too quickly. You will need to add less water than indicated on the material directions to make a mixture that resembles thick pancake batter.
2. The mixture is stirred quickly and completely to achieve a semismooth consistency (a few lumps are expected); air bubbles will be tapped out as the mixture is poured.
3. The mixture is then poured into shallow receptacles large enough to accommodate the baby 's hand or foot. The receptacles can be anything available; (e.g., drinking cups (cut to size), specimen bottle lids, denture cups, soap dishes).
4. The infant's hand or foot is gently placed in the impression material. The limb will need to be supported, allowing it to suspend and not come in contact with the bottom of container. The limb is held in place until the material "sets up" (usually within 5 minutes). The material becomes "rubbery" to touch.
5. The hand or foot is carefully removed, taking care not to tear mold. The molds need to be moistened with a few drops of water or a moist paper towel inside the zip-lock bag and refrigerated.
6. The next phase is the pouring of the impressions: simple plaster of paris or porcelain can be used. Mix it according to package directions and then pour it into the molds of the hands and/or feet. When pouring the plaster into the molds, gently tap the mold to eliminate trapped air bubbles. Take care not to let molds sit too long once poured because the plaster will adhere to the mold.
7. Unmolding the impressions is done when they have air-dried and hardened. When individual hands and feet are completely dry, the rough edges can be sanded with a nail file.
8. The final step is the mounting process. The hands and feet impressions are set in plaster-filled containers such as sea shells or shaped hearts.

Additional plaster is mixed and poured to fill the final container. When the plaster begins to thicken or partially "set-up" the impressions are carefully placed in the plaster material. If the plaster has not set up enough the hands/feet will sink down too far.

Note: Always wear disposable gloves when working with these materials because they can irritate the skin.

### Ordering Information for Impression Materials:
Leventhal and Sons, Inc.
711 Davis Street
P.O. Box 5150
Scranton, PA 18505
717-342-9106
1-800-982-4312
Price: $6.55 per 1-pound can

## Care Plan · Nursing Care of the Intrapartum Woman with Diabetes Mellitus

NURSING DIAGNOSIS  **Risk for injury (maternal or fetal)** related to hyperglycemia or hypoglycemia
GOALS/OUTCOMES  Mother/baby will remain free of injury; baby will be born in healthy state

**NOC Suggested Outcomes**
- Risk Control (1902)
- Blood Glucose Control (2300)
- Vital Sign Status (0802)
- Fluid Balance (0601)
- Tissue Perfusion: Cerebral (0406)

**NIC Priority Interventions**
- Hyperglycemia Management (2130)
- Electronic Fetal Monitoring: Intrapartum (6772)
- Fluid Monitoring (4130)
- Cerebral Perfusion Promotion (2550)
- Fluid Management (4120)
- Acid-Base Monitoring (1920)
- Acid-Base Management: Metabolic Acidosis (1911)

**Nursing Activities and Rationale**
- Obtain a baseline blood glucose and monitor every 1 to 2 hours *to provide data for future comparisons to prevent hyperglycemia or hypoglycemia.*
- Assess and monitor woman's current state of blood glucose control *to identify risk for fetal and maternal morbidity and mortality.*
- Maintain prescribed insulin infusion or intermittent subcutaneous insulin injections *to maintain glucose level between 70 and 90 mg/dl throughout labor.*
- Monitor uterine placement and contractility *to identify overdistention and/or displacement of uterus due to complications such as macrosomia (birth weight above the 90th percentile on intrauterine growth curve).*
- Monitor for clinical manifestations of PIH. *Women with pregnancy-induced DM are at increased risk for PIH.*
- Monitor FHR, variability, and response to contractions *to provide data regarding the baby's physical state throughout the birth process.*
- Monitor for indications of dystocia or arrest of descent of the fetus down the birth canal. *If progression of the labor process is inhibited, the woman may need to have a surgical abdominal birth.*
- Monitor fluid status and acid-base balance *to prevent hypovolemia secondary to osmotic diuresis or metabolic acidosis secondary to hyperglycemia and elevated ketones.*

**Evaluation Parameters**
- Blood gluocose levels within range of 70 to 90 mg/dl.
- Fluid balance and acid-base status within normal limits.
- No evidence of fetal distress.
- Vital signs within normal limits.
- Normal progression of labor.

NURSING DIAGNOSIS  **Anxiety (or Fear)** related to real or imagined threat to maternal and/or fetal well-being
GOALS/OUTCOMES  Woman will exhibit anxiety/fear control *(See "Evaluation Parameters.")*

**NOC Suggested Outcomes**
- Fear Control (1404)
- Anxiety Control (0704)

**NIC Priority Interventions**
- Anxiety Reduction (5820)
- Coping Enhancement (5230)
- Security Enhancement (5380)

**Nursing Activities and Rationale**
- Assess woman's reaction and understanding of her disease process and correct misconceptions *to establish a baseline for care planning and determine the degree of intervention needed. Correcting misconceptions and supplying factual information may reduce fear and anxiety.*
- Encourage verbalization of feelings, concerns and fears. *Verbalization of fears can help relieve them and provide insight into the woman's individual needs.*
- Encourage the woman with preexisting DM to participate in making decisions about own care during the birth process. *Focuses on the woman's knowledge of her disease and provides a sense of power over the situation.*
- Stay with the woman without requiring verbal interactions *to promote feelings of security while fostering physical and emotional rest.*

## Care Plan · Nursing Care of the Intrapartum Woman with Diabetes Mellitus—cont'd

- Explain all tests and procedures. *Knowledge can reduce fear and anxiety.*
- Provide reinforcement for use of positive coping strategies and relaxation techniques. *Such techniques allow the woman to gain control over her fears. Reinforcement increases the possibility that positive coping strategies and relaxation will be used again.*
- Use a calm, reassuring approach *to prevent transference of anxiety to the woman during stressful situations and to help the woman maintain control when feeling stressed.*
- Convey acceptance of the woman's perception of fear *to encourage open communication with the woman regarding the source of her fear.*
- Encourage an attitude of realistic hope *to help the woman focus on a positive, but realistic outcome.*

### Evaluation Parameters
- Participates in self-care and decision making.
- Seeks information to reduce fears.
- Uses relaxation techniques and positive coping strategies.
- Freely verbalizes fears and concerns.
- Verbalizes feelings of hope.

NURSING DIAGNOSIS **Knowledge deficit** related to lack of previous experience or lack of recall of information
GOALS/OUTCOMES Will adhere to prescribed regimens throughout birth process

### NOC Suggested Outcomes
- Knowledge: Disease Process (1803)
- Knowledge: Labor and Delivery (1817)
- Knowledge: Treatment Procedures (1814)

### NIC Priority Interventions
- Teaching: Disease Process (5602)
- Teaching: Procedure/Treatment (5618)

### Nursing Activities and Rationale
- Teach the woman about the risks involved in the birth process when complicated by diabetes *to enhance the woman's understanding, correct misconceptions, and gain compliance with prescribed therapies.*
- Explain treatments and procedures and the reason for their performance *to increase the woman's understanding and decrease her fears and anxiety during a stressful situation.*
- Prepare the woman regarding the need for constant monitoring of her blood glucose levels *to alleviate her anxiety about frequent glucose monitoring and assure her that frequent monitoring does not indicate the presence of a complication.*
- Teach the woman about continuous fetal monitoring *to alleviate her anxiety and assure her that monitoring her baby's response to labor is a precautionary measure.*
- Teach the woman and her partner about surgical delivery if possibility is anticipated *to prepare her for the possibility of surgical abdominal delivery intervention should it become necessary.*

### Evaluation Parameters
- Describes monitoring procedures.
- Describes birth process and possible alterations caused by her disease.

## CASE STUDY

Raeanne is a 25-year-old woman, G 3, P 2. She delivered her first baby 5 years ago with abdominal surgery after reaching 32 weeks of gestation and starting labor. The little girl's development has progressed within normal limits. Last year Raeanne delivered a boy after 26 weeks of gestation. He died within 48 hours because of respiratory distress syndrome. She is pregnant again and has completed 25 weeks of gestation. This morning she started cramping and her doctor had her admitted to the hospital. She has experienced no vaginal discharge or bleeding. The FHR is 138 with variability.

- Why is Raeanne considered at risk for a preterm labor?

## CASE STUDY

- What assessments are critical when caring for Raeanne at this time? Why?

- What diagnostic tests may be ordered?

- What factors determine whether to intervene with the contractions?

The decision is made with Raeanne and her husband to attempt to suppress the labor.

- What information will she require about the treatment plan?

- How can side effects be reduced?

- What specifically must be monitored if she is given magnesium sulfate?

- Why can a much higher dose of magnesium be given to stop preterm labor than to prevent the possibility of seizures from preeclampsia?

- Why won't you give narcotics or sedatives concurrently?

- What assessments will be ongoing while she is receiving the drug?

- What findings will lead to immediate termination of magnesium sulfate before the contractions are suppressed?

Raeanne's contractions stop and she is discharged. She is placed in a home uterine monitoring program and receives visits from a visiting nurse every other day. To comply with these directives she has to take an unpaid leave of absence from her job. The family health insurance policy will continue because it is through her husband's employment.

- If you were providing the follow-up care at home, what assessments would you focus on during your visits?

- What limitations may be suggested for Raeanne's activities within the home?

- What strategies will increase Raeanne's ability to follow those suggestions?

When doing a home visit at 34 weeks, you detect uterine contractions. They are mild and Raeanne cannot feel them. When you tell her she says, "I feel so bad. I should have tried harder then this wouldn't be happening."

- How do you respond?

Arrangements are made for the care of her 5-year-old daughter, and Raeanne is readmitted to the hospital.

- What are the concerns about delivering a fetus of 34 weeks' gestation?

- How will some of the risks to the fetus of early delivery be minimized?

- How should Raeanne and her husband be prepared for the events that will follow this readmission?

## Scenarios

1. Haley is a 28-year-old woman, G 1, P 0, in early labor. She has a history of cardiac disease caused by rheumatic fever. You have just assumed her care with the change of shifts. You know that cardiac output gradually increases during labor and peaks at a 65% increase at 5 minutes after the birth and continues at a 40% increase at 1 hour after birth. Haley has just become fully dilated and is now pushing with the second stage of labor.

- What assessments are critical during this birth? Why?

- What medical technology or interventions may you be required to administer or monitor during the birthing process?

- What nursing diagnoses could apply? How will you validate these?

- What are the goals of the critical care she is receiving? Why?

- What other goals may be developed?

- What interventions are critical because of Haley's preexisting medical condition?

- What interventions are necessary because Haley is in labor?

- How will you evaluate the effectiveness of your interventions?

---

2. Shannon, age 34, G 2, P 1, has developed asthma since the birth of her first child. She is now in labor with her second child and is very concerned about how this may affect her labor and birth.

- What assessments are critical during this birth? Why?
- What medical technology or interventions may you be required to administer or monitor during the birthing process?
- What nursing diagnoses could apply? How will you validate these?
- What are the goals of the critical care she is receiving? Why?
- What other goals may be developed?
- What interventions are critical because of Shannon's preexisting medical condition?
- What interventions are necessary because Shannon is in labor?
- How will you evaluate the effectiveness of your interventions?

---

3. Genevieve is a 28-year-old woman, G 1, P 1, who learned during this pregnancy that she has SLE. She has not yet developed a full understanding of her disease and now she is trying to deal with the effect of the disease on her labor experience.

- What assessments are critical during this birth? Why?
- What medical technology or interventions may you be required to administer or monitor during the birthing process?
- What nursing diagnoses could apply? How will you validate these?
- What are the goals of the critical care she is receiving? Why?
- What other goals may be developed?
- What interventions are critical because of Genevieve's preexisting medical condition?
- What interventions are necessary because Genevieve is in labor?
- How will you evaluate the effectiveness of your interventions?

---

4. Celeste, a 15-year-old girl, G 1, P 1, developed PIH during her pregnancy. She is now in early labor and her blood pressure is within normal limits. Celeste has no family and friends with her in labor. She says she expects to be given something for the pain—her doctor promised. You will be providing her one-to-one care during her labor and the delivery process.

- What assessments are critical during this birth? Why?
- What medical technology or interventions may you be required to administer or monitor during the birthing process?
- What nursing diagnoses could apply? How will you validate these?
- What are the goals of the critical care she is receiving? Why?
- What other goals may be developed?
- What interventions are critical because of Celeste's preexisting medical condition?
- What interventions are necessary because Celeste is in labor?
- How will you evaluate the effectiveness of your interventions?

---

5. Gyna, a 29-year-old woman, G 4, P 3, came in with small amounts of dark vaginal bleeding and uterine cramping earlier this afternoon. She is 37 weeks' pregnant and is concerned because this is different than her other pregnancy experiences. It is determined that Gyna is experiencing mild abruptio placentae. The baby is in a cephalic presentation and the FHR is 136 with variability. There is no evidence of fetal tachycardia, bradycardia, or late or variable decelerations. Gyna is started on continuous fetal monitoring and intravenous Pitocin and the cramping evolves into contractions.

- What assessments are critical during this birth? Why?
- What medical technology or interventions may you be required to administer or monitor during the birthing process?
- What nursing diagnoses could apply? How will you validate these?
- What are the goals of the critical care she is receiving? Why?
- What other goals may be developed?
- What interventions are critical because of Gyna's preexisting medical condition?

- What interventions are necessary because Gyna is in labor?
- How will you evaluate the effectiveness of your interventions?

---

6. Tamar is 40 years old, G 2, P 1. She has been pregnant for 31 weeks and has been sent to the labor and delivery unit by her physician because she reported over the telephone an almost steady stream of fluid from her vagina for the last 4 hours. You take her vital signs and find the following: blood pressure, 112/62; pulse, 68; respirations, 20; and temperature, 98.6° F. You place Tamar on an external fetal monitor for an hour to record fetal and uterine activity as well as the FHR.

- What assessments are critical during this birth? Why?
- What assessment will you not perform?
- What medical technology or interventions may you be required to administer or monitor?
- What nursing diagnoses could apply? How will you validate these?
- What are the goals of the critical care she is receiving? Why?
- What other goals may be developed?
- What interventions are critical because of Tamar's preexisting medical condition?
- What interventions are necessary because Tamar is in labor?
- How will you evaluate the effectiveness of your interventions?

---

7. Katia is a 26-year-old healthy woman, G 1, P 0, who has received no prenatal care because she has no health insurance at her job, and if she took time off from work to go for care, she would lose pay. She has had a history of regular menses in a 28-day cycle. Based on her recall of her last regular menstrual period and the date of quickening, she is at 42 weeks of gestation. A nonstress test is ordered and a biophysical profile is completed.

- What assessments are critical during this birth? Why?
- What assessment will you not perform?
- What medical technology or interventions may you be required to administer or monitor?
- What nursing diagnoses could apply? How will you validate these?
- What are the goals of the critical care she is receiving? Why?
- What other goals may be developed?
- What interventions are critical because of Katia's preexisting medical condition?
- What interventions are necessary because Katia is in labor?
- How will you evaluate the effectiveness of your interventions?

---

8. Aisha is a 28-year-old woman who has a history of DM (Class B). She is a G 2, P 0, and is currently at 32 weeks of gestation. As you might expect, she has been concerned during this pregnancy and has been doing "kick counts" twice a day every day. She has been sent into the hospital for an evaluation after calling her physician and reporting that she hasn't felt any movement in 6 hours. Her partner will be joining her as soon as he can be relieved at work. You have been assigned as her primary nurse for the duration of her admission.

- What assessments are critical at this time? Why?
- What do you think may have happened? How will you respond to Aisha's questions?
- What nursing diagnoses could apply? How will you validate these?
- What are the goals of the critical care she is receiving? Why?
- What other goals may be developed?
- What interventions are critical because of Aisha's preexisting medical condition?
- What interventions are critical because of Aisha's obstetric history?
- How will you evaluate the effectiveness of your interventions?

## REFERENCES

American College of Obstetricians and Gynecologists (ACOG): *Premature labor,* Technical Bulletin, Washington, DC, 1994, The College.

American Diabetes Association (ADA): *Medical management of pregnancy complicated by diabetes,* ed 2, Alexandria, Va, 1995, The Association.

Brown C: The crises of pregnancy loss: a team approach to support, *Birth* 19(1):82-91, 1992.

Brown C and Kozick P: Impressioning: a way to preserve memories, *Matern Child Nurs* 19(5):285-287, 1994.

Crowley P: Elective induction of labor at or beyond term. In Enkin M and others, editors: *A guide for effective care in pregnancy and childbirth,* ed 2, Oxford, 1995, Oxford University Press.

Cunningham F and Lindheimer M: Hypertension in pregnancy, *N Engl J Med* 326:427-432, 1992.

Cunningham F and others: *Williams obstetrics,* ed 20, Norwalk, Conn, 1997, Appleton and Lange.

Enkin M and others: *A guide for effective care in pregnancy and childbirth,* ed 2, Oxford, 1995, Oxford University Press.

Gabbe S, Neibyl J, and Simpson J: *Obstetrics: normal and problem pregnancies,* ed 3, New York, 1996, Churchill Livingstone.

Gilbert ES and Harmon JS: *Manual of high risk pregnancy and delivery,* ed 2, St Louis, 1998, Mosby.

Grub D, Rabello Y, and Paul R: Post-term pregnancy: fetal death rate with antepartum surveillance, *Obstet Gynecol* 70:1024-1026, 1992.

Harr B and Thistlethwaite J: Creative intervention strategies in the management of perinatal loss, *Matern Child Nurs J* 19(2):135-141, 1990.

Iams J: Premature labor and birth. In Gabbe S, Neibyl J, and Simpson J, editors: *Obstetrics: normal and problem pregnancies,* ed 3, New York, 1996, Churchill-Livingstone.

Janke J: The effect of relaxation therapy on preterm labor outcomes, *J Obstet Gynecol Neonatal Nurs* 28(3):255-263, 1999.

Knupple R: High-risk pregnancy: a team approach, Philadelphia, 1993, WB Saunders.

Limbo R and Wheeler S: *When a baby dies: a handbook for helping and healing,* La Crosse, 1998, Gunderson Lutheran Affiliate.

Mattson S and Smith J: *Core curriculum for maternal-newborn nursing,* ed 2, Philadelphia, 2000, WB Saunders.

Pagel M and others: Psycosocial influences on newborn outcomes: a controlled prospective study, *Soc Sci Med* 30(5):597-604, 1990.

Rubin R: *Maternal identity and the maternal experience,* New York, 1984, Springer.

Seeds J and Walsh M: Malpresentations. In Gabbe S, Neibyl J, and Simpson J, editors: *Obstetrics: normal and problem pregnancies,* ed 3, New York, 1996, Churchill-Livingstone.

Simpson K and Creehan P: *AWHONN perinatal nursing,* Philadelphia, 1996, Lippincott.

# CHAPTER 19

# Care of the Woman with Postpartum Complications in the Hospital

*All my worries seem less important,*
*because in the center,*
*there is always Sam. And he's what's*
*most important.*

— A POSTPARTUM MOTHER
(*OUR BODIES, OURSELVES*, 1998)

*How can we help normalize a complicated postpartum for a woman?*

*What assistance can we offer women whose lives are complicated by preexisting health issues (e.g., addictions, domestic violence, homelessness)?*

*What assistance can we offer women whose lives are complicated by preexisting health concerns (e.g., anemia, diabetes, infections)?*

*What assistance can we offer women whose lives are complicated by events of the pregnancy and birth?*

For healthy women, the normal postpartum period presents a series of challenges. As explained in Chapters 14 and 15, after a baby is born many physical and emotional adjustments occur simultaneously, creating various specific care needs for the mother, the baby, and their family.

For women who are dealing with these same postpartum adjustments *in addition to* requiring extended care for complications from preexisting health issues or concerns or complications due to the pregnancy or birth, the process is even more challenging. This chapter focuses on the supplementary care some women may need to receive in a hospital beyond the basic postpartal care because of complications or health problems. Keep in mind that whatever complications the new mother experiences, they do not negate her need for holistic postpartum care. Whatever else is occurring or

threatening to occur, she is still adapting to a new role or a familiar role with a new baby.

Women are better able to successfully navigate the many challenges of pregnancy, birth, and parenting with guidance and care. The challenge for us is to provide that guidance in a caring, concise manner when the average length of stay is 1.5 days for a vaginal delivery and 2.5 days for a surgical delivery (Clinical Classifications for Health Policy Research: Hospital Inpatient Statistics, 1995). Not only must we assess women's needs and provide interventions during their hospitalization, but also we must empower them to take on their new role by anticipating their needs and providing them with appropriate guidance and referrals. In this chapter, we explore some of the conditions that may require special assessments and discharge planning and possibly a postpartum stay of more than 48 hours.

## CULTURAL CONSIDERATIONS

For some women, hospitalization may be an unsettling thought. For others, it is what they expect in the American culture. When speaking of the postpartal period, every mother voices several "normal" expectations. Some of these may conflict with what the hospital staff expects. Some anticipated or cautionary behaviors are based on personal beliefs, while others come from cultural expectations. Women who believe that pregnancy has caused them to "lose heat" may fear that cold air and water will have harmful effects; this belief can cause conflict if we tell her she has to get up and take a shower. We must learn a woman's attitudes and beliefs about bathing, showering, shampooing, ambulating, and other self-care practices before prescribing what she is to do. Realistically, women may pretend to follow the activities we suggest, even to the extent of going into the shower, running the water, and pretending to follow instructions, all the while avoiding the water. Learn from the woman what hygienic measure she would like to use.

Helping the woman wear the clothing she desires and providing extra blankets as requested demonstrates cultural sensitivity. Some women may wish to have air conditioners and fans turned off in their room. The routine distribution of ice water can be replaced with hot fluids or by offering the woman the choice of room temperature water; warm tea—regular, decaffeinated, or herbal; broth; or other beverages of her choice. This demonstrates respect for her while providing the desired fluid intake.

## MATERNAL-INFANT ATTACHMENT

The process of maternal-infant attachment can be adversely affected when the mother cannot care for her infant because of her own health problems. If the woman's condition prevents her from being with the infant during this part of the postpartum, take photographs of the infant and then give them to the mother. Encourage and facilitate family contact with the infant. Requests for services from the social worker and/or the chaplain's office also may be appropriate to assist with the woman's psychosocial and spiritual needs.

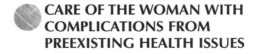

## CARE OF THE WOMAN WITH COMPLICATIONS FROM PREEXISTING HEALTH ISSUES

Women live their lives confronting multiple issues that affect their health. Three situations that compromise their health and the health of their newborn and may af-

fect their discharge from the hospital are addiction, domestic violence, and homelessness. To provide appropriate, supportive care we must first identify the situation, gain the mother's trust to talk about it, know how to connect her with services in the community, and collaborate with her in addressing these issues that affect her health and well-being.

### Addiction

The terms *abuse, dependence,* and *addiction* are sometimes used interchangeably, but they have different meanings. **Abuse** is the use of psychoactive substances in a manner not consistent with the legal or medical guidelines; an example is the nonmedical use of prescription medications. **Dependence** is the physical and/or psychologic need for repeated doses of a psychoactive substance to feel good or to avoid feeling bad. **Addiction** is a chronic adherence—a compulsive, uncontrollable dependence on a substance, habit, or practice to such a degree that cessation causes severe emotional, mental, or physiologic reactions (Anderson, 1994; Smith and Maurer, 2000). Components of the addiction status include tolerance, physical dependence, and psychologic dependence (Kolander, Ballard, and Chandler, 1999). "It is important to remember that addiction is a process that includes the stages of abuse and dependence" (Smith and Maurer, 2000).

#### Anticipated Issues

The postpartum period serves as a critical time for providing interventions with addicted women. "Alcoholism is by far the most common disorder, despite the tendency of many to abuse multiple drugs" (Smith and Maurer, 2000). Addicting drugs, such as amphetamine and cocaine, act on the dopamine system directly. Alcohol and nicotine indirectly activate the dopamine system, also giving the biochemical reward that causes an intense sense of well-being and pleasurable feelings, reinforcing more drug use (Allen and Feeney, 1997). Many patients will have coexisting or dual diagnoses. For example an alcoholic also may have a mental health diagnosis such as antisocial personality disorder, mania, or schizophrenia. When this occurs, finding a facility for treatment becomes problematic because a facility for one disorder may reject the client based on the other diagnosis (Smith and Maurer, 2000).

The postpartum period provides the time to explore the causes of addiction with a woman and ways to deal with it. Although this time frame is a window of opportunity, barriers complicate the process. Stigma is attached to substance abuse during pregnancy and may prevent a woman from disclosing substance abuse until the delivery. Once she sees the infant, she may become overwhelmed with concern for it (Coletti and Donaldson, 1996). If overwhelmed by guilt and shame, the woman may be unable to cope. This could lead either to a relapse in a recovering woman or increased dependencies. The infant's presence does offer hope and a focus of renewal, but at the same time, there is the possibility that she will be unable to care for herself and her infant.

If the alcohol or drugs have negatively affected the infant, it may be a difficult child to console. After birth, newborns go through a withdrawal period because the drugs that have been supplied through the placenta are no longer available. Even if the mother has been in a drug treatment program with methadone, the newborn will go through withdrawal. Wakefulness, irritability, tremors, hyperactivity, hypertonus, a high-pitched cry, and diarrhea are additional challenges that may complicate the normal tasks of infant care. When a new mother cannot provide adequate care to a difficult infant it can produce strong feelings of inadequacy and frustration in the mother (Kaye and Chasnoff, 1993).

Women with histories of substance abuse often have concomitant social issues. When they also are dealing with sexual abuse, domestic violence, HIV infection, or homelessness, providing care to an infant becomes a more complex issue. Her support systems may be limited or nonexistent because of a nomadic existence or the social isolation that is common among people with addictions. We may provide needed care and referrals, but we must do so in an open and accepting manner (Coletti and Donaldson, 1996).

View the woman as an individual who is coping with her life in the only way she sees possible. Remain nonjudgmental about her situation while finding programs or facilities that support her, believe that with intervention change is possible, and believe that she is a human being worthy of this care.

### Ethical Considerations

Ethical issues strongly influence care provided to women with addictions. Examples of ethical questions that may arise when we provide care to a woman with an addiction problem include the following: When we learn that the woman has been deceitful about her drug-free status before delivery, do we continue to care for her health concerns or do we notify the proper authorities to have them remove the baby? How do we make the choice between referring the woman for treatment or threatening to report her to authorities? Are maternal urine tests that include toxicology screening a violation of a patient's right of confidentiality? Whose rights are more important—the mother's or the infant's? When managed care only pays for outpatient treatment and the woman requires inpatient care, how do we support her request for help? (Allen and Buppert, 1996).

### Legal Issues

The mother does not have to be tested directly to learn about drug use. Maternal drug use close to the time of labor may be detected in a newborn urine sample.

Meconium drug testing gives longer-term information about drug use during the pregnancy. Newborn hair analysis also provides accurate information about substance exposure in utero. Meconium testing and hair sampling, although accurate, are expensive and not routinely used. Research has shown that maternal substance abuse may lead to both mental and physical problems for newborns. If we are aware of substance abuse by a mother, we may be required to report it. Some states including Florida, Massachusetts, and Minnesota, require the reporting of a positive drug screen. This requirement was put in place to allow social services to investigate and refer women.

Women need to trust their health care providers to do their best to help them and not to just point the finger of accusation. However, some mothers who were reported by their health care provider to have used drugs while they were pregnant have been criminally prosecuted. Women may not trust us because they have heard of cases in which mothers have been charged with providing an illegal substance to their infants via the umbilical cord. Because the main thrust of our care is toward prevention and treatment, we are left to decide between what is ethically right and what is legally required. We also need to consider why a woman would seek assistance with an abuse problem if instead of care she is charged as a criminal? How do we uphold the law while meeting the health needs of our clients? Future court decisions may change these laws and our responsibilities.

### Nursing Assessment

The postpartum assessment follows the prescribed hospital protocol for all postpartum women, with the additional focus on understanding the woman's status in relation to drug withdrawal and current use. Be aware that sometimes drugs are brought into the hospital by family members and friends and are used by the mother.

Recognition of the layered context of need in the addicted mother requires special attention to both her prenatal and addiction histories, nutritional and diet status, previous attempts to overcome addictions, current support systems, housing and environmental conditions, and psychologic concerns. Gather this information through interviewing and reviewing her medical records (Box 19-1).

Shannon and Hill (1999) state that we need to be alert to the following signs and symptoms of withdrawal in all women:

- Woman is disoriented
- Lethargy
- Extremes of mood
- Tremors or jitteriness
- Tachycardia
- Fasciculations (small involuntary muscular contractions under the skin)
- Increased temperature

If withdrawal symptoms are identified, assessment of vital signs and orientation is required every hour. Information related to the type of drug used must be obtained because each drug has different levels of withdrawal and side effects. Once the drug or drugs are identified, appropriate care may be given. Documenting the type of drug used may be based on what the woman reports or may be determined or verified by urine testing.

After a thorough assessment, develop nursing diagnoses and a plan of care with the woman. The plan must be goal directed, culturally sensitive, and individualized to the woman and her family situation. In addition, other professionals will be involved because a multidisciplinary team approach provides the most comprehensive care for a mother with an addiction.

### Possible Nursing Diagnoses

When working with a postpartum woman that has a problem with addiction, various nursing diagnoses, in addition to the regular diagnoses for a woman who has just delivered an infant either vaginally or surgically, may be applicable. Learn from the woman about her vision of herself and her situation because this will help make her needs clearer. Keep in mind that in addition to her own physical care, she also may need assistance with the factors that have led to her addiction, the possible legal ramifications of her use, the possible need for assistance in caring for her infant, or the placement of her child by state authorities.

### Goals of Care

Goals are developed with the woman, using a nonjudgmental, proactive approach that (1) enhances communication, (2) fosters an understanding that the health care team is concerned about the woman, and (3) shows the providers believe that there can be positive outcomes for mother, infant, and family. All expected outcomes are based on the woman's individual needs. Sample goals are that by discharge the woman will:

* Identify supports and resources that would assist with her recovery from addiction
* Identify appropriate skin maintenance techniques
* Communicate her level of discomfort due to withdrawal symptoms
* Verbalize an understanding of alternative pain relief

---

### BOX 19-1   *Areas to Assess with the Woman Who Is Experiencing Addiction*

The following are samples of some questions you might ask a woman when you are assessing her unique needs because of addiction. They do not have to be asked in this order or in these words. Use words and phrases that both the woman and you are comfortable with. Follow up her answers with the next logical area so that her train of thought is not interrupted. During this assessment conversation, cover these areas and any additional ones of concern to her.

**HOUSING**
Where do you live?
With whom do you live?

**DAILY ACTIVITY**
What do you do during your daytime hours?
What activities do your family and friends expect you to participate in?
Are you comfortable with their expectations?
Would you like to do something different?

**FOOD**
Who obtains the food for your family?
Who does the planning and preparation?
Are there ever any problems in obtaining the food you want?

**SELF-CARE**
How do you take care of your self?
Are you sexually active? Is this by choice or is it expected?

How do you protect yourself from sexually transmitted infection?
How do you protect yourself from pregnancy?

**SAFETY**
Do you feel safe in your environment?
What could be done to improve your sense of security?
Will your infant be safe?
(If there are other children) Are your children safe?

**STORAGE**
Where do you keep your things that are important to you?
Do you think they are safe there?
Will you be able to easily get to them if you need them?

**COMMUNITY SERVICES**
What people, services, or agencies have you found helpful?
How have they helped?
What people, services, or agencies have you found not helpful?
How have they not helped?
Where would you like to go with your baby when you are discharged from the hospital?
How would you like us to help you and your baby (family)?

- Demonstrate infant care techniques
- State plans for infant care if she enters treatment (Shannon and Hill, 1999)

### Self-Care

All change has to start with the woman herself. The hospital setting can serve as a haven and a positive place to start to empower and strengthen the woman who would like to be relieved of her addiction. While hospitalized, she is removed from personal and environmental factors that may have led to or supported her addiction. The process of recovery can be started and then sustained through referral to an appropriate facility. Women may find it easier to interact in a positive manner with the multidisciplinary health care team in the hospital, unencumbered by the complexities of her external environment (French and others, 1998). Giving her competent care and offering support if she decides to enter a treatment program will foster resiliency of her spirit (Stump, 1992).

### Interventions

***Care of the Woman.*** Mothers with addictions require the same type of physical care that all mothers need, but they have additional needs that must also be met. First and foremost is the emphasis on admission to and continuation in drug treatment therapy. Women with severe problems with addictions are counseled regarding an inpatient treatment setting. Efforts to obtain a placement should include the possibility of bringing their infant with them. Women already in treatment can continue on an outpatient basis, but emphasis is focused on an intense multiweekly program that also provides child care (Bragg, 1997).

Because a disproportionate number of women identified with addictions are minorities, it is incumbent that our care be culturally competent (Louie, 1995). Communication skills that are culturally sensitive are critical in interactions between provider and patient. Culturally appropriate verbal and nonverbal patterns of communication acknowledge and validate individual cultures. Before discharge, ask the woman how she relates to her community and what her community's understanding and values are in relationship to drug use and motherhood. Will the members of her community expect her to continue use or will they expect her to quit?

Before referring a woman to programs, services, and institutions that provide the necessary care, examine them for cultural bias. We will lose our credibility with a client and she will be less successful in overcoming her addiction if we refer her to a program that is culturally inappropriate.

***Mother-Infant Interaction.*** Emphasize enhancing mother-infant interaction. Negative feelings associated with guilt and shame can interfere with the initial relationship between mother and infant. Even women with other children often lack the knowledge of basic newborn care because either they were in an addictive state when their older child was born or prior infants have been removed by court order (Davis, 1997).

When infants undergo withdrawal, they can be irritable and fussy. This behavior may reinforce a mother's guilt about the drug use. It also becomes a barrier to the bonding process. Mothers who are experiencing withdrawal symptoms and/or heightened pain as a result of ineffective analgesia due to a drug use–induced tolerance to medication levels do not tolerate infants with poor temperaments.

When the mother can tolerate it, rooming-in should be encouraged. Teach her ways to soothe and calm her infant. Having the child in her room offers more teaching moments during which we can enhance and reinforce positive maternal activity. It also allows the mother to become acquainted with her child during both quiet moments and fussy moments. Remind the mother that all infants can be fussy and that this fussiness is not exclusively related to maternal drug use. Provide for positive infant care experiences because they are an opportunity for enhancement of mother-infant interaction (French and others, 1998).

***Health Promotion.*** Infections as a result of poor nutrition, lack of prenatal care, history of sexually transmitted diseases, and intravenous drug use are treated with appropriate drug therapy specific to the causative agent. Teaching is focused on promotion of drug-free health behaviors. Women need assistance in learning how to practice safer sex, learning possible ways to approach a partner to get them to participate in condom use, and understanding the relationship between risk behaviors and infection. Contraception methods that are realistic for the woman and individualized for her lifestyle have a greater chance of being used successfully (Matteson, 1995). When possible, partners should be included in the teaching plan so that their needs and concerns also are considered. This relieves the woman from the full responsibility of trying to teach the partner about why and how past behaviors must be changed.

***Nutrition.*** Diet counseling may be done by a 24-hour recall of food intake before the onset of the birth experience. However, a more realistic approach is to use the "typical day" approach. In a typical day what does she eat? What does she like to eat? When does she eat? Who shops and who prepares the food?

Anemia and vitamin deficiencies secondary to drug addiction are common. Any nutritional plans must suit the home environment and community. We need to collaborate with the patient in identifying neighborhood stores and financial resources. It is not enough to know the food pyramid if no options are available or what is available is beyond the woman's financial resources. If she is eligible, provide her with information about neighborhood food banks and governmental programs such as the Women, Infants, and Children (WIC) program, food stamps, and Medicaid.

***Discharge Planning.*** Discharge planning is prioritized to meet the needs of the woman. Evaluation of the hospital course of care and her agreement with the discharge plan is required. A collaborative meeting among nurses, social workers, physicians, community outreach workers, and others pertinent to the care of the woman is held to identify questions and formulate an appropriate plan.

- Where is the woman going?
- Will the mother and infant be together?
- What are the woman's health concerns?
- Who will the mother see for her postpartum care?
- Who is responsible for implementing or facilitating her health care?
- Are there appropriate resources in her community?
- What is the addiction treatment plan? Who is supporting the woman in these efforts?

## Evaluation

Evaluation of interventions are based on the achievement of the short-term goals for the woman's postpartum recovery while hospitalized. Because the woman will require ongoing care, it also involves the identification of and connection with appropriate referrals within the community for continuing care for the mother and her baby after discharge and the woman's capacity to understand and state her role in following through with those referrals.

## Summary

With appropriate care and timely intervention, women dealing with addiction can be successful in reconstructing their lives. Because of the brevity of the postpartum hospital stay, we can only initiate the process and make appropriate referrals. We can start to rebuild a woman's sense of self-esteem by praising her appropriate care of the new infant. In addition, we must connect her with community resources, such as food stamps and safe housing. All interventions to assist women in overcoming addictions must be multifaceted and individualized to the needs of a woman and her infant.

# Domestic Violence

Domestic violence, which includes physical, mental, and/or emotional abuse, may first be suspected or documented during the prenatal period or during the labor and delivery experience. However, with the lack of continuity of care by nurses as a childbearing woman progresses through the health care continuum and the reluctance to put a suspicion in the chart where the abuser might find it, a woman may arrive on a postpartum unit without being documented as at risk. All postpartum women, regardless of race, ethnicity, age, or financial status, must be screened for the physical, mental, and emotional aspects of domestic violence. This postpartum period in the hospital provides a woman with the opportunity to learn her options and determine for herself what it is she would like to do.

## Anticipated Concerns

Women who are victims of domestic violence may be late entrants to prenatal care. They may have been prevented from seeing a health care provider by their partner, or they may have been afraid of questions that health care professionals would ask regarding their condition. They often don't know their options if they leave the relationship or they are fearful to do so (McFarlane, Parker, and Soeken, 1996). Abuse during pregnancy and depression and drug use are strongly correlated (Christian, 1995).

During the postpartum period, we may help a woman identify her resources. As women consider their children and learn what their options are, they may, with appropriate support, be able to remove themselves and their children from danger.

## Ethical and Legal Considerations

State laws consider an adult woman capable of making her own decisions about whether to report her abuse or not. This may not be true if the injury involved a weapon or if the postpartum woman is under the age of adulthood. Know your state laws concerning child abuse, so that you will know your legal responsibility regarding mandated reporting for adolescent mothers.

You may not understand why a woman makes the decisions she does concerning her relational situation. However, ethically you are bound to support her in her decisions. Do not attempt to "fix" the situation by intervening with the abuser. This will only make things worse for the woman after she leaves the protection of the hospital.

## Nursing Assessment

Hospitalization during the postpartum period affords a window of opportunity to provide interventions in an emotionally safe environment to victims of domestic violence and/or sexual abuse. It is a time to empower the woman and encourage her strengths. If the partner desires to be with the woman all the time, there are ways to remove her from his presence under the pretence of doing something with her or for her. If he refuses to leave her alone, this is a clear indicator that control of her is a major issue with him and the situation should be investigated further.

Assessment begins with very simple, subjective questions. Even if it is charted that the woman was asked about domestic violence during the prenatal or intrapartum, she should be asked again. Data support that repeated questioning often leads to disclosure. Women who have been abused often state that they do not report it because no one seemed interested. They didn't see the nurse as someone who was concerned or could do anything to help them. They state that they would have felt permitted to disclose the abuse if the nurse had given them an opening such as "Sometimes childbirth brings up a lot from a person's past . . ." or "Now that you are thinking about going home with a baby, we need to talk about your safety. Do you feel safe in your home?" (Daddario, 1999) (Box 19-2).

Inadequate prenatal care or late entry into prenatal care, evidence of bruising, and abdominal trauma are objective findings that might suggest domestic violence. We should also investigate the possibility with women who are overly concerned about people touching their body or demonstrate revulsion at touching their "private parts" or breastfeeding. This type of response may be suggestive of disdain for their body, which can be the result of prior abuse as a child or adult (Burian, 1995).

### Possible Nursing Diagnoses

When working with a postpartum woman who experiences physical or emotional abuse in her home, various additional nursing diagnoses, beyond the regular concerns for a postpartum woman, may be applicable. Talk with the woman who is experiencing periodic violence to gain a clearer understanding of her vision of herself and her situational needs. Her collaboration is essential to develop accurate and appropriate nursing diagnoses and related goals.

### Goals of Care

Discuss with the woman what she would like to happen. Develop both short- and long-term goals. Because most victims of abuse have very low self-esteem, it is most helpful if they set what seem like small goals at first so that they may achieve a measure of success before moving on to more difficult goals. Many emotionally abused women have lost the ability to determine their own preferences, so a first goal may be for her to determine what she would like to eat for breakfast.

Examples of possible goals beyond her normal postpartum needs are the following:

- Identify ways to keep herself and her infant safe.
- Identify what personal papers and items she needs to have if she decides to leave. (See Chapter 6 for more details on developing an escape plan.)

---

### BOX 19-2  *Areas to Assess with the Woman Who Is Experiencing Domestic Violence*

The following are samples of some questions you might ask a woman when you are assessing her unique needs because of domestic violence. They do not have to be asked in this order or in these words. Use words and phrases that both the woman and you are comfortable with. Follow up her answers with the next logical area so that her train of thought is not interrupted. During this assessment conversation, cover these areas and any additional ones of concern to her.

**HOUSING**
Where do you live?
With whom do you live?

**DAILY ACTIVITY**
What do you do during your daytime hours?
Do you have restrictions as to whom you may see or what you may do?

**FOOD**
Who obtains the food for your family?
Who does the planning and preparation?
Are there ever any problems about the choices you make or how you prepare the food?

**SELF-CARE**
How do you take care of your self?
Are you sexually active? Is this by choice or is it expected?

Are you ever in pain or hurt during sexual activity?
How do you protect yourself from sexually transmitted infection?
How do you protect yourself from pregnancy?

**SAFETY**
Do you feel safe in your environment?
What could be done to improve your sense of security?
Will your infant be safe?
(If there are other children) Are your children safe?

**STORAGE**
Do you have a set of personal papers and some money set aside?
Where do you keep them?
Do you think that they are safe there?
Will you be able to get to them easily if you need them?

**COMMUNITY SERVICES**
What people, services, or agencies have you found helpful?
How have they helped?
What people, services, or agencies have you found not helpful?
How have they not helped?
Where would you like to go with your baby when you are discharged from the hospital?
How would you like us to help you and your baby (family)?

- Identify resources available to her in the community.
- Identify a possible support network among friends and/or family members. (Remember that family and friends may side with the abuser so this may not be an option.)

### Self-Care

Sensitivity by nursing personnel may provide a woman the impetus and opportunity to disclose a history of abuse during the postpartum period. Her acknowledgment of the abuse is the first step toward receiving help and ensuring survival. Women may then choose to change their environment if provided information and a sufficient support system. If she is not yet able to leave the situation, she can learn that she has options and be given reinforcement for thinking positive thoughts about herself, realizing the necessity for self-care, and using positive decision making. These are the first small steps to being able to take charge of her life.

### Interventions

*Moving Toward Safety.* Safety is the primary concern in strategizing care for women involved in domestic violence issues. Women may choose to accept help in making plans for discharge into a safe environment when they understand the risk of escalation of the violence. When a woman has a history of being abused, she needs to be counseled that she is at constant risk for escalation in the severity of the abuse and death (Campbell, 1995).  She also needs to be aware that her infant is now also at risk. Women should be told of the possibility of safe, alternative living arrangements and the availability of secret shelters. If the woman cannot leave now, she should be told how to contact assistance at a later date.

Women with decisional conflict require empathetic understanding and counseling to help them move toward positive decision making and the ultimate goal of safety. Keep in mind that she wants the abuse to end, not the relationship. She will not be able to uproot her life and walk away from her partner just because we tell her it is possible. She has to perceive for herself that she or her child is in real danger.

Women may leave a relationship many times before being able to make the permanent break. A woman becomes more at risk for being killed when she does leave the relationship. Leaving is therefore a decision that must be left up to the woman because she is the only one who can weigh the cost and benefits and who will ultimately experience the outcome, negative or positive.

*Previous Sexual Abuse.* Birth and the postpartum period may bring to the surface a previous history of sexual abuse. This can interfere with mother-infant interaction and requires interventions provided by a specialist on the health care team to help women through this time. Some women will have negative feelings toward their girl in-

fants because they fear that they will not be able to protect the girl from abuse. Other women harbor intense feelings against their male child, seeing that gender as the cause of their pain (Heritage, 1998). In addition to arranging counseling, we can assist a woman in understanding that her infant is a unique person, with no responsibility for the mother's past. Rooming-in with the infant and our reinforcement of her mothering skills foster healthy interactions.

*Physical Needs.* Interventions for health issues are provided as they arise. Trauma during pregnancy can lead to postpartum hemorrhage. Women with a history of abuse are carefully monitored through frequent pad checks, laboratory studies, and assessment of vital signs.  Increased temperature may signal an infection. Discharge teaching includes danger signs such as increased bleeding, dizziness, and fatigue. Reinforcement of teaching is provided with the use of instruction sheets.

Because of the risk of being assaulted, the woman is at greater risk of hemorrhage from the placental site or the birth canal. Her partner may not agree to wait until she is healed before penetrating her vagina. An argument may develop and she may be punched in the abdomen.

*Discharge Planning.* Because of the association between domestic violence and other social problems, nurses must be proactive in promoting a holistic healthy lifestyle. Interventions aimed at smoking and substance abuse also may be offered. A woman with related issues may be helped with counseling from social services to see the relationship and how to start to address these risks to her health. If the woman wants them, referrals to community programs should be initiated to help support and reinforce her selected behavioral changes.

For interventions to be successful, we must be sensitive to the cultural context of the woman's life. What does her partnership or marriage mean to her? How does her community view this relationship? What support will there be if she chooses to leave the partner? How does the community feel about the involvement of health professionals in the privacy of a family?

Education and sensitivity by health care professionals regarding these issues is critical (Campbell, 1995). Women learn that violence in the home is a problem that affects more than just them when posters and literature are displayed within the facility. When information is placed within bathrooms or toilet stalls each woman has the time and privacy to read the information, learn about the services in her community, and memorize the emergency phone numbers. Given the opportunity and a listening ear, you will learn from the woman herself what further assistance she requires.

### Evaluation

Evaluation of the effectiveness of care involves an assessment of the status of the woman and her infant at the time of discharge. Is she currently comfortable with the plans made to deal with the issue of violence in her life? Does she have the means to follow up on the referrals to the social service organizations that will offer her continued support? Does she know that help is available when she is able to accept it? Does she know that she is not alone? Does she have the means to call for help and know where to call 24 hours a day?

### Summary

Helping a woman with a new infant deal with the violence in her life is complicated and often frustrating. Part of her ability to escape from a violent situation in which she has been disempowered is to be allowed to become empowered and make her own decisions. This includes the decision as to when to stay and when to leave.

## Homelessness

The lack of low-income housing has been and continues to be a primary factor in the number of homeless families and individuals (Smith and Maurer, 2000). A homeless person is defined as (1) a person who lacks a fixed, regular, and adequate nighttime residence or (2) an individual who has a primary nighttime residence that is a shelter, including welfare hotels, congregate shelters, and transitional housing for the mentally ill; an institution that provides a temporary residence for individuals intending to be institutionalized; or a public or private place not designated for nor ordinarily used as a regular sleeping accommodation (Stewart, 1987). Despite an increase in shelter beds during the last 20 years, there are not enough shelters and transitional housing spaces for the homeless population (National Coalition for the Homeless, 1998). Very few beds are available to women, women with children, and families.

Homeless people comprise a heterogeneous group with variations in personal characteristics, the length of time they are homeless, and the extent of their disabilities. Rather than categorize them by their various characteristics (e.g., employment status, mental illness, veteran, substance abuser), it is more meaningful to use the stages of homelessness. The homeless may be classified as experiencing episodic, temporary, or chronic homelessness (Belcher, Scholler-Jaquish, and Drummond, 1991). Learning her stage of homelessness is the first step to understanding a woman's situation (Box 19-3).

Women represent approximately 25% of the homeless population, and the largest group of homeless women have children with them (Vissing, 1996; Waxman and Henderliter, 1996). Women with children are the fastest-growing subgroup of the homeless nationally. They tend to be young and their rates of mental illness and substance abuse are low. "Homeless mothers have less education and lower employment rates and appear to have fewer friends than other homeless persons" (Smith and

Maurer, 2000). They have a greater prevalence of unwanted pregnancies, adverse birth outcomes, and histories of domestic abuse (McNamee and Lindsey, 1998). "Women often stay in abusive relationships to avoid becoming homeless until they feel forced to move into the streets to avoid the domestic violence. Domestic abuse has been cited as the primary cause for homelessness for mothers with children" (Smith and Maurer, 2000).

The woman that you see in postpartum care may have had the infant because of a planned pregnancy with a long-term, loving partner; she may have had the child because of an unintended pregnancy and be in an intermittent relationship, or she may have become pregnant because of a sexual assault on the street or when she sought protection from the weather. She may or may not plan on keeping the infant.

### Anticipated Issues

The experience of being homeless affects a woman physically, psychologically, socially, and economically. It is more than living in poverty; it means being uprooted and losing valued objects and places. It is a life situation over which the person has little, if any, control (Smith and Maurer, 2000). When a woman is homeless, she exists in a nomadic state. She has difficulty receiving assistance with finances, food, or health care because she has no mailing address. "There is widespread hunger and malnutrition among the nation's growing number of homeless women" (Brown, 2000). She is viewed negatively because she doesn't have the resources to care for her children as others do (Kozol, 1988). Just getting them clean and dressed appropriately becomes a major task without a home and facilities.

During the postpartum period, instead of concentrating her energy on recovery and providing care to her newborn she will be concerned about where she is going next. If she was living in a shelter, she may have lost her space either because she left to come to the hospital or because she cannot return with a child. If she has other children, she may be concerned about their care while she remains in the hospital. Women who have lived with parents may find themselves put out because of the child and, unable to find affordable housing, seek shelters as a place for themselves and their newborns (Beal and Redlener, 1995).

### Ethical and Legal Issues

The ethical and legal issues related to the care of a homeless woman encompass her right for self-determination, just as the woman who experiences violence or the woman with an addiction. The reality that a woman is homeless cannot be the sole basis for removing a child from her care. Her ability to provide for the health and well-being of that child in what may be considered a nontraditional living arrangement is what takes precedence. Our role during the postpartum period is to help

## BOX 19-3 Stages of Homelessness

**STAGE 1: EPISODIC HOMELESSNESS**

The first stage of homelessness consists of people who live below or slightly above the poverty line, are socially stigmatized, and are constantly vulnerable to the harsh realities of homelessness. Their connection to a home is tenuous and may be episodic as they move in and out of intense poverty.

**STAGE 2: TEMPORARY HOMELESSNESS**

The second stage of homelessness consists of people who have recently become homeless. They still identify themselves with the mainstream of their communities rather than with other homeless people; display symptoms of anxiety and depression; may abuse alcohol or drugs; view living on the streets or relying on shelters as an unacceptable lifestyle; and are attempting to regain a lost home, job, and social standing.

**STAGE 3: CHRONIC HOMELESSNESS**

The third stage of homelessness consists of people who have been homeless for longer periods. They accept their life experiences on the streets as normative, are more easily and clearly identifiable as homeless, are extremely suspicious of interacting with members of the mainstream of society, and are generally socially decompensated.

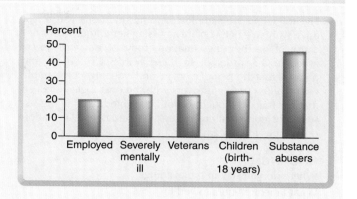

Estimated subgroups of the urban homeless, United States. Note that categories are not mutually exclusive. (Data from Waxman L and Henderliter S: *Status report on hunger and homelessness in America's cities: 1996,* Washington, DC, 1996, U.S. Conference of Mayors.)

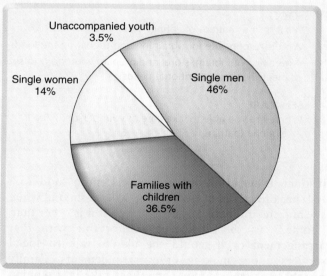

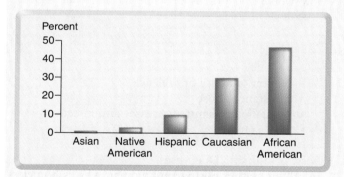

Estimated racial composition of urban homeless, United States. (Data from Waxman L and Henderliter S: *Status report on hunger and homelessness in America's cities: 1996,* Washington, DC, 1996, U.S. Conference of Mayors.)

Estimated composition of urban homeless, United States. (Data from Waxman L and Henderliter S: *Status report on hunger and homelessness in America's cities: 1996,* Washington, DC, 1996, U.S. Conference of Mayors.)

From Belcher JR, Scholler-Jaquish A, and Drummond M: Three stages of homelessness: a conceptual model for social workers in health care, *Health Soc Work* 16(2):87-93, 1991.

her be as successful as possible by connecting her and the infant with the support services they require (Box 19-4).

### Nursing Assessment

Women who are homeless may not be apparent to you or identify themselves as such. Some homeless women have jobs. Some have advanced skills and graduate de-

grees. They just don't have housing. There will be an address on her hospital record; however, it may be a shelter, it may not exist, or it may not be where she lives. She may be afraid to let the staff know about her situation for fear that she will lose custody of the baby.

Be alert to clues of personal neglect in her overall grooming and health. Pay attention to your intuitive

**BOX 19-4** *Areas to Assess with the Woman Who Is Experiencing Homelessness*

The following are samples of some questions you might ask a woman when you are assessing her unique needs because of her housing situation. They do not have to be asked in this order or in these words. Use words and phrases that both the woman and you are comfortable with. Follow up her answers with the next logical area so that her train of thought is not interrupted. During this assessment conversation, cover these areas and any additional ones of concern to her.

**HOUSING**
Where do you stay in the evening?
What time are you allowed in?
What time do you have to be out by?
Is there a limited amount of time that you may stay there?
When will you have to move?

**DAILY ACTIVITY**
What do you do during your daytime hours?

**FOOD**
What is your pattern of eating? Where do you eat?
Who is responsible for obtaining and preparing the food?
Where do you obtain, store, and prepare your food? (if she meets her own nutritional needs)

**SELF-CARE**
Where are you able to take care of your personal needs for hygiene (bathing)?

Where are you able to take care of your elimination needs?
How are you able to take care of your menstrual needs?
Are you sexually active?
How do you protect yourself from sexually transmitted infection?
How do you protect yourself from pregnancy?

**PERSONAL SAFETY**
Do you feel safe in your environment?
What could be done to improve your sense of security?

**STORAGE**
Where do you keep your things? Do you think that they are safe there?

**COMMUNITY SERVICES**
What people, services, or agencies have you found helpful?
How have they helped?
What people, services, or agencies have you found not helpful?
How have they not helped?
Where would you like to go with your baby when you are discharged from the hospital?
How would you like us to help you and your baby (family)?

---

instincts if her information doesn't seem to "add up." Ask her directly about where she will be staying when she and the infant leave the hospital. If it is other than "home," ask her if she is comfortable with that arrangement or if would she like to talk to social services about making other arrangements. Family members or friends may sometimes take in a woman and her infant after the birth of the baby. However, these arrangements may not last more than a few months.

Because women in a homeless state are on the move and are often ineligible for health care, they come into prenatal care late in the pregnancy or not at all. Labor and delivery may have been the first point of contact she had with the health care system.

The assessment in the postpartum period follows the normal postpartum protocols. In addition to her housing status, gather subjective and objective data information about other possible health issues:

- Smoking
- Nutritional needs
- Victim of abuse or violence
- Substance abuse
- Sexually transmitted diseases and infection
- HIV status

**Possible Nursing Diagnoses**
In talking with a postpartum woman who is homeless, various nursing diagnoses, in addition to the regular diagnoses for a postpartum woman, may be applicable. By talking with the woman, her vision of herself and her situational needs may become clearer to you. Issues of safety, nutrition, options for assistance, and the care of her child should be explored

**Goals of Care**
Discuss with the woman what she would like to happen. Is she able to return to her prior living arrangements? Does she want to do so? Is she aware of other options she would like to pursue? Would she like the assistance of hospital social services to help her with her situation? What are her goals for personal care and arrangements for the care of the infant? Together you

will establish goals. Examples of some that may be agreed upon are that by discharge, the woman will:

- Collaborate with health care professionals to find housing
- Identify her postpartum concerns
- Understand where she may receive health care for herself and her child
- Strategize self-care ways to increase personal safety
- Verbalize her plans for the baby
- Verbalize who she will contact if she experiences a fever; a foul-smelling discharge; excessive vaginal bleeding; red vaginal bleeding after having been brown; pain or a warm, swollen area in her leg; burning on urination; or pelvic pain.

### Self-Care

Homeless women face many daily adversities. The survival skills and strengths that have sustained them thus far are foundations on which each may build. Helping them recognize their incredible strengths and connecting them with supportive services that they understand and trust starts them on their way to self-care. Through active listening, we can discover what has worked in the past, why it stopped being helpful, and what they need and would accept for assistance now (Cook, 1995).

Explore with the woman how she deals with the stressors in her life. Being homeless doesn't necessarily mean that she doesn't have a support network. Who does she turn to for help and support? Can she turn to them now? (Killion, 1995).

### Interventions

Purposeful strategies stand a greater chance of success in planning interventions for women and their families who are homeless. Giving birth is a powerful incentive, which, if she has been empowered during the birthing process, can help the woman revive her sense of control. Children can remotivate women who have given up to try again to seek assistance in searching for solutions to problems (Killion, 1995). Scheduling specific times during the day to collaborate with social service personnel allows the new mother the remainder of the brief time of hospitalization to relax and get to know her infant.

**Mother-Infant Interaction.** Rooming-in allows the woman to focus on her newborn. They may spend quiet time alone just getting to know one another. These opportunities enhance the interactions between mother and infant through contact, feeding, and eye-to-eye gazing.

"Seizing the moment" for teaching regarding newborn care is critical. Provide the mother time to demonstrate her caring abilities. This gives us the opportunity to offer positive input that will increase her self-esteem. While she cares for the baby, have her talk about how she will continue to care for the baby once discharged. Provide reinforcement for decisions that improve the health and safety of the woman and her child.

**Health Promotion.** Because the pregnancy rate for homeless women is estimated to be twice as high as the national rate, contraception teaching for homeless women is a priority (Killion, 1995). As a result of moving from place to place and needing to keep personal items at a minimum, birth control that is cumbersome and requires a specific routine (e.g., the pill is taken at the same time every day) may not be practical. Women who are homeless may not be in the same place or be able to obtain their method. We need to provide practical information about how to access free or inexpensive birth control methods and how to use them.

**Nutrition.** Nutritional counseling based on shelter living can be taught. Identification of typical foods available can provide us with the information we need to assist the mother in food selection. Resources regarding places where wholesome food is offered at reasonable prices can be provided. Attention to normal growth and development of infants and children and their nutritional requirements is considered from the viewpoint of what will be available. If WIC cannot be accessed because of legal issues of residency, alternatives must be found.

**Discharge Planning.** The time in the hospital provides safety and a brief period when a woman might find rest and nurturing. Release from worry is not a reality, but active pursuit of possible solutions in conjunction with caring, nonjudgmental health care professionals is a rational approach. Nurses and social workers need to have viable options to propose. Identification of community resources that keep families together is paramount. Because of various social problems, sometimes including domestic violence and substance abuse, homeless women may be aware of few options and require assistance in maneuvering through the bureaucracy to find appropriate care. Referral to a community health nurse and supportive programs within the community can help.

### Evaluation

Ongoing evaluation is difficult because once a woman leaves the hospital there is no guarantee that she will be able to return for follow-up care or have a phone for postpartum contact. Without overwhelming the woman, we must collaborate with other health care professionals to coordinate services to maximize meeting the mother's health care needs. We can provide the woman 24-hour hotline numbers; concise written explanations of danger signs; and a compact, prioritized summary of the most important information. Her statements and responses to questions can indicate her understanding of the information.

## Summary

Postpartum care of the homeless woman is, of necessity, multifaceted and often more complex than the care of the woman with an addiction or the woman who is experiencing domestic violence. The homeless woman can only be helped through a collaborative effort of the health care providers within the hospital and the available local and regional community services. Because of the limited number of spaces to house homeless women, and homeless women with children in particular, it is not only an issue of care for women on our postpartum floors but also an area for advocacy. Based on what we learn about the reality of their lives while providing care for women with addictions, women in violent relationships, and women who are homeless, we can speak with conviction to community and governmental programs and the legislature to develop more supportive programs.

## CARE OF THE WOMAN WITH HEALTH DISORDERS COMPLICATING THE POSTPARTUM

Women may become pregnant and deliver a child while they also are dealing with health disorders. Some of these disorders require hospitalization and special care during the postpartum. Some women may gain an extra day or two of hospitalized care, while others will have to receive this extra information and care within the now standard 2-day postpartum stay.

### Anemia

Anemia may be discovered with postpartum screening. Anemia is defined either as a reduction in red blood cell (RBC) volume measured by the hematocrit (Hct) or a decrease in the percent concentration of hemoglobin (Hgb) in the peripheral blood. Woman with anemia who come to prenatal care late or not at all will not have had the condition diagnosed and treated during pregnancy.

### Areas of Concern

*Iron Deficiency Anemia.* Iron deficiency anemia (IDA) is the most common type seen in the postpartum woman, accounting for approximately 90% of the cases of anemia. IDA occurs when hemoglobin production is inadequate as the result of insufficient dietary intake of iron during pregnancy or loss of blood through bleeding during the delivery process. The remaining 10% of the cases include folic acid deficiency anemia (the second most common cause of anemia), thalassemia, sickle cell anemia, or other acquired or hereditary anemias (Youngkin and Davis, 1998; Brown, 2000; Mattson and Smith, 2000).

*Folic Acid Deficiency Anemia.* Folic acid deficiency (FAD) anemia may result from poor intake of folate, malabsorption of folate from the intestines, liver damage, or depletion of stores through frequent pregnancies. It can be treated with diet and supplementation after the woman is discharged home. The anticipatory guidance and self-care measures needed to treat IDA and FAD anemia may be given to the woman while on the postpartum unit. Assistance and teaching may be incorporated into her meal selection while there. However, the long-term dietary changes and supplementation process will be most successful when the woman is assisted during a home visit. These interventions are addressed in Chapter 20.

*Inherited Anemia.* Thalassemia and sickle cell anemia are inherited, lifelong conditions that may affect the parents' health. In addition, the infant may have inherited this problem. Thalassemia occurs primarily among people descended from the Mediterranean area, North Africa, the Middle East, India, Pakistan, China, and Southeast Asia. It is a group of hereditary anemias caused by decreased or defective production of RBCs. "Individuals who are heterozygous for $\alpha$- or $\beta$-thalassemia have thalassemia minor; those who are homozygous have thalassemia major" (Youngkin and Davis, 1998). Thalassemia minor is benign and often is diagnosed by abnormal laboratory findings during the pregnancy or postpartum. Women with thalassemia major rarely become pregnant.

Sickle cell trait and sickle cell anemia are caused by genetic defects in the hemoglobin chains. It is among the most prevalent of genetic diseases in the United States. The conditions are seen primarily in clients of African or Caribbean descent, and from South and Central America. It also occurs in Native Americans, Hispanic Americans, whites, and persons of Mediterranean, Arabian, or East Indian descent (Sickle Cell Disease Guideline Panel, 1993).

If the woman has the sickle cell trait she may have no symptoms. However, some women do experience hematuria, increased bacteriuria, and pyelonephritis during pregnancy.

### Anticipated Concerns

Pregnancy predisposes all women to depletion of their iron stores. In addition, if a woman is experiencing substance abuse, domestic violence, or homelessness she is more likely to experience the nutritional inadequacies that increase her risk for anemia (Perry, Yip, and Zyrkowski, 1995).

When women are anemic, they are at a higher risk for infection, pregnancy-induced hypertension, and postpartum hemorrhage. If even a small postpartum hemorrhage occurs, the loss of blood will make the woman's anemia even more critical (Engstrom and Sittler, 1994).

### Nursing Assessment

The postpartum assessment begins with reviewing a woman's history, physical examination, and laboratory results during the prenatal period if available. In addition, any laboratory work obtained once she was admitted in labor should be reviewed. If her laboratory work indicates that the postpartum woman has a hemoglobin of less than 10 g/dl, consider it a low value and reflective of an anemic state (Brown, 2000).

Monitor all postpartum women closely for early signs or symptoms of postpartum hemorrhage. However, because women with anemia do not tolerate well the loss of blood experienced at birth, they should be watched even more closely during the initial period after birth. Assess her uterus, check her flow, do a pad count, and take her vital signs every hour. Also evaluate her for abnormal fatigue, pale skin, and pallor of the conjunctiva, which are all symptoms associated with anemia (Henly and others, 1995) (Box 19-5).

### Possible Nursing Diagnoses

Nursing diagnoses for a woman diagnosed with anemia focus on nutritional interventions to restore iron levels, injury prevention so that she doesn't lose any more blood, and anticipatory guidance to prevent infection. If the woman has a newly diagnosed genetically caused anemia, she will require education and guidance about what this means for her health.

### Expected Outcomes

Most often a woman with IDA or FAD anemia is sent home after a mean length of stay of 1.5 days. However, if she has thalassemia or experiences a hemorrhage during childbirth or the postpartum period, her stay may be extended to an average length of 1.9 to 2.5 days (Clinical Classifications for Health Policy Research: Hospital Inpatient Statistics, 1995). The longer stay is helpful to the woman because the initial fatigue and malaise of a person with severe anemia make it difficult for her to learn self-care measures. The extra time can allow for more effective provision of anticipatory guidance. Expected outcomes might be that by the time of discharge the woman will:

- Identify ways to continue to monitor the amount of her vaginal bleeding
- Identify foods on the hospital menu that will provide her with iron and folic acid
- If prescribed, identify how to take her iron supplement most effectively
- Describe how she will care for her fatigue while caring for a new infant

### Self-Care

The birth of an infant can serve as a powerful motivator for a woman to become more interested in learning about eating a proper diet and how to select foods that support it. However, at this time, a woman with anemia may just be too tired to be able to learn how to implement change for herself. Use practical teaching and small changes to help her while she is making selections of food in the hospital.

Once discharged, the woman will be responsible for assessing the amount of her vaginal flow on an ongoing basis and notifying her health care provider if the flow increases. Even if the discharge plan includes home nursing visits, the woman must still be able to assess her own flow. She begins to build self-confidence in her ability to do so by assessing her own flow while still hospitalized.

### Interventions

***Care of the Woman.*** The primary goal of medical intervention is to identify and treat the problem causing the anemia. The cause of the anemia determines the type of medical treatments and nursing interventions that are needed. IDA or FAD anemia respond to iron therapy and folate supplementation. If the woman has thalassemia, iron therapy is not recommended, even if the stress of pregnancy may have worsened her condition. Supplementing her diet with iron tablets is a needless expense and may even be dangerous to her health. If she has severe anemia, a transfusion may be ordered before she is discharged (Table 19-1).

***Health Promotion.*** Nursing interventions include teaching the woman about nutrition, medication, lifestyle, activity, and rest to accommodate the needs of her body. Teach the woman about her specific condition and the interventions that will be most helpful to her.

---

### BOX 19-5   *Summary of Assessment of the Woman with Anemia*

*Blood pressure, respirations, and pulse*: q 15 min × 4, q 30 min × 2, q 1 hr until stable

*Evaluate lochia*: q 15 min × 4, q 30 min × 2, q 1 hr until stable

*Assess uterus*: q 15 min × 4, q 30 min × 2, q 1 hr until stable

*Intake and output*: q hr × 2, q 8 hr until stable

*Hemoglobin and hematocrit*: immediately after delivery

   If Hct is <10% lower than predelivery, take no further action

   If Hct is >10% lower than predelivery, obtain HcT at 24 hr and review actions

Assess woman for pallor, fatigue, decreased tolerance for exercise, anorexia, weakness, malaise, dyspnea, and edema.

From Hyashi R and Castillo MS: Bleeding in pregnancy. In Knuffel R and Drukker J, editors: *High risk pregnancy: a team approach*, ed 2, Philadelphia, 1993, WB Saunders; Mattson S and Smith JE: *Core curriculum for maternal newborn nursing*, ed 2, Philadelphia, 2000, WB Saunders.

## TABLE 19-1 *Administering a Blood Transfusion*

The physician orders blood products to restore circulatory blood volume, improve hemoglobin, or correct serum protein levels. Administration of blood or blood components is a nursing procedure.

**POTENTIAL NURSING DIAGNOSES**
Client data derived during assessment reveal defining characteristics to support the following nursing diagnoses in clients requiring this skill:
Fluid volume deficit, high risk for
Cardiac output, decreased

**EQUIPMENT**
In addition to that used to initiate an IV infusion:
Normal saline IV solution, 0.9%
Infusion set with inline filter (Figure A)
Large catheter (18- or 19-gauge)
Correct blood product
Another nurse to double-check correct blood product with correct client
Disposable gloves

| Steps | Rationale |
|---|---|
| 1. Wash hands. | Reduces transmission of microorganisms. |
| 2. Apply disposable gloves. | Reduces transmission of bloodborne pathogens. Gloves should be worn when handling items soiled by body fluids. |
| 3. Explain procedure to client. Determine if there has been any previous transfusion and note reactions, if any. | Clients who have had a blood transfusion in the past may have greater fear of transfusion. |
| 4. Ask client to immediately report any of following symptoms: chills, headache, itching, rash. | These can be signs of a transfusion reaction. Prompt reporting and discontinuation of transfusion will help minimize reaction. |
| 5. Be sure that client has signed any necessary consent forms. | Some agencies require clients to sign consent forms before receiving any blood component transfusions. |
| 6. Establish IV line with large (18- or 19-gauge) catheter. | Permits infusion of whole blood and prevents hemolysis. |
| 7. Use infusion tubing that has in-line filter; tubing should also be Y-type administration set (Figure B). | Filter removes any debris and tiny clots from blood. Using Y-type set permits (1) administration of additional products or volume expanders easily and (2) immediate infusion of 0.9% sodium chloride solution after completion of initial infusion. |

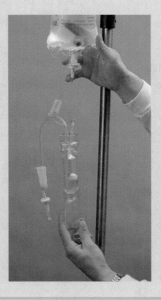

Figure A

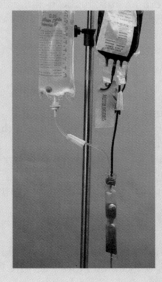

Figure B

From Perry AC and Potter PA: *Pocket guide to basic skills and procedures,* ed 3, St Louis, 1994, Mosby.

TABLE 19-1  *Administering a Blood Transfusion—cont'd*

| Steps | Rationale |
|---|---|
| 8. Hang solution container of 0.9% normal saline to be administered after blood infusion. | Prevents hemolysis of red blood cells. |
| 9. Follow agency protocol in obtaining blood products from blood bank. Request blood when you are ready to use it. | Whole blood or packed red blood cells must remain in a cold (1°-6° C) environment. |
| 10. With another nurse, correctly identify blood product and client: | One nurse reads out loud while other nurse listens and double-checks information. |
| • Check compatibility tag attached to blood bag and information on bag itself. | Verifies that ABO group, Rh type, and unit number match. |
| • For whole blood, check ABO group and Rh type (on client's chart). | Verifies that they match those on compatibility tag and blood bag. |
| • Double-check blood product with physician's order. | Verifies correct blood component. |
| • Check expiration date on bag. | After 21 days, blood has only 70% to 80% of its original cells and 23 mEq/L of potassium. |
| • Inspect blood for clots. | Anticoagulent citrate-phosphate-dextrose (CPD) is added to blood and permits preserved blood to be stored for 21 days. Newer anticoagulant citrate-phosphate-dextrose-adenine (CPD-A) allows storage for 35 days. If clots are present, return blood to blood bank. |
| 11. Obtain baseline vital signs within 30 minutes before administering transfusion. Report any temperature elevation to the physician. | Verifies client's pretransfusion temperature, pulse, blood pressure, and respirations and allows detection of reaction by noting changes in vital signs. |
| 12. Have client void or empty urine drainage collection container. | If a transfusion reaction occurs, the urine specimen obtained needs to be urine produced after the initiation of the transfusion. |
| 13. Open blood administration set. | Prepares blood administration tubing. |
| a. For Y-tubing administration, set all three roller clamps to "off" position. | Moving roller clamp(s) to "off" position prevents accidental spilling and wasting of blood. |
| b. For single tubing administration, set roller clamp to "off" position. | |
| 14. For Y-tubing: | Use of Y-tubing permits nurse to quickly switch from infusion of 0.9% normal saline to blood unit. Dextrose solutions are never used because they can cause coagulation of the donor blood. When unit is finished, nurse is able to maintain patency of vein by infusing normal saline. Y-tubing administration sets should be used when multiple blood transfusions are anticipated. Follow manufacturer's guidelines regarding number of units that can be given before tubing is changed. |
| a. Spike 0.9% normal saline IV bag. | |
| b. Prime tubing with 0.9% normal saline. | |
| • Open roller clamp on Y-tubing connected to normal saline bag and release roller clamp on unused inlet tube until tubing from normal saline bag is filled. | Allows fluid to flow from normal saline bag to drip chamber. |
| • Close clamp on unused tubing. | Prevents waste of IV solution. |
| • Squeeze sides of drip chamber. Allow filter to be partially covered. | Prevents air bubbles from entering system. |
| • Open lower roller clamp and allow infusion tubing to fill with normal saline. | Removes all air from system. |
| • Close lower roller clamp. | Prevents waste of IV fluid. |
| c. Gently invert blood bag 1 to 2 times to equally distribute cells. Spike blood or blood component container, open clamps on inlet tube and lower tubing, and fill tubing, completely covering the filter with blood. | Prevents clumping of cells, which can block outlet of bag or lead to clotting. Fragile blood cells may be damaged if they hit an uncovered filter. |
| d. Close lower clamp. | |
| 15. For single tubing administration: | Prepares administration filter and tubing with blood. Promotes quick connection of prepared infusion tubing to IV catheter. |
| a. Spike blood unit. | |
| b. Squeeze drip chamber; allow filter to be filled with blood. | |

*Continued*

## TABLE 19-1 *Administering a Blood Transfusion—cont'd*

| Steps | Rationale |
|---|---|
| c. Open roller clamp and allow infusion tubing to fill with blood. | |
| d. When a single tubing administration set is used, another IV tubing with 0.9% normal saline infusing is piggybacked to the blood administration set. Use tape to secure all connections. | The blood product should not be piggybacked into the normal saline line to avoid forcing fragile blood cells through both a needle and an IV catheter, which could cause mechanical trauma to cells. |
| 16. Attach blood transfusion tubing to IV catheter maintaining sterility. Open lower clamp. | Initiates infusion of blood product into the client's vein. |
| 17. Remain with client during first 15 to 30 minutes of transfusion. Initial flow rate during this time should be 2 to 5 ml/min. | Most reactions occur during the first 15 to 30 minutes of a transfusion. Infusing a small amount initially minimizes the volume of blood to which the client is exposed, which limits the severity of the reaction. This also allows prompt treatment of a transfusion reaction. |
| 18. Monitor client's vital signs: every 5 minutes for first 15 minutes; every 15 minutes for next hour; hourly until unit of blood is infused; for 1 hour after the infusion is completed. | Be alert for any change in vital signs that could be early warning of transfusion reaction. |
| 19. Regulate infusion according to physician's orders. Packed cells usually run over $1\frac{1}{2}$ to 2 hours while whole blood runs over 2 to 3 hours. | Client's condition dictates rate at which blood should be infused. Drop factor for blood tubing is 10 gtt/ml. |
| 20. After blood has infused, clear IV tubing with 0.9% normal saline and place blood bag in plastic bag to return to the laboratory. | Infuses remainder of blood in IV line; 0.9% normal saline prevents hemolysis of red cells. |
| 21. Dispose of all supplies appropriately. Remove gloves and wash hands. | Reduces transmission of microorganisms. |
| 22. Record type and amount of blood component administered and client's response to blood therapy. A separate transfusion record is usually used. | Documents administration of blood component and client's reaction. |

**NURSE ALERT**
Never inject any medication into an IV line with blood or a blood product infusing because of possible incompatibility and bacterial contamination of the blood product. When client requires rapid infusion of multiple units of blood, the infusion tubing itself should be warmed with a special blood warmer. A unit of blood and blood filter should not be allowed to hang longer than 4 hours because of danger of bacterial growth.

**TEACHING CONSIDERATIONS**
Client is instructed to notify nurse of signs of itching, swelling, dizziness, dyspnea, or chest pain. Clients and caregivers are taught signs of long-term reactions, such as delayed hemolysis, so they can notify their doctor and receive treatment.

*Mother-Infant Interaction.* While hospitalized, assist the woman with her activities of daily living and ambulation, allowing her to rest as much as possible while she also spends time with the infant. Because anemia with its associated fatigue levels may interfere with the establishment of breastfeeding, help the woman who wants to breastfeed find ways to rest and be successful. Once home, having others care for the house and other family members while providing some infant care at the beginning allows the mother to obtain her rest while establishing breastfeeding with her infant. Women without supports will need links to community services because the overwhelming fatigue will present a barrier to either selecting or continuing breastfeeding (Henly and others, 1995).

*Nutrition.* When a woman experiences the effects of anemia she may become more attuned to dietary changes that help her. Schedule time to do realistic diet planning based on her personal preferences, family and cultural preferences, and ability to obtain and prepare the foods that she wants that would be beneficial to her health.

*Discharge Planning.* Help her modify her expectations about caring for herself and her family after discharge. Explain her limitations and the assistance she will need to her support network. Assistance also may be gained from members of her church or other community groups. Teach her to space her activities so that she may have frequent rest periods during the day and longer periods of sleep at night.

### Evaluation

Before discharge, assess the level of the woman's understanding of her condition and her treatment plan. Have her explain how she will implement the instructions. If during this postpartum period she has learned that she carries a genetic trait or disease, provide her with written information about this condition. Make the appropriate referrals. Explain that within 1 week after the start of therapy she may be asked to have her hemoglobin levels checked. Explain that this may be done by a visiting nurse so that the woman does not have to leave her home.

### Summary

Postpartum care of the woman with anemia is multifaceted and becomes more complex if she learns that she has passed an inherited condition onto her infant. The woman needs physical care and assistance from others for a condition that she and her family cannot see. This in itself can be difficult because there does not appear to be anything wrong with her. In addition, the woman is learning self-care for the treatment of her anemia, and if she or her infant have a newly diagnosed inherited condition, she will be coming to terms with this and its implications for her health.

## Diabetes Mellitus

Diabetes mellitus is a chronic, systemic endocrine disorder characterized by abnormal metabolism of carbohydrates, fats, and proteins. Diabetes is classified as (1) type I diabetes, insulin-dependent diabetes mellitus (IDDM), (2) type II diabetes, noninsulin-dependent diabetes mellitus (NIDDM), or (3) gestational diabetes mellitus (GDM). "GDM is being recognized as little more than a form of type II, with a development that is condensed into a shorter frame" (Burrow and Duffy, 1999). Native Amer-

---

**BOX 19-6** *Classification of Diabetes in Pregnancy*

**PREGESTATIONAL DIABETES ("OVERT" DIABETES)**

*1. Type I Diabetes*
a. Complicated by retinopathy
b. Complicated by nephropathy
c. Complicated by coronary artery disease

*2. Type II diabetes*
a. Complicated by retinopathy
b. Complicated by nephropathy
c. Complicated by coronary artery disease

**GESTATIONAL DIABETES**

*1. Diet-Controlled*

*2. Insulin-Requiring*

From Burrow GN and Duffy TP: *Medical complications during pregnancy,* Philadelphia, 1999, WB Saunders.

---

icans, African-Americans, Hispanic Americans, Asian Americans, and Pacific Islanders have a greater risk for developing gestational diabetes that may evolve into type II diabetes later in life (Dacus and others, 1994; Burrow and Duffy, 1999).

With the delivery of the baby, most women who have developed GDM have the problem disappear. Some women with NIDDM may be able to gradually control their condition with diet, weight loss, exercise, and possibly oral medications. To provide the appropriate guidance and care to a woman with diabetes, the type and nature of her condition must be fully understood (Box 19-6).

### Anticipated Concerns

The pregnant women with diabetes is more likely to have had a surgical delivery because of concurrent complications, have worried about the baby because of fetal distress or fetal macrosomia (great body size), or have been induced before she had completed 38 to 40 weeks of pregnancy.

Postpartum women who have been insulin dependent to control their GDM or IDDM share a common problem during the postpartum period. At delivery there is an abrupt cessation of the antagonistic placental hormones and suppression of the anterior pituitary growth hormone, creating a significant decrease in the need for insulin (Gilbert and Harmon, 1998). Women who have maintained tight control of their glycemic levels during pregnancy now find their insulin requirements have dropped and if they take the same level of insulin as when pregnant they risk hypoglycemia. For at least the first 72 hours after delivery the woman with type I diabetes may require small doses of insulin as determined by her blood glucose levels. For the woman with type II diabetes the insulin dose, if necessary, is typically minimal. By the third or fourth postpartum day the woman who has IDDM will generally require about two thirds of her prepregnancy dose of insulin (Gilbert and Harmon, 1998). This monitoring often necessitates a longer postpartum stay than generally is allowed. No data are available on the length of postpartum stay for a woman with IDDM; however, according to the AHCPR, the average length of stay for a person with diabetes mellitus with complications is 6.7 days (Clinical Classifications for Health Policy Research: Hospital Inpatient Statistics, 1995).

"The incidence of postpartum thyroiditis is increased in women with type I diabetes, with approximately 25% of women affected, which is a threefold increase over that observed in the nondiabetic population. Nearly half require treatment for the thyroid dysfunction. Therefore women with type I diabetes should be vigilantly followed postpartum for any sign or symptoms of either thyrotoxicosis or hypothyroidism" (Burrow and Duffy, 1999).

### Nursing Assessment

Whether the woman has type I, type II, or gestational diabetes, monitor her blood glucose levels for the first 48 hours, take her vital signs, and monitor her intake and output, in addition to the other postdelivery protocols. "Women who were not insulin dependent before pregnancy most likely will not need insulin" (Gilbert and Harmon, 1998).

During the immediate postpartum period, learn from the mother any concerns she may have about her diabetic condition. If she experienced GDM she may wonder about its effect on the baby and the long-term implications for herself. If she was not an insulin user before pregnancy but had to use it during pregnancy, she may wonder what the future holds for her. Learn if the mother wishes to breastfeed or bottle feed her child.

### Possible Nursing Diagnoses

The diagnoses that will direct the care of the woman, depend on the type of diabetes the woman has and her body's return to a state of homeostasis. In addition educational needs and interventions help allay anxiety about her future health needs and abilities.

### Goals of Care

The goals are developed in collaboration with the woman and may vary. Some examples are that by discharge the woman will:

- Report a decrease in anxiety levels
- Identify eating choices that contribute to the management of glycemia

- Identify ways to maintain glycemic control when breastfeeding an infant.
- Report a plan of regular exercise to be undertaken while also caring for the infant

### Self Care

Women with IDDM have had the responsibility for monitoring their blood sugar and insulin requirements on a routine basis for some time. They are to be respected as the experts of their body and their program of care. If changes are necessary, we need to recognize their autonomy and build upon their control and maintenance of their health in our teaching in the postpartum period. Women may want more detailed explanations as they are empowered to be directors of their own care.

Woman who are not insulin dependent in the postpartum also will be assuming their own care with regard to maintaining an ideal body weight, eating an appropriate diet, and participating in a regular program of exercise. Using these skills, they may delay or prevent the need for further intervention later in life (Avery and Rossi, 1994). Motivation to change dietary habits, lose weight, and increase exercise are high right after delivery, and we can reinforce a new mother's interest.

### Interventions

***Care of the Woman.*** With resumption of normal dietary intake and decrease in insulin sensitivity, her insulin requirements generally return to prepregnancy levels (Brown and Hare, 1995). Review the nurse-midwife's or the physician's instruction regarding resumption of self-care with the woman.

The woman who developed gestational diabetes during this pregnancy should be advised that she has an increased risk (50%) of developing type II diabetes mellitus. Inform  her of the importance of an ongoing screening program for detection. The screening will start with a 75-g, 2-hour oral glucose tolerance test at her 6-week postpartum checkup. If her health insurance or personal income covers the cost, she should plan on having a random or fasting blood glucose test annually. Explain the benefits of early detection and intervention to her long-term health (Gilbert and Harmon, 1998).

If the woman had a surgical delivery, provide interventions for pain, anxiety, and her increased risk for infections as they will complicate her post delivery care. Pain control management and education about the course of recovery can decrease her anxiety. Careful monitoring of the surgical incision and maintaining good aseptic technique promote proper wound healing. Medical therapy will be instituted if an infection develops.

***Mother-Infant Interaction.*** Changing blood sugar levels combined with hormonal alterations can lead to labile moods. Proper preparation of the woman and her family can help them understand this part of the process of recovery (Kay, 1995). Encouraging her to verbalize her feelings and providing support for her concerns help her stabilize her emotions.

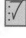

Breastfeeding is encouraged among women with diabetes. Breastfeeding decreases her fasting and postprandial blood glucose levels and increases her high-density lipoprotein blood glucose levels. Therefore, during breastfeeding, the woman's insulin requirements are usually considerably less. During weaning, she will need to closely monitor her glucose levels because they will fluctuate, and if she has IDDM, she will have to adjust her insulin accordingly. The woman who requires pharmocologic therapy for glycemic control will be switched to insulin instead of oral agent therapy. Oral agents may be excreted in the breast milk and affect the infant's blood glucose levels, whereas injected insulin secreted in the mother's breast milk is digested by the infant and does not affect his or her blood glucose levels (Mattson and Smith, 1993; Gilbert and Harmon, 1998). A woman with diabetes is at increased risk for nipple infections and mastitis. Teach her about the early symptoms of these conditions and how to respond to them. (Refer to Chapter 15.) If her sore nipples do not respond to the nonspecific treatments mentioned, tell her to contact her nurse-midwife or physician. An antifungal, nystatin ointment will be prescribed for application on the nipples and a nystatin suspension prescribed for the infant to take as well (Gilbert and Harmon, 1998).

**Health Promotion.** Obesity in combination with gestational diabetes increases by 70% a woman's risk of developing type II diabetes later in life (Avery and Rossi, 1994). Her weight makes a difference in the amount of insulin the pancreas must produce. For example the pancreas of an active thin person may only have to produce 35 to 40 U/day as compared with a person who is overweight, especially with abdominal fat, whose pancreas may be required to produce 150 U/day to clear the same amount of glucose. Even a 10-pound weight loss can make a major difference (Gilbert and Harmon, 1998). The postpartum period is a time when most women are receptive to learning about the benefits of diet change and exercise.

Birth control information for women with diabetes needs special consideration. Women who are obese, hypertensive, and smoke are not advised to take oral contraceptives because of risk of blood clots. Diabetic women are at risk for infections because of poor circulation and are cautioned regarding IUDs (Avery and Rossi, 1994). "The barrier methods of contraception are very safe for the woman with diabetes. Oral contraceptives have been reported to alter carbohydrate metabolism by causing insulin resistance. Therefore in the past the diabetic woman has been encouraged to avoid oral contraception. Recent research has indicated that the current low-progestin and low-estrogen preparations have minimal effect on carbohydrate metabolism" (Gilbert and Harmon, 1998). In the discussion of options available to her, the woman and her nurse-midwife or physician will balance her choice between the risk of the method to prevent pregnancy and the risk of a pregnancy. Once the decision is made, our role is to help the woman understand how to use the method to obtain the greatest efficacy.

**Lifestyle Changes.** The postpartum period is a time when most women are receptive to learning about the benefits of lifestyle changes. Nutritional guidance focuses on increasing caloric intake from lean meats, fruits, and vegetables. For women who are not used to eating this way or who have a family who may not choose to change, developing a strategic plan with them on how to incorporate the changes into their lifestyles is important. Providing specific guidelines and ideas, such as placing cut-up bagged vegetables and fruits in the refrigerator, gives women more helpful assistance than just telling them to increase consumption of fruits and vegetables. Use the same process to explore how they may incorporate more exercise into her lifestyle. Support of dietary changes with a prescribed postpartum exercise program affords women a better opportunity for weight loss and establishing a healthy lifestyle.

**Grieving.** Women who lose their infant because of complications of diabetes will not only grieve the death but also feel that maybe if they had done something different it would have survived. The women and their families require a multidisciplinary team follow-up. A bereavement team should offer the woman and her partner all available support. With experience in this situational crisis, we can assist the family in the grieving process by helping with the selection of burial arrangements, as well as obtaining spiritual guidance, physical and emotional care, and referrals to postpartum grief groups.

**Discharge Planning.** Discharge plans are centered on follow-up referrals given with specific instructions for postpartum home care. Women are advised to report any abnormal signs and symptoms to their health provider or given a phone number to call the clinic.

### Evaluation

Evaluation of the plan of care and discharge plans are centered on the woman's stability of blood glucose levels; insulin regulation; recovery from birth, either surgical or vaginal; grieving process; knowledge of contraception; and her verbalization of an acceptable and practical dietary and exercise plan. Determine if the woman understands how to access the referrals that have been given and her specific instructions for postpartum home care.

### Summary

Pregnant women with diabetes who receive prenatal care attend more prenatal visits and are closely monitored during the entire period. They become aware of the risks to themselves and the developing fetus and worry about how long they will be able to carry the pregnancy, what method of delivery they will have, and the health and well-being of the infant. The postpartum period provides a chance to return to their prepregnant health status and regain a sense of control of their body. In addition, they generally are receptive to health maintenance teaching and learning ways they can care for their new infant. If their infant died because of complications of diabetes, the woman and her family will require care that facilitates their grief process. In addition, she will worry about the possible outcomes of future pregnancies.

## Cardiac Disease

When you encounter a woman with heart disease during the postpartal period, she may have rheumatic fever (50%), valve deformities, congenital heart disease, developmental abnormalities, congestive cardiomyopathies, or cardiac dysrhythmias.

### Anticipated Issues

The first hours after the delivery of the baby are critical for maternal safety because of the high risk for fluid volume overload as the large blood volume of pregnancy shifts vascular compartments (Gilbert and Harmon, 1998). The pressure that had been exerted by the fetus and placenta no longer exists after birth, allowing improved blood flow from the lower extremities to the heart. After the delivery of the placenta, the uterine vessels constrict, preventing hemorrhage but shunting blood from the uterus to the systemic circulation. This creates an autotransfusion of approximately 1,000 ml of blood and an increase in cardiac output to about 65% higher than prelabor values (Simpson and Creehan, 1996).

### Nursing Assessment

Assess blood pressure, apical and radial pulses, lung sounds, and weight loss. Assess for presence of edema. Ask the woman if she is feeling any chest pain. Assess each leg for Homan's sign. If the woman has calf pain with a positive Homan's sign, it may indicate a blood clot in one of the deep veins, an inflammation of one of the superficial veins, or an inflammation of a tendon in the leg. To avoid confusing this calf pain with Achilles tendon pain, a common complaint with athletes who stress the tendon and women who wear high-heeled shoes and shorten the tendon, be sure to keep the knee flexed when you dorsiflex the foot (Seidel and others, 1999) (Figure 19-1).

Learn the type and amount of help the mother will have when she goes home. Determine if the woman wishes to breastfeed her infant. Assess knowledge of methods and desired choices for pregnancy prevention.

### Possible Nursing Diagnoses

Because of the cardiac compromise, the woman will have concerns about her own physical health, concerns about how this problem will affect her ability to care for her child, and concerns about the possibility of future pregnancies.

### Goals of Care

Keep her as comfortable as possible to reduce the cardiac workload. Based on her concerns and the physical difficulties involved, the goals of care for a woman with a cardiac condition could be as follows:

The complications the woman experiences will be minimized because of early assessment.

The woman and her family will verbalize understanding of the need for providing the woman with assistance.

The woman and her partner will agree on using a method of contraception that has high efficacy and does not endanger the woman's health.

### Self-Care

The best self-care that the woman may give herself is to allow herself to be taken care of by others as her body readjusts to being nonpregnant. Rest and gradual resumption of care of self and baby allow her to progress without becoming overtired. Encouragement to follow a plan of good nutrition is also beneficial to her recovery. Encourage her to be patient and over the first 6 weeks of postpartum gradually resume her former activities.

### Interventions

Be cautious during the administration of intravenous fluids or oxytocin after the delivery because either one may compromise the woman's cardiac condition. The rapid addition of intravenous fluids to her circulatory system places her at risk of fluid overload (Gilbert and Harmon, 1998).

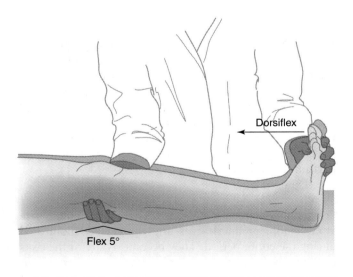

Dorsiflex

Flex 5°

FIGURE 19-1 ● Assessment of Homan's Sign.

***Continuing Assistance of the Woman.*** Discuss with the woman and her family their plans for care after discharge. Help them understand that the woman will need assistance for several weeks until she can gradually resume her previous level of activity. Planning for someone to prepare nutritious meals for her and assist with the care of the baby will be necessary at first. Inquire about the amount and type of care the network of family and friends will be able to provide. Provide information and referrals if additional resources are needed.

***Breastfeeding of Infant.*** If the woman is not on medications that contraindicate breastfeeding, she may choose to do so. In addition to the regular teaching and assistance given to breastfeeding mothers, help her determine additional ways to conserve her energy. Feeding while in a side-lying position and having someone else prepare and then burp the baby will be helpful as she tries to rest.

***Pregnancy Prevention.*** Prevention of another pregnancy before the woman is fully recovered is essential. Ensure that the woman understands the directions for the use of the method of contraception provided by her nurse-midwife or physician. Explore with her the implications that this may have for her relationship with her partner. Respond to her need for assistance in explanation and implementation of this self-care.

### Evaluation

Evaluation of interventions is based on the achievement of the short-term goals for the woman's postpartum recovery while hospitalized. Evaluate the woman's understanding about the need for pregnancy prevention until she is fully recovered and her ability to implement that measure of self-care. Also determine the level of understanding and willingness of her partner to cooperate.

Because the woman will require ongoing self-care and assistance, it also involves the assessment of her understanding about the need for assistance and connection with appropriate resources within her family and referrals within her community.

### Summary

As more women with cardiac conditions reach childbearing age and find themselves with energy and a sense of well-being, more may choose to become pregnant. Their care during the postpartal period is the last step in assisting them to regain their prepregnancy level of health.

## Human Immunodeficiency Virus

Human immunodeficiency virus type 1 (HIV-1) infection, although not the rapid death sentence it once was, causes a slow and relentless destruction of the woman's immune system, eventually resulting in acquired immunodeficiency syndrome (AIDS). The pregnant woman

with HIV-1 is not only facing this downhill process for herself but knows that she may pass the virus on to her child. Unable to learn the status of her child for months after the birth, the woman during the postpartum period will need honest information and support as she interacts with her child and wonders if she has infected it.

### Anticipated Concerns

Women with HIV face many questions and concerns in the postpartum period. In addition to the normal recovery from the pregnancy and delivery, she will have concerns about her own health and future. In addition, she may wonder about the health and future of her infant. "Who will care for my child if I get too sick?" (Boston Women's Health Book Collective, 1999).

Some women learn they are HIV positive during the routine blood work of prenatal care. Pregnancy can in fact mask the symptoms of HIV infection because the clinical manifestations of HIV—fatigue, nausea, and weight loss—are also common complaints of pregnancy. A woman's pregnancy delays the diagnosis, but contrary to what was previously thought, pregnancy by itself does not appear to accelerate the course of the HIV infection (Lindberg, 1995).

### Ethical Considerations

Nurses, nurse-midwives, and physicians often find they have strong feelings about caring for women who have exposed their infants to a possible death sentence through vertical transmission of the virus. The woman may wonder, "How do I deal with health care providers who don't respect me because I use drugs or sell sex, or because they think I do?" (Boston Women's Health Book Collective, 1999). Remember that women are infected in various ways, including by partners who refuse to wear condoms, from blood transfusions given between 1977 and 1985, as a result of infection while caring for a person who has HIV, or as the result of a date rape or sexual assault. When working with women infected with the HIV-1 virus be aware of your own values and beliefs. This is necessary to provide competent unbiased care and true concern for the mother who also is infected and facing a terminal illness (Allen and Buppert, 1996).

### Collaborative Medical Management

An increasing array of therapeutic agents and the ways in which they are used are complex and evolving. It is vital that an HIV/AIDS specialist participates in all care. Until the delivery, the treatment plan focuses on the dual responsibility of optimizing therapy for the mother while reducing the possibility of transmission of HIV from the mother to the infant. During the postpartum period, medical therapy with HIV drug protocols continues for a woman who has been taking the drugs. The infant also may be placed on antiretroviral therapy. Care during and after discharge is managed by specialists in pediatric HIV for the infant and a gynecologist and an HIV specialist for the mother.

### Nursing Assessment

HIV infection has a minimal effect on causing pregnancy complications and a negative birth experience. Problems occur if the woman drinks, smokes, or uses IV drugs during the gestational period. Our postpartum nursing assessment is individualized and focuses on other health problems present during the prenatal period or from the delivery experience.

Learn from the mother what concerns she may have about her HIV status and the treatments required during the postpartum period for both herself and her child. Does she anticipate any difficulties in adjusting to her own care and the care of her newborn? Does she have a support network of family and friends on whom she may depend? How will she manage providing both herself and her infant with the necessary medications? The infant will probably receive medication for the next 6 weeks to reduce the risk of perinatal transmission (Gilbert and Harmon, 1998).

Explore how she feels about the CDC recommendation that she not breastfeed her infant. Is she willing and able to bottle feed? Assess how she is bonding with the baby. Does she seem to be holding back in developing an attachment? Does she understand that it is very difficult to determine if the infant has acquired an HIV infection because of the presence of passive acquired maternal antibodies until 12 to 14 months? How will she cope with not knowing until then? (Box 19-7)

### Possible Nursing Diagnoses

Nursing diagnoses for the care of a woman experiencing a postpartum complicated by HIV reflect all the regular concerns of the postpartum period plus a possibility for altered parent-infant attachment because of the physical effects of the virus on the mother, her worry about the baby, the loss of not being able to breastfeed the infant, and concern about how long and how well she may live and be able to care for her child.

---

**BOX 19-7** *Possible Concerns of the Woman with HIV*

Infection
Medical needs for HIV
Contraception
Health practices
Assessment of current psychosocial needs
Social service needs
Infant feeding care teaching

---

### Goals of Care

The goals are developed in collaboration with the woman and may vary. Some examples are that by discharge the woman will do the following:

- Describe a daily plan for rest periods to decrease fatigue
- Identify ways to obtain daily nutritional requirements
- Identify support links
- Make decisions regarding care for herself and infant in collaboration with health care professionals
- Seek appropriate external resources as needed
- Demonstrate mother-infant attachment behaviors
- Demonstrate proper bottle-feeding techniques
- Demonstrate universal blood and body fluid precautions
- Describe the plan of treatment for herself and her child

### Self-Care

The birth of an infant is a source of joy for women who see this event as something that gives meaning to life. Women infected with the HIV virus may view this as an opportunity to care for themselves and achieve as optimal a level of health as possible for themselves and their infants. Identifying and reinforcing the strengths the women possess will help support and motivate them. They now will be responsible not only for maintaining their own health and treatment regimens but also caring for their infant.

### Interventions

Interventions not only focus on preventing the spread of the virus but also on improving the quality of life for persons living with HIV/AIDS and their family members and friends who also may be affected by the stigma. Women with HIV frequently feel isolated. Connections to others are important to provide a sense that they are not alone. When women feel that their health care providers are not afraid of them and regard their welfare as important, they are more likely to want to collaborate in their treatment.

***Care of the Woman.*** The woman with HIV requires the same postpartum care as other women who experience either a vaginal or surgical delivery. With universal precautions, all bodily fluids of all clients are treated in the same manner. Mothers with HIV are reminded to protect the infant from coming in contact with their body fluids. Mothers will be using universal precautions when interacting with their own child as well as other persons.

***Feeding the Infant.*** Breast milk is a body fluid, so breastfeeding is not recommended. Women who live where formula feeding is a safe alternative can be taught proper bottle-feeding techniques and how to safely prepare formula. Women with positive HIV status in undeveloped parts of the world need guidance in evaluating the risks posed by breastfeeding versus bottle feeding. In undeveloped areas where formula's properties cannot be guaranteed and a safe water supply may not be available, a directive not to breastfeed is problematic. In these regions, breast milk provides the infant significant protection against life-threatening gastrointestinal (GI) and respiratory tract infections. Thus the decision to avoid breastfeeding in favor of bottle feeding also can have serious and even fatal consequences (Shannon, 1994; Lindberg, 1995; Burrow and Duffy, 1999).

**Health Promotion.** Because of the compromised immune status, interventions to decrease the chances of contacting infection are a priority. Handwashing, aseptic techniques in any invasive procedure, and proper perineal care and sterile wound care as applicable to lacerations or surgical incisions are required standards of care. These are also teaching opportunities for women with HIV to learn how to protect themselves. Women are also taught the immunization schedule for their infant and their ongoing care needs (Lindberg, 1995).

To facilitate her health, instruct the woman in ways to enhance her immune system. These include: adequate sleep; decreasing stress; a diet with adequate protein, vitamin E, zinc, vitamin A, pyridoxine, pantothenic acid, folic acid and decreased polyunsaturated fatty acid; and avoidance of infections.

Because of the complexities of the diet recommendations, nutritional teaching is specifically necessary. It should include guidelines for fulfilling daily requirements with the types of food that women prefer and have available to them. When the woman is involved in selecting foods she likes and understands why she needs them, she is more able to adhere to the plan. Innovative ways to find high-calorie foods of appropriate nutritional composition that are readily available and affordable will help her nutrition and her resulting energy level.

Anticipatory guidance also includes teaching early signs of infection that women should note and report to their nurse practitioner, nurse-midwife, or physician. Women are cautioned about the following:

* Worsening fatigue
* Anorexia
* Weight loss
* Cough
* Skin lesions
* Vaginitis (Ropka and Williams, 1998)

Contraceptive practices must emphasize the need for informing partners of the women's status, using condoms (male or female), and preventing pregnancy. Women and their partners need to understand the implications linked with transmission of the disease. Identify places women may obtain free or inexpensive condoms.

Both written and verbal instructions offer the best way to maximize a woman's understanding and implementation of her own care. After hospital discharge various community based services will provide the woman's care, so provide her with written lists of the names and phone numbers of the nurse practitioners, nurse-midwives, physicians, social workers and other professionals who will guide that care.

### Evaluation

Evaluation of interventions are based on the achievement of the short-term goals for the woman's postpartum recovery while hospitalized. Because the woman who is HIV positive requires ongoing care, it also involves the identification of and connection with appropriate referrals within the community for her continuing care and that of her baby after discharge and the woman's capacity to understand and state her role in following through with those referrals.

### Summary

A woman who is HIV positive and has a child faces more than the usual challenges in the postpartum. Although an HIV-1 infection is increasingly seen as a chronic infection, the woman faces the stigma of having contracted the virus. In addition, she now has to deal with the possible guilt of having a child who also is infected. The women and their families require nonjudgmental information about their condition and health care needs and a supportive environment within which they may care for themselves so that they also may care for their child.

## Sexually Transmitted Infections

Sexually transmitted infections (STIs) are usually detected and most cases are treatable during the prenatal period. A woman with an undetected or untreated STI may deliver an infant if she has received inadequate or insufficient prenatal care. Postpartum assessment is key to identifying and treating infections before discharge.

### Anticipated Concerns

If untreated, STIs may result in postpartum complications in the mother, and some may be transmitted to the infant during the birth. Treatment during the postpartal period for bacterial vaginosis (BV), herpes simplex virus (HSV-2), hepatitis B virus (HBV) and trichomoniasis may interfere briefly with a woman's plan for breastfeeding.

### Nursing Assessment

If the woman has no prenatal history, all pertinent information is gathered during the postpartum evaluation, including a careful and sensitive sexual history. Laboratory values are obtained, including swabs of fluid if infection is suspected plus a complete blood count (CBC) and tests for specific STIs. A physical assessment includes the following:

- Assess skin for color, rash, capillary refill, and body temperature
- Inspect lochia for color, odor, and consistency
- Inspect episiotomy, if present, and/or any lacerations
- Inspect surgical incision if present for edema, redness, and drainage (Clark and others, 1996).

### Possible Nursing Diagnoses

Based on the individual woman's history, physical findings, laboratory results, and her concerns, nursing diagnoses are developed. In addition to the normal postpartum concerns, nursing diagnoses designed to respond to knowledge deficits, physical discomfort, self-esteem issues, and concerns about how and where the infection was contracted may be applicable.

### Goals of Care

The goals of care are developed in collaboration with the woman and may vary. Some examples are that by discharge the woman will be able to do the following:

- Identify who infected her and who she might have passed the infection on to.
- Identify her infection and the necessary regimen of treatment.
- Identify when and where she should go for care after discharge.
- Describe the signs and symptoms of STIs.
- State where she may obtain condoms (male and female) and how she might convince her partner to accept condom use.
- State the benefit of wearing cotton underwear.
- State the precautions she must follow so as to not infect her infant.
- State how she may still breastfeed and complete the use of medication.

### Self-Care

The self-care that a woman must assume to regain her health is the completion of all medication. Reduction in the possibility of receiving infectious organisms from future intimate encounters requires the use of condoms.

### Interventions

Based on the nursing assessment and medical diagnosis, a collaborative nursing and medical treatment plan is developed. Nursing interventions are aimed at management of the woman's medical therapy, support of her physical condition, infection control, education, and health promotion.

Rest, antipyretic therapy, and comfort measures help the mother regain her strength during the postpartum and assume her role as the infant's caretaker. In addition, many of the pharmacologic agents required to treat infection require that the woman not give the baby breast milk while the drugs are in her system. Assist the woman in reconciling herself both physically and emotionally during this time period. Teach her how to maintain her milk supply during the treatment period if desired.

***Bacterial Vaginosis.*** Women with bacterial vaginosis are treated with one dose of metronidazole, 2 g orally, and are instructed to pump and discard their breast milk for the next 24 hours. Explain the reason for this procedure, teach them how to use the breast pump, and assist them with the process. Then supply the bottles of formula that the infant needs during that time. Depending on the reasons a woman has chosen to breastfeed, she may prefer that the baby receive soy-based formula rather than cow's milk–based formula. If the woman is discharged before the 24 hours are completed, help her determine how she can still pump and discard the milk as required (Gilbert and Harmon, 1998).

***Candidiasis.*** Candidiasis is resistant to treatment in pregnancy, so even though she may have been treated, the condition may not have resolved and may require treatment again after the delivery. If she is breastfeeding, teach her the signs and symptoms of neonatal thrush and that any nipple soreness should be evaluated by her nurse, nurse practitioner, nurse-midwife, or physician (Gilbert and Harmon, 1998).

***Herpesvirus.*** If a woman is diagnosed with active genital herpes, mother and baby are placed together in a private room so the infection is not transmitted to babies in the nursery. A woman with HSV should be counseled about the importance of good handwashing and hygiene so that she does not transmit the virus to her infant. No therapy will cure HSV. Acyclovir is the treatment that is used to lessen a woman's symptoms and decrease viral shedding. However, a woman who is breastfeeding may not take acyclovir. Comfort measures for the pain include keeping lesions dry and clean, using a topical lotion such as Campho-Phenique on lesions, or using compresses of cold milk or colloidal oatmeal or a boric acid sitz bath (Gilbert and Harmon, 1998).

***Hepatitis B Virus.*** If a woman has been diagnosed with HBV, she may pass it to her infant after delivery through blood contact or breast milk. Breastfeeding is contraindicated, unless the infant was immunized. Teach the mother how to implement safe practices so that her infant is not exposed to her blood (Gilbert and Harmon, 1998).

***Human Papillomaviruses.*** Human papillomaviruses (HPVs) are human wart viruses. Ninety percent of cases of condylomata acuminata, known as genital warts, are caused by HPV types 6 and 11 (Gilbert and Harmon, 1998). No treatment eradicates HPV, so even though the lesions are removed and the signs and symptoms are alleviated, the virus remains. The woman's natural immune response may then control the replication of the virus. "There is an increased risk of poor episiotomy healing in the presence of condylomata. This risk becomes greater if the woman smokes" (Gilbert and Harmon, 1998).

***Trichomoniasis.*** Trichomoniasis is generally contracted through sexual activity. "However, it may be contracted by swimming in contaminated water, using contaminated towels, or sitting in hot tubs" (Gilbert and Harmon, 1998). When a woman is breastfeeding, symptomatic relief is gained if she takes clotrimazole. If eradication of the protozoa is desired, she may be treated with metronidazole (Flagyl), 2 g orally for one dose. However, if Flagyl is used she must pump and discard her breast milk for the next 24 hours (Lawrence and Lawrence, 1998). Work with the woman so that if Flagyl is prescribed, she can successfully pump her breasts and discard the milk. Also ensure that she has appropriate formula to feed the infant.

### Evaluation

Women are discharged from postpartum care after a short-term stay. An evaluation of their health status and the acceptance of an ongoing treatment plan for an infection are important.

For those infections that may have recurring episodes (i.e., herpesvirus) or are conditions that she may pass to others (i.e., hepatitis B), she should verbalize how she will reduce the risk of infecting her baby and other family members. The woman should also be able to state how she can prevent the occurrence of future infections of STIs. Written instruction should be given about the use of medication and appointments for follow-up care. The reasons for completing an antibiotic schedule must be emphasized and understood by the woman. If she is discharged from the hospital with a supply of the entire dose of medication she requires, she will be more successful in following the plan. Trying to take care of her postpartum needs and the needs of the new baby and travel to fill a prescription may be just too much, even for a woman with a support network.

### Summary

Women with STIs have to deal with several concerns: (1) the possible humiliation of having such an infection and (2) the concern about who they contracted it from and why. If it is an infection that has injured their infant or that they risk passing on to their infant, even in the postpartum period, there may be continuing worry or anger. Identification of infections, treatment, and education for protection from future infections in a nonjudgmental environment are the major interventions we may offer.

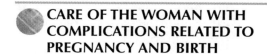

## CARE OF THE WOMAN WITH COMPLICATIONS RELATED TO PREGNANCY AND BIRTH

### Pregnancy-Induced Hypertension

The terminology for hypertensive disorders of pregnancy is inconsistent and causes confusion. Basically there are two etiologic disorders involved. One disorder is related to a woman that has a preexisting condition of hypertension who then becomes pregnant. The other disorder develops during pregnancy, labor, or the early postpartum period in a woman who has not previously had hypertension or protein in her urine. This is pregnancy-induced hypertension (PIH).

PIH is hypertension or proteinuria that develops after 20 weeks of gestation or within 7 days postpartum (Gilbert and Harmon, 1998). It complicates pregnancy, childbirth, and the puerperium and may extend the mean length of stay for a woman to 3.7 days (Clinical Classifications for Health Policy Research: Hospital Inpatient Statistics, 1995). This section focuses on the postpartum care of a woman with PIH.

### Anticipated Concerns

When women develop PIH during pregnancy, the condition resolves during the first postpartum week. However, some women will experience a continuing rise in blood pressure after delivery and the hypertension may persist for 2 to 4 weeks postpartum (Atterbury and others, 1998). "It is recommended that systolic blood pressure levels greater than or equal to 150 mm Hg and diastolic levels greater than or equal to 100 mm Hg be treated" (Burrow and Duffy, 1999).

The HELLP syndrome develops 30% of the time during the postpartum period. It is characterized by *h*emolysis of red blood cells, *e*levated *l*iver enzymes, and *l*ow *p*latelets. Clinical manifestations of the syndrome usually occur within the first 48 hours postpartum (Gilbert and Harmon, 1998) (Box 19-8).

### Postpartum Monitoring of Woman with Preeclampsia

Postpartum preeclampsia or eclampsia is uncommon but may appear late in the first postpartum week or afterward. There are no standard protocols for the medical management of these late postpartum syndromes (Burrow and Duffy, 1999).

### Nursing Assessment

***Physical Assessment.*** During the postpartal period, careful assessment of each of the following areas is initiated:

- Vital signs
- Uterus

- Lochia
- Complaints of headache or blurry vision
- Reflexes
- Intake and output
- Response to magnesium sulfate, if given
- Level of consciousness
- Hemodynamics (Sisson and Sauer, 1996).

The following are signs of the HELLP syndrome:

- Epigastric pain or right upper quadrant tenderness
- Nausea or vomiting
- Headache
- Malaise
- Jaundice
- Hematuria (Gilbert and Harmon, 1998).

The first 24 hours is the most critical phase for the woman who experiences PIH, but monitoring is continued through 48 hours or the duration of the woman's hospitalization.

During the first 48 hours, neurologic assessment includes checking the reflexes, level of consciousness, and responsiveness to stimuli every 4 hours. Hyperreflexia or hyporeflexia indicates an abnormal state and is documented as 4+, 3+, 2+ (normal value), 1+, or 0. Vital signs are evaluated every 4 hours for the first 48 hours. Ask about headaches, visual disturbances, and dizziness (Lubarsky and others, 1994; Atterbury and others, 1998).

During the immediate postpartum, pulmonary edema may occur periodically as a result of the normal fluid shift from the extravascular cells to the intravascular chambers. A decrease in colloid pressure from pregnancy to the postpartum period may correlate with a rising hydrostatic pressure pushing fluid into the lungs. Coughing, shortness of breath, tachycardia, cyanosis, and pink frothy sputum signal the onset of pulmonary edema (Surratt, 1993).

Because women with PIH are at risk for developing disseminated intravascular coagulation (DIC), watch IV sites, surgical sites (cesarean incision or episiotomy), and lochia for excessive bleeding (Surratt, 1993). Monitor her uterus for continuing firmness. Laboratory results including CBC, blood type and antibody screen, clotting profile, liver and renal function, and a 24-hour urine sample, are used to document DIC (Surratt, 1993).

If the woman has been receiving medical therapy during the antepartal or intrapartal period, including the use of a continuous infusion of magnesium sulfate or another anticonvulsant to prevent eclampsia; this is usually continued for 24 to 48 hours following delivery. If the woman also has the HELLP syndrome, it may be continued longer. We need to be alert to signs of drug toxicity, including decreased or absent reflexes, a decreased level of consciousness, and oliguria (Gilbert and Harmon, 1998).

***Psychosocial Assessment.*** The mother's psychosocial needs during the postpartum are great. Assess her need to resolve the events of pregnancy and labor. Assess her concerns regarding the close monitoring she is experiencing due to an actual or potential health crisis. If her condition is critical, she may have her neuromuscular stimulation limited by being kept in a dark, quiet environment with limited visitors, including her baby.

Assess her concerns regarding her infant's well-being. The baby may have been born prematurely or have intrauterine growth retardation (IUGR) and be in an intensive care nursery (ICN). The mother also may have concerns about the effect of her medication on her baby and if she will be able to breastfeed.

### Possible Nursing Diagnoses

The situation of each woman with PIH differs depending on the onset of and severity of her condition. Some women are improving during the postpartum period, while others are in crisis. Each woman has an individual physical and emotional response to her health condition, the health of her baby, and the impact of their conditions on the family. Your assessment provides important data about her physical condition. In addition, learn from the woman how this is affecting her and her family.

### Goals of Care

The goals of care are developed in collaboration with the woman and may vary a great deal. Some examples are that by discharge the woman will do the following:

- Understand her current condition and be able to state symptoms that require immediate medical care.
- Understand the follow-up monitoring that may be required and the community resource that will provide this care.

- Have a supportive care network of family and friends to help her during the first postpartal week.
- Be reassured that, because she is no longer receiving magnesium sulfate, she may breastfeed.
- Understand the possible implications for her future pregnancies and blood pressure status.

### Self-Care

As the woman's medical condition improves, she will take on more of her self-care (Figure 19-2). When she is discharged she will then be responsible for assuming the ongoing assessment of her condition and deciding when and whom to call for care.

### Interventions

**Care of the Woman.** Stabilizing the woman's medical condition is the collaborative goal of the health care team during the first 24 hours after delivery and longer as her condition warrants. Providing her with anticipatory guidance about her condition and the condition of her infant keeps her informed and decreases her anxiety.

Each woman must be monitored as closely as before delivery because her condition can still deteriorate rapidly. Protocols as to physical assessment vary from institution to institution and as determined by the individual woman's condition (Box 19-9).

As her condition improves, we are able to decrease our critical care monitoring and shift the emphasis to establishing health promotion of the parturition period. Having been fearful that she might not survive, some women will find it difficult to now be sure that they may move from a critical care state to a normative state. They will need support from partners, family members, and the nursing staff to consider themselves healthy. They may need help in refocusing attention to what is healthy about them and their infant. Because PIH is a disorder that occurs in higher frequency in a woman having her first pregnancy, the attention now shifts to learning about and caring for the newborn (Suratt, 1993).

**Nutrition Education.** Nutritional counseling is an important aspect of care. Obese women are at a higher risk of developing PIH. Weight gain during pregnancy also contributes to the problem. Establishing guidelines for weight loss and an exercise program that is realistic provides the woman with a self-care plan she can initiate after discharge. Acknowledging cultural beliefs and customs that influence her eating habits and determining how they may be modified for her health are important. Support from her family and friends is a vital aspect of diet change and success in weight loss (Morin, 1995).

**Anticipatory Guidance.** In counseling women and their families about the long-term effects and recur-

---

**BOX 19-9   Interventions for a Woman with PIH during Postpartum**

- Monitor MgSo₄ infusion
- Take vital signs
- Check reflexes every 4 hours and record data
- Administer oxygen as needed
- Measure intake and output every 4 hours
- Monitor IV solutions
- Document headache and visual disturbances
- Check her uterus and massage if not firm
- Check perineal pads on a frequent basis
- Change underpads (Chux) and keep the woman comfortable

---

ring incidence of preeclampsia and hypertension the following should be made clear:

1. If the woman developed PIH, she has a high possibility of developing chronic hypertension later in life.
2. If this was the woman's first pregnancy and she developed preeclampsia, she has a low risk of PIH in subsequent pregnancies and no greater risk of developing chronic hypertension.
3. If this is not the woman's first pregnancy and she developed preeclampsia, she has a high risk of developing it during future pregnancies. She is also at higher risk for abruptio placentae, preterm labor, and IUGR of the fetus (Burrow and Duffy, 1999).

**Discharge Planning.** When discharged, the woman needs a written list of reportable symptoms and specific instructions as to when and whom to inform. The woman and her family members should be cautioned that women have experienced symptoms including seizures up to 3 weeks postpartum (Atterbury and others, 1998) and are advised to keep in close contact with their health care provider.

### Evaluation

Evaluation of interventions are based on the achievement of the short-term goals for the woman's postpartum recovery while hospitalized. Because the woman requires ongoing self-monitoring and care, it also involves identification that the woman and her family understand the signs and symptoms that indicate she requires immediate care.

### Summary

PIH is a serious condition that frightens the woman and her family and has serious repercussions for the health and well-being of the woman and her infant. Careful monitoring of the woman's physiologic and psychologic responses is necessary to assist her through the crises. Once the woman's condition becomes stable, the development of the mother-infant dyad is important. The woman and community caregivers continue ongoing monitoring of the woman's condition after discharge.

## Early Postpartum Hemorrhage

Maternal hemorrhage in the early postpartum period is a significant cause of mortality and morbidity for women. Approximately one third of maternal deaths are related to postpartum hemorrhage (Brown, 2000; Mattson and Smith, 2000).

Postpartum hemorrhage is defined as a blood loss of more than 500 ml during the first 24 hours after vaginal delivery. "Hemorrhage is defined objectively as a decrease in hematocrit of at least 10% or a need for blood cell transfusion. The hemoglobin value will decrease 1 to 1.5 g/dl and the hematocrit will decrease 2 to 4 percent for each 450 to 500 ml of blood loss" (Simpson and Creehan, 1996).

### Anticipated Concerns

Postpartum hemorrhage is not always predictable, and careful consideration of risk factors is critical to maintaining appropriate assessment. Immediate postpartum hemorrhage occurs within 24 hours of delivery while the woman is generally still hospitalized. The greatest risk is in the first hour after birth when the venous areas of the placental site are exposed. Under normal conditions after the placenta has separated from the uterine wall, the uterus contracts and myometrium fibers act as ligatures to prevent excessive bleeding in the arterial bed (Brown, 2000; Mattson and Smith, 2000). The two most common causes of immediate postpartum hemorrhage are uterine atony and laceration of the cervix, vagina, and/or perineum.

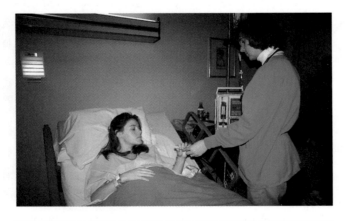

FIGURE 19-2 • A call button ensures communication as the woman assumes self-monitoring. *(Courtesy of Caroline E. Brown.)*

**Uterine Atony.** "Eighty to ninety percent of immediate postpartum hemorrhage results from uterine atony, reported as complicating 1 in 20 births" (Dildy and Clark, 1993). When uterine atony occurs the ligatures of the muscles of the uterus relax, allowing bleeding to continue. Factors that may increase a woman's risk of uterine atony are conditions that create overdistention of the uterus or excessive tension on the fibers. If the woman has retained placental fragments within the uterus, it is prevented from contracting. The uterus remains large and the bleeding is painless and bright red.

**Hematoma.** Trauma to the soft tissues due to the baby's presenting part, forceps manipulation, a prolonged second stage, an epidural regional anesthesia, or excessive pressure on the fundus of the uterus may contribute to the formation of a hematoma and the risk of hemorrhage. A hematoma is created when blood vessels are damaged and bleed into the tissue. They may occur in various locations including the vagina, the vulva, and the soft tissues of the peritoneum. Hematomas may be the result of excessive fundal pressure on the uterus, the pressure of the fetus on pelvic structures, or forceps manipulation (Ridgeway, 1995; Mattson and Smith, 2000).

**Lacerations.** During the delivery of the infant the cervix, vagina, and/or perineum may be lacerated. This is more common if the woman has received Pitocin to initiate or augment her contractions or forceps have been used in the delivery process.

Lacerations of the cervix may be extensive within the lower uterine segment. Longitudinal tears may occur in the upper vagina. The lower vagina and vulva may have superficial tears or deep lacerations that extend into the urethra, labia minora, clitoris, or bladder. Lacerations of the perineum are classified from first to fourth degree:

- First degree are superficial and extend through the skin.
- Second degree extend through the muscles of the perineum.
- Third degree extend to the anal sphincter.
- Fourth degree extend through the anal sphincter and involve the wall of the rectum.

**Abnormalities of the Placenta.** Placental abnormalities also may cause a life-threatening hemorrhage. **Placenta accreta** is an uncommon condition in which the chorionic villi adhere to the myometrium of the uterus. It becomes **placenta increta** if the chorionic villi invade the myometrium and **placenta percreta** when the chorionic villi grow through the myometrium, causing the placenta to adhere abnormally to the uterus. The abnormal growth may involve one cotyledon of the placenta (focal), several cotyledons (partial adherence), or all the cotyledons (total adherence). These problems of placental attachment are usually diagnosed soon after delivery when the placenta fails to separate spontaneously from the uterine wall. Each of the conditions can lead to profuse hemorrhage, with the mother possibly losing so much blood that she may go into shock or die. Partial or total adherence generally leads to immediate blood replacement therapy and hysterectomy (Gilbert and Harmon, 1998).

***Altered Clotting Mechanisms.*** If a woman has experienced an obstetric or medical complication, disseminated intravascular coagulation (DIC) can cause postpartum hemorrhage by altering her blood clotting mechanisms. Abruptio placentae, placenta previa, uterine infection, placenta accreta, uterine inversion, trauma during birth, and fetal demise may precipitate this condition (Clark and others, 1997) (Box 19-10).

## Medical Intervention

Standard therapy for problems with the uterus begins with manual exploration or uterine ultrasound to determine if placental fragments remain; if found, they are removed. Pharmacologic agents may be administered to stimulate uterine contractions. If medications are unsuccessful, ligation of the uterine artery and the hypogastric artery may be considered.

If the bleeding is from lacerations, these are sutured. If the hematoma is large, it may need to be opened surgically, drained, and the blood vessels litigated. Small hematomas may resolve on their own.

The occurrence of placental abnormalities generally creates an emergency situation necessitating the removal of the woman's uterus. Because of the amount of blood lost, Ringer's lactate solution, plasma expanders, or blood transfusions usually are required.

## Nursing Assessment

Check the woman's delivery record for any risk factors as well as notations related to her estimated blood loss. If she has experienced any of the risk factors, her vaginal bleeding and vital signs must be checked every 15 minutes until it is apparent that her condition is stable. Pay particular attention to the mean arterial pressure (MAP) because the first blood pressure response to hypovolemia may be a pulse pressure decrease to 30 mm Hg or less. Do not relax your vigilance when her vital signs are normal. Because vasoconstriction shunts the available blood to vital organs during the initial phase of hypovolemic shock, she may be becoming hypovolemic and it not yet be measurable (Simpson and Creehan, 1996).

Palpation of a soft or boggy uterus indicates that the woman is probably bleeding into her vagina. If she is lying down, it usually is not apparent on the perineal pad, but if she stands the blood that has pooled in the vagina may gush out. Signs and symptoms such as perspiration, tachycardia, decreasing BP (especially systolic blood pressure), reduced pulse pressure and/or a thready pulse, and other indications of shock do not appear until the hemorrhage is advanced (Akins, 1994; Brown, 2000).

A hematoma is a hemorrhage that is unseen because she is bleeding into a pocket created in the tissues. As the woman continues to bleed and the hematoma grows it becomes increasingly painful as it puts pressure on surrounding tissues. If it is located next to the urethra it may become painful for the woman to void. With a hematoma, she may exhibit signs of a firm uterus, while also experiencing hypotension or tachycardia.

Assessment of an undiagnosed laceration may occur with the observation that the woman has a firm uterus but is still experiencing a steady trickle of bright red, unclotted blood when she reclines or that a large amount of blood is discharged when she moves to an upright position.

Also be alert to the occurrence of petechiae, ecchymosis, prolonged bleeding from venipuncture sites, tachycardia, or oliguria because these may indicate the development of DIC (Box 19-11).

Assess vaginal blood loss by weighing her perineal pads or the chux. When compared to the weight of a clean pad, a weight increase of 1 g is equal to 1 ml of fluid.

---

### BOX 19-10   *Causes of Early Postpartum Hemorrhage*

Early postpartum hemorrhage most commonly occurs following:
- Uterine atony
  Multiple gestation
  A large fetus
  Polyhydramnios
  Prolonged labor
- Trauma due to fetus or forceps delivery
  Hematoma of cervix and/or vagina
  Laceration of cervix and/or vagina
- Difficult third stage
  Aggressive external fundal pressure
  Uterine inversion
  Excessive pressure on umbilical cord
  Retained placenta
  Placenta accreta
- Use of some types of drugs in labor
  Pitocin to start or augment labor
  Anticonvulsants (magnesium sulfate), β-adrenergic tocolytic agents, antihypertensives (e.g., Diazoxide), calcium channel blockers (e.g., nifedipine), and anesthetics (Halothane)
- Bleeding disorders such as DIC

From Simpson KR and Creehan PA: *Perinatal nursing.* Philadelphia, 1996, Lippincott; Clark S and others, editors: *Critical care obstetrics,* ed 3, Boston, Mass, 1996, Blackwell Science; Morey SS: ACOG releases report on risk factors, causes and management of postpartum hemorrhage, *Am Fam Phys* 58(4):1002-1004, 1998; Brown K: *Management guidelines for women's health nurse practitioners,* Philadelphia, 2000, FA Davis; Mattson S and Smith JE: *Core curriculum for maternal newborn nursing,* ed 2, Philadelphia, 2000, WB Saunders.

Measure her intake and output. "Ringer's lactate solution, other plasma expanders, or blood components are usually given in amounts necessary to counteract hypovolemia. These amounts should produce at least 30 ml/hr (60 ml preferred) of urine output and hematocrit values of >30 percent" (Simpson and Creehan, 1996).

### Possible Nursing Diagnoses

The woman may experience not only the physical changes in her body related to hemorrhage but also be fearful about what is happening to her and wonder if she will survive. Nursing diagnoses may relate to her

---

**BOX 19-11   Signs and Symptoms of Postpartal Hemorrhage**

**Signs and Symptoms of Uterine Atony**
Boggy, large uterus
Bright red bleeding
Expelled clots

**Signs and Symptoms of Lacerations**
Firm uterus
Bright red bleeding
Steady stream or trickle of blood

**Signs and Symptoms of Retained Placental Fragments**
Placenta not intact
Uterus remains large
Bright red bleeding (painless)

**Signs and Symptoms of a Hematoma**
Firm uterus
Bright red bleeding
Extreme perineal or pelvic pain
Tense, sensitive mass covered by discolored skin or mucous membrane
Difficulty voiding
Unexplained tachycardia
Hypotension
Anemia

**Signs and Symptoms of DIC**
Petechiae
Ecchymosis
Prolonged bleeding from injection or intravenous sites
Tachycardia
Oliguria
Signs of acute renal failure
Convulsions and coma

From Brown K: *Management guidelines for women's health nurse practitioners*, Philadelphia, 2000, FA Davis; Mattson S and Smith JE: *Core curriculum for maternal newborn nursing*, ed 2, Philadelphia, 2000, WB Saunders.

---

physical needs due to the loss of the blood, her fears about herself, and the separation from her infant as she receives care. If the emergency occurred during the delivery, she may not yet have seen or held her infant.

### Goals of Care

Hemorrhage is a medical emergency that is stabilized through the collaborative interventions of nurses, nurse-midwives and/or physicians. Some examples of goals are that after the woman is stable and by discharge, she will do the following:

- Report decreased anxiety
- Demonstrate a normal lochia pattern
- Demonstrate a return of vital signs to normal levels
- Demonstrate attachment behaviors with her infant
- State the signs and symptoms of hemorrhage and when to call her provider

### Nursing Interventions

***Physical Care of the Mother.*** Stabilization of the mother's medical condition is the first priority. Monitoring vital signs, providing for adequate hydration, continually observing of the uterus, maintaining intravenous access, monitoring administration of intravenous solutions and/or blood products, obtaining necessary blood samples, and measuring intake and output are collaborative measures designed to support the medical regimen.

Enhance uterine contraction with appropriate uterine massage and by preventing bladder distention, which displaces the uterus. Anticipate the need for conscious relaxation, labor breathing, or other pain management before providing uterine massage. "Place one hand pointing toward the woman's head with the thumb resting on the side of the uterus and fingers along the other side. Use the other hand to massage with only the force needed to effect contraction or expulsion of clots" (Simpson and Creehan, 1996). Once accumulated clots are expelled, the uterus will contract more efficiently. Do not provide uterine massage unless necessary because the muscle may become fatigued and relax, creating increased atony. Do not be too vigorous with the massage because ligament damage may occur or the uterus may become inverted, an emergency situation that creates great blood loss and possible death (Box 19-12).

***Emotional Support.*** Because of fear and anxiety, women require a great deal of support until they are stabilized.  Careful explanation to the mother and her family, when available, decreases anxiety levels. Women want to know what is happening to their bodies, why it is happening, and what they should expect. Uncontrolled bleeding or large clots are frightening. Changing a woman's perineal pad, bed pad, and her clothing frequently will enhance her comfort. Offer her a sponge bath and clean sheets to make her feel more comfortable.

If the woman is separated from her infant because of her medical status, she may feel negligent. If the mother is in a critical care unit, contact the nursery staff and arrange for a visit from the infant. Touching and seeing her infant will provide the woman with reassurance that the child is alive and doing well. Once the woman is stable, encourage rooming-in with assistance. Add a cot to her room or a large chair and extra pillow and blanket for a partner, family member, or friend so they may stay with the new mother.

To provide self-assessment and care, the woman must learn about the involution process and how to evaluate where the fundus of her uterus is. She can gently massage the fundus of the uterus to maintain or increase the muscle tone. If she is breastfeeding, explain to her how the contractions that come with each feeding are helpful to her.

In preparation for discharge, teach her about the changes that will occur in her lochia and when to expect the discharge to stop. Until that time, ensure that she knows how to apply the perineal pad appropriately and the signs of infection.

***Support of Breastfeeding.*** If the woman wishes to breastfeed but must delay starting until she is better, provide interventions that support her production of breast milk. Breastfeeding may be useful in her recovery because it aids in contracting the uterus and decreases postpartum bleeding (Figure 19-3).

***Discharge Planning.*** Before discharge the woman's vital signs and laboratory values should have returned to within normal limits. However, the woman will still feel fatigued and need assistance so that she may continue to recover at home. Determine from her the type of support she will be receiving when she returns home. Help her strategize to obtain the assistance she will need.

The woman must have complete written instructions on follow-up care and signs and symptoms of late postpartum hemorrhage as well as directions on when to call her health care provider. Make the appropriate referrals for community-based care so that a home visit will be provided within the next 24 hours.

### Evaluation

To evaluate the nursing interventions, determine that the short-term goals for physical and emotional care have been met. In addition, confirm that the woman understands how to continue self-assessment and care when she is at home continuing her recovery. It is vitally important that she understands which situations require that she contact her health care provider and which require that she go to an emergency room immediately.

### Summary

An early postpartum hemorrhage can be frightening for the woman and her family. The blood loss may leave her fatigued and unable to provide adequate care for herself, much less her infant. With appropriate guidance, the woman's support system should be able to offer her care, and community services can monitor her recovery.

---

### BOX 19-12   *Monitoring for Hemorrhage*

To provide adequate monitoring of the woman's condition, medical orders may include the following:

- Monitor vital signs every 15 minutes (normal vital signs do not mean a woman is not in shock)
- Assess blood loss by weighing perineal pads or Chux (1 g of added weight = 1 ml of fluid)
- Maintain accurate measurement of intake and output
- Draw blood for CBC, platelets, PT, PTT, and arterial gases
- Monitor intravenous infusion of:
  5% dextrose in Ringer's lactate solution, or
  Fresh whole blood or packed red blood cells, or
  Platelets and FFP (fibrin, fibrinogen split products)
- Use invasive hemodynamic monitoring if woman fails to respond to therapy
- Administer oxygen as indicated
- Administer prescribed drugs to contract uterus: oxytocin IV infusion; methylergonovine IM; prostaglandin IM, intramyometrial or as vaginal suppository
- Insert an indwelling urinary catheter to empty bladder and keep an accurate measurement of output

From Akins S: Postpartum hemorrhage: a 90's approach to an age-old problem, *J Nurse Midwifery* 39(suppl 2):123s-133s, 1994; Hyashi R and Castillo MS: Bleeding in pregnancy. In Knuffel R and Drukker J, editors: *High risk pregnancy: a team approach,* ed 2, Philadelphia, 1993, WB Saunders; Simpson KR and Creehan PA: *Perinatal nursing.* Philadelphia,1996, Lippincott.

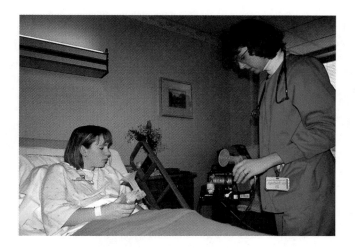

FIGURE 19-3 • Breast pump teaching for a mother who must delay starting. *(Courtesy of Caroline E. Brown.)*

## Complications of Abdominal Delivery

A surgical delivery through the abdominal and uterine walls is a major surgical event that adds stressors beyond the normal vaginal birth. The postpartum woman is simultaneously recovering from the surgical procedure and the anesthesia for the surgery, while dealing with the pain of the incision, a customary blood loss of 1000 to 1200 ml (this is twice as much as a normal uncomplicated vaginal delivery), and the care of a newborn.

### Anticipated Concerns

Significant postoperative complications may occur in six bodily systems: cardiovascular, pulmonary, gastrointestinal, genitourinary, skin, and reproductive. Some may occur more immediately than others (Table 19-2).

### Nursing Assessment

A mother who delivers by abdominal surgery receives both postsurgical assessments and postpartum assessments. These are easily integrated so that she does not become overly fatigued.

**Physical Assessment.** After an abdominal delivery, it is important to monitor vital signs and check her perineal pads and all dressings for bleeding. The close monitoring should continue until the woman is bleeding minimally, passing at least 30 ml of urine per hour, and maintaining a satisfactory blood pressure (Compendium of Postpartum Care, 1996).

When the woman appears to be stable, a typical assessment protocol may be to monitor for signs of hemorrhage by taking vital signs every 15 minutes for 8 times, every 30 minutes for 2 times, every 4 hours for 2 times and then routinely.

The firmness of the uterus and the nature and amount of vaginal flow are checked during each vital signs check. The flow of lochia should be moderate and without large or excessive clots. A pad count is kept in order to have a measure of the flow. Bleeding is considered excessive after a surgical delivery if more than two perineal pads are saturated within 60 minutes. Check the lochia every shift for unusual odor, an early sign of infection (Compendium of Postpartum Care, 1996; Phillips, 1996; Gilbert and Harmon, 1998).

Assess her temperature every 4 hours during the first 48 hours. If it is more than 38° C (100.4° F), monitor it every 2 hours. A rise in temperature may be an indication of infection (Gilbert and Harmon, 1998).

Monitor intravenous flow. Maintain an accurate intake (intravenous and oral) and output record. Note if she is experiencing any vomiting and record how much.

Assess the amount, color, and clarity of her urine. A Foley catheter may be kept in place for up to 48 hours until the bladder resumes its normal functioning. Once her Foley catheter is removed, measure the amount of the next two voids. If the woman is successfully ambulating on her own, she may be taught how to do this. Ask her if she is experiencing burning on urination and if blood is present in the urine.

Every 4 hours assess for the presence of bowel sounds in all four quadrants of her abdomen. Their presence will determine when the intravenous is removed, when she will be able to resume eating, and what she will be allowed to eat.

Monitor the condition of the surgical dressings and evaluate the incision using the REEDA scale. This scale provides a means to assess the healing process by evaluating for *r*edness, *e*dema, *e*cchymosis, *d*rainage, and *a*pproximation. Each attribute is rated on a scale of 0 to 3. The points in the 5 areas are then added. The lower the score, the better the healing process. Scores should range from 0 to 6 on the first day after surgery, 0 to 8 on the second day, 0 to 7 after 7 days, and 0 to 1 after 14 days (Davidson, 1974) (Table 19-3).

Women react to pain differently, so a thorough pain assessment is necessary. Ask the woman what sensations she is experiencing, where she is feeling the sensations, and if she would like relief from these sensations. In addition to the pain from the surgery, some women experience an itching sensation due to anesthesia.

Assess the woman's ability to move and reposition herself more comfortably. Assess her ability to begin to perform light abdominal contractions within the first 24 hours. Assess the woman's readiness for ambulation when ordered.

**Psychosocial Assessment.** Assess the woman's response to having undergone surgery. If it was unplanned, determine if she understands the reasons for the surgery and how the surgery was performed. Encourage her to verbalize her feelings about the surgery. Assess for feelings of guilt or failure in not having had a vaginal delivery.

---

**TABLE 19-2** *Significant Postoperative Complications following Abdominal Delivery*

| System | Significant complication |
|---|---|
| Cardiovascular | Hemorrhage, hypovolemic shock, deep vein thrombosis |
| Pulmonary | Pulmonary embolus, pneumonia |
| Gastrointestinal | Paralytic ilius |
| Genitourinary | Renal failure, hematuria, urinary tract infection, oliguria |
| Integumentary | Wound infection, wound dehiscence |
| Reproductive | Endometritis, septic pelvic emboli |

Adapted from Phillips CR: *Family-centered maternity-newborn care: a basic text,* ed 3, St Louis, 1991, Mosby.

## Possible Nursing Diagnoses

Nursing diagnoses for the care of a postpartum woman after a surgical delivery reflect all the regular concerns of the postpartum period plus issues created by the surgical experience. The woman may express grief over the method of delivery and exhibit a disturbance in her self-esteem because of the change in birth plan. She may be concerned because her own physical condition interferes with her ability to care for her child and she wonders how she will care for herself and her child when discharged.

## Goals of Care

Goals of care are that no surgical complications will develop, or if they do develop the signs and symptoms will be minimized and managed appropriately. Other goals include that the woman will:

* Have a temperature below 38° C.
* Urinate without pain.
* Have the incision approximate and heal without pain or swelling.
* Maintain stable vital signs.
* Experience active bowel sounds.
* Report passing flatus.
* Ambulate within 24 hours of surgery.
* Assume care of the infant within her postsurgical limits.
* Verbalize a positive birth experience despite the alternative birth process (Gilbert and Harmon, 1998).

## Self Care

Encourage the woman to assess her uterus and massage it to keep it firm. Until she is allowed to get up and walk, encourage her to do abdominal tightening exercises to decrease her risk of experiencing gas pains.

Teach the mother to turn, cough, and do deep breathing exercises every 2 hours to decrease her risk of respiratory infection. Once she can ambulate on a regular basis, this becomes less important.

Wound infections do not usually become apparent until 3 to 8 days after the surgery. Teach the woman about the signs of infection so that she can monitor the healing process and notify providers if infection occurs.

## Interventions

***Care of the Woman.*** Women often experience tremors soon after giving birth. Placing warmed blankets on her will help relieve this discomfort.

Pain management should be ongoing. Use nonpharmacologic methods as appropriate. Assist her in finding and changing positions frequently and support her knees with a pillow or rolled blankets. Teach her to splint her abdomen by pressing a pillow against it to cushion the operative area and incision. The pressure of the pillow also makes moving about and coughing less uncomfortable. Offer analgesia as ordered (Phillips, 1996; Mattson and Smith, 2000).

If her uterus becomes relaxed, manually massage it very gently until it is firm. Maintain the flow of the oxytocics and intravenous fluids as ordered. It is important not to infuse the fluids more rapidly than ordered because it may create a fluid overload.

Once bowel sounds are heard, she will be allowed a full liquid diet. Once she passes flatus, she will be allowed either a soft or a regular diet (Gilbert and Harmon, 1998).

Early ambulation is important, so new mothers are helped to ambulate within 24 hours of surgery. Walking helps prevent thrombophlebitis and facilitates normal bowel and bladder function. It also helps minimize the development of intestinal gas (flatus) and reduce the amount of pain the woman may experience from it. If the pain from the flatus becomes too great, a rectal suppository, a rectal tube, or an enema may be prescribed to provide relief to the woman.

Women who undergo a surgical delivery may be given antibiotics prophylactically just after the cord is

### TABLE 19-3   REEDA Scale

| Points | Redness | Edema | Ecchymosis | Discharge | Approximation |
|---|---|---|---|---|---|
| 0 | None | None | None | None | Closed |
| 1 | Within 0.25 cm of incision bilaterally | <1 cm from incision | Within 0.25 cm bilaterally or 0.5 cm unilaterally | Serum | Skin separation 3 mm or less |
| 2 | Within 0.5 cm of incision bilaterally | 1-2 cm from incision | 0.25-1 cm bilaterally or 0.5-2 cm unilaterally | Serosanguinous | Skin and subcutaneous fat separation |
| 3 | Beyond 0.5 cm of incision bilaterally | >2 cm from incision | >1 cm bilaterally or 2 cm unilaterally | Bloody, purulent | Skin, subcutaneous fat, and fascial separation |

**SCORE**

**TOTAL**

Adapted from Davidson N: REEDA: evaluating postpartum healing, *J Nurse-Midwifery* 19(2):6-8, 1974.

clamped. Endomyometritis occurs in 35% to 40% of women, but with prophylactic antibiotics the number is reduced to 5% (Gilbert and Harmon, 1998).

Notify the woman's physician if her uterus fails to contract or stay contracted, her temperature rises to more than 38° C, her lochia develops an unusual odor, the incision shows signs of an infection, or the woman complains of burning on urination.

*Anticipatory Guidance.* Women who have had a surgical delivery often produce less lochia than women who have given birth vaginally. The lochia will pass through the same stages of rubra, serosa, and finally alba, but it will occur more rapidly.

Reiterate the reasons for the surgical birth and explain that it does not mean that the next pregnancy also will be a surgical delivery. Each pregnancy is a different event because the "passenger" (infant), position (of the baby), passageway (vagina), and power (strength of contractions) are variables.

*Maternal-Infant Interaction.* Keep in mind that this woman recovering from surgery is most importantly a new mother. She has the same needs and desires as a mother who has delivered vaginally. Help her be with and interact with her child and be successful in assuming the parts of the mothering role she can accomplish while recovering from surgery.

If the mother is breastfeeding, coordinate the offer of pain medication with breastfeeding, so that the mother will be more comfortable when the uterus contracts. Also encourage her to use relaxation exercises and breathing techniques in pain management during the contractions of involution. She may be most comfortable breastfeeding the baby in a side-lying position at first. When in the sitting position, using a football hold or placing a pillow on her lap to support the baby will increase her comfort.

*Nutrition.* Good nutrition is a requirement for wound healing. Review with the woman how to achieve a balanced diet without requiring a lot of food preparation. Encourage her to drink 3000 ml of water and other liquids every 24 hours.

*Discharge Planning.* Women who experience surgical deliveries are discharged home within 3 to 4 days. The woman will need assistance and support for her own care as well as the care of the baby. Arrangements for assistance by family and friends must be made before she leaves the hospital. Give her partner information on arranging for additional help at home, how to incorporate frequent rest periods, adequate levels of nutrition and fluids, and an explanation of how to differentiate between the postpartum blues and postpartum depression (Simpson and Creehan, 1996).

With discharge the woman becomes responsible for assessing her recovery from the pregnancy and the surgery. Specific written instructions should be reviewed and given to her regarding the signs and symptoms of hemorrhage, infection, or wound separation.

### Evaluation

Evaluation of nursing care is based on the attainment of the established goals. The woman will be hydrated, her vital signs will remain within normal limits, and excessive blood loss will not occur. She will not experience an infection, and her temperature and white blood cell count will be within normal limits. The woman will provide care for her child, verbalize self-confidence, and express a positive attitude toward her body.

 **SUMMARY**

Mothers and families who have experienced surgical delivery have special needs. Mothers and families who undergo planned, scheduled surgical deliveries are able to use coping mechanisms to prepare for the experience. Women who have an unplanned experience cannot prepare and may have a more difficult time afterwards (Phillips, 1996). Women may be happy and excited about having a healthy baby but disappointed about having a surgical birth (Simpson and Creehan, 1996).

Providing postpartal care and postsurgical care simultaneously is a challenge. Help the woman achieve a level of comfort and ability for self-assessment and care before discharge. Simultaneously support her in caring for and developing a bond with her child. All too soon she will be on her own providing the care for them both.

## Care Plan · Nursing Care Plan for the Woman with Early Postpartum Hemorrhage

NURSING DIAGNOSIS   **Fluid volume deficit** related to excessive blood loss secondary to uterine atony or laceration
GOALS/OUTCOMES   Fluid volume deficit (blood loss) will be eliminated

**NOC Suggested Outcomes**
- Fluid Balance (0601)
- Hydration (0602)

**NIC Priority Interventions**
- Bleeding Reduction: Postpartum Uterus (4026)
- Fluid Management (4120)

## Care Plan · Nursing Care Plan for the Woman with Early Postpartum Hemorrhage—cont'd

- Coagulation Status (0409)
- Fear Control (1404)

- Shock Management (4250)
- Hypovolemia Management (4180)
- Blood Products Administration (4030)
- Anxiety Reduction (5820)
- Electrolyte Management (2000)

### Nursing Activities and Rationale

- Monitor and record type, amount, and location of bleeding *to provide an estimate of blood loss and to determine treatment need and a baseline for treatment effectiveness.*
- Gently massage boggy uterus while maintaining mild pressure with second hand above symphysis pubis until clots are expelled *to decrease or control blood loss while preventing uterine inversion. The uterus contracts more efficiently when clots have been expelled.*
- Apply ice pack to hematoma or laceration. *Ice decreases blood flow and aids with clotting.*
- Encourage voiding or catheterize distended urinary bladder (NIC) *to prevent displacement of the uterus.*
- Monitor for trends in vital signs, capillary refill, mucous membranes and nailbeds *to detect impending shock related to continued blood loss and hypovolemia.*
- Maintain accurate intake and output *to estimate the extent of fluid loss and detect complications such as acute renal failure.*
- Maintain patent intravenous access *to provide an accessible route for administration of fluids and emergency medications.*
- Administer fluid and electrolyte resuscitation as prescribed *to support circulation and prevent the development of hypovolemic shock and electrolyte imbalances.*
- Administer medications as prescribed and monitor for potential side effects (oxytocin, methylergonovine maleate) *to increase contractility of uterus and halt hemorrhage when uterine atony is present.*
- Promote bed rest, limit activity, and elevate legs 20 to 30 degrees *to decrease metabolic demands, increase venous return, protect blood flow to vital organs, and maintain client safety.*
- Monitor coagulation studies, CBC, and differential *to determine amount of blood loss, replacement needs, and effect of collaborative interventions.*
- Monitor for indications of fluid volume excess *to prevent fluid volume overload related to fluid revascularization as the client improves and fluid resuscitation efforts.*
- Use a calm, reassuring approach *to prevent transference of anxiety to client during a stressful situation.*
- Explain all care and procedures. *Keeping the client informed reduces anxiety and fear of the unknown.*

### Evaluation Parameters

- No evidence of active bleeding.
- Uterus remains contracted.
- Pulse, blood pressure, color, capillary refill, and mucous membranes within normal limits.
- CBC, differential, coagulation studies, and serum electrolytes within normal limits.
- Verbalizes reduced fear.

NURSING DIAGNOSIS   **Altered tissue perfusion** related to hypovolemia and hypotension

GOALS/OUTCOMES   Demonstrates effective cardiac, cerebral, renal, and peripheral tissue perfusion

### NOC Suggested Outcomes

- Electrolyte and Acid-Base Balance (0600)
- Hydration (0602)
- Urinary Elimination (0503)
- Tissue Perfusion: Cardiac (0405)
- Tissue Perfusion: Cerebral (0406)
- Fluid Balance (0601)
- Vital Sign Status (0802)
- Energy Conservation (0002)
- Anxiety Control (1402)

### NIC Priority Interventions

- Oxygen Therapy (3320)
- Emergency Care (6200)
- Shock Management, Volume (4258)
- Fluid Resuscitation (4140)
- Hypovolemia Management (4180)
- Fluid/Electrolyte Management (2080)
- Acid/Base Management: Metabolic Acidosis (1912)
- Medication Administration: Intravenous (2314)
- Energy Management (0180)
- Emotional Support (5270)

*Continued*

## Care Plan • Nursing Care Plan for the Woman with Early Postpartum Hemorrhage—cont'd

### Nursing Activities and Rationale
- Administer oxygen as prescribed to *maximize available oxygen and prevent or reverse tissue hypoxia related to blood loss or poor perfusion.*
- Monitor hydration status (e.g., of mucous membranes, skin turgor, urinary output) *to determine the effect and extent of blood loss and effectiveness of fluid resuscitation.*
- Monitor Hgb and Hct levels *to determine the extent of blood loss and effectiveness of treatment.*
- Obtain and maintain intravenous access *to provide route for administration of emergency medications, fluid replacement, and blood products.*
- Administer fluids and/or blood products as prescribed *to support circulation and tissue perfusion.*
- Monitor for signs of fluid overload *to prevent fluid volume overload related to fluid resuscitation efforts and fluid revascularization as the client improves.*
- Monitor serum electrolytes *to detect alterations, determine the need for electrolyte replacement, and monitor effectiveness of treatment.*
- Monitor acid-base status *to detect alterations, determine the need for intervention, and monitor effectiveness of treatment.*
- Monitor urinary output *to determine the degree of tissue hypoxia and effectiveness of fluid resuscitation.*
- Implement cardiopulmonary resuscitation *to support airway, breathing, and circulation until treatment measures are implemented.*

### Evaluation Parameters
- Systolic and diastolic blood pressure, heart rate, and pulse pressure within normal limits.
- Urinary output within normal limits.
- Serum electrolytes and acid-base parameters within normal limits.
- Peripheral pulses strong.
- No evidence of peripheral edema.
- No evidence of orthostatic hypotension.
- Mentally alert.

NURSING DIAGNOSIS **Fear** related to threat to one's own well-being and/or powerlessness

GOALS/OUTCOMES Reports anxiety at a manageable level and reduced fear; no behavioral manifestations of anxiety *(See "Evaluation Parameters")*

### NOC Suggested Outcomes
- Anxiety Control (1402)
- Coping (1302)
- Fear Control (1404)
- Hope (1201)
- Social Support (1504)

### NIC Priority Interventions
- Anxiety Reduction (5820)
- Coping Enhancement (5230)
- Emotional Support (5270)
- Presence (5340)

### Nursing Activities and Rationale
- Assess woman's reaction to postpartal hemorrhage and correct misconceptions *to establish a baseline for care planning. Correcting misconceptions and supplying factual information may reduce fear and anxiety.*
- Use a calm, reassuring approach (NIC) *to prevent transference of anxiety to client during stressful situation to help client maintain control during stressful event.*
- Encourage verbalization of feelings, fears, and anxiety *to help client identify fears and concerns. Allows nurse to correct misunderstandings.*
- Support the use of appropriate defense mechanisms that have been successful in the past *to build on present strengths.*
- Stay with the woman without requiring verbal interactions *to promote feelings of security while fostering physical and emotional rest.*

### Evaluation Parameters
- Reports decreased anxiety appropriate to situational crisis (hemorrhage).
- Uses breathing and relaxation techniques.
- No change in vital signs (blood pressure and pulse).

## Care Plan · Nursing Care Plan for the Woman with Early Postpartum Hemorrhage—cont'd

- Able to focus and follow directions.
- Able to communicate needs.

**NURSING DIAGNOSIS**   **Pain** related to uterine contractions, distention from blood between uterine wall and placenta, trauma, or surgery

**GOALS/OUTCOMES**   Maintains optimal level of comfort *(See "Evaluation Parameters")*

**NOC Suggested Outcomes**
- Comfort Level (2100)
- Pain Control (1605)
- Pain: Disruptive Effects (2101)
- Pain Level (2102)

**NIC Priority Interventions**
- Analgesic Administration (2210)
- Pain Management (1400)

**Nursing Activities and Rationale**
- Ask the woman what pain relief measure she prefers; provide information as needed. *This allows her to have control over her pain and use measures she feels will benefit her.*
- Monitor effectiveness of pain relief measures *(See "Evaluation Parameters"). Different pain relief measures may be needed if pain is not well controlled.*
- Provide basic comfort measures, such as maintaining dry linens and using a cool cloth to the forehead or lip balm. *If basic needs are being met, client can focus on relaxation techniques.*
- Monitor for side effects of pharmacologic agents (e.g. respirations, level of consciousness, blood pressure). *Close monitoring is needed for the client who is at risk for shock related to hemorrhage in order to achieve a balance between pain relief and dosages that create unwanted or dangerous side effects.*

**Evaluation Parameters**
- No change in pulse, blood pressure, or respirations.
- Reports acceptable comfort level.
- Demonstrates minimal restlessness and muscle tension.

**NURSING DIAGNOSIS**   **Risk for infection** related to traumatized tissues, blood loss, and invasive procedures

**GOALS/OUTCOMES**   Woman will remain free of infection

**NOC Suggested Outcomes**
- Risk Control (1902)
- Risk Detection (1908)

**NIC Priority Interventions**
- Infection Protection (6550)
- Infection Control (6540)
- Surveillance (6650)
- Wound Care (3660)

**Nursing Activities and Rationale**
- Use proper handwashing techniques *to prevent the spread of infections from one client to another or from health care worker to client.*
- Maintain medical and surgical asepsis *to decrease the potential for infection in a client who is at increased risk because of decreased hemoglobin and hematocrit.*
- Promote fluid and nutritional intake. *Adequate nutrition and fluid intake are essential to maintain normal immune function.*
- Administer antibiotics as prescribed. *Organism-specific antibiotics reduce pathogenic cell counts when constant blood levels of antibiotics are maintained.*
- Monitor for indications of infection (e.g., fever, tachycardia, tachypnea, lochia, wound drainage, pain or tenderness at site of suspected infection) *to determine presence of localized or systemic infection.*
- Obtain cultures of purulent drainage *to determine causative organism and select appropriate antibiotic therapy.*
- Monitor white blood cell count *to support the presence of infection.*
- Obtain cultures of purulent drainage *to determine causative organism and appropriate antibiotic therapy.*
- Teach woman wound care procedures *to decrease the potential for self-contamination of wound with pathogenic organisms.*

*Continued*

## Care Plan  ·  Nursing Care Plan for the Woman with Early Postpartum Hemorrhage—cont'd

**Evaluation Parameters**
- Temperature, pulse, and respirations within normal limits.
- No inflammation or drainage from wound sites.
- Lochia free of odor.
- WBC count within normal limits.

**NURSING DIAGNOSIS**  **Anticipatory grieving** related to possible effect of hemorrhage on future childbearing abilities

**GOALS/OUTCOMES**  Demonstrates ability to make decisions regarding anticipated loss; expresses feelings of self-worth, productivity, and usefulness

**NOC Suggested Outcomes**
- Coping (1302)
- Grief Resolution (1304)

**NIC Priority Interventions**
- Active Listening (4920)
- Emotional Support (5270)
- Grief Work Facilitation (5300)
- Hope Instillation (5310)
- Support System Enhancement (5440)

**Nursing Activities and Rationale**
- Establish trusting relationship. *Women must trust in order to share personal concerns and feelings. Our demeanor and actions can facilitate or establish barriers to communication.*
- Provide positive affirmation of worth. *Focus on strengths because the woman may feel that she is useless or of little worth if she loses her ability to bear children.*
- Encourage woman to focus on what is known rather than what may occur *to provide hope for a positive outcome. Focusing on what may happen rather than what is known increases anxiety.*
- Encourage woman to identify her own strengths. *Focusing on those areas in which the woman feels in control will increase her sense of power over the current situation.*
- Assess the woman's knowledge of community resources. *Knowledge of available resources and how to obtain those resources increases the woman's feeling of power and/or control over her situation.*
- Assess the amount of emotional support provided by the woman's partner. *An adequate support system facilitates developmental tasks and adaptation; if partner support is not adequate, the nurse can make other recommendations for support.*
- Involve partner and other family members (as client desires) in care planning to *strengthen family ties and provide emotional support for client.*
- Explain to partner and family members how they can help. *Many times the partner and family members want to be helpful but need concrete suggestions for ways in which to do so.*

**Evaluation Parameters**
- Relates fears and concerns about possible loss of childbearing ability.
- Woman and partner express feelings freely with one another.
- Expresses optimism about outcome of current situation.
- Verbalizes self-acceptance and self-worth.
- Maintains eye contact.
- Communicates openly.
- Woman verbalizes realistic appraisal of her situation.
- Couple is involved in making decisions about treatment options.

**Other Possible Nursing Diagnoses**
- **Risk for altered family processes** related to change in family roles, inability to assume usual role, or prolonged recovery secondary to hemorrhage or surgery.
- **Breastfeeding, interrupted** related to maternal illness (hemorrhage).
- **Family processes, altered** related to woman's inability to assume family role secondary to prolonged recovery or surgery.

# CASE STUDY

Sarah, a 32-year-old woman, arrived at the emergency department 4 hours ago, fully dilated and pushing. She delivered a 5-lb infant girl within 15 minutes of admission with Apgar scores of 7 and 9. Sarah has no prenatal record. She reports that she has been pregnant three times and has two other children.

She is now being admitted to the postpartum unit. During your intake interview and assessment you learn the following data:

SUBJECTIVE DATA: "I've lived in 3 shelters with my 2 kids for the past 7 months. They are not safe for my kids, so I leave. My husband beat me, but I can't take no more of these shelters. I'm just thinking about going home. I'm tired. I've been dragging these kids everywhere and I can't do it."

SOCIAL DATA: 2 male children, ages 3 and 5. Newborn female, age 4 hours

No insurance

No public assistance

No family except for husband, from whom she is hiding

OBJECTIVE DATA: G 3, P 3

T, P, R within normal limits; BP 185/ 95

Spontaneous vaginal delivery with no episiotomy

Perineum clean

Lochia: rubra

Breasts: soft

Fundus: firm at umbilicus

Lochia: heavy flow

Urine: bright yellow.

LABORATORY DATA:

Urine: no trace of illicit drugs

Hct: 34%

Hgb: 10 g/dl

CBC: Within normal limits (WNL)

PHYSICAL EXAMINATION: Pale and very thin

Wgt: 110

Hgt: 5' 7"

Body odor

REVIEW OF SYSTEMS: WNL with exception of old healed injuries on arms

Based on the available data, develop a list of Sarah's strengths and health risks.

- What nursing diagnoses could apply? How will you validate these?
- Develop a plan of care with Sarah: What short-term goals might the two of you develop? How will these be prioritized?
- What long-term goals might the two of you develop? How will these be prioritized?
- What interventions may be possible? Provide a rationale for the interventions.
- How will you evaluate the effectiveness of your care when Sarah is discharged from the hospital?

# Scenarios

1. You are caring for Helene in the labor/delivery/recovery (LDR) room 2 hours after she gave birth to a 9-lb baby girl. This is her fifth child. You find that her vaginal flow is very light. Her uterus feels soft and you measure it at 2 cm above her umbilicus.

- What will be your initial response? Why? What do think might be happening?
- What other subjective and/or objective data do you need immediately?
- What nursing diagnoses could apply? How will you validate these?
- What goals are appropriate? How will these be prioritized?

- What nursing interventions will you do? Why?
- What are the expected outcomes?
- How will you evaluate the effectiveness of your interventions?

2. You are assigned to do postpartum follow-up interviews with all women who experience a surgical birth. You are visiting Tamara, a 31-year-old, G 1, P 1, with cardiac disease. Tamara had a cesarean delivery 8 hours ago because of cardiac decompensation. The baby is in the special care nursery.

You explain that you would like to ask her questions that everyone is asked after a surgical delivery.

Is that okay with her? She says "fine," so you begin reading the questions on the form. "Is this your first section? Has anyone else in your family been sectioned? Why weren't you able to have a normal vaginal birth? Did your husband stay with you for your section?"

You look up from your clipboard and see that Tamara is quietly crying.

- What will be your initial response? Why? What do think might be happening?
- What other information will help you determine why she might be crying?
- What nursing diagnoses could apply? How will you validate these?
- What short-term goals are appropriate?
- What nursing interventions will you do? Why?
- What are the expected outcomes?
- What long-term goal is appropriate? Why?
- How will you evaluate the effectiveness of your interventions, both short-term and long-term?

---

3. Henrietta, age 20 years, has given birth to a 10-lb, 12-oz baby. Henrietta is 5' 7" tall; during her pregnancy she gained 60 pounds. She was overweight by 30 pounds when she became pregnant. During the pregnancy she developed gestational diabetes and required insulin to control her glucose levels.

While you assess her knowledge of nutrition and dietary patterns, Henrietta tells you that she is glad that the gestational diabetes is going away, but she is worried about developing diabetes later in life. She explains that she has been on diets all her life and they never seem to work.

Henrietta's mother is sitting in her room listening to the conversation. She interrupts Henrietta and explains that they are from Brazil and that in their culture a full-bodied woman is more desirable. She does not understand why her daughter will need to lose any more weight than the weight she gained in pregnancy.

- What will be your initial response? Why? What do think might be happening?
- What other information will help you understand the Brazilian culture?
- What nursing diagnoses could apply? How will you validate these?
- What goals are appropriate? Why?
- What interventions will you provide Henrietta?
- What interventions will you supply her mother?

- How will you evaluate the effectiveness of your interventions?

---

4. Rebecca is a 38-year-old woman who has delivered a 7-lb girl. She was diagnosed with PIH during the last trimester of her pregnancy. During labor she experienced a grand mal seizure. A magnesium sulfate drip is continuing.

At 1 PM Rebecca's BP was 180/90. When you took it again at 1:15 PM it was 140/80. Over the last hour her urine output has been 30 cc and the urine is 2+ for protein. Her reflexes are 1+. When you talk to Rebecca she responds in a soft whisper that she is very sleepy.

- What will be your initial response? Why?
- What is your nursing assessment of her condition?
- What subjective and objective data is that based on?
- What is your first nursing diagnosis?
- What goal is a priority? Why?
- What interventions will you provide? When?
- How will you evaluate the effectiveness of your interventions?

---

5. Leah is 18 years old, G 2, P 1. She has a history of substance abuse. She delivered a 4-lb premature infant 6 hours ago who is being evaluated in the special care nursery. You are conducting Leah's assessment on the postpartum unit. Based on this information:

- What do you expect Leah to be at high risk for?
- What subjective data do you need?
- What objective data do you need?
- What nursing diagnoses could apply? How will you validate these?
- What goals may be desired by Leah? How will these be prioritized?
- What nursing interventions can you provide?
- What are the expected outcomes?
- How will you evaluate the effectiveness of your interventions?

---

6. Mary Ann is a 39-year-old woman who entered her pregnancy with extensive varicose veins. Now 2 days postpartum and about to be discharged, you notice red streaks on her right leg running along these veins. In addition, she experiences pain with the dorsiflexion of her foot. Mary Ann tells you that she

is fine. Her leg looks like that periodically and the pain when she moves her leg is from the activities of labor and delivery.

- What will be your initial response? Why? What do think might be happening?
- What other subjective and objective data should you obtain?
- What nursing diagnoses could apply? How will you validate these?
- What will you report to her nurse-midwife or physician?
- What will be the goals of care?
- What nursing interventions will you provide? Why?
- What will you not do? Why?
- How will you evaluate the effectiveness of your interventions?

---

7. Philomena is a 25-year-old, G 3, P 2, sab 2, who has just given birth to dizygotic twins weighing 8 lbs, 7 oz and 6 lbs, 12 oz, respectively, after an 8-hour labor. You are providing her care on the postpartum floor 4 hours after delivery. Your initial assessment determines that her vital signs are stable. Her lochia flow is bright red and moderate to heavy, and when she sits up, she expels a clot about 2 cm in diameter.

Philomena tells you that she put the infants to breast soon after delivery and would like to do it again if either one of them is awake.

- What will be your initial response? Why?
- What other subjective and objective data should you obtain?
- Based on the information given, what risks does Philomena face during the postpartum? Why?
- What nursing diagnoses could apply? How will you validate these?

- What will you report to her nurse-midwife or physician?
- What will be the goals of care?
- What nursing interventions will you provide? Why?
- What will you not do? Why?
- How will you evaluate the effectiveness of your interventions?

---

8. Marissa is a 25-year-old woman, G 1, P 1. She was in active labor when fetal distress led to an emergency abdominal delivery 48 hours ago. She delivered a 7-lb, 12-oz boy in relatively good health. The fetal distress appeared to have been caused by cord compression.

Her vital signs have been stable, her lochia flow is red and consistently slight, and there are no large clots. The dressing over the abdominal incision is clean and dry. A Foley catheter was inserted before the surgery and remained in place until removed during the last shift. You are assuming the care of Marissa this morning and have just completed your assessment of her vital signs. Her pulse and respirations are within normal limits; however, she has an oral temperature of 100.4° F. You check it again in 2 hours and it is 100.8° F.

- What will be your initial response? Why?
- What do think might be happening?
- What other subjective and objective data should you obtain?
- What nursing diagnoses could apply? How will you validate these?
- What will you report to her nurse-midwife or physician?
- What will be the goals of care?
- What nursing interventions will you provide? Why?
- How will you evaluate the effectiveness of your interventions?

## REFERENCES

Akins S: Postpartum hemorrhage: a 90's approach to an age-old problem, *J Nurse Midwifery* 39(suppl 2):123s-133s, 1994.

Allen AB and Buppert C: Legal issues in the care of addicted clients. In Allen KM, editor: *Nursing care of the addicted client,* New York, 1996, Lippincott.

Allen KM and Feeney E: Alcohol and other drug use, abuse, and dependence. In Allen KM and Phillips JM, editors: *Women's health across the lifespan.* Philadelphia, 1997, Lippincott.

Anderson KN: *Mosby's medical, nursing and allied health dictionary,* ed 4, St Louis, 1994, Mosby.

Atterbury JL and others: Clinical presentation of women readmitted with postpartum severe preeclampsia or ecclampsia, *J Obstet Gynecol Neonatal Nurs* 27(2)134-141, 1998.

Avery MD and Rossi MA: Gestational diabetes, *J Nurse Midwifery* 39(2):9s-19s, 1994.

Beal AC and Redlener I: Enhancing outcomes in homeless women: the challenge of providing comprehensive health care, *Semin Perinatol* 19(4):307-313, 1995.

Belcher JR, Scholler-Jaquish A, and Drummond M:. Three stages of homelessness: a conceptual model for social workers in health care, *Health Soc Work* 16(2):87-93, 1991.

Boston Women's Health Book Collective: *Our bodies, ourselves,* New York, 1999, Touchstone.

Bragg EJ: Pregnant adolescents with addictions, *J Obstet Gynecol Neonatal Nurs* 26(5):577-584, 1997.

Brown FM and Hare JW: Medical management. In Brown FM and Hare JW, editors: *Diabetes complicating pregnancy: the Joslin Clinic method,* New York, 1995, Wiley & Sons.

Brown K: *Management guidelines for women's health nurse practitioners,* Philadelphia, 2000, FA Davis.

Burian J: Helping survivors of sexual abuse through labor, *MCN Am J Matern Child Nurs* 20(Sept-Oct) 252-256, 1995.

Burrow GN and Duffy TP: *Medical complications during pregnancy,* Philadelphia, 1999, WB Saunders.

Campbell JC: Addressing battering during pregnancy: reducing low-birth weight and ongoing abuse, *Semin Perinatol* 19(4) 301-306, 1995.

Christian A: Home care of the battered pregnant woman: one battered woman's pregnancy, *J Obstet Gynecol Neonatal Nurs* 24(9): 836-847, 1995.

Clark S and others, editors: *Critical care obstetrics,* ed 3, Boston, Mass, 1996, Blackwell Science.

Clinical Classification for Health Policy Research: Hospital Inpatient Statistics, 1995. HCUP-3 Research Note. Agency for Health Care Policy and Research, Rockville, Md. Available at http://www.ahcpr.gov/data/his95/clinclas.htm.

Coletti S and Donaldson P: Maternal-child nursing. In Allen K, editor: *Nursing care of the addicted client,* New York, 1996, Lippincott.

*Compendium of postpartum care,* Skillman, NJ, 1996, Johnson and Johnson Consumer Products, Inc.

Cook M: Substance-abusing homeless mothers in Rx programs: a question of knowing, *Contemp Drug Problems* 22(2):297-316, 1995.

Dacus JV and others: Gestational diabetes: postpartum glucose tolerance testing, *Am J Obstet Gynecol* 171:927-931, 1994.

Daddario J: Trauma in pregnancy. In Mandeville LK and Troiano M, editors: *AWHONN high risk and critical care: intrapartum nursing,* New York, 1999, Lippincott.

Davidson N: REEDA: evaluating postpartum healing, *J Nurse Midwifery* 19(2):6-8, 1974.

Davis SK: Comprehensive interventions for affecting the parenting effectiveness of chemically dependent women, *J Obstet Gynecol Neonatal Nurs* 26(5):604-610, 1997.

Dildy GA and Clark SL: OB emergencies, *Contemp Obstet Gynecol* 38(5):21-29, 1993.

Engstrom L and Sittler CP: Nurse midwifery management of iron-deficiency anemia during pregnancy, *J Nurse Midwifery* 39(2):20-32, 1994.

French ED and others: Improving interactions between substance-abusing mothers and their substance exposed newborns, *J Obstet Gynecol Neonatal Nurs* 27(3):262-268, 1998.

Gilbert ES and Harmon JS: *Manual of high risk pregnancy and delivery,* St Louis, 1998, Mosby.

Hayashi R and Castillo MS: Bleeding in pregnancy. In Knuffel R and Drukker J, editors: *High risk pregnancy: a team approach,* ed 2, Philadelphia, 1993, WB Saunders.

Henly SJ and others: Anemia and insufficient milk in first-time mothers, *Birth* 22(2) 87-92, 1995.

Heritage C: Working with childhood sexual abuse: survivors during pregnancy, labor and birth, *J Obstet Gynecol Neonatal Nurs* 27(6): 671-677, 1998.

Kay E: Psychosocial responses to pregnant women with diabetes. In Brown FM and Hare JW, editors: *Diabetes complicating pregnancy: the Joslin Clinic method,* New York, 1995, John Wiley & Sons.

Kaye M and Chasnoff I: Substance abuse in pregnancy. In Knuppel RA and Drukker JE, editors: *High-risk pregnancy: a team approach,* ed 2, Philadelphia, 1993, WB Saunders.

Killion C: Special health care needs of homeless pregnant women, *ANS Adv Nurs Sci* 18(2):44-56, 1995.

Kolander CA, Ballard DJ, and Chandler CK: *Contemporary women's health,* Boston, 1999, McGraw-Hill.

Kozol J: *Rachel and her children: homeless families in America,* New York, 1988, Crown Publishers

Lawrence R and Lawrence R: *Breastfeeding: a guide for the medical profession,* ed 5, St Louis, 1998, Mosby.

Lindberg C: Perinatal transmission of HIV: how to counsel women, *MCN Am J Matern Child Nurs* 20(4):207-212, 1995.

Louie KB: Cultural competence. In Allen KM, editor: *Nursing care of the addicted client,* New York, 1995, Lippincott.

Lubarsky SL and others: Late postpartum eclampsia revisited, *Obstet Gynecol* 83:502-505, 1994.

Mattson S and Smith JE: *Core curriculum for maternal newborn nursing,* ed 2, Philadelphia, 2000, WB Saunders.

Matteson P: *Advocating for self—women's decisions concerning contraception,* New York, 1995, Harworth Press.

McFarlane J, Parker B, and Soeken K: Abuse during pregnancy: association with maternal health and infant birthweight, *Nurs Res* 45(1):36-41, 1996.

McNamee MJ and Lindsey AM: Homeless health. In Fitzpatrick JJ, editor: *Encyclopedia of nursing research,* New York, 1998, Springer.

Morey SS: ACOG releases report on risk factors, causes and management of postpartum hemorrhage, *Am Fam Phys* 58(4):1002-1004, 1998.

Morin K: Obese and non-obese postpartum women: complications, body image and perceptions of the intrapartal experience, *Appl Nurs Res* 8(2):81-87, 1995.

National Coalition for the Homeless (NCH): *How many people experience homelessness?* Fact sheet #2, Washington, DC, 1998, The Coalition.

Perry Y, Yip R, and Zyrkowski C: Nutritional risk factors among low-income pregnant US women: the Centers for Disease Control and Prevention (CDC) pregnancy nutrition surveillance system, 1979 through 1993, *Semin Perinatol* 19(3):211-221, 1995.

Phillips CR: *Family-centered maternity-newborn care: a basic text,* ed 3, St Louis, 1991, Mosby.

Phillips CR: *Family-centered maternity-newborn care: a basic text,* ed 4, St Louis, 1996, Mosby.

Queenan J, editor: *Management of high-risk pregnancy,* ed 4, Malden, Mass, 1999, Blackwell Science, Inc.

Ridgeway LE: Puerpera emergency: vaginal and vulvar hemaotmas, *Obstet Gynecol Clin North Am* 22(2):275, 1995.

Ropka M and Williams A: *HIV nursing and symptom management,* Boston, 1998, Jones and Bartlett.

Seidel H and others: *Mosby's guide to physical examination,* ed 4, St Louis, 1999, Mosby.

Shannon D and Hill MK: The chemically dependent pregnant woman. In Troiano N and Mandeville L, editors: *AWHONN high-risk and critical care: intrapartum nursing,* Philadelphia, 1999, Lippincott

Shannon M: Clinical issues and therapeutic interventions in the care of pregnant woman infected with HIV, *J Perinatal Neonatal Nurs* 7(4):25-26, 1994.

Sickle Cell Disease Guideline Panel: *Sickle cell disease: comprehensive screening and management in newborns and infants. quick reference guide for clinicians,* No 6, AHCPR Pub. No. 93-0563. Rockville, Md, 1993, AHCPR, Public Health Service, Dept. of Health and Human Services.

Simpson KR and Creehan PA: *Perinatal nursing.* Philadelphia, 1996, Lippincott.

Sisson MC and Sauer PM: Pharmacologic therapy for pregnancy-induced hypertension, *J Perinatal Neonatal Nurs* 9(4):1-12, 1996.

Smith CM and Maurer FA: *Community health nursing,* ed 2, Philadelphia, 2000, WB Saunders.

Stewart B: McKinney Homeless Assistance Act (PL 100-77), 1987.

Stump J: *Our best hope: early interventions with prenatally drug-exposed infants and their families,* Washington, DC, 1992, Child Welfare League.

Surratt N: Severe pre-eclampsia: implications for critical-care obstetric nursing, *J Obstet Gynecol Neonatal Nurs* 22(6):500-506, 1993.

Vissing Y: *Out of sight, out of mind: homeless children and families in small town America,* Lexington, Ky, 1996, The University Press of Kentucky.

Waxman L and Henderliter S: *Status report on hunger and homelessness in America's cities: 1996,* Washington, DC, 1996, US Conference of Mayors.

Worthington-Roberts: Mineral needs during pregnancy. In Worthington B, Williams SR, editors: *Nutrition in pregnancy and lactation,* Boston, 1997, McGraw-Hill.

Youngkin EQ and Davis MS: *Women's health—a primary care clinical guide,* Stamford, Conn, 1998, Appleton & Lange.

# CHAPTER 20

# Care of the Woman with Postpartum Complications at Home

*Celebration and change surround the birth of a baby.*
*But the new life isn't just the baby's —*
*it's yours, too.*

— A. LoCicero and D. Issakson
(Our Bodies, Ourselves)

---

*What are the additional health care requirements for new mothers with complications?*

*What psychologic impact may complications have on the new mother?*

*In what ways can we assist mothers and their families in attaining optimal health?*

*What is our responsibility in the care of women with specific complications?*

---

Coming home with a new baby is an exciting and exhausting time for both the new mother and her family. Some experts agree that the postpartum period may be a time of crisis, even when the outcome of the birth process was normal for mother and baby. If this is true, what must the postpartum experience be for the new mother when her health is compromised by a preexisting health concern or a complication related to the pregnancy and birth? In times past, a new mother was hospitalized until she and her physician believed she was ready to go home and able to independently care for her newborn. Now discharge from the hospital to home is occurring within days for women with or without complications. This change in health care has profound implications for the woman who has experienced a complication. Once home, the woman and her family and friends must deal with the normal postpartum crises, plus the added health care concerns of the mother and, possibly, the newborn.

In situations when the woman is separated from extended family or is without a supportive network of friends, the woman may find herself on her own trying to "do it all." Professional care and support often are necessary and may be provided in the form of ambulatory care services that the mother must go to or home care nursing visits.

This chapter provides information about how to assist in providing follow-up care once the postpartum woman is in her home. Not all areas have supportive services available and, when available, the extent of the services differs from one area to the next. However, supportive home care during the postpartum recovery is part of the continuum of care required for recovery after a complicated postpartum.

## CARE OF THE WOMAN WHO EXPERIENCES COMPLICATIONS

Whether occurring immediately after childbirth or after initial discharge, a complication severe enough to necessitate hospitalization is a very frightening situation for the new mother and her family because it causes them to face the mother's mortality and fractures the family. All of the dreams of parenthood and grandparenthood are put on hold during the time that the mother's life is in danger, yet the care of the dependent newborn must still be maintained.

Arrangements must be made for care of the newborn. The times when a newborn could remain in the hospital with the mother are gone. It now becomes the family's responsibility to assume care of the newborn at home when the baby is discharged. The family will need assistance with this process because they are dealing with multiple factors. Provide those assuming primary care for the infant with the same teaching and accompanying literature that you would provide to the parents after childbirth. Refer the family to support services within the community that can help families through this time. Volunteers may be available from the family's church, neighborhood, or other community connections.

Facing one's mortality does not fade quickly. Once the physiologic condition is resolved, it is not uncommon for these women to suffer continued emotional turmoil for a time. Although excitement over being discharged to home initially may mask these feelings in the mother, family members should be prepared. The mother has probably not had a chance to become acquainted with her infant in the way she desired. Her feelings may swing between gratefulness toward and jealousy of the people who were caregivers for her newborn during her crisis. She may feel incompetent or insecure and lack confidence that she is able to provide care for her baby.

To assist in maternal adaptation, every effort should be made during the mother's hospitalization to facilitate visits with her newborn. The mother's feelings should be explored. Assurance that what she is feeling is normal and will decrease with time can be comforting. The desired outcome is for the mother and her family to have a clear understanding of the events surrounding this childbirth and subsequent complications. The ultimate goal is successful adaptation of an expanded family.

## CARE OF THE WOMAN WITH COMPLICATIONS FROM PREEXISTING HEALTH CONCERNS

### Anemia

When anemia is diagnosed during pregnancy, it may be the normal physiologic anemia anticipated during pregnancy or an indication of a more critical condition found through the hemoglobin and hematocrit screening that a woman receives during antepartal and intrapartal care.

### Anticipated Issues

By 2 or 3 days postpartum, the natural process of postpartum diuresis will have reversed the hemodilution of pregnancy, and the woman's blood plasma levels will return to her prepregnancy state (Simpson and Creehan, 1996). If the woman is still anemic at her 4- or 6-week postpartal examination, further evaluation and treatment may be necessary to rule out other causes.

### Nursing Assessment

Differentiating between fatigue due to childbirth and care of an infant and fatigue due to anemia is difficult at best. Determine from the woman the amount and type of her lochia flow. Also learn about her rest and activity patterns, diet, fluid intake, and ability to obtain and use nutritional supplements.

Review the discharge plan developed with the woman and her family before she returned home. Evaluate the degree to which that plan has been successfully implemented. Determine if the plan is still appropriate or if changing circumstances require a revision.

### Possible Nursing Diagnoses

Based on the woman's description of what she is feeling and is capable of doing for herself and her baby, develop nursing diagnoses with her. Depending on her specific needs, the diagnoses may focus on nutrition, nutritional supplementation, or the possible negative ramifications of inadequate nutrition. Other diagnoses may focus on her ability to provide appropriate care for herself or to assume the parenting role and the care of her child.

### Goals of Care

Work with the woman to develop mutual goals of care. Sample goals for 4 to 6 weeks postpartum include the following:

- The woman will have obtained a level of energy sufficient to care for her infant and herself.
- The woman will have increased her laboratory values of hemoglobin and hematocrit.
- A more long-term goal may be that by 6 months postpartum, the woman will have returned to her prepregnant status with regard to anemia.

### Self-Care

To cope effectively, the woman with anemia generally needs some assistance with her activities of daily living, care of the infant, and household management until her iron levels are replenished and her energy level improves. Problem solving with the woman to locate volunteers or services that may help her with her responsibilities, obtaining nutritional foods and supplementation, and then scheduling them appropriately are useful forms of assistance.

## Interventions

The interventions vary depending on the cause of the woman's anemia and the degree to which she is anemic. Educational materials and guidance must be individualized and specific.

***Iron-Deficiency Anemia.*** The condition of iron-deficiency anemia (IDA) may occur at any time in a woman's life. To determine who should receive iron supplementation, the woman's hemoglobin, hematocrit, and serum ferritin values are measured. The serum ferritin values reflect her iron reserves (Gilbert and Harmon, 1998).

The symptoms of IDA include activity intolerance, fatigue, malaise, pallor, tachycardia, dyspnea, and changes in pulse rate. They are expected to improve fairly quickly with treatment; however, periodic monitoring may be necessary. Treatment includes an iron-rich diet and possible oral iron supplementation (Box 20-1).

Iron replacement or supplementation is easily achieved in most women with oral administration of ferrous sulfate or gluconate tablets. These tablets are better absorbed on an empty stomach, but intolerance is common when taken this way. Because ingestion of iron is better tolerated with food, the woman may prefer to take it with meals. Another way to improve tolerance is to gradually increase the medication from 1 to 3 tablets daily. Iron may cause constipation that may lead some women to stop taking it. Duration of the therapy should continue through the postpartum period and for at least 3 to 6 months. Encourage her to continue to take the iron even after she feels better. Serum ferritin levels may be checked monthly until the anemia is no longer a concern.

The supplemental dosage that may be ordered is a 325-mg tablet of ferrous sulfate 3 times a day with 500 mg of vitamin C for a 6-month period. Gastrointestinal side effects from ferrous sulfate may be nausea; constipation; and tarry, black stools. These effects may be minimized by taking the iron tablet with food, starting the implementation process slowly and gradually increasing the dosage, as well as increasing the intake of fluids and dietary fiber. Occasionally parenteral iron is used when oral iron causes severe nausea and vomiting (Youngkin and Davis, 1998). Once the anemia is resolved, the woman should be encouraged to take a daily multivitamin supplement that includes iron and to maintain a diet that is high in iron.

***Folic Acid Deficiency.*** Folic acid deficiency (FAD) also is treated with supplements and is expected to quickly resolve. Folic acid deficiency is associated with an increased occurrence of neural tube defects, so it is recommended that all women of childbearing age who may become pregnant consume 400 µg of folic acid daily or take a daily supplement (Gilbert and Harmon, 1998). Even though this woman has just had a child, she should pay attention to her folic acid intake in case of an unintended pregnancy (Box 20-2).

***Thalassemia.*** Thalassemia can leave the new mother very tired and weak. Because this anemia does not respond well to iron therapy, she may receive a transfusion before leaving the hospital. Folic acid and vitamin B complex may be prescribed for her to take at home.

***Sickle Cell Anemia.*** Sickle cell anemia is aggravated by the normal anemia that occurs in pregnancy. Treatment includes periods of rest, analgesics, comfort measures, and maintenance of hydration and good nutrition.

---

**BOX 20-1** *Foods High in Iron*

***Choose:***
Lean meats

Egg yolk

Plant foods such as legumes; dried fruits; whole grains; and dark, green leafy vegetables (iron from plant foods is absorbed better when eaten with a food high in vitamin C)

Enriched breads and cereals

Dried fruits (e.g., raisins, apricots, peaches)

Shellfish

Molasses

***Avoid:***
Beverages with caffeine (e.g., cola, coffee, tea)

Dairy products

Antacids

From Gilbert ES and Harmon JS: *High risk pregnancy and delivery,* ed 2, St Louis, 1998, Mosby; Youngkin EQ and Davis MS: *Women's health—a primary care clinical guide,* ed 2, Stamford, Conn, 1998, Appleton & Lange.

---

**BOX 20-2** *Foods High in Folic Acid*

***Choose***
Dark, green leafy vegetables

Citrus fruits

Eggs

Legumes

Whole grains (since 1998, specified grain products are now fortified with folic acid)

***Avoid***
Cigarette smoking and extensive use of drugs or alcohol (these increase the need for folic acid)

From Gilbert ES and Harmon JS: *High risk pregnancy and delivery,* ed 2, St Louis, 1998, Mosby; Youngkin EQ and Davis MS: *Women's health—a primary care clinical guide,* ed 2, Stamford, Conn, 1998, Appleton & Lange.

*Health Promotion.* In educating the mother about caring for herself and her anemia, we must not only ensure that the mother understands the importance of following the treatment regimen, but also that the treatment regimen is appropriate for the mother's situation.

Although other family members may be helpful at times, the new mother might find herself in a situation in which receiving help with activities of daily living and care of the newborn is impossible. The woman may find herself alone for long periods of time or most of the day  as she cares for her child. The mother can be instructed to stand up slowly and not pick up the newborn until she is stable. She also can be instructed to use aids whenever possible, such as using walls and countertops for support while walking and using a stroller to move the newborn from one place to another.

*Nutrition.* Women and members of their support network also require nutritional counseling to supplement their medical therapy. Menu planning and shopping for foods rich in iron is an important aspect of diet teaching. A family member may need to explore where culturally appropriate foods rich in iron may be obtained at affordable prices. Women may live in a neighborhood where small stores with high prices and poor selections exist, and they may not have transportation to larger stores. You may provide the women with the best opportunity to identify these issues and collaborate with problem solving for the solutions.

*Discharge Planning.* Some insurance companies allot women only one postpartum home visit; others may allot two or three. Discharge planning starts during the first encounter with the woman to ensure that she may successfully regain her health after the nursing visits stop.

The mother should be told of the importance of completing any medications or nutritional supplements ordered. She should understand that until she starts to recover from her anemia she is more susceptible to infection due to decreased systemic resistance resulting from the loss of antibodies. Be sure she is aware of the signs and symptoms of infection and how to receive assistance (Box 20-3).

Questions and concerns may arise after the final home visit. Leave information with the mother about who to contact and how to make that contact. Ensure that she has the information and the means, both with financial coverage and transportation, to make contact with providers as needed. Community-based assistance programs may be found to assist her.

### Evaluation

Assess the level of a woman's understanding of her specific condition and her treatment plan. Have the woman verbalize her understanding of all instructions for her therapy so that she does not develop more serious complications. Her recovery is determined in part by the support she receives from family members and friends, so evaluate the functioning of her support system. Assessment of her ability to connect with a supportive environment, ongoing health care, and community services is vital as she gradually resumes care for herself and her newborn. Make the appropriate referrals as necessary.

## Diabetes

A woman with preexisting diabetes is likely familiar with diabetic dietary needs, blood glucose monitoring, and insulin administration; however, it is our responsibility to review this information and ensure that she is knowledgeable and capable of meeting her diabetic needs.

### Anticipated Issues

By the third or fourth postpartum day, insulin requirements in a woman with type 1 diabetes, as determined by her blood glucose levels, are usually about two thirds of her prepregnancy dosage. If she is not breastfeeding, a balance is usually attained by 7 to 10 days postpartum (Gilbert and Harmon, 1998).

While a mother is breastfeeding, her insulin requirements are usually less than her prepregnancy needs. Breastfeeding is encouraged in diabetic mothers, not just because breastfeeding is personally satisfying and the newborn is better nourished, but also because glucose levels are easier to control when lactating. Once weaning is complete, the insulin requirement usually returns to prepregnancy levels.

### Nursing Assessment

Once home, the woman is responsible for monitoring and maintaining her blood glucose levels. "To continue normal blood glucose levels after delivery, ongoing self-monitoring of blood glucose (SMBG), comprehensive meal planning, and regular exercise along with possible

---

**BOX 20-3** *Expectations of a Woman with Anemia*

The woman with anemia and her support system will:
- Understand her specific problem with anemia and her responsibilities in its management.
- Verbalize how her current physiologic status may compromise her ability to care for her newborn.
- Develop a plan of care that supports her physical needs while also allowing her to gradually take on her other roles.
- Verbalize the potential complications she faces because of her type of anemia and how she may minimize the occurrence.
- Understand the potential of inheritance if the anemia is a genetic condition.

oral hypoglycemic agents and/or insulin regimen are required" (Gilbert and Harmon, 1998).

Review the discharge plan that was developed with the woman and her family in the hospital. Evaluate the degree to which the woman believes she has been able to successfully implement the plan. Determine if she feels the plan is still appropriate or if changing circumstances require a revision.

### Possible Nursing Diagnoses

The woman's blood glucose readings will indicate how successfully she is keeping them within normal limits. The nursing diagnoses will focus on the factors that are helping or hindering her in this process.

### Goals of Care

The goal of nursing care for a woman with diabetes is to enable her to maintain the most consistent control of her blood glucose as she can in order to reduce complications. "Keeping blood glucose levels within normal limits reduces the risk of diabetic complications such as retinopathy by 76%, nephropathy by 50%, and cardiac problems by 35%" (Gilbert and Harmon, 1998). Short-term goals may focus on understanding the process and the need to maintain control and being able to implement the necessary self-care.

### Self-Care

The women are to be respected as the experts of their body and the feasibility of their program of care. If changes are necessary, recognize her autonomy and build upon her control and maintenance of her health. Women who see themselves as directors of their own care will want more detailed explanations.

Women will be assuming their own care with regard to maintaining an ideal body weight, eating an appropriate diet, and participating in an acceptable program of exercise. Motivation to change dietary habits, lose weight, and increase exercise through activities like walking the baby is high right after delivery. Reinforce this area of interest and help her set realistic goals.

### Interventions

**Nutrition.** All women with diabetes should have an individualized dietary prescription developed with a nutritionist knowledgeable in the needs of people with diabetes, the dietary guidelines for people with diabetes, and the cultural and economic realities of the woman. Once blood glucose levels are established, postpartum women with type 2 diabetes may be able to maintain normal glucose levels with diet alone.

 All diabetic mothers should quickly establish and maintain a regulated diet. At times a crying baby or ringing phone may distract the mother, yet she must strive to eat correct amounts of appropriate foods at established times. In this way, she will be healthier to care

for her family. It could be disastrous for a mother to check her blood glucose, administer her insulin, and then become distracted before she eats the necessary amount of food.

 **Health Promotion.** Nutritional guidance should focus on increasing caloric intake from lean meats, fruits, and vegetables. Determine her preferences in these areas and learn if they are readily available. Determine if she can afford them or will need assistance in obtaining them.

For women who are not used to eating this way or who have a family who may not choose to change their eating habits, develop a strategic plan with her on how to incorporate change that supports her health. Providing specific guidelines and ideas, such as placing cut-up bagged vegetables and fruits in the refrigerator, gives women more helpful assistance than just directing her to increase her consumption of fruits and vegetables.

Use the same process to explore how she may incorporate an appropriate level of exercise into her lifestyle. When exercise is incorporated in the activities of the day rather than requiring a "set aside time," the woman will be more successful in establishing a healthy lifestyle. Walking rather than riding and going up stairs rather than using escalators or elevators are often the most time effective ways to increase a woman's level of exercise.

**Pregnancy Prevention.** Review with the woman the pregnancy prevention information she has received. In general, women with diabetes do not use oral contraception or IUDs. However, the provider will have balanced her choice between the risk of the method to prevent pregnancy with the risk of becoming pregnant. Be sure that she understands the proper use of her selected method and the signs and symptoms of possible problems that should be reported immediately.

Also ensure that she understands why other methods may not be offered as options to her. Oral contraception is often not suggested because of the reported alteration in carbohydrate metabolism that causes insulin resistance. Recent research indicates that the low-progestin and low-estrogen pills have minimal effect on carbohydrate metabolism (Gilbert and Harmon, 1998). Because women with diabetes are at increased risk of infections when they have poor circulation, caution is used in inserting an IUD. The methods that have the least chance of compromising the woman's health are the barrier methods. Knowledge, guidance, and access to supplies help the woman and her partner successfully prevent pregnancy.

**Anticipatory Guidance.** When a new mother feels good, she may tend to resume her activity level faster than she should and suffer a setback. Encourage the woman to hold back some of her energy, keeping it in reserve for when she has to meet unexpected demands of the baby or her family.

Remind the woman that every postpartum woman experiences hormonal alterations that may create labile moods. When a woman is also dealing with changing blood glucose levels, mood changes can become even more apparent. Prepare her and her family so that they can recognize the process and understand when and if this occurs (Box 20-4).

### Evaluation

Assess the level of a woman's understanding of her specific condition and her treatment plan. Have the woman verbalize her understanding of all instructions for her therapy so that she does not develop more serious complications. Her recovery will be determined in part by the support she receives from family members and friends, so the functioning of her support system must be evaluated. Assessment of her ability to connect with a supportive environment, ongoing health care, and community services is vital as she gradually resumes care for herself and her newborn. Make the appropriate referrals as necessary.

### Summary

A postpartum woman has many adjustments to make. Faced with fluctuating sleeping and possibly eating schedules and the care of the newborn, a woman with diabetes may have a difficult time. Encouragement and anticipatory guidance for the woman, while engaging the family members in assisting her, may help her maintain blood glucose levels within a normal range.

## Cardiovascular Disease

### Anticipated Issues

Follow-up home care for a postpartum woman with a cardiac condition is important so that ongoing monitoring may occur without the woman experiencing the fatigue created by having to leave her home. Women may experience cardiac decompensation late in the first week postpartum; thus ongoing care is critical.

### Nursing Assessment

A woman with cardiac problems may report increasing fatigue, shortness of breath, frequent cough, and palpitations. She may exhibit cyanosis of the lips and nailbeds. The physical assessment includes blood pressure, apical/radial pulses, lung sounds, weight gain or loss, and Homan's sign as indicated. Ask about the presence of chest pain and assess for edema. If she is experiencing cardiac decompensation, her respirations may be greater than or equal to 25 breaths/min. Her pulse may be rapid and/or irregular at greater than or equal to 100 beats/min. Auscultation may reveal crackles in the lung bases that do not clear with coughing. Determine what medications she is on and her pattern of use.

Review the discharge plan that was developed with the woman and her family before she returned home. Evaluate the degree to which that plan has been implemented successfully. Determine if the plan is still appropriate or if changing circumstances require a revision.

### Possible Nursing Diagnoses

Nursing diagnoses may focus on health maintenance and knowledge development. A woman may have limitations in her activity level and ability to care for herself and her child because of a cardiac condition. She also may not understand how she can evaluate and manage her condition.

### Goals of Care

The goals of care are that the woman understands her condition and accepts and is able to implement a plan of management that will enable her to achieve the highest level of wellness possible.

### Self-Care

The best self-care that the woman can provide is to allow herself to be taken care of by others as her body adjusts to not being pregnant. Caring for her infant as she is able, while following a plan of rest, good nutrition, and gradual resumption of former activities creates the best outcomes.

Help her determine how she can get the most rest possible. She will probably require at least 10 hours of sleep per night and periodic rests during the day.

The woman monitors herself for early signs of cardiac difficulties. Instruct her to weigh herself daily, if she has access to a scale, so that she can monitor sudden fluid retention. If she doesn't have a scale or doesn't want to weigh herself, instruct her on how to observe her face, hands, and ankles for fluid retention

Help her establish a medication regimen that she can maintain consistently from one day to the next.

---

**BOX 20-4  Expectations of a Woman with Diabetes**

The woman with diabetes and her support system will:

- Understand her disease process and her responsibilities in its management.
- Describe her dietary, insulin, and exercise needs and strategies she will use to maintain these while caring for a newborn.
- Verbalize potential complications and actions she will take should any complication occur.
- Understand the impact the newborn will have on her life and her ability to meet the demands of her diabetes.
- Understand that most new mothers become somewhat depressed after childbirth and that her susceptibility to depression may be worse because of her additional physical fluctuations.
- Understand that it is possible to continue life in a stable diabetic state while resuming her prepregnancy responsibilities and caring for a newborn but that it will take time.

Determine who will fill her prescriptions for her and if she has the insurance or economic means to obtain the necessary medications.

### Interventions

***Care of Woman.*** A plan of care must be individualized and adapted to the type and severity of the new mother's cardiac condition and her functional ability. Once she returns home, it is not unusual for her recovery to be several weeks to months longer than a woman who experiences a normal postpartum. The length of recovery time is usually determined by the effects of the pregnancy and birth on the heart muscle.

Family- and community-based support of a mother with cardiac conditions is imperative. It is possible that the mother may need help with activities of daily living such as hygiene, eating, and bathing and may qualify for the services of a home health aide. Ongoing nursing visits may be ordered for a period of time to continue to assess the woman's physical adaptation and help organize her care within the family.

***Nutrition.*** Determine who will be doing the shopping and food preparation and involve them in the process of nutrition counseling. Review with the woman and her support network the information that was provided before discharge from the hospital. Help them problem solve about how the information can now become a practical part of their life.

It is important that the woman have a well-balanced diet to lessen stress on the heart and decrease her risk of edema. Her risk of fluid retention will be increased if she has a protein deficiency or excess sodium. If she has inadequate amounts of iron, her heart will have to work harder. Her risk of constipation increases if she doesn't have sufficient fiber in her diet. If a diuretic is part of her pharmacologic management, she should eat foods high in potassium, such as bananas, citrus fruits, and whole grains.

*Maternal-Infant Interaction.* Cardiac output is not compromised by lactation, so the mother may breastfeed her infant. However, the safety of the woman's cardiac medications for the infant must be evaluated because some are inappropriate. When the woman feeds her child, have her sit well supported in a chair or lie down so that she may conserve energy. Others may help her by burping and changing the baby.

***Anticipatory Guidance.*** A woman may become indifferent and apathetic as a result of her inability to assume her own care and that of her newborn as quickly as other mothers. Usually once progressive ambulation and increasing care of the newborn are allowed, the mother is less likely to exhibit this depression.

***Pregnancy Prevention.*** Sexual activity may be resumed after the woman has recovered from the pregnancy and when she has the means to prevent a pregnancy. Assess the couple's knowledge about the risk a pregnancy poses to the woman's health. Determine the methods they believe will best fit their sexual activities and that they can obtain and use regularly. Oral contraception may not be an option because of the thromboembolic potential. Barrier methods used in combination, such as the diaphragm and male condom, may provide the highest level of protection with the least compromise of health risk to the woman (Box 20-5).

### Evaluation

Assess the level of a woman's understanding of her specific condition and understanding of her treatment plan so that she may achieve the highest level of wellness possible. Have the woman verbalize her understanding of all instructions for her therapy so that she does not develop more serious complications. Her recovery will be determined in part by the support she receives from family members and friends, so evaluate the functioning of her support system. Assessment of her ability to connect with a supportive environment, ongoing health care, and community services is vital as she gradually assumes care for herself and her newborn. Make the appropriate referrals as necessary.

### Summary

Women with cardiac disease are, with medical supervision, increasingly able to survive pregnancy and childbirth. Supportive care must continue after their return home because they experience an extended postpartal recovery period. With assistance, women with cardiac conditions can regain their former level of health. The women's needs, both physical and emotional, and the needs of their families must be addressed.

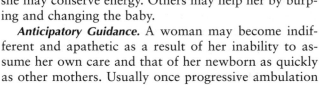

**BOX 20-5** *Expectations of a Woman with Cardiovascular Disease*

The woman with cardiovascular disease and her support system will:
- Understand her disease process and her responsibilities in its management.
- Monitor her physiologic status, including her pulse, respirations, edema, skin color, and blood pressure.
- Verbalize the physical limitations related to her cardiac condition and describe strategies that will maintain these limitations while caring for a newborn.
- Verbalize potential complications and actions to take if they occur.
- Understand the impact the newborn will have on her life and her ability to meet the demands of her cardiac condition.
- Describe her dietary and exercise needs.
- Understand that it is possible to continue life in a stable cardiac state while managing her prepregnancy responsibilities and caring for a newborn, but it will take time.

# CARE OF THE WOMAN WITH COMPLICATIONS RELATED TO PREGNANCY AND BIRTH

## Late Postpartum Hemorrhage

Postpartal hemorrhage continues to be a leading cause of maternal morbidity and mortality in the United States (Berg and others, 1996). **Late postpartal hemorrhage** occurs in 0.1% to 1% of new mothers. By definition, late postpartal hemorrhage occurs after the first 24 hours following delivery and as late as 4 to 6 weeks into the postpartum period (Norris, 1997).

Much of the literature implies that early discharge has contributed to the potential for acute episodes of hemorrhage to occur outside of the hospital or birthing center. However, since the possibility of hemorrhage exists for 4 weeks or more, the occurrence is not simply related to early postpartum discharge. It is therefore important to educate every mother and her family regarding this life-threatening condition.

The primary causes of late postpartum hemorrhage include retained placenta, subinvolution of the uterus, and endometritis. **Retained placenta** is a condition in which a piece or pieces of the placenta do not completely separate from the uterus after birth. Generally this is recognized when the placenta is inspected after delivery. Although rare, bleeding associated with retained placenta may occur after discharge.

**Subinvolution of the uterus** is a condition in which the uterus does not return to normal size or function in the time expected. Two causes may be retained placenta and infection. The signs and symptoms of subinvolution include outright hemorrhage, irregular bleeding, or prolonged lochial discharge. It might be hard for a mother to determine that she has experienced a prolonged lochial discharge if she doesn't understand the normal progression of recovery. Some new mothers report that they believe they went right from postpartal bleeding into a menstrual period when actually they are experiencing a postpartum hemorrhage from subinvolution.

**Endometritis,** an infection of the uterine lining, is covered in detail under postpartal infections.

### Anticipated Issues

Many women who are unsure about how much bleeding is too much wait before reporting or seeking help; thus when they finally present to the health care facility, their well-being is often compromised. Late postpartum hemorrhage can be one of the most frightening complications for a woman and her family because it creates an ominous feeling of doom for everyone involved. The woman should seek care immediately.

### Nursing Assessment

As with any bleeding after childbirth, it is important that the mother and her family understand the possible causes and the necessary treatments to ensure the health and well-being of the mother. All mothers and their families should be instructed to get to a hospital immediately if bleeding becomes heavier than a heavy period.

When doing a home visit evaluate the woman's ability to assess what an abnormal flow of lochia would be and how she would respond if it occurred.

### Possible Nursing Diagnoses

All women who experience postpartal hemorrhage will have anxiety and possibly fear related to the bleeding. This also applies to family members and friends. In addition, they will require education about the interventions she will experience. Although the emergency involves saving the woman's life, other needs that may need to be addressed are the care of the baby and possibly other children both during the emergent period and during the woman's recovery.

### Goals of Care

The primary goal of care is to enable the woman to regain a healthy state and resume her activities of daily living. To do this she will require information, appropriate medical intervention, and assistance with the care of herself and her family as she recovers.

### Self-Care

Review with the woman how to monitor the height of her uterine fundus. Each woman must also be aware of what constitutes normal and abnormal lochia. If she thinks she may be experiencing abnormal lochia or abnormal involution, she must alert her health care provider (Box 20-6).

### Nursing Interventions

***Anticipatory Guidance.*** If a woman experiences a hemorrhage, quick recognition and rapid aggressive treatment

---

**BOX 20-6   *Expectations of the Woman with Late Postpartum Bleeding***

The woman who has experienced an episode of postpartum bleeding and her family will:
- Understand the signs and symptoms of abnormal bleeding.
- Verbalize the physical limitations related to treating postpartum bleeding.
- Describe strategies that will support the woman's rest while caring for her newborn.
- Verbalize the nutritional needs of the woman.
- Verbalize action the woman will take should bleeding recur.

are the most important aspects in saving the woman's life. Maternal exsanguination is possible if the hemorrhage process is unrecognized and untreated (Knuppel and Hatangadi, 1995). Teach all women about the possibility of abnormal postpartal bleeding. However, don't offer the false reassurance of, "You will know when it happens." This explanation is bewildering and does not support the woman's ability to provide appropriate self-care. Give specific ways to evaluate lochia flow and directions for seeking care.

***Care of the Woman.*** If the bleeding is minimal and due to subinvolution, after an evaluation, the woman may be allowed to remain at home on bedrest and self-medicate with an oral oxytocic such as methylergonovine maleate (Methergine). If pieces of retained placenta are preventing the uterus from contracting, the woman will be readmitted to the hospital for a dilation and curettage to remove the tissue and stabilize her condition. In rare cases, the woman may have to undergo a hysterectomy to stop the bleeding. If endometritis is the cause she may be hospitalized for intravenous antibiotic therapy.

In today's world, new mothers are often left alone to care for their family within days of birth or return to work soon after giving birth. Yet it remains common to instruct new mothers not to lift heavy objects or overexert themselves during the recovery period. Although the basic principle of this information is sound and the information still needs to be presented to new mothers, the belief that mothers can and will heed the instruction is not always realistic.

If the woman experiences a hemorrhage that requires hospitalization, when she returns home she must be able to follow the instructions for rest, fluid intake, and adequate nutrition. Arranging and accepting assistance for herself and her child or children is important.

***Mother-Infant Interaction.*** Once the emergency is passed, the infant and mother should be reunited as much as possible. However, the woman must regain her strength before she assumes full care of the baby.

## Evaluation

Assess the level of a woman's understanding of her condition and the treatment plan. Have the woman verbalize her understanding of all instructions. Her success will be determined in part by the support she receives from family members and friends, so evaluate the functioning of her support system. Assessment of her ability to connect with a supportive environment, ongoing health care, and community services is vital as she gradually resumes care for herself and her newborn.

## Summary

A late postpartal hemorrhage can be very frightening for a woman and her family. It may come at an unexpected time when they have moved from thinking of the delivery experience to the integration of the new family member. It is not only potentially life threatening for the mother, but also unexpected for the family unit. Quick identification of the problem by the woman and rapid intervention provides the best outcomes. The woman's needs, both physical and emotional, and the needs of her family must be addressed.

## Postpartum Eclampsia

Eclampsia is generally thought of as a condition that occurs during pregnancy and disappears with delivery. However, some women develop it during the postpartum period.

### Anticipated Issues

Because eclampsia is not readily identified with the postpartum period, it can be overlooked easily. "Postpartum eclampsia may occur within 10 days of delivery, but cases have been reported as late as 23 days' postpartum" (Youngkin and Davis, 1998).

### Nursing Assessment

The woman may complain of a severe and persistent headache in the occipital region. Her vision may be blurred or she may have an unusual intolerance for light (photophobia). She may have pain in the epigastric area or right upper quadrant of the abdomen.

Examination may reveal proteinuria, pedal edema, and/or hypertension. Any diastolic pressure above 90 mm Hg is to be considered abnormal. The woman's reflexes should be assessed for clonus. Diagnostic tests that may be ordered are urinalysis, serum uric acid, blood urea nitrogen (BUN), plasma glucose, liver function enzymes (including SGOT, PT, and PTT), electrolytes, serum creatinine, and fibrinogen (Youngkin and Davis, 1998).

### Possible Nursing Diagnoses

The nursing diagnoses focus on helping the woman become comfortable and assisting her in understanding her medical diagnosis and the treatment plan that is developed. The family will have concerns about the health of the woman and the care of the infant.

### Goals of Care

Goals of care include early identification of the condition and implementation of appropriate treatment so that the woman does not suffer a seizure or other complications. Additional goals include alleviating the woman's discomfort and establishing a normal diastolic blood pressure as soon as possible.

### Self-Care

The woman must identify that what she is experiencing is abnormal and refer herself for care. After the cause of her discomfort is determined, she will be responsible for following the treatment plan.

### Nursing Interventions

The woman may require admission to the hospital for initial therapy. She will require education about the nature of her condition and the need for medical management and hospitalization. The medical management is identical to that given to a pregnant woman with hypertension—anticonvulsant and antihypertensive therapy.

The woman and her family will require emotional support and assistance in addressing concerns about her care and safety and the care of her infant.

### Evaluation

Assess the woman's level of understanding of her condition and the treatment plan. Have the woman verbalize her understanding of the need for hospitalization and all instructions. Her ability to leave her family and be admitted for hospitalization without great concern will be determined in part by the support she receives from family members and friends, so evaluate the functioning of her support system. Once she returns home, assessment of the ongoing support of her family and her ability to connect with a supportive environment, ongoing health care, and community services are vital as she gradually resumes care for herself and her newborn.

### Summary

The diagnosis of postpartum eclampsia can be very frightening for a woman and her family. It may come at an unexpected time when they have moved from thinking of the delivery experience to the integration of the new family member. It is not only potentially life threatening for the mother, but also unexpected for the family unit. The woman's quick identification of the problem and rapid intervention provide the best outcomes. The needs of the woman, both physical and emotional, and the needs of her family must be addressed.

## Postpartum Infection

Postpartum infection remains a major cause of maternal morbidity and mortality throughout the world and occurs in approximately 6% of births in the United States. The most common organisms are anaerobic streptococcus, *Clostridium*, group A or G hemolytic streptococcus, *Escherichia coli*, *Klebsiella*, *Gardnerella vaginalis*, and *Chlamydia trachomatis* (Mattson and Smith, 2000). These infections are categorized as either **endogenous** (resulting from bacteria commonly originating in the vagina) or **exogenous** (resulting from pathogens introduced from outside the vagina).

### Anticipated Issues

A woman is more apt to develop a postpartum infection if before or during pregnancy she experienced a venous thrombosis, a UTI, mastitis, chorioamnionitis, or pneumonia. Chronic conditions such as diabetes mellitus, anemia, immunosuppression, drug abuse, alcoholism, and malnutrition also place her at higher risk.

Incidents that destroy the normal barriers to infiltration by organisms may occur during labor and delivery, increasing her risk of an infection. Factors that increase the risk of infection are prolonged labor, especially with a prolonged rupture of membranes; introduction of instruments with bladder catheterization, internal fetal monitoring, or intrauterine pressure monitoring; epidural anesthesia; surgical interventions of cesarean birth or episiotomy; or tissue damage such as a hematoma or laceration.

Although it is expected that in the United States when a postpartal infection occurs it will be resolved with no residual problems, it should be remembered that postpartal infections can lead to death. It is imperative that women and their families be educated regarding the signs of infection.

### Nursing Assessment

A woman may experience an elevated temperature in the postpartal period due to dehydration, breast engorgement, or the trauma of a surgical delivery. A woman is determined to have a postpartum infection if for no known reason she experiences a temperature of 38° C (100.4° F) or higher, on two or more occasions, for longer than 24 hours more than 2 days after the delivery.

***Mastitis.*** **Mastitis** is caused when bacterial infection occurs in a woman's breast because of a cracked nipple, plugged milk duct, or inadequate emptying of the breast. Symptoms include a reddened and painful area, generally occurring in only one breast and usually accompanied by a fever and flulike symptoms (Figure 20-1).

***Localized Infections.*** Wound infections include infections at the site of a repaired laceration, episiotomy, or incision for abdominal delivery. Incisions should be monitored using the REEDA scale (see Table 19-3). Signs of a wound infection include discomfort, erythema, edema, warmth, drainage, and wound separation.

***Endometritis.*** The most common type of genital tract infection during the postpartum period is endometritis, the inflammation of the endometrium. The inflammation is caused by a bacterial invasion and may be acute or subacute or become chronic in nature. When such an infection begins in the uterus, if not recognized and treated, it may continue moving through the system, involving the fallopian tubes, the ovaries, and other organs. **Pelvic cellulitis** can occur when the infection spreads into the broad ligament. Abscesses can develop that require draining to prevent rupture. **Salpingitis** and/or **oophoritis** occurs when the infection spreads to the fallopian tubes and/or ovaries. **Generalized peritonitis** can occur when infection spreads from the uterus via the lymphatics to the abdominal cavity. **Bacteremia** occurs when the organism invades the blood system. With virulent organisms septic shock occurs.

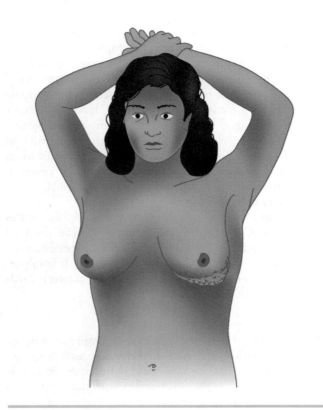

FIGURE 20-1 • Mastitis.

The infection usually begins at the placental site and then spreads to the endometrium. Symptoms usually occur on postpartum days 3 through 5. If the infectious agent is β-hemolytic streptococci, the onset is earlier. Assessment for signs of infection include fever, increased pulse, chills, anorexia, nausea, fatigue, lethargy, pelvic pain, enlarged uterus, uterine tenderness, or foul-smelling profuse lochia (Calhoun and Brost, 1995). Pathogens usually are identified within 36 to 48 hours through intracervical or intrauterine aerobic or anaerobic cultures. Infection in one or more sites should be viewed as a life-threatening condition in the postpartum woman and should be treated aggressively.

Be alert to the absence of bowel sounds, abdominal distention, and nausea or vomiting. These may be indications that the infection has spread.

### Possible Nursing Diagnoses

The woman's response to an infection will lead to diagnoses that reflect her need for physical comfort, education, and emotional support. In addition diagnoses that reflect the understanding and needs of the family during this time of crises will be made.

### Goals of Care

The goal of care is that once the infection is identified, it is treated as required, minimizing the damage to the woman's reproductive organs and minimizing the risk to her life. In addition, the woman and her family, including the newborn, will receive the necessary guidance, support, and physical care required to successfully negotiate this crisis.

### Self-Care

Localized infection often develops after the woman is providing her own assessments and care within her home. A postpartum visit assesses the current status of a woman regarding the possibility of an infection and ensures that she knows how to assess for it and how to respond if she thinks it may be occurring.

Educate women about the early signs of infection within their breasts, perineum, or abdomen. If the infection is located in the perineal region, it is not as easily observed and can go undetected for a longer period of  time. Women often believe that any discomfort experienced in the perineal area is normal healing; therefore they do not report it to their health care provider until the symptoms of infection become unbearable.

Encourage them to use a mirror and observe the perineal area for abnormal drainage, separation of the episiotomy if they had one, swelling, or hematoma. If the infection is at a cesarean incision site, it can be spotted by looking at the site daily during bathing.

### Interventions

***Mastitis.*** After ensuring good hygiene, treatment includes bedrest for 24 to 48 hours, analgesics for discomfort, and warm compresses and massage of the  breast before feeding. Antibiotics may be required.

The mother is usually relieved to find that she can continue to breastfeed. She should be encouraged to vary the baby's position on the breast; breastfeed every 2 to 3 hours; and to express, by hand or pump, any milk left in the breasts after a feeding.

Advising a new mother to stay in bed for 24 to 48 hours may be an impossible requirement. Any home care or teaching should be done with the understanding that each mother's situation is different and the mother's situation should be assessed and the treatment regimen adapted accordingly.

***Localized Infections and Endometritis.*** It is imperative that infections such as these be medically treated immediately. Some infections will require admission to an inpatient facility for care. Other women will be cared for in the home with daily or twice daily visits by a visiting nurse. Care includes monitoring the mother's condition and carrying out physician's orders for antibiotic therapy and other medical interventions.

Assistance with psychologic adaptation is also a focus of nursing care. Mothers will be better able to cope with an episode of infection if they:

* are encouraged and supported in efforts to maintain lactation

- understand the plan of treatment,
- are reassured about their recovery and ability to resume care of the baby,
- have opportunities for resuming mothering activities as her condition improves,
- have family members included in the care process, and
- have continued nursing support after hospital discharge (Box 20-7).

### Evaluation

Assess the level of a woman's understanding of the effect the infectious process has had on her postpartum recovery and her treatment plan. Have the woman verbalize her understanding of all instructions. Her success will be determined in part by the support she receives from family members and friends, so evaluate the functioning of her support system. Assessment of her ability to connect with a supportive environment, ongoing health care, and community services is vital as she gradually resumes care for herself and her newborn.

### Summary

Postpartum infection does not pose the risk of death to new mothers as it did in the past. However, it does still occur, and with its associated pain, discomfort, damage to internal organs, and risk of future infertility, it must be managed. In addition, the woman and her family must deal with an interruption in normal activities because care must now be provided for the woman and the infant.

## Thromboembolic Disease

A thrombosis (blood clot within a blood vessel) can lead to **thrombophlebitis** (inflammation of the lining of a blood vessel) and a possible thromboembolism. The most common time for a thrombophlebitis to develop is between postpartum days 10 to 20.

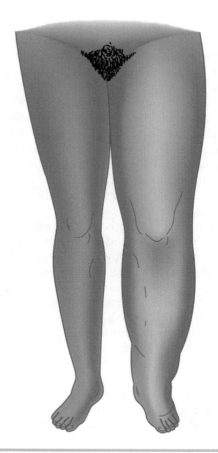

FIGURE 20-2 ● Deep vein thrombosis.

### Anticipated Issues

A postpartum thrombophlebitis may occur in the veins of the leg, thigh, or pelvis. It may be either a superficial venous thrombosis or a deep venous thrombosis (DVT) (Figure 20-2). If part or all of a clot from a DVT detaches, it may cause a **pulmonary embolism,** obstructing the blood flow through a pulmonary artery to the lungs, which may be fatal.

The incidence of thrombolitic conditions has decreased as a result of early ambulation after birth, but it still occurs in approximately 1 in 1000 to 2000 births (Cunningham, 1997). The major causes are the result of venous stasis and hypercoagulation, both fairly common in the postpartum period. A woman is at increased risk if she is obese, used oral contraception before pregnancy, has a history of circulatory problems or infections, smokes, is more than 35 years of age, has had other pregnancies, or has an abdominal delivery.

### Nursing Assessment

The woman may report pain and tenderness in her pelvis or a lower extremity. She may experience chills or have an elevated body temperature, an elevated pulse, and/or hypotension. If pain or tenderness occurs in her leg, visualization may reveal a warm, red, enlarged or hardened vein of a superficial venous thrombosis. If the calf appears swollen she may be experiencing DVT.

A positive Homan's sign may indicate a DVT, but this is not conclusive because it also may be attributed to other causes such as muscle strain from childbirth. Objective and subjective information provide information but not specific data to determine the diagnosis.

To reach a conclusive diagnosis the nurse midwife or physician may order blood work to determine hemoglobin and hematocrit values, a phlebography (study of the structure and function of the veins), a Doppler ultrasound, or a contrast venography (a radiographic procedure to visualize veins).

A pulmonary embolism is a thrombolic complication in which a clot dislodges and is carried to the pulmonary artery, obstructing blood flow to the lungs. Most of these originate as thrombi in the deep leg veins and dislodge spontaneously. This condition occurs without warning and is life-threatening. Signs and symptoms range from shortness of breath, fever, and productive blood-tinged cough, to shock, pallor, severe dyspnea, and crushing chest pain.

## Possible Nursing Diagnoses

Because of the blockage of the vein, the woman will have physiologic needs due to the decreased tissue perfusion and the pain caused by the inflammation. The treatment of the condition will lead to nursing diagnoses that reflect how she has to change her role within the family. In addition, she may become anxious about her own well-being and the care and well-being of her infant and other family members.

## Goals of Care

The goals of care are to increase the woman's comfort and prevent a thrombolitic accident. In addition, the

### BOX 20-8 Expectations of a Woman with a Thromboembolic Disorder

The woman with a thromboembolic disorder and her support system will:
• Understand her thromboembolic disorder and her responsibilities in its management, including bedrest, taking oral anticoagulants, and wearing elastic stockings.
• Understand the impact this disorder will have on the woman's ability to care for herself and her newborn.
• Identify family or friends who will help care for her newborn while she achieves the necessary bedrest to recover from this disorder.
• Verbalize potential complications and actions she will take should any complication occur.
• Verbalize signs of further complication such as a pulmonary embolism, which may be indicated by chest pain, coughing, dyspnea, and tachypnea.

woman's support system will need to understand what is happening to her and be involved in providing for the needs of the family until the woman is able to resume her role.

### Self-Care

Because this condition most often occurs after the immediate postpartum period, the woman must identify and report problems to her health care provider. Prevention of further problems will be enhanced if the woman wears support hose correctly, keeps her legs uncrossed, refrains from doing a deep flexion of her legs at the groin, and rests her legs in a way that keeps the pressure off the back of the knees.

If she is put on anticoagulant therapy, she will have to be monitored for signs of excessive anticoagulation. These would include nosebleeds, easy bruising, tarry or black stools, hematuria, or uterine hemorrhage.

### Interventions
Medical management of this condition includes administration of analgesia; rest; elevation of the extremity; and intravenous administration of an anticoagulant, usually heparin for 5 to 7 days. The mother usually continues oral anticoagulants for several months. Antibiotics may be given for an infectious process. When the mother is allowed to resume ambulation, she is instructed to wear elastic stockings until the threat of further coagulation is past.

In addition to monitoring her condition and administering appropriate medications, you need to educate the woman about anticoagulant therapy, recognition of warning signs and symptoms of further complications, activity restrictions, and strategies for coping with emotions after this life-threatening event (Box 20-8).

### Evaluation
Assess the level of a woman's understanding of her treatment plan. Have the woman verbalize her understanding of all instructions. Her success will be determined in part by the support she receives from family members and friends, so evaluate the functioning of her support system. Assessment of her ability to connect with a supportive environment, ongoing health care, and community services is vital as she gradually resumes care for herself and her newborn.

### Summary
A thrombophlebitis and possible thromboembolism remain risks to the comfort and well-being of new mothers. Early identification and treatment depend on the woman reporting the occurrence and seeking care. Once the problem is identified, treatment is generally successful. The woman's needs, both physical and emotional, and the needs of her family must be addressed.

## Thyroiditis

**Thyroiditis** is the inflammation of the thyroid gland. Postpartum thyroidistis is an autoimmune thyroid disease that may result following delivery or abortion because of a transient rebound of the autoimmune process. It is different from other forms of hyperactivity of the thyroid in that thyroid pain is absent, it has transient symptoms with spontaneous remission, and serum antibody and thyroid hormone levels are elevated (Youngkin and Davis, 1998).

### Anticipated Issues

Symptoms of postpartum thyroiditis may manifest at any time during the first postpartum month, but mostly during weeks 3 and 4. A thyroid-toxic storm or crises may occur, creating a life-threatening emergency. This involves a sudden and dangerous increase in the symptoms of thyrotoxicosis, a condition caused by excessive levels of thyroid hormones.

### Nursing Assessment

If the woman is experiencing thyrotoxicosis, she may report a fever, marked weakness, and extreme restlessness with wide emotional swings. Family members may describe behaviors that indicate confusion, psychosis, and even coma. This condition has a rapid onset during the third or fourth postpartum week and is usually resolved by the fourth month. The woman may also experience weight loss, heat intolerance, palpitations, and/or hand tremors.

During thyrotoxicosis, the woman experiences sinus tachycardia. Her eyes are fixed in a stare or she may have lid lag. Her reflexes are brisk. On palpation her thyroid is firm and nontender. Fifty percent of women will have a normal size thyroid.

If the woman is experiencing transient hypothyroidism, she will report progressive and pronounced fatigue and weight gain during months 3 through 6 of the postpartum year. Her hair will become coarse and her skin will be dry. Her affect will be one that mimics depression. Because of the nature of this problem any complaint of fatigue, palpitations, impaired memory, depression, or loss of attention span during the postpartum year needs further evaluation. During the transient phase, the woman will exhibit delayed reflexes and psychomotor retardation.

Assessment of the woman's condition includes venipuncture for blood tests to measure the levels of thyroid stimulating hormone (TSH), an antithyroglobulin antibody assay (ATA), and antithyroid peroxidase antibodies (antiTPOAB) assay (Youngkin and Davis, 1998).

### Possible Nursing Diagnoses

Attention will be paid to the physical and emotional care of the woman and support for the care of her family. Education about the nature and treatment of her illness is important to both the woman and her family.

### Goals of Care

Goals of care are to assist the woman in understanding her disease process, to provide supportive care until she is able to resume the care for herself and her family, and to prevent the disease from becoming life threatening (Youngkin and Davis, 1998).

### Self-Care

The woman should report the symptoms she is feeling and follow the directions for testing and treatment.

### Nursing Interventions

Reassure the woman about the validity of her symptoms and her concerns. Explain to her and her family the etiology of postpartum thyroiditis. Provide anticipatory guidance that even though the condition will resolve spontaneously, it can recur with future births.

Explain the reason for the blood tests and the venipuncture procedure. If the woman is to undergo a radioactive iodine uptake test and thyroid scan, she will have to alter her diet and medication regimen for 1 to 3 weeks before the test. Be sure she understands how to do that safely for her own health and appropriately for the best test results.

If medical treatment is prescribed, ensure that the woman is able to obtain the necessary type and amounts of medication, knows how and where she should store it, and understands how to take it (i.e., in the morning on an empty stomach). Explain the possible side effects of the medication and how she should respond.

### Evaluation

Assess the level of a woman's understanding of her treatment plan. Have the woman verbalize her understanding of all instructions. Her success will be determined in part by the support she receives from family members and friends, so evaluate the functioning of her support system. Assessment of her ability to connect with a supportive environment and community services is vital as she gradually resumes care for herself and her newborn. Determine her ability to maintain ongoing health care, because she will need follow-up physical and laboratory assessments for 2 years. The thyroid may recover after the first year of treatment and gradually return to normal function by 2 years postpartum (Youngkin and Davis, 1998).

### Summary

A postpartum thyroiditis poses a risk to the comfort and well-being of new mothers. Early identification and treatment depends on the woman reporting the symptoms and seeking care. Once the problem is identified, treatment, although long, is generally successful. The woman's needs, both physical and emotional, and the needs of her family must be addressed.

## Urinary Tract Infection

### Anticipated Issues

Urinary tract infections (UTIs) occur in 2% to 4% of postpartum women because of urinary catheterization or frequent pelvic examinations, in which bacteria normally present at the opening of the urethra are pushed up the urethra or enter the bladder. The experience of a genital tract injury is also related to increased frequency. Women who have a history of UTI, urinary retention for any reason, or urinary calculus are more susceptible to UTIs.

### Nursing Assessment

Women with UTIs are often febrile and describe painful urination associated with frequency. If the organism has ascended into her kidneys, she may develop a high fever, tremors, nausea and vomiting, or pain in the costovertebral angle (CVA) or flank. The woman may experience suprapubic tenderness on examination.

### Possible Nursing Diagnoses

With a UTI discomfort becomes an issue for the woman. She also may need information about fluid intake, perineal hygiene, and the correct use of antibiotic therapy. She is at risk for the infection moving into the kidneys

### Goals of Care

The goal of care is for the woman to receive appropriate treatment as quickly as possible so that she becomes comfortable and the progression of the infection is stopped. In addition, the woman should understand the infection process and know how to reduce her risk of developing a UTI in the future.

### Self-Care

The key is recognizing the signs and symptoms of infections and seeking treatment quickly. Toileting care, in which the woman wipes her perineum with clean toilet paper from front to back, is vital. When changing perineal pads, they should also be placed from front to back. A high fluid intake, up to 3 liters a day, and the consumption of foods that increase the acidity of urine, such as cranberries, apricots, plums, and prunes also help.

### Nursing Interventions

Broad-spectrum antibiotics usually are prescribed immediately. Verification that the appropriate antibiotic is being given is then confirmed through urine culture and sensitivity analysis. Although prophylactic antibiotics are not justified, prompt diagnosis and treatment are important.

Instruct the woman to take all of the medication. It is not unusual for patients to stop taking the medication once the symptoms disappear. Be sure she understands that just because she becomes asymptomatic, this does not mean the bacteria are gone. Explain that if the full course of medication is not taken, some of the bacteria may survive and the infection will regrow. Each time it returns it becomes more and more difficult to treat.

### Evaluation

Assess the level of a woman's understanding of her treatment plan. Have the woman verbalize her understanding of all instructions for antibiotic therapy, elimination of pain, and the need to complete the course of treatment so that the infection does not lead to more serious complications. Have the woman state the activities she may use to reduce her risk of developing a UTI in the future.

Her recovery will be determined in part by the support she receives from family members and friends, so evaluate the functioning of her support system. Assessment of her ability to connect with a supportive environment, ongoing health care, and community services is vital as she gradually resumes care for herself and her newborn.

### Summary

Women may experience a UTI at any point in their lives. The adoption of preventive practices is important. Early identification and treatment when an infection occurs decreases the amount of pain and stress experienced by the woman and the possibility of her sustaining permanent damage. The woman's needs, both physical and emotional, and the needs of her family must be addressed.

## Structural Disorders of the Uterus or Vagina

### Anticipated Issues

Prolonged labor, precipitous birth, abnormalities in fetal presentation, or traumatic birth from forceps or vacuum extractor application can create structural problems within a woman's reproductive system. Structural disorders of the uterus and vagina may lead to pelvic relaxation and urinary incontinence; uterine displacement and prolapse; or the development of a cystocele, rectocele, or genital fistulas.

***Pelvic Relaxation.*** Pelvic relaxation with urinary incontinence can be an annoying complication of childbearing. Some women experience leakage of urine when coughing, sneezing, laughing, or straining to lift objects. It is estimated that this affects about 20% of all women between 25 and 54 years of age, with the highest percentage occurring in women who have given birth vaginally (Sampselle and others, 1997).

When a woman experiences urinary incontinence, diagnostic strategies will be followed to establish the correct etiology. In addition to trauma to the tissues during birth, urinary incontinence may be caused by the following:

- Bladder or urethral disorders (e.g., urethritis, urethral stricture, cystitis)
- Neurologic problems as seen in multiple sclerosis or diabetic neuritis

- Pathologic conditions of the spinal cord
- Congenital or acquired urinary conditions

***Uterine Displacement and Prolapse.*** Uterine displacement and prolapse occur when the normal action of the round ligaments holding the uterus in anteversion or the ability of the uterosacral ligaments to hold the cervix up and back in the pelvis is disrupted. In some cases the prolapse is so severe, the uterus protrudes through the vagina.

Congenital or acquired weakness of the pelvic support structures can cause this condition. Sometimes this condition is noted and repaired after childbirth. Pelvic radiation or surgery can also cause pelvic weakness. The most common type of displacement is retroversion, in which the uterus is tilted posteriorly and the cervix is rotated anteriorly. In approximately two thirds of all women, normal placement returns by the third month postpartum. Although rarely symptomatic, the other one third of women have a uterus that remains retroverted. Difficulties that may arise from this continued retroversion include the following:

- Difficulty conceiving
- Deep pelvic pressure and low back pain

- Difficulty with elimination
- Increased premenstrual tension
- Dyspareunia (Figures 20-3 to 20-5)

***Cystocele and Rectocele.*** Cystocele and rectocele are protrusions of the bladder and rectum, respectively, into the vagina. The **cystocele** occurs when the supporting structures in the vesicovaginal septum are injured, allowing the bladder to protrude downward into the vagina. When a woman stands the weight of the urine in the bladder pushes against the weakened anterior vaginal wall, forcing the vesicovaginal septum downward. The bladder is stretched and its capacity is increased. Over time, the cystocele enlarges until it protrudes into the vagina. This makes complete emptying of the bladder difficult. **Rectocele** occurs when the anterior rectal wall herniates through the relaxed vaginal fascia and rectovaginal septum. This often can be seen as a large bulge through the relaxed introitus (Figures 20-5 and 20-6).

***Genital Fistulas.*** Genital fistulas are abnormal openings between one genital tract organ and another. They can develop after labor's compression of the genital tract tissues or can result from a congenital anomaly, gynecologic surgery, cancer, radiation therapy, infection

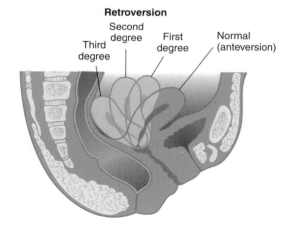

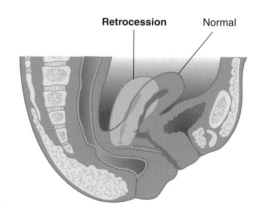

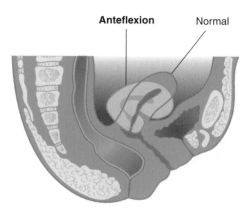

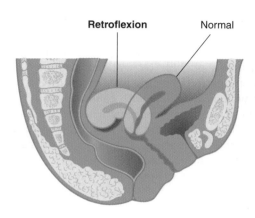

*FIGURE* 20-3 • Variations in uterine positions.

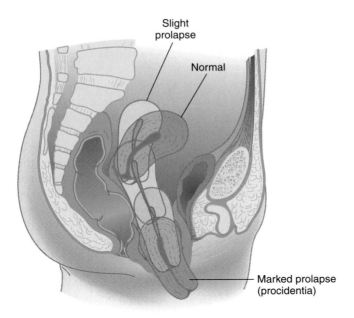

*FIGURE 20-4* • Prolapsed uterus.

at a surgical site such as an episiotomy, or obstetric trauma. Approximately 75% of all fistulas follow gynecologic surgery. Common types of fistulas are those that occur between the following:

- bladder and genital tract—called **vesicovaginal**
- urethra and vagina—called **urethrovaginal**
- rectum or sigmoid colon and vagina—called **rectovaginal** (Figure 20-7)

### Nursing Assessment

Nursing intervention should focus on encouraging the mother to acknowledge the problem and seek diagnosis and treatment. Many women think that this is a normal outcome of pregnancy or are embarrassed by these symptoms and therefore delay seeking care for the condition. Many incontinence centers for women are now available. They provide successful treatment for lingering urinary incontinence resulting from childbirth. Ask every woman if she is having this problem. This provides the opportunity not only to assist her with education and a possible referral but also enables her to spread the word that this isn't necessarily a condition that a woman must live with constantly.

Although some women experience no symptoms from uterine displacement and prolapse, others will report an uncomfortable sensation of fullness or that they can feel something in their vagina.

Women with a cystocele or rectocele also may not have any symptoms. Others report annoying sensations of fullness in the vagina, urinary frequency, urinary retention, urinary incontinence, recurrent cystitis, or UTIs. Rectoceles, while causing some women no difficulty, cause other women a disturbance in bowel function.

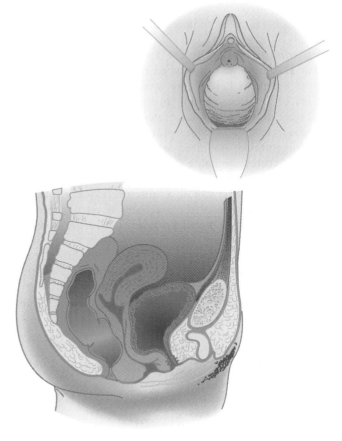

*FIGURE 20-5* • Cystocele.

Signs and symptoms of fistulas are related to the type of fistula. If the opening involves the rectum, feces will leak through the vagina. If it involves the bladder, urine will leak from the vagina. Depending on the placement and size of the fistula, the woman may or may not experience discomfort.

### Possible Nursing Diagnoses

For a woman with this condition, nursing diagnoses may focus on knowledge development that will affect her comfort and body image. Knowledge deficit related to exploration of cause and selection of possible interventions is common.

### Goals of Care

With guidance, support, and information, the woman may be able to learn the true origin of her condition. With appropriate intervention, she will regain control of her urinary incontinence.

### Self-Care

If the urinary incontinence is due to tissue trauma during the birth process the situation may improve as the tissues heal. To assist in the process the woman may do pelvic floor exercises to strengthen the muscles in the pelvis.

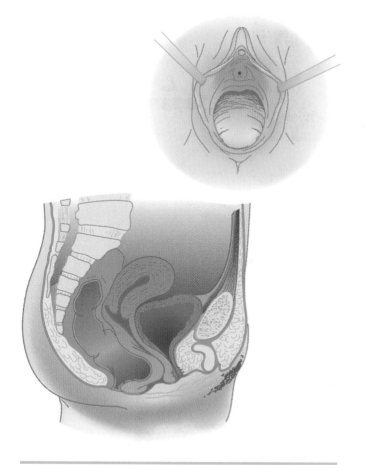

FIGURE 20-6 • Rectocele.

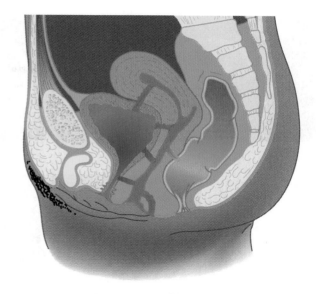

FIGURE 20-7 • Locations of fistulas.

Some women find that holding weights in the vagina helps strengthen the muscles. These weights are shaped like a tampon and are coated with Teflon. The woman inserts the lightest weight into her vagina and holds it in place as she goes through her day. Over time she gradually uses heavier and heavier weights, rebuilding the strength of the muscles.

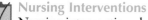 Nursing Interventions

Nursing interventions begin with ensuring that the woman understands her anatomy and a history of the changes she is experiencing. Often the woman will have to be convinced that what she is experiencing is not a normal side effect of the birth process—something to be endured as a "badge of courage." What she has been taught by her family members and friends and the expectations of her cultural group will have a strong effect on what she reports and how she responds to offered care.

If the problem is pelvic floor relaxation, the woman will need a review of the process of how to do pelvic floor exercises correctly. If the nurse-midwife or physician determines that the vaginal weights would be helpful, she will need to learn how to use them appropriately. The weights are expensive and are not always covered by insurance, so they may not be an option for the woman.

If the diagnostic workup determines that the cause is something other than birth trauma, the woman will need additional support, information, and interventions. This may range from the use of medication to further testing and treatment plans for her specific condition.

Treatment for uterine displacement includes educating the woman about the condition and teaching her that pelvic floor exercises and assuming a knee-chest position may be used to increase her comfort and encourage recovery from a mild retroversion.

Treatment for a cystocele includes use of a pessary or surgical repair. In an anterior surgical repair, the pelvic muscle is shortened to provide better bladder support.

Small rectoceles may be treated with a high-fiber diet, increase in fluid intake, stool softeners, and/or mild laxatives. Large rectoceles causing major symptoms are surgically repaired. A posterior surgical repair similar to the anterior repair for the cystocele is the usual procedure. Often the anterior and posterior repairs are done at the same time, either with or without vaginal hysterectomy.

Treatment for a prolapse depends on the degree of prolapse. If it is determined that a pessary would be helpful to hold the uterus in correct position, the woman will require education concerning the hygiene related to use of a pessary and how and when to wear it (Figure 20-8).

For some women with a severe prolapse, the recommended treatment may be a hysterectomy. If it is determined that surgical intervention may correct the problem, the woman requires information about the procedure, including the actual expectations of improvement and the risks of undergoing surgery.

Small fistulas may heal spontaneously without treatment. Large fistulas often require surgical repair that cannot take place until the edema or inflammation in

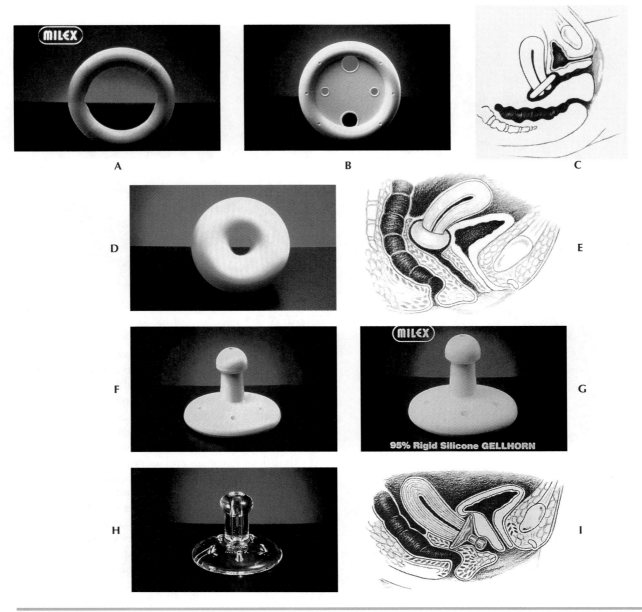

*FIGURE 20-8* • Pessaries for prolapsed uterus. **A,** Ring pessary for first and second degree mild prolapse. **B,** Ring with support for mild prolapse complicated by mild cystocele. **C,** Ring pessary in position. **D,** The donut pessary offers effective support for third degree prolapse/procidentia. **E,** Donut pessary in position. **F,** The flexible Gellhorn offers effective support in third-degree prolapse/procidentia. Its flexibility allows for easier insertion and removal. **G,** The Gellhorn provides greater comfort and similar support, and **H,** offers effective support in third-degree prolapse/procidentia. **I,** Gellhorn pessary in position. *(Courtesy of Milex Products, Inc., Chicago.)*

the surrounding tissues has dissipated. That process may take months. In difficult cases, it may be necessary for the surgery to include an ileal conduit or temporary colostomy (Lewis, Heitkemper, and Dirksen, 1999) (Box 20-9).

### Evaluation

Assess the level of a woman's understanding of her specific conditions and the choices available to her. Have the woman verbalize her understanding of all instructions for the therapy she chooses so that the condition

does not lead to more serious complications. Her recovery will be determined in part by the support she receives from family members and friends, so evaluate the functioning of her support system. Assessment of her ability to connect with a supportive environment, ongoing health care, and community services is vital as she gradually resumes care for herself and her newborn.

### Summary

Because many women don't understand the structure and placement of their internal organs, they also do not understand when the integrity of the organs is damaged. Shame and fear may delay the reporting of symptoms or the desire for intervention. Sensitivity and knowledge of the situation are required for effective diagnosis and offering of treatment interventions. Women vary a great deal in the choices they make and the interventions they choose. The woman's needs, both physical and emotional, and the needs of her family must be addressed.

## Psychologic Conditions

Fatigue, role changes, and an unforeseen future all have an impact on a family trying to adjust to a new baby. For the new mother, who is also experiencing hormonal changes and the return of her body to a nonpregnant state, the times are even more trying.

**Postpartum depression (PPD)** tends to manifest insidiously within 2 weeks postpartum to 1 year following childbirth. Symptoms may range from mild to severe and are distinguished from the "baby blues" by their intensity and degree. Additionally, new symptoms consistent with a diagnosis of depression manifest (Herz, 1992).

The etiology of PPD is multifactorial and is thought to include a complex interplay of cultural, social, psychologic, and biologic factors (Dunnewold and Sanford, 1994). Social factors include social isolation or a lack of social support (Collins and others, 1993), discord in the primary relationship (Sheppard, 1994; O'Hara, 1995), and recent life stressors (Carsoni, David, and Berthiaume, 1993). Cultural factors include a lack of rituals that support and recognize the new mother (Harkness, 1987; Kruckman, 1992). Biologic factors include adverse responses to biochemical and hormonal shifts (Epperson, 1999). Psychologic factors may include an infant with a difficult temperament (Gelfano and Teti, 1990; Carsoni, David, and Berthiaume, 1993); the mother's perceptions

about the birth experience as problematic or as an experience in which she felt helpless and disempowered (Edwards, Porter, and Stein, 1994); and a vulnerability to depression (Campbell and others, 1992; O'Hara, 1995). Further, contemporary economic conditions, the increased mobility of the family, and changes in childbirth practices have been proposed as possible etiologic factors in the development of PPD (Locicero, Weiss, and Issokson, 1997).

### Anticipated Issues

Mental health disorders have implications not only for the mother and baby but also for all family members. New mothers can shift between euphoria and depression. Family members may downplay the signals the mother is giving in hopes that the changes go away. Alternatively, the mother's behavior may be confusing to the family and cause them to withdraw.

**Postpartum "Blues."** The most common condition is "postpartum blues," a mild and transient depression that occurs in 50% to 80% of postpartum women on the third to eighth day after childbirth and may last from a few hours to several weeks. For many women and their families, it is considered a "normal" part of the adjustment during the postpartum period. It is covered in more detail in Chapter 15.

**Postpartum Depression.** Postpartum depression differs from postpartum blues in that it is an intense pervasive sadness with subtle changes in personality. There are no periods of happiness, just degrees of sadness. Women with PPD experience increasing sleep disturbances that result in a loss of energy and an inability to function. They experience eating problems, feelings of inadequacy with regard to the maternal role, dysphoria, preoccupation with self-deprecatory thoughts, overconcern or a lack of concern for the infant, possible suicidal ideation and withdrawal and social isolation that is accompanied by complaints about a lack of emotional support. When these feelings of despondency and anxiety continue, this is not a normal part of postpartum blues (Shrock, 1994).

About 10% to 15% of all mothers experience postpartum depression. It can occur at anytime during the first postpartum year; however, 60% to 70% of the women with this condition have it occur between 3 weeks and 3 months (Beck, 1999). As many as 25% of these women will develop chronic depression (Youngkin and Davis, 1998).

Maternal depression also has been shown to have a moderate to large adverse effect on children's behavior and developmental functioning (Beck, 1995b). In the postpartum period, depression may limit the mother's ability to read and respond to her infant's verbal and behavioral cues. Further, women with postpartum depression have been reported to have less verbal and physical interaction with their infants (Sameroff, Siefer, and Zax, 1982). Women that are moderately to severely depressed have been reported to demonstrate aggression towards their children (Zuravin, 1989). Additionally, studies have demonstrated that infants of depressed mothers tend to be fussier, less content, avoidant, and make fewer positive facial expressions and vocalizations than infants of nondepressed mothers (Field, 1984; Field and others, 1988).

***Postpartum Psychosis.*** Postpartum psychosis has the same traits as postpartum depression but with the added feature of delusions, hallucinations, and phobias with possible thoughts of harming either the infant or herself. Onset may occur at any time during the postpartum year. A much rarer disorder, this occurs in 1 to 2 per 1000 births (Kaplan, Sadock, and Grebb, 1994). A woman who experiences postpartum depression with psychosis once has a 35% to 60% likelihood of recurrence during subsequent births (APA, 1994).

### Nursing Assessment

Assessment is based on perceived changes in the new mother's behaviors, reports from her, or reports from the members of her support system. The symptoms may initially be similar for all three conditions. However, the length of time the symptoms are present and the inten-

sity of the woman's response increases with the more serious conditions.

***Baby Blues.*** A woman with "baby blues" may report feeling fine 1 minute and sad the next. Mothers may be weepy, irritable, feel anxious or fatigued, have difficulty sleeping, and have headaches. Some women may express feeling depersonalized or deserted as they and their contribution are ignored while the new baby is showered with attention. When asked, some will say that they felt like they had done all of the work for 9 months and after the birth it was like they didn't even exist.

***Postpartum Depression.*** New mothers with a major depression feel incompetent and inadequate in their parenting ability. According to Fishel (1995) at least five of the following components must be present every day for diagnosis of major depression:

* Depressed mood, often with spontaneous crying
* Markedly diminished interest in all activities
* Insomnia or hypersomnia
* Weight changes

---

**TABLE 20-1** *Assessment of Postpartum Depression*

| Symptoms | Assessment questions |
|---|---|
| Dysphoria | Describe any changes you have experienced in your mood since the birth of your infant? How strong is this feeling? |
| Appetite | How has your appetite been lately? |
| Sleep disturbances | Describe what a typical night's sleep has been like since the birth of your infant? Are you sleeping longer or more than usual? |
| Fatigue | What has your energy level been like since the birth of your infant? How does this compare to your usual energy level? |
| Loss of interest | What kinds of things do you typically do that bring you pleasure and enjoyment? When was the last time you did one of those things? What are your current goals? |
| Lack of positive emotions | When caring for your infant what kinds of emotions do you feel? |
| Loss of self | Describe yourself before the birth of your infant. How does that person compare to the person you have become since the birth of your infant? How do you feel about your current life? |
| Loneliness | When was the last time you had an outing with your friends? How many people do you feel you can confide in who really understand what you have been experiencing as a new mother? How often have you felt lonely lately? |
| Insecurity | How insecure, fragile, or vulnerable do you feel? How overwhelmed are you by the responsibility of motherhood? |
| Loss of control | How "in control" of your emotions and thoughts are you feeling? |
| Guilt feelings | Many new mothers experience feelings of guilt or blame. Do you blame yourself for anything or feel guilty? |
| Concentration | How difficult is it for you to concentrate? How difficult has it been for you to make decisions? |
| Anxiety | How often have you experienced anxiety attacks? Chest pains? Palpitations? |
| Obsessive thinking | How often have you experienced having repetitive thoughts? (e.g., "What's wrong with me?" "Am I going crazy?" "Why can't I enjoy being with my baby?") |
| Suicidal ideation | How often have you had thoughts about harming yourself or your infant? How appealing is the thought of leaving this world to you? |

Adapted by Westcott J and Havener JE from Beck C: Screening methods for postpartum depression, *J Obstet Gynecol Neonatal Nurs,* 24:308-312, 1995b; and O'Hara MW and Engeldinger J: Postpartum mood disorders, *The Female Patient,* 14:136-141, 1989.

- Psychomotor retardation or agitation
- Fatigue or loss of energy
- Feelings of worthlessness or inappropriate guilt
- Diminished ability to concentrate
- Suicidal ideation with or without a plan

Shrock (1994) also noted that these mothers are irritable and may escalate to having outbursts that seem unwarranted. They can sob violently and aim their outbursts at their baby or other family members. One of the predominant features of this disorder may be jealousy and possible rejection of the baby. Women who experience postpartum depression with a psychosis may also express thoughts of harming their child.

***Postpartum Psychosis.*** Unlike postpartum depression, psychosis may have an early onset, occurring within days after delivery, and may initially be confused with postpartum blues. If a woman is experiencing postpartum depression with psychosis, symptoms of fatigue, insomnia, and restlessness may begin at any time from a few days after birth to 8 weeks, with the mean at 2 to 3 weeks postpartum.

Distinguishing features include severe functional impairment, confused thought processes, vivid hallucinations, and delusions. Further, some women may have psychotic depression and display symptoms congruent with PPD and psychosis. Delusions are present in approximately 50% and hallucinations in 25% (Kaplan, Saddock, and Grebb, 1994). In women with psychotic depression, the delusional and hallucinatory episodes may alternate with periods of apparently lucid thought. In those women who are psychotic, the potential for suicide and infanticide are high (Harberger, Berchtold, and Honikman, 1992). Mothers with this condition sometimes relate that they believe their baby is possessed by the devil and voices tell them to kill the baby.

The Postpartum Depression Checklist (Beck, 1995b) is an easy format with which to assess for depression. Assess all women and identify those with beginning symptoms because if PPD remains untreated, it may have long-term sequelae for the mother and infant (Table 20-1).

Assessment may be done through follow-up telephone calls or home visits to postpartum mothers. Other times it occurs during the woman's postpartum physical examination. It should also occur when the woman takes her infant for pediatric visits. Assessment includes making observations and asking specifically about sadness, loneliness, emptiness, or inability to find joy in things that would normally bring new mothers joy. Based on the information provided and intuition, it also may be necessary to ask the mother if she has had thoughts about harming herself or her baby. How these questions are phrased is important. To develop trust, say, "Some mothers say that they have felt like it wasn't worth living. Have you ever felt like that?" If the mother says "yes" the answer should be explored further. Appropriate follow-up care and referral should follow (Box 20-10).

### Possible Nursing Diagnoses

For women experiencing depression during the postpartum a quick correct diagnosis is an essential aspect of caring. This is based on astute observations and intuition that something might be wrong with the mother (Beck, 1995a). Nursing diagnoses focus on the impairment the postpartum depression may be creating for the woman and her family. If the depression is a major mood disorder, the risk of harm to the mother or the infant must be considered. Knowledge about the possible range of depression in the postpartum period and how to respond is a focus for intervention with the woman's support network.

---

### BOX 20-10   *Assessment Interview for Postpartum Depression*

Heed the following points during the conduction of an assessment interview for postpartum depression:

- Pay attention to your own emotions. Our own experiences shape our attitudes and receptivity to a woman who is depressed about having a baby. It is important for her to experience a nonjudgmental response.
- Ask questions in an open-ended manner that does not presume an answer (e.g., "Tell me how you feel when you see the baby smile at you"). Leading questions make it more difficult for the new mother to communicate any negative emotions that she might be feeling (e.g., "It must be great to see him smile at you").
- Mirror the patient's language. For example, if the mother describes the infant as difficult, ask her to describe the ways in which the infant is difficult. This will

make the woman feel listened to and make her more likely to place trust in you as a caregiver.

- Questions should reflect an understanding that each birth experience is unique and brings certain contextual challenges.
- Watch for overly rigid or limited answers that may indicate that you may have moved in too close, either spatially or psychologically.
- Disorganized, tangential, or unrestrained answers may require some structuring or classifying of issues through use of communication techniques such as validation and reiteration. Physical grounding—a touch on the arm and eye contact—may be helpful in refocusing the woman, but do not touch the woman without her permission to do so.

Adapted by Westcott J and Havener JE from Issoksen D: *Postpartum depression.* Presented at Medical Grand Rounds, Bassett Healthcare, Cooperstown, New York, December 9, 1998.

### Self-Care

Understanding the mood changes possible during the postpartum period provides women with the ability to do a self-assessment. When experiencing "the blues" a woman and her family can take comfort in the fact that this is within the range of normal and that it will pass. Recognition of the less common postpartum experience of depression by the woman or her family and seeking care are also forms of self-care.

### Nursing Interventions

Women must become aware that the feelings they are having may be dealt with and that there is hope that her living nightmare will end. Being with the woman, understanding her experience, and sharing valuable time with her is an important sign of care.

*Postpartum Depression.* Women who have been diagnosed with postpartum depression benefit from an integrated approach to treatment that acknowledges its multicausal nature. An integrated network of services that includes sensitive health care for the mother and infant, postpartum exercise classes, home-visiting services, parenting education, family support programs and lactation support may provide the best intervention (Locicero, Weiss, and Issoksen, 1997). Additionally, services for the woman with depression might include mother-infant psychiatric units, a mutual support group, pregnancy loss groups, and postcesarean support. Most women live in communities that have a variety of these services available; however, the degree of integration of services varies. Identify the woman in need of services and then put together the appropriate network of care. To optimize care a collaborative model that makes possible multiple points of entry and freedom of movement within the network works best.

During the time that a woman is receiving care for her depression, facilitate to the extent possible her maternal attachment. Encourage family support for the woman and ongoing assessment of her condition. This disorder has a favorable outcome when diagnosis is made early in the disorder and treatment is implemented.

*Postpartum Psychosis.* Postpartum psychosis is a psychiatric emergency that requires antidepressant therapy and hospitalization. If diagnosed and treated early on, the prognosis for these women is good, although they may experience subsequent episodes of psychosis.

Although contact with the baby should be maintained while the woman is in treatment, the interactions should be closely supervised until the threat of infanticide passes. Preferably these mothers can be placed on mother-baby units or units that allow unrestricted visitation of the infant. Removal of the infant should be done only in extreme cases when the infant's safety is an issue and cannot be guaranteed.

Regardless of whether the mother experiences inpatient or outpatient treatment, the use of psychotropic medications along with counseling and supports is required. Antidepressant medications such as tricyclic antidepressants and selective serotonin reuptake inhibitors (SSRIs) most frequently are prescribed for women with moderate to severe depressive symptoms. Clinical improvement can generally be expected within 2 to 4 weeks.

Women choosing to use the drug fluoxetine (Prozac) while breastfeeding should be encouraged to have the infant's blood tested after 6 weeks to rule out toxic accumulations of the drug (Epperson, 1999). Haloperidol (Haldol) also may be used in treatment of postpartum psychosis and usually is considered compatible with breastfeeding. Although the American Academy of Pediatrics (AAP) (1997) lists these medications as usually compatible with breastfeeding, they should be used with caution (Box 20-11).

### Considerations for Future Care

Women who experience postpartum depression are at a higher risk of having it occur with subsequent pregnancies. Lithium may be used preventively for those with a previous history of affective psychosis. These women will require close and frequent follow-up through the first 2 months postpartum. Sichel and others (1995) report that oral administration of high-dose estrogen immediately after birth can reduce the rate of postpartum depression to 9%.

### Evaluation

Assess the level of a woman's understanding of her treatment plan. Have the woman verbalize her understanding of all instructions and where she may seek resources within the community. Make the appropriate referrals as necessary. Her success will be determined in part by the support she receives from family members and friends, so the functioning of her support system

---

**BOX 20-11**    *Expectations of a Woman with Postpartum Depression*

The woman and her support system will:
- Understand the signs and symptoms of depression and the need to seek help when evidence of depression is observed.
- Understand the etiology and management of the psychiatric disorder.
- Verbalize the limitations she may experience related to her postpartum depression.
- Understand the woman's need for social support and be able to name the people that she will contact to provide this support.

Her support system will:
- Understand the effect their patience, care, and positive support can have on the mother's recovery.

must be evaluated. In addition, her ability to connect with a supportive environment, ongoing health care, and community services is vital.

## Summary

The postpartum period is generally negotiated without many serious mental health problems. However, for the new mothers and their families that must confront clinical depression, the experience can be unsettling. Dealing with the mental health issues robs them of the precious beginnings of family life with their new baby, and in the most serious cases, may remove the women from the family situation. By understanding the warning signs, women and their families may be assisted in determining the difference between expected postpartum blues and indications of serious depression and responding appropriately. The women's needs and the needs of their families must be addressed.

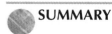

## SUMMARY

Most women come through the experience of pregnancy and birth without health problems. The minority that do experience threats to their health are often at home providing their own care when these potentially life-threatening changes occur. Women must feel empowered to make their own determination that they are in need of health services and then seek out the necessary resources. They do this while still considering and attempting to arrange how others will take on the role they fill within their family and the care of the infant. Care of the woman with postpartum complications must be multifaceted and inclusive of the woman, her infant, and her support network.

## Care Plan • Nursing Care Plan for the Woman with Postpartum Infection

NURSING DIAGNOSIS    **Risk for puerperal infection (metritis, wound infection, urinary tract infection)** related to multiple risk factors (abdominal birth, vaginal birth, necrosis of endometrial lining, lacerations, episiotomy)

GOALS/OUTCOMES    Infection will not occur

**NOC Suggested Outcomes**
- Infection Status (0703)
- Maternal Status: Postpartum (2511)
- Knowledge: Infection Control (1807)
- Risk Detection (1908)
- Risk Control (1902)

**NIC Priority Interventions**
- Infection Protection (6550)
- Incision Site Care (3440)
- Postpartal Care (6930)

**Nursing Activities & Rationale**
- Maintain careful hand washing. *Hand washing is the most important method of controlling the spread of microorganisms.*
- Teach woman to maintain asepsis of incisions or lacerations. *Aseptic practices reduce or eliminate pathogenic contamination of wounds, lacerations, or others breaches in the skin or mucous membranes.*
- Assess for risk factors (e.g., incision, lacerations, presence of known infection, depressed immune state). *To detect factors that place the woman at increased risk for the development of infection.*
- Monitor incisions/lacerations using REEDA scale. *To detect developing or existing localized infection* (e.g., discomfort, erythema, edema, warmth, drainage, wound seperation).
- Monitor for signs of systemic infection (e.g., elevated temperature, increased heart rate, increased respirations). *To detect the presence of systemic infection for early treatment and prevention of complications.*
- Monitor character and odor of lochia. *Foul odor and increased amount of lochia suggest endometrial infection.*
- Monitor for uterine subinvolution. *Subinvolution may indicate the presence of endometrial infection.*
- Monitor urine appearance, smell, and quantity. *To detect the presence of UTI. Dysuria, urinary frequency and urgency, and foul smelling urine indicates the presence of infection.*
- Encourage woman to maintain perineal hygiene. *To reduce the number of microorganisms, prevent wound contamination, and prevent infection.*
- Obtain specimens for laboratory tests when ordered for indications of infection (e.g., white blood cell count, differential). *To detect the presence of a localized or systemic infection.*

*Continued*

## Care Plan · Nursing Care Plan for the Woman with Postpartum Infection—cont'd

- Encourage adequate fluid intake. *Hydration helps prevent urinary stasis, which contributes to urinary tract infection.*
- Confer with nurse practitioner, nurse-midwife or physician regarding abnormal laboratory values. *To promote the initiation of early treatment measures to prevent the spread of infection or complications associated with infection.*
- Teach woman signs and symptoms of infection that must be reported. *To make the woman aware of the need to self-monitor for infection, report signs of infection, and access treatment in a timely manner should an infection develop.*

### Evaluation Parameters
- No evidence of localized or systemic infection.
- Surgical margins are well-approximated and without drainage, redness, swelling, pain.
- No reported difficulty with urination.
- WBC and differential within normal limits.
- Woman demonstrates appropriate perineal care.
- Normal uterine involution observed.
- Woman verbalizes understanding of methods to reduce risks for infection after returning home.

NURSING DIAGNOSIS  **Potential complications of postpartum infection: sepsis, septic shock**

GOALS/OUTCOMES  Resolution of infection; complications of infection will not occur

### NOC Suggested Outcomes
- Infection Status (248)
- Tissue Perfusion: cardiac (0405)
- Tissue Perfusion: cerebral (0406)
- Vital Sign Status (0802)

### NIC Priority Interventions
- Surveillance (6650)
- Infection Control (6540)
- Medication Management (2380)
- Shock Prevention (4260)

### Nursing Activities & Rationale
- Monitor for changes in the woman's infection status (e.g., fever, incision, urinary elimination). *To determine effectiveness of collaborative interventions.*
- Collaborate with nurse practitioner, nurse-midwife, or physician to implement treatment protocols. *To provide early and appropriate treatment interventions to quickly reduce the presence of infection.*
- Use careful hand washing procedures. *Hand washing is one of the most effective means of preventing the spread of infection.*
- Assess woman's ability to take prescribed antibiotics. *Determine if she has ever had a negative reaction to the prescribed antibiotic. Be sure that she has access to the prescribed medication.*
- Teach woman to take antibiotics as prescribed. *To maintain blood levels and increase the potential for infection elimination.*
- Monitor for prescribed antibiotic effectiveness. *To determine the appropriateness of treatment and the need for discontinuing an ineffective drug.*
- Monitor culture and sensitivity reports. *To identify infectious pathogen and assist with selection of appropriate antibiotic therapy.*
- Monitor for trends in vital signs, capillary refill, mucous membranes, and nail beds. *To detect impending shock related to sepsis.*
- Monitor for indications of inadequate tissue perfusion (e.g., hypotension, narrowing of pulse pressure, tachycardia, hyperthermia, tachypena, confusion, cyanosis). *To detect the presence of sepsis and developing septic shock.*
- Teach woman how to identify potential complications of infection and where and when health care should be sought. *Woman will be monitoring her own progress between nurse visits. She must know the signs and symptoms indicating a possible problem and be able to respond appropriately.*

### Evaluation Parameters
- Heart rate, blood pressure, temperature, color, capillary refill, and mucous membranes within normal limits.
- WBC and differential within normal limits.

## Care Plan · Nursing Care Plan for the Woman with Postpartum Infection—cont'd

**NURSING DIAGNOSIS**   **Nutrition: less than body requirements** related to anorexia, nausea/vomiting secondary to localized or systemic infection

**GOALS/OUTCOMES**   Woman will maintain optimal nutritional and fluid status (*See "Evaluation Parameters"*)

### NOC Suggested Outcomes
- Nutritional Status (1004)
- Nutritional Status: Food and Fluid Intake (1008)
- Nutritional Status: Nutrient Intake (1009)

### NIC Priority Interventions
- Nutritional Monitoring (1160)
- Nutrition Management (1100)
- Fluid Monitoring (4130)

### Nursing Activities & Rationale
- Monitor woman's weight. *To assess effect of anorexia, nausea, and vomiting and need for intervention.*
- Monitor laboratory values when tests are ordered. *To detect negative nitrogen balance, electrolyte balance, etc.*
- Monitor skin turgor, oral mucous membranes, and urinary output. *To detect adequacy of hydration.*
- Monitor dietary intake. *To determine adequacy of nutritional content and calories.*
- Consult with dietitian to establish protein requirements resulting from protein loss secondary to infection. *To assist with planning for protein replacement.*
- Ascertain woman's food preferences. *Women are more likely to eat foods they enjoy.*
- Serve small, frequent meals rather than large meals. *To maintain stable blood glucose levels. Smaller meals are more readily consumed in their entirety than large meals.*
- Monitor woman's fluid intake. *Sufficient fluid intake is necessary for production of adequate breast milk.*
- Monitor woman's ability to provide adequate breast milk for her baby during recovery. *To prevent nutritional deficit for baby during the woman's recovery, supplementation may be necessary.*

### Evaluation Parameters
- Woman tolerates prescribed diet.
- Woman maintains body mass and weight within normal limits.
- Moist oral mucous membranes.
- Elastic skin turgor.
- Laboratory values (e.g., transferrin, albumin, electrolytes) within normal limits.
- Woman reports adequate energy levels.
- Woman denies anorexia or nausea.

**NURSING DIAGNOSIS**   **Fear** related to threat to one's own well-being secondary to presence of infection

**GOALS/OUTCOMES**   Reports anxiety is at a manageable level and reduced fear; no behavioral manifestations of anxiety (*See "Evaluation Parameters"*)

### NOC Suggested Outcomes
- Anxiety Control (1402)
- Coping (1302)
- Fear Control (1404)
- Social Support (1504)

### NIC Priority Interventions
- Anxiety Reduction (5820)
- Coping Enhancement (5230)
- Emotional Support (5270)
- Presence (5340)

### Nursing Activities & Rationale
- Assess woman's reaction to presence of infection and correct misconceptions. *To establish a baseline for care planning. Correcting misconceptions and supplying factual information may reduce fear and anxiety.*
- Use a calm, reassuring approach (NIC). *To prevent transference of anxiety to woman during stressful situation. To help woman maintain control when feeling stressed.*
- Encourage verbalization of feelings, fears and anxiety. *To help woman identify fears and concerns. Enables the correction of misunderstandings.*
- Support the use of appropriate defense mechanisms that have been successful in the past. *To build on present strengths.*

*Continued*

## Care Plan · Nursing Care Plan for the Woman with Postpartum Infection—cont'd

- Assess for anxiety on the part of the woman or her family members. *The woman and/or family members may be concerned about the possibility of hospitalization or serious health risk related to infection.*

### Evaluation Parameters
- Reports decreased anxiety appropriate to situational crisis (infection).
- No change in vital signs (blood pressure and pulse) related to anxiety/fear.
- Able to focus and follow directions.
- Able to communicate needs.

NURSING DIAGNOSIS    **Pain** related to localized or systemic infection
GOALS/OUTCOMES    Maintains optimal level of comfort (*See "Evaluation Parameters"*)

### NOC Suggested Outcomes
- Comfort Level (2100)
- Pain Control (1605)
- Pain: Disruptive Effects (2101)
- Pain Level (2102)

### NIC Priority Interventions
- Analgesic Administration (2210)
- Pain Management (1400)

### Nursing Activities & Rationale
- Ask woman what pain-relief measure she prefers; provide information as needed. *Allows her to have control over her pain and use measures she feels will benefit her.*
- Monitor effectiveness of pain-relief measures (see "Evaluation Parameters"). *Different pain relief measures may be needed if pain is not well-controlled.*
- Ask the family to assist with basic comfort measures (e.g., maintaining dry linens, applying a cool cloth to forehead or providing lip balm). *If basic needs are being met, woman can focus on relaxation technique to increase level of comfort.*
- Monitor for side effects of pharmacologic agents (e.g., respirations, level of consciousness, blood pressure). *Close monitoring is needed for the woman who is at risk for shock from sepsis in order to achieve a balance between pain relief and dosages that create unwanted or dangerous side effects.*

### Evaluation Parameters
- No change in pulse, blood pressure, or respirations (or return to normal).
- Reports acceptable comfort level.
- Demonstrates minimal restlessness and muscle tension.

### Other Possible Nursing Diagnoses
- **Activity intolerance** related to fatigue secondary to postpartum infection.
- **Risk for altered family processes** related to change in family roles, inability to assume usual role, or prolonged recovery secondary to postpartum infection.
- **Breastfeeding, interrupted** related to maternal illness (e.g., infection, sepsis).
- Family processes, altered **related to client's inability to assume family role secondary to prolonged recovery from infection.**

## CASE STUDY

Suzie and Steve had waited to conceive until they could afford a child. Suzie delivered a healthy baby boy after an uneventful pregnancy. She had a normal postpartum physiologic course. Friends and family visited her during her hospitalization and she seemed happy to be going home. The student nurse who cared for her remembered her as taking an active part in learning about care for herself and her baby. She asked appropriate questions and provided hands-on care to her infant.

The student nurse did a home visit when Sammy was 7 days old. Suzie and Steve were both in attendance and both seemed attentive to their baby. They talked about the help provided by Steve's parents who worked next door.

The student nurse received a call from the emergency room about 5 weeks later asking if she could come be with a patient she had previously cared for. Suzie had been brought to the emergency room having overdosed on an antidepressant. She had arrived by ambulance

## CASE STUDY

with her husband, baby, and both sets of parents following in their cars. Once she was stabilized it was noted that she was dirty and extremely thin. Her hair was matted, and she was wearing a sanitary napkin that was extremely odorous with thick dried matter. Her perineum appeared not to have been washed for some time. In contrast, her baby was spotless and calmly sleeping in an infant seat. The baby looked well-nourished.

The family related that Suzie had become more and more isolated over the past couple of weeks. Her obstetrician had prescribed a mild antidepressant at her 6-week visit for mild depression. Before her overdose, Suzie was staying in her room most of the time and had refused to cook or eat. During that time she was providing all of the care for the baby, feeding, bathing, dressing, and changing it. She was obsessive about the baby's care, but was doing nothing for herself.

Once she awoke she would not talk to anyone but kept asking for the student nurse by name. Once alone with the student nurse, initially Suzie would do nothing but hold the student's hand and cry. Slowly she began to talk about her feelings and her life over the past weeks. During the next few days Suzie related her need to have the student be with her to support her.

Over the next couple of months Suzie received extensive professional counseling. As she recovered she talked at length about her feelings of depression that just got deeper and deeper. She felt that she was of no value to anyone, even though she was providing almost all of her baby's care. At 6 months, Suzie was weaned from her antidepressants and resumed a normal life. The experience was so devastating, she and her husband chose not to have more children. Suzie has not experienced any further bouts with depression in the 20 years since that incident but she remembers her anguish vividly.

# Scenarios

1. Pamela and Peter came home with their full-term daughter 3 days ago; she is now 5 days old. The vaginal delivery was uncomplicated. Pamela was discharged with a diagnosis of iron-deficiency anemia. You are doing a well-baby visit in the home. Peter tells you that Pam seems really tired. He wants to know what is wrong and what he may do to help.

- What subjective and objective data do you need before you answer?
- What nursing diagnoses could apply for Pam? For Peter?
- What goals are necessary? How will these be prioritized?
- What nursing interventions can you provide?
- How will you evaluate the effectiveness of your interventions?

2. You are visiting Kimberly and her 1-week-old son at home. It says in her referral that she developed gestational diabetes during her pregnancy. Kimberly says that she is fine now; they just told her to "watch her diet and exercise" and to "call with any problems." She asks you, "What exactly does that all mean?"

- What subjective and objective data do you need before you answer?
- What nursing diagnoses could apply for Kimberly?
- How will you validate these?
- What goals are necessary? How will these be prioritized?
- What nursing interventions can you offer?
- How will you evaluate the effectiveness of your interventions?

3. Carlotta and James are the parents of a 4-day-old baby girl. Carlotta has a cardiac condition that necessitated her being hospitalized for the last month of her pregnancy. James is glad to have his partner and daughter at home now. He is assuming the care of the baby during the evening and night, and friends and family members are coming in during the day to help. James asks two questions: "What would be the best way for us to help while Carlotta regains her strength?" and "How long will the friends and relatives have to keep coming in?"

- What subjective and objective data do you need before you answer?

- What nursing diagnoses could apply for James? For Carlotta?
- How will you validate these?
- What goals are necessary? How will these be prioritized?
- What nursing interventions can you offer?
- How will you evaluate the effectiveness of your interventions?

---

4. Linda and Caroline are at home with their 15-day-old infant. Linda received her prenatal care at the women's health clinic and she calls you with an urgent question. "This is my first baby and I just don't know what is normal. I seem to be bleeding an awful lot. Is there something wrong with me?"

- What subjective and objective data do you need before you answer?
- What nursing diagnoses could apply for Linda?
- How will you validate these?

- What goals are necessary? How will these be prioritized?
- What nursing interventions can you offer?
- How will you evaluate the effectiveness of your interventions?

---

5. Fiona delivered a baby boy 14 days ago and is now the sole care provider of him and her 4-year-old daughter. She has come into the clinic for a new-baby visit. When you ask her how she is doing she says that for the last 2 days she has had a severe headache at the back of her head but other than that she is okay. Does this alarm you?

- What subjective and objective data do you need to further your assessment?
- What nursing diagnoses could apply to Fiona?
- How will you validate these?
- What nursing interventions are necessary?
- How will you evaluate the effectiveness of your interventions?

## REFERENCES

American Academy of Pediatrics and The American College of Obstetricians and Gynecologists: *Guideline for perinatal care,* ed 4, Washington, DC, 1997, The Association.

American Psychiatric Association (APA): *Diagnostic and statistical manual of mental disorders: DSM-IV,* ed 4, Washington, DC, 1994, The Association.

Beck CT: Perceptions of nurses caring by mothers experiencing postpartum depression, *J Obstet Gynecol Neonatal Nurs* 27:29-36, 1995a.

Beck CT: Screening methods for postpartum depression, *J Obstet Gynecol Neonatal Nurs* 24(4):308, 1995b.

Beck CT: Postpartum depression: stopping the thief that steals motherhood, *AWHONN Lifelines* 3(4):41-44, 1999.

Berg CJ and others: Pregnancy-related mortality in the United States, 1987-1990, *Obstet Gynecol* 88(2):161-167, 1996.

Calhoun BC and Brost B: Emergency management of sudden puerperal fever, *Obstet Gynecol Clin North Am* 22(2):357-367, 1995.

Campbell S and others: Course and correlates of postpartum depression during the transition to parenthood, *Dev Psychopathol* 4:29-47, 1992.

Carsoni D, David H, and Berthiaume M: *Psycho-social correlates of postpartum depression,* Paper presented at the 101st annual meeting of the American Psychological Association, Toronto, Canada, August, 1993.

Collins NL and others: Social support in pregnancy: psychosocial correlates of birth outcomes and postpartum depression, *Personality Social Psych* 65:1243-1258, 1993.

Cunningham FG: *Williams obstetrics,* ed 20, Stamford, Conn, 1997, Appleton & Lange.

Dunnewold A and Sanford D: *Postpartum survival guide,* Oakland, Calif, 1994, New Harbinger Publications.

Edwards D, Porter SM, and Stein GS: A pilot study of postnatal depression following cesarean section using two retrospective self-rating instruments, *J Psychosomatic Res* 38:111-117, 1994.

Epperson CN: Postpartum major depression: detection and treatment, *Am Fam Physician* 59(8):2247-2254, 1999.

Field T: Early interactions between infants and their postpartum depressed mothers, *Infant Behavior Dev* 7:517-522, 1984.

Field T and others: Infants of depressed mothers show "depressed" behavior even with nondepressed adults, *Child Dev* 59:1569-1579, 1988.

Fishel A: Mental health. In Fogel C and Woods N, editors: *Women's health care,* Thousand Oaks, Calif, 1995, Sage Publications.

Gelfano D and Teti D: The effects of maternal postpartum depression on children, *Clin Psychol Rev* 10:329-3, 1990.

Gilbert ES and Harmon JS: *High risk pregnancy and delivery,* ed 2, St Louis, 1998, Mosby.

Harberger P, Berchtold N, and Honikman J: Cries for help. In Hamilton JA and Harberger PN, editors: *Postpartum psychiatric illness: a picture puzzle,* Philadelphia, 1992, University of Pennsylvania Press.

Harkness S: The cultural mediation of postpartum depression, *Med Anthropol Q* 1:194-209, 1987.

Herz EK: Prediction, recognition, and prevention. In Hamilton JA and Harberger PN, editors: *Postpartum psychiatric illness: a picture puzzle,* Philadelphia, 1992, University of Pennsylvania Press.

Kaplan HI, Sadock BJ, and Grebb JA: *Kaplan and Sadock's synopsis of psychiatry: behavioral sciences, clinical psychiatry,* ed 7, Baltimore, Md, 1994, Williams & Wilkins.

Knuppel RA and Hatangadi SB: Acute hypotension related to hemorrhage in the obstetric patient, *Obstet Gynecol Clin North Am* 22(1):111-129, 1995.

Kruckman LD: Rituals and support: an anthropological view of postpartum depression. In Hamilton JA and Harberger PN, editors: *Postpartum psychiatric illness: a picture puzzle,* Philadelphia, 1992, University of Pennsylvania Press.

Lewis S, Heitkemper M, and Dirksen S: *Medical surgical nursing: assessment and management of clinical problems,* ed 5, St Louis, 1999, Mosby.

Locicero AK, Weiss DM, and Issokson D: Postpartum depression: proposal for prevention through an integrated care and support network, *Appl Prevent Psychol* 6:169-178, 1997.

Mattson S and Smith JE, editors: *Core curriculum for maternal newborn nursing*, ed 2, Philadelphia, 2000, WB Saunders.

Norris TC: Management of postpartum hemorrhage, *Am Fam Physician* 55:635-640, 1997.

O'Hara MW: Postpartum depression: causes and consequences, New York, 1995, Springer.

Sameroff J, Siefer R, and Zax M: Early development of children at risk for emotional disorders, *Mono Soc Res Child Dev* 47:1-74, 1982.

Sampselle CM and others: Continence for women: evidence-based practice, *J Obstet Gynecol Neonatal Nurs* 26(4), 375-385, 1997.

Sheppard M: Postnatal depression, child care and social support: a review of findings and their implications for practice, *Soc Work Soc Sci Rev* S(1):24-26, 1994.

Shrock P: More than baby blues, *Adv Nurse Pract* 2(6):24, 1994.

Sichel DA and others: Prophylactic estrogen in recurrent postpartum affective disorder, *Biolog Psych* 38(12):814-818, 1995.

Simpson KR and Creehan PA: *AWHONN perinatal nursing*, Philadelphia, 1996, Lippincott.

Youngkin EQ and Davis MS: *Women's health—a primary care clinical guide*, ed 2, Stamford, Conn, 1998, Appleton & Lange.

Zuravin S: Severity of maternal depression and three types of mother-to-child aggression, *Am J Orthopsychiatry* 59:377-389, 1989.

# Pregnant Patient's Bill of Rights

The Pregnant Patient has the right to participate in decisions involving her well-being and that of her unborn child, unless there is a clear-cut medical emergency that prevents her participation. In addition to the rights set forth in the American Hospital Association's "Patient's Bill of Rights," the Pregnant Patient, because she represents two patients rather than one, should be recognized as having the following additional rights*:

1. The Pregnant Patient has the right, before the administration of any drug or procedure, to be informed by the health care professional caring for her of any potential direct or indirect effects, risks, or hazards to herself or her unborn or newborn infant that may result from the use of a drug or procedure prescribed for or administered to her during pregnancy, labor, birth, or lactation.

2. The Pregnant Patient has the right, before the proposed therapy, to be informed not only of the benefits, risks, and hazards of the proposed therapy but also of any known alternative therapies, such as available childbirth education classes that could help prepare the Pregnant Patient physically and mentally to cope with the discomfort or stress of pregnancy and the experience of childbirth, thereby reducing or eliminating her need for drugs and obstetric intervention. She should be offered such information early in her pregnancy so that she may make a reasoned decision.

3. The Pregnant Patient has the right, before the administration of any drug, to be informed by the health care professional who is prescribing or administering the drug to her that any drug that she receives during pregnancy, labor, and birth, no matter how or when the drug is taken or administered, may adversely affect her unborn infant, directly or indirectly, and that there is no drug or chemical that has been proven safe for an unborn child.

4. The Pregnant Patient has the right, if cesarean birth is anticipated, to be informed before the administration of any drug, and preferably before her hospitalization, that minimizing her and, in turn, her infant's intake of nonessential preoperative medicine will benefit her infant.

5. The Pregnant Patient has the right, before the administration of a drug or procedure, to be informed of the areas of uncertainty if there is no properly controlled follow-up research that has established the safety of the drug or procedure with regard to its direct or indirect effects on the physiologic, mental, and neurologic development of the child exposed, via the mother, to the drug or procedure during pregnancy, labor, birth, or lactation (this would apply to virtually all drugs and the vast majority of obstetric procedures).

6. The Pregnant Patient has the right, before the administration of any drug, to be informed of the brand and generic names of the drug so that she may advise the health care professional of any past adverse reaction to the drug.

7. The Pregnant Patient has the right to determine for herself, without pressure from her attendant, whether she will accept the risks inherent in the proposed therapy or refuse a drug or procedure.

8. The Pregnant Patient has the right to know the name and qualifications of the individual administering a medication or procedure to her during labor or birth.

9. The Pregnant Patient has the right to be informed, before the administration of any procedure, whether that procedure is being administered to her for her or her infant's benefit (medically indicated) or as an elective procedure (for convenience, teaching purposes, or research).

*From Haire DB: The pregnant patient's bill of rights, *J Nurse Midwifery* 20:29, 1975. (From Committee on Patient's Rights, Box 1900, New York, NY 10001.)

10. The Pregnant Patient has the right to be accompanied during the stress of labor and birth by someone she cares for and someone to whom she looks for emotional comfort and encouragement.
11. The Pregnant Patient has the right after appropriate medical consultation to choose a position for labor and birth that is the least stressful to her infant and to herself.
12. The Obstetric Patient has the right to have her infant cared for at her bedside if her infant is normal and to feed her infant according to her infant's needs rather than according to the hospital regimen.
13. The Obstetric Patient has the right to be informed in writing of the name of the person who actually delivered her infant and the professional qualifications of that person. This information should also be provided on the birth certificate.
14. The Obstetric Patient has the right to be informed if there is any known or indicated aspect of her or her infant's care or condition that may cause her or her infant later difficulty or problems.
15. The Obstetric Patient has the right to have her and her infant's hospital medical records complete, accurate, and legible and to have their records, including nurses' notes, retained by the hospital until the child reaches at least the age of majority or to have the records offered to her before they are destroyed.
16. The Obstetric Patient has the right, both during and after her hospital stay, to have access to her complete hospital medical records, including nurses' notes, and to receive a copy of her records upon payment of a reasonable fee and without incurring the expense of retaining an attorney.

It is the Obstetric Patient and her infant, not the health care professional, who must sustain any trauma or injury resulting from the use of a drug or obstetric procedure. The observation of the rights listed will not only permit the Obstetric Patient to participate in the decisions involving her and her infant's health care but also will help to protect the health care professional and the hospital against litigation arising from resentment or misunderstanding on the part of the mother.

# Abbreviations Used in Women's Health and Maternal-Newborn Nursing

| | | | |
|---|---|---|---|
| ABC | Alternative birth center | BSE | Breast self-examination |
| ABC | Airway, breathing, circulation | BST | Breast stimulation test (see MST) |
| ABCD | Acronym for skin cancer assessment | BUN | Blood urea nitrogen |
| AC | Abdominal circumference | BV | Bacterial vaginosis |
| Accel | Accelerations of fetal heart rate | CAGE | Alcoholism screening test |
| ACHES | Acronmyn for assessment of oral contra- | CAPD | Continuous ambulatory peritoneal dialysis |
| | ceptive side effects | CAT | Computerized axial tomography |
| ADH | Antidiuretic hormone | CBC | Complete blood count |
| ADLs | Activities of daily living | CBE | Clinical breast examination |
| AF | Amniotic fluid | cc | Chief complaint |
| AFDC | Aid to Families with Dependent Children | cc | Cubic centimeter |
| AFI | Amniotic fluid (volume) index | CC | Chest circumference; cord compression |
| AFP | Alpha-fetoprotein | CDC | Centers for Disease Control and |
| AFV | Amniotic fluid volume | | Prevention |
| AGA | Appropriate for gestational age | C-H | Crown-to-heel length |
| AID | Artificial insemination by donor | CH | Congenital hypothyroidism |
| AIDS | Acquired immunodeficiency syndrome | CHF | Congestive heart failure |
| AIH | Artificial insemination by husband | CHN | Community Health Nurse |
| AMOL | Active management of labor | CID | Cytomegalic inclusion disease |
| AP | Anterior-posterior | CIS | Carcinoma in situ |
| ARDS | Adult respiratory distress syndrome | cm | Centimeter |
| AROM | Artificial rupture of membranes | CMV | Cytomegalovirus |
| ART | Assisted reproduction technique | CNM | Certified nurse-midwife |
| ASB | Asymptomatic bacteriuria | CNS | Central nervous system |
| ASD | Atrial septal defect | CNS | Clinical nurse specialist |
| BAT | Brown adipose tissue (brown fat) | CPAP | Continuous positive airway pressure |
| BBT | Basal body temperature | CPD | Cephalopelvic disproportion |
| Beats/min | Beats per minute | CPR | Cardiopulmonary resuscitation |
| BL | Baseline (fetal heart baseline) | CRH | Corticotrophin-releasing hormone |
| BMI | Body mass index | CRL | Crown-rump length |
| BMR | Basal metabolic rate | C/S | Cesarean section (C section), surgical |
| BOW | Bag of waters | | birth |
| BP | Blood pressure | CSE | Combined spinal-epidural block |
| BPD | Biparietal diameter | CST | Contraction stress test |
| BPD | Bronchopulmonary dysplasia | CT | Computed tomography |
| BPP | Biophysical profile | CVA | Cerebrovascular accident |
| BPS | Biophysical profile score | CVA | Costo-vertebral angle tenderness |

| | | | | |
|---|---|---|---|---|
| CVP | Central venous pressure | | FSP | Fibrin split products |
| CVS | Chorionic villus sampling | | FVC | Forced vital capacity |
| D&C | Dilation and curettage | | G or grav | (Gravida) pregnant |
| D&E | Dilation and evacuation | | G6PD | Glucose-6-phosphate dehydrogenase deficiency |
| decels | Deceleration of fetal heart rate | | | |
| DES | Diethylstilbestrol | | GBS | Group B streptococcal |
| DFMR | Daily fetal movement response | | GC | Gonorrhea |
| DIC | Disseminated intravascular coagulation | | GDM | Gestational diabetes mellitus |
| dil | Dilation (of cervix) | | GFR | Glomerular filtration rate |
| DM | Diabetes mellitus | | GH | Growth hormone |
| DMPA | Depo-Provera (medroxyprogesterone) | | GI | Gastrointestinal |
| DNA | Deoxyribonucleic acid | | GIFT | Gamete intrafallopian transfer |
| DOB | Date of birth | | GLT | Glucose load test |
| DPL | Diagnostic peritoneal lavage | | GnRH | Gonadotropin-releasing hormone |
| DRG | Diagnosis-related group | | GTD | Gestational trophoblastic disease |
| DTR | Deep tendon reflexes | | GTT | Glucose tolerance test |
| DUB | Dysfunctional uterine bleeding | | GYN | Gynecology |
| DVT | Deep vein thrombosis | | H/A | Head-abdomen ratio |
| Dx | Diagnosis | | Hb, HgB, Hbg | Hemoglobin |
| ECG | Electrocardiogram (see FECG) | | | |
| ECMO | Extracorporeal membrane oxygenation | | $HbA_{1c}$ | Glycosylated hemoglobin test |
| ECV | External cephalic version | | HBV | Hepatitis B virus |
| EDB | Estimated date of birth | | HC | Head circumference |
| EDC | Estimated date of childbirth | | HC | Head compression |
| EDD | Estimated date of delivery | | hCG | Human chorionic gonadotropin |
| EFM | Electronic fetal monitoring | | hCS | Human chorionic somatomammotropin |
| EFW | Estimated fetal weight | | Hct | Hematocrit |
| EGA | Estimation of gestational age | | HELLP | Syndrome of hemolysis, elevated liver enzymes, low platelets |
| ELF | Elective low forceps | | | |
| ELISA | Enzyme-linked immunosorbent assay | | HIV | Human immunodeficiency virus |
| ENT | Ears, nose, and throat | | HMD | Hyaline membrane disease |
| EOAE | Evoked otoacoustic emissions | | hMG | Human menopausal gonadotropin |
| epis | Episiotomy | | hPL | Human placental lactogen |
| FAD | Fetal activity diary | | HPV | Human papillomavirus |
| FAE | Fetal alcohol effect | | HRT | Hormone replacement therapy |
| FAS | Fetal alcohol syndrome | | HSG | Hysterosalpingography |
| FAST | Fetal acoustic stimulation test | | HSV | Herpes simplex virus |
| FB | Fingerbreadth | | Hx | History |
| FBD | Fibrocystic breast disease | | ICS | Intercostal space |
| FBM | Fetal breathing movements | | ICSI | Intracytoplasmic sperm injection |
| FBS | Fetal blood sample | | IDDM | Insulin-dependent diabetes mellitus |
| FBS | Fasting blood sugar | | IDM | Infant of diabetic mother |
| FECG | Fetal electrocardiogram | | Ig | Immunoglobulin |
| FFN | Fetal fibronectin | | IGT | Impaired glucose tolerance |
| FFP | Fresh frozen plasma | | IGTT | Intravenous glucose tolerance test |
| FHR | Fetal heart rate | | IM | Intramuscularly |
| FHT | Fetal heart tones | | IRMA | Immunoradiometric assay pregnancy test |
| FIA | Fluoroimmunoassay pregnancy test | | ISAM | Infant of substance-abusing mother |
| FM | Fetal movement | | ITP | Immune thrombocytopenia |
| FMLA | Family and Medical Leave Act | | IUD | Intrauterine contraceptive device |
| FMR | Fetal movement record | | IUFD | Intrauterine fetal death |
| FPG | Fasting plasma glucose | | IUGR | Intrauterine fetal growth retardation |
| FRC | Female reproductive cycle | | IUI | Intrauterine insemination |
| FRC | Functional residual capacity | | IUPC | Intrauterine pressure catheter |
| FSE | Fetal spiral (or scalp) electrode | | IV | Intravenously |
| FSH | Follicle-stimulating hormone | | IVF | In vitro fertilization |

| | | | | |
|---|---|---|---|---|
| IVF-ET | In vitro fertilization-embryo transfer | | OTC | Over-the-counter (drugs) |
| IVH | Intraventricular hemorrhage | | P | Para, parity |
| JVP | Jugular venous pressure | | PAC | Premature atrial contractions |
| L&W | Living and well | | Paco₂ | Carbon dioxide pressure (tension), arterial |
| LBW | Low birth weight (i.e., neonate weight less than 2500 g at birth) | | Pao₂ | Oxygen pressure (tension), arterial |
| LCM | Left costal margin | | PAP | Pulmonary artery pressure |
| LDH | Lactate dehydrogenase | | Pap smear | Papanicolaou smear |
| LDL | Low-density lipoprotein | | PAT | Paroxysmal atrial tachycardia |
| LDR | Labor-delivery-recovery room | | PCO | Polycystic ovary disease |
| LGA | Large for gestational age | | Pco₂ | Carbon dioxide pressure (tension) |
| LH | Luteinizing hormone | | PCR | Polymerase chain reaction |
| LHRH | Luteinizing hormone–releasing hormone | | PCWP | Pulmonary capillary wedge pressure |
| LICS | Left intercostal space | | PDA | Patent ductus arteriosus |
| LLQ | Left lower quadrant | | PEEP | Positive end expiratory pressure |
| LML | Left mediolateral (episiotomy) | | PEFR | Peak expiratory flow rates |
| LMP | Last menstrual period | | PFC | Persistent fetal circulation |
| LOA | Left occipitoanterior presentation | | PG | Prostaglandin |
| LOP | Left occipitoposterior presentation | | PI | Present illness |
| LOT | Left occipitotransverse presentation | | PID | Pelvic inflammatory disease |
| L/S | Lecithin-sphingomyelin ratio | | PIH | Pregnancy-induce hypertension |
| LTV | Long-term variability (of FHR) | | Pit | Pitocin (oxytocin) |
| LUL | Left upper lobe | | PKU | Phenylketonuria |
| LUQ | Left upper quadrant | | PMI | Point of maximal impulse |
| MAP | Mean arterial pressure | | PMI | Point of maximum intensity |
| MAS | Meconium aspiration syndrome | | PMS | Premenstrual syndrome |
| mec | Meconium | | PMS | Premenstrual symptoms |
| mec st | Meconium stained | | Po₂ | Oxygen pressure (tension) |
| ml | Milliliter | | PPH | Postpartal hemorrhage |
| ML | Midline (episiotomy) | | PPHN | Persistent pulmonary hypertension |
| M/P | Milk/plasma ratio | | PPP | Prenatal Psychologic Profile |
| MPA | Medroxyprogesterone acetate | | PPV | Postpartum visit program |
| MRI | Magnetic resonance imaging | | Primip | Primipara |
| MS | Multiple sclerosis | | PRL | Prolactin |
| MSAFP | Maternal serum alpha-fetoprotein | | PROM | Premature rupture of membranes |
| multip | Multipara | | PT | Prothrombin time |
| MVP | Mitral valve prolapse | | PTL | Preterm labor |
| NANDA | North American Nursing Diagnosis Association | | PTSD | Post-traumatic stress disorder |
| NEC | Necrotizing enterocolitis | | PTT | Partial thromboplastin time |
| NGU | Nongonoccocal urethritis | | PUBS | Percutaneous umbilical blood sampling |
| NICU | Neonatal intensive care unit | | PVC | Premature ventricular contractions |
| NIDDM | Non–insulin-dependent diabetes mellitus | | RBC | Red blood cells |
| NP | Nurse practitioner | | RDA | Recommended Dietary Allowances |
| NPH | Neutral protamine Hagedorn insulin | | RDS | Respiratory distress syndrome |
| NST | Nonstress test | | REEDA | Redness, edema, ecchymosis, discharge (drainage), approximation (wound healing recording system) |
| NST | Nonshivering thermogenesis | | | |
| NSVD | Normal spontaneous vaginal delivery | | REM | Rapid eye movements |
| NTD | Neural tube defect | | Rh | Rh factor |
| NVP | Nausea and vomiting of pregnancy | | RhoGAM | Rh immune globulin |
| OA | Occiput anterior | | RIA | beta-subunit radioimmunoassay pregnancy test |
| OB | Obstetrics | | | |
| OC | Oral contraceptive | | RLF | Retrolental fibroplasia |
| OD | Optical density | | RLQ | Right lower quadrant |
| OGTT | Oral glucose tolerance test | | ROA | Right occipitoanterior presentation |
| OP | Occiput posterior | | ROM | Rupture of membranes |
| | | | ROP | Right occipitoposterior presentation |

| | | | | |
|---|---|---|---|---|
| ROT | Right occipitotransverse presentation | | TPAL | Term infants (number), preterm infants (number), abortions (number), living (number) |
| RRA | Radioreceptor assay pregnancy test | | | |
| RRR | Regular rate and rhythm | | | |
| RU 486 | Mifepristone | | TPN | Total parenteral nutrition |
| RUQ | Right upper quadrant | | TSH | Thyroid-stimulating hormone |
| RV | Residual volume | | TSS | Toxic shock syndrome |
| S/D | Systolic/diastolic ratio | | TTN | Transient tachypnea of newborn |
| SAB | Spontaneous abortion | | U | Umbilicus |
| SGA | Small for gestational age | | u/a | Urinalysis |
| SIDS | Sudden infant death syndrome | | UA | Uterine activity |
| SLE | Systemic lupus erythematosus | | UA | Umbilical artery |
| SMBG | Self-monitoring of blood glucose | | UAC | Umbilical artery catheter |
| SROM | Spontaneous rupture of membranes | | UC | Uterine contractions |
| STD | Sexually transmitted disease | | UE3 | Unconjugated estriol |
| STI | Sexually transmitted infection | | UPI | Uteroplacental insufficiency |
| STS | Serologic test for syphilis | | U/S | Ultrasound |
| STV | Short term variability (of FHR) | | UTI | Urinary tract infection |
| SVE | Sterile vaginal examination | | VBAC | Vaginal birth after cesarean |
| SVT | Supraventricular variability | | VDRL | Venereal Disease Research Laboratory (syphilis) |
| $T_3$ | Triiodothyronine | | | |
| $T_4$ | Thyroxine | | VLBW | Very low birth weight, neonate weight less than 1500 g at birth |
| TAB | Therapeutic abortion | | | |
| TB | Tuberculosis | | VSD | Ventricular septal defect |
| TCA | Trichloroacetic acid | | VST | Vibroacoustic stimulation test |
| TCOM | Transcutaneous oxygen monitoring | | VT | Tidal volume |
| TDI | Therapeutic donor insemination | | VVC | Vulvovaginal candidiasis |
| TENS | Transcutaneous electrical nerve stimulation | | WBC | White blood cell |
| | | | WIC | Supplemental food program for Women, Infants, and Children |
| TGA | Transposition of great vessels | | | |
| TOL | Trial of labor | | ZDV | Zidovudine |
| TORCH | Toxoplasmosis, rubella, cytomegalovirus, herpes-virus testing | | ZIFT | Zygote intrafallopian transfer |

# Effect of Food on Common Antiinfectives

| Antiinfective | Effect of Food | Management |
|---|---|---|
| Amoxicillin (e.g., *Amoxil*) | Delayed absorption. | May take without regard to food. |
| Amoxicillin/Potassium Clavulanate (*Augmentin*) | No effect on absorption. | Take with food to decrease gastric irritation. |
| Ampicillin (e.g., *Omnipen*) | Decreased absorption. | Take on an empty stomach. |
| Atovaquone (*Mepron*) | Decreased absorption. | Take with food. |
| Azithromycin (*Zithromax*) | Increased absorption. | Take on an empty stomach.* |
| Bacampicillin (*Spectrobid*) | | |
|    Tablets | No effect. | May take without regard to food. |
|    Suspension | Decreased absorption. | Take on an empty stomach. |
| Carbenicillin (e.g., *Geopen*) | Decreased absorption. | Take on an empty stomach.* |
| Cefaclor (*Ceclor*) | No significant effect. | May take without regard to food. |
| Cefadroxil (e.g., *Duricef*) | No effect. | May take without regard to food. |
| Cefpodoxime (*Vantin*) | Increased absorption. | Take with food. |
| Cefradine (*Velosef*) | Delayed absorption. | May take without regard to food. |
| Cefuroxime (*Ceftin*) | Increased bioavailability. | Take with food. |
| Cephalexin (*Keflex*) | Delayed absorption. | May take without regard to food. |
| Chloramphenicol (e.g., *Chloromycetin*) | Decreased absorption. May cause gastric irritation. | Take on an empty stomach.* |
| Chloroquine (*Aralen*) | Increased absorption. | Take with food to decrease gastric irritation. |
| Ciprofloxacin (*Cipro*) | Delayed absorption. | Take on an empty stomach.* |
| Clarithromycin (*Biaxin*) | Increased absorption. | May take without regard to food. |
| Clindamycin (*Cleocin*) | Delayed absorption. | May take without regard to food. |
| Clofazamine (*Lamprene*) | Increased absorption. | Take with food. |
| Cloxacillin (e.g., *Tegopen*) | Decreased absorption. | Take on an empty stomach.* |
| Colistin (*Coly-Mycin S*) | No effect. | May take without regard to food. |
| Cycloserine (*Seromycin*) | No effect. | May take without regard to food. |
| Dicloxacillin (*Dynapen*) | Decreased absorption. | Take on an empty stomach.* |
| Didanosine (*Videx*) | Decreased absorption. | Take on an empty stomach. |
| Doxycycline (e.g., *Vibramycin*) | Slightly decreased absorption. | May take with food or milk. |
| Enoxacin (*Penetrex*) | Decreased absorption. | Take on an empty stomach.* |
| Erythromycin base Enteric-coated (e.g., *E-Mycin*) | No effect. | May take with food if gastric upset occurs. |

Reprinted with permission from *Prescriber's Letter*. *Prescriber's Letter* is a totally independent newsletter providing unbiased drug information to physicians and other prescribers who subscribe.

*1 hour before or 2 hours after food.

| Antiinfective | Effect of Food | Management |
|---|---|---|
| Uncoated | Decreased absorption due to degradation. | May take with food if gastric upset occurs. |
| Erythromycin estolate (e.g., *Ilosone*) | Increased or no effect on absorption. | May take with food if gastric upset occurs. |
| Erythromycin ethylsuccinate (*EES, EryPed*) | No effect. | May take with food if gastric upset occurs. |
| Erythromycin stearate (e.g., *Erythrocin*) | Decreased absorption. | Take on an empty stomach.* If gastric upset occurs, take with food. |
| Ethambutol (*Myambutol*) | No effect. | May take with food if gastric upset occurs. |
| Ethionamide | | May take with food to decrease gastric irritation. |
| Furazolidone (*Furoxone*) | Furazolidone is a potent MAO inhibitor. | Avoid tyramine-containing foods while taking furazolidone and for several weeks after stopping. |
| Griseofulvin (e.g., *Gris-PEG*) | Fatty meals increase absorption. | Take with food. |
| Hydroxychloroquine (*Plaquenil*) | | Take with food to decrease gastric irritation. |
| Isoniazid (*Nydrazid*) | Decreased absorption. Isoniazid may cause pyridoxine deficiency. | Take on an empty stomach.* If gastric irritation occurs, take with food. |
| Itraconazole (*Sporanox*) | Increased absorption. | Take with food. |
| Ketoconazole (*Nizoral*) | Decreased absorption. | Take with food to decrease gastric irritation. |
| Lincomycin (*Lincocin*) | Decreased absorption. | Take on an empty stomach.* |
| Lomefloxacin (*Maxaquin*) | No effect. | May take without regard to food. |
| Loracarbef (*Lorabid*) | Slowed absorption. | Take on an empty stomach.* |
| Mebendazole (*Vermox*) | Increased absorption. | Chew or crush tablet and take with food. |
| Mefloquine (*Lariam*) | | Take with food and a full glass of water. |
| Methenamine (e.g., *Mandelamine*) | | Take with food to decrease gastric irritation. |
| Metronidazole (*Flagyl*) | Delayed absorption. | Take with food to decrease gastric irritation. |
| Minocycline (*Minocin*) | No effect. | May take with food or milk. |
| Nafcillin (e.g., *Unipen*) | Decreased absorption. | Take on an empty stomach.* |
| Nalidixic acid (e.g., *NegGram*) | | Take with food to decrease gastric irritation. |
| Neomycin (e.g., *Mycifradin*) | Chronic use may decrease fat-soluble vitamin absorption. | Vitamins A, D, E and K supplements may be needed. |
| Niclosamide (e.g., *Niclocide*) | | Take with a light meal to decrease gastric upset. |
| Nitrofurantoin (e.g., *Macrodantin*) | Increased absorption. | Take immediately after food. Food will also decrease gastric irritation. |
| Norfloxacin (*Noroxin*) | Decreased absorption. | Take on an empty stomach.* |
| Novobiocin (*Albamycin*) | Delayed absorption. | May take without regard to food. |
| Ofloxacin (*Floxin*) | Decreased absorption. | Take on an empty stomach.* |
| Oxacillin (e.g., *Prostaphlin*) | Decreased absorption. | Take on an empty stomach.* |
| Penicillin G | Decreased absorption. | Take on an empty stomach.* |
| Penicillin V | Delayed absorption. | May take without regard to food. |
| Piperazine (e.g., *Antipar*) | Contact between drug and parasite decreased by food. | Take on an empty stomach.* |
| Praziquantel (e.g., *Biltricide*) | | Bitter taste may cause gagging or vomiting. Take with liquid during meals. |
| Primaquine | | May take with food if gastric upset occurs. |

| Antiinfective | Effect of Food | Management |
|---|---|---|
| Pyrimethamine (*Daraprim*) | | Take with food to decrease gastric irritation. |
| Quinacrine (*Atabrine*) | | Take after meals with a full glass of water to decrease gastric irritation. |
| Quinine | | Take with food to minimize gastric irritation. |
| Rifabutin (*Mycobutin*) | | Take with food to decrease gastrointestinal distress. |
| Rifampin (e.g.,*Rimactane*) | Decreased absorption. Rifampin may decrease vitamin D absorption. | Take on an empty stomach.* Give vitamin D if needed. |
| Sulfonamides    Sulfisoxazole (*Gantrisin*)    Sulfmethoxazole (*Gantanol*) | Delayed absorption. | Take on an empty stomach with a full glass of water. |
| Sulfasalazine (e.g., *Azulfidine*) | Sulfasalazine may decrease folate absorption. | Give folic acid if needed. Take with food if gastric irritation occurs. |
| Tetracycline | Decreased absorption of most tetracyclines. | Take on an empty stomach and 3 hours before or after dairy products. |
| Thiabendazole (*Mintezol*) | | May take with food to decrease gastric irritation. |
| Trimethoprim (e.g., *Proloprim*) | No effect. | May take without regard to food. |
| Troleandomycin (*Tao*) | No effect. | May take without regard to food. |
| Vancomycin (e.g., *Vancocin*) | No effect. | May take without regard to food. |
| Zalcitabine (*Hivid,* ddc) | Decreased absorption. | Take on an empty stomach. |
| Zidovudine (*Retrovir, AZT*) | Fatty foods decrease absorption. | Avoid taking with fatty foods. |

# Oral Contraceptive Drug Interactions*

| Drug Class | Generic (Trade) | Effect | Recommendation |
|---|---|---|---|
| Anticonvulsants | Carbamazepine (*Tegretol,* etc.) Felbamate (*Felbatol*) Phenobarbital Phenytoin (*Dilantin,* etc.) Primidone (*Mysoline,* etc.) | OC action may be decreased due to increased metabolism. | Use alternative method of contraception or consider a higher dose product (e.g., ethinyl estradiol 50 mg daily). Sodium valproate (*Depakene*) does not appear to interact with OCs. |
| Antiinfectives | Troleandomycin (*Tao*) Erythromycin (*E-Mycin,* etc) Griseofulvin (*Grisactin,* etc.) Penicillins Rifampin (*Rifadin,* etc.) Tetracycline (*Achromycin V,* etc.) | Increased risk of cholestasis. OC action may be decreased. Erythromycin, penicillins, and tetracyclines may kill GI bacteria, which decreases serum levels of OC by interfering with enterohepatic recirculation. Griseofulvin or rifampin may increase OC metabolism. | Use alternative antibiotic. Use alternative method of contraception during the antiinfective course of treatment and for at least one week after stopping the antiinfective (and for one month after stopping rifampin). |
| Antiviral | Ritonavir (*Norvir*) | Action of OC may be decreased due to increased metabolism. | Use alternative method of contraceptive. |
| Azole Antifungal Agents | Fluconazole (*Diflucan*) Itraconazole (*Sporanox*) Ketoconazole (*Nizoral*) | OC action may be decreased. | Use alternative method of contraception. |
| Benzodiazepines | Alprazolam (*Xanax,* etc.) Chlordiazepoxide (*Librium,* etc.) Diazepam (*Valium,* etc.) Flurazepam (*Dalmane,* etc.) Triazolam (*Halcion,* etc.) | Metabolism of benzodiazepines that undergo oxidation may be decreased, increasing their CNS effects. | It may be necessary to decrease the dose of the benzodiazepine if the CNS effects are increased |

*David S. Tatro, Pharm.D., Drug Information Analyst

Reprinted with permission from *Prescriber's Letter*. *Prescriber's Letter* is a totally independent newsletter providing unbiased drug information to physicians and other prescribers who subscribe.

References: Tatro DS: Oral contraceptive drug interactions; *Drug Newsletter* 15:66-69, 1996; Bolt HM: Interactions between clinically used drugs and oral contraceptives, *Environ Health Perspect* 102(suppl 9):35-38, 1994; Fazio A: Oral contraceptive drug interactions: important considerations; *South Med J* 84:997-1002, 1991; Baciewicz AM: Oral contraceptive drug interactions, *Ther Drug Monit* 7:26-35, 1985; Back DJ and others: Pharmacokinetic drug interactions with oral contraceptives, *Clin Pharmacokinet* 18:472-484, 1990.

| Drug Class | Generic (Trade) | Effect | Recommendation |
|---|---|---|---|
| Bronchodilator | Theophylline | The metabolism of theophylline may be decreased, increasing theophylline side effects. | Monitor serum theophylline levels when starting or stopping OCs and adjust the dose as needed. |
| Corticosteroids | Hydrocortisone Methylprednisolone (*Medrol*, etc.) Prednisolone (*Delta-Cortef*, etc.) Prednisone (*Deltasone*, etc.) | The effects of the corticosteroid may be increased due to inhibition of metabolism by the OC. | Monitor the response of the patient for several weeks after starting or stopping the contraceptive. Adjust the dose of the corticosteroid as needed. |
| Lipid-Lowering Agent | Clofibrate (*Atromid-S*) | Metabolism of clofibrate may be increased, decreasing the effect. | Monitor serum lipoprotein when starting or stopping OCs. Adjust clofibrate dose as needed. |
| Tricyclic Anti-depressants (TCAs) | Amitriptyline (*Elavil*, etc.) Imipramine (*Tofranil*, etc.) | The metabolism of the TCA may be decreased, increasing the side effects. | Monitor TCA levels and decrease the dose if needed. |

# APPENDIX V

# Standard Laboratory Values: Women and Pregnant Women

| | Nonpregnant | Pregnant |
|---|---|---|
| **HEMATOLOGIC VALUES** | | |
| **COMPLETE BLOOD COUNT (CBC)** | | |
| Hemoglobin, g/dl | 12 to 16* | >11* |
| Hematocrit, PCV, % | 37 to 47 | >33* |
| Red blood cell (RBC) volume, per ml | 1600 | 1500 to 1900 |
| Plasma volume, per ml | 2400 | 3700 |
| RBC count, million/mm³ | 4.2 to 5.4 | 5 to 6.25 |
| White blood cells, total per mm³ | 5000 to 10,000 | 5000 to 15,000 |
| Polymorphonuclear cells, % | 55 to 70 | 60 to 85 |
| Lymphocytes, % | 20 to 40 | 15 to 40 |
| Erythrocytes sedimentation rate, mm/hr | 20/hr | Elevated second and third trimesters |
| MCHC, g/dl packed RBCs (mean corpuscular hemoglobin concentration) | 32 to 36 | No change |
| MCH (mean corpuscular hemoglobin) per picogram (less than a nanogram) | 27 to 31 | No change |
| MCV/$\mu$m³ (mean corpuscular volume) per cubic micrometer | 80 to 95 | No change |
| | | |
| **BLOOD COAGULATION AND FIBRINOLYTIC ACTIVITY†** | | |
| Factors VII, VIII, IX, X | | Increase in pregnancy; return to normal in early puerperium; factor VIII increases during and immediately after birth |
| Factors XI, XIII | | Decrease in pregnancy |
| Prothrombin time (PT) | 11 to 12.5 sec | Slight decrease in pregnancy |
| Partial thromboplastin time (PTT) | 60 to 70 sec | Slight decrease in pregnancy and again during second and third stage of labor (indicates clotting at placental site) |
| Bleeding time | 1 to 9 min (Ivy) | No appreciable change |
| Coagulation time | 6 to 10 min (Lee/White) | No appreciable change |
| Platelets | 150,000 to 400,000/mm³ | No significant change until 3 to 5 days after birth and then a rapid increase (may predispose woman to thrombosis) and gradual return to normal |

From Pagana K and Pagana T: *Mosby's diagnostic and laboratory test reference*, ed 3, St Louis, 1997, Mosby.

*At sea level. Permanent residents of higher levels (e.g., Denver) require higher levels of hemoglobin.

†Pregnancy represents a hypercoagulable state.

|  | Nonpregnant | Pregnant |
|---|---|---|
| **HEMATOLOGIC VALUES—cont'd** | | |
| **BLOOD COAGULATION AND FIBRINOLYTIC ACTIVITY†—cont'd** | | |
| Fibrinolytic activity | | Decreases in pregnancy and then abrupt return to normal (protection against thromboembolism) |
| Fibrinogen | 200 to 400 mg/dl | Increased levels late in pregnancy |
| **MINERAL/VITAMIN CONCENTRATIONS** | | |
| Vitamin $B_{12}$, folic acid, ascorbic acid | Normal | Moderate decrease |
| Serum proteins | | |
|    Total, g/dl | 6.4 to 8.3 | 5.5 to 7.5 |
|    Albumin, g/dl | 3.5 to 5.0 | Slight increase |
|    Globulin, total, g/dl | 2.3 to 3.4 | 3 to 4 |
| Blood glucose | | |
|    Fasting, mg/dl | 70 to 105 | Decreases |
|    2-hour postprandial, mg/dl | <140 | Under 140 after a 100 g carbohydrate meal is considered normal |
| **HEPATIC VALUES** | | |
| Bilirubin total | Not more than 1 mg/dl | Unchanged |
| Serum cholesterol | 120 to 200 mg/dl | Increases from 16 to 32 weeks of pregnancy; remains at this level until after birth |
| Serum alkaline phosphatase | 42 to 128 U/L | Increases from week 12 of pregnancy to 6 weeks after birth |
| Serum globulin albumin | 2.3 to 3.4 g/dl | Slight increase |
| **RENAL VALUES** | | |
| Bladder capacity | 1300 ml | 1500 ml |
| Renal plasma flow (RPF), ml/min | 490 to 700 | Increases by 25% |
| Glomerular filtration rate (GFR), ml/min | 88 to 128 | Increases by 50% |
| Nonprotein nitrogen (NPN), mg/dl | 25 to 40 | Decreases |
| Blood urea nitrogen (BUN), mg/dl | 10 to 20 | Decreases |
| Serum creatinine, mg/dl | 0.5 to 1.1 | Decreases |
| Serum uric acid, mg/dl | 2.0 to 6.6 | Decreases |
| Urine glucose | Negative | Present in 20% of pregnant women |
| Intravenous pyelogram (IVP) | Normal | Slight-to-moderate hydroureter and hydronephrosis; right kidney larger than left kidney |

# Standard Laboratory Values of the Neonatal Period

| | Neonatal | |
|---|---|---|
| **1. HEMATOLOGIC VALUES** | | |
| Clotting factors | | |
| Activated clotting time (ACT) | 2 min | |
| Bleeding time (Ivy) | 2 to 7 min | |
| Clot retraction | Complete 1 to 4 hr | |
| Fibrinogen | 125 to 300 mg/dl* | |

| | **Term** | **Preterm** |
|---|---|---|
| Hemoglobin (g/dl) | 14.5 to 22.5 | 15 to 17 |
| Hematocrit (%) | 44 to 72 | 45 to 55 |
| Reticulocytes (%) | 0.4 to 6 | Up to 10 |
| Fetal hemoglobin (% of total) | 40 to 70 | 80 to 90 |
| Red blood cells (RBCs)/mm³ | $4.0^6$ to $6.0^6$ | |
| Platelet count/mm³ | 84,000 to 478,000 | 120,000 to 180,000 |
| White blood cells (WBCs)/mm³ | 9000 to 30,000 | 10,000 to 20,000 |
| Neutrophils (%) | 54 to 62 | 47 |
| Eosinophils and basophils (%) | 1 to 3 | |
| Lymphocytes (%) | 25 to 33 | 33 |
| Monocytes (%) | 3 to 7 | 4 |
| Immature WBC (%) | 10 | 16 |

*dl refers to deciliter (1 dl = 100 ml); this conforms to the SI system (standardized international measurements).

| | | | Neonatal |
|---|---|---|---|
| **2. BIOCHEMICAL VALUES** | | | |
| Bilirubin, direct | | | 0 to 1 mg/dl |
| Bilirubin, total | Cord: | | <2 mg/dl |
| | Peripheral blood: | 0 to 1 day | 6 mg/dl |
| | | 1 to 2 days | 8 mg/dl |
| | | 3 to 5 days | 12 mg/dl |
| Blood gases | | Arterial: | pH 7.31 to 7.45 |
| | | | $Pco_2$ 33 to 48 mm Hg |
| | | | $Po_2$ 50 to 70 mm Hg |
| | | Venous: | pH 7.28 to 7.42 |
| | | | $Pco_2$ 38 to 52 mm Hg |
| | | | $Po_2$ 20 to 49 mm Hg |
| $\alpha_1$-Fetoprotein | | | 0 |
| Fibrinogen | | | 150 to 300 mg/dl |
| Serum glucose | | | 40 to 60 mg/dl |

| | Neonatal |
|---|---|
| **3. Urinalysis** | |
| Color | Clear, straw |
| Specific gravity | 1.001 to 1.018 |
| pH | 5 to 7 |
| Protein | Negative |
| Glucose | Negative |
| Ketones | Negative |
| RBCs | Rare |
| WBCs | 0 to 4 |
| Casts | Rare |
| 17-Ketosteroids | Under 1 |
| 17-Hydroxycorticosteroids | Same |
| Urinary calcium | 5 mg/kg of body weight |
| Urinary sodium | 20% of adult values |
| Urinary vanillylmandelic acid (VMA) | <1.0 mg/24 hr |

*Volume:* 20 to 40 ml excreted daily in the first few days; by week 1, 24-hr urine volume close to 200 ml
*Protein:* may be present in first 2 to 4 days
*Osmolarity* (mOsm/L): 100 to 600

## 4. Urine Screening Tests For Inborn Errors of Metabolism
*Benedict's test:* for reducing substances in the urine—glucose, galactose, fructose, lactose; phenylketonuria (PKU), alkaptonuria, tyrosyluria, and tyrosinosis may give a positive Benedict's test result.
*Ferric chloride test:* an immediate green color for PKU, histidinemia, and tyrosinuria; a gray to green color for presence of phenothiazines, isoniazid; red to purple color for presence of salicylates or ketone bodies.
*Dinitrophenylhydrazine test:* for PKU, maple syrup urine disease, Lowe's syndrome.
*Cetyltrimethylammonium bromide test:* for mucopolysaccharides: immediate positive reaction in gargoylism (Hurler syndrome); delayed, moderately positive reaction for Marfan, Morquio-Ullrich, and Murdoch syndromes.
*Metachromatic stain (or urine sediment):* granules (free or as inclusion bodies in cells) are seen in metachromatic leukodystrophy; may also be seen rarely in Tay-Sachs and other lipid diseases of central nervous system.
*Amino acid chromatography:* aminoaciduria may be normal in newborns; chromatography may be helpful to detect hypophosphatasia and argininosuccinicaciduria.
*Diaper test, Phenistix test, and Dinitrophenylhydrazine (DNPH) test:* simple, inexpensive tests for PKU; used for screening; most useful when infant is at least 6 weeks of age.

## 5. Blood Serum Phenylalanine Tests
*Guthrie inhibition assay methods:* drops of blood placed on filter paper; laboratory uses bacterial growth inhibition test; phenylalanine level above 8 mg/dl blood: diagnostic of PKU. Effective in newborn period; used also to monitor PKU diet; blood easily obtained by heel or finger puncture; inexpensive; used for wide-scale screening.

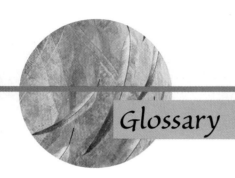

# Glossary

**24-hour recall** In the course of the interview, the client is asked to relate foods (and amounts) consumed during the previous 24 hours.

**abdominal** Belonging or relating to the abdomen and its functions and disorders.

  **a. birth** Birth of a child through a surgical incision made into the abdominal wall and uterus; cesarean birth.

  **a. gestation** Implantation of a fertilized ovum outside the uterus but inside the peritoneal cavity.

**ABO incompatibility** Hemolytic disease that occurs when the mother's blood type is O and the newborn's is A, B, or AB.

**abortion** Termination of pregnancy before the fetus is viable and capable of extrauterine existence, usually at less than 20 weeks of gestation (or when the fetus weighs less than 500 g).

  **complete a.** Abortion in which the fetus and all related tissue have been expelled from the uterus.

  **habitual (recurrent) a.** Loss of three or more successive pregnancies for no known cause.

  **incomplete a.** Loss of pregnancy in which some but not all the products of conception have been expelled from the uterus.

  **induced a.** Intentionally produced loss of pregnancy by woman or others.

  **inevitable a.** Threatened loss of pregnancy that cannot be prevented or stopped and is imminent.

  **missed a.** Loss of pregnancy in which the products of conception remain in the uterus after the fetus dies.

  **spontaneous a.** Loss of pregnancy that occurs naturally without interference or known cause; preferred term is *miscarriage*.

  **therapeutic a.** Pregnancy that has been intentionally terminated.

  **threatened a.** Possible loss of a pregnancy; early symptoms are present (e.g., the cervix begins to dilate).

**abruptio placentae** Partial or complete premature separation of a normally implanted placenta.

  **complete separation** Causes massive vaginal bleeding and hypoxia for the fetus.

  **marginal separation** Least risky because bleeding is evident and provides an earlier indication that there is a problem.

  **partial separation** Bleeding is trapped under the placenta and is therefore not noticeable. Abruption may continue with more of the placenta becoming detached.

**abstinence** Refraining from sexual intercourse periodically or permanently.

**accreta, placenta** See *placenta accreta*.

**acidosis** Increase in hydrogen ion concentration resulting in a lowering of blood pH below 7.35.

**acini cells** Milk-producing cells in the breast.

**acme** Highest point (e.g., of a contraction).

**acoustic stimulation test** Antepartum test to elicit fetal heart rate response to sound; performed by applying sound source (laryngeal stimulator) to maternal abdomen over the fetal head.

**acrocyanosis** Peripheral cyanosis; blue color of hands and feet in most infants at birth that may persist for 7 to 10 days.

**active listening** Skill of understanding what another is saying and feeling.

**acupressure** Massage technique applied to specific points along certain energy pathways of the body called meridians. A form of treatment based in the theories of traditional Chinese medicine.

**acupuncture** A form of treatment using slender needles to stimulate points along energy pathways to correct, enhance, and rebalance the flow of body energy.

**adaptation** A change or response to stress of any kind. It may be normal, protective, and developmental; or it may be all-encompassing, creating further stress.

**adnexa** Adjacent or accessory parts of a structure.

  **uterine a.** Ovaries and uterine (fallopian) tubes.

**adoption** To take voluntarily a child of other parents as one's own child; to release one's own child to be parented by others.

  **agency a.** An agency specializing in adoption selects and performs background screens on the potential adoptive couple.

  **closed a.** Full confidentiality on the identity of the birth mother is maintained. Information cannot be accessed except through legal channels and not before the child is of age to understand the ramifications.

  **open a.** Some relationship between the adoptive family and the birth mother may be maintained. This may range from simply meeting with each other before or after the birth to periodic updates on the child's progress or allowing occasional visits from the birth mother.

private a. The adoption is arranged between the birth mother and the adoptive parents without the involvement of an agency. The adoption records may be open or closed.

adolescence The period of an individual's transformation from a child to an adult.

adverse outcome A pregnancy that does not result in a live birth. The adverse outcomes reported for ART procedures are miscarriages, ectopic (tubal) pregnancies, induced abortions, and stillbirths.

advocacy Speaking on behalf of another to help him or her achieve what he or she desires or needs.

affective domain An area of learning that deals with changes in attitude and values and the development of appreciation and adequate adjustment.

affirmations Positive statements that can be used as support tools. They may be based on religious statements or Scripture or just a simple statement that the woman finds encouraging.

afibrinogenemia Absence or decrease of fibrinogen in the blood such that the blood will not coagulate. In obstetrics, this condition occurs from complications of abruptio placentae or retention of a dead fetus.

afterbirth Lay term for the placenta and membranes expelled after the birth of the child.

afterbirth pains (afterpains) Painful uterine cramps that occur intermittently for approximately 2 or 3 days after birth and that result from contractile efforts of the uterus to return to its normal involuted condition.

AGA Appropriate (growth) for gestational age.

age A stage of development at which the body has arrived, as measured by physical and laboratory standards of what is normal for a male or female of the same chronologic span of life.

aggregate Any total or whole considered with reference to its constituent parts; an assemblage or group of distinct particulars massed together; a gross amount.

agonal cesarean Performed as the mother is dying if she is not responding well to resuscitative efforts. On occasion, the maternal response to resuscitation improves after the infant's birth.

albuminuria Presence of readily detectable amounts of albumin in the urine.

alkalosis Abnormal condition of body fluids characterized by a tendency toward an increased pH, such as from an excess of alkaline bicarbonate or a deficiency of acid.

allopathic, standard, or Western medicine Interchangeable terms used to describe the current U.S. health care system. With foundations in germ theory and reductionism, standard medical practice often focuses on one body system or disease complex. Treatments are often pharmaceutic or surgical and produce effects that are different from those of the disease complex.

alpha-fetoprotein (AFP) Fetal antigen; elevated levels in amniotic fluid are associated with neural tube defects.

Ambivalence A state in which a person concomitantly experiences conflicting feelings, attitudes, drives, desires, or emotions. Common among women who have just discovered they are pregnant.

amenorrhea Absence or suppression of menstruation.
primary a. The failure of menstrual cycles to begin.
secondary a. The cessation of menstrual cycles once established.

American Society for Reproductive Medicine (ASRM) A professional society whose affiliate organization, the Society for Assisted Reproductive Technology (SART), reports annual fertility clinic data to the CDC.

amniocentesis Procedure in which a needle is inserted through the abdominal and uterine walls into the amniotic fluid; used for assessment of fetal health and maturity.

amnioinfusion Infusion of normal saline warmed to body temperature through an intrauterine catheter into the uterine cavity in an attempt to increase the fluid around the umbilical cord and prevent compression during uterine contractions.

amnion Inner membrane of two fetal membranes that form the sac and contain the fetus and the fluid that surrounds it in utero.

amnionitis Inflammation of the amnion, occurring most frequently after early rupture of membranes.

amniotic Pertaining or relating to the amnion.
a. band An abnormal condition of fetal development characterized by the development of fibrous bands within the uterus that entangle the fetus, leading to deformities in structure and function.
a. fluid Fluid surrounding fetus derived primarily from maternal serum and fetal urine.
a. fluid embolism Embolism resulting from amniotic fluid entering the maternal bloodstream during labor and birth after rupture of membranes; this is often fatal to the woman if it is a pulmonary embolism.
a. sac Membrane "bag" that contains the fetus and fluid before birth.

amniotomy Artificial rupture of the fetal membranes (AROM) using a plastic Amnihook or surgical clamp.

analgesia Absence of pain without loss of consciousness.

analgesic Any medication or agent that relieves pain.

anaphylaxis Immediate hypersensitivity reaction characterized by local reactions such as urticaria or by systemic reactions; may be fatal.

anemia A decrease in hemoglobin in the blood to levels below the normal range. It may be caused by a decrease in red cell production, an increase in red cell destruction, or a loss of blood.
physiologic a. Anemia caused by pregnancy as the red blood cell volume increases.

anesthesia Partial or complete absence of sensation with or without loss of consciousness.

**ankyloglossia** An oral defect, characterized by an abnormally short lingual frenum that limits tongue movement and impairs speech. It may be surgically corrected by a frenotomy or frenectomy.

**anomaly** Organ or structure that is malformed or in some way abnormal with reference to form, structure, or position.

**anorexia nervosa** A disorder characterized by a prolonged refusal to eat, resulting in emaciation, amenorrhea, emotional disturbance concerning body image, and fear of becoming obese. The condition is seen primarily in adolescents, predominantly in girls, and is usually associated with emotional stress or conflict, such as anxiety, irritation, anger, and fear, which may accompany a major change in the person's life.

**anovulatory** Failure of the ovaries to produce, mature, or release eggs.

**anoxia** Absence of oxygen.

**antenatal** Occurring or formed before birth (newborn).

**antepartal** Before labor (maternal).

**anticipatory grief** Grief that predates the loss of a beloved object.

**antigen** Protein foreign to the body that causes the body to develop antibodies (e.g., bacteria, dust, Rh factor).

**anuria** The cessation of urine production or a urinary output of less than 100 ml per day. Anuria may be caused by kidney failure or dysfunction, a decline in blood pressure below that required to maintain filtration pressure in the kidney, or an obstruction in the urinary passages.

**Apgar score** The evaluation of an infant's physical condition, usually performed 1 minute and again 5 minutes after birth, based on a rating of five factors that reflect the infant's ability to adjust to extrauterine life.

**aphrodisiacs** Herbs, drugs, or other agents thought to enhance a person's sexual desire or pleasure.

**areola** Pigmented ring of tissue surrounding the nipple.

**ART cycle** One full attempt to conceive, beginning with the production of eggs, either naturally or by medication, leading to egg retrieval, combination of eggs with sperm in the laboratory, transfer of the embryo to the woman's ovary, clinical pregnancy (attachment of the embryo to the uterus), and live birth.

**arterial pressure catheter** A Teflon intravenous catheter, usually 20 gauge, that is placed in an artery and connected to a hemodynamic monitor by means of a pressure line to provide continuous measurements of the systolic, diastolic, and mean arterial blood pressures.

**asphyxia** Decreased oxygen with or without excess of carbon dioxide in the body.

**asset mapping** The process of locating and inventorying a the assets, resources, gifts, and capacities of individuals, associations, and institutions within a community.

**assisted reproductive technology (ART)** Treatments for infertility, including in vitro fertilization procedures, embryo adoption, embryo hosting, and therapeutic insemination.

**atony** Absence of muscle tone.

**attachment** A specific and enduring affective tie to another person.

**attitude** Body posture or position.

  **fetal a.** Relation of fetal parts to each other in the uterus (e.g., all parts flexed, all parts flexed except neck is extended).

**auditory learners** Persons who learn using their sense of hearing. Debates, discussions, stories, or audio tapes are most useful for them.

**augmentation of labor** Stimulation of ineffective uterine contractions after labor has started spontaneously but is not progressing satisfactorily.

**authentic** Genuine, true to oneself and one's word, not pretending to be someone or something different.

**autoimmune disease** Body produces antibodies against itself, causing tissue damage.

**autoimmunization** Development of antibodies against constituents of one's own tissues (e.g., a man may develop antibodies against his own sperm).

**autosomal dominant inheritance** A pattern of inheritance in which the transmission of a dominant gene on an autosome causes a characteristic to be expressed. Each child, whether male or female, has a 50% chance of having the same condition if the parent has the gene for a dominant condition. Some examples are achondroplasia, Marfan syndrome, high cholesterol, or glaucoma.

**autosomal inheritance** Characteristics transmitted by genes on the autosomes, not the sex chromosomes.

**autosomal recessive inheritance** A pattern of inheritance in which the transmission of a potentially harmful recessive gene occurs if both parents are carriers. A carrier is someone with one copy of the recessive disorder. Cystic fibrosis, sickle cell anemia, and Tay-Sachs disease are some examples.

**autosomes** Any of the paired chromosomes other than the sex (X and Y) chromosomes.

**axilla** A pyramid-shaped space forming the underside of the shoulder between the upper arm and the side of the chest. The armpit.

**azoospermia** Absence of sperm in the semen.

**β-sympathomimetic** Denoting a pharmacologic agent that mimics the effects of stimulation of organs and structures by the sympathetic nervous system. It functions by occupying adrenergic receptor sites and acting as an agonist or by increasing the release of the neurotransmitter norepinephrine at postganglionic nerve endings.

**bacterial vaginosis** A chronic inflammation of the vagina caused by a bacterium.

**bag of waters** Lay term for the sac containing amniotic fluid and fetus.

**ballottable** Pertaining to a use of palpation to detect movement of objects suspended in fluid, such as a fetus in amniotic fluid.

**ballottement** (1) Movability of a floating object, such as a fetus. (2) Diagnostic technique using palpation: a floating object, when tapped or pushed, moves away and then returns to touch the examiner's hand.

**Bandl's ring** Abnormally thickened ridge of uterine musculature between the upper and lower segments that occurs after a mechanically obstructed labor, with the lower segment thinning abnormally.

**barrier method** Any contraception strategy that places a barrier between the sperm and the ova. These include male or female condoms, the diaphragm, and the cervical cap.

**Bartholin's glands** Two small glands situated on either side of the vaginal orifice that secrete small amounts of mucus during coitus and that are homologous to the bulbourethral glands in the male.

**basal body temperature** Lowest body temperature of a healthy person taken immediately after awakening and before getting out of bed.

**basal body temperature method** Fertility awareness contraception method based on changes in the temperature of the woman's body at rest, first thing in the morning.

**basal cell carcinoma** A malignant epithelial cell tumor that begins as a papule and enlarges peripherally, developing a central crater that erodes, crusts, and bleeds.

**behavioral assessment** Assessment of activity, feeding and sleeping patterns, and responsiveness.

**bereavement** The feelings of loss, pain, desolation, and sadness that occur after the death of a loved one.

**bicornuate uterus** Anomalous uterus that may be either a double or single organ with two horns.

**bilateral tubal ligation** Abdominal procedure in which the uterine tubes are tied off and a section is removed to interrupt tubal continuity and thus sterilize the woman.

**bilirubin** Yellow or orange pigment that is a breakdown product of hemoglobin. It is carried by the blood to the liver, where it is chemically changed and excreted into the bile or is conjugated and excreted by the kidneys.

**Billings method** See *ovulation method*.

**bimanual** Performed with both hands.

    **b. palpation** Examination of a woman's pelvic organs done by placement of one hand on the abdomen and one or two fingers of the other hand into the vagina.

**binding-in** The progressive and formative maternal-child relationship that occurs over a 12- to 15-month period, spanning from pregnancy to 6 months postpartum.

**binge-eating/purging subtype** A particular manifestation of anorexia nervosa in which the woman may restrict food intake, but she also experiences periods of binge eating followed by purging.

**biofeedback** Technique that teaches the client to consciously control certain body functions usually thought of as unconscious (e.g., breathing, heart rate). Often involves electronic instrumentation that provides immediate visual and auditory feedback to assist the learning process.

**biophysical profile (BPP)** Noninvasive assessment of the fetus and its environment using ultrasonography and uterine fetal monitoring; includes fetal breathing movements, gross body movements, fetal tone, reactive fetal heart rate, and qualitative amniotic fluid volume.

**biopsy** Removal of a small piece of tissue for microscopic examination and diagnosis.

**biparietal diameter** Largest transverse diameter of the fetal head; extends from one parietal bone to the other.

**birth defect** Any abnormality present at birth, particularly a structural one, which may be inherited genetically, acquired during gestation, or inflicted during parturition.

**birth plan** A tool by which parents can explore their childbirth options and choose those that are most important to them.

**birth rate** Number of live births per 1000 women per year. See also *fertility*.

**Bishop score** Rating system to evaluate inducibility of the cervix; a higher score increases the rate of successful induction of labor.

**blastocyst** Stage in the development of a mammalian embryo, occurring after the morula stage, that consists of an outer layer, or trophoblast, and a hollow sphere of cells enclosing a cavity.

**blood pressure** The pressure exerted by the circulating volume of blood on the walls of the arteries and veins and the chambers of the heart. Overall blood pressure is maintained by the complex interaction of the homeostatic mechanisms of the body. During labor, blood pressure may vary from 100/60 to 140/90.

**bloody show** Vaginal discharge that originates in the cervix and consists of blood and mucus; increases as cervix dilates during labor.

**body boundaries** Boundaries that serve to separate the self from the nonself and provide a feeling of safety.

**body image** A person's subjective concept of his or her physical appearance.

**bonding** A process by which parents, over time, form an emotional relationship with their infant.

**Bradley method** Husband-coached childbirth using labor breathing techniques.

**Braxton-Hicks contractions** Mild, intermittent, painless uterine contractions that occur during pregnancy.

These contractions occur more frequently as pregnancy advances but do not represent true labor.

**breakthrough bleeding** Escape of blood occurring between menstrual periods; may be noted by women using oral contraception (birth control pills).

**breast abscess** An abscess of a mammary gland, usually during lactation or weaning.

**breast augmentation** Surgical procedure that uses silicone sheaths filled with saline to increase the size of a woman's breasts.

**breast self-examination (BSE)** Self-examination of the breasts.

**breast shells** Rigid plastic cups that are worn inside a bra to put pressure on the areola to help a nipple protrude or to protect sore nipples from the pressure of clothing.

**breech presentation** Presentation in which buttocks or feet are nearest the cervical opening and are born first; occurs in approximately 3% of all births.

    **complete or full b.p.** Simultaneous presentation of buttocks, legs, and feet.

    **footling (incomplete) b.p.** Presentation of one or both feet.

    **frank b.p.** Presentation of buttocks, with hips flexed and legs extended over the anterior surface of the body.

**bulimia nervosa** A disorder characterized by an insatiable craving for food, often resulting in episodes of continuous eating and often followed by purging, depression, and self-deprivation.

**café-au-lait spot** A pale tan macule the color of coffee with milk. Simultaneous development of several café-au-lait spots is associated with neurofibromatosis, but occasional café-au-lait spots occur normally.

**calcaneovalgus** A less-severe type of clubfoot characterized by lateral deviation and dorsiflexion either outward from or inward toward the midline of the body.

**calcium channel blocker** A drug that inhibits the flow of calcium ions across the membranes of smooth muscle cells. By reduction of the calcium flow, smooth muscle tone is relaxed and the risk of muscle spasms is diminished.

**calendar method** See *rhythm method*.

**canceled cycle** An ART cycle in which ovarian stimulation was carried out but was stopped before eggs were retrieved, or in the case of frozen embryo cycles, before embryos were transferred.

**candida vaginitis** Vaginal, fungal infection; formerly called moniliasis.

**candidiasis** Infection of the skin or mucous membrane by a yeastlike fungus, *Candida albicans;* see *thrush*.

**caput** Occiput of fetal head appearing at the vaginal introitus preceding birth of the head.

**carcinoma in situ** A premalignant neoplasm that has not invaded the basement membrane but shows cytologic characteristics of cancer.

**cardiac decompensation** A condition of heart failure in which the heart is unable to maintain a sufficient cardiac output.

**cardiac output (CO)** Volume of blood ejected from the left ventricle in 1 minute, measured in liters per minute. Cardiac output is the product of stroke volume and heart rate ($SV \times HR = CO$).

**cardinal movements of labor** The mechanism of labor in a vertex presentation; includes engagement, descent, flexion, internal rotation, extension, external rotation (restitution), and expulsion.

**carpal tunnel syndrome** Pressure on the median nerve at the point at which it goes through the carpal tunnel of the wrist. It causes soreness, tenderness, and weakness of the muscles of the thumb.

**carrier** Individual who carries a gene that does not exhibit itself in physical or chemical characteristics but that can be transmitted to children (e.g., a female carrying the trait for hemophilia, which is expressed in male offspring).

**cascade** Any process that develops in stages, with each stage dependent on the preceding one, often producing a cumulative effect.

**catecholamines (adrenalin)** Any one of a group of sympathomimetic compounds composed of a catechol molecule and the aliphatic portion of an amine. Some catecholamines are produced naturally by the body and function as key neurologic chemicals.

**Centers for Disease Control and Prevention (CDC)** A government agency within the U.S. Department of Health and Human Services responsible for publishing annual fertility clinic success rates.

**cephalhematoma** (NOTE: This is spelled cephalohematoma in some sources.) Extravasation of blood from ruptured vessels between a skull bone and its external covering, the periosteum. Swelling is limited by the margins of the cranial bone affected (usually parietals).

**cephalic presentation** A classification of fetal position in which the head of the fetus is at the uterine cervix. Cephalic presentation is usually further qualified by an indication of the part of head presenting, such as the occiput, brow, or chin.

**cephalocaudal development** Principle of maturation that development progresses from the head to tail (rump).

**cephalopelvic disproportion (CPD)** Condition in which the infant's head is of such a shape, size, or position that it cannot pass through the mother's pelvis.

**cerclage** Use of nonabsorbable suture to keep a premature dilating cervix closed; released when pregnancy is at term to allow labor to begin.

**Certified Nurse Midwife (CNM)** Has postgraduate training in the care of normal pregnancy and delivery and is certified by the American College of Nurse Midwives (ACNM).

**cervical cancer** A neoplasm of the uterine cervix that can be detected in the early stage by the Papanicolaou (Pap) test. Factors that may be associated with the development of cervical cancer are coitus at an early age, relations with many sexual partners, genital infections, multiparity, and poor obstetric and gynecologic care.

**cervical cap** Individually fitted contraceptive barrier for the cervix.

**cervical cauterization** Destruction (usually by heat or electric current) of the superficial tissue of the cervix.

**cervical conization** Excision of a cone-shaped section of tissue from the endocervix.

**cervical intraepithelial neoplasm (CIN)** Uncontrolled and progressive abnormal growth of cervical epithelial cells.

**cervical mucus method** See *ovulation method.*

**cervical os** "Mouth" or opening to the cervix.

**cervical ripening** Process of effecting physical softening and distensibility of the cervix in preparation for labor and birth

**cervicitis** Inflammation of the cervix.

**cervix** Lowest and narrow end of the uterus; the "neck." The cervix is situated between the external os and the body, or corpus, of the uterus, and its lower end extends into the vagina.

**cesarean birth** Birth of a fetus by an incision through the abdominal wall and uterus.

**cesarean hysterectomy** Removal of the uterus immediately after the cesarean birth of an infant.

**Chadwick's sign** Violet color of vaginal mucous membrane that is visible from about the fourth week of pregnancy; caused by increased vascularity.

**chancroid** A highly contagious sexually transmitted disease caused by infection with the bacillus *Haemophilus ducreyi.* It characteristically begins as a papule, usually on the skin of the external genitalia; it then grows and ulcerates, other papules form, and, if untreated, the bacillus spreads, causing buboes in the groin.

**chief complaint** Primary reason for a client seeking care.

**chlamydia** A sexually transmitted infection caused by the organism *chlamydia trachomatis.* Symptoms may include cervical motion tenderness or adnexal pain; however, many women have no symptoms at all. The consequences include PID, infertility, salpingitis, chronic pelvic pain, and transmittal of the infection to the neonate during vaginal birth.

**chloasma** Increased pigmentation over bridge of nose and cheeks of pregnant women and some women taking oral contraceptives; also known as mask of pregnancy.

**cholecystitis** Acute or chronic inflammation of the gallbladder.

**cholelithiasis** Presence of gallstones in the gallbladder.

**chorioamnionitis** Inflammatory reaction in fetal membranes to bacteria or viruses in the amniotic fluid, which then become infiltrated with polymorphonuclear leukocytes.

**choriocarcinoma** An epithelial malignancy of fetal origin that develops from the chorionic portion of the products of conception. The primary tumor usually appears in the uterus; it may invade and destroy the uterine wall; and it may metastasize through lymph or blood vessels, forming secondary hemorrhagic and necrotic tumors in the vaginal wall, vulva, lymph nodes, lungs, liver, and brain.

**chorion** Fetal membrane closest to the intrauterine wall that gives rise to the placenta and continues as the outer membrane surrounding the amnion.

**chorionic villus (villi)** Tiny vascular protrusions on the chorionic surface that project into the maternal blood sinuses of the uterus and that help form the placenta and secrete human chorionic gonadotropin.

**chorionic villus sampling (CVS)** Removal of fetal tissue from placenta for genetic diagnostic studies.

**chromosome** Element within the cell nucleus carrying genes and composed of DNA and proteins.

**chronic fatigue syndrome (CFS)** An autoimmune condition characterized by disabling fatigue, accompanied by a constellation of symptoms, including muscle pain, multijoint pain without swelling, painful cervical or axillary adenopathy, sore throat, headache, impaired memory or concentration, unrefreshing sleep, and postexertional malaise. The diagnosis is one of exclusion; the cause remains obscure.

**circumcision**

**female c.** Religious or cultural removal of a portion of the clitoris and labia; practiced in some Third World countries but illegal in the United States. This mutilating procedure can cause problems with intercourse, infection and childbirth.

**male c.** Excision of the prepuce (foreskin) of the penis, exposing the glans; may be done for religious or cultural reasons.

**cleansing breath** A deep and deliberate inhalation and exhalation that gives the mother a boost of oxygen which indicates the beginning and completion of a contraction. It is also called a welcoming or greeting breath.

**cleft lip** Incomplete closure of the lip. Lay term used is harelip.

**cleft palate** Incomplete closure of the palate or roof of mouth; a congenital fissure.

**climacteric** The period of a woman's life when she is passing from a reproductive to a nonreproductive state, with regression of ovarian function. The cycle of endocrine, physical, and psychosocial changes that occurs during the termination of the reproductive years. Also called climacterium.

**clitoris** Female organ analogous to male penis; a small, ovid body of erectile tissue situated at the anterior junction of the vulva.

clonus (ankle) Spasmodic alternation of muscular contraction and relaxation; counted in beats.

clubfoot Congenital deformity in which portions of the foot and ankle are twisted out of a normal position.

cocaine A bitter crystalline alkaloid obtained from coca leaves used medically as a topical anesthetic and illicitly for its euphoric effects and that may result in a compulsive psychologic need.

cognitive domain An area of learning that deals with the recall or recognition of knowledge and the development of intellectual abilities and skills.

coitus Penile-vaginal intercourse.

cold stress Excessive loss of heat that results in increased respirations and nonshivering thermogenesis to maintain core body temperature.

colostrum The fluid in the breast from pregnancy into the early postpartal period. It is rich in antibodies, which provide protection from many diseases; high in protein, which binds bilirubin; and laxative acting, which speeds the elimination of meconium and helps loosen mucus.

colposcopy Examination of vagina and cervix with a colposcope to identify neoplastic or other changes.

columnar epithelial cells The major cell group found in the endocervical canal; they appear long, narrow, and hexagonal in a one-cell layer along the papillae found in the canal.

combined oral contraceptives Oral hormone medication for contraception. The two major hormones used are progestin and a combination of progestin and estrogen. The hormones act by inhibiting the productivity of gonadotropin-releasing hormone by the hypothalamus, and therefore the pituitary does not secrete gonadotropins to stimulate ovulation. Also called oral contraceptives.

commercially prepared formula Cow's milk modified to more closely resemble the nutritional content of human milk. They are available in ready-to-use, concentrated, and powdered forms.

communication The exchange of thoughts, messages, or the like, as by speech, signals, or writing.

community A social group characterized by people within a geographic place and/or having common goals and interests.

community forum A meeting of members within the community with the express purpose of discussing or addressing particular issues that impact the community.

conception Union of the sperm and ovum resulting in fertilization; formation of the one-celled zygote.

conceptional age In fetal development the number of completed weeks since the moment of conception. Because the moment of conception is almost impossible to determine, conceptional age is estimated at 2 weeks less than gestational age.

conceptus Embryo or fetus, fetal membranes, amniotic fluid, and the fetal portion of the placenta.

condom, female A loose-fitting sheath with flexible rings that fit the top of the vagina and form a protective barrier for the external genitalia.

condom, male Mechanical barrier worn on the penis for contraception or to protect against STIs; a "rubber."

condyloma acuminatum Wartlike growth on the skin usually seen near the anus or external genitals caused by human papillomavirus (HPV); genital warts. (Must be differentiated from condyloma latum seen in secondary syphilis.) (Plural, condylomata acuminata.)

confinement Forced retirement from employment and/or home seclusion during pregnancy.

congenital Present at or existing before birth as a result of either hereditary or prenatal environmental factors.

congenital lymphedema A primary or secondary condition characterized by the accumulation of lymph in soft tissue and the resultant swelling caused by inflammation, obstruction, or removal of lymph channels.

congenital rubella syndrome Complex of problems, including hearing defects, cardiovascular abnormalities, and cataracts, caused by maternal rubella in the first trimester of pregnancy.

conjugate

diagonal c. Radiographic measurement of distance from inferior border of symphysis pubis to sacral promontory; may be obtained by vaginal examination; usually about 12.5 to 13 cm.

true c. (conjugata vera) Radiographic measurement of distance from upper margin of symphysis pubis to sacral promontory; generally 1.5 to 2 cm less than diagonal conjugate.

conscious relaxation Technique used to release the mind and body from tension through conscious effort and practice.

consultant A person who gives expert or professional advice.

contact dermatits Skin rash resulting from exposure to a primary irritant or to a sensitizing antigen. In the first, or nonallergic, type, a primary irritant, such as an alkaline detergent or an acid, causes a lesion similar to a thermal burn. In the second, or allergic type, sensitizing antigens cause an immunologic change in certain lymphocytes. Poison ivy is an example.

contraception Prevention of impregnation or conception.

contraction ring See *Bandl's ring.*

contractions

duration Period from the beginning of the contraction to the end.

frequency How often the contractions occur—the period from the beginning of one contraction to the beginning of the next.

**intensity** Strength of the contraction at its peak.

**interval** Period between uterine contractions, timed from the end of one contraction to the beginning of the next.

**resting tone** The tension in the uterine muscle between contractions.

**contraction stress test (CST)** Test to stimulate uterine contractions for the purpose of assessing fetal response; a healthy fetus does not react to contractions, whereas a compromised fetus demonstrates late decelerations in the fetal heart rate that are indicative of uteroplacental insufficiency.

**Coombs' test** Indirect: determination of Rh-positive antibodies in maternal blood; direct: determination of maternal Rh-positive antibodies in fetal cord blood. A positive test result indicates the presence of antibodies or titer.

**cordocentesis** Fetal blood analysis using fetal blood obtained through percutaneous umbilical cord sampling.

**cotyledon** One of the 15 to 28 visible segments of the placenta on the maternal surface, each made up of fetal vessels, chorionic villi, and an intervillous space.

**counterpressure** Pressure to sacral area of back during uterine contractions.

**couvade syndrome** The phenomenon of expectant fathers' experiencing pregnancy-like symptoms

**crack** Highly purified cocaine in small chips used illicitly (usually smoked).

**Crohn's disease** A chronic inflammatory bowel disease of unknown origin, usually affecting the ileum, the colon, or another part of the gastrointestinal tract. Diseased segments may be separated by normal bowel segments, which give it the characteristic "skip lesions."

**crowning** Stage of birth when the top of the fetal head can be seen at the vaginal orifice as the widest part of the head distends the vulva.

**cryosurgery** Local freezing and removal of tissue without injury to adjacent tissue and with minimum blood loss, done with special equipment.

**culdocentesis** Puncture of cul-de-sac of Douglas through the vagina for aspiration of fluid.

**cultural teachings** Beliefs and procedures valued and passed within a culture.

**culture** Setting in which one considers the individual's and the family's beliefs and practices (cultural context).

**curettage** Scraping of the endometrium lining of the uterus with a curet to remove the contents of the uterus (as is done after an incomplete miscarriage or induced abortion) or to obtain specimens for diagnostic purposes.

**cutis marmorata** Skin that has a "marbled" appearance caused by conspicuous dilation of small vessels.

**cyanosis** Bluish discoloration of the skin and mucous membranes caused by an excess of deoxygenated hemoglobin in the blood or a structural defect in the hemoglobin molecule, such as in methemoglobin.

**cyclic breast changes** Swelling, tenderness, or pain related to the menstrual cycle before and sometimes during the menstrual period.

**cycle of violence** Pattern of three phases: period of increasing tension, the abusive episode, and a period of contrition and kindness.

**cyst** A closed sac or pouch in or under the skin containing fluid or semisolid material.

**cystitis** An inflammatory condition of the urinary bladder and ureters, characterized by pain, urgency, frequency of urination, and hematuria. It may be caused by a bacterial infection, calculus, or tumor. Depending on the diagnosis, treatment may include anitbiotics, increased fluid intake, bed rest, medications to control bladder wall spasms, and, when necessary, surgery.

**daily fetal movement counts (DFMCs)** Maternal assessment of fetal activity; the number of fetal movements within a specific time are counted.

**date rape** A sexual assault or rape by a person known to the victim, such as a date, employer, friend, or casual acquaintance.

**decidua** Mucous membrane, lining of uterus, or endometrium of pregnancy that is shed after giving birth.

**deep tendon reflexes (DTRs)** Reflex caused by stimulation of tendons, such as elbow, wrist, knee, triceps, and ankle jerk reflexes.

**defecation** The elimination of feces from the digestive tract through the rectum.

**deformation** Abnormalities occurring during the second or third trimester.

**deformity** A condition of being distorted, disfigured, flawed, malformed, or misshapen, which may affect the body in general or any part of it. The deformity may be a result of disease, injury, or birth defect.

**delivery (birth)** Expulsion of the child with placenta and membranes by the mother or their extraction by the birth attendant.
  **abdominal d.** See *abdominal birth.*

**deoxyribonucleic acid (DNA)** Intracellular complex protein that carries genetic information, consisting of two purines (adenine and guanine) and two pyrimidines (thymine and cytosine).

**Depo-Provera (DMPA)** An injectable contraceptive, it is given intramuscularly in 150-mg doses every 12 weeks.

**DES** Diethylstilbestrol; female fetus is predisposed to reproductive tract malformations and (later) dysplasia if her mother ingested this medication during pregnancy.

**developmental dysplasia of the hip (Congenital dislocation of the hip)** An orthopedic defect, present at birth, in which the head of the femur does not articulate with the acetabulum as a result of an abnormal shallowness of the acetabulum. Treatment consists of maintaining continuous adduction of the thigh so that the head of the femur presses into the center of the shallow cavity, causing it to deepen.

developmental theory Theoretic approach for viewing the family. The developmental perspective sees family members pass through phases of growth from dependence through active independence to interdependence.

diabetes mellitus Systemic disorder of carbohydrate, protein, and fat metabolism; caused by deficient insulin production or ineffective use of insulin at the cellular level.

diabetogenic state A health condition manifested by signs and symptoms of diabetes.

diaphoresis The secretion of sweat, especially the profuse secretion associated with an elevated body temperature, physical exertion, exposure to heat, and mental or emotional stress.

diastasis recti abdominis Separation of the two rectus muscles along the median line of the abdominal wall. This is often seen in women with repeated childbirths or with a multiple gestation (e.g., triplets). In the newborn it is usually attributable to incomplete development.

Dick-Read method An approach to childbirth based on the premise that fear of pain produces muscular tension, producing pain and greater fear. The method includes teaching physiologic processes of labor, exercise to improve muscle tone, and techniques to assist in relaxation and prevent the fear-tension-pain mechanism.

dilation of cervix Stretching of the external os from an opening a few millimeters in size to an opening large enough to allow the passage of the infant.

diploid number Having two sets of chromosomes; found normally in somatic (body) cells; 23 sets or 46 chromosomes.

disseminated intravascular coagulation (DIC) Pathologic form of coagulation in which clotting factors are consumed to such an extent that generalized bleeding can occur; associated with abruptio placentae, eclampsia, intrauterine fetal demise, amniotic fluid embolism, and hemorrhage.

diuresis Increased formation and secretion of urine. It occurs in conditions such as diabetes mellitus, diabetes insipidus, or acute renal failure, and is normal in the first 48 hours after delivery.

dizygotic Related to or proceeding from two zygotes (fertilized ova).

domain A particular sphere of concern or function.

domestic violence Interpersonal violence, including child, elder, sibling, and spouse.

dominant trait Gene that is expressed whenever it is present in the heterozygous gene state (e.g., brown eyes are dominant over blue).

donor egg cycle An embryo formed from the egg of one woman (the donor) and then transferred to another woman who is unable to conceive with her own eggs (the recipient). The donor relinquishes all parental rights to any resulting offspring.

Doppler blood flow analysis Device for noninvasive measurement of blood flow between the fetus and placenta to assess for intrauterine growth restriction.

doula Experienced assistant hired to give the woman support during labor and birth.

Down syndrome Abnormality involving the occurrence of a third chromosome, rather than the normal pair (trisomy 21), that characteristically results in a typical picture of mental retardation and altered physical appearance. This condition was formerly called mongolism.

drug dependence (addiction) Physical or psychologic dependence or both on a chemical substance.

ductus arteriosus In fetal circulation an anatomic shunt between the pulmonary artery and arch of the aorta. It is obliterated after birth by a rising $PO_2$ and a change in intravascular pressures in the presence of normal pulmonary function. It normally becomes a ligament after birth but in some instances remains patent.

ductus venosus In fetal circulation, a blood vessel carrying oxygenated blood between the umbilical vein and the inferior vena cava, bypassing the liver. It is obliterated and becomes a ligament after birth.

dysfunctional labor Abnormal uterine contractions that prevent normal progress of cervical dilation and effacement.

dysfunctional uterine bleeding (DUB) Abnormal bleeding from the uterus for reasons that are not readily established.

dysmenorrhea Pain associated with menstruation.
   primary d. Painful menstruation beginning 2 to 6 months after menarche, related to ovulation.
   secondary d. Painful menstruation related to organic disease such as endometriosis, pelvic inflammatory disease, or uterine neoplasm.

dyspareunia Painful sexual intercourse.

dysplasia Any abnormal development of tissues or organs.

dystocia Prolonged, painful, or otherwise difficult birth because of mechanical factors produced by the passenger (the fetus) or the passage (the pelvis and soft tissues of the birth canal of the mother), inadequate powers (uterine and other muscular activity), or maternal position.

Ebstein anomaly A congenital heart defect in which the tricuspid valve is displaced downward into the right ventricle. The abnormality is often associated with right-to-left atrial shunting and Wolff-Parkinson-White syndrome.

ecchymosis Bruise; bleeding into tissue caused by direct trauma, serious infection, or bleeding disorder.

eclampsia Severe complication of pregnancy of unknown cause and occurring more often in the primigravida; characterized by tonic and clonic convulsions, coma, high blood pressure, albuminuria, and oliguria occurring during pregnancy or shortly after birth.

**economic abuse** Making a woman dependent by maintaining total control over financial resources.

**economic support** A pregnant woman's source, level, and stability of income, as well as degree of dependence on another person for economic support.

**ectopic** Out of normal place.

e. **pregnancy** Implantation of the fertilized ovum outside of its normal place in the uterine cavity. Locations include the abdomen, uterine tubes, and ovaries.

**edema** Generalized accumulation of interstitial fluid.

dependent e. Edema of lower or most dependent parts of body where hydrostatic pressure is greater.

**educational level** The degree of formal schooling a woman has received.

**effacement** Thinning and shortening or obliteration of the cervix that occurs during late pregnancy or labor or both.

**effleurage** Gentle stroking used in massage.

**egg** A female reproductive cell, also called an oocyte or ovum.

**egg retrieval** The first stage in the ART cycle; a surgical procedure in which the woman's eggs are collected from the woman's ovaries for combination with sperm in the laboratory. Also called oocyte retrieval.

**egg transfer** The transfer of retrieved eggs into a woman's fallopian tubes through laparoscopy (see definition). This procedure is used only in GIFT (see definition).

**Eisenmenger syndrome** Pulmonary hypertension characterized by elevated pulmonary vascular resistance and right-to-left (or bidirectional) shunting in either atria or ventricles.

**emancipated minor** A person who is not legally an adult but who, because he or she is married, in the military, or otherwise no longer dependent on the parents, may not require parental permission for medical or surgical care. State and national laws vary in specific interpretations of the rule.

**embolus** Any undissolved matter (solid, liquid, or gaseous) that is carried by the blood to another part of the body and obstructs a blood vessel.

**embryo** Conceptus from the second or third week of development until about the eighth week after conception, when mineralization (ossification) of the skeleton begins. This period is characterized by cellular differentiation and predominantly hyperplastic growth.

**embryo transfer** Placement of embryos into a woman's uterus through the cervix after in vitro fertilization.

**emotional abuse** The debasement of a person's feelings that causes the individual to perceive himself or herself as inept, not cared for, and worthless.

**emotional lability** Rapid mood changes from irritability to anger or sadness to joy and cheerfulness; often seen in the first trimester of pregnancy.

**empowerment** To enable, permit, or invest another with power.

**endocervical** Pertaining to the interior of the canal of the cervix of the uterus.

**endometriosis** Endometrial tissue located outside the uterine cavity. Symptoms may include pelvic pain or pressure, dysmenorrhea, dyspareunia, abnormal bleeding from the uterus or rectum, and sterility.

**endometritis** Postpartum uterine inflammation, often beginning at the site of the placental implantation.

**endometrium** Inner lining of the uterus that undergoes changes caused by hormones during the menstrual cycle and pregnancy; decidua.

**endorphins** Endogenous opioids secreted by the pituitary gland that act on the central and peripheral nervous systems to reduce pain.

**en face** Face-to-face position in which the parent's and infant's faces are approximately 20 cm apart and on the same plane.

**engagement** In obstetrics, the entrance of the fetal presenting part into the superior pelvic strait and the beginning of the descent through the pelvic canal.

**engorgement** Distention or vascular congestion. In obstetrics, the process of swelling of the breast tissue brought about by an increase in blood and lymph supply to the breast, which precedes true lactation. It lasts about 48 hours and usually reaches a peak between the third and fifth postbirth days.

**engrossment** A parent's absorption, preoccupation, and interest in his or her infant; term typically used to describe the father's intense involvement with his newborn.

**enzyme-linked immunosorbent assay (ELISA)** A pregnancy test that uses an enzyme to identify the antigen to be measured; hCG amounts as low as 25mIU/ml may be registered. The most common test, it is also the basis of most of the over-the-counter home pregnancy tests.

**epicanthus** Fold of skin covering the inner canthus and caruncle that extends from the root of the nose to the median end of the eyebrow; characteristically found in certain races but may occur as a congenital anomaly.

**epidemiology** The study of the determinants of disease events in populations.

**epidural block** Type of regional anesthesia produced by injection of a local anesthetic into the epidural (peridural) space.

**epidural blood patch** A patch formed by a few millimeters of the mother's blood occluding a tear or hole in the dura mater around the spinal cord.

**episiotomy** Surgical incision of the perineum at the end of the second stage of labor to facilitate birth.

   **mediolateral e.** The incision is made at about 4:00 and goes across the natural longitudinal pattern of the musculature of the perineum. They are more difficult to repair and heal, but there is much less danger that it will extend to the rectum.

   **midline e.** The incision is made straight down from the vaginal os. It is easier to repair and heal, but there is a danger that it will extend to the rectum.

**epispadias** Defect in which the urethral canal terminates on the dorsum of the penis or above the clitoris (rare).

**Epstein's pearls** Small, white blebs found along the gum margins and at the junction of the soft and hard palates. They are a normal manifestation and are typically seen in the newborn. Similar to Bohn's nodules.

**epulis** Tumorlike benign lesion of the gingiva seen in pregnant women.

**Erb-Duchenne paralysis** Paralysis caused by physical injury to the upper brachial plexus, occurring most often in childbirth from forcible traction during birth. The signs of Erb-Duchenne paralysis include loss of sensation in the arm and paralysis and atrophy of the deltoid, the biceps, and the branchialis muscles. Also called Erb's palsy.

**ergot** Drug obtained from Claviceps purpurea, a fungus, which stimulates the smooth muscles of blood vessels and the uterus, causing vasoconstriction and uterine contractions.

**erythema toxicum neonatorum** Innocuous pink papular neonatal rash of unknown cause, with superimposed vesicles appearing within 24 to 48 hours after birth and resolving spontaneously within a few days.

**erythroblastosis fetalis** Hemolytic disease of the newborn usually caused by isoimmunization resulting from Rh incompatibility or ABO incompatibility.

**erythropoietin** A glycoprotein hormone synthesized mainly in the kidneys and released into the bloodstream in response to anoxia. The hormone acts to stimulate and to regulate the production of reythrocytes and thus increases the oxygen-carrying capacity of the blood.

**essential vulvodynia** Chronic pain, itching or discomfort in the female external genitals without an identified cause.

**estimated date of confinement (EDC)** An antiquated term from when women were generally confined or separated from the public for childbirth.

**estimated date of delivery (EDD)** Approximate date of birth. Usually determined by calculation using Nägele's rule; "due date."

**estradiol** The most potent naturally occurring human estrogen.

**estriol** Major metabolite of estrogen that increases during the second half of pregnancy with an intact fetoplacental unit (normal placenta, normal fetal liver and adrenals) and normal maternal renal function.

**estrogen** Female sex hormone produced by the ovaries and placenta.

**estrogen replacement therapy (ERT)** Exogenous estrogen given to women during and after menopause to prevent hot flashes, mood changes, osteoporosis, and genitourinary symptoms.

**ethnic group** A population of individuals organized on the basis of an assumed common cultural origin.

**ethnicity** The condition of belonging to a particular ethnic group; a social group within a cultural and social system that claims or is accorded special status on the basis of complex, often variable traits including religious, linguistic, ancestral, or physical characteristics.

**euglycemia** A normal concentration of glucose in the blood.

**evaluation** A category of nursing behavior in which the extent to which the established goals of care have been met is determined and recorded.

**evaporated milk formula** Homogenized whole milk from which 50% to 60% of the water content has been evaporated. It is fortified with vitamin D, canned, and sterilized. When it is diluted with an equal amount of water, its nutritional value is comparable to that of fresh whole milk.

**exchange transfusion** Replacement of 75% to 85% of circulating blood by withdrawal of the recipient's blood and injection of a donor's blood in equal amounts, the purposes of which are to prevent an accumulation of bilirubin in the blood above a dangerous level, to prevent the accumulation of other byproducts of hemolysis in hemolytic disease, and to correct anemia and acidosis.

**external genitalia** The vulva or pudenum; collective term for the labia majora, labia minora, clitoris, urinary meatus, and vaginal introitus.

**extrauterine** Occurring outside the uterus.

**failure to progress (FTP)** An arrest in the dilation process that places the fetus or mother in danger; an indication that a cesarean section may be required.

**fallopian tubes** Two canals or oviducts extending laterally from each side of the uterus through which the ovum travels, after ovulation, to the uterus; also called uterine tubes.

**false labor** Uterine contractions that do not result in cervical dilation, are irregular, are felt more in front, often do not last more than 20 seconds, and do not become longer or stronger. Also called Braxton-Hicks contractions.

**false negative** Test results that indicate that a person does not have a condition when in fact he or she does have it.

**false pelvis** Part of the pelvis superior to a plane passing through the linea terminalis (brim or outlet).

**false positive** Test results that indicate that a person has a condition when in fact he or she does not have it.

**false positive pregnancy test** Generally rare, they may occur if there was an error, a misreading, drug use, hormonal changes related to menopause, tumors, or other medical conditions.

**family** A group of two or more persons related by birth, marriage, or adoption and residing together.

**family functions** Activities carried out within families for the well-being of family members, including biologic, economic, educational, psychologic, and sociocultural aspects.

**family-interactional approach** A therapy model that views the family as a communication system comprising interlocking subsystems of family members. Family dysfunction occurs when the rules governing family interaction become vague and ambiguous. The therapeutic goal is to help the family clarify the rules governing their relationships.

**family nurse practitioner (FNP)** Has advanced preparation and is certified in the promotion of health and prevention of illness in all persons across the lifespan.

**family structural-functional theory** A model of family therapy that views the family as an open system and identifies subsystems within the family that carry out specific family functions.

**family structure** Self-defined pattern of family makeup.

**family systems theory** Theory that conceptualizes the family as a unit and focuses on observing interactions among family members.

**fat necrosis** A condition caused by trauma or infection in which neutral tissue fats are broken down into fatty acids and glycerol.

**feedback** Process by which the system gains information that aids in establishing equilibrium.

**female genital mutilation (FGM)** Any procedure that involves partial or total removal of the external female genitalia or other injury to the female genital organs whether for cultural or any other non-therapeutic reasons.

**female reproductive cycle (FRC)** A complex set of events involving the sequential occurrence of the ovarian cycle, during which ovulation occurs, and the menstrual cycle, during which menstruation occurs.

**fern (arborization) test** The appearance of a fernlike pattern found on microscope slides of certain fluids.

   **ovulation f.t.** Test in which cervical mucus, placed on a slide, dries in a branching pattern in the presence of high estrogen levels at the time of ovulation.

**fertile period** Period before and after ovulation during which the human ovum can be fertilized; usually 3 days before and 4 days after ovulation.

**fertility** Quality of being able to reproduce; also number of births per 1000 women ages 15 through 44 years. See also *birth rate.*

**fertility awareness methods** Contraception based on abstinence during ovulation is identified by natural changes in a woman's body.

**fertilization** The penetration of the egg by the sperm and the resulting combining of genetic material that develops into an embryo.

**fetal** Pertaining or relating to the fetus.

   **f. age** The age of the conceptus computed from the time elapsed since fertilization. It is 2 weeks less than the gestational age in a woman who has regular 28-day menstrual cycles.

   **f. alcohol effect (FAE)** Lesser set of the same symptoms that make up fetal alcohol syndrome.

   **f. alcohol syndrome (FAS)** Congenital abnormality or anomaly resulting from excessive maternal alcohol intake during pregnancy. It is characterized by typical craniofacial and limb defects, cardiovascular defects, intrauterine growth restriction, and developmental delay.

   **f. asphyxia** A condition of hypoxemia, hypercapnia, and respiratory and metabolic acidosis that may occur in the uterus. Among possible causes are uteroplacental insufficiency, abruptio placentae, placenta previa, uterine tetany, maternal hypotension, and compression of the umbilical cord.

   **f. attitude** See *attitude, fetal.*

   **f. compromise** Evidence such as a nonreassuring fetal heart rate pattern that indicates the fetus may be in jeopardy.

   **f. heart rate (FHR)** Beats per minute of the fetal heart. Normal range is 110 to 160 beats per minute.

   **f. lie** Relation of the fetal spine to the maternal spine; that is, in vertical lie, maternal and fetal spines are parallel and the fetal head or breech presents; in transverse lie, fetal spine is perpendicular to the maternal spine and the fetal shoulder presents.

   **f. presentation** The part of the fetus that enters the pelvic inlet first.

   **f. scalp (or spiral) electrode** Internal signal source for electronically monitoring the fetal heart rate.

**fetal heart rate**

   **acceleration** Increase in fetal heart rate, usually seen as a reassuring sign.

   **baseline** Average fetal heart rate between uterine contractions.

   **bradycardia** Baseline fetal heart rate below 110 beats per minute.

   **deceleration** Slowing of fetal heart rate attributed to a parasympathetic response and described in relation to uterine contractions.

   **early deceleration** Onset corresponding to onset of uterine contraction, related to fetal head compression.

late deceleration Onset after peak of contraction, continuing into interval after contraction; caused by uteroplacental insufficiency.

prolonged deceleration Slowing of fetal heart rate lasting longer than 2 minutes.

tachycardia Baseline fetal heart rate above 160 beats per minute.

variable deceleration Onset at any time unrelated to contraction; caused by cord compression.

fetal well-being An area of assessment during the labor process considering the status of the fetal heart rate.

fetus The unborn offspring from approximately the eighth week after conception until birth.

fibroadenoma A benign tumor composed of dense epithelial and fibroblastic tissue. A fibroadenoma of the breast is nontender, encapsulated, round, movable, and firm. It occurs most frequently in women under 25 years of age.

fibroid Fibrous, encapsulated connective tissue tumor, especially of the uterus.

fibromyalgia A form of nonarticular rheumatism characterized by musculoskeletal pain, spasm and stiffness, fatigue, and severe sleep disturbance. Common sites of pain are called trigger points. Physical therapy, nonsteroidal antiinflammatory drugs, and muscle relaxants provide temporary relief.

flaccid Having relaxed, limp, or absent muscle tone.

flexion Opposite of extension. In obstetrics, resistance to the descent of the baby down the birth canal causes the head to flex, or bend, so that the chin approaches the chest. Thus the smallest diameter (suboccipitobregmatic) of the vertex presents.

focal seizure A transitory disturbance in motor, sensory, or autonomic function that results from abnormal neuronal discharges in a localized part of the brain, most frequently motor or sensory areas adjacent to the central sulcus.

follicle A structure in the ovaries that contains a developing egg.

follicle-stimulating hormone (FSH) Hormone produced by the anterior pituitary during the first half of the menstrual cycle. Stimulates development of the graafian follicle.

follicular cysts A type of functional ovarian tumor, follicular cysts are caused by the failure of the ovarian follicle to rupture at the time of ovulation.

folliculitis Inflammation of hair follicles, forming small abscesses.

fontanel Broad area, or soft spot, consisting of a strong band of connective tissue contiguous with cranial bones and located at the junctions of the bones.

anterior f. Diamond-shaped area between the frontal and two parietal bones just above the baby's forehead at the junction of the coronal and sagittal sutures.

mastoid f. A posterolateral area that is not palpable.

posterior f. Small, triangular area between the occipital and parietal bones at the junction of the lambdoidal and sagittal sutures.

sagittal f. Soft area located in the sagittal suture, halfway between the anterior and posterior fontanels; may be palpated in normal newborns and in some neonates with Down syndrome.

sphenoid f. Anterolateral fontanel, usually not palpable.

food frequency questionnaire (FFQ) Identifies food intake over a specific period of time. It provides a list of foods and a scale for identifying how often each is consumed over a given period of time. The list may be all-inclusive or it may focus only on foods specifically related to the particular chronic illness.

food record An account of food eaten and an estimate of amounts within a certain period of time, usually 3 to 7 days.

footling (incomplete) breech presentation See *breech presentation, footling*.

forceps Curved-bladed instruments used to protect head of fetus during birth and to apply traction to assist birth.

forceps-assisted birth Birth in which forceps are used to assist in delivery of the fetal head.

foreskin Prepuce, or loose fold of skin covering the glans penis.

formative evaluation Feedback incorporated into an ongoing class for the purpose of focusing the content of the specific class and subsequent classes within the series.

fornix of the vagina Anterior and posterior spaces, formed by the protrusion of the cervix into the vagina, into which the upper vagina is divided.

fourth trimester Another term for the 3-month interval after the birth of the newborn that includes return of the reproductive organs to their nonpregnant state and psychologic adaptation to parenthood.

frank breech presentation See *breech presentation, frank*.

fraternal twins See *twins, dizygotic*.

free-standing birth center A center that provides prenatal care, labor and birth, and postbirth care outside of a hospital setting.

frenulum Thin ridge of tissue in midline of undersurface of tongue extending from its base to varying distances from the tip of the tongue.

fresh eggs, sperm, or embryos Eggs, sperm, or embryos that have not been frozen. However, fresh embryos may have been conceived using fresh or frozen sperm.

friability Easily broken. May refer to a fragile condition of the cervix, especially during pregnancy, that causes the cervix to bleed easily when touched.

Friedman's curve Labor curve; pattern of descent of presenting part and of dilation of cervix; partogram.

frozen cycle A cycle in which embryos are preserved through freezing (cryopreservation) for transfer at a later date.

**FSH** See *follicle-stimulating hormone.*

**function** Activities that a group, organization, or community use to achieve goals.

**fundus** Dome-shaped upper portion of the uterus between the points of insertion of the uterine tubes.

**funic souffle** See *souffle, funic.*

**galactorrhea** Lactation not associated with childbirth or breastfeeding; a symptom of a pituitary gland tumor.

**galactosemia** Inherited, autosomal recessive disorder of galactose metabolism, characterized by a deficiency of the enzyme galactose-1-phosphate uridyltransferase.

**gamete** Mature male or female germ cell; the mature sperm or ovum.

**gamete intrafallopian transfer (GIFT)** A human fertilization technique in which male and female gametes are transferred to the fallopian tubes.

**gastroenteritis** Inflammation of the stomach and intestines accompanying numerous gastrointestinal disorders. Symptoms are anorexia, nausea, vomiting, fever (depending on causative factor), abdominal discomfort, and diarrhea.

**gate control theory** Proposed in 1965 by Melzack and Wall, this theory explains the neurophysical mechanism underlying the perception of pain: the capacity of nerve pathways to transmit pain is reduced or completely blocked by using distraction techniques.

**gender** Sense or awareness of knowing to which sex one belongs. The process begins in infancy, continues throughout childhood, and is reinforced during adolescence.

**gene** Factor on a chromosome responsible for hereditary characteristics of offspring.

**genetic** Dependent on the genes. A genetic disorder may or may not be apparent at birth.

**genetic counseling** Process of determining the occurrence or risk of occurrence of a genetic disorder within a family and of providing appropriate information and advice about the courses of action that are available, whether care of a child already affected, prenatal diagnosis, termination of a pregnancy, sterilization, or artificial insemination is involved.

**genitalia** Organs of reproduction.

**genital warts** A small soft moist pink or red swelling that becomes pedunculated. The growth may be solitary, or a cauliflower-like group may be present in the same area. It is caused by a human papilloma virus (HPV) and is contagious.

**genome** Complete copy of genetic material in an organism.

**genotype** Hereditary combinations in an individual determining physical and chemical characteristics. Some genotypes are not expressed until later in life (e.g., Huntington's chorea); some hide recessive genes, which can be expressed in offspring; and others are expressed only under the proper environmental conditions (e.g., diabetes mellitus appearing under the stress of obesity or pregnancy).

**geopolitical communities** Social groups based on geographic boundaries, common governance or association (i.e., apartment complex or fire protection district).

**gestation** Period of intrauterine fetal development from conception through birth; the period of pregnancy.

**gestational age** In fetal development, the number of completed weeks counting from the first day of the last normal menstrual cycle.

**gestational carrier** (Also called a gestational surrogate.) A woman who carries an embryo that was formed from the egg of another woman. The gestational carrier usually has a contractual obligation to return the infant to its intended parents.

**gestational diabetes** Glucose intolerance first recognized during pregnancy.

**gestational hypertension** Hypertension or proteinuria that develops during pregnancy, generally after 20 weeks of gestation in the absence of a molar pregnancy and subsides after delivery.

**gestational proteinuria** The finding of protein in a woman's urine after 20 weeks of gestation when she has no history of it prior to the pregnancy and she does not have hypertension.

**gestational sac** A fluid-filled structure that develops within the uterus early in pregnancy. In a normal pregnancy, a gestational sac contains a developing fetus.

**gestational trophoblastic disease** A spectrum of neoplastic disorders that have common clinical findings (e.g. abnormal proliferative tissues) and abnormally high HCg levels.

**gestational trophoblastic neoplasia (GTN)** Persistent trophoblastic tissue that is presumed to be malignant.

**glans penis** Smooth, round head of the penis, analogous to the female glans clitoris.

**glomerulonephritis** Noninfectious disease of the glomerulus of the kidney, characterized by proteinuria, hematuria, decreased urine production, and edema.

**glucose tolerance test** A test of the body's ability to use carbohydrates; used as a screening measure for gestational diabetes.

**glycosuria** Presence of glucose (a sugar) in the urine.

**glycosylated hemoglobin (Ghb)** Glycohemoglobin, a minor hemoglobin with glucose attached. Ghb A1c concentration represents the average blood glucose level over the previous several weeks and is a measurement for glycemic control in diabetic therapy.

**goal** Statement of intent and purpose that helps to focus planning toward long-range outcomes.

**gonad** Gamete-producing, or sex, gland; the ovary or testis.

**gonadotropic hormone** Hormone that stimulates the gonads.

gonadotropin-releasing hormone (GnRH) Hormone released from hypothalamus that stimulates pituitary gland to produce FSH and LH.

gonorrhea A common sexually transmitted disease that most often affects the genitourinary tract and occasionally the pharynx, conjunctiva, or rectum. Infection results from contact with an infected person or with secretions containing the causative *Neisseria gonorrhoeae*.

Goodell's sign Softening of the cervix, a probable sign of pregnancy, occurring during the second month.

granuloma inguinale A sexually transmitted disease characterized by ulcers of the skin and subcutaneous tissues of the groin and genitalia. It is caused by infection with *Calymmatobacterium granulomatis*, a small, gram-negative, rod-shaped bacillus.

gravida Pregnant woman.

gravidity Number of times a woman has been pregnant.

grief process A complex of somatic and psychologic symptoms associated with some extreme sorrow or loss, specifically the death of a loved one.

growth The increase in the size of an organism or any of its parts, as measured in increments of weight, volume, or linear dimensions, that occurs as a result of hyperplasia or hypertrophy.

grunt, expiratory Sign of respiratory distress (hyaline membrane disease [respiratory distress syndrome, or RDS] or advanced pneumonia) indicative of the body's attempt to hold air in the alveoli for better gaseous exchange.

guided imagery The use of imagination and thought processes in a purposeful way to change certain physiologic and emotional conditions.

gustatory movements Part of the first period of reactivity just after birth. The infant pushes his or her tongue out, indicating he or she is ready to feed.

gynecology Study of the diseases of the female, especially of the genital, urinary, and rectal organs.

habituation An acquired tolerance from repeated exposure to a particular stimulus. Also called negative adaptation; a decline and eventual elimination of a conditioned response by repetition of the conditioned stimulus.

harlequin sign Rare color change of no pathologic significance occurring between the longitudinal halves of the neonate's body. When infant is placed on one side, the dependent half is noticeably pinker than the superior half.

hashish The concentrated resin from the flowering tops of the female hemp plant that is smoked, chewed, or drunk for its intoxicating effect.

hash oil Resins and other juices from the hemp plant that are often spread onto tobacco cigarettes.

healing The integrating and balancing of the body, mind, and spirit. May or may not affect physical healing from illness. Often perceived as improved sense of well-being, acceptance, and inner peace and harmony.

healing touch A combination of energetic healing techniques used by nurses and other health care professionals.

heart rate The first and most important parameter in the Apgar score. The rate varies from 120 to 190 bpm in the first 15 minutes of extrauterine life. After 15 minutes, the average is between 120 and 140 bpm with a possible range of 90 to 175 bpm. Consistently low rates may indicate a pathologic condition.

Hegar's sign Softening of the lower uterine segment that is classified as a probable sign of pregnancy and that may be present during the second and third months of pregnancy and is palpated during bimanual examination.

helix The tip of the ear.

HELLP syndrome Condition characterized by hemolysis, elevated liver enzymes, and low platelet count; a form of severe preeclampsia.

hematocrit Volume of red blood cells per deciliter (dl) of circulating blood; packed cell volume (PCV).

hematoma Collection of blood in a tissue; a bruise or blood tumor.

hemodilution An increase in fluid content of blood, resulting in diminution of the proportion of formed elements.

hemoglobin Component of red blood cells consisting of globin, a protein, and hematin, an organic iron compound.

   h. electrophoresis Test to diagnose sickle cell disease in newborns. Cord blood is used.

hemolytic disease of the newborn Breakdown of fetal red blood cells by maternal antibodies, usually from an Rh-negative mother.

hemorrhage A loss of a large amount of blood in a short period, either externally or internally. The blood loss may be arterial, venous, or capillary.

hemorrhoid A varicosity in the lower rectum or anus caused by congestion in the veins of the hemorrhoidal plexus.

hepatitis A A form of infectious viral hepatitis caused by the hepatitis A virus (HAV), characterized by slow onset of signs and symptoms. The virus may be spread by direct contact through fecally-contaminated food or ward. The infection most often occurs in young adults and is usually followed by complete recovery.

hepatitis B A form of viral hepatitis caused by the hepatitis B virus (HBV). The virus is transmitted in contaminated serum in blood tranfusion, by sexual contact with an infected person, or by the use of contaminated needles and instruments. Severe infection may cause prolonged illness, destruction of liver cells, cirrhosis, or death. A vaccine is available and recommended for those at risk for exposure.

**hermaphrodite** Person having genital and sexual characteristics of both sexes.

**heroin** A strongly physiologically addictive narcotic that is made by acetylation of morphine resulting in a more potent drug. It is prohibited for medicinal use in the United States but is used illicitly for its euphoric effects.

**herpes** Indicates vesicular eruptions caused by a virus, usually herpes simplex.

**herpes simplex virus (HSV)** An infection caused by herpes simplex virus type 1 or type 2, which has an affinity for the skin and nervous system and usually produces small, transient, irritating and sometimes painful fluid-filled blisters on the skin and mucous membranes. HSV-1 infections tend to occur in the facial area, partiuclarly around the mouth and nose; HSV-2 infections are usually limited to the genital region.

**heterozygous** Having two dissimilar genes at the same site, or locus, on paired chromosomes (e.g., at the site for eye color, one chromosome carrying the gene for brown, the other for blue).

**hiatal hernia** Protrusion of a portion of the stomach upward through the diaphragm.

**holism** Philosophy that states that the whole is greater than the sum of its parts. In healing, refers to consideration and treatment of the whole client as a unified being. May include alternative and complementary modalities, but it is more a philosophic base than a modality in and of itself.

**holistic medicine** Health care treatment with techniques not commonly taught in U.S. medical schools or widely available in U.S. hospitals. May include a variety of disciplines involving diet, exercise, vitamin and nutritional supplements, bodywork, or alternative pharmacologic agents. Philosophy of medicine that encompasses holism.

**holistic nursing** Nursing practice that stems from the philosophy of holism, one that views the client as an integrated whole, and influenced by a variety of internal and external factors, including the biopsychosocial and spiritual dimensions of the person.

**Homans' sign** Early sign of phlebothrombosis of the deep veins of the calf in which there are complaints of pain when the leg is in extension and the foot is dorsiflexed.

**home birth** Planned birth of the child at home.

**homeopath** A physician practicing a system of therapeutics based on the theory that "like cures like." A large amount of a particular drug may cause symptoms of a disease and moderate dosage may reduce those symptoms; thus some disease symptoms could be treated with very small doses of medicine.

**homologous insemination** Insemination in which the semen specimen is provided by the husband. The procedure is used primarily in cases of impotence or when the husband is incapable of sexual intercourse because of some physical disability.

**homosexual family** Family in which parents form a homosexual union. Children may be the offspring of a previous heterosexual union, adopted, or conceived by one or both members of a homosexual couple through artificial insemination.

**homozygous** Having two similar genes at the same locus, or site, on paired chromosomes.

**hormone** Chemical substance produced in an organ or gland that is conveyed through the blood to another organ or part of the body, stimulating it to increased functional activity or secretion.

**hormone therapy** The treatment of diseases with hormones obtained from endocrine glands or substances that simulate hormonal effects.

**household** All persons who occupy a housing unit (house, apartment, etc.), including related members and unrelated persons.

**householder** The one in whose name the household is owned or rented.

**human chorionic gonadotropin (hCG)** Hormone that is produced by chorionic villi; the biologic marker in pregnancy tests.

**human gestational period** The average length of gestation; either 266 days from fertilization or 280 days from the first day of the woman's last true menstrual period.

**husband-coached childbirth** A method of psychophysical preparation for childbirth, comprising education about the physiologic characteristics of childbirth, exercise and nutrition during pregnancy, and techniques of breathing and relaxation for control and comfort during labor and delivery. The father is extensively involved in the classes and acts as the mother's "coach" during labor. Among the advantages of the method are its simplicity, the father's involvement, and the realistic approach to the efforts and discomfort of labor.

**hyaline membrane disease (HMD)** See *respiratory distress syndrome (RDS)*.

**hydatidiform mole (molar pregnancy)** Gestational trophoblastic neoplasm usually resulting from fertilization of egg that has no nucleus or an inactivated nucleus.

**hydralazine** A vasodilator used in hypertension.

**hydramnios (polyhydramnios)** Amniotic fluid in excess of 1.5 liters; often indicative of fetal anomaly and frequently seen in poorly controlled, insulin-dependent, diabetic pregnant women even if there is no coexisting fetal anomaly.

**hydrocephalus** Accumulation of fluid in the subdural or subarachnoid spaces.

**hydrops fetalis** Most severe expression of fetal hemolytic disorder, a possible sequela to maternal Rh isoimmunization; infants exhibit gross edema (anasarca), cardiac decompensation, and profound pallor from anemia, and seldom survive.

hydrotherapy The use of water in the treatment of various disorders. Hydrotherapy may include continuous tub baths, wet sheet packs, or shower sprays.

hymen Membranous fold that normally partially covers the entrance to the vagina.

hyperbilirubinemia Elevation of unconjugated serum bilirubin concentrations.

hyperemesis gravidarum Abnormal condition of pregnancy characterized by protracted vomiting, weight loss, and fluid and electrolyte imbalance.

hyperemia An excess of blood in part of the body, caused by increased blood flow, as in the inflammatory response, local relaxation of arterioles, or obstruction of the outflow of blood from an area. Skin overlying a hyperenic area usually becomes reddened and warm.

hyperglycemia Excess glucose in the blood.

hyperreflexia Increased action of the reflexes.

hyperthyroidism Excessive functional activity of the thyroid gland.

hyperventilation Rapid, shallow (or prolonged, deep) respirations resulting in respiratory alkalosis: a decrease in $H^1$ concentration and $PCO_2$ and an increase in the blood pH and the ratio of $NaHCO_3$ to $H_2CO_3$. Symptoms may include faintness, palpitations, and carpopedal (hands and feet) muscular spasms.

hypervolemia An increase in the amount of intravascular fluid, particularly in the volume of circulating blood or its components.

hypofibrinogenemia Deficient level of a blood-clotting factor, fibrinogen, in the blood; in obstetrics, it occurs after complications of abruptio placentae or retention of a dead fetus.

hypoglycemia Less than normal amount of glucose in the blood, usually caused by administration of too much insulin, excessive secretion of insulin by the islet cells of the pancreas, or dietary deficiency.

hypospadias Anomalous positioning of urinary meatus on undersurface of penis or close to or a urethrl opening into the vagina.

hypothermia Temperature that falls below normal range, that is, below 35° C, usually caused by exposure to cold.

hypothyroidism Deficiency of thyroid gland activity with underproduction of thyroxine.

hypotonic uterine dysfunction Weak, ineffective uterine contractions usually occurring in the active phase of labor; often related to cephalopelvic disproportion (CPD) or malposition of the fetus.

hypoxemia Reduction in arterial $PO_2$ resulting in metabolic acidosis by forcing anaerobic glycolysis, pulmonary vasoconstriction, and direct cellular damage.

hypoxia Insufficient availability of oxygen to meet the metabolic needs of body tissue.

hysterectomy Surgical removal of the uterus.

hysterotomy Surgical incision into the uterus.

ICSI (intracytoplasmic sperm injection) A procedure in which a single sperm is injected directly into an egg; this procedure is most commonly used to overcome male infertility problems.

illicit drugs Illegal to obtain or use. Some may be legal for research purposes within the United States and some may be used in other countries because the laws vary.

immunity
    acquired i. Protection against microorganisms that develops in response to actual infection or transfer of antibody from an immune donor.
    active i. Protection against specific microorganisms that develops in response to actual infection or vaccination.
    natural i. Nonspecific protection against microorganisms. Natural immunity is the first line of defense and includes skin and phagocytic cells.
    passive i. Protection against specific microorganisms that develops in response to the transfer of antibody or lymphocytes from an immune donor.

immunoassay A test for pregnancy that depends on an antibody reaction between hCG-coated particles and a first morning urine specimen from a woman. A woman is considered pregnant if no particle agglutination takes place because of the presence of the hCG in the woman's urine.

immunocompetent Ability of the immune system to respond appropriately to foreign antigens and to develop antigen-specific antibodies.

immunoglobin
    IgA Primary immunoglobulin in colostrum.
    IgG Transplacentally acquired immunoglobulin that confers passive immunity to the fetus against the infections to which the mother is immune.
    IgM Immunoglobulin neonate can manufacture soon after birth. Fetus produces it in the presence of amnionitis.

impaired fertility Inability to conceive or to carry fetus to live birth at a time a couple chooses to do so.

implantation Embedding of the fertilized ovum in the uterine mucosa; nidation.

impotence Term designating a man's inability, partial or complete, to perform sexual intercourse or to achieve orgasm; erectile dysfunction.

inborn error of metabolism Hereditary deficiency of a specific enzyme needed for normal metabolism of specific chemicals (e.g., deficiency of phenylalanine hydroxylase results in phenylketonuria [PKU]; a deficiency of hexosaminidase results in Tay-Sachs disease).

incompetent cervix Cervix that is unable to remain closed until a pregnancy reaches term because of elasticity in the cervix resulting in dilation and effacement usually during the second or early third trimester of pregnancy. Premature dilation of the cervix is the preferred term.

incomplete abortion See *abortion, incomplete.*

induced abortion See *abortion, induced.*

induction Stimulation of uterine contractions before the spontaneous onset of labor.

inevitable abortion See *abortion, inevitable.*

infant Child who is under 1 year of age.

infertility Decreased capacity to conceive.

primary i. Women who have never been able to become pregnant or carry the pregnancy to term.

secondary i. Women who have difficulty becoming pregnant after they have had a baby.

informational exchange Sharing content about childbearing and related community resources with a pregnant woman.

input Information, environmental influences, or diseases that affect the community.

insemination Introduction of semen into the vagina or uterus for impregnation.

therapeutic donor i. Introduction of donor semen by instrument injection into the vagina or uterus for impregnation.

insulin Hormone produced by the beta cells of the pancreatic islets of Langerhans; promotes glucose transport into the cells; aids in protein and lipid synthesis.

internal monitoring Monitoring the status of the baby by inserting monitors into the uterus.

internal os See *os.*

intervention Any act performed to prevent harming of a patient or to improve the mental, emotional, or physical function of a patient.

interview A face-to-face meeting in order to gain particular facts.

intervillous space Irregular space in the maternal portion of the placenta filled with maternal blood and serving as the site of maternal-fetal gas, nutrient, and waste exchange.

intraductal papilloma A small, wartlike growth that projects into breast ducts near the nipple. Any slight bump or bruise in the area of the nipple can cause the papilloma to bleed.

intrapartum During labor and birth.

intrauterine device (IUD) Small plastic and or metal form placed in the uterus to prevent pregnancy.

intrauterine growth restriction (IUGR) Fetal undergrowth of any cause, such as deficient nutrient supply or intrauterine infection, or associated with congenital malformation; birth weight below population 10th percentile corrected for gestational age.

intrauterine pressure catheter (IUPC) Catheter inserted into uterine cavity to assess uterine activity and pressure by electronic means.

intrauterine resuscitation Interventions initiated when nonreassuring fetal heart rate patterns are noted and are directed at improving intrauterine blood flow.

introitus Entrance into a canal or cavity such as the vagina.

invasive mole A more severe manifestation of the hydatiform mole in which the chorionic villi of the mole penetrate into the myometrium and parametrium of the uterus and metastasize to distant parts of the body, most commonly the lungs.

in vitro fertilization Fertilization in a culture dish or test tube.

inversion Turning end for end, upside down, or inside out.

involution (1) Rolling or turning inward. (2) Reduction in size of the uterus after birth and its return to its nonpregnant condition.

ischemic phase of menstrual cycle Final phase (days 27 and 28) in which levels of estrogen and progesterone fall, causing the spiral arteries to undergo vasoconstriction, cutting off the blood supply, and necrotizing the endometrium as it prepares to slough.

isoimmunization Development of antibodies in a species of animal with antigens from the same species (e.g., development of anti-Rh antibodies in an Rh-negative person).

IUI (intrauterine insemination) A medical procedure that involves placing sperm into a woman's uterus to facilitate fertilization. IUI is not considered an ART procedure because it does not involve the manipulation of eggs.

IVF (in vitro fertilization) An ART procedure that involves removing eggs from a woman's ovaries and fertilizing them outside her body. The resulting embryos are then transferred into the woman's uterus through the cervix.

jaundice Yellow discoloration of the body tissues caused by the deposit of bile pigments (unconjugated bilirubin); icterus.

breast milk j. Term used by some clinicians to describe late-onset (after day 5) jaundice in the breastfed infant. A cause for this phenomenon has not been conclusively identified. See *physiologic j.*

pathologic j. Jaundice usually first noticeable within 24 hours after birth; caused by some abnormal condition such as an Rh or ABO incompatibility and resulting in bilirubin toxicity (e.g., kernicterus).

physiologic j. Yellow tinge to skin and mucous membranes in response to increased serum levels of unconjugated bilirubin; not usually apparent until after 24 hours; also called neonatal jaundice, physiologic hyperbilirubinemia.

Kegel exercises Pelvic muscle exercises to strengthen the pubococcygeal muscles.

kernicterus Bilirubin encephalopathy involving the deposit of unconjugated bilirubin in brain cells, resulting in death or impaired intellectual, perceptive, or motor function and adaptive behavior.

ketoacidosis The accumulation of ketone bodies in the blood as a consequence of hyperglycemia; leads to metabolic acidosis.

kinesthetic learners People who use all of their senses to learn. Practice sessions, role playing, and demonstrations are most useful for them.

kinship The state of being kin or related by blood.

labia majora Two folds of skin containing fat and covered with hair that lie on either side of the vaginal opening and form each side of the vulva. (Singular, labium majus.)

labia minora Two thin folds of delicate, hairless skin inside the labia majora. (Singular, labium minus.)

labor Series of processes by which the fetus is expelled from the uterus; parturition; childbirth.

active phase of l. Phase in first stage of labor from 4 to 7 cm in dilation.

first stage of l. Stage of labor from the onset of regular uterine contractions to full dilation of the cervix.

fourth stage of l. Initial period of recovery from childbirth. It is usually considered to last for the first 1 to 2 hours after the expulsion of the placenta.

latent phase of l. Phase in first stage of labor from 0 to 3 cm in dilation.

second stage of l. Stage of labor from full dilation of the cervix to the birth of the baby.

third stage of l. Stage of labor from the birth of the baby to the expulsion of the placenta.

transition phase of l. Phase in first stage of labor from 8 to 10 cm in dilation.

labor, delivery, recovery (LDR) A single room where all steps of the birth process occur. Avoids having to move the woman to different rooms for each phase of the birth process. The woman is moved to a postpartum room after recovery.

labor, delivery, recovery, postpartum (LDRP) A single room where all steps of the birth process and hospitalization occur. The woman stays in the same room throughout her hospitalization.

laceration Irregular tear or wound of tissue; in obstetrics, it usually refers to a tear in the perineum, vagina, or cervix during childbirth.

lactase Enzyme necessary for the digestion of lactose.

lactation Function of secreting milk or period during which milk is secreted.

lactogenesis stage I Initial synthesis of milk components (colostrum) that begins during pregnancy.

lactogenesis stage II Beginning of milk production 2 to 5 days postpartum.

lacto-ovo vegetarian One whose diet consists primarily of foods of vegetable origin but also includes some animal products such as eggs, milk, and cheese, but no meat, fish, or poultry.

lactose intolerance Inherited absence of the enzyme lactose.

lacto-vegetarian One whose diet consists of milk or milk products in addition to foods of vegetable origin but does not include eggs, meat, fish, or poultry.

Lamaze (psychoprophylaxis) method Method of preparation for childbirth developed in the 1950s by a French obstetrician, Fernand Lamaze, that gained popularity in the United States in the 1960s. It requires practice at home and coaching during labor and birth. The goals are to minimize fear and the perception of pain and to promote positive family relationships by using both mental and physical preparation.

laminaria Cone of dried seaweed that swells as it absorbs moisture. Used to dilate the cervix nontraumatically in preparation for an induced abortion or in preparation for induction of labor.

lanugo Downy, fine hair characteristic of the fetus between 20 weeks of gestation and birth that is most noticeable over the shoulder, forehead, and cheeks but is found on nearly all parts of the body except the palms of the hands, soles of the feet, and the scalp.

laparoscopy Examination of the interior of the abdomen by insertion of a small telescope through the anterior abdominal wall.

laparatomy Any surgical incision into the peritoneal cavity, usually performed under general or regional anesthesia, often on an exploratory basis.

large for gestational age (LGA) Exhibiting excessive growth for gestational age.

last normal menstrual period (LNMP) Date of the first day of the last normal menstrual bleeding.

latch on Attachment of the infant to the breast for feeding.

lavage The process of washing out an organ, usually the bladder, bowel, paranasal sinuses, or stomach for therapeutic purposes.

lecithin A phospholipid that decreases surface tension; surfactant.

lecithin/sphingomyelin ratio (l/s ratio) The ratio of two components of amniotic fluid, used for predicting fetal lung maturity. The normal ratio in amniotic fluid is 2.1 or greater when fetal lungs are mature.

leiomyoma Benign smooth muscle tumor.

leg cramps Sudden, intense gripping contractions of the calf muscle that may occur when a woman rests or awakens from sleep. They are caused by a lowered serum ionized calcium and increased phosphates, or inadequate calcium intake.

Leopold's maneuvers Four maneuvers for diagnosing the fetal position by external palpation of the mother's abdomen.

lesbian A female homosexual; a woman whose primary emotional, social, and sexual relationships are with other women.

letdown reflex (or milk ejection reflex [MER]) Release of milk caused by the contraction of the myoepithelial cells within the milk glands in response to oxytocin.

**letting-go phase** Interdependent phase after birth in which the mother and family move forward as a system with interacting members.

**leukocytosis** An abnormal increase in the number of circulating white blood cells. The normal range is 5,000 to 10,000 per cubic millimeter of blood.

**leukorrhea** White or yellowish mucous discharge from the cervical canal or the vagina that may be normal physiologically or caused by pathologic states of the vagina and endocervix (e.g., *Trichomonas vaginalis* infections).

**libido** Sexual drive or desire.

**lichen planus** A nonmalignant, chronic, pruritic skin disease of unknown cause that is characterized by small flat purplish papules or plaques with fine gray lines on the surface.

**lichen sclerosis** A chronic skin disease characterized by white flat papules, tending to coalesce into large white patches of thin pruritic skin in advanced cases.

**licit drug** Any drug (e.g., tobacco, alcohol, OTC medications, prescription medications) accepted by society and legal to use, with some restrictions for age.

**life expectancy** The probable number of years a person will live after a given age, as determined by mortality in a specific geographic area. It may be individually qualified by the person's condition or race, sex, age, or other demographic factors.

**lightening** Sensation of decreased abdominal distention produced by uterine descent into the pelvic cavity as the fetal presenting part settles into the pelvis. It usually occurs 2 weeks before the onset of labor in nulliparas.

**linea nigra** Line of darker pigmentation seen in some women during the latter part of pregnancy that appears on the middle of the abdomen and extends from the symphysis pubis toward the umbilicus.

**lithotomy position** Position in which the woman lies on her back with her knees flexed and with abducted thighs drawn up toward her chest.

**live birth** Birth in which the neonate, regardless of gestational age, manifests any heartbeat, breathes, or displays voluntary movement.

**live birth per cycle** Average chances of having a live born infant by ART; the percentage of cycles started that result in a live birth.

**live birth per egg retrieval** The percentage of cycles in which live births resulted from eggs that were retrieved. It is generally higher than the live birth per cycle statistic because cycles that were canceled before egg retrieval began are not counted.

**live birth per transfer** The percentage of cycles in which live births resulted from embryos transferred from the laboratory. This is the highest reported rate of success because it does not include eggs that were not fertilized, abnormal embryos, or other unsuccessful transfer attempts.

**living arrangements** Where the pregnant woman is living, what kind of housing she is in, where she will live after the baby is born, who she lives with, and how stable these arrangements are will make a difference in the prenatal diagnosis.

**local infiltration anesthesia** Process by which a substance such as a local anesthetic drug is deposited within the tissue to anesthetize a limited region.

**locality development model** Emphasizes self-direction of community members as they determine their own needs and find their own solutions. Also called community development, this model depends on "grass roots" initiatives.

**lochia** Vaginal discharge during the puerperium consisting of blood, tissue, and mucus.

    **l. alba** Thin, yellowish to white, vaginal discharge that follows lochia serosa on about the tenth day after birth and that may last from 2 to 6 weeks postpartum.

    **l. rubra** Red, distinctly blood-tinged vaginal flow that follows birth and lasts 2 to 4 days.

    **l. serosa** Serous, pinkish brown, watery vaginal discharge that follows lochia rubra until about the tenth day after birth.

**low birth weight (LBW)** An infant birth weight of less than 2500 g.

**low spinal (saddle) block anesthesia** Type of regional anesthesia produced by injection of a local anesthetic solution into the cerebrospinal fluid intrathecal (subarachnoid) space in the spinal canal.

**L/S ratio** See *lecithin/sphingomyelin ratio.*

**lunar month** Four weeks (28 days).

**lung surfactant** A detergent-like agent that reduces the surface tension of the liquid film covering the lining of the pulmonary alveoli. As an alveolus becomes smaller during expiration, the surfactant becomes more concentrated, further reducing the surface tension and preventing alveolar collapse.

**lutein cysts** A result of the corpus luteum becomes cystic or hemorrhagic and fails to break down after 14 days.

**luteinizing hormone (LH)** Hormone produced by the anterior pituitary that stimulates ovulation and the development of the corpus luteum.

**lymphogranuloma venereum** A sexually transmitted disease caused by a strain of the bacterium *chlamydia trachomatis.* It is characterized by ulcerative genital lesions, marked swelling of the lymph nodes in the groin, headache, fever, and malaise. The infection is cured with an antibiotic, but the tissue damage remains and buboes may need to be aspirated.

**maceration** (1) Process of softening a solid by soaking it in a fluid. (2) Softening and breaking down of fetal skin from prolonged exposure to amniotic fluid as seen in a postterm infant. Also seen in a dead fetus.

**macrosomia** Large body size as seen in neonates of diabetic or prediabetic mothers.

**magnesium sulfate** A salt of magnesium. Also called Epsom salt.

magnetic resonance imaging (MRI) Noninvasive nuclear procedure for imaging tissues with high fat and water content; in obstetrics, uses include evaluation of fetal structures, placenta, and amniotic fluid volume.

malattachment Rejection of the infant in the early postpartum period.

male factor Any cause of infertility due to deficiencies in sperm quantity or that make it difficult for a sperm to fertilize an egg under normal conditions.

malformation An anomalous structure in the body, usually genetic in nature and developing during the first trimester before birth.

malignant melanoma See *melanoma.*

mammary gland Compound gland of the female breast that is made up of lobes and lobules that secrete milk for nourishment of the young. Rudimentary mammary glands exist in the male.

marijuana The dried leaves and flowering tops of the pistillate hemp plant that yield THC and are smoked in cigarettes for their intoxicating effect.

Marfan's syndrome An inherited disorder that is an autosomal dominant trait resulting in an abnormal condition characterized by elongation of the bones, causing significant musculoskeletal disturbances. Also usually associated with cardiovascular and eye abnormalities.

marital rape Forcible sexual intercourse by a man with his wife.

married couple A husband and wife living together in the same household, with or without children and other relatives.

mask of pregnancy See *melama.*

mastectomy Excision, or removal, of the mammary gland.

    modified radical m. Removal of breast tissue, skin, and axillary nodes.

masterbation Sexual activity in which the penis or clitoris is stimulated, usually to orgasm, by means other than coitus. It is performed at least occasionally by most people and is considered to be normal and harmless.

mastitis Inflammation in a breast, usually confined to a milk duct, characterized by influenza-like symptoms and redness and tenderness in the affected breast.

maternal adaptation Process that a woman goes through in adjusting to her version of the maternal role; includes three phases: taking in, taking hold, and letting go.

maternal mortality Death of a woman related to childbearing.

maternal well-being An area of assessment during the labor process considering the physical, psychosocial, and spiritual status of the mother.

McBurney's point A site of extreme sensitivity in acute appendicitis, situated in the normal area of the appendix about 2 inches from the right anterosuperior spine of the ilium, on a line between the spine and the umbilicus.

McDonald's sign Easy flexion of the fundus on the cervix.

mean arterial pressure (MAP) Average of systolic and diastolic blood pressures. A MAP of greater than 90 mm Hg in the second trimester is associated with an increase in the incidence of pregnancy-induced hypertension in the third trimester.

meconium First stools of infant: viscid, sticky; dark greenish brown, almost black; sterile; odorless.

meditation Any activity that focuses the attention in the present moment and quiets and relaxes the mind and body in the process.

melama Increased pigmentation over bridge of nose and cheeks of pregnant women and some women taking oral contraceptives; previously termed chloasma. Also known as mask of pregnancy.

melanoma Any of a group of malignant neoplasms that originate in the skin and that are composed of melanocytes. A melanocytic nevus may be acquired or congenital. The congenital melanocytic nevus is regarded as more likely to develop into a malignant melanoma, primarily because of its larger size. Smaller melanomas tend to develop from a pigmented nevus over several months or years.

membrane(s) Thin, pliable layer of tissue that lines a cavity or tube, separates structures, or covers an organ or structure; in obstetrics, the amnion and chorion surrounding the fetus.

    artificial rupture of m. (AROM) Ruptue of amniotic sac with an instrument.

    premature rupture of m. (PROM) Rupture of amniotic sac and leakage of amniotic fluid beginning at least 1 hour before onset of labor at any gestational age.

    spontaneous rupture of m. (SROM) Rupture of membranes by natural means.

menarche Onset, or beginning, of menstrual function.

menopause From the Greek word mewn (month) and Greek word pausis (cessation), the actual permanent cessation of menstrual cycles; so diagnosed after 1 year without menses.

    post m. The time after menopause, including the first 12 months of amenorrhea.

menorrhagia Abnormally profuse or excessive menstrual flow.

menses (menstruation) Latin plural of mensis "month." Periodic vaginal discharge of bloody fluid from the nonpregnant uterus that occurs from the age of puberty to menopause.

menstrual phase The final of the three phases of the menstrual cycle, the one in which menstruation occurs, comprising days 1 through 5 of the female reproductive cycle (FRC).

menstruation The periodic discharge through the vagina of a bloody secretion containing tissue debris from the shedding of the endometrium from the nonpregnant uterus.

mentum Chin, a fetal reference point in designating position (e.g., "left mentoanterior" [LMA], meaning that the fetal chin is presenting in the left anterior quadrant of the maternal pelvis).

meralgia paresthetica A condition characterized by pain, paresthesia, and numbness on the lateral surface of the thigh in the region supplied by the lateral femoral cutaneous nerve. The cause of the condition is ischemia of the nerve caused by its entrapped position in the inguinal ligament.

metatarsus adductus A congenital deformity of the foot in which the forepart rotates inward toward the midline of the body and the heel remains straight.

methadone A synthetic addictive narcotic drug used especially in the form of hydrochloride for the relief of pain and as a substitute narcotic in the treatment of heroin addiction.

methyldopa An antihypertensive.

metrorrhagia Abnormal bleeding from the uterus, particularly when it occurs at any time other than the menstrual period.

midwife One who practices the art of helping and aiding a woman to give birth.

    certified nurse m. Registered nurse with advanced education in midwifery.

    lay m. Independent or direct-entry provider for pregnancy and birth. Some states have provisions to license lay midwives.

milia Unopened sebaceous glands appearing as tiny, white, pinpoint papules on forehead, nose, cheeks, and chin of a neonate that disappear spontaneously in a few days or weeks.

milk-leg Thrombophlebitis of femoral vein resulting in edema of leg and pain; may occur after difficult vaginal birth.

mini pill An oral contraceptive containing only progesterone; it does not contain estrogen. Women who cannot use combined pills because of the risk for major side effects may be candidates for this pill. It inhibits ovulation, suppresses midcycle peaks of FSH and LH, and alters the configuration of the endometrium.

minority A racial, religious, political, national, or other group regarded as different from the larger group of which it is a part.

miscarriage Lay term for spontaneous abortion; a pregnancy ending in the spontaneous loss of the embryo or fetus before 20 weeks of gestation.

missed abortion See *abortion, missed.*

mitral valve stenosis Narrowing of the opening of the mitral valve caused by stiffening of valve leaflets, obstructing the blood flow from the atrium to the ventricle.

mittelschmerz Abdominal pain in the region of an ovary during ovulation that usually occurs midway through the menstrual cycle. Present in many women, mittelschmerz is useful for identifying ovulation, thus pinpointing the fertile period of the cycle.

molar pregnancy A hydatiform mole.

    complete m. No fetus or amnion is present.

    partial m. A fetus or amnion is present.

molding Overlapping of cranial bones or shaping of the fetal head to accommodate and conform to the bony and soft parts of the mother's birth canal during labor.

mongolian spot Bluish gray or dark nonelevated pigmented area usually found over the lower back and buttocks present at birth in some infants, primarily nonwhite. The spot usually fades by school age.

monitrice A nurse with clinical skills to provide both nursing care and labor support.

monozygotic Originating or coming from a single fertilized ovum, such as identical twins.

monozygotic twins See *twins, monozygotic.*

Montgomery's glands (tubercles) Small, nodular prominences (sebaceous glands) on the areolas around the nipples of the breasts that enlarge during pregnancy and lactation.

mood disorders Disorders that have as the dominant feature a disturbance in the prevailing emotional state. Cause is unknown.

morbidity (1) Condition of being diseased. (2) Number of cases of disease or of sick persons in relationship to a specific population; incidence.

morning sickness Nausea and vomiting that affect some women during the first few months of their pregnancy; may occur at any time of day.

Moro's reflex Normal, generalized reflex in a young infant elicited by a sudden loud noise or by striking the table next to the child, resulting in flexion of the legs, an embracing posture of the arms, and usually a brief cry. Also called startle reflex.

mortality (1) Quality or state of being subject to death. (2) Number of deaths in relation to a specific population; incidence.

    fetal m. Number of fetal deaths per 1000 births (or per live births).

    infant m. Number of deaths per 1000 children 1 year of age or younger.

    maternal m. Number of maternal deaths per 100,000 births.

    neonatal m. Number of neonatal deaths per 1000 births (or per live births). See also *neonatal mortality.*

    perinatal m. Combined fetal and neonatal mortality.

motor maturity A category of evaluating an infant's behavioral response. It evaluates posture, tone coordination, and movements during the alert state.

mucous plug A collection of thick mucus in the uterine cervix that is often expelled at the onset of dilation of the cervix, just before labor begins or in its early hours. The plug may be dry and firm, following the shape of the endocervical canal, but more often it is semifluid and mucoid, streaked with blood. During pregnancy, it serves as a barrier from bacteria and other substances for the cervix.

**multifetal pregnancy reduction** Originally called selective reduction or selective abortion, the procedure involves reducing the pregnancy to a singleton or twin gestation by stopping the development of fetuses most accessible to the provider. This enhances the odds of a successful term gestation with normal-birth-weight infants, but the emotional cost to the parents may be high.

**multigenerational family** Family form that includes extended family across generational lines (i.e., grandparents, parents, and children).

**multigravida** Woman who has been pregnant two or more times.

**multipara** Woman who has carried two or more pregnancies to viability, whether they ended in live infants or stillbirths.

**multiple birth** A pregnancy that results in the birth of more than one infant.

**multiple gestation** A pregnancy with multiple fetuses.

**muscle tone** The fourth factor in the Apgar score. It evaluates the degree to which the newborn returns a stretched-out foot or hand from extension to flexion.

**mutation** Change in a gene or chromosome in gametes that may be transmitted to offspring.

**myoclonic seizure** Twitching or spasm of a muscle or a group of muscles.

**nabothian cyst** A cyst formed in a nabothian gland of the uterine cervix. It is a common finding on routine examinations of women of reproductive age, especially in women who have borne children. Pearly white and firm, the cysts seldom result in adverse or pathologic effects.

**Nägele's (or Naegele's) rule** Method for calculating the estimated date of birth (EDB) or "due date."

**NANDA (North American Nursing Diagnosis Association)** A professional organization of registered nurses created in 1982 in order to develop, refine, and promote a taxonomy of nursing diagnostic terminology of general use to the professional.

**narcotic antagonist** A compound such as naloxone (Narcan) that promptly reverses the effects of narcotics such as meperidine (Demerol).

**natural childbirth** Labor and parturition accomplished by a mother with little or no medical intervention. It is generally considered the optimal way of giving birth and being born, safest for the baby and most satisfying for the mother. Prerequisites include normal gestation, an adequate birth canal, strong maternal motivation, physical and emotional preparation, and constant and intensive support of the mother during labor and birth.

**necrosis** Localized tissue death that occurs in groups of cells in response to disease or injury.

**neighborhood** A district considered in regard to its inhabitants or distinctive characteristics; the people who live in a particular vicinity.

**neonatal mortality** Statistical rate of infant death during the first 28 days after live birth, expressed as the number of such deaths per 1000 live births in a specific geographic area or institution in a given period of time.

**neonate** An infant from birth to 28 days of age.

**neoplastic tumors** Growth of new tissue; tumor that serves no physiologic function; may be benign or malignant.

**nesting instinct** A burst of energy some women experience about 24 hours before labor commences; many women apply this energy toward cleaning house or preparing for the baby, although they should be encouraged to rest so they can conserve the energy for the impending process of labor.

**neural tube** Tube formed from fusion of the neural folds from which develop the brain and spinal cord.

**nevus** Natural blemish or mark; a congenital circumscribed deposit of pigmentation in the skin; mole.

    **faun tail n.** A tuft of hair overlying the spinal column in the lumbosacral area which may be an indication of spina bifida occulta.

    **n. flammeus** Port-wine stain; reddish, usually flat, discoloration of the face or neck. Because of its large size and color, it is considered a serious deformity.

    **n. vasculosus (strawberry hemangioma)** Elevated lesion of immature capillaries and endothelial cells that regresses over a period of years.

**nipple discharge** Spontaneous exudation of material from the nipple. It may be normal, such as colostrum in pregnancy, or it may be a sign of endocrinologic, neoplastic, or infectious disease.

**nitrazine test** A test to determine whether discharge is amniotic fluid (alkaline) or a vaginal secretion (acidic).

**nonpurging type** A particular manifestation of bulimia nervosa which occurs as binge eating only.

**non-stress test (NST)** Evaluation of fetal response (fetal heart rate) to natural contractile uterine activity or to an increase in fetal activity.

**Norplant implant (or system)** Trademark for a method of implanting flexible rods filled with levonorgestrel, beneath the skin of the upper arm of a woman. A set of six rods is inserted in a fan-shaped pattern through an incision about 10 cm above the elbox crease. The levonorgestrel diffuses through the walls of the rods, maintaining a blood level of the progestin that can prevent pregnancy for up to 5 years, depending on individual differences in metabolism and body weight.

**nuchal cord** Encircling of fetal neck by one or more loops of umbilical cord.

**nuclear family** Family form consisting of mother, father, and their dependent children.

**nulligravida** Woman who has never been pregnant.

**nullipara** Woman who has not yet carried a pregnancy to viability.

**nurse-practitioner** Registered nurse who has additional education to practice nursing in an advanced role.

**nursing diagnosis** A statement of a health problem or a potential problem in the client's health status that a nurse is licensed and competent to treat.

**nursing process** The process that serves as an organizational framework for the practice of nursing. It encompasses all of the steps taken by the nurse in caring for a patient: assessment, nursing diagnosis, planning, implementation, and evaluation. The rationale for each step is grounded in nursing theory.

**obese** Pertaining to a corpulent or excessively heavy individual. Generally a person is regarded as medically obese if he or she is 20% above desirable body weight for the person's age, sex, height, and body build. Because the 'average' human body is 25% fat, the proportion may be doubled for a medically defined obese person.

**objective data** The process in which data relating to the client's problem are obtained by an observer through direct physical examination, including observation, palpation, and auscultation, and by laboratory analyses and radiologic and other studies.

**occipital frontal circumference (OFC)** Measurement around the newborn's head from just above the eyebrow and around the most prominent part of the occipital bone on the back of the head. Average measurement ranges from 31 to 38 cm and is plotted on a growth chart in comparison to the weight and height of the infant.

**occiput** Back part of the head or skull.

**oligohydramnios** Abnormally small amount or absence of amniotic fluid; often indicative of fetal urinary tract defect.

**oliguria** Urine output below 25 to 30 ml by the kidneys for 2 consecutive hours (in adults).

**Omaha Classification System** Provides a framework in which problems can be categorized. It includes three components: a Problem Classification Scheme (environmental, psychologic, physiologic, health-related behaviors); an Intervention Scheme (nursing activities to address the problem), and a Problem Rating Scale (a Likert-type scale which evaluates client outcomes).

**omphalitis** Inflammation of the umbilical stump characterized by redness, edema, and purulent exudate in severe infections.

**oocyte** Primordial or incompletely developed ovum; the female reproductive cell, also called an egg.

**ophthalmia neonatorum** A purulent conjunctivitis and keratitis of the newborn resulting from exposure of the eyes to chemical, chlamydial, bacterial, or viral agents. Chemical conjunctivitis usually occurs as a result of the instillation of silver nitrate in the eyes of a newborn to prevent a gonococcal infection.

**oral contraceptives** See *combined oral contraceptives.*

**oral glucose tolerance test** Test for blood glucose after oral ingestion of a concentrated sugar solution.

**orthostatic hypotension** Abnormally low blood pressure occurring when an individual assumes the standing posture. Also called postural hypotension.

**Ortolani maneuver** A procedure used to evaluate the stability of the hip joints in newborns and infants. The baby is placed on his back, and the hips and knees are flexed at right angles and abducted until the lateral aspects of the knees are touching the table. The examiner's fingers are extended along the outside of the thighs, with the thumbs grasping the insides of the knees. Internal and external rotation are attempted, and symmetry of mobility is evaluated. A click or popping sensation may be felt if the joint is unstable, because the head of the femur moves out of the acetabulum under pressure from the examiner's hands during rotation and abduction.

**os** Mouth, or opening.
   **external o. (o. externum)** External opening of the cervical canal.
   **internal o. (o. internum)** Internal opening of the cervical canal.
   **o. uteri** Mouth, or opening, of the uterus.

**osteopath** A physician who specializes in osteopathy, a therapeutic approach to the practice of medicine that uses all the usual forms of medical diagnosis and therapy but that places greater emphasis on the influence of the relationship between the organs and the musculoskeletal system than traditional medicine does.

**osteoporosis** Deossification of bone tissue resulting in structural weakness; decreased bone mass increasing risk of fractures, especially after menopause.

**outcome objectives** Focused on changing or affecting health status or behaviors of community members.

**outlet** Opening by which something can leave.
   **pelvic o.** Lower aperture, or opening, of the true pelvis.

**ovarian stimulation** The use of drugs to stimulate the ovaries to develop follicles and eggs.

**ovarian tumors**
   **functional ot.** One of several different kinds of cysts (follicular, lutein, theca lutein, or polycystic ovary syndrome).
   **inflammatory ot.** Inflammation or infection of the ovaries (e.g., PID) that can lead to abscess formation.

metaplastic ot. A form of endometriosis in which the affected sites of endometrial implantation include the ovary.

ovary One of two glands in the female situated on either side of the pelvic cavity that produces the female reproductive cell, the ovum, and two known hormones, estrogen and progesterone.

over-the-counter (OTC) Any drug available to the consumer without a prescription.

ovulation Periodic ripening and discharge of the ovum from the ovary, usually 14 days before the onset of menstrual flow.

ovulation method A natural method of family planning that uses observation of changes in the character and quantity of cervical mucus to determine the time of ovulation during the menstrual cycle. Because pregnancy occurs with fertilization of an ovum extruded from the ovary at ovulation, the method is used to increase or decrease the woman's chance of becoming pregnant by causing or avoiding insemination by spontaneous or artificial means during the fertile period associated with ovulation.

ovulatory dysfunction A cause of infertility due to problems with egg production by the ovaries.

ovum Female germ, or reproductive cell, produced by the ovary; egg.

oxytocics Drugs that stimulate uterine contractions, thus accelerating childbirth and preventing postbirth hemorrhage. They may be used to increase the letdown reflex during lactation.

oxytocin Hormone produced by the posterior pituitary that stimulates uterine contractions and the release of milk in the mammary gland (letdown reflex).

   o. challenge test (OCT) Evaluation of fetal response (fetal heart rate) to contractile activity of the uterus stimulated by exogenous oxytocin (Pitocin).

PaCO$_2$ Partial pressure of carbon dioxide in arterial blood.

palmar erythema Rash on the surface of the palms sometimes seen in pregnancy.

palsy Permanent or temporary loss of sensation or ability to move and control movement; paralysis.

   Bell's p. Peripheral facial paralysis of the facial nerve (cranial nerve VII), causing the muscles of the unaffected side of the face to pull the face into a distorted position.

   Erb's p. See *Erb-Duchenne paralysis.*

pancretitus An inflammatory condition of the pancreas that may be acute or chronic.

panic disorder An acute, psychobiologic reaction manifested by intense anxiety and panic. Symptoms vary according to the individual and the intensity of the attack. Attacks usually occur suddenly, last from a few seconds to an hour or longer, and vary in frequency from several times a day to once a month.

PaO$_2$ Partial pressure of oxygen in arterial blood.

Papanicolaou (Pap) smear Microscopic examination using scrapings from the cervix, endocervix, or other mucous membranes that will reveal, with a high degree of accuracy, the presence of premalignant or malignant cells.

para A woman who has given birth, regardless of whether the fetus was born alive or dead.

paracervical block Type of regional anesthesia produced by injection of a local anesthetic into the lower uterine segment just beneath the mucosa adjacent to the outer rim of the cervix (3 and 9 o'clock positions).

parity Number of past pregnancies that have reached viability, regardless of whether the infant or infants were alive or stillborn. See *para.*

participant observation Assessment of a community by observing participants in key community events or settings (i.e. a board meeting, a street fair or block party).

parturition Process or act of giving birth.

passage The maternal pelvis and soft tissue the baby must pass through.

passenger In labor, the infant, with its size, position, and presentation influencing the process.

patent ductus arteriosus (PDA) An abnormal opening between the pulmonary artery and the aorta caused by failure of the fetal ductus arteriosus to close after birth. It is seen primarily in premature infants and is usually corrected during early childhood.

pathologic nipple discharge Spontaneous, intermittent, and persistent discharge from one breast that is bloody, serous, serosanguinous, watery, or green. The woman must be examined thoroughly for the possibility of cancer.

pattern A composite of traits or features characteristic of an individual.

peau d'orange Orange peel-like skin secondary to cancerous lesions and seen over edematous breasts.

pedagogy The art and science of teaching children, based on a belief that the purpose of education is the transmittal of knowledge.

pelvic Pertaining or relating to the pelvis.

   p. exenteration Surgical removal of all reproductive organs and adjacent tissues

   p. inflammatory disease (PID) Nonspecific immune response of internal reproductive structures and adjacent tissues usually secondary to sexually transmitted infections.

   p. inlet The inlet to the true pelvis, bounded by the sacral promontory, the horizontal rami of the pubic bones, and the top of the symphysis pubis. Because the infant must pass through the inlet to enter the true pelvis and to be born vaginally, the anteroposterior, transvers, and the oblique dimensions of the inlet are important measurements to be made in assessing the pelvis in pregnancy.

p. outlet See *outlet, pelvic.*

p. relaxation Refers to the lengthening and weakening of the fascial supports of pelvic structures.

p. relaxation syndrome Lengthening and weakening of the musculature of the pelvic floor, causing the pelvic organs to lose their support, descend toward the vaginal canal, and possibly prolapse.

p. tilt (rock) Exercise used to help relieve low back discomfort during menstruation and pregnancy.

pelvimetry Measurement of dimensions and proportions of the pelvis to determine its capacity and ability to allow the passage of the fetus through the birth canal.

pelvis Bony structure formed by the sacrum, coccyx, innominate bones, and symphysis pubis and the ligaments that unite them.

percutaneous umbilical blood sampling (PUBS) Procedure during which the fetal umbilical vessel is accessed for blood sampling or for transfusions.

perimenopause Period of transition of changing ovarian activity before menopause and through first year of amenorrhea.

perinatal Of or pertaining to the time and process of giving birth or being born.

perinatal period Period extending from the twentieth or twenty-eighth week of gestation through the end of the twenty-eighth day after birth.

perineum Area between the vagina and rectum in the female and between the scrotum and rectum in the male.

peripartum cardiomyopathy A primary disease of the heart muscle with no apparent cause, occurring during the peripartum period.

pescetarian One whose diet consists of fish in addition to foods of vegetable origin but does not include eggs, meat, or poultry.

pessary Device placed inside the vagina to function as a supportive structure for the pelvic organs.

petechiae Pinpoint hemorrhagic areas caused by numerous disease states involving infection and thrombocytopenia and occasionally found over the face and trunk of the newborn because of increased intravascular pressure in the capillaries during birth.

phenylketonuria (PKU) Recessive hereditary disease that results in a defect in the metabolism of the amino acid phenylalanine caused by the lack of an enzyme, phenylalanine hydroxylase, that is necessary for the conversion of the amino acid phenylalanine into tyrosine. If PKU is not treated, brain damage may occur, causing severe mental retardation.

phlebitis Inflammation of a vein with symptoms of pain and tenderness along the course of the vein, inflammatory swelling and acute edema below the obstruction, and discoloration of the skin because of injury or bruise to the vein, possibly occurring in acute or chronic infections or after procedures or childbirth.

phlebothrombosis Formation of a clot or thrombus in the vein; inflammation of the vein with secondary clotting.

phototherapy Utilization of lights to reduce serum bilirubin levels by oxidation of bilirubin into water-soluble compounds that are then processed in the liver and excreted into bile and urine.

physical abuse One or more episodes of aggressive behavior, usually resulting in physical injury with possible damage to internal organs, sense organs, the central nervous system, or the musculoskeletal system of another person.

physiologic addiction A result of the body's need for a drug to maintain physical equilibrium. If the drug is not available, the individual will experience physical symptoms such as tremors, diaphoresis, and lacrimation. With continued use, the individual will experience higher levels of tolerance. Narcotics, opiates, benzodiazepines, and amphetamines can result in addiction.

physiologic discharge A normal response of the breast to stimulation. It is bilateral, serous in color, and does not occur spontaneously.

physiologic jaundice See *jaundice, physiologic.*

physiologic leukorrhea Leukorrhea that occurs during the course of pregnancy.

pica Unusual craving during pregnancy (e.g., of laundry starch, dirt, red clay).

placenta Specialized vascular disk-shaped organ for maternal-fetal gas and nutrient exchange. Normally it implants in the thick muscular wall of the upper uterine segment. In postpartum may be referred to as afterbirth.

abruptio p. See *abruptio placentae.*

battledore p. Umbilical cord insertion into the margin of the placenta.

circumvallate p. Placenta having a raised white ring at its edge.

p. accreta Invasion of the uterine muscle by the placenta, thus making separation from the muscle difficult if not impossible.

p. increta Deep penetration in myometrium by placenta.

p. percreta Perforation of uterus by placenta.

p. previa Placenta that is abnormally implanted in the thin, lower uterine segment and that is typed according to proximity to cervical os: total–completely occludes os; partial–does not occlude os completely; and marginal–placenta encroaches on margin of internal cervical os.

complete p.p. A placenta that has grown to cover the internal cervical os completely.

low p.p. A placenta that is just within the lower uterine segment. Also called marginal previa.

partial p.p. A placenta previa in which the placenta is implanted in the lower uterine segment and partially covers the internal os of the uterine cervix. The part of the placenta that lies over the cervix is separated as the cervix dilates in labor, causing bleeding from the villous spaces of the uterine wall. Depending on the degree of separation, the bleeding may be scant or severe, varying the impact on the mother and the baby. If it is serious enough, cesarean section may be required.

**p. succenturiata** Accessory placenta and main placenta.

**placental** Pertaining or relating to the placenta.

**p. infarct** Localized, ischemic, hard area on the fetal or maternal side of the placenta.

**plethora** Deep, beefy-red coloration of a newborn caused by an increased number of blood cells (polycythemia) per volume of blood.

**PLISSIT counseling model** An aid for health care providers who are not mental health specialists, the model consists of four stages of counseling: permission giving, limited information giving, specific suggestions, and intensive therapy.

**plugged ducts** Milk ducts blocked by small curds of dried milk.

**polarization** Process by which the mother comes to see herself physically, socially, and conceptually as a separate entity from the infant. This ability also aids her in seeing the infant in a similar fashion.

**polycystic ovary syndrome** *(PCOS or Stein-Leventhal syndrome)* Associated with androgen excess, anovulation, and secondary amenorrhea.

**polydactyly** Excessive number of digits (fingers or toes).

**polyhydramnios** See *hydramnios.*

**polyp** Small tumorlike growth that projects from a mucous membrane surface.

**polyuria** Excessive secretion and discharge of urine by the kidneys.

**population** All of the individuals in a particular geographical area or all of the individuals sharing a particular race, class, or other specific characteristic.

**population projection** Assumptions about future demographic trends developed by the Census Bureau.

**position** Relationship of an arbitrarily chosen fetal reference point, such as the occiput, sacrum, chin, or scapula on the presenting part of the fetus to its location in the front, back, or sides of the maternal pelvis.

**positive pregnancy test** Indicates that hCG is in the woman's system.

**positive signs of pregnancy** Definite indication of pregnancy (e.g., hearing the fetal heartbeat, visualization with and palpation of fetal movement by the examiner).

**postcoital contraception** A pharmocologic or mechanical intervention that inhibits fertilization or implantation, it is available after unintended, unexpected, or unprotected intercourse has occurred, or the contraceptive method used has failed.

**posterior** Pertaining to the back.

**postmature infant** Infant born after the 42 weeks of gestation or later and exhibiting signs of dysmaturity.

**postpartum** Happening or occurring after birth (mother).

**p. blues** A letdown feeling, accompanied by irritability and anxiety, that usually begins 2 to 3 days after giving birth and disappears within a week or two. Sometimes called the "baby blues."

**p. depression** Depression occurring within 6 months of childbirth, lasting longer than postpartum blues and characterized by a variety of symptoms that interfere with activities of daily living and care of the baby.

**p. hemorrhage** Excessive bleeding after childbirth; traditionally defined as a loss of 500 ml or more after a vaginal birth

**p. psychosis** Symptoms begin as postpartum blues or depression but are characterized by a break with reality. Delusions, hallucinations, confusion, delirium, and panic can occur.

**postterm pregnancy** Pregnancy prolonged past 42 weeks of gestation (also called postdate pregnancy).

**posttraumatic stress disorder** An anxiety disorder characterized by an acute emotional response to a traumatic event or situation such as sexual abuse.

**poverty** The state or condition of being poor; lack of the means of providing material needs or comforts.

**power** Provided by the contractions that provide the expulsive efforts of labor and birth.

**precipitous labor** Rapid or sudden labor of less than 3 hours beginning from onset of cervical changes to completed birth of neonate.

**preconception health care** Care designed for health attainment and maintenance before pregnancy.

**preeclampsia** Disease encountered after 20 weeks of gestation or early in the puerperium; a vasospastic disease process characterized by increasing hypertension, proteinuria, and hemoconcentration.

**preembryonic stage** The first stage of human development occurring the day the ovum is fertilized and continuing for 14 days afterward.

**pregestational diabetes** Diabetes mellitus type 1 or type 2 that exists before pregnancy.

**pregnancy** Period between conception through complete birth of the products of conception. The usual duration of pregnancy in the human is 280 days, 9 calendar months, or 10 lunar months.

**clinical p.** Pregnancy documented by the presence of a gestational sac on ultrasound. For ART data collection purposes, pregnancy is defined as a clinical pregnancy rather than a chemical pregnancy (i.e., a positive pregnancy test).

**pregnancy-induced hypertension (PIH)** Hypertensive disorders of pregnancy including preeclampsia, eclampsia, and transient hypertension.

**pregnancy per cycle** Number of ART cycles that produce a pregnancy.

**premature dilation of the cervix** See *incompetent cervix.*

**premature infant** Infant born before completing week 37 of gestation, irrespective of birth weight; preterm infant.

**premature rupture of membranes (PROM)** See *membrane(s)*.

**premenstrual syndrome** Syndrome of nervous tension, irritability, weight gain, edema, headache, mastalgia, dysphoria, and lack of coordination occurring during the last few days of the menstrual cycle preceding the onset of menstruation.

**premonitory signs** An early sign or symptom preceding a more major event.

**prenatal** Occurring or happening after conception and before birth.

**preparation for childbirth** A program of instruction based on a theoretic framework, with specific objectives, structured content, and an integrated, flexible approach.

**prepuce** Fold of skin, or foreskin, covering the glans penis of the male.

**presence** Being available with the whole of oneself and open to the experience of another through a reciprocal interpersonal encounter.

**presentation** That part of the fetus that first enters the pelvis and lies over the inlet: may be head, face, breech, or shoulder.

 breech p. See *breech presentation*.

 cephalic p. See *cephalic presentation*.

**presumptive signs of pregnancy** Manifestations that are suggestive of pregnancy but are not absolutely positive. These include the cessation of menses, Chadwick's sign, morning sickness, and quickening.

**preterm birth** Birth occurring before 37 weeks of gestation.

**preterm labor (or premature labor)** Labor that occurs earlier in pregnancy than normal, either before the fetus has reached a weight of 2000 to 2500 g or before the thirty-seventh or thirty-eighth week of gestation. No single measure of fetal weight or gestational age is used universally to designate preterm birth; local or institutional policy dictates which of several standards is applied. Prematurity is a concomitant of 75% of births that result in neonatal mortality.

**previa, placenta** See *placenta previa*.

**primary level of prevention** Activities directed toward decreasing the probability of becoming ill.

**primary source** Data about the client is collected directly from that client.

**primigravida** Woman who is pregnant for the first time.

**primipara** Woman who has carried 1 pregnancy to viability whether the child is dead or alive at the time of birth.

**probable signs of pregnancy** Manifestations or evidence that indicates that there is a definite likelihood of pregnancy. Among the probable signs are enlargement of abdomen, Goodell's sign, Hegar's sign, Braxton Hicks sign, and positive hormonal tests for pregnancy.

**process evaluation** Examines as how the planning and interventions occurred, how effective the communication between parties was, and how timely and efficient each step were during a program.

**prodromal** Serving as an early symptom or warning of the approach of a disease or condition.

 **p. labor** The early period in parturition before uterine contractions become forceful and frequent enough to result in progressive dilation of the uterine cervix.

**progesterone** Hormone produced by the corpus luteum and placenta whose function is to prepare the endometrium of the uterus for implantation of the fertilized ovum, develop the mammary glands, and maintain the pregnancy.

**progress of labor** An area of assessment during the labor process that considers status of the cervix, contractions, the position of the fetus in utero, and the maternal pelvis.

**prolactin** A pituitary hormone that triggers milk production.

**prolapsed cord** Protrusion of the umbilical cord in advance of the presenting part of the baby.

**proliferative phase of menstrual cycle** Preovulatory, follicular, or estrogen phase of the menstrual cycle.

**prolonged latent phase** A stage of labor that lasts more than 14 hours in the multiparous woman and more than 20 hours in the primiparous woman.

**prolonged labor** Labor that lasts longer than expected.

**proscription** Forbidden; taboo.

**prostaglandin (PG)** Substance present in many body tissues; has a role in many reproductive tract functions; used to induce abortions, cervical ripening for labor induction.

**prostaglandin synthase inhibitor** An agent that prevents the production of prostaglandins.

**proteinuria** Presence of protein in urine.

**protracted active phase** Cervical dilation in a nullipara of less than 1.2 cm per hour and of less than 1.5 cm per hour in the multipara. Secondary arrest of cervical dilation is defined as no cervical changes for 2 hours during active labor.

**pruritus** Itching.

**pseudocyesis** Condition in which the woman has all the usual signs of pregnancy (e.g., enlargement of the abdomen, cessation of menses, weight gain, and morning sickness) but is not pregnant; phantom or false pregnancy.

**psoriasis** A common chronic skin disorder characterized by circumscribed red patches covered by thick, dry silvery adherent scales that are the result of excessive development of epithelial cells.

psyche Considers the energy, anxiety, and fears the woman brings to the event as well as the support she perceives from the network that surrounds her.

psychologic abuse Aimed at controlling the woman's behavior, it instills fear or threatens physical harm to the individual, her children, loved ones, or pets.

psychologic addiction An individual needs the drug to feel normal and to help cope with daily events. A diagnosis can be made in the absence of physical symptoms. It is most common with cocaine and its derivatives.

psychologic strength A balance between interrelated behaviors, attitudes, beliefs, and experiences such as vulnerability and safety or emotion and logic. Also known as "inner strength."

psychomotor domain An area of learning that deals with the development of manipulative skills involving tools, machinery, procedures, and techniques.

psychoprophylactic method A system of prenatal education for giving birth using the Lamaze method of natural childbirth.

ptyalism Excessive salivation.

puberty Period in life in which the reproductive organs mature and one becomes functionally capable of reproduction.

pubic Pertaining to the pube, innominate pubis bone forming the front of the pelvis.

pudendal block Injection of a local anesthetizing drug at the pudendal nerve root to produce numbness of the genital and perianal region.

puerperal infection Infection of the pelvic organs during the postbirth period; childbed fever.

puerperium Period after the third stage of labor and lasting until involution of the uterus takes place, usually about 3 to 6 weeks.

pulse oximetry Noninvasive method of monitoring oxygen levels by detecting the amount of light absorbed by oxygen-carrying hemoglobin.

pulse rate The number of beats per minute as measured on the radial, carotid, femoral, and pedal arteries. In labor, a rate higher than 100 bpm indicates stress, pain, dehydration, infection, or possible hemorrhagic shock.

purging type A particular manifestion of bulimia nervosa that takes the form of self-induced vomiting and indiscriminate use of laxatives, emetics, and/or diuretics.

pyelonephritis A diffuse pyogenic infection of the pelvis and parenchyma of the kidney.

pyrosis A burning sensation in the epigastric and sternal region from stomach acid (heartburn).

quickening Maternal perception of fetal movement; usually occurs between weeks 16 and 20 of gestation.

race A group of genetically related people who share certain physical characteristics.

radioimmunoassay Pregnancy test that tests for the beta subunit of human chorionic gonadotropin using radioactively labeled markers.

radioreceptor assay (RRA) A pregnancy test that measures the ability of the suspected hCG in the woman's blood sample to inhibit the binding of radio-labeled hCG to receptors. A false-positive reading may be received by women in menopause because the test fails to distinguish between hCG and luteinizing hormone (LH).

rape-trauma syndrome Characteristic symptoms seen in victims of rape and consisting of several phases; similar to posttraumatic stress syndrome.

reanastamosis Surgical repair of tubal ligation on the woman's fallopian tubes.

recessive trait Genetically determined characteristic that is expressed only when present in the homozygotic state.

recommended dietary allowances (RDAs) Recommended nutrient intakes estimated to meet the needs of almost all (97% to 98%) of the healthy people in the population.

rectocele Herniation or protrusion of the rectum into the posterior vaginal wall.

referred pain Discomfort originating in a local area such as cervix, vagina, or perineal tissues but felt in the back, flanks, or thighs.

reflex Automatic response built into the nervous system that does not need the intervention of conscious thought (e.g., in the newborn, rooting, gagging, grasp).

reflex irritability The third factor in the Apgar score, judged by reaction to touch or temperature change resulting in a robust cry.

reflexology A system of treating certain disorders by massaging the soles of the feet, using principles similar to those of acupuncture.

regional anesthesia Anesthesia of an area of the body by injection of a local anesthetic to block a group of sensory nerve fibers.

relational communities A social group based on associations or connections between people based on common goals or interests.

relaxation techniques A method of reducing tension that increases the descending inhibitory activity in the higher brain centers while it lowers heart rate, respiratory rate, blood pressure, and level of blood lactates.

progressive r.t. A technique for combating tension and anxiety by systematically tensing and relaxing muscle groups.

tension r.t. Active relaxation in response to a noxious stimulus.

touch r.t. Combines massage and touch with breathing awareness and active relaxation.

religious framework A system of belief, worship, or conduct that may be followed to help satisfy a person's spiritual needs.

residual urine Urine that remains in the bladder after urination.

**RESOLVE** A national, nonprofit consumer organization offering education, advocacy, and support to those experiencing infertility. Services include a national HelpLine, quarterly newsletter, extensive literature list, member-to-member contact systems, and local support groups through a network of over 50 chapters nationwide.

**respiratory distress syndrome (RDS)** Condition resulting from decreased pulmonary gas exchange, leading to retention of carbon dioxide (increase in arterial $PCO_2$). Most common neonatal causes are prematurity, perinatal asphyxia, and maternal diabetes mellitus; hyaline membrane disease (HMD).

**restitution** In obstetrics, the turning of the fetal head to the left or right after it has completely emerged from the introitus as it assumes a normal alignment with the infant's shoulders.

**restricting subtype** A particular manifestation of anorexia nervosa in which the woman simply restricts food intake.

**restrictive belief** Statements based on a woman's religion or culture about what should not be done during the pregnancy. Not having your picture taken, avoiding cold air, or not attending funerals are some examples.

**resuscitation** Restoration of consciousness or life in one who is apparently dead or whose respirations or cardiac function or both have ceased.

**retained placenta** Retention of all or part of the placenta in the uterus after birth.

**retraction** (1) Drawing in or sucking in of soft tissues of chest, indicative of an obstruction at any level of the respiratory tract from the oropharynx to the alveoli. (2) Retraction of uterine muscle fiber. After contracting, the muscle fiber does not return to its original length but remains slightly shortened, a unique attribute of uterine muscle that aids in preventing postdelivery hemorrhage and results in involution.

**retroflexion** Bending backward.

**retroversion of uterus** Backward displacement.

**review of systems** A system-by-system review of the body functions begun during the initial interview with the patient and completed during the physical examination as physical findings prompt further questions. Included in the health history.

**rheumatic fever** An inflammatory disease that may develop as a delayed reaction to inadequately treated group A beta-hemolytic streptococcal infection of the upper respiratory tract. This disorder usually occurs in young school-age children and may affect the brain, heart, joints, skin, or subcutaneous tissues.

**rheumatic heart disease** Permanent damage of the heart muscle and valves secondary to an autoimmune reaction in the heart tissue precipitated by rheumatic fever.

**rheumatoid arthritis** A chronic, inflammatory, destructive, sometimes deforming, collagen disease that has an autoimmune component. Most commonly appearing in early middle-aged women (aged 36 to 50 years), it is characterized by symmetric inflammation of the synovium and increased synovial exudate, leading to thickening of the synovium and swelling of the joint.

**Rh factor** Inherited antigen present on erythrocytes. The individual with the factor is known as positive for the factor.

**Rh immune globulin (RhIG)** Solution of gamma globulin that contains Rh antibodies. Intramuscular administration of Rh immune globulin (trade name RhoGAM) prevents sensitization in Rh-negative women who have been exposed to Rh-positive red blood cells.

**rhythm method** Contraceptive method in which a woman abstains from sexual intercourse during the ovulatory phase of her menstrual cycle; calendar method.

**risk factors** Situations or issues that cause a person or a group of people to be particularly vulnerable to an unwanted, unpleasant, or unhealthful event. In pregnancy, risk factors are any assessment findings that suggests the pregnancy may have negative outcomes for either the mother or the fetus.

**rite of passage** Significant life event indicating movement from one maturational level to another.

**rooting reflex** Normal response of the newborn to move toward whatever touches the area around the mouth and to attempt to suck. This reflex usually disappears by 3 to 4 months of age.

**rotation** In obstetrics, the turning of the fetal head as it follows the curves of the birth canal downward.

**rubella vaccine** Live attenuated rubella virus given to clients who have not had rubella or who are serologically negative. Exposure to the rubella virus through vaccination causes the client to form antibodies, producing active immunity.

**Rubin's test** Transuterine insufflation of the uterine tubes with carbon dioxide to test their patency; infrequently used.

**rugae** Folds in the vaginal mucosa and scrotum.

**sacrum** Triangular bone composed of five united vertebrae and situated between L5 and the coccyx; forms the posterior boundary of the true pelvis.

**scleroderma** Chronic hardening and thickening of the skin caused by new collagen formation, with atrophy of pilosebaceous follicles. Most common in middle-aged women, it may occur in a localized form or as a systemic disease.

**sclerosing adenosis** A benign condition involving excessive growth of tissues in the breast's lobules. It often causes breast pain or lumps and may show up on a mammogram.

scrotum Pouch of skin containing the testes and parts of the spermatic cords.

sebaceous gland hyperplasia White or yellow macules and papules at the opening of pilosebaceous follicles, most common on the forehead, cheeks, nose, and chin, probably as a result of androgen stimulation.

seborrheic dermatitis A common chronic inflammatory skin disease characterized by dry or moist greasy scales and yellowish crusts. In acute stages there may be exudate and infection resulting in secondary furunculosis.

secondary level of prevention Screening for disease so that early treatment may be given.

secondary source Any secondhand or indirect data source, such as health department records or epidemiologic studies.

secretory phase of menstrual cycle Postovulatory, luteal, progestational, premenstrual phase of menstrual cycle; 14 days in length.

self-assessment (self-examination) A person's ability to determine and evaluate changes in his or her own body.

self-care Client provides care for self as part of plan of care.

self-quieting ability A category of assessing the infant's behavioral response that considers the newborn's ability to stop crying on its own whether through oral stimulation or in response to visual or auditory stimuli.

semen Thick, white, viscid secretion discharged from the urethra of the male at orgasm; the transporting medium of the sperm.

semen analysis Examination of semen specimen to determine liquefaction, volume, pH, sperm density, and normal morphology.

sensitivity The proportion of persons with a condition that will be correctly identified as having it by a screening test.

sensitization Development of antibodies to a specific antigen.

sepsis Bacterial infections of the bloodstream.

septal defect An abnormal, usually congenital defect in the wall separating two chambers of the heart. Depending on the size and the site of the defect, various amounts of oxygenated and deoxygenated blood mix, causing a decrease in the amount of oxygen carried in the blood to the peripheral tissues.

atrial s.d. (ASD) A congenital cardiac anomaly characterized by an abnormal opening between the atrial. The severity of the condition depends on the size and location of the defect.

ventricular s.d. (VSD) An abnormal opening in the septum separating the ventricles. It permits blood to flow from the left to the right ventricle and to re-circulate through the pulmonary artery and lungs. It is the most common congenital heart defect.

sex chromosome Chromosome associated with determination of gender: the X (female) and Y (male) chromosomes. The normal female has two X chromosomes, and the normal male has one X and one Y chromosome.

sex-linked recessive inheritance A pattern of inheritance in which a disorder is transmitted by one of the X chromosomes (a sex-determining chromosome). Hemophilia, red-green color blindness, and Duchenne's muscular dystropy are examples of sex-linked recessive inheritance.

sexual abuse The sexual mistreatment of another person by fondling, rape, or forced participation in sex acts or other perverted behavior. Victims tend to experience a traumatic feeling of loss of control of themselves.

sexual equilibrium Balance of psychologic forces between partners resulting in sexual comfort or decreased anxiety for each partner.

sexual health Freedom from sexual diseases or disorders and a capacity to enjoy and control sexual behavior without fear, shame, or guilt.

sexual history Past and present health conditions, lifestyle behaviors, knowledge, and attitudes related to sex and sexuality.

sexual intention How a person chooses to participate in sexual behavior (i.e., celibacy, masturbation, or with a partner).

sexuality The part of life that has to do with being male or female.

sexually transmitted infections (STIs) Infections transmitted as a result of sexual activity with an infected individual; also called sexually transmitted diseases (STDs).

sexual orientation The clear, persistent desire of a person for affiliation with one sex rather than the other.

sexual response cycle The phases of physical changes that occur in response to sexual stimulation and sexual tension release. These include excitement, plateau, orgasm, and resolution.

shake test "Foam" test for lung maturity of fetus; more rapid than determination of lecithin/sphingomyelin ratio.

sibling mutuality A pattern of interaction between siblings characterized by sensitivity and empathy. A focus on the feelings, behavior, and needs of the baby rather than on critiquing the older child's behavior. Older siblings are included in planning for the baby, sharing in the care of, and entertaining the baby.

sibling rivalry Negative behaviors exhibited by siblings in response to the addition of a new baby in the family.

sickle cell hemoglobinopathy Abnormal crescent-shaped red blood corpuscles in the blood.

**Sims' position** Position in which the client lies on the left side with the right knee and thigh drawn upward toward the chest.

**single-parent family** Family form characterized by one parent (male or female) in the household. This may result from loss of spouse by death, divorce, separation, desertion, or birth of a child to a single woman.

**sitz bath** Application of moist heat to the perineum by sitting in a tub or basin filled with warm water.

**Sjogren's syndrome (SS)** An immunologic disorder characterized by deficient moisture production of the lacrimal, salivary, and other glands, resulting in abnormal dryness of the mouth, eyes, and other mucous membranes. The symptoms primarily affect women over 40 years of age.

> **secondary SS** Symptoms of SS accompanying rheumatoid arthritis.

**skin tags** A small brown or flesh-colored outgrowth of skin. Also called cutaneous papilloma.

**small for gestational age (SGA)** Inadequate growth for gestational age.

**smegma** Whitish secretion around labia minora and under foreskin of penis.

**social action model** Change is implemented through debate and discussion between community members who are polarized around an issue or issues. The center of power is located within the community as they develop support for their position on the issue.

**social behavior** A category for assessing an infant's behavioral response that evaluates the infant's relationships with those around it, such as snuggling into the arms of a parent or crying to be fed.

**socialization** The process by which an individual learns to live in accordance with the expectations and standards of a group or society, acquiring the beliefs, habits, values, and accepted modes of behavior primarily through imitation, family interaction, and educational systems; the procedure by which society integrates the individual.

**social planning model** Change is implemented through an emphasis on rational decision making by "expert" planners using factual documentation of needs.

**Society for Assisted Reproductive Technology (SART)** An affiliate of the American Society for Reproductive Medicine composed of clinics and programs that provide ART. SART reports annual fertility clinic data to CDC.

**sonogram** See *ultrasonography.*

**souffle** Soft, blowing sound or murmur heard by auscultation.

> **funic s.** Soft, muffled, blowing sound produced by blood rushing through the umbilical vessels and synchronous with the fetal heart sounds.

> **uterine s.** Soft, blowing sound made by the blood in the arteries of the pregnant uterus and synchronous with the maternal pulse.

**specificity** Proportion of people without the condition who correctly test negative on a screening text.

**sperm** Male reproductive cell. Also called spermatozoon, spermatozoa.

**spermatogenesis** Process by which mature spermatozoa are formed, during which the diploid chromosome number (46) is reduced by half (haploid, 23).

**spermicide** Chemical substance that kills sperm by reducing their surface tension, causing the cell wall to break down by a bactericidal effect or by creating a highly acidic environment. Also called spermatocide.

**spider angiomas** A form of telangiectasis characterized by a central elevated red dot the size of a pinhead from which small blood vessels radiate.

**spina bifida occulta** Congenital malformation of the spine in which the posterior portion of laminas of the vertebrae fails to close but there is no herniation or protrusion of the spinal cord or meninges through the defect. The newborn may have a dimple in the skin or growth of hair over the malformed vertebrae.

**spinnbarkheit** Formation of a stretchable thread of cervical mucus due to the estrogen influence at time of ovulation.

**spirituality** The individual's connection to his or her own values, purpose, and meaning of life. May encompass organized religion or belief in higher power or authority. Recognition of wisdom, imagination, spirit, intuition. A perception of the unity of nature and the interconnectedness of all beings; inner strength.

**spontaneous abortion** See *abortion, spontaneous.*

**spontaneous rupture of membranes (SROM)** See *membrane(s).*

**squamocolumnar junction** Site in the endocervical canal where columnar epithelium and squamous epithelium meet; also called transformation zone.

**squamous cell** A flat, scalelike epithelial cell.

**squamous cell carcinoma** A slow-growing malignant tumor of squamous epithelium, frequently found in the lungs and skin and occurring also in the anus, cervix, larynx, nose, and bladder. The neoplastic cells characteristically resemble prickle cells and form keratin pearls.

**squamous intraepithelial lesion (SIL)** Term used to describe neoplastic changes of the cervix.

**squamous metaplasia** The process in which columnar cells are transformed into squamous cells in the squamocolumnar junction.

**station** Relationship of the presenting fetal part to an imaginary line drawn between the ischial spines of the pelvis.

**stenosis** An abnormal condition characterized by the constriction or narrowing of an opening or passageway in a body structure.

> **aortic s.** A cardiac anomaly characterized by a narrowing or stricture of the aortic valve. It is sec-

ondary to congenital malformation or of fusion of the cusps, as may result from rheumatic fever.

pulmonic s. An abnormal cardiac condition, generally characterized by concentric hypertrophy of the right ventricle with relatively little increase in diastolic volume.

sterile vaginal examination Assessment of cervical effacement, dilation, and fetal station during labor by feeling the cervix and fetal presenting part with gloved fingers.

sterilization Process or act that renders a person unable to produce children.

female s. The occlusion of the fallopian tubes through a variety of means in order to render the woman unable to bear children.

male s. Each vas deferens is cut between two ligated sections, thus preventing the sperm from becoming part of the ejaculate.

stillborn The birth of a baby after 20 weeks of gestation and 1 day or weighing 350 g (depending on the state code) that does not show any signs of life.

stimulated cycle An ART cycle in which a woman receives oral or injected fertility drugs to stimulate ovaries to produce more follicles.

stork bites See *telangiectatic nevi.*

strawberry hemangioma (also called nevus vasculosus) Elevated lesion of immature capillaries and endothelial cells that regresses over a period of years.

stress Any emotional, physical, social, economic, or other factor that requires a response or change; a disruptive or disquieting influence or occurrence.

stress urinary incontinence (SUI) Loss of urine occurring with increased abdominal pressure (e.g., with coughing or sneezing).

striae ("stretch marks") Shining reddish lines caused by stretching of the skin, often found on the abdomen, thighs, and breasts during pregnancy. These streaks turn to a fine pinkish white or silver tone in time in fair-skinned women and brownish in darker-skinned women.

structural-functional stroke volume Volume of blood ejected from the left ventricle during one cardiac cycle.

subcutaneous terbutaline pump Provides continuous subcutaneous infusion of small amounts of terbutaline.

subfamily A couple and their children, if any, living in a household where neither adult is the householder.

subinvolution Failure of a part (e.g., the uterus) to reduce to its normal size and condition after enlargement from functional activity (e.g., pregnancy).

subjective data The process in which data relating the problem are elicited from a patient. The interviewer encourages a full description of the onset, the course, and the character of the problem and any factors that aggravate or ameliorate it.

subsystem Smaller elements or groups within the system (i.e., the family unit).

summative evaluation Feedback addressing the level of satisfaction participants have at the end of a class; it serves as a reference for future revisions of the program.

supernumerary nipples An excessive number of nipples, which are usually not associated with underlying glandular tissue. They may vary in size from small pink dots to that of normal nipples.

supine hypotension Shock; fall in blood pressure caused by impaired venous return when gravid uterus presses on ascending vena cava, when woman is lying flat on her back; vena cava syndrome.

support To emotionally sustain, hold up, or maintain patients under stress.

support system Social network from which women receive help during their pregnancy.

suprasystem Larger unit or context of the system (i.e., the county or national association of the local association).

surfactant Phosphoprotein necessary for normal respiratory function that prevents the alveolar collapse (atelectasis). See also *lecithin* and *lecithin/sphingomyelin ratio.*

survey To examine or look at in a comprehensive way.

suture (1) Junction of the adjoining bones of the skull. (2) Procedure uniting parts by their being sewn together.

symphysis pubis Fibrocartilaginous union of the bodies of the pubic bones in the midline.

symptothermal method Fertility awareness contraception method based on cervical mucus, the basal body temperature, and other bodily signs.

synchrony Fit between an infant's cues and the parent's response.

syphilis A sexually transmitted disease caused by the spirochete *Treponema pallidum,* characterized by distinct stages of effects over a period of years. Any organ system may become involved. The spirochete is able to pass through the human placenta, producing congenital syphilis.

congenital s. Neonates who have had the spirochete transmitted through the placentas of their infected mothers. Of these pregnancies, 60% end in stillbirth or neonatal death; of those that survive, half will have a variety of problems.

primary s. Appearance of a small painless red pustule on the skin or mucous membrane between 10 and 90 days after exposure. The lesion may appear anywhere on the body but it is seen most often in the anogenital region. It quickly erodes, forming a painless, bloodless ulcer, called a *chancre,* exuding a fluid that swarms with spirochetes. The *chancre* may not be noticed by the patient and many people may become infected. Its spontaneous healing within 10 to 40 days may create the impression that it was not a serious symptom.

secondary s. Occurs about 2 months later, after the spirochetes have spread throughout the body. It is characterized by the appearance of a morbilliform rash that does not itch, flat white sores in the mouth and through, or condylomata lata papules on the moist areas of the skin. The disease remains highly contagious at this stage and can be spread by kissing.

tertiary s. May not develop for 3 to 15 years. It is characterized by the appearance of soft rubbery tumors, called *gummas*, that ulcerate and heal by scarring. They may develop anywhere on the surface of the body and in the eye, liver, lungs, stomach, or reproductive organs.

systems theory perspective A holistic medical concept in which the patient is viewed as an integrated complex of opens systems rather than as semi-independent parts. The health care approach in this perspective requires the incorporation of family, community, and cultural factors as influences to be considered in the diagnosis and treatment of the patient.

systemic lupus erythematosus (SLE) A chronic inflammatory connective tissue disease affecting many systems, caused by a buildup of immune complexes within those systems.

taboo Proscribed (forbidden) by society as improper and unacceptable; a proscription.

TACO An acronym used for assessing an amniotomy. It stands for *Time* the amniotic sac was ruptured; *Amount* of amniotic fluid present; *Color* of the fluid; and presence of an *Odor*.

taking-hold phase Period after birth characterized by a woman becoming more independent and more interested in learning infant care skills; learning to be a competent mother is an important task.

taking-in phase Period after birth characterized by the woman's dependency; maternal needs are dominant, and talking about the birth is an important task.

telangiectasia Permanent dilation of groups of superficial capillaries and venules.

telangiectatic nevi ("stork bites") Clusters of small, red, localized areas of capillary dilation frequently seen in neonates at the nape of the neck or lower occiput, upper eyelids, and nasal bridge that can be blanched with pressure of a finger.

temperament The features of a persona that reflect an individual's emotional disposition, or the way he or she behaves, feels, and thinks.

temperature A relative measure of sensible heat associated with the metabolism of the human body, normally maintained at a constant level of 98.6° F by the thermotaxic nerve mechanism that balances heat gains and losses. During labor, temperature should be checked every 4 hours or every 2 hours if the amniotic sac is ruptured. Slightly elevated temperature indicates dehydration and any temperature over 100.3° F may indicate infection.

teratogenic agent Any drug, virus, or irradiation, the exposure to which can cause malformation of the fetus.

teratogens Nongenetic factors that cause malformations and disorders in utero.

term infant Live infant born between weeks 38 and 42 of completed gestation.

term pregnancy Gestation that continues until at least 38 weeks.

testis One of the glands contained in the male scrotum that produces the male reproductive cell, or sperm, and the male hormone, testosterone; testicle.

tetany, uterine Extremely prolonged uterine contractions.

tetralogy of Fallot A congenital cardiac anomaly that consists of four defects: pulmonic stenosis, ventricular septal defect, malposition of the aorta so that it arises from the septal defect or the right ventricle, and right ventricular hypertrophy.

tetratogen Nongenetic factors that can produce malformations of the embryo or fetus.

thalassemia A Mediterranean group of hereditary anemias occurring in and Southeast Asian populations in which there is an insufficient amount of globin produced to fill the red blood cells.

thawed cycle A cycle in which frozen embryos are thawed for transfer.

theca lutein cysts Associated with polycystic ovary syndrome (PCOS), clomiphene therapy, and others.

therapeutic abortion See *abortion, therapeutic*.

thermoregulation Control of temperature.

threatened abortion See *abortion, threatened*.

thrombocytopenia Abnormal hematologic condition in which the number of platelets is reduced, usually by destruction of erythroid tissue in bone marrow because of certain neoplastic diseases or an immune response to a drug.

thromboembolism Obstruction of a blood vessel by a clot that has become detached from its site of formation.

thrombophlebitis Inflammation of a vein with secondary clot formation.

thrombosed Pertaining to a blood vessel where a blood clot has formed.

thrombosis An abnormal vascular condition in which a clot (thrombus) develops within a blood vessel of the body.

thrush Fungal infection of the mouth or throat that is characterized by the formation of white patches on the mucous membrane, caused by *Candida albicans*.

thyroid storm a crisis in uncontrolled hyperthyroidism caused by the release into the bloodstream of increased amounts of thyroid hormones. The storm may occur spontaneously or be precipitated by infection, stress, or a thyroidectomy performed on a patient who is inadequately prepared with antithyroid drugs.

**tinea cruris** A superficial fungal infection of the groin caused by species of *Trichophyton* or *Epidermophyton floccosum.*

**tocodynamometer** An electronic device for monitoring and recording uterine contractions in labor.

**tocolysis** See *tocolytic therapy.*

**tocolytic** Medications used to relax the uterus, to suppress preterm labor, or for version.

**tonic-clonic seizure** An epileptic seizure characterized by a generalized involuntary muscular contraction and cessation of respiration followed by tonic and clonic spasms of the muscles. Breathing resumes with noisy respirations. The teeth may be clenched, the tongue bitten, and control of the bladder or bowel lost. As this phase of the seizure passes, the person may fall asleep or experience confusion. Usually the person has no recall of the seizure on awakening.

**TORCH infections** Infections caused by organisms that damage the embryo or fetus; acronym for Toxoplasmosis, Other (e.g., syphilis), Rubella, Cytomegalovirus, and Herpes simplex.

**toxemia** Term previously used for hypertensive states of pregnancy.

**toxicology screen** Laboratory analysis of blood or urine to test for alcohol or drug content. Urine drug screening is the most common because it is noninvasive.

**toxic shock syndrome** A severe acute disease usually caused by *Staphylococcus aureus;* associated with high-absorbency tampon use during menstruation.

**toxoplasma gondii** An intracellular parasite of cats and other hosts that causes toxoplasmosis in humans. The acquired form is characterized by rash, fever, malaise, myocarditis, and central nervous disorders. In acute infection of the mother, transplacental transmission occurs and the disease is very serious in the fetus, possibly leading to miscarriage, stillbirth, or premature labor.

**transcutaenous electrical nerve stimulation (TENS)** Stimulation of skin and underlying tissues with controlled low-voltage electrical vibration via electrodes.

**transfer** The second stage of the ART cycle; a viable embryo resulting from laboratory fertilization is transferred into the woman's uterus, usually through her cervix (IVF).

**transformation zone** See *squamocolumnar junction.*

**transient hypertension** High blood pressure in late pregnancy without other signs of preeclampsia.

**transition period–newborn** Period from birth to 4 to 6 hours later; infant passes through period of reactivity, sleep, and second period of reactivity.

**first stage of t.** From 0 to 30 minutes old. If not experiencing the effects of maternal medication, the baby is alert and moving and may experience a startle reaction when it moves or is moved abruptly. Also called the "first period of reactivity."

**second stage of t.** From 30 minutes to 2 hours old. The baby either sleeps or significantly decreases motor activity. Also called "period of decreased responsiveness."

**third stage of t.** From 2 hours to 6 or 8 hours old. The baby becomes more responsive to exogenous and endogenous stimuli. Also called the "second period of reactivity."

**trial of labor (TOL)** Period of observation to determine if a laboring woman with health concerns is likely to be successful in progressing to a vaginal birth.

**trichomonas vaginitis** Inflammation of the vagina caused by *Trichomonas vaginalis,* a parasitic protozoon, and characterized by persistent burning and itching of the vulvar tissue and a profuse, frothy, white discharge.

**trimester** One of 3 periods of about 3 months each into which pregnancy is divided.

**trisomy** Condition whereby any given chromosome exists in triplicate instead of the normal duplicate pattern.

**trophoblast** Outer layer of cells of the developing blastodermic vesicle that develops the trophoderm or feeding layer, which will establish the nutrient relationships with the uterine endometrium.

**trophoblastic disease** A condition in which trophoblastic cells covering the chorionic villi proliferate and undergo cystic changes, which may be malignant.

**tubal factor** Structural or functional damage to one or both fallopian tubes that reduces fertility.

**twins** Two neonates developed within the same uterus at the same time.

**conjoined t.** Twins who are physically united; Siamese twins.

**disparate t.** Twins who are different (e.g., in weight) and distinct from one another.

**dizygotic t.** Twins developed from two separate ova fertilized by two separate sperm at the same time; fraternal twins.

**monozygotic t.** Twins developed from a single fertilized ovum; identical twins.

**type I diabetes** An autoimmune disease in which insulin levels are very low. The immune system attacks the insulin-producing cells of the pancreas so that carbohydrates are unable to be metabolized. Individuals must be given insulin for life.

**type II diabetes** Patients are not insulin-dependent or ketosis prone, although they may use insulin for correction of symptomatic or persistent hyperglycemia. Onset is usually after 40 years of age; about 60% to 90% of patients are obese.

**ulcerative colitis** A chronic, episodic, inflammatory disease of the large intestine and rectum. It is characterized by profuse watery diarrhea containing varying amounts of blood, mucus, and pus. Some of the many systemic complications of ulcerative colitis include peripheral arthritis; ankylosing spondylitis; kidney and liver disease; and inflammation of the eyes, skin, and mouth.

**ultrasonography** Use of high-frequency sound waves for a variety of obstetric diagnoses and for fetal surveillance.

**ultrasound** A technique used for visualizing the follicles in the ovaries and the gestational sac or fetus in the uterus.

**ultrasound transducer** External signal source for monitoring fetal heart rate electronically.

**umbilical cord (funis)** Structure connecting the placenta and fetus and containing two arteries and one vein encased in a tissue called Wharton's jelly. The cord is ligated at birth and severed; the fetal stump falls off in 4 to 10 days.

**umbilicus** Navel, or depressed point in the middle of the abdomen that marks the attachment of the umbilical cord during fetal life.

**unconjugated bilirubin** Bound to albumin in blood and builds up in the body creating hyperbilirubinemia when uridyl diphosphoglucuronyl transferase (UDPGT) is insufficient to break down the bilirubin and allow it to be excreted via the bile to the intestines.

**unintended pregnancy** Occurs to a woman who is not intending to get pregnant at this time.

**unstimulated cycle** An ART cycle in which the woman does not receive drugs to stimulate her ovaries to produce more follicles. Instead, follicles develop naturally.

**unwanted pregnancy** Occurs to a woman who, for whatever reason, does not want to be pregnant.

**urethra** Small tubular structure that drains urine from the bladder.

**urinary frequency** Need to void often or at close intervals.

**urinary meatus** Opening, or mouth, of the urethra.

**uterine** Referring or pertaining to the uterus.

    **u. factor** A disorder in the uterus (e.g., fibroid tumors) that reduces fertility.

    **u. prolapse** Falling, sinking, or sliding of the uterus from its normal location in the body.

**uteroplacental insufficiency (UPI)** Decline in placental function—exchange of gases, nutrients, and wastes—leading to fetal hypoxia and acidosis; evidenced by late fetal heart rate decelerations in response to uterine contractions.

**uterus** Hollow muscular organ in the female designed for the implantation, containment, and nourishment of the fetus during its development and expulsion of fetus during labor and birth; also organ of menstruation.

**vaccination** Intentional injection of antigenic material given to stimulate antibody production in the recipient.

**vacuum-assisted birth** Birth involving attachment of vacuum cup to fetal head and using negative pressure to assist in birth of the fetus.

**vacuum curettage** Uterine aspiration method used in early abortion.

**vagina** Normally collapsed musculomembranous tube that forms the passageway between the uterus and the entrance to the vagina.

**vaginal birth after cesarean (VBAC)** Giving birth vaginally after having had a previous cesarean birth.

**vaginal discharge** Any discharge from the vagina. A clear or pearly-white discharge occurs normally. Throughout the reproductive years the amount varies greatly from woman to woman, and the amount and character vary in each woman at different times in her menstrual cycle.

**vaginismus** Intense, painful spasm of the muscles surrounding the vagina.

**vaginitis** An inflammation of the vaginal tissues, generally leading to the production of a discharge.

**vaginosis** An often symptomless mild inflammation of the vaginal tissues involving fewer white blood cells than vaginitis.

**Valsalva maneuver** Any forced expiratory effort against a closed airway such as holding one's breath and tightening the abdominal muscles (e.g., pushing during the second stage of labor).

**variability** Normal irregularity of fetal cardiac rhythm; short term—beat-to-beat changes; long term—rhythmic changes (waves) from the baseline value.

**varicosity (varicose veins)** Swollen, distended, and twisted veins that may develop in almost any part of the body but are most commonly seen in the legs, caused by pregnancy, obesity, congenital defective venous valves, and occupations requiring much standing.

**vasectomy** Ligation or removal of a segment of the vas deferens, usually done bilaterally to produce sterility in the male.

**vasoocclusive crisis (sickle cell crisis)** An acute episodic condition that occurs in children with sickle cell anemia. The crisis may be vasoocclusive, resulting from the aggregation of misshapen erythrocytes, or anemic, resulting from bone marrow aplasia, increased hemolysis, folate deficiency, or splenic sequestration of erythrocytes.

**vegan (strict vegetarian)** A vegetarian whose diet excludes the use of all foods of animal origin. Such diets, unless adequately planned, may be deficient in many essential nutrients, particularly vitamin $B_{12}$.

**VDRL test** Abbreviation for Venereal Disease Research Laboratories test, a serologic flocculation test for syphilis.

**ventricular hypertrophy** An abnormal enlargement of the heart ventricles. It is often caused by hypertension or a valvular disease.

**vernix caseosa** Protective gray-white fatty substance of cheesy consistency covering the fetal skin.

**version** Act of turning the fetus in the uterus to change the presenting part and facilitate birth.

external cephalic v. See *external cephalic version.*

podalic v. Shifting of the fetus' position so as to bring the feet to the outlet during birth.

vertex Crown or top of the head.

v. presentation Presentation in which the fetal head is nearest the cervical opening and is born first.

very–low-birth weight (VLBW) Refers to infant weighing 1500 g or less at birth.

viable, viability Capable, capability of living, as in a fetus that has reached a stage of development, usually more than 22 menstrual weeks (20 weeks of gestation), which will permit it to possibly live outside the uterus when it receives intensive support.

visual learners Persons who learn by using their eyes. Pictures, demonstrations, models, and being able to take notes or surveys are most useful for them.

visualization An effective means of deepening relaxation and desensitizing a real-life situation that is generally met with stress and tension. The imagery combines positive experiences with actual or perceived negative events or situations in an effort to desensitize the person to the trauma.

vitiligo A benign acquired skin disease of unknown cause, consisting of irregular patches of various sizes totally lacking in pigment and often having hyperpigmented borders. Exposed areas of skin are most often affected.

vulnerability Susceptible to injury; unprotected from physical, psychologic, or spiritual danger.

vulva External genitalia of the female that consist of the labia majora, labia minora, clitoris, urinary meatus, and vaginal introitus.

vulvar self-examination (VSE) Systematic examination of the vulva by the client.

vulvar vestibulitis Pain with touch or pressure at the vestibule while the only physical finding is erythema in the area.

Wharton's jelly White, gelatinous material surrounding the umbilical vessels within the cord.

windshield survey Assessment of a community by making observations while driving or walking through the geographic area.

withdrawal (1) Physiologic or cognitive changes that occur after removal of the substance in the substance-dependent person; (2) removing penis from vagina before ejaculation (coitus interruptus).

withdrawal bleeding The passage of blood from the uterus, associated with the shedding of endometrium that has been stimulated and maintained by hormonal medication.

women's health care Women supported by nurses in their journey to attain, maintain, or regain an optimal sense of health and well-being throughout life.

Women's Health Nurse Practitioner (WHNP) Has advanced preparation and is certified in the promotion of health and prevention or treatment of illness in women.

womb See *uterus.*

wound approximation How well wound edges come together.

X chromosome Sex chromosome in humans existing in duplicate in the normal female and singly in the normal male.

X linkage Genes located on the X chromosome.

Y chromosome Sex chromosome in the human male necessary for the development of the male gonads.

ZIFT (Zygote intrafallopian transfer) An ART procedure in which eggs are collected from a woman's ovary and fertilized outside her body. It is similar to IVF in that the oocytes are fertilized in the laboratory; however here the resulting fertilized oocytes are transferred to the fallopian tubes at an earlier stage in their development than in IVF. A laparoscope is used to place the resulting zygote (fertilized egg) into the woman's fallopian tube through a small incision in her abdomen.

zygote Cell formed by the union of two reproductive cells or gametes; the fertilized ovum resulting from the union of a sperm and an ovum.

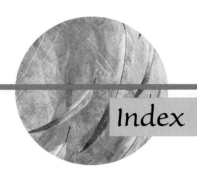

# Index